P9-CRO-651

MILADY'S STANDARD COSMETOLOGY

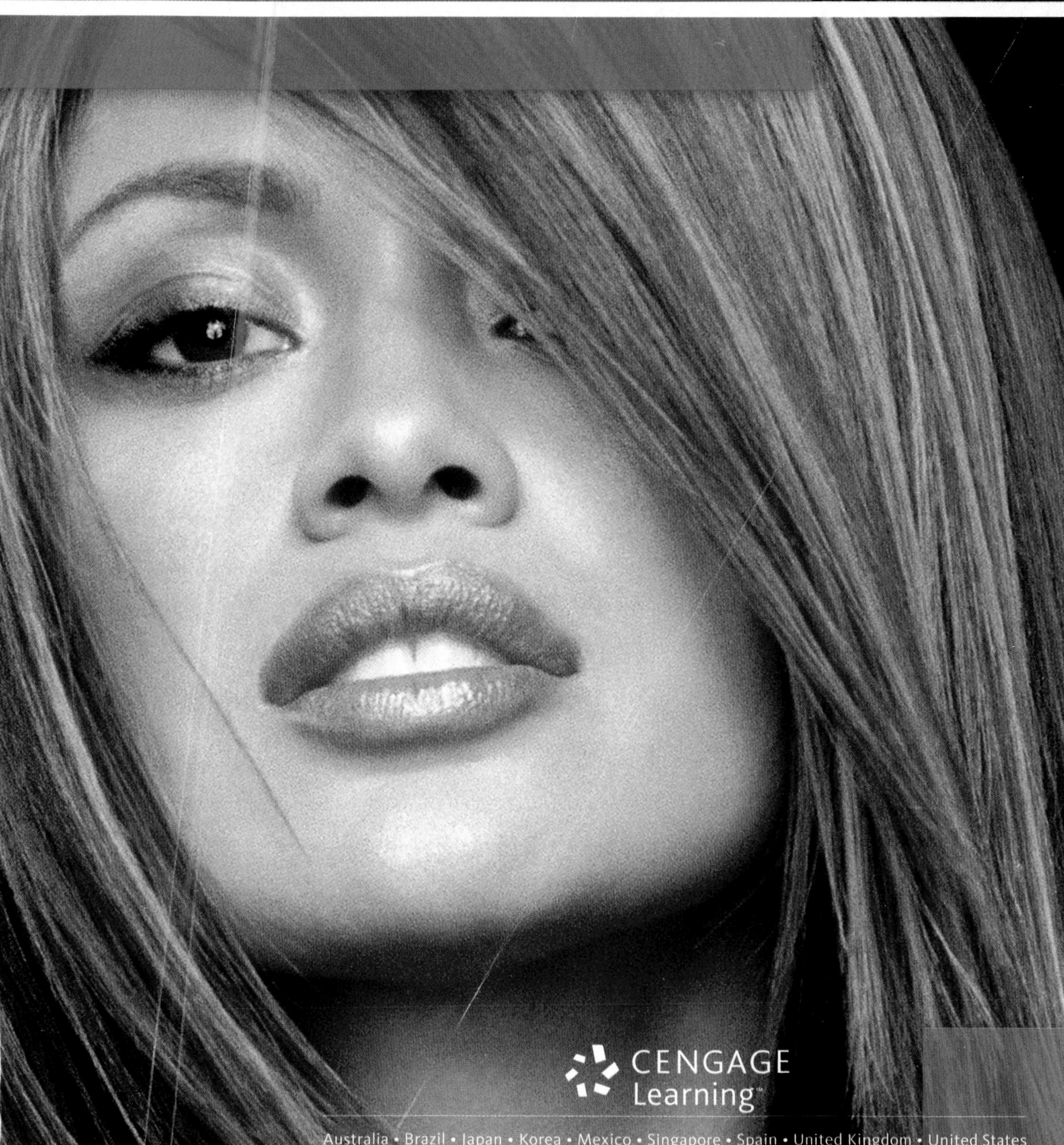

Arlene Alpert
Margrit Altenburg
Diane Carol Bailey
Letha Barnes
Lisha Barnes
Deborah Beatty
Mary Brunetti
Jane Crawford
Robert Cromeans
Alyssa Evirs
Catherine Frangie
John Halal
Colleen Hennessey
Mary Beth Janssen
Nancy King
Mark Lees
Toni Love
Vivienne Mackinder
Carey Nash
Ruth Roche
Teresa Sammarco
Sue Sansom
Douglas Schoon
Sue Ellen Schultes
Frank Shipman
Jeryl Spear

CENGAGE Learning™

Australia • Brazil • Japan • Korea • Mexico • Singapore • Spain • United Kingdom • United States

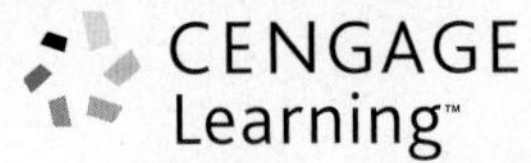

Milady's Standard: Cosmetology

President, Milady: Dawn Gerrain

Director of Editorial: John Fedor

Managing Editor: Robert Serenka

Product Manager: Jessica Burns

Editorial Assistant: Michael Spring

Director of Content and Media Production: Wendy A. Troeger

Content Project Manager: Nina Tucciarelli

Composition: Graphic World Inc.

Director of Marketing: Wendy Mapstone

Director of Industry Relations Milady and Salon Training International: Sandra Bruce

Marketing Coordinator: Nicole Riggi

Text Design: Studio Montage

Library of Congress Control Number: 2006033202

Softcover Book:
ISBN-13: 978-1-4180-4936-2
ISBN-10: 1-4180-4936-0

Hardcover Book:
ISBN-13: 978-1-4180-4935-5
ISBN-10: 1-4180-4935-2

Milady
Executive Woods
5 Maxwell Drive
Clifton Park, NY 12065
USA

Cengage Learning is a leading provider of customized learning solutions with office locations around the globe, including Singapore, the United Kingdom, Australia, Mexico, Brazil, and Japan. Locate your local office at **international.cengage.com/region**

Cengage Learning products are represented in Canada by Nelson Education, Ltd.

To learn more about Milady, visit **www.milady.cengage.com**

Purchase any of our products at your local college store or at our preferred online store **www.ichapters.com**

Printed in the United States of America
10 11 12 13 14 15 13 12 11 10

CONTENTS IN BRIEF

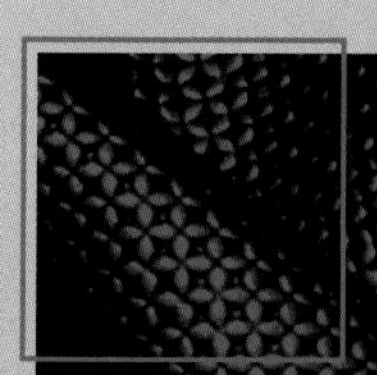

PROCEDURES

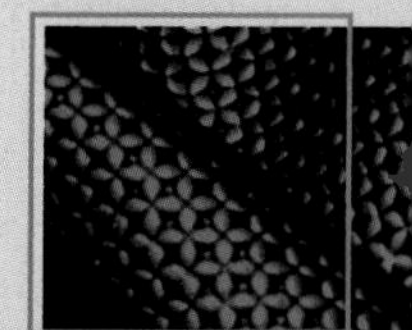

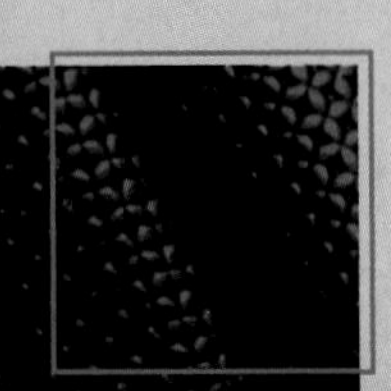

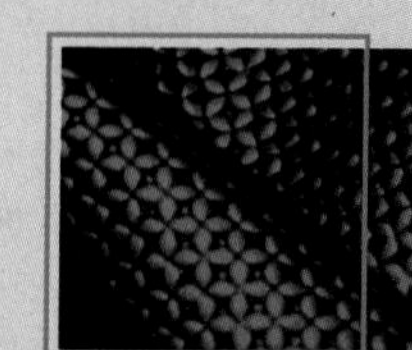

PREFACE

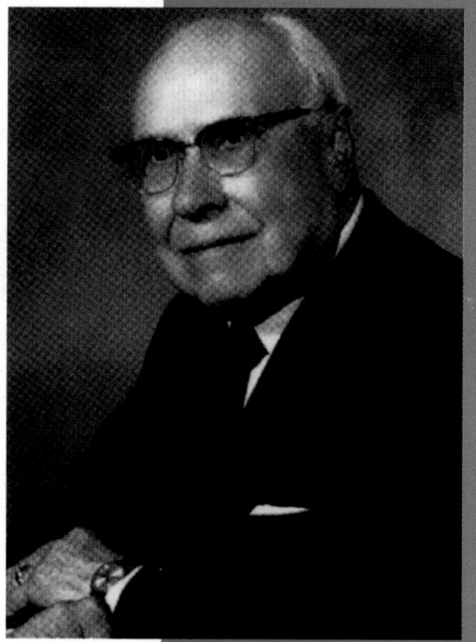

MILADY'S STANDARD COSMETOLOGY

Congratulations! You are about to start on a journey that can take you in many directions and holds the potential to make you a confident, successful professional in cosmetology. As a cosmetologist, you will become a trusted professional, the person your clients rely on to provide them with ongoing service, enabling them to look and feel their best. You will become as personally involved in your clients' lives as their physicians or dentists are, and with study and practice, you can be as much in demand as a well-regarded medical provider.

Milady's Standard Textbook of Cosmetology was the creation of Nicholas F. Cimaglia, founder of Milady Publishing Company, which he established 80 years ago, in 1927. He began his career in the beauty business as a salesman for a beauty supply distributor, selling his book, the *New York State Barbering Exam,* along with hair tonics and razors, door to door to barber shops in New York City. In 1938, Nick Cimaglia published the first edition of *Milady's Standard Textbook of Cosmetology,* and it has since been the textbook of choice for cosmetology education, undergoing many revisions.

Throughout its lifetime, it has consistently been the most-used cosmetology textbook in the world. With the many changes in the field of cosmetology, new editions of the text are needed periodically, and Milady is committed to making it the best cosmetology educational tool available.

THE INDUSTRY STANDARD

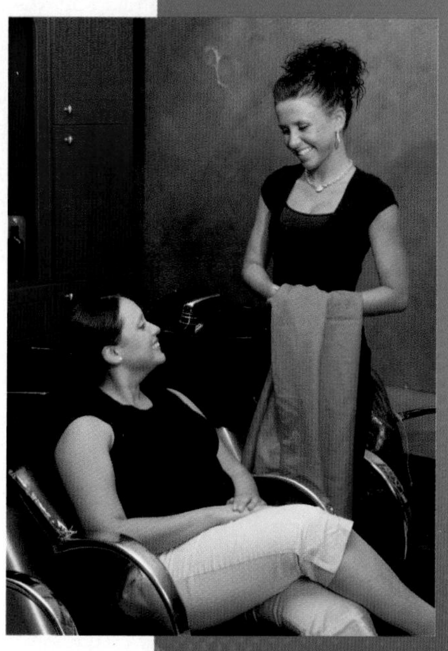

This edition of *Milady's Standard Cosmetology* provides you with the information you will need to pass the licensure exams as well as the most contemporary techniques to ensure your success once you are on the job. Before beginning this revision, Milady surveyed hundreds of educators and professionals, held focus groups, and received in-depth comments from dozens of reviewers to learn what needed to be changed, added, or deleted. Next we consulted with educational experts to learn the best way to present the material, so that all types of learners could understand it and remember it. Then we went to several experts in various cosmetology-related fields to write or revise the chapters. Finally, we sent the finished manuscripts to yet more subject experts to ensure the accuracy and thoroughness of the material. What you hold in your hands is the result.

Milady's Standard Cosmetology contains new information on many subjects, including sanitation and infection control, and haircoloring. As a part of your cosmetology education, this book will serve as a valuable guide, and you'll refer to it again and again throughout your career.

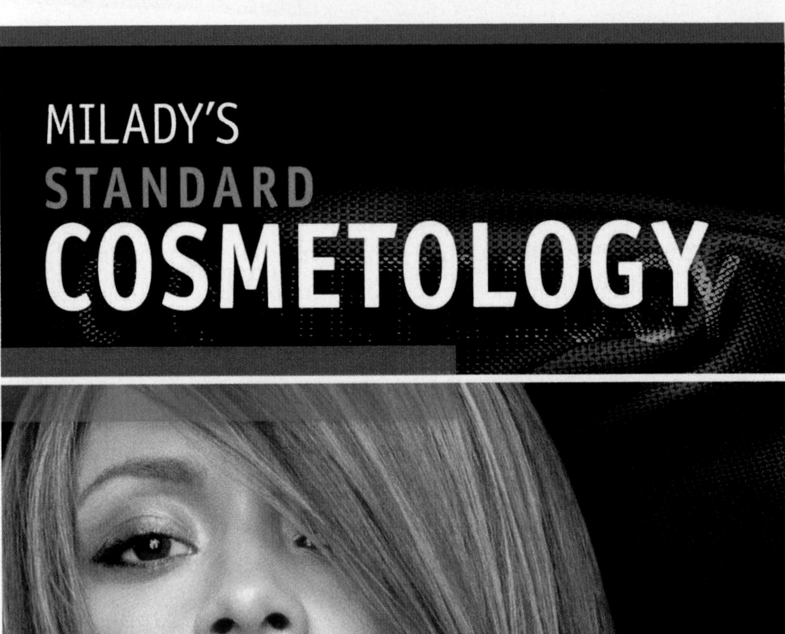

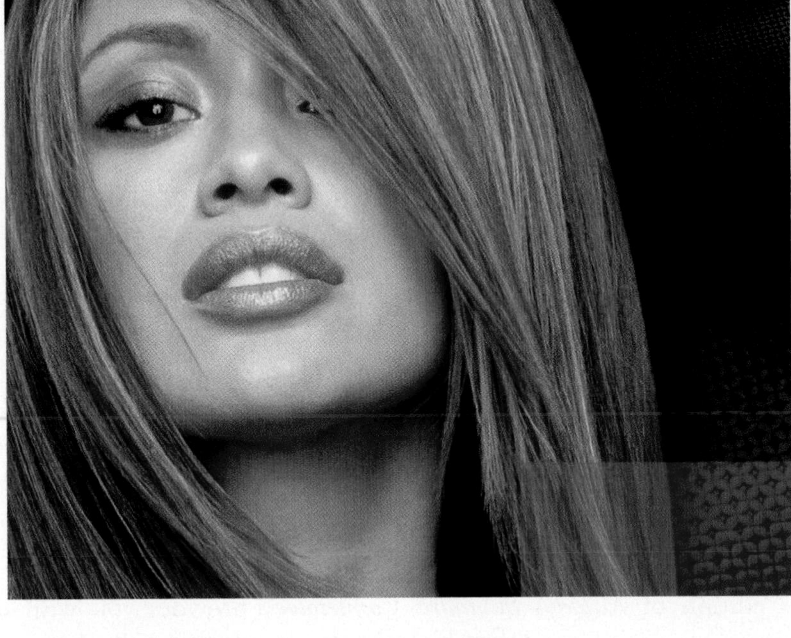

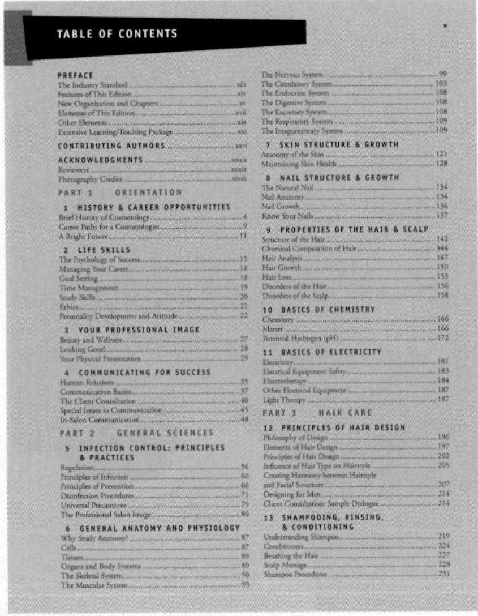

TABLE OF CONTENTS

v

FEATURES OF THIS EDITION

In response to the suggestions of the cosmetology educators and professionals who reviewed the *Milady's Standard Cosmetology* and to those submitted by the students who use this text, this edition includes many new chapters. We've aligned our core textbooks so that information appearing in any book that is also in another text, whether it be cosmetology, nail technology, or esthetics, now matches from one book to another.

Milady has also dramatically changed the design of the textbook to reflect the innovative and unique energy and artistry found in a career within the beauty business and we've included new photography and illustrations to bring you the most valuable, effective educational material available.

To get the most out of the time you will spend studying, take a few minutes first to learn about the textbook and how to use it before you begin. Use the Preface information that follows as a guide to lead you through the special features the textbook provides to help you learn, understand, and retain the important information within.

NEW ORGANIZATION AND CHAPTERS

By learning and using the tools in this text along with your teachers' instruction, you will develop the abilities you need to build a loyal and satisfied clientele. To help you locate information more easily, the chapters are grouped in six main parts.

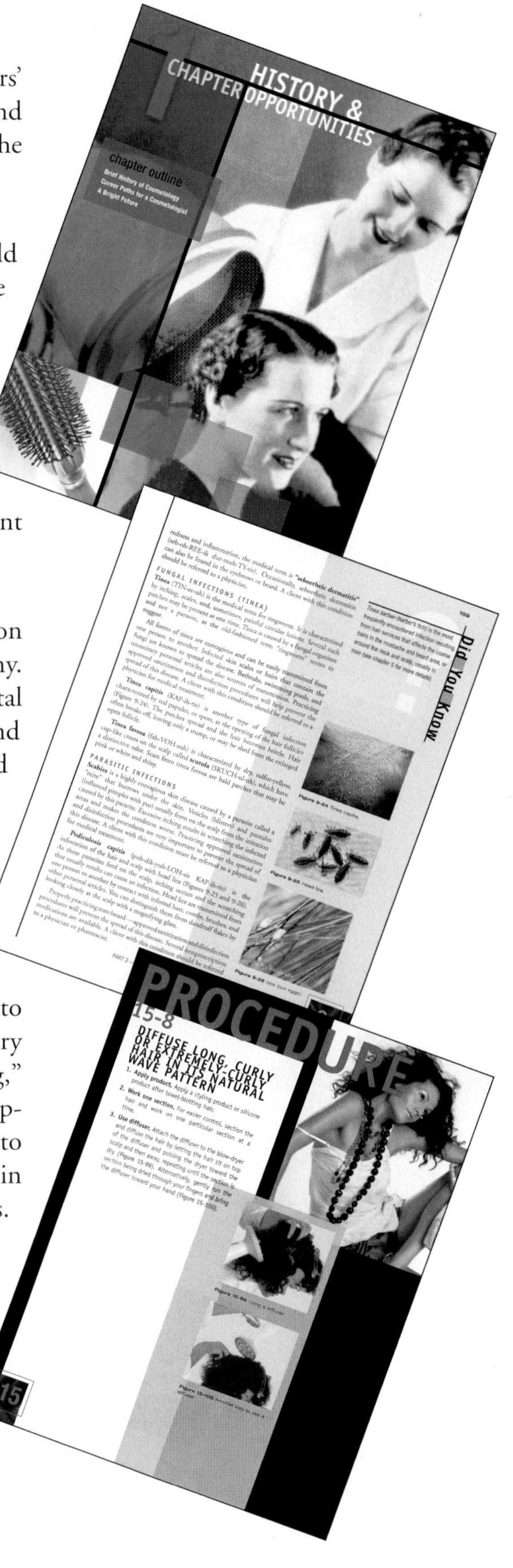

Part 1: Orientation consists of four chapters that cover the field of cosmetology and the personal skills you will need to become successful. The first chapter, "History & Opportunities," outlines where cosmetology came from and where it can take you. In "Life Skills," the second chapter, the ability to set goals and maintain a good attitude are emphasized along with the psychology of success. "Your Professional Image" stresses the importance of inward beauty and health as well as outward appearance, and "Communicating for Success" describes the important process of building client relationships based on trust and effective communication.

Part 2: General Sciences includes important information you need to know to keep yourself and your clients safe and healthy. "Infection Control: Principles & Practice" offers the most current, vital facts about hepatitis, HIV, and other infectious viruses and bacteria and tells how to prevent their spread in the salon. "General Anatomy and Physiology," "Skin Structure & Growth," "Nail Structure & Growth," "Properties of the Hair & Scalp," "Basics of Chemistry," and "Basics of Electricity" provide essential information that will affect how you work with clients, service products, and tools.

Part 3: Hair Care offers information on every aspect of hair. "Principles of Hair Design" explores the ways hair can be sculpted to enhance a client's facial shape. The foundation on which almost every hair service is built is covered in "Shampooing, Rinsing, & Conditioning," followed by a totally updated "Haircutting" chapter, complete with step-by-step procedures for core cuts with fantastic new glamour shots to show the finished look. Step-by-step procedures are also found in "Hairstyling," along with information on new tools and techniques. Another revised chapter, "Braiding & Braid Extensions," is followed by "Wigs & Hair Enhancements," and both "Chemical Texture Services" and "Haircoloring" reflect the most recent advances in these areas.

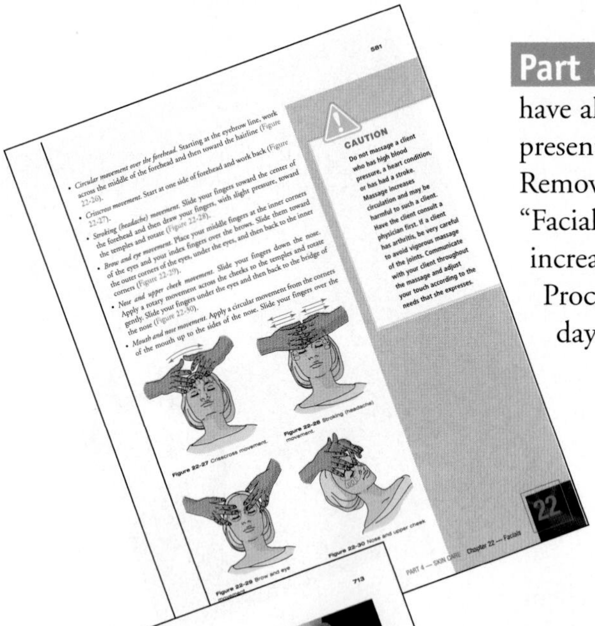

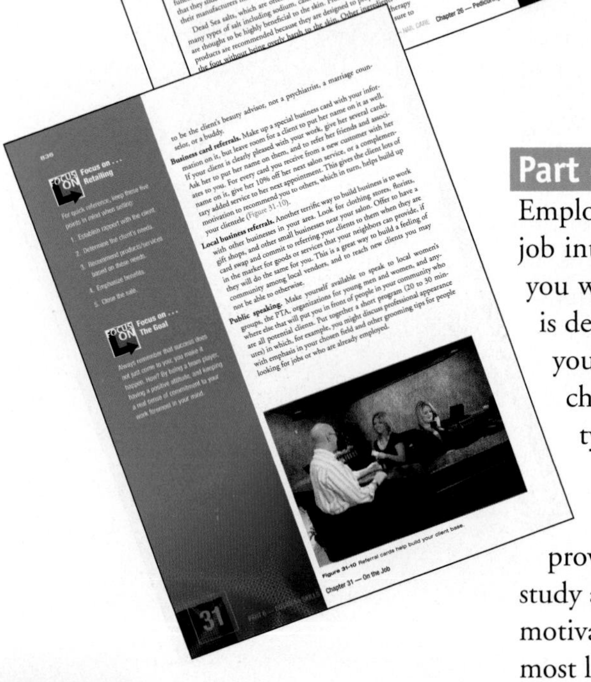

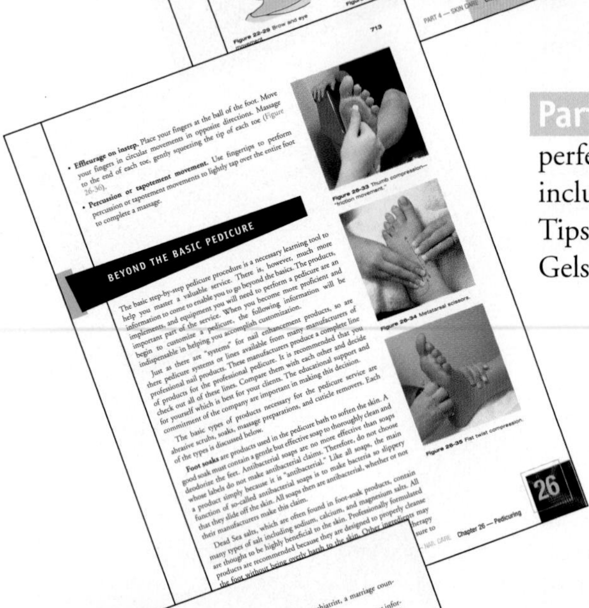

Part 4: Skin Care focuses on another area in which new advances have altered the way students must be trained. The basics about skin are presented in "Skin Diseases & Disorders." The popular topic of "Hair Removal" covers waxing, tweezing, and popular methods. "Facials" and "Facial Makeup" offer the critical information you'll need for these increasingly requested services in the expanding field of esthetics. Procedures are included for many of the services needed in salons and day spas.

Part 5: Nail Care contains completely revised chapters that are also perfectly aligned with *Milady's Standard Nail Technology.* These chapters include "Nail Diseases & Disorders," "Manicuring," "Pedicuring," "Nail Tips, Wraps & No-Light Gels," "Acrylic (Methacrylate) Nails," and "UV Gels."

Part 6: Business Skills opens with the updated chapter "Seeking Employment" which prepares students for licensure exams as well as for job interviews and explains how to create a resume and portfolio. What you will be expected to know and do as a newly licensed cosmetologist is described in "On the Job." It offers tips on how to make the most of your first job and how to learn the most from it, too. And the final chapter "The Salon Business," exposes students to the numerous types of salons and salon ownerships available to them.

"In Closing," written by Robert Cromeans, one of the most widely recognized personalities in today's professional hair industry, provides a message to students who have completed their course of study and are ready to enter the professional world. Robert's message will motivate and encourage you and send you off to what can be one of the most lucrative and fun careers available today.

ELEMENTS OF THIS EDITION

As part of this edition, many features are available to help you master key concepts and techniques.

FOCUS ON Throughout the text are short paragraphs in the outer column that draw attention to various skills and concepts that will help you reach your goal. The "Focus On . . ." pieces target sharpening technical skills, sharpening personal skills, ticket upgrading, client consultation, and building your client base. These topics are key to your success as a student and as a professional.

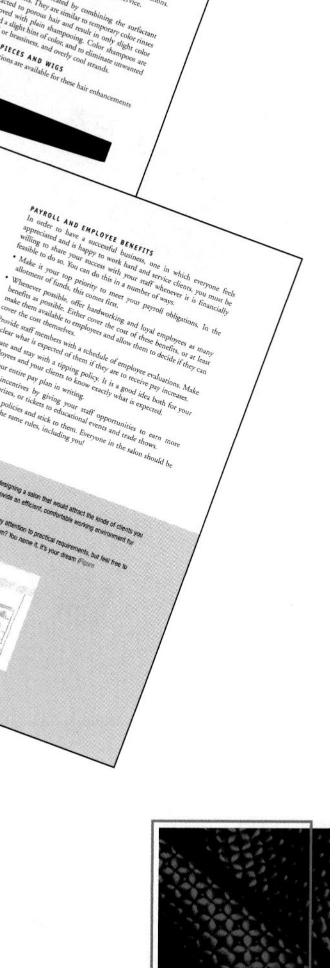

Did You Know These features provide interesting information that will enhance your understanding of what you are learning in the text and call attention to a special point.

ACTIVITY The "Activity" boxes describe classroom exercises that will help you understand firsthand the concepts being explained in the text.

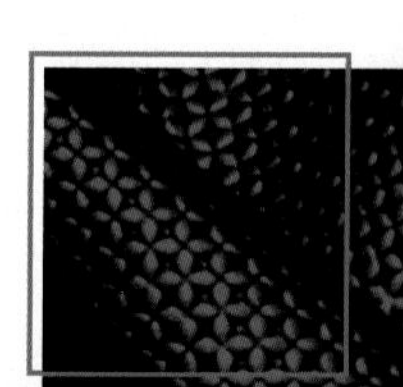

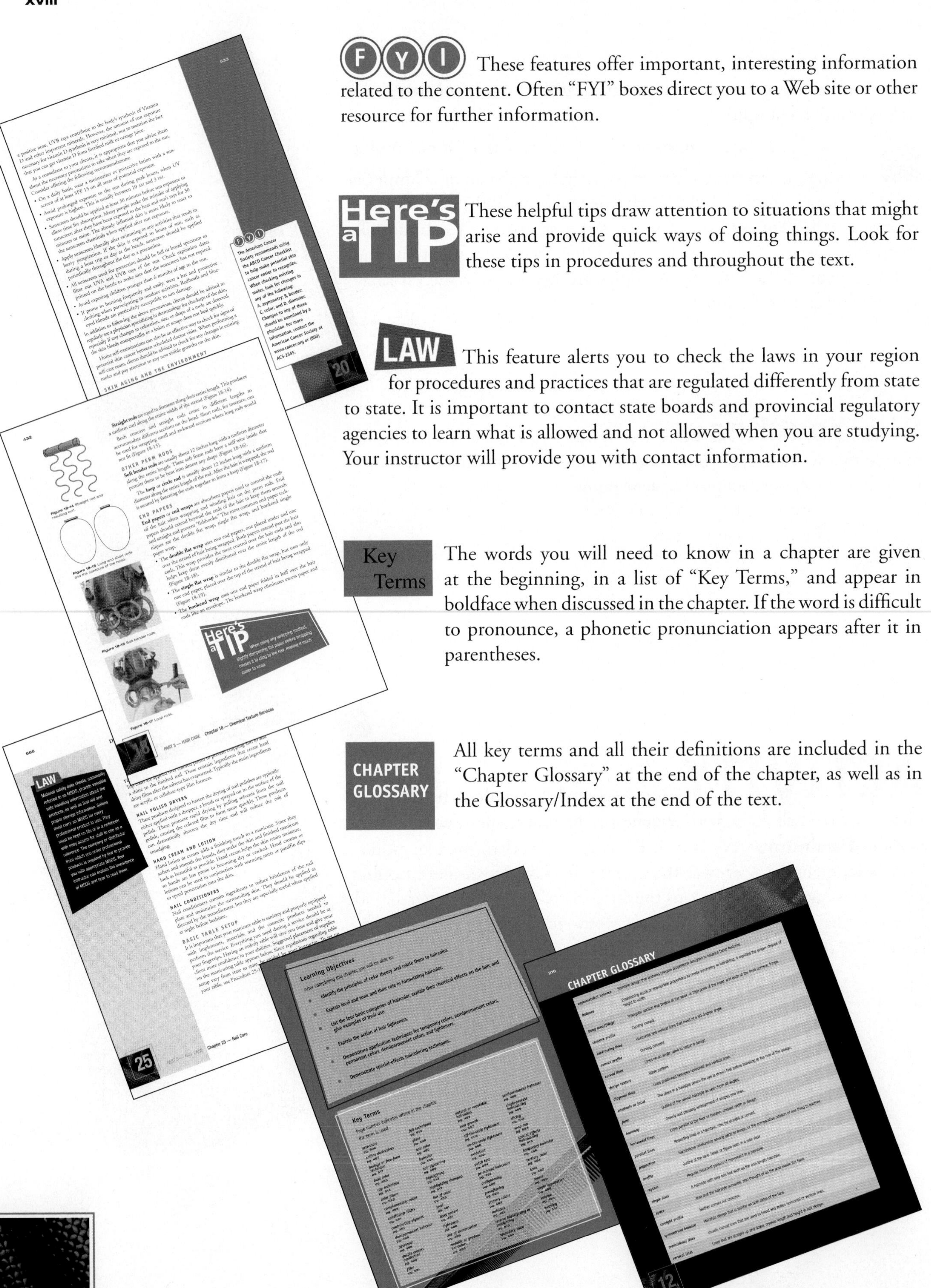

FYI These features offer important, interesting information related to the content. Often "FYI" boxes direct you to a Web site or other resource for further information.

Here's a TIP These helpful tips draw attention to situations that might arise and provide quick ways of doing things. Look for these tips in procedures and throughout the text.

LAW This feature alerts you to check the laws in your region for procedures and practices that are regulated differently from state to state. It is important to contact state boards and provincial regulatory agencies to learn what is allowed and not allowed when you are studying. Your instructor will provide you with contact information.

Key Terms The words you will need to know in a chapter are given at the beginning, in a list of "Key Terms," and appear in boldface when discussed in the chapter. If the word is difficult to pronounce, a phonetic pronunciation appears after it in parentheses.

CHAPTER GLOSSARY All key terms and all their definitions are included in the "Chapter Glossary" at the end of the chapter, as well as in the Glossary/Index at the end of the text.

OTHER ELEMENTS

Many features from previous editions of *Milady's Standard* have been retained in this new edition.

Learning Objectives

At the beginning of each chapter is a list of learning objectives that will tell you what important information you will be expected to know from the chapter.

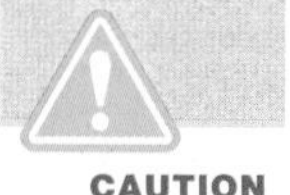
CAUTION

Some information is so critical for your safety and the safety of your clients that it deserves special attention. The text directs you to this information in the "Caution" boxes found in the margins.

REVIEW QUESTIONS Each chapter ends with questions designed to test your understanding of the information in it. Your instructor may ask you to write the answers to these questions as an assignment or to answer them orally in class. If you have trouble answering a question, go back to the chapter to review the material and try again. The answers to the "Review Questions" are in your instructor's *Course Management Guide*.

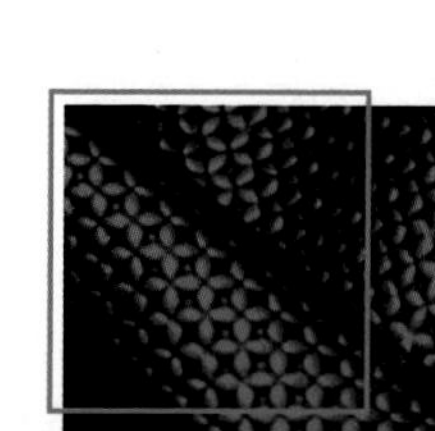

All step-by-step procedures offer clear, easy-to-understand directions and multiple photographs for learning the techniques.

Step-by-step instructions occur in Parts 2, 3, 4, and 5 of the text.

A list of the needed implements and materials appears at the start, along with any preparation that must be completed before the procedure, and the finished result appears at the end.

Clear, precise instructions make following the procedure easy. Specific steps for cleanup and sanitation appear at the end of the procedure.

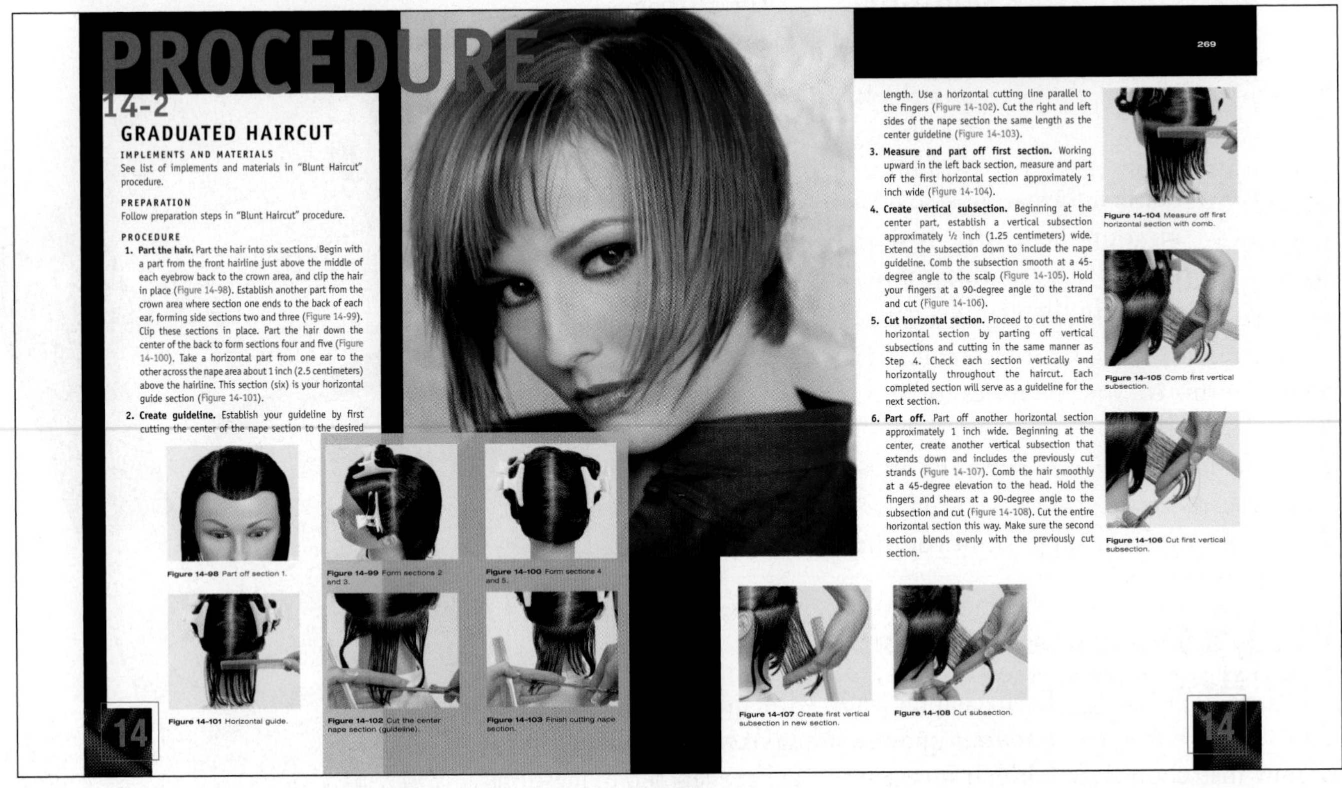

PROCEDURE 14-2

GRADUATED HAIRCUT

IMPLEMENTS AND MATERIALS
See list of implements and materials in "Blunt Haircut" procedure.

PREPARATION
Follow preparation steps in "Blunt Haircut" procedure.

PROCEDURE

1. **Part the hair.** Part the hair into six sections. Begin with a part from the front hairline just above the middle of each eyebrow back to the crown area, and clip the hair in place (Figure 14-98). Establish another part from the crown area where section one ends to the back of each ear, forming side sections two and three (Figure 14-99). Clip these sections in place. Part the hair down the center of the back to form sections four and five (Figure 14-100). Take a horizontal part from one ear to the other across the nape area about 1 inch (2.5 centimeters) above the hairline. This section (six) is your horizontal guide section (Figure 14-101).
2. **Create guideline.** Establish your guideline by first cutting the center of the nape section to the desired length. Use a horizontal cutting line parallel to the fingers (Figure 14-102). Cut the right and left sides of the nape section the same length as the center guideline (Figure 14-103).
3. **Measure and part off first section.** Working upward in the left back section, measure and part off the first horizontal section approximately 1 inch wide (Figure 14-104).
4. **Create vertical subsection.** Beginning at the center part, establish a vertical subsection approximately ½ inch (1.25 centimeters) wide. Extend the subsection down to include the nape guideline. Comb the subsection smooth at a 45-degree angle to the scalp (Figure 14-105). Hold your fingers at a 90-degree angle to the strand and cut (Figure 14-106).
5. **Cut horizontal section.** Proceed to cut the entire horizontal section by parting off vertical subsections and cutting in the same manner as Step 4. Check each section vertically and horizontally throughout the haircut. Each completed section will serve as a guideline for the next section.
6. **Part off.** Part off another horizontal section approximately 1 inch wide. Beginning at the center, create another vertical subsection that extends down and includes the previously cut strands (Figure 14-107). Comb the hair smoothly at a 45-degree elevation to the head. Hold the fingers and shears at a 90-degree angle to the subsection and cut (Figure 14-108). Cut the entire horizontal section this way. Make sure the second section blends evenly with the previously cut section.

Figure 14-98 Part off section 1.

Figure 14-99 Form sections 2 and 3.

Figure 14-100 Form sections 4 and 5.

Figure 14-101 Horizontal guide.

Figure 14-102 Cut the center nape section (guideline).

Figure 14-103 Finish cutting nape section.

Figure 14-104 Measure off first horizontal section with comb.

Figure 14-105 Comb first vertical subsection.

Figure 14-106 Cut first vertical subsection.

Figure 14-107 Create first vertical subsection in new section.

Figure 14-108 Cut subsection.

14 269 14

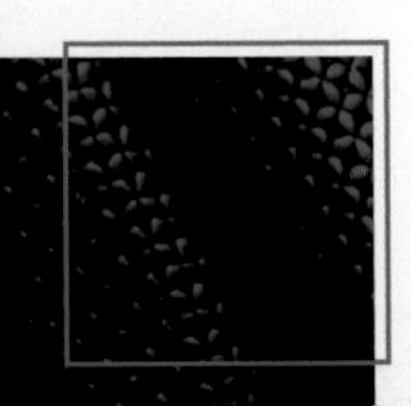

EXTENSIVE LEARNING/TEACHING PACKAGE

While *Milady's Standard Cosmetology* is the center of the curriculum, students and educators have a wide range of supplements from which to choose. All supplements have been revised and updated to complement the new edition of the textbook.

STUDENT SUPPLEMENTS

In addition to the textbook, Milady has created many supplements to meet every student's needs. All supplements have been revised, including the following:

Milady's Standard Cosmetology Study Guide

The *Study Guide* is a colorful new study guide to help students recognize, understand, and retain the key concepts presented in each chapter of *Milady's Standard Cosmetology*. The student-led exercises require minimal educator assistance. *The Essential Companion* provides six easy-to-follow features for each chapter—Essential Objectives, Essential Subjects, Essential Concepts, Essential Review, and Essential Discoveries and Accomplishments. Each one presents the key content in a different manner to help all students comprehend and remember it. A great new feature added to this edition is rubrics to be used as self-assessment by students. The attractive color design will engage all types of students so they can learn the important theory and practical aspects necessary for licensure and professional success. Answers are supplied in your instructor's *Course Management Guide.*

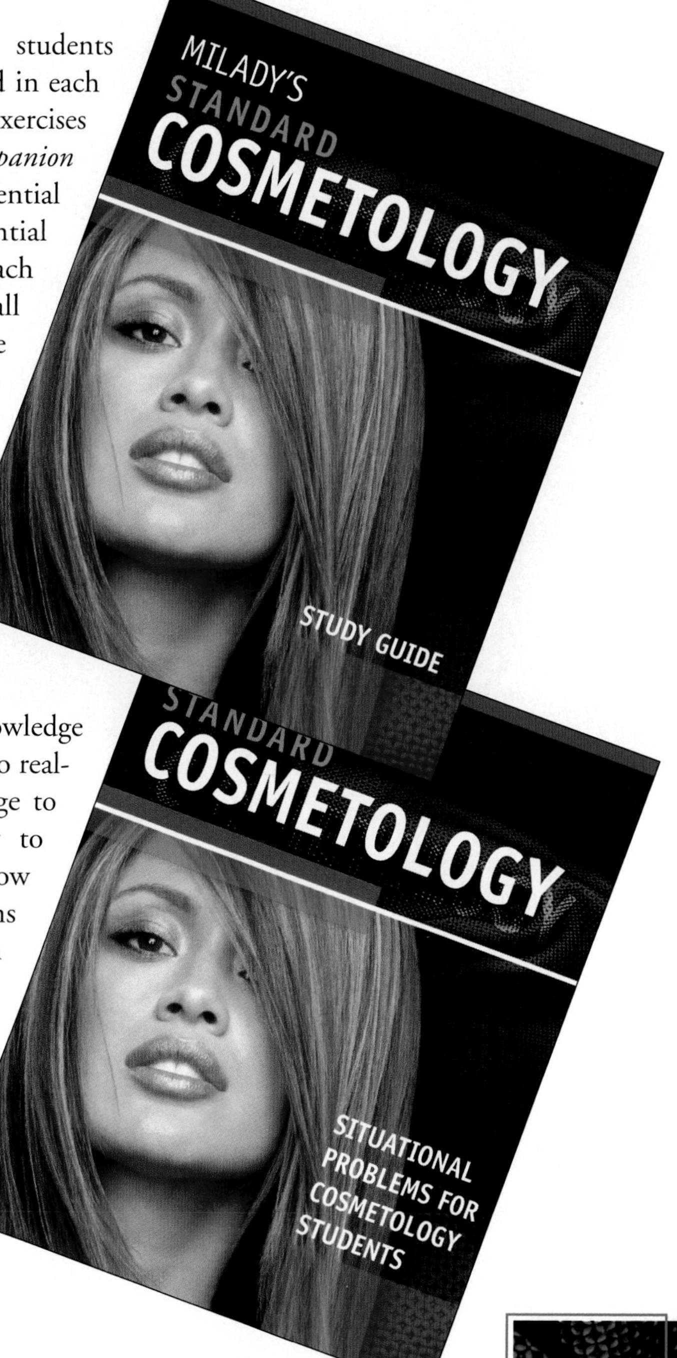

Milady's Situational Problems for Cosmetology Students

Situational Problems for Cosmetology Students tests students' knowledge of how they should apply the information they have learned to real-life situations. This text asks that they apply that knowledge to situations that more closely reflect what they are likely to encounter as a salon employee, demonstrating that they know how to use the information they have learned. The questions are more complex than Exam Review questions, often describing a salon stylist or other professional who has a client with a combination of conditions, problems, or attitudes. The student will have to take desired results, both from a technical and a communication perspective. Answers are included in the back of the book.

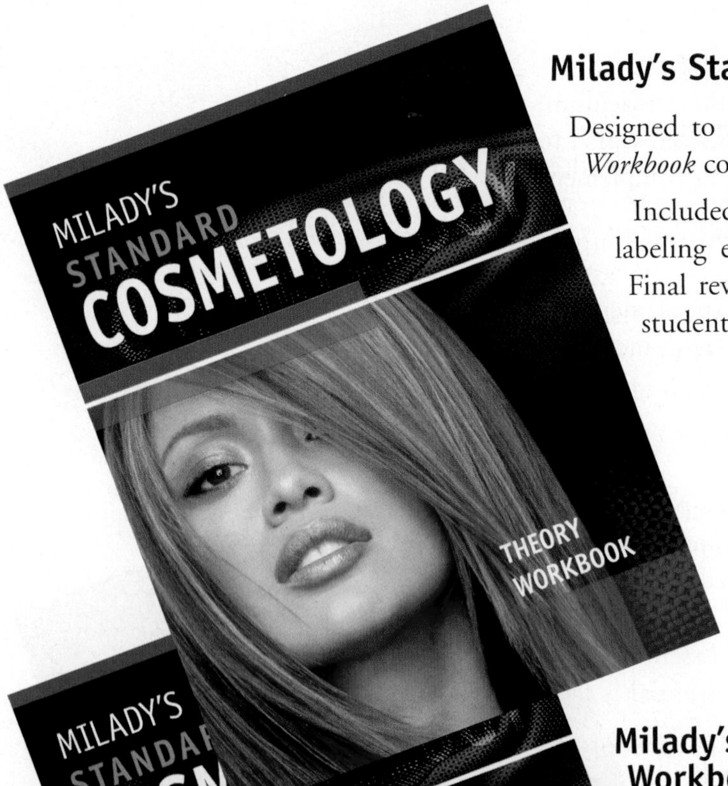

Milady's Standard Cosmetology Theory Workbook

Designed to reinforce classroom and textbook learning, the *Theory Workbook* contains chapter-by-chapter exercises on theory subjects.

Included are fill-in-the-blank, multiple-choice, matching, and labeling exercises, all coordinated with material from the text. Final review examinations at the end of the workbook prepare students for testing.

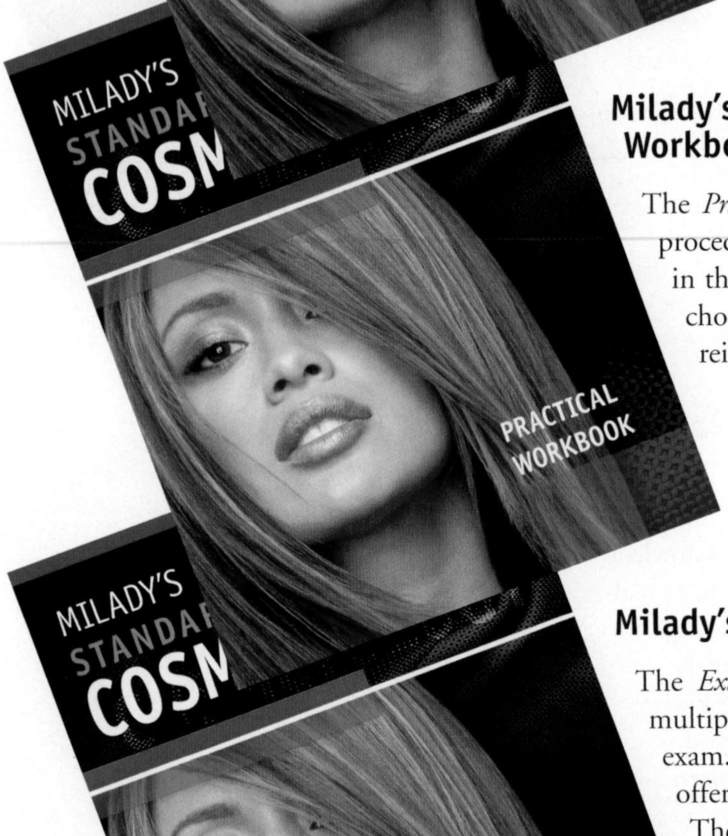

Milady's Standard Cosmetology Practical Workbook

The *Practical Workbook* helps students master the techniques, procedures, and product usage needed for licensure as covered in the textbook. Using fill-in-the-blank, matching, multiple-choice, and labeling exercises, students will benefit from the reinforcement of practical applications.

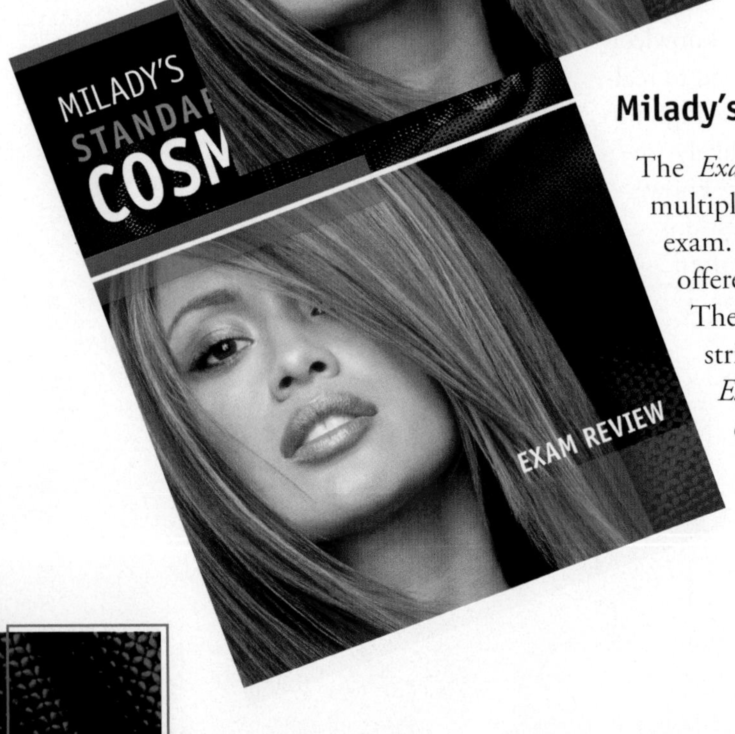

Milady's Standard Cosmetology Exam Review

The *Exam Review* contains chapter-by-chapter questions in a multiple-choice format to help students prepare for the licensure exam. While not intended to be the only form of review offered to students, it aids in overall classroom preparation. The *Exam Review* has been revised to meet the most stringent test-development guidelines. The questions in the *Exam Review* are for study purposes only and are not the exact questions students will see on the licensure exams.

Milady's Standard Cosmetology Student CD-ROM

Milady's Standard Cosmetology Student CD-ROM is an interactive student product designed to reinforce classroom learning, stimulate the imagination, and aid in preparation for board exams. Featuring more than 100 helpful video clips to demonstrate practices and procedures, this exciting educational tool also contains a test bank with 1,200 chapter-by-chapter or randomly accessed multiple-choice and matching questions to help students study for the exam. Another feature is the game bank, which offers games to strengthen knowledge of terminology, and a glossary that pronounces and defines each term. The content follows and enhances *Milady's Standard Cosmetology.*

The technology of the program is interactive, allowing the learner to be surrounded or "pulled into" the content, and it tracks the student's progress through the program. The CD-ROM is also available as a networkable product for schools.

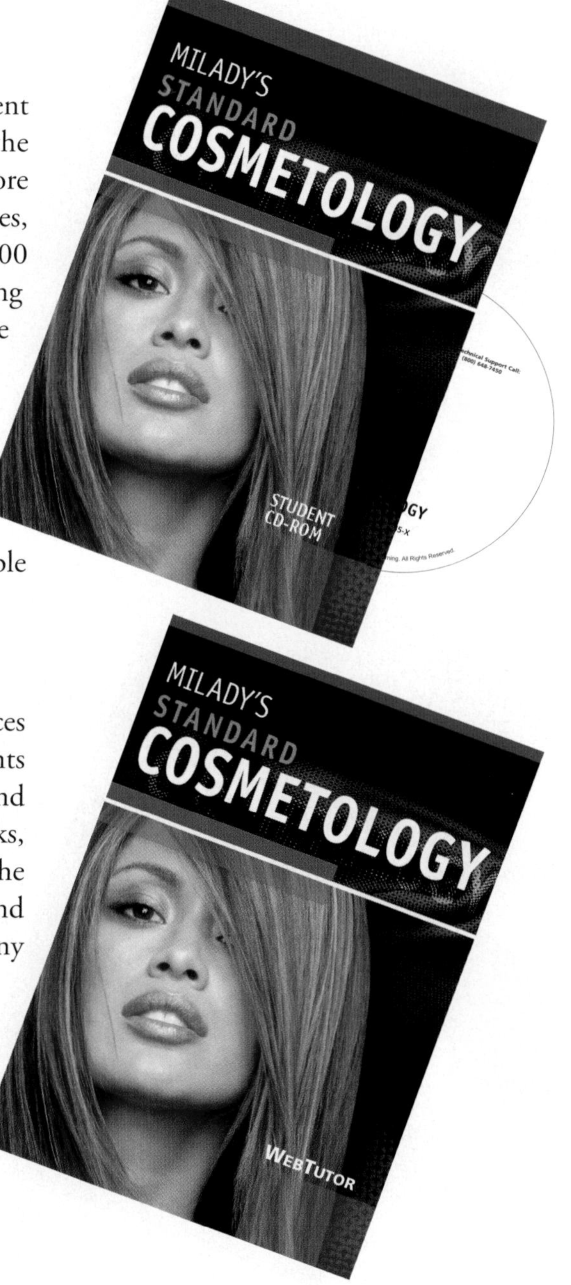

Milady's Standard Cosmetology WebTutor

The *WebTutor* is a content-rich, Web-based learning aid that reinforces and clarifies complex concepts in the textbook. *WebTutor* presents information in a new and different way, making it easier to understand material as well as allowing easier management of time, progress checks, exam preparation, and organization of notes. Available on either the WebCT or Blackboard platform, *WebTutor* is fully customizable and includes a course calendar, chat, e-mail, threaded discussions, and many more features custom designed to your individual course.

Features:

- Chapter Learning Objectives
- Online Course Preparation
- Study Sheets
- Online Chapter Quizzes
  - Fill-in-the-Blank
  - Multiple Choice
  - True/False
  - Matching
- Flash cards
- Discussion Topics
- Web Links
- FAQs
- Glossary

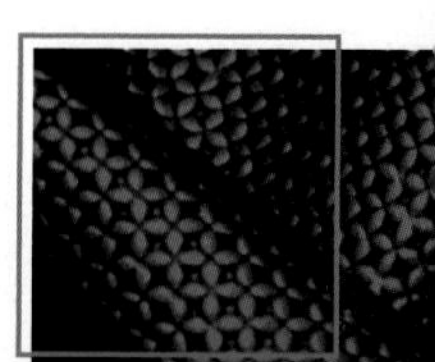

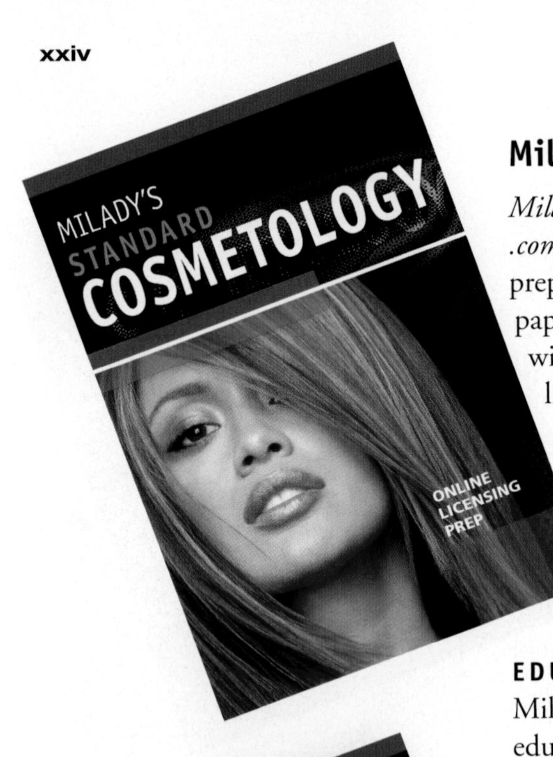

Milady's Online Licensing Preparation: Cosmetology

Milady's Online Licensing Preparation: Cosmetology, www.MiladyOnline .com, provides students with a technology study alternative to better prepare them for licensure exams, whether taken on a computer or on paper. Over 1,000 multiple-choice questions for cosmetology appear with rationales for correct and incorrect choices, and the correct answer links to the portion of *Milady's Standard Cosmetology* in which the information is given. Students have the flexibility to study from any computer, whether at home or at school. Because exam review preparation is available to students at any time of day or night, class time can be used for other activities. Students gain familiarity with a computerized test environment as they prepare for licensure.

EDUCATOR SUPPLEMENTS

Milady offers a full range of products created especially for cosmetology educators to make classroom preparation and presentation simple, effective, and enjoyable.

Course Management Guide

The *Course Management Guide* contains all the materials educators need in one package. This innovative instructional guide is written with cosmetology educators in mind and is designed to make exceptional teaching easy. With formatting that provides easy-to-use material for use in the classroom, it will transform classroom management and dramatically increase student interest and understanding. Included in the three-ring binder are: Transition Tools, Instructor Support Forms, Lesson Plan Index, Chapter Tests, and Resources. The binder is accompanied by the answer keys to the *Theory and Practical* workbooks and the *Study Guide*.

Added features you will find on the *Course Management Guide* CD-ROM version:

- Every page from the *Course Management Guide* can be printed to appear exactly like the page from the print product.
- A Computerized Test bank contains new multiple-choice questions that instructors can use to create random tests from a single chapter or the whole book. In this new edition, Computerized Test bank questions are not the same questions in the *Exam Review.* Answer keys are automatically created. A gradebook feature to track students' progress is also included.
- An Image Library of 1,000 photos and illustrations from *Milady's Standard Cosmetology* can be added to PowerPoint® presentations or printed onto paper or acetate for overheads. They can even be imported into other documents.

DVD Series

The 2004 edition of *Milady's Standard Cosmetology DVD Series* is complete with five hours of video content that continues to correlate

with the 2008 edition of the textbook. This three-DVD set offers interactive content with features for classroom use that provides instructors with easy search features, easy-to-use student assessment exercises, and optional Spanish subtitles. More than just video on DVD, this series creates the option of viewing a procedure from several camera angles. Milady also offers Professional Barber DVDs, Nail Tech DVDs, and Soft Skills DVDs as supplemental visual aids for the correlating content in the *Standard Cosmetology* textbook.

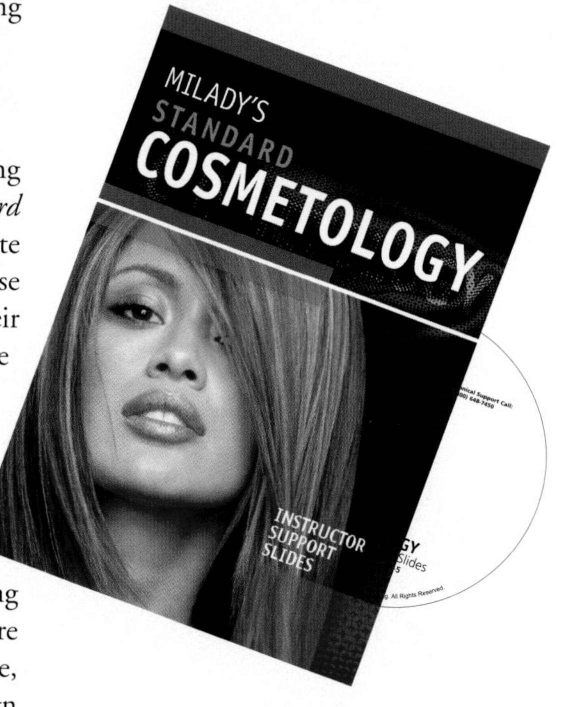

Instructor Support Slides

The new Instructor Support Slides use PowerPoint® technology, offering instructors pre-designed presentations to accompany the *Standard Cosmetology*, making lesson plans simple yet incredibly effective. Complete with photos and art, this chapter-by-chapter CD-ROM has ready-to-use presentations that will help engage students' attention and keep their interest through its varied color schemes and styles. Instructors can use it as is or adapt it to their own classrooms by importing photos they have taken, changing the graphics, or adding slides.

Procedure Posters

This poster series was created with the 2004 edition of *Milady's Standard Cosmetology.* The posters feature key procedures, including haircuts, haircoloring, permanent waves, manicures, and skin care techniques to use for repeated reference on the clinic floor. Large in size, each poster contains photos and text in a step-by-step format. The design complements the 2008 revision of the textbook.

Wall Charts

Milady's Standard Wall Charts include a transparent overlay with lines for terminology or directional arrows that will improve presentations to cover all topics needed for Cosmetology, Esthetics, and Nail Technology. Each of the 17 charts is 26.5″ × 36″ and will feature, on average, five color drawings depending on the topic. The charts are printed in full color on a tear-resistant, coated paper and two metal grommets make hanging easier.

Charts:

- Anatomy of the Hand and Arm
- Bones of the Head and Face
- Circulation of the Blood
- Histology of the Hair, Follicles
- Histology of the Skin, Hair, Glands
- Motor Points of the Face
- Muscles of the Head, Face, and Neck
- Nerves of the Head, Face, and Neck
- Foot and Ankle Massage
- Foot Reflexology
- Lymphatic System
- Anatomy of the Nail
- Facial Movements and Manipulations
- Face Shapes
- Facial Areas for Product Application
- Anatomy of the Foot and Ankles
- Hand and Arm Massage

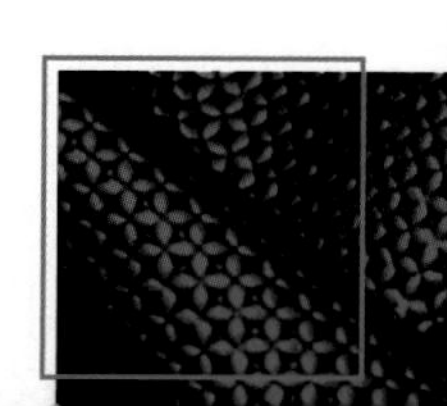

CONTRIBUTING AUTHORS

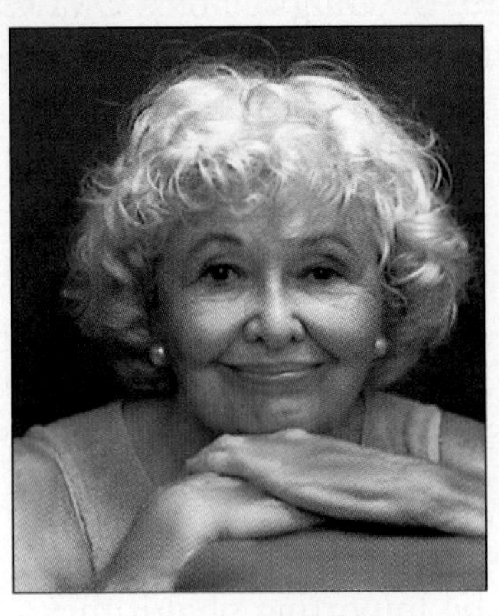

ARLENE ALPERT

Arlene Alpert, MS, LMHC, is President/CEO of Jupiter Consulting & Training Institute. Ms. Alpert has been a licensed Psychotherapist/Counselor in private practice for almost 30 years. In addition, her expertise includes Business Relationships Consultant, Coach, Educator, Professional Speaker, and Workshop Leader in the United States, Canada, and Europe, and is past president of the Florida Speakers Association. Ms. Alpert has advanced degrees in psychology and counseling and is considered an authority on "The Business of Relationships." Her latest books are *Traveling Beyond Life's Roadblocks: Creating A Life Of Choice* and *The Aha Experience: How One Sentence Has The Power To Change Your Life.* She offers coaching and consulting on the telephone, as well as in her office or yours. She focuses on advancing professional and personal development, increasing self-esteem and confidence, and providing emotional re-education to clear up "trouble spots" that prevent creating remarkable relationships and being effective communicators and decision-makers.

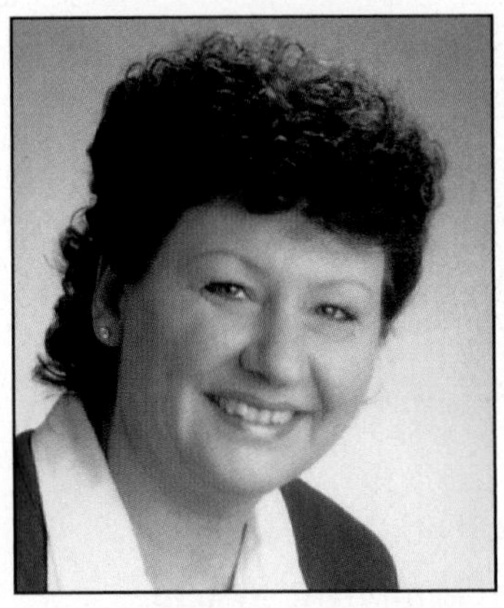

MARGRIT ALTENBURG

Educated and licensed in Switzerland, Margrit Altenburg has been working in the beauty industry since 1976. She owned her own skin care clinic for 17 years and obtained her Master's in Skin and Body Care in 1990. Altenburg received her CIDESCO international board certification in 1991, and served as General Secretary from 1992 to 1998. She spent the early 1990s working in a Swiss dermatologist's clinic and moved to Houston in 1999 to accept the esthetics department head teacher position at the first CIDESCO-accredited school in the United States–the Institute of Cosmetology & Esthetics–where she became the director a year later. Altenburg is active organizing educational workshops in Switzerland and Germany, has taught several classes for the National Cosmetology Association in the United States, and is a CIDESCO international examiner worldwide.

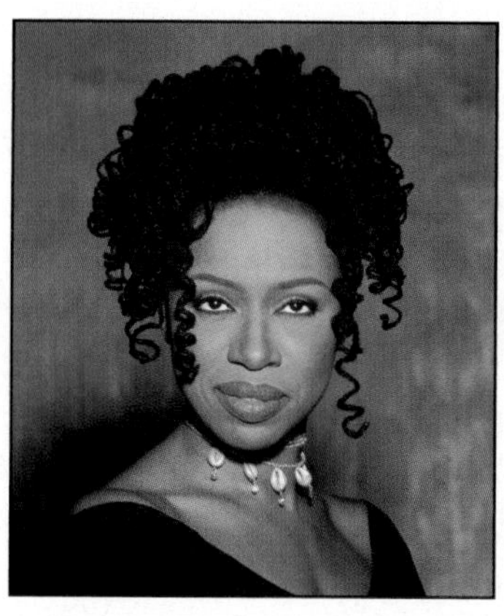

DIANE CAROL BAILEY

At 21, Diane Carol Bailey graduated from Hunter College and entered beauty school, but her calling first began at age nine, when she started experimenting with her own hair. She began braiding at home and was frustrated by the bias and lack of education for the care and treatment of natural hair. Bailey became involved in the natural hair care movement in 1987, and helped found the International Braiders Network (IBN) in 1992, whose members drafted and adopted the first natural hair care license in July 1994. Today, as President of IBN, she works to promote and establish professional standards, procedures, and training for natural hair care stylists and braiders.

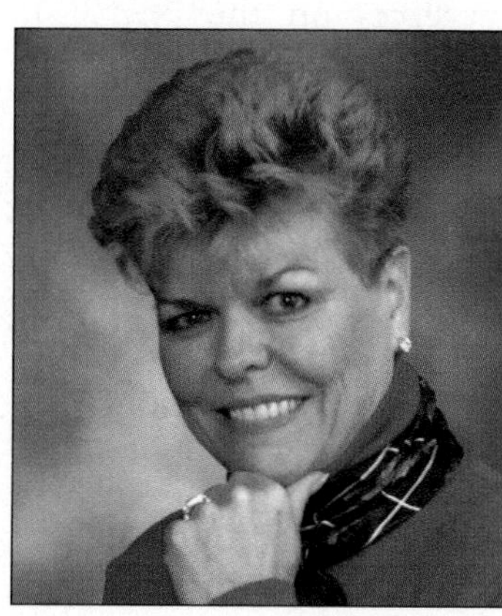

LETHA BARNES

Commitment toward cosmetology education is what Letha Barnes is all about. In her 39 years of industry experience, she served as President of AACS, where she helped revive and expand the mission of their educational arm, the Cosmetology Educators of America (CEA). She also gained recognition for her service as Vice-Chairman of the National Accrediting Commission of Cosmetology Arts and Sciences. She served as a NACCAS evaluator and taught accreditation workshops for years. She is the former owner of three cosmetology schools and former Vice President of Education for thirty-two others. She became the Director of Milady's Career Institute in January 2000. She has authored three editions of *Milady's Standard Cosmetology Course Management Guide* and *Milady's Standard Cosmetology Study Guide—The Essential Companion* as well as *Milady's Master Educator,* all receiving positive feedback from educators in the industry.

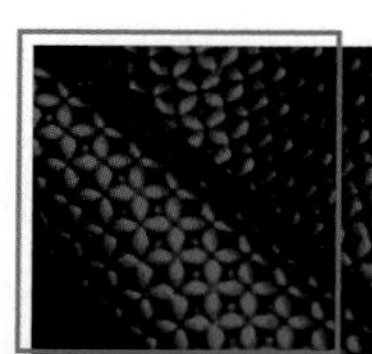

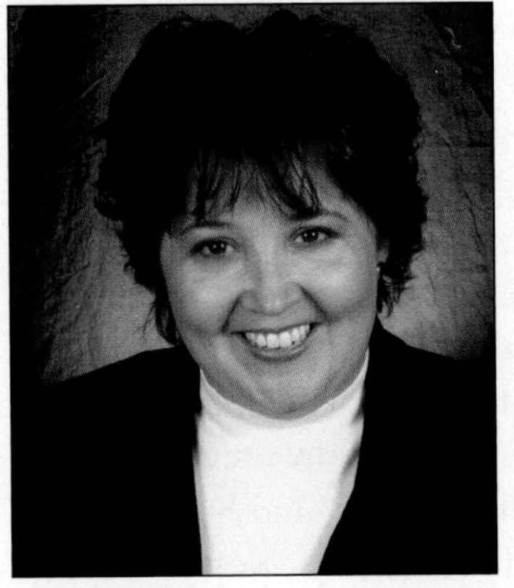

LISHA BARNES

A licensed cosmetologist, instructor, and barber, Lisha Barnes is committed to improving the quality of cosmetology education. She received a B.S. in Communications from Eastern New Mexico University in 1990 and completed her cosmetology training at Olympian University of Cosmetology. She currently serves as the Corporate Director of Education for the Milan Institute of Cosmetology campuses located in the western United States. Barnes is a member of Cosmetology Educators of America and has worked on numerous projects for Milady and The Career Institute, where her experience in education, communications, and administration add insight to her presentations. She currently serves on the NACCAS Advisory Committee on the Standards and Criteria.

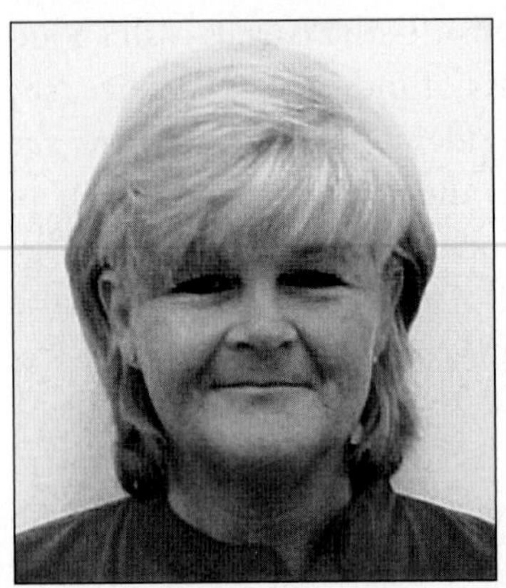

DEBORAH BEATTY

Deborah Beatty has over 32 years of industry experience, which has allowed her to gain and develop a wealth of knowledge that she shares during her educational seminars as well as in her classrooms. With 15 years' experience in the educational sector, she enlightens and motivates cosmetologists, instructors, and students with her energetic and interactive approach to teaching. She is presently the Program Manager for the Cosmetology Department at a post-secondary college. In addition to being a Master Cosmetologist and Licensed Instructor, she also holds her Master Barber License, is a Licensed Practical Nurse, and is licensed by the Georgia Professional Standards Commission. Deborah is a book and product reviewer for CengageLearning and is an educator for Milady's Career Institute. She is also a contributing editor for the revision of *Milady's Standard Cosmetology Textbook* and *Milady's Standard Nail Technology.* She is the author of the popular book *Preparing for the Practical Exam: Cosmetology;* for students and instructors, as well as the author of *Preparing for the Practical Exam: Nail Technology* for students and instructors.

Deborah holds her B.S. in Education for Technological Studies from the University of Georgia.

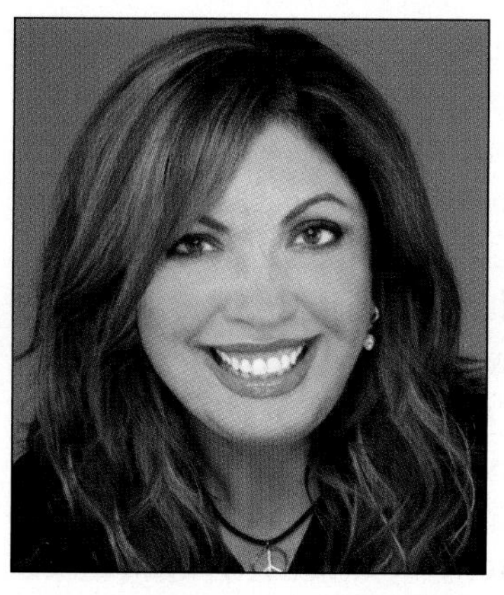

MARY BRUNETTI

Thirty focused years of fashion shoots have made Mary Brunetti an expert in the photography studio. This accomplished session stylist divides her time between fashion shoots for such magazines as *Elle, Town & Country,* and *New York Magazine,* as well as designing hair for runway shows during Fashion Week and educating on stages across the country.

She was the first woman to be awarded the prestigious title of North American Hairstylist of the Year in 1991 and has since served as a judge and consultant for the awards. She authored the book, *The Inside Track to NAHA,* and most recently art directed the DVD *How to Do a Successful Photo Shoot and Win at NAHA.*

Currently Mary is the Director of Education at a high, profile salon in New York City and is the co-owner of Brunetti Hair & Beauty in Westhampton Beach, New York, along with her husband, Michael.

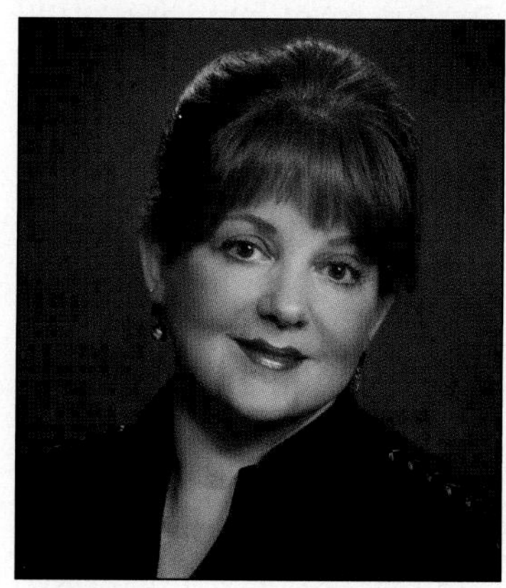

JANE CRAWFORD

As CEO of Jane Crawford Associates, this entrepreneur pioneered the first Med-Spa in the United States and earned the title of "America's foremost Med-Spa consultant." Ms. Crawford is on the faculty of the American Society of Aesthetic Plastic Surgeons, is a founding member of the International Medical Spa Association, and is a former board member of the American Aestheticians Education Association. She consults nationally and internationally to physicians. Ms. Crawford is co-owner of Carolina Aesthetics, a dermatological-based medical skin care clinic in Greenville, South Carolina. She is also a freelance writer for numerous medical and skin care magazines. Ms. Crawford presents seminars, educates physicians on successful ancillary service/product offerings, and trains nurses and estheticians about clinical skin care, chemical peels, and marketing.

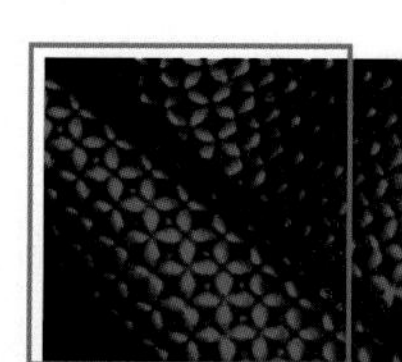

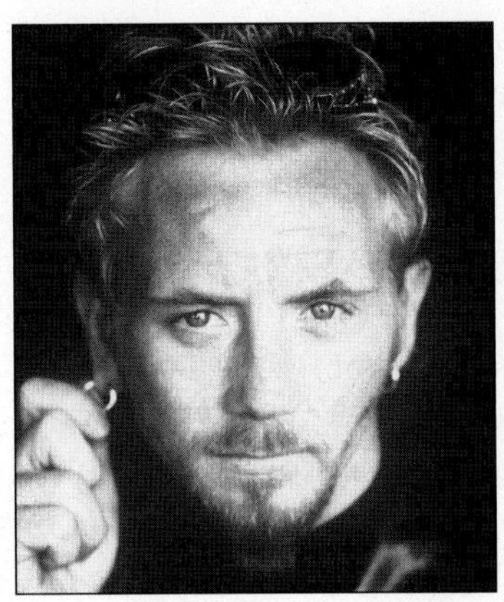

ROBERT CROMEANS

Robert Cromeans is the artistic director for John Paul Mitchell Systems and the owner of four successful salons. As a hairdresser, he is known for his daring and innovative designs. He has made guest appearances on national and international television an radio shows and has appeared in numerous publications such as *Vogue, Bazaar,* and *Glamour,* and other beauty industry magazines. Cromeans was named Platform Artist of the Year for *behindthechair.com's* Stylists Choice Awards. Known for his wit, wisdom, and great sense of personal sytle, Robert Cromeans is widely respected and in demand globally as an educator, motivator, and hairdresser.

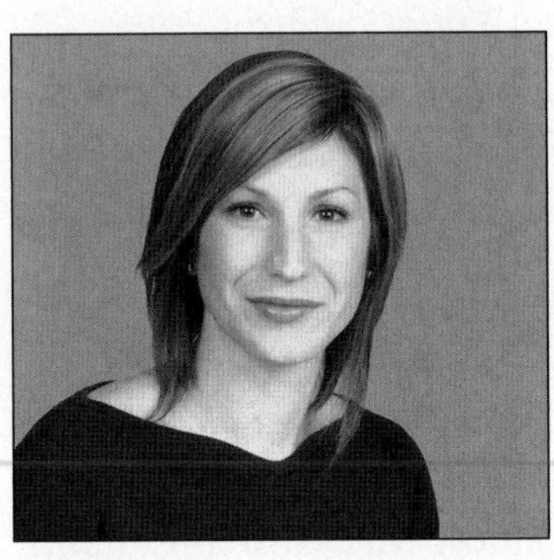

ALYSSA EVIRS

Beginning her career in the esthetics field in 1996, Alyssa Evirs has continuously worked to provide quality education and technical instruction to estheticians of all skill levels around the Untied States. Beyond holding licenses as an esthetician; she is a certified Esthetics Instructor and currently employed as the West Coast Spa Sales and Education Manager for the Aveda Corporation. Having great passion for holistic esthetics, Alyssa has worked with and for the Aveda Corporation for the past 11 years and continues to dedicate her time to the study and science of natural skin care.

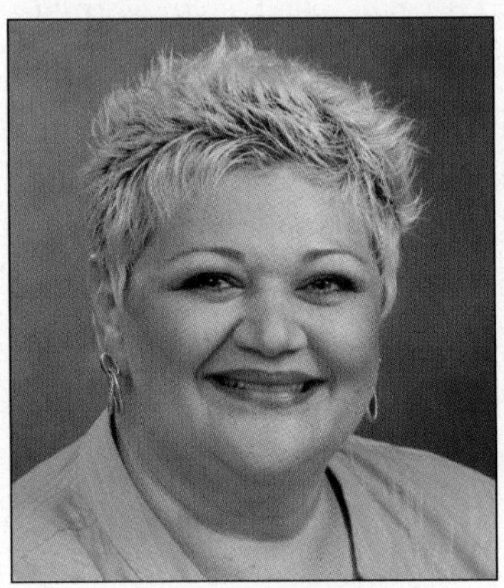

CATHERINE FRANGIE

Catherine M. Frangie has been a dedicated and passionate beauty professional since 1982 when she first began her career as a licensed cosmetologist, salon owner, and beauty school instructor. Since then, Catherine has held prominent and dynamic positions throughout many facets of the professional beauty industry, including Marketing, Communications, and Education Vice President for a leading product company; Communications Director, Trade Magazine Editor/Publisher; and Textbook Editor and Author.

Catherine has addressed her beauty colleagues numerous times as a guest lecturer at the International Beauty Show in New York City and in other national venues. She has personally authored more than 125 feature-length trade and consumer magazine articles and several books on beauty trends, fashion, and the business of the professional salon. Catherine holds a graduate degree in communications as well as undergraduate degrees in marketing and advertising.

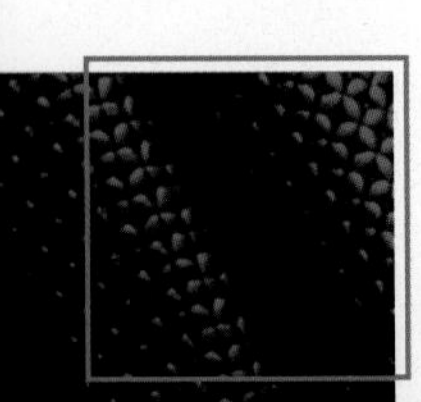

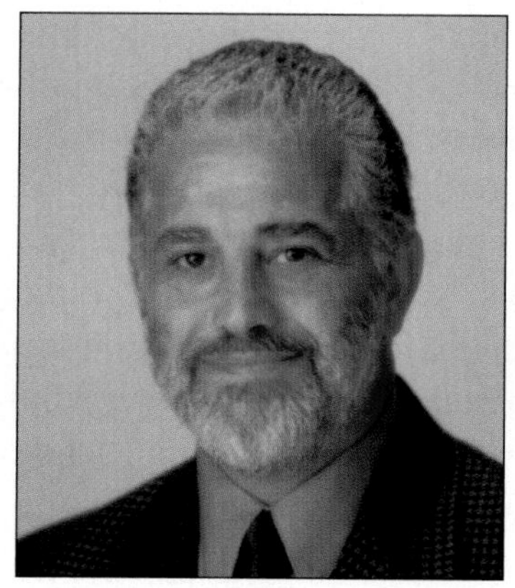

JOHN HALAL

A hairstylist, licensed instructor, and president of Honors Beauty College, Inc., John Halal is an active member of the National Cosmetologist Association (NCA), the Salon Association (TSA), the Beauty & Barber Supply Institute (BBSI), and the Society of Cosmetic Chemists (SCC). He serves as a Vice President and Executive Director for the American Association of Cosmetology Schools (AACS) and is the Past-President of the Indiana Cosmetology Educators Association (ICEA). Halal has published several books and numerous articles on hair structure and product chemistry. Halal obtained his associate's degree, with highest distinction, from Indiana University and is a member of The Golden Key National Honor Society and Alpha Sigma Lambda.

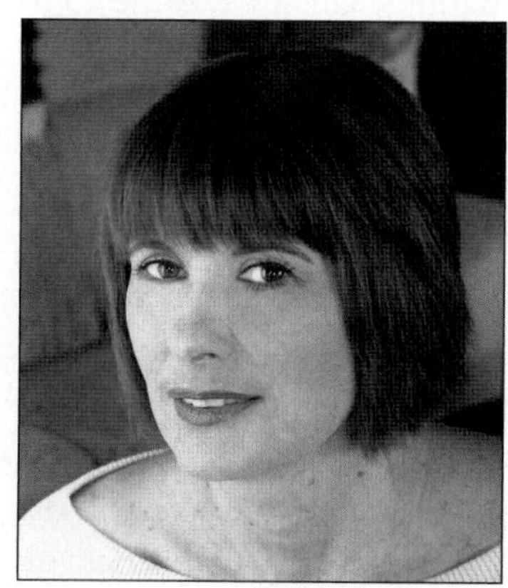

COLLEEN HENNESSEY

Recognized nationally as a Master Hair Colorist, Platform Artist, and Technical Educator, Colleen Hennessey bring years of hands-on coloring experience to the industry. She spent eight years at the renowned Adam Broderick Salon and Spa as a colorist and a manager.

Colleen's rare skills as an educator make her a sought-after resource throughout the professional arena. For the past six years she has serviced as Senior Technical Editor for *Hair Color and Design Magazine,* where she writes an editorial called "The Hair Color Department."

Formerly, Clairol Professional's exclusive color designer and Senior Manager of Clairol's Education Department, Colleen has brought techniques and color corrective advice to all licensed cosmetologists. Her work has also been featured in *Color & Style, Matrix News, Modern Salon,* and *Passion* magazines.

As an artist of many talents, Colleen is an established platform artist performing throughout the United States, including Hair Color USA, Long Beach, Mid-west, and IBS.

Wherever she teaches—on platform, in salons, or in textbooks and magazines—Colleen communicates her love of hair color by teaching others precise, technical, artistic, and communication skills that have earned her the prestigious title of Master Colorist.

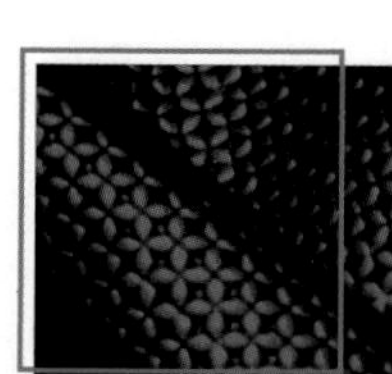

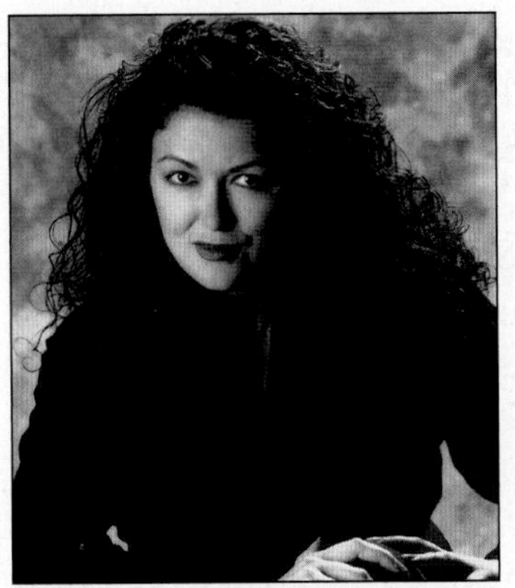

MARY BETH JANSSEN

Mary Beth Janssen is an internationally acclaimed educator and designer with over 25 years as a licensed cosmetologist and teacher. She's produced and directed numerous projects for the beauty industry, and her expertise has graced magazine editorials, television shows, and commercials. She's a regular beauty industry speaker and has authored several books on beauty and wellness. Janssen currently oversees and directs all activities of The Janssen Source, Inc., a Chicago-based company integrating Janssen's message of beauty and wellness. Because Janssen believes "real beauty begins with health – and true wellness is directly related to how we nurture our mind, body, and spirit," she inspires cosmetologists and clients alike to tap into their higher consciousness through educational seminars, on-site visits, and one-on-one consultations. Janssen was the 1996 recipient of the Rocco Bellino Award for outstanding contributions in education, and is also a certified herbalist, aromatherapist, massage therapist, and yoga teacher.

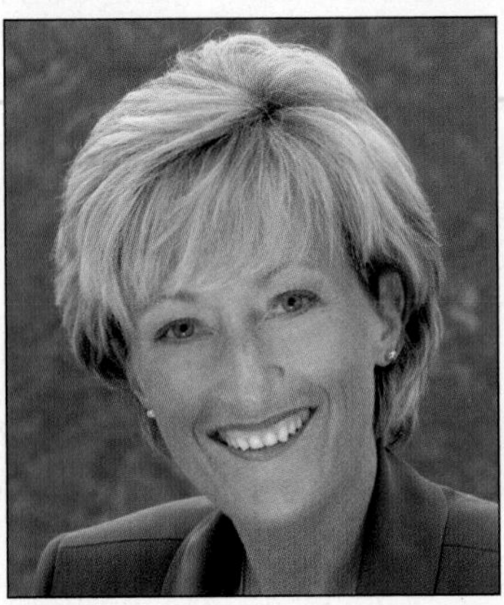

NANCY KING

Nancy King is an internationally recognized expert on safe salon practices and regulation. She has been an industry spokesperson to the media and was the technical advisor to the producers of the ABC's *20/20* and CNN nail stories on pedicure infections and salon chemical safety. A licensed nail technician, educator, and industry consultant, she has written articles and has been a cover artist for international trade publications. In 2000, Nancy became the Director of the AEFM, and took that organization to new heights in setting the industry standard for electric file education, both in the United States and internationally. Nancy is currently the Director of Education for *Nailpro Magazine.*

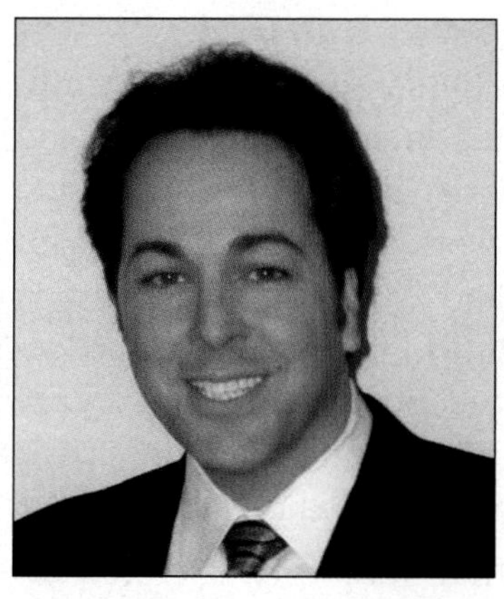

MARK LEES

Mark Lees, Ph.D., M.S., is an award-winning speaker and product developer, specializing in products for acne-prone and sensitive skin, and has been actively practicing clinical skin care for over 20 years at his multi-award winning CIDESCO-accredited Florida salon.

Dr. Lees is author of the popular book, *Skin Care: Beyond the Basics,* and contributing science author of *Milady's Comprehensive Training for Estheticians.* He holds a Ph.D. in Health Sciences, a Master of Science in Health, and a CIDESCO International Diploma. He is licensed to practice in both Florida and Washington State.

Dr. Lees is former Chairman of the Board of the Esthetics Manufacturers and Distributors Alliance, and is a member of the Society of Cosmetic Chemists. Dr. Lees is former Chairman of EstheticsAmerica and currently serves on the Board of Directors of the National Cosmetology Association.

His line of products is available through skin care professionals throughout the United States.

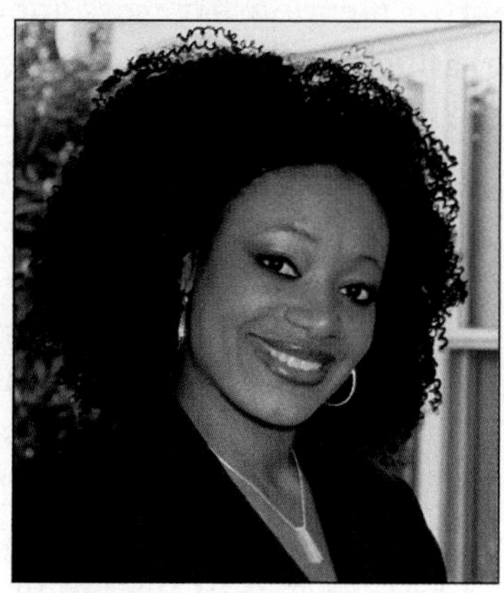

TONI LOVE

Toni Love is the daughter of a cosmetologist, (Mrs. Theresa Burroughs) and began working in her mother's salon at age 14. She is a veteran of the U.S. Army Reserves and a graduate of Hair Design Academy. She obtained a B.S. in Business Management and a Master's Degree in Continuing Education and is pursuing an Educational Specialist Degree in Career and Technical Education.

Toni has taught in the Greene County School Systems in Eutaw, Alabama, and she has taught at Shelton State Community College in Tuscaloosa, Alabama. She served as Director of Continuing Education for Dudley Products Company in Kernersville, North Carolina.

Today, Toni owns Toni Love's Cosmetology Training Center in Moundville, Alabama (basic and advanced classes), and is the author of a self-published book, *Tips to Passing the Cosmetology Exam,* and *Wigs, Weaves, and Extensions,* published by Thomson Learning. She has released several videos, including *Interlocking and Net Weaving, Hair Replacement,* and *Keeping Cutting Simple.* She travels abroad, teaching classes at hair shows and seminars. For more information, please visit www.tonilove.com.

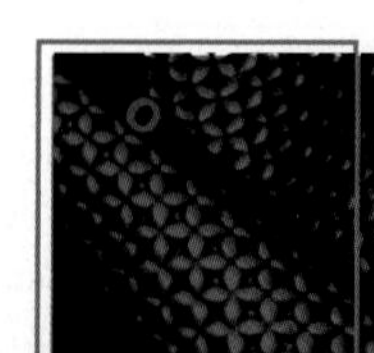

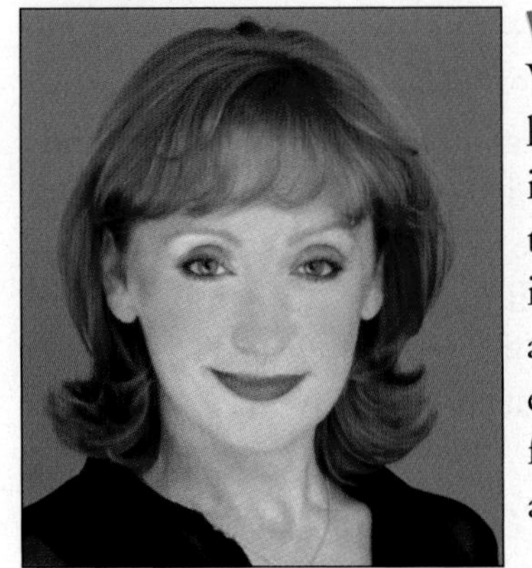

VIVIENNE MACKINDER

Vivienne Mackinder is one of the most highly respected international leaders and innovators in the hairdressing profession today. In her work as Artistic Director for industry "Grand Masters" Vidal Sassoon and Trevor Sorbie, Vivienne developed an expertise for precision cutting and an eye for original hair design, from the classic and the commercial, to the avant-garde.

Based in New York City, she grew up in London and subsequently opted to "spread her wings" to the United States. She has been honored with numerous awards, including the much coveted North American Hairstyling Awards (NAHA) (five times), the most recent being "Masters," and the prestigious IBS "Editors" Choice Awards (three times).

Vivienne is an "in-demand" featured guest artist-educator for premier international events worldwide, and her work is consistently published in the international press. She founded the "Roots and Wings" educational program in New York City to much acclaim.

Vivienne's career, as a master stylist, is divided between her salon clientele, editorial and advertorial shoots, advertising campaigns, and countless special events as featured artist, not to mention her work for entertainment entities, MTV, and the VH-1 Fashion Awards.

As a session stylist, she has collaborated and designed hair collections for runway fashion collections in New York, Paris, and London.

Vivienne's newest and most rewarding project to date, *I'm Not Just a Hairdresser,* is an exciting, informative, and inspirational documentary film series that will inspire a new generation of professionals and re-inspire the seasoned stylist who may be facing "burn out" syndrome, or questioning what's next in their career.

"Legends," the first episode in the series, was released in the spring of 2005, and "Empires," the second episode, was released in the fall of the same year. "Stars Behind The Chair," the third episode profiling the leading ladies of hair, released in the spring of 2006.

I'm Not Just A Hairdresser has a mission to: "Uplift the spirit and image of our profession," one stylist at a time.

For more detailed information, please visit the Web site: www.ImNOTJUSTaHairdresser.com. A portion of the proceeds will be donated to Movement of the Heart a non-profit organization. www.movementoftheheart.org.

CAREY NASH

Carey Nash received her cosmetology license in 1958 and a year later received her instructor's license at the age of 20. She worked full- and part-time in a salon for 6 years and was an instructor at the Bartmore Beauty Colleges until 1970. At that time, she joined the Marinello Schools of Beauty and has held various titles, including Instructor, Assistant Supervisor, Supervisor, Registrar, Manager, Accreditation Specialist, Director of Education, and her current title, Director of Compliance. She has also served as an expert witness and test analyst, where she helped validate the written examination for the California State Board of Cosmetology.

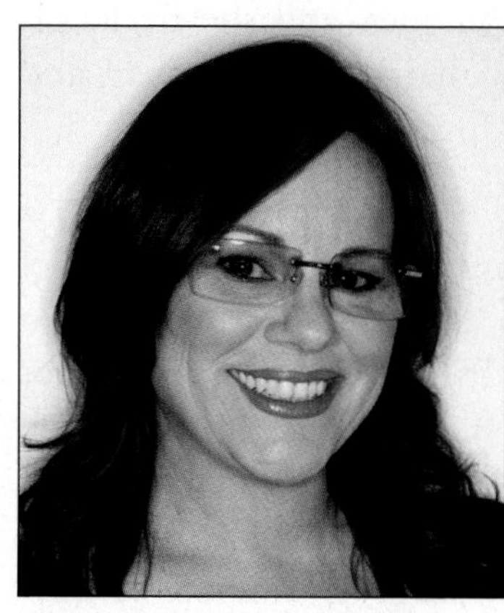

RUTH ROCHE

Since arriving in New York City in 1990, Ruth Roche has reached the top of her profession as a hairstylist. Salon owner, editorial stylist, platform artist, and educator, Ruth's work has appeared in magazines such as *Harper's Bazaar, Elle, Vanity Fair, Interview, Self, More,* and *Cosmopolitan,* to name a few. Represented by Artists by Timothy Priano, Ruth maintains a busy freelance career.

Her celebrity clients have included Sheryl Crow, Claire Danes, Lindsay Lohan, Kelly Ripa, Laura Linney, Sharon Stone, Mischa Barton, Amerie, Antigone Rising, Natalie Maines (Dixie Chicks), Lake Bell, and Beverley Mitchell. She has worked with renowned photographers such as Annie Liebovitz, Gilles Bensimon, Terry Richardson, Timothy White, Rod Spicer, and Mike Ruiz. Her creations have been seen on runways of many designers during New York's famed Fashion Week.

In 2003 Ruth opened RARE Salon in NYC's downtown hotspot, Tribeca, marking another milestone in her career. She and the RARE team have quickly become a neighborhood favorite. Ruth also created the RARE Academy, the perfect place for fellow stylists from around the country to learn, grow, and fuel their creative fire.

With almost two decades in beauty, Ruth has been honored multiple times by the North American Hairstyling Awards, including Master Stylist of the Year. She raised the bar at Redken as Global Artistic Director of Design and previously for renowned British hairdresser Trevor Sorbie. She has travelled the world for both companies, and now RARE, sharing her experience and new techniques with fellow professionals.

If that wasn't enough, she also writes a monthly column for *American Salon Magazine.* Through her column she inspires many fellow hairdressers with her stories and brings freshness to the craft. She has become a master in her field, with a following unlike any other!

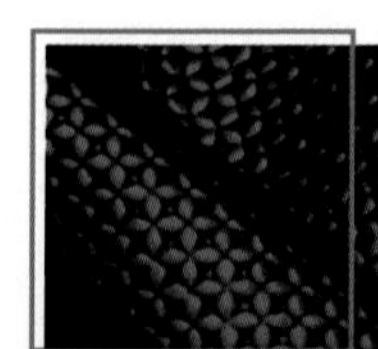

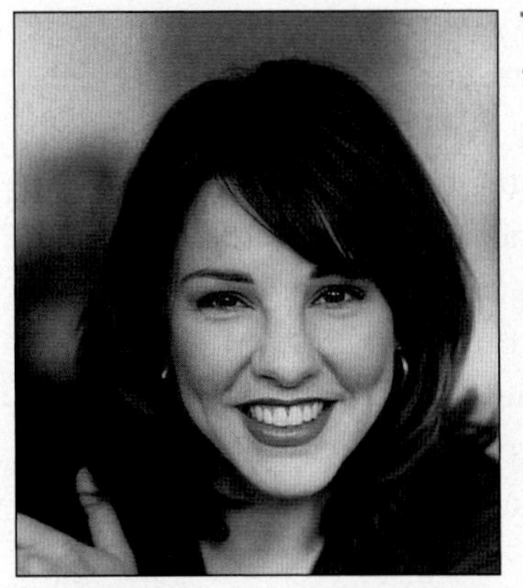

TERESA SAMMARCO

The last decade has provided makeup artist Teresa Sammarco with a strong foundation in the industry. As a dual makeup artist and hairstylist, she has created looks for top fashion designers, photographers, print advertisements, television commercials, and theater productions. She's even known to frequently appear in front of the camera herself. Sammarco is a regular on the lecture circuit, providing both tips and techniques, and she freelances nationwide, performing makeup and hairstyling looks and consultations.

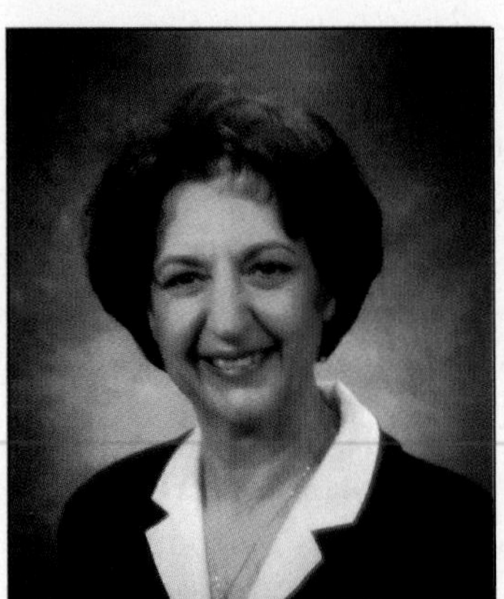

SUE SANSOM

When Sue Sansom received a high school scholarship to attend beauty school in 1963, she saw it as a way to help pay for law school. After a year in a salon, however, she discovered a love for cosmetology that led her to become Arizona's youngest licensed cosmetology instructor of that time at age 19. Rather than pursue a law degree, Sue instead applied her passion for administrative law to the cosmetology field and became the first Executive Director of the Arizona State Board of Cosmetology in 1984. She has spent 22 years involved with the National Interstate Council of Cosmetology Boards (NIC) actively promoting regulation, education, and examinations with respect to health and safety in the cosmetology industry. Sue is a graduate of Arizona State University (ASU) Certified Public Managers and is Certified as a Public Vocational Education Teacher. She is the recipient of the NIC Nick Cimaglia Award 1993 and Arizona Administrator of the year 1994, and she led the Arizona Board to receive the AACS/TSA State Excellence award in the year 2000.

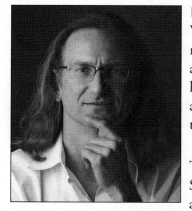

DOUGLAS SCHOON

With over thirty years' experience as a research scientist, international lecturer, author, and educator, Douglas Schoon heads up the most extensive nail research and development laboratory in existence today.

As the Vice President of Science & Technology for Creative Nail Design, Schoon spends much of his time leading a team of scientists working with high-tech, computerized testing equipment to produce state-of-the-art nail enhancement products and natural nail treatments, as well as, world-renown spa products. With all of this expertise and technology, Creative Nail Design's research capabilities exceed even those found in many university laboratories.

For over sixteen years Schoon has led the Creative Nail Design's Research and Development program. He directs the Quality Assurance, Technical Services, and Field Testing department, as well. Schoon is the author of many books and video and audio training programs, as well as dozens of magazine articles on salon chemicals, chemical safety, and disinfection. He often serves as an expert witness in legal cases involving cosmetic safety and health. Additionally, dermatologists frequently call upon Schoon to assist them in writing books and scientific papers concerning fingernails, proving without a doubt, he is a world leading experts on natural and artificial nail product, services, and salons. He is also a strong advocate for salon safety and represents the entire nail industry on scientific and technical issues in Europe, Canada, the United States. Schoon first entered the nail industry in 1986 as the founder of Chemical Awareness Training Service, CATS, the beauty industries first company focused on safety training programs for salons. He has a long history of educating safe practices to nail professionals.

As a writer and speaker, Mr. Schoon is especially popular with the nail technicians because of his unique ability to make complex chemical theories and ideas seem simple, even easy to understand. His natural nail health, safety, and disinfection lectures are also invaluable to anyone interested in product chemistry, safety, and health issues, as is his most popular book, *Nail Structure & Product Chemistry—Simplified,* Second Edition, Delmar, Cengage Learning.

In addition, Schoon is a Co-chair of the Safety and Standards Committee of Nail Manufacturers Council (NMC), as well as the holder of a Master's Degree in Chemistry from the prestigious University of California–Irvine. He currently resides in Dana Point, California.

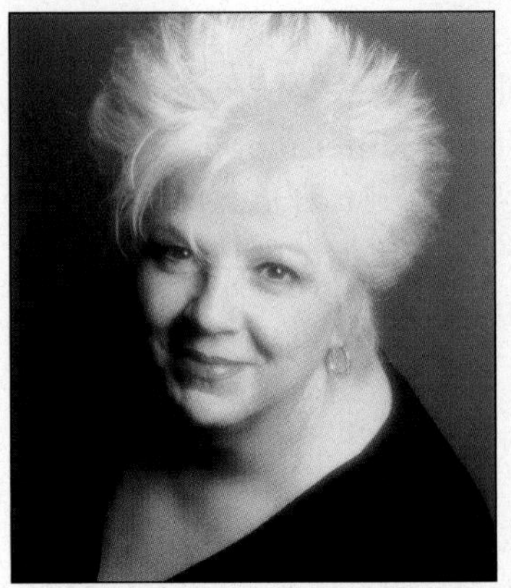

SUE ELLEN SCHULTES

Sue Ellen Schultes is an award-winning nail artist, a licensed nail technician, and a former salon owner whose business was recognized as one of the top 100 nail salons in the country by *Nails* magazine ten years running. Sue is recognized as one of the leading nail art technology authorities in the U.S. and has taught extensively throughout the United States, conducting workshops and seminars via Notorious Nails Seminars. Sue serves as Competition Judge for various trade shows, both nationally and internationally. Besides acting as series editor and contributing author for Delmar, Cengage Learning, Sue also contributes special interest articles to *Nails* magazine and several other publications. Sue was commissioned by the Smithsonian Institute's National Museum of American History to create a full set of nails commemorating the United States Presidential Inauguration.

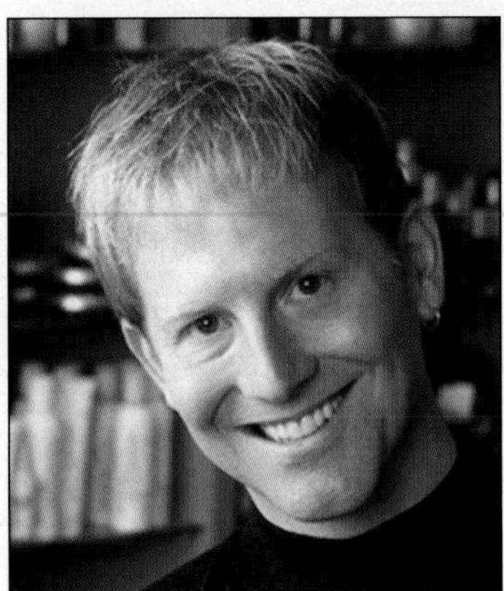

FRANK SHIPMAN

Frank Shipman has been making hair look great for more than two decades. As the owner of the nationally recognized Technicolor/TC Salon Spas, Frank is proud to have the privilege of working behind the chair. He also continues to be a beauty educator, writer, and speaker, bringing his own unique perspective to the industry. In 2005, Frank received the prestigious Diamond Award from *Day Spa Magazine* to add to his many professional awards and honors. Frank has a graduate degree in art from Boston University and has had his art exhibited nationally and internationally. Today he no longer creates "precious objects" but creates "experiences." Frank is happy to be in a profession, that, as he states "what I do is make people feel good."

JERYL SPEAR

Jeryl E. Spear is a veteran stylist and salon owner who perfected her craft over a 17-year stint in the beauty business. She has been contributing for several years, having had her work published in *Modern Salon, Salon News,* and *DaySpa* magazines, plus consumer writing for magazines such as *Self, Healing Lifestyles and Spas,* and *Spa.* Loving all things beauty and fashion, she is now the executive editor of *Launchpad* magazine.

ACKNOWLEDGMENTS

Many cosmetologists and educators have contributed to the development of this book since its initial publication in 1938. *Milady's Standard Textbook of Cosmetology* owes its creation to the lifetime dedication of Nicholas F. Cimaglia, founder of Milady Publishing Company. Mr. Cimaglia was also one of the founders of the National Association of Accredited Cosmetology Schools and the Teachers' Education Council, and helped form the National Accrediting Commission for Cosmetology Art and Sciences.

The standard set by Mr. Cimaglia has been carried on in the beauty education industry by his son, Thomas Severance, and by two gentlemen whose tireless efforts have established the success of *Milady's Standard:* Jacob Yahm, the father of accreditation in our industry and a driving force behind the National Interstate Council of State Boards of Cosmetology, and Arnold DeMille, founding editor of the *National Beauty School Journal* and continuing education specialist.

Milady recognizes with gratitude and respect the many professionals who have offered their time to contribute to this edition of the *Standard.* Milady wishes to extend enormous thanks to the following people who have played a part in this edition.

SPECIAL THANKS:

- Kimberley Comiskey, owner of Kimberley's . . . A Day Spa, Ltd., located in Latham, New York, and her incredible staff for allowing us use of their location, equipment, and participating as models in the photo shoot.
- Fernando Fischbach of CinderellaHair, Inc. (www.cinderellahair.com) and Golden Supreme (www.goldensupreme.com) for supplying hair extensions and product photos for our Braiding and Braid Extensions chapter.
- Tom Carson Photography for allowing us use of his extensive photo collection for glamour shots throughout the new edition.

REVIEWERS:

Betty Abernethy, Wyoming Board of Cosmetology, WY

Michael Adams, Coshocton County Career Center, OH

Sharon Lee Adebimpe, Ailano School of Aesthetics, MA

Jennifer Adler, Hill College, TX

Jessie Aki, Honolulu Community College, HI

Marlene Alfman, National Beauty College, OH

Kristin Allison, Four Seasons Salon & Day Spa, Inc., WI

Karen Altavela, Monroe #1 BOCES, NY

Rae Ann Amacher, Orleans/Niagara BOCES, NY

Marjorie Amorosi-Farinha, Capri Institute, NJ

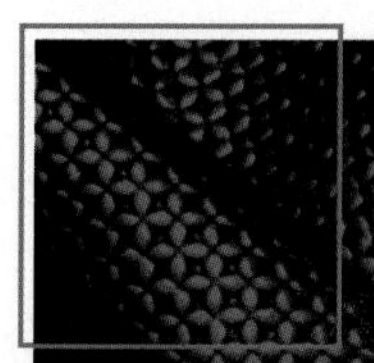

Joan Armistead, Northwest-Shoals Community College, AL

Margie Arnold, First Coast Technical Institute, FL

Paula Askew, Vance Granville Community College, NC

LaFaye Austin, National Interstate Council, Chairman, OK

Kimberly Avery, Navarro College, TX

Darlene Azadnia, Greater New Bedford Regional Vocational Technical High School, MA

Maria Baca, Socorro High School, TX

Essie Baldwin, Fairfield High Preparatory School, AL

Brenda Baker, New England Institute of Technology, FL

Joan Bannister, College of the North Atlantic, NL

Petra-Ann Baptiste, Chaconia Spa Essentials/Kingwood College, TX

Rita Barger, Scott County Career & Technical Center, VA

Harry Barney, International College of Hospitality Management, CT

Lisa Baron, Questar III BOCES, NY

Paullett Barton, Birdville Independent School District, TX

Daniel Basto-Gurwell, Guam Community College, GU

Rita Baumgartl, Cuyahoga Valley Career Center, OH

Deborah Beatty, Columbus Technical College, GA

Stephen Beers, Venango Technology Center, PA

Paul Berry, Stewart County High School, TN

Sharon Bethel, Eastland Career Center, OH

Laurie Biagi, Skyline College, CA

Andrea Blankinship, Transitions School of Cosmetology Careers/Mott Community College, MI

Patricia Blanusa, CA

Cathy Bonaccorso, Orleans Niagara BOCES, NY

Marcia Bonawitz, Sacramento City College, CA

Betty Boully, Traviss Career Center, FL

Ross Briggs, Champion Beauty and Massage Schools, TX

Neva Brode, Auburn Career Center, OH

Jerry D. Brown, Vincennes University/Wabash Valley School of Barbering, IN

Mary Brown, Cape Fear Community College, NC

Shandy Brown, Flawless Institute De Beaute Enhancement, FL

Chris Browne, Kaskaskia College, IL

Jennie Bubloni, Lake County High Schools Technology Campus, IL

Mary Buker, Century College, MN

Larry Bulechek, Protégé of Arizona-Phoenix Union High School, AZ

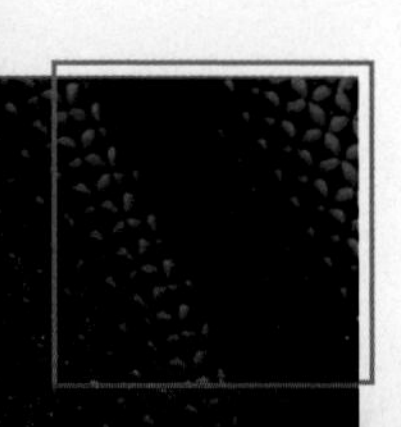

Anita Burleson, Riverwalk Salon, AL
Paullett Burton, Texas A&M University, TX
James Butina, Warren Woods Public Schools, MI
Patricia Butler, Powhatan High School, VA
Tracy Caddy, Colorado Northwestern Community College, CO
Judith Cardin, Conlee's College of Cosmetology, TX
Gerri Cevetillo, Ultronics Inc., NJ
Antoinette Chambers, TNT University, NC
Donna Charron, Eastern Wyoming College, WY
Gayle Cherry, R.D. Anderson Applied Technology Center, SC
Carla Chin, Traviss Career Center, FL
Chaconne Christiansen, Innovative Balance School of Esthetics, UT
Diane Cingel, Lake County Tech Campus, IL
Betty R. Clawson, Dudley Beauty College, IL
Robin Cochran, Gadsden State Community College-Ayers Campus, AL
Nikki Cole, Academy of Cosmetology, PA
Betty Coleman, Hephzibah High School, GA
Linda Colley, TN
Kay Collins, Prater Way College of Beauty, NV
Patricia D. Collins, Truman College, IL
Karen Comer, Gateway Technical College, WI
Bonnie Conkle, Tennessee Technical Center at Hohenwald, TN
Ruth Cosmopoulos, Pathfinder Regional Vocational Technical High School, MA
Thom Costa, Century College, MN
Carolyn Cox, Vogue College of Cosmetology, TX
Fern Cox, Hill Community College, TX
Norma Curl, The Hair Design School, KY
Jackie Dahlquist, National Interstate Council (NIC) Executive Board, SD
Janet D'Angelo, J.Angel Communications, Marketing & PR Consultant, MA
Jenae Davei, John Paul Mitchell, IL
Cindy Lee Davidson, Beauty First, OR
Sandra Davis, Coffee County Central High School, TN
Susan Day, Vocational School, PA
Carol DeLong, Fiser's College of Cosmetology, MI
Anthony De Sando, Natural Motion Institute of Hair Design, NJ
Robert Diaz, East San Gabriel Valley ROP & Tech Center, CA

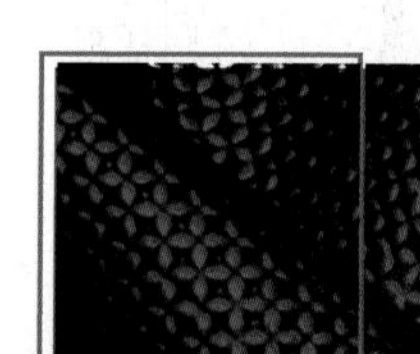

Wanda Duncan, Eastern Hills Academy of Hair Design, Batavia, Ohio

Patricia Dunn, C.H. McCann Technical School, MA

Kathy Earl, Apollo Career Center, OH

Corrine (Denise) Edwards, Hair Duo, Co-owner, MD

Debbie Elliott, Antioch, ME

Amy Ellison, Butler County Area Vocational-Technical School, PA

Amy Enzweiler, Instructor, Eastern Hills Academy of Hair Design, KY

Kelly Ferguson, Ashland County-West Holmes Career Center, OH

Susanne Ferkingstad, Minnesota School of Cosmetology, MN

Flora Finch, Northland Pioneer College, AZ

Mary Finnegan, Saint Paul College—A Community & Technical College, MN

Jerri Franco, SBCC Cosmetology Academy, CT

Wilbert Frazier, Bessemer Center for Technology, AL

Mary Frilot, Aspen Beauty Academy, MD

Rick Fuger, I.S.U. College of Technology, ID

Cathy Fultz, Arkansas Valley/ATU, AZ

Gabriela Gagnier, Knoxville Institute of Hair Design, TN

Becky Gant, Sunstate Hairstyling Academy, FL

Sylvia Garcia, Spokane Community College, WA

Roberta Garner, Louisiana Technical Collage, LA

Zora Garner, Gadsden State Community College, AL

Bonnie Garrity, NCOC–Suny Oswego, NY

Denise Gaston, Miss Marty's Hair Academy & Esthetics Institute, CA

Sandra Gay, Oehrlein School of Cosmetology, IL

Sheryl George, LCM High School, TX

Lisa Gibson, Stafford High School, VA

Ruth Gibson, Orleans Niagara Boces, NY

Sharon Gill, Somerset County Vocational and Technical institute, NJ

Patty Glover, Citrus College, CA

Myssi Goldsmith, The Hair Design School, KY

Hector Gonzalez, Hi-Tech The School of Cosmetology, FL

Gloria Greene, Houston Community College, TX

Crystal Grier, White County High School, GA

Shonell Griffith, Lee College, TX

Jane Guenzer, Camden County Technical School, NJ

Martin Gugliotti, International Institute of Cosmetology, CT

Crystal Gutshall, Sun Area CTC, PA

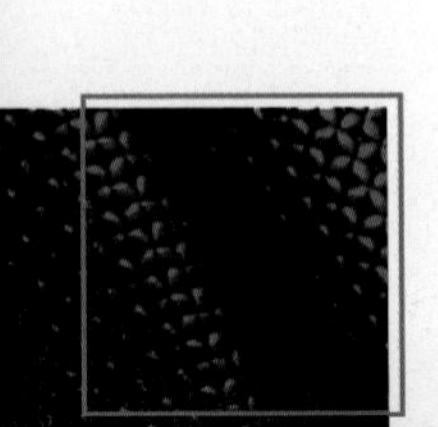

Connie Hackmann, Vatterott College, MO

John Halal, Honors Beauty College, Inc., IN

Mary Ann Haley, Solano Community College, CA

Esther Halley, Sundial School, St. Maarten (Ned. Ant.)

Pamela Hamilton, Rob Roy Academy, MA

Farzana Hanif, Country Clipper, AZ

Sandy Hansert, Western Hills School of Beauty & Hair Design, Hornsby Group, OH

Gloria Harding, Tranquility Day Spa & Salon, VA

Ollie Harkleroad, Okefenokee Technical College, GA

Laura Harnden, Ulster Career & Tech Center, NY

Dara Harrell, College of the Albemarle, NC

Kenneth Harris, Halifax Community College, NC

Pamela Harris, Riverdale High School, GA

Beverly Jo Hart, Toledo Academy of Beauty Culture, OH

Joyce Hawkins, Johnston Community College, NC

Ronald Hawkins, Albany Technical College, GA

Jennifer Hayes, Tennessee Technology Center at Paris, TN

Andria Haynes, Advanced Cosmetology–College of San Mateo, CA

Dayna Heath, Earl's Academy of Beauty, AZ

Patricia Heitz, Dermatech Academy, NY

Suzanne (Sue Marie) Hemming, Minnesota School of Cosmetology, MN

Gail Henderson, Coosa Valley Technical College, GA

Louise Hester, PJ's College of Cosmetology, KY

Michael Hill, National-Interstate Council of State Boards of Cosmetology, Inc., AR

Kathe Holley, Sidney Lanier High School, TX

Stephanie Holtz, Polaris Career Center, OH

Robin Hometchko, A Place in the Sun, MT

Delores Hunt, Central Florida Community College, FL

Tanya Huyard, Unicoi County Vocational School, TN

Judith A. James, Western Hills School of Beauty and Hair Design, OH

Carol Jeter, Valdosta Technical College, GA

Caryl Ann Johnson, Olympian University of Cosmetology/International Academy/I.T.S. Academy of Beauty/Aladdin Beauty College, AZ

Jeanne Johnson, Cerritos College, CA

Linda Johnson, Carver Beauty Academy, WV

Cathy Jones, Tri-County Technical High School, MA

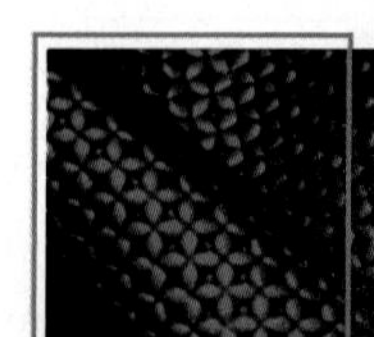

Gwen Jordan, Garrett Academy of Technology High School, SC
Myra Jowers, Florida Community College at Jacksonville, FL
Jane Juliano, Burlington County Institute of Technology, NJ
Darlene Kajs, Vernon College, TX
Dianna Kenneally, Proctor & Gamble, OH
Donn Kerr, Esthetics International, SC
David Kile, Bates Technical College, WA
Cynthia King, Lamar State College–Port Arthur, TX
Nancy King, Nail Care Consulting, Director of AEFM, CO
Rosanne Kinley, National Interstate Council (NIC) of State Boards of Cosmetology, SC
Jen Knight, U.P. Academy of Hair, MI
Susan Kolar, Transitions/Mott Community College, MI
Karen Kraus, Milwaukee Area Technical College, WI
May Lahham, West Valley Occupational Center, CA
Angela LaMorte, Morris County School of Technology, NJ
Helen LeDonne, Santa Monica College, CA
May Lee, Skyline Community College, CA
Suzanne Lehmkuhl, Protégé of Arizona, AZ
Robert LeJeune II, Demmon's School of Beauty, LA
Caroline Lerette, Citrus College, CA
Patricia Leslie, Indianapolis Public School CTC, IN
Carolyn Lewis, Barbara Jordan High, TX
Lisa Lewis, Lee County Career and Technical Center, VA
Teresa Lewis, MonMouth College, IL
Shirley Lipscomb, Lanier Technical College, GA
Liz Linard, Northeast Career Center, OH
Julie Linville, Winston-Salem Forsyth County School System—Career Center, NC
Barbara Litavecz, Excel Academies of Cosmetology, IN
Camille Lloyd, Shawsheen Vocational Tech High School, MA
Stacia Lowrie, Old Town Barber & Beauty College, KS
Karen Lynn, LCHSTC/College of Lake County, IL
Juanita Mace, Academy of Nail, Skin and Hair, MT
Sharon MacGregor, JC Penney Salon, NY
Felicia Maienza-Trusevitch, Clairol Professional, VA
Marilyn Maine, Los Angeles Trade Technical College, CA
Betty Martinez, Sam Houston High School/HCCS, TX
Thomas Maya, Maya's School of Beaute, Inc., FL

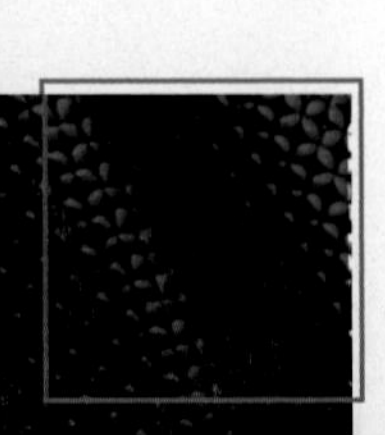

Nancy Mays, MPISD, TX
G'Marie McCollum, Harmon's Beauty School, MD
Dorothy McKinley Soressi, Empire Beauty School, NY
Julie Mead, HFM Career & Technical Center, NY
Shirley Meek, North Central Texas College, TX
Angela Mike, Westinghouse High School, PA
Catherine Minkler, Plainfield High School, NJ
Wendy Mitchell, Erwin Technical Center, FL
Andrina Monte, Brio Academy, CT
Leah Morgan, Instructor, OH
Kerrie Morris, Hill College, TX
Linda Mottishaw, The School of Hairstyling, ID
Connie Moyher, Portland High School, TN
Lisa Nave, Bradley Central High School, TN
Debbie Neatock, Center for Arts & Technology, PA
Linda Newman, Senior Instructor, Tri County Beauty College, OH
Trudy Nicholson, North Fayette Area Vocational-Technical School, PA
Linda Nicodemus, Spring Branch ISD Guthrie Center, TX
Stan Nielson, Snow College Richfield, UT
Stacey Noelting, Western Hills School of Beauty and Hair Design, OH
Kimber Novak, Crown College of Cosmetology Inc., IN
Marlene Nucifora, Artistic Academy Morris Plains, NJ
Susan O'Brien, Poplar Bluff Technical Career Center, MO
Diana Orndorff, Region 2 Director of NIC, PA
Cimarron Owens, Dtotal Woman Beauty and Nail Academy, VA
Jerri Paige, Howard College, TX
Mary Ann Parish, Pioneer Career and Technology Center, OH
Marisa Peach, DermAware Bio-Targeted Skincare, PA
Ernestine Peete, Tennessee Technology Center, TN
Regina Pelayo, Skyline Community College, CA
Maria Penn, Eastern Hills Academy of Hair Design, OH
Sandra Peoples, Pickens Tech, CO
Jonathan Perkins, SUNY Brockport Rochester Educational Opportunity Center, NY
Pam Perondi, Western Nevada Community College, NV
Kathrine Phelps, Moore Norman Technology Center, OK
Lynn Phillips, Lurleen B. Wallace Community College, AL
Nina Pierce, Jonesboro High School, GA
Brenda Porter, Polytech High School, DE

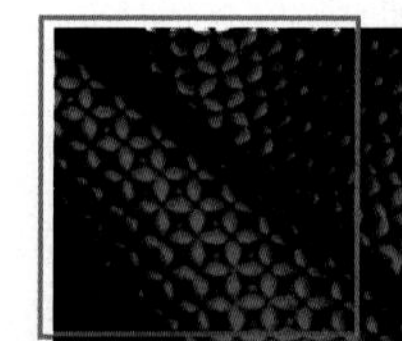

Robert Powers, Pinellas Technical Education Center, FL
Phyllis Pratt, Botetourt Technical Ed Center, VA
Erin Price, Instructor, Eastern Hills Academy of Hair Design, OH
Vivian Price, A Cut Above Beauty College, IN
Nancy Quick, Berks Career and Technology Center, PA
Ventura Ramirez, Houston Community College, TX
Kathryn Ray, Powder Springs Beauty College, GA
Lynette Reeves, Otero Junior College, CO
J Dale Reino, Davidson County Community College, NC
Lynn Reyes, Coastal Carolina Community College, NC
Lin Rice, Athens Technical College, GA
Judy Rickstrew, Amarillo High School, TX
Heidi Riley, Northwest MS Community College–Oxford Campus, MS
Susan Rineer, Lancaster County Brownstown Campus, PA
Patty Roberts, State School, MS
Ron Robinson, McLennan Community College, TX
Sharon Roctz, Raphael's Beauty School, OH
Nina Rogers, San Jacinto College Central Spencer, TX
Barbara Romerhausen, McLinney High School, TX
Linda Ronspiez, Howard College, TX
Tammy Rouse, Gateway Community and Tech College, KY
Judith Rousseau, Northern Michigan University, MI
Marilyn Rovelli, Springfield Technical Community College, MA
Rosa Sanchez, Americas High School, TX
Terry Sanders, Byng High School, OK
Jo-Ann Saporito, John Amico School of Hair Design, IL
Helen Scalise, St. Joseph Secondary School, Ontario
Sheila Scheib, Seward County Community College of Cosmetology, KS
Evelyn Schenk, Kirtland Community College, MI
Linda Schierbaum, Margate School of Beauty, Inc., FL
Rita Schimelpfening, Coastal Bend College/Pleasanton Campus, TX
Cathie Schmerse, Highland Community College, IL
Donna Schneider, Western Hills School of Beauty, OH
Clare Scott, Northeast Technology Center, OK
Mary Seong, MA
Vickie Servais, New Horizons Regional Education Center, VA
Alice Sharp, Questar III—Rensselaer Educational Center, NY
Judy Sikes, Griffin Technical College, GA
Gloria Smith, Institute of Cosmetic Arts, SC

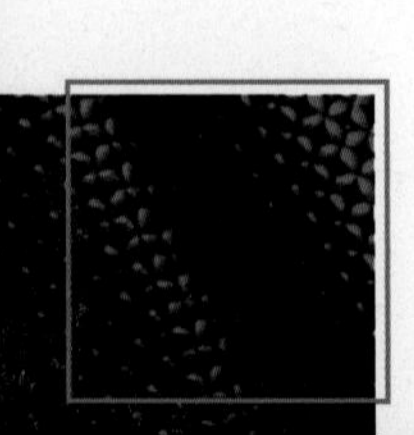

Darlene Smolko, Clearfield County Career and Technology Center, PA
Tom Sollock, Metro Area Vo-Tech, OK
Deanne Speer, Arkansas Beauty School, AR
Monica Stacy, Tricounty Beauty College, The Hornsby Group, OH
D. Stallman, The Haskana Institute of Hair Design, IL
Helene (Tina) Stanley, The County Alternative High School, PA
Mary Starling, South Florida Community College, FL
Dolores Stemwedel, Lake Area Technical Institute, SD
Jamie Sterle, Tranquility Design Academy, VA
Hope Strawder, East Central Technical College, GA
Hilda Sustaita, Houston Community College System, TX
Barbara Taylor, Carlisle School District, PA
Joyce Thomas, Central Carolina Community College, NC
Sydney Thomas, Laney College, CA
Lori Thorsen, MBIT, PA
Wanda Tidwell, Traviss Career Center, FL
Mary Todaro, PA
Laura Todd, Institute of Advanced Medical Esthetics & Health Sciences, VA
Starlette Tolver, Legends International School, BC
Charlene Treier, Miller-Motte Technical College, TN
Stephen Ukes, Prometric, Cosmetology Subject Matter Expert, MN
Michael Vanacore, Learning Institute for Beauty Sciences/Empire Beauty Schools, NY
Theresa Vaughn, Odessa College, TX
Maria Vick, New Mexico Junior College, NM
Therese Vogel, Tiffin Academy of Hair Design, OH
Nicki Vrooman, St. Law-Lewis BOCES, NY
Connie Wallace, Wallace Community College, AL
Nancy Walters, Milwaukee Area Technical College, WI
Regena Walters, Ehove Career Center, OH
Linda Ward, Mecosta Osceola Career Center, MI
David Waters, San Jacinto College South, TX
Faye Wells, Dodge City Community College, KS
Michele Werni, Lebanon County Career and Technology Center, PA
Patricia White, Caddo-Kiowa Tech Center, OK
Mary Jo Wiggins, Cuyahoga Falls High School, OH
Pier Wilkerson, Lawson State Community College, AL
Ken Young, Region 3 Director, NIC, OK

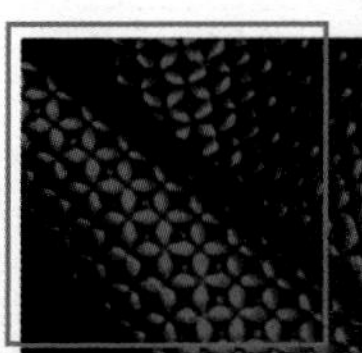

Sharon Young-Wester, University of the District of Columbia, DC

Alexandra J. Zani, Academy of Hair Technology, SC

PHOTOGRAPHY CREDITS:

Cover photo provided by Clairol Professional and Q Management in New York, NY. Photographer, Rod Spicer and Artist is Sharon Dorram.

Part 1: photo from Fred Goldstein/Shutterstock; hair dryer, © Getty Images; hair brush, © Paul Castle, Castle Photography.

Chapter 1: chapter opener photo courtesy of Tony Kendall, French Lick Hair Museum, Figures 1-1, 1-2: Corbis. Figures 1-3 and 1-6: PhotoDisc. Figure 1-5: Paul Castle.

Chapter 2: chapter opener photo, © Eric Bean/Getty Images. Figure 2-1: Paul Castle. Figures 2-2 and 2-5: Corbis. Figure 2-3: Paul Castle. Figure 2-4 and 2-6: Photodisc. Figure 2-7: Ed Hille. Figure 2-9: Paul Castle.

Chapter 3: chapter opener photo, © Ariel Skelley/CORBIS. Figures 3-1 to 3-3, 3-5, 3-8 to 3-10: Paul Castle. Fig. 3-7, Larry Hamill.

Chapter 4: chapter opener, © Paul Castle/Castle Photography. Figures 4-1, 4-3, 4-5, 4-7, 4-8, 4-9: Paul Castle. Figure 4-2: Michael Dzaman. Figure 4-6: Getty Images.

Part 2: photo provided by Scott Rothstein/Shutterstock. H_20 molecule, Dan Collier/Shutterstock.

Chapter 5: chapter opener, Figures 5-13 thru 5-19, 5-21, 5-22, Procedure 5-4: Paul Castle, Castle Photography. Beaker, © Jan Kaliciak/Shutterstock. Figure 5-2: Tom Stock. Figure 5-11: Courtesy of Godfrey F. Mix, DPM Sacramento, CA. Figure 5-12: Courtesy of The National Pediculosis Association®, INC. Figure 5-20: Michael Dzaman. Procedure 5-2 and 5-3: photos courtesy of Tranquility Day Spa & Salon, Manassas, VA.

Chapter 6: chapter opener, Sebastian Kaulitzki/Shutterstock.

Chapter 7: chapter opener, Inspirestock. Figure 7-6: Getty Images.

Chapter 8: chapter opener, Getty Images. Figure 8-2: Courtesy of Godfrey F. Mix, DPM, Sacramento, CA.

Chapter 9: chapter opener, Jerome Tisne/Getty Images. Figures 9-4, 9-21, and 9-22: Courtesy of P&G Beauty from John Grey's, The World of Hair Care. Figures 9-5, 9-6: Graphic World. Figures 9-8, 9-9, 9-10, 9-12 thru 9-14, 9-23: The Gillette Research Institute. Figures 9-11, 9-15, 9-16: Paul Castle. Figs. 9-17 thru 9-19: courtesy of Pfizer Inc. Figures 9-20, 9-24: courtesy of Robert A. Silverman, MD, Clinical Associate Professor, Department of Pediatrics, Georgetown University. Figure 9-25: Courtesy of The National Pediculosis Association®, Inc. Figure 9-26: Courtesy of Hogil Pharmaceutical Corporation.

Chapter 10: chapter opener, Jan Kaliciak/Shutterstock.

Chapter 11: chapter opener, Juriah Mosin/Shutterstock. Figures 11-9, 11-10: Larry Hamill.

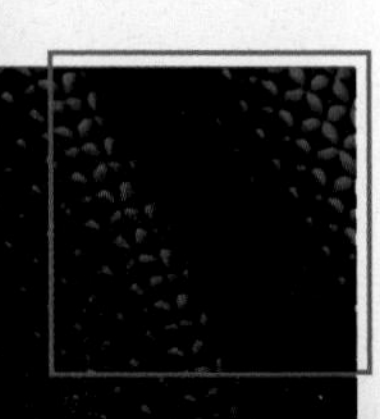

Part 3: part opener photo by James Mosley/Getty Images.

Chapter 12: chapter opener, courtesy of Clairol Professional and Q Management, NY. Figure 12-1: Courtesy of "Silents are Golden" (www.silentsaregolden.com). Figure 12-2: Scruples Professional Salon Products, Inc. Figure 12-84, Paul Castle.

Chapter 13: chapter opener photo, Figures 13-1, 13-8 thru 13-35 by Paul Castle. Procedure 13-1 (top right photo), Alfred Wekelo/Shutterstock.

Chapter 14: chapter opener, Simon Taplin/Getty Images. Figures 14-11, 14-12, 14-13, 14-21, 14-24, 14-28, 14-32, 14-91, 14-93, 14-129, 14-162, 14-166, 14-174, 14-176: photos used with the permission of the authors, Martin Gannon and Richard Thompson, as featured in their book, Mahogany; Steps to Cutting, Colouring and Finishing Hair. Copyright © Martin Gannon and Richard Thompson, 1997. Figure 14-20: John Paul Mitchell Systems, hair by John Chadwick, photo by Alfred Tolot. Figure 14-30: John Paul Mitchell Systems, hair by People & Schumacher, photo by Andreas Elsner. Figure 14-168: John Paul Mitchell Systems, hair by Jeanne Braa, photo by Alberto Tolot. Figure 14-23, 14-178: John Paul Mitchell Systems, The Relaxer Workshop, photo by Sean Cokes. Figures 14-26 and 14-90: Gebhart International, hair by Dennis & Sylvia Gebhart, makeup by Rose Marie, production by Purely Visual, photo by Winterhalter. Figure 14-34: Mario Tricoci Hair Salons & Day Spa, hair by Mario Tricoci, makeup by Shawn Miselli. Figures 14-64, 14-210: Tom Carson Photography, Bon Vivant Salon, Woodstock, GA. Figures 14-65, 14-126, 14-127: Tom Carson Photography, Salon Visage, Knoxville, TN. Top right photo of Procedure 14-1, Figures 14-149, 14-150, 14-167, 14-212: Tom Carson, Yellow Strawberry Global Salon, Sarasota, FL. Procedure 14-2 (top right), Tom Carson, Hair Benders Internationale', Chattanooga, TN. Procedure 14-3: Tom Carson. Figure 14-130: Tom Carson, Shortino's Salon, York, PA. Procedure 14-4 (top right): Yellow Strawberry Global Salon, Ft. Lauderdale, FL. Figures 14-211, 14-214, Tom Carson, Tangles Salon, Wichita Falls, TX. Figure 14-213: Tom Carson, Salon 124, Snellville, GA. Figure 14-215: Tom Carson, Kathy Adams Salon, Buford, GA. Figure 14-92: Getty Images. Figure 14-97: hair by Brian & Sandra Smith, makeup by Rose Marie, wardrobe by Victor Paul, photo by Taggart/Winterhalter, production by Purely Visual. All other photos provided by Paul Castle, Castle Photography.

Chapter 15: chapter opener, Getty Images. Figure 15-1: Sculpt Salon, hair by George Alderete. Makeup by Rose Marie, production by Purely Visual, photo by Taggart/Winterhalter. Procedure 15-1 (top right corner): Leah-Anne Thompson/Shutterstock. Procedure 15-2 (top right), courtesy of Rumors Inc. Procedure 15-3 (top right), Figure 15-94: Tom Carson, Hair Benders Internationale', Chattanooga, TN. Procedure 15-6 (top right), Tom Carson, Yellow Strawberry Global Salon, Sarasota, FL. Procedure 15-7 (top right),

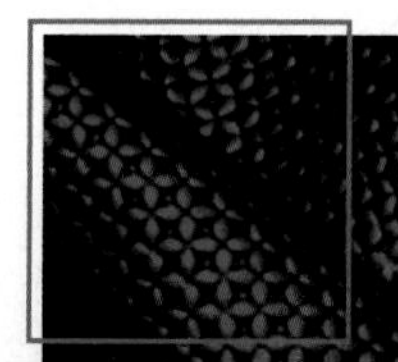

Iryna Kurhan/Shutterstock. Procedure 15-8 (top right). Ana Blazic/Shutterstock. Procedure 15-9 (top right), Joanne Verspuij/Shutterstock. Procedure 15-10 (top right), Penka Uzunova/Shutterstock. Procedure 15-12, Carly Rose Hennigan/Shutterstock. Procedure 15-13, Cris Calhoun/Shutterstock. Procedure 15-14 (top right), Tom Carson, Bob Steele Salon, Atlanta, GA. Procedure 15-15 (right top corner), Anton Albert/Shutterstock. Procedure 15-16 (right top corner), JupiterImages. All other photos by Paul Castle. Figures 15-118, 15-119: Courtesy of Golden Supreme, Inc. (www.goldensupreme.com).

Chapter 16: chapter opener, Getty Images. Figures 16-1, 16-70, 16-90: courtesy of Preston Phillips. Figures 16-3 thru 16-9: Graphic World. Figure 16-16: Barry Fletcher. Procedure 16-5 (top right corner), Carlin Photo/Shutterstock. Procedure 16-6 (right corner), Jason Stitt/Shutterstock. Figures 16-12, 16-13, 16-14: Photography by Paul Castle, products from Cinderella Hair. Procedure 16-7, MAT/Shutterstock. All other photos provided by Paul Castle, Castle Photography.

Chapter 17: chapter opener, Figures 17-4, 17-5: Hair by Vivienne Mackinder, Photograph by Jill Wachter. Figures 17-34, 17-35, 17-36: photography from the Gabor Collection, supplied by Eva Gabor International. Figures 17-37, 17-38: photography from American Hairlines, supplied by Eva Gabor International. Figure 17-63: photography from Great Lengths USA, supplied by Eva Gabor Collection.

Chapter 18: chapter opener, Image State. Figure 18-1: photo used with the permission of the authors, Martin Gannon and Richard Thompson, as featured in their book, Mahogany; Steps to Cutting, Colouring and Finishing Hair. Copyright © Martin Gannon and Richard Thompson, 1997. Figures 18-2, 18-3: Courtesy of P&G Beauty from John Grey's, The World of Hair Care. Figures 18-4 thru 18-9, 18-39: Graphic World. Figure 18-99: hair by Geri Mataya, makeup by Mary Klimeck, photo by Jack Cutler. All other photos provided by Paul Castle, Castle Photography.

Chapter 19: chapter opener, Paul Castle. Figures 19-1, 19-86: photos used with the permission of the authors, Martin Gannon and Richard Thompson, as featured in their book, Mahogany; Steps to Cutting, Colouring and Finishing Hair. Copyright © Martin Gannon and Richard Thompson, 1997. Figure 19-2: reprinted with permission of Clairol, Inc. Procedure 19-5 (top right corner), Tom Carson, Bon Vivant Salon, Woodstock, GA. Procedure 19-7 (top right), Tom Carson, Dante Lucci Salon, Rocky River, OH. Procedure 19-9 9(top right), Tom Carson, Yellow Strawberry Global Salon, Sarasota, FL.

Part 4: opener photo provided by Big Cheese Photo.

Chapter 20: chapter opener: Phil Date/Shutterstock. Figures 20-2, 20-3, 20-6, 20-7, 20-8, 20-10, 20-12 thru 20-20: Reprinted with permission from the American Academy of Dermatology. All rights reserved. Figure 20-4: Timothy Berger, MD, Associate Clinical Professor, University of California San Francisco. Figure 20-9: Larry Hamill. Figure 20-11: Center for Disease Control and Prevention.

Chapter 21: chapter opener, Larry Hamill. Figure 21-1: Larry Hamill. All other photos by Paul Castle.

Chapter 22: chapter opener, Adam Borkowski/Shutterstock. Figure 22-46: Courtesy of Revitalight. Procedure 22-1 (top right corner), Leah-Anne Thompson/Shutterstock. Figure 22-70: Michael Dzaman. All other photos in this chapter by Larry Hamill Photography, Columbus, OH.

Chapter 23: chapter opener, Tracy Siermachesky/Shutterstock. Figure 23-1: Stephen Ciuccoli. Figures 23-2 thru 23-10, 23-16, 23-17, 23-18, 23-77 thru 23-81: Larry Hamill. Procedure 23-1(right corner), Andrew Taylor/Shutterstock. Figures 23-19 thru 23-35: Paul Castle.

Part 5: part opener, Creative Nail Design

Chapter 24: chapter opener, Creative Nail Design. Figures 24-2, 24-14, 24-17, 24-22: Robert Baran, MD (France). Figures 24-4, 24-5, 24-7, 24-8, 24-10, 24-13: Courtesy of Godfrey F. Mix, DPM, Sacramento, CA. Figures 24-6, 24-12: Paul Castle. Figure 24-16: Michael Dzaman. Figure 24-21: Reprinted with permission from the American Academy of Dermatology. All rights reserved.

Chapter 25: chapter opener, Paul Castle. Figures 25-6, 25-10, 25-15: Paul Castle. Figure 25-45: Courtesy of Paul Rollins. Procedure 25-10 (top right), John Clines/Shutterstock. Procedure 25-11, Shutterstock. All other photos by photographer, Michael Dzaman.

Chapter 26: chapter opener, ImageSource. Figures 26-2, 26-28: Paul Castle. Procedure 26-2 (top right), Svetlana Larina/Shutterstock. Figure 26-27: Tihis/Shutterstock. Procedure 26-5 (top right), PhotoDisc. All other photos in this chapter by photographer, Michael Dzaman.

Chapter 27: chapter opener, iStock International Inc. Figures 27-1, Procedure photo 27-6, 27-13 thru 27-19: NSI (Nail Systems International). Figures 27-2, 27-5: Paul Castle. Procedure 27-2 (top right), Konstantin Tavrov/Shutterstock. All other photos by photographer, Michael Dzaman.

Chapter 28: chapter opener, Kateryna Govorushchenko/iStock International Inc. Figures 28-1, Procedure 28-1 (right top), 28-5, 28-7, 28-9, 28-11 thru 28-22: NSI (Nail Systems International). Figures 28-4, 28-24, 28-34: Paul Castle. Figure 28-6: Michael Dzaman

Chapter 29: chapter opener courtesy of Light Elegance Nail Products. Figures 29-1, 29-3 thru 29-12, 29-14 thru 29-16: NSI (Nail Systems International). Figure 29-2: Paul Castle. Figure 29-13: Michael Dzaman.

Part 6: photo by Kulezma Maxim & Krashenninnikova Alina/Shutterstock.

Chapter 30: chapter opener, Comstock Images. Figure 30-2: Getty Images. Figure 30-5: Jerry Kelon Carter, CC's Cosmetology College, Tulsa, OK. Figure 30-6: Tom Stock. Figure 30-7: Ed Hille. All other photos by Paul Castle.

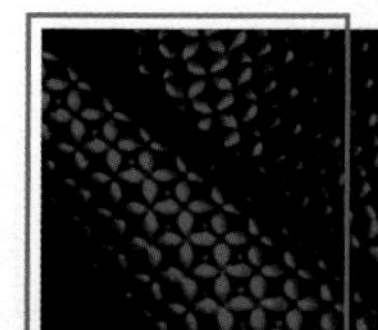

Chapter 31: chapter opener: Getty Images. All other photos from Paul Castle.

Chapter 32: Figure 32-4: Getty Images. Figure 32-9: Tom Stock. Chapter opener and all other photos by Paul Castle, Castle Photography Inc., Troy, NY.

ORIENTATIO

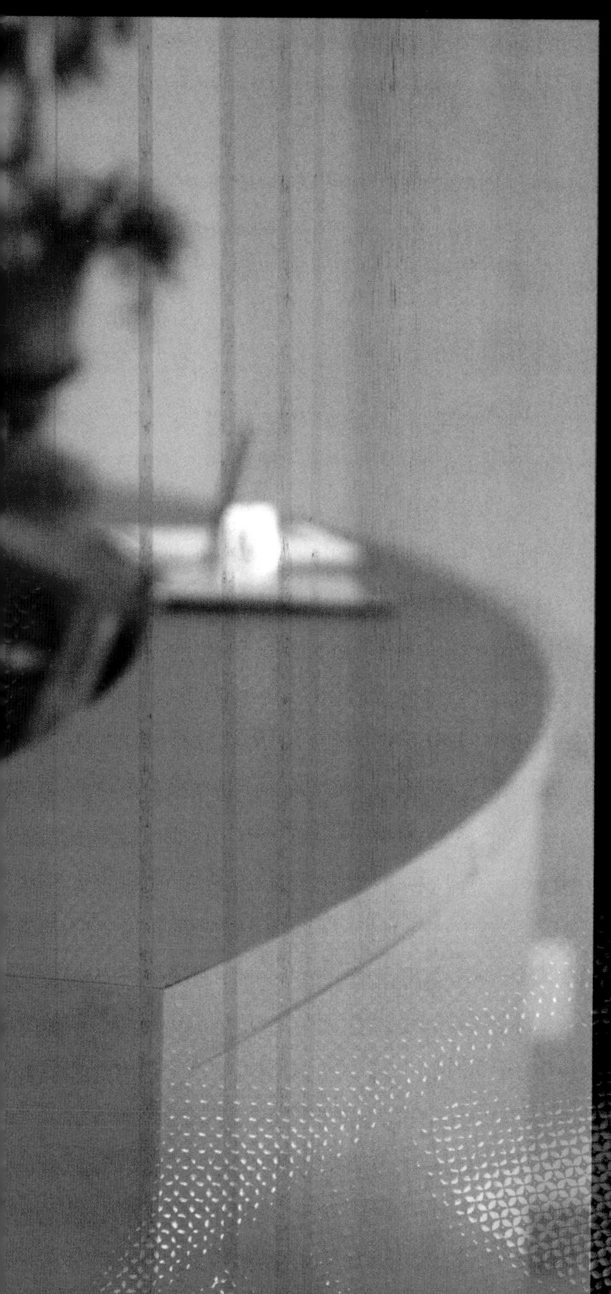

PART 1

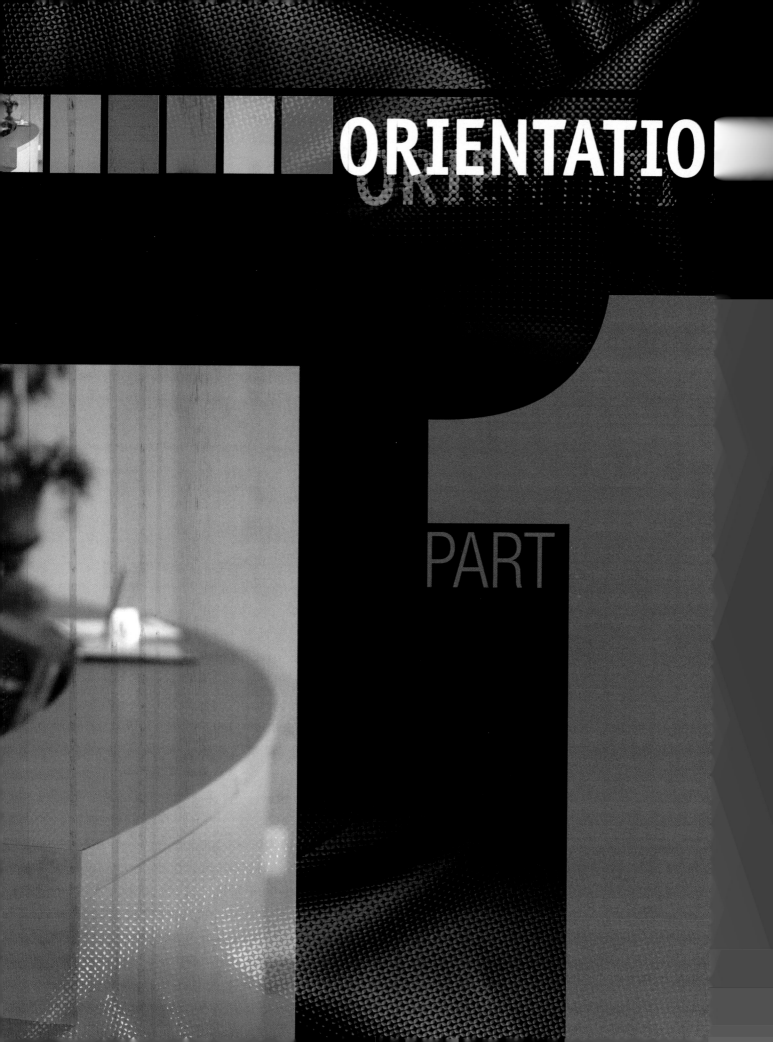

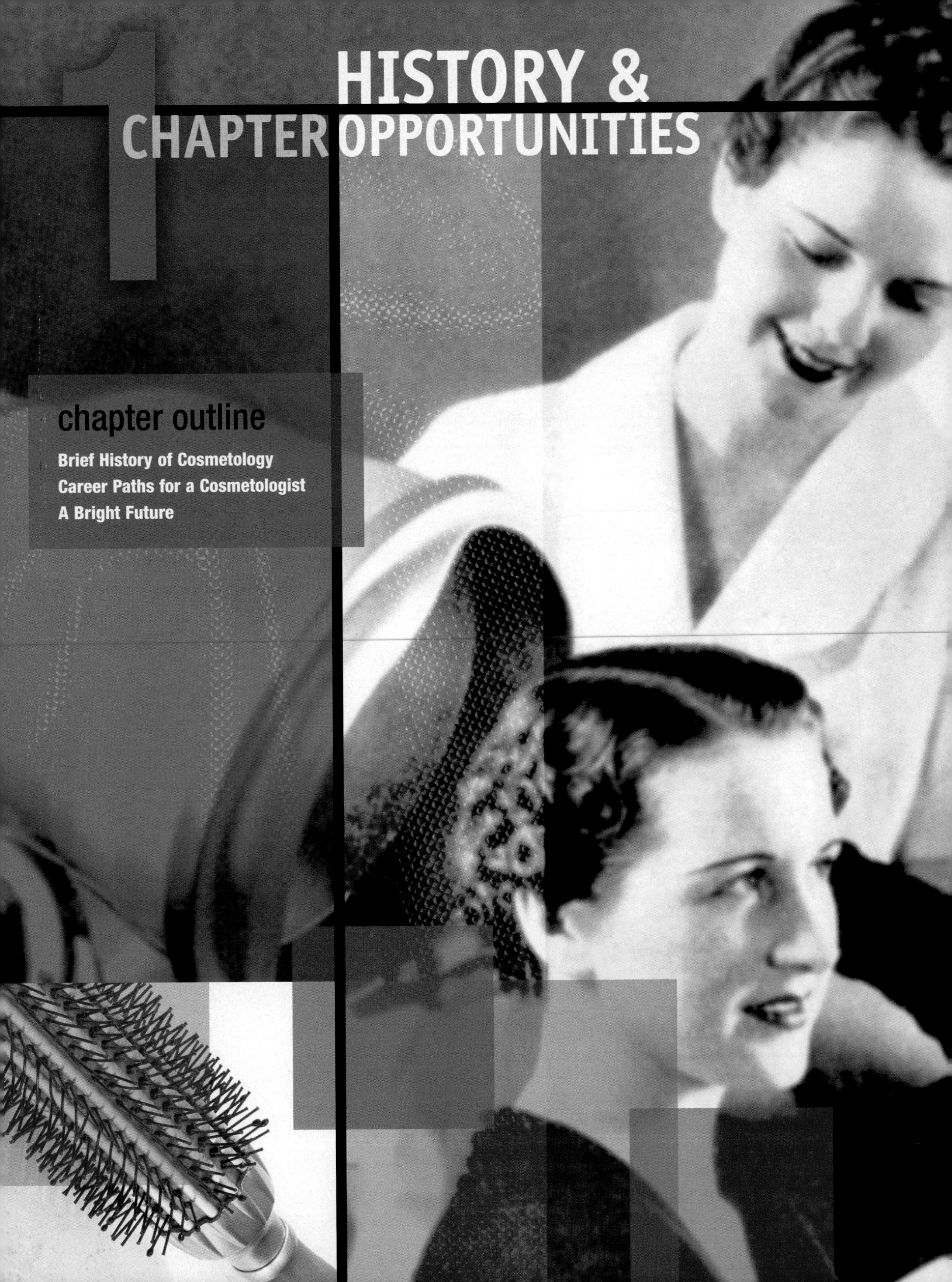

CHAPTER 1 HISTORY & OPPORTUNITIES

chapter outline

Learning Objectives

After completing this chapter, you will be able to:

- Describe the origins of appearance enhancement.
- Describe the advancements made in cosmetology during the 19th, 20th, and early 21st centuries.
- List the career opportunities available to a licensed beauty practitioner.

Key Terms

Page number indicates where in the chapter the term is used.

cosmetology
pg. 4

BRIEF HISTORY OF COSMETOLOGY

Cosmetology is a term used to encompass a broad range of specialty areas, including hairstyling, nail technology, and esthetics. Cosmetology defined is "the art and science of beautifying and improving the skin, nails, and hair, and the study of cosmetics and their application." The term comes from the Greek word *kosmetikos,* meaning "skilled in the use of cosmetics." Archaeological studies reveal that haircutting and hairstyling were practiced in some form as early as the Ice Age.

The simple but effective implements used at the dawn of history were shaped from sharpened flints, oyster shells, or bone. Animal sinew or strips of hide were used to tie the hair back or as adornment. Ancient people around the world used coloring matter on their hair, skin, and nails, and practiced tattooing. Pigments were made from berries, tree bark, minerals, insects, nuts, herbs, leaves, and other materials. Many of these colorants are still used today.

THE EGYPTIANS

The Egyptians were the first to cultivate beauty in an extravagant fashion, and to use cosmetics as part of their personal beautification habits, religious ceremonies, and preparing the deceased for burial.

As early as 3000 B.C., Egyptians used minerals, insects and berries to create makeup for their eyes, lips and skin, and henna to stain their hair and nails a rich, warm red. They were also the first civilization to infuse essential oils from the leaves, bark and blossoms of plants for use as perfumes and for purification purposes. Queen Nefertiti (1400 B.C.) stained her nails red by dipping her fingertips in henna, wore lavish makeup designs and used custom-blended essential oils as signature scents. Queen Cleopatra (50 B.C.) took this dedication to beauty to an entirely new level by erecting a personal cosmetics factory next to the Dead Sea.

Ancient Egyptians are also credited with creating kohl makeup—originally made from a mixture of ground galena (a black mineral), sulfur and animal fat—to heavily line the eyes, alleviate eye inflammations and protect the eyes from the glare of the sun.

In both ancient Egypt and Rome, military commanders stained their nails and lips in matching colors before important battles (Figure 1-1).

CHINESE

History also shows that during the Shang Dynasty (1600 B.C.), Chinese aristocrats rubbed a tinted mixture of gum arabic, gelatin, beeswax and egg whites onto their nails to turn them crimson or ebony. Throughout the Chou Dynasty, (1100 B.C.) gold and silver were the royal colors. During this early period in Chinese history, nail tinting was so closely tied to social status that commoners caught wearing a royal nail color faced a punishment of death.

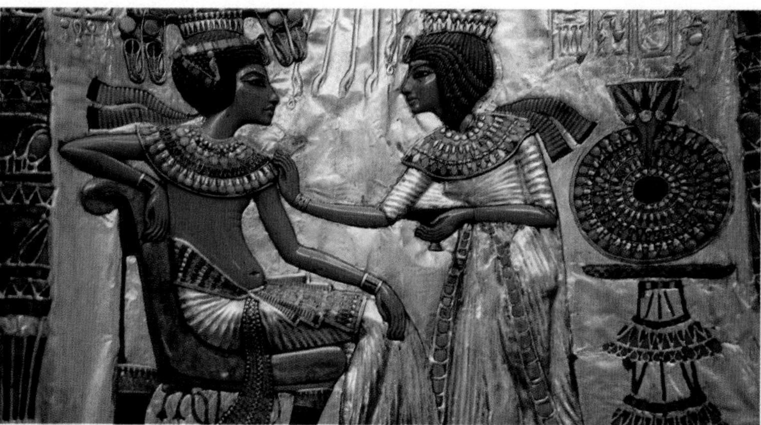

Figure 1–1 The Egyptians wore elaborate hairstyles and cosmetics.

THE GREEKS

During the golden age of Greece (500 B.C.), hairstyling became a highly developed art. The ancient Greeks made lavish use of perfumes and cosmetics in their religious rites, in grooming, and for medicinal purposes. They built elaborate baths and developed excellent methods of dressing the hair and caring for the skin and nails. Greek women applied preparations of white lead on their faces, kohl on their eyes, and vermillion on their cheeks and lips. The brilliant red pigment was made by grinding cinnabar, a mineral that is the chief source of mercury, to a fine powder. It was mixed with ointment or dusted on the skin in the same way as modern cosmetics are applied today.

THE ROMANS

Roman women made lavish use of fragrances and cosmetics. Facials made of milk and bread or fine wine were popular. Other facials were made of corn, flour, and milk, or flour and fresh butter. A mixture of chalk and white lead was used as a facial cosmetic. Women used hair color to indicate their class in society. Noblewomen tinted their hair red, middle-class women colored their hair blond, and poor women colored their hair black.

MIDDLE AGES

The Middle Ages is the period of European history between classical antiquity and the Renaissance, beginning with the downfall of Rome in 476 A.D., and lasting until about 1450. Beauty culture is evidenced by tapestries, sculptures, and other artifacts from this period. All show towering headdresses, intricate hairstyles, and the use of cosmetics on skin and hair. Women wore colored makeup on their cheeks and lips, but not on their eyes. Around 1000 A.D., a Persian physician and alchemist named Avicenna refined the process of steam distillation. This ushered in the modern era of steam distilled essential oils that we use today.

RENAISSANCE

This is the period in history during which Western civilization made the transition from medieval to modern history. Paintings and written records tell us a great deal about the grooming practices of the time. One

Did You Know

The barber pole—symbol of the barber surgeon—has its roots in a medical procedure called bloodletting that was once thought to strengthen the immune system. The pole is believed to represent the staff that patients held tightly to make the veins in their arms stand out during the procedure. The bottom-end cap represents the basin used to catch the blood. The white bandages that stopped the bleeding were hung on the pole to dry. As the wind blew, these bandages would become twisted around the pole, forming a red-and-white pattern. Up until the 19th century, many barbers also performed minor surgeries and practiced dentistry.

The modern barber pole, then, was originally the symbol of the barber surgeon, and is believed to represent the bandages (white), blood (red), and veins (blue) involved in bloodletting (Figure 1-2).

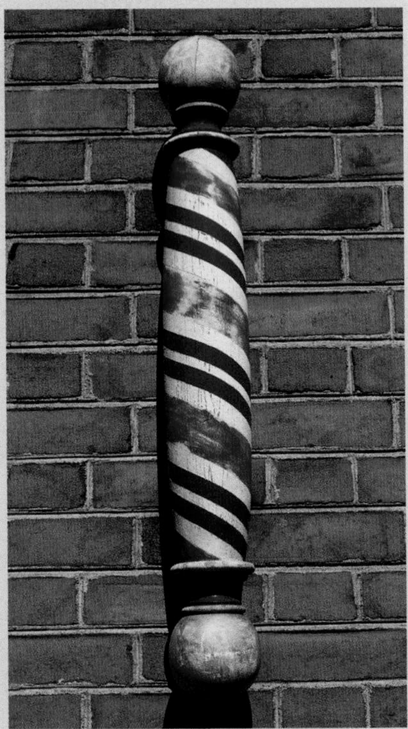

Figure 1-2 A traditional barber pole.

of the most unusual practices was the shaving of the eyebrows and the hairline to show a greater expanse of forehead. A bare brow was thought to give women a look of greater intelligence. During this period, both men and women took great pride in their physical appearance and wore elaborate elegant clothing. Fragrances and cosmetics were used, although highly colored preparations of lips, cheeks, and eyes were discouraged.

VICTORIAN AGE

The reign of Queen Victoria of England between 1837 and 1901 was known as the Victorian Age. Fashions in dress and personal grooming were drastically influenced by the social mores of this austere and restrictive period in history. To preserve the health and beauty of the skin, women used beauty masks and packs made from honey, eggs, milk, oatmeal, fruits, vegetables, and other natural ingredients. Victorian women are said to have pinched their cheeks and bitten their lips to induce natural color rather than use cosmetics such as rouge or lip color.

20TH CENTURY

In the early 20th century, the invention of motion pictures coincided with an abrupt shift in American attitudes. As viewers saw pictures of celebrities with flawless complexions, beautiful hairstyles, and manicured nails, standards of feminine beauty began to change. This era also signaled the onset of industrialization, which brought a new prosperity to the United States, and all forms of beauty began to follow trends.

1901-1910

In 1904 Max Faktor emigrated from Lodz, Poland to the United States. By 1908, he had Americanized his name to Max Factor and moved to Los Angeles, where he began by making and selling to movie stars makeup that wouldn't cake or crack, even under hot studio lights.

On October 8, 1905, Charles Nessler invented a heavily wired machine that supplied electrical current to metal rods around which hair strands were wrapped. These heavy units were heated during the waving process. They were kept away from the scalp by a complex system of counterbalancing weights, suspended from an overhead chandelier mounted on a stand.

Two methods were used to wind hair strands around the metal units. Long hair was wound from the scalp to the ends in a technique called spiral wrapping. After World War I, when women cut their hair into the short bobbed style, the croquignole wrapping technique was introduced. In this method, shorter hair was wound from the ends toward the scalp. The hair was then styled into deep waves with loose end curls.

One of the most notable success stories of the cosmetology industry is that of Sarah Breedlove. She was the daughter of former slaves and was orphaned at age seven when she went to work in the cotton fields of the Mississippi delta. In 1906, Sarah married her third husband, C. J. Walker, and became known as Madame C. J. Walker. Sarah had suffered from a scalp condition and began to lose her hair which caused her to experiment with store-bought products and homemade remedies. She began to sell

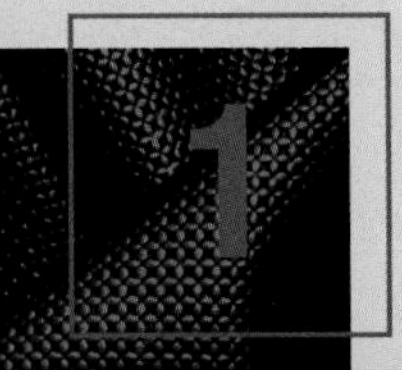

her scalp conditioning and healing treatment called "Madam Walker's Wonderful Hair Grower." Devising sophisticated sales and marketing strategies, she traveled extensively giving product demonstrations. In 1910, she moved her company to Indianapolis where she built a factory, hair salon, and training school. As she developed new products, her empire grew. She devoted much time and money to a variety of causes including the National Association of the Advancement of Colored People (NAACP) and the YMCA in Indianapolis. In 1917, she organized a convention for her Madam C. J. Walker Hair Culturists Union of America. This was one of the first national meetings for businesswomen ever held. By the time of her death, she had established herself as a pioneer of the modern black hair care and cosmetics industry.

1920'S

The cosmetics industry grew rapidly during the 1920s. Advertising expenditures in radio alone went from $390,000.00 to $3.2 million between 1927 and 1930. At first, many women's magazines refused advertisements for cosmetics—deeming them improper—but by the end of the 1920s, cosmetics provided one of their largest sources of advertising revenue.

1930'S

In 1931, the preheat perm method was introduced. Hair was wrapped using the croquignole method. Then clamps, preheated by a separate electrical unit, were placed over the wound curls. An alternative to the machine perm was introduced in 1932 when chemists Ralph L. Evans and Everett G. McDonough pioneered a method that used external heat generated by chemical reaction. Small, flexible pads containing a chemical mixture were wound around hair strands. When the pads were moistened with water, a chemical heat was released that created long-lasting curls. Thus the first, machineless permanent wave was born. Salon clients were no longer subjected to the dangers and discomforts of the Nessler machine.

In 1932—nearly 4,000 years after the first recorded nail color craze—Charles Revson of Revlon fame marketed the first nail polish—as opposed to a nail stain—using formulas that were borrowed from the automobile paint industry. This milestone marked a dramatic shift in nail cosmetics, as women finally had an array of nail lacquers available to them. Early screen sirens, Jean Harlow and Gloria Swanson glamorized this hip new nail fashion in silent pictures and early talkies by appearing in films wearing matching polish on their fingers and toes.

Also in 1932, Lawrence Gelb, a New York Chemist, introduced the first permanent haircolor product and founded a company called Clairol. In 1935, Max Factor created pancake makeup to make actors' skin look natural on color film. In 1938, Arnold F. Willatt invented the cold wave that used no machines or heat. The cold wave is considered to be the precursor to the modern perm.

1940'S

In 1941, scientists developed another method of permanent waving that used waving lotion. Because this perm did not use heat, it was called a

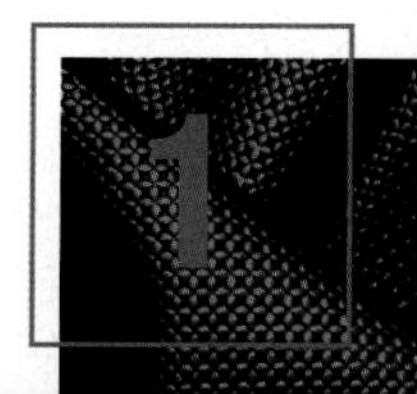

cold wave. Cold waves replaced virtually all predecessors and competitors, and the terms cold waving and permanent waving became almost synonymous. Modern versions of cold waves, usually referred to as alkaline perms, are very popular today. The term *texture services* is used today to refer to the variety of permanent wave services available for different hair types and conditions.

1951-2000

The second half of the 20th century saw the introduction of tube mascara, improved hair care and nail products, and the boom and then death of the weekly salon appointment. In the late 1960's, Vidal Sassoon turned the hairstyling world on its ear with his revolutionary geometric cuts. The 1970's saw a new era in highlighting when French hairdressers introduced the art of "hair weaving," using aluminum foil. In the 1980's makeup went full circle, from being barely there to cat-eyes and the heavy use of eye shadows and blush. In the 1990's hair color became gentler, allowing all ethnicities to enjoy being blonds, brunettes, or redheads. In 1998, Creative Nail Design introduced the first spa pedicure system to the professional beauty industry.

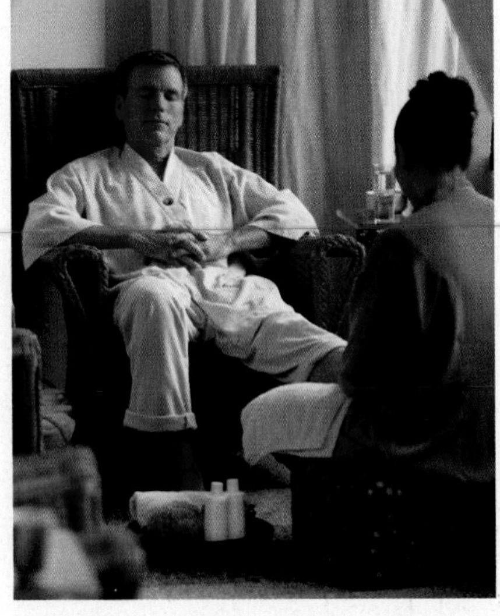

Figure 1-3 Spas are increasing in number and popularity.

21ST CENTURY

Today, hairstylists have far gentler, no-fade hair color, and estheticians can noticeably rejuvenate the face, as well as keep disorders such as sunspots and mild acne at bay. The beauty industry has also entered the age of specialization, where cosmetologists frequently specialize in either hair color or haircutting; estheticians specialize in esthetic or medical-esthetic services; and nail technicians can either offer a full array of services, or specialize in artificial nail enhancements, natural nail care, or even pedicures.

Since the late 1980's, the salon industry has evolved to include day spas, a name that was first coined by beauty legend Noel DeCaprio. Day spas now represent an excellent employment opportunity for beauty practitioners (Figure 1-3).

Men's-only specialty spas and barber spas have also grown in popularity, providing new opportunities for men's nail care specialists.

CAREER PATHS FOR A COSMETOLOGIST

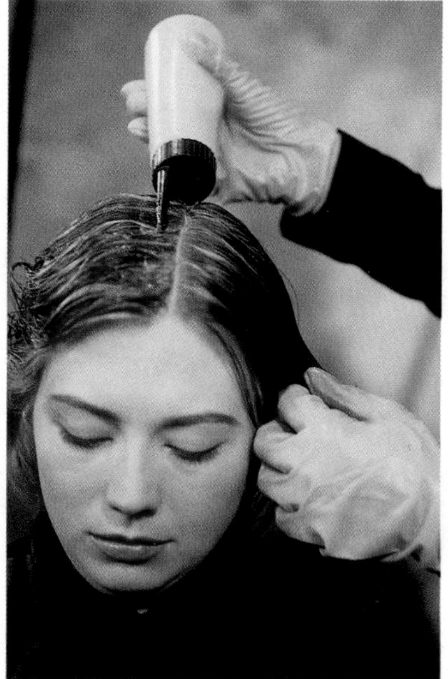

Figure 1-4 Haircolor specialists are in great demand.

Once you have completed your schooling and are licensed, you will be amazed at how many career opportunities will open up for you. The possibilities can be endless for a hard-working professional cosmetologist who approaches her or his career with a strong sense of personal integrity. Within the industry there are numerous areas you may wish to specialize in, such as the following:

- Haircolor specialist. This may include training yourself or others to perform color services in the salon or working for a product manufacturer, where you will be expected to train others in how best to perform color services according to the company's guidelines and product instructions (Figure 1-4).
- Texture specialist. This may include training yourself or others to perform texture services in the salon, or working for a manufacturer where you will be expected to train others on how best to perform texture services according to your company's guidelines and product instructions.
- Cutting specialist. This type of position requires a dedicated interest in learning various cutting styles and techniques. After perfecting your own skills and developing your own method of cutting (everyone develops their own unique way of cutting hair), you may want to study with other reputable haircutters in the business to learn and adopt their systems and techniques. This training will allow you to perform top-quality haircutting in your own salon as well as coach those around you how to hone their skills (Figure 1-5).
- Salon trainer. Many companies such as manufacturers and salon chains hire experienced salon professionals and train them to train others. This kind of training can take many forms, from technical training to management and interpersonal relationship training. A salon trainer can work with small salons as well as large organizations and trade associations to help develop the beauty industry's most valuable resource—salon staff and personnel.
- Distributor sales consultant. The salon industry depends heavily on its relationships with its product distributors to learn about new products, new trends, and new techniques to stay abreast of what is occurring in the marketplace. This relationship provides an excellent opportunity for a highly skilled and trained cosmetology professional to become a distributor sales consultant (DSC). The DSC is the salon and salon staff's link with the rest of the industry, and this person is the most efficient method outside companies have to reach the salon stylist.

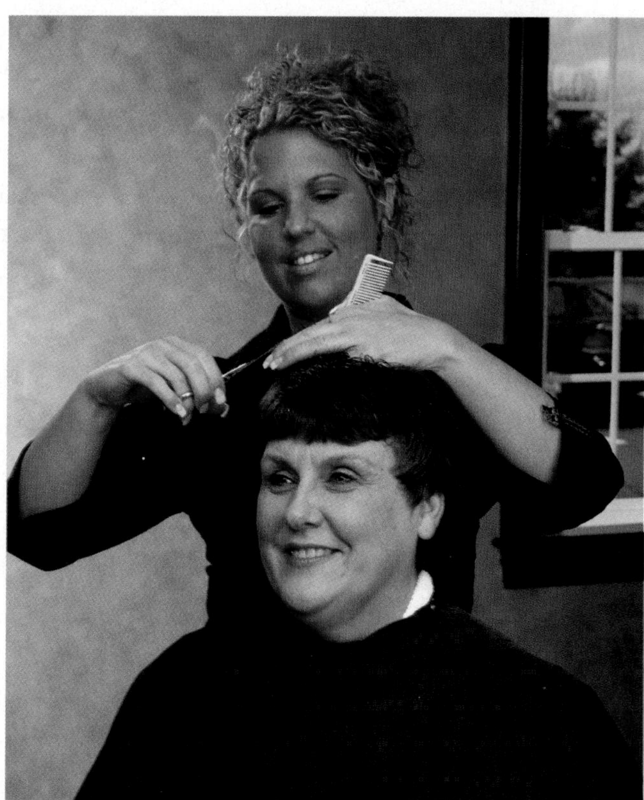

Figure 1-5 Cutting hair in a salon is one of the many choices open to you.

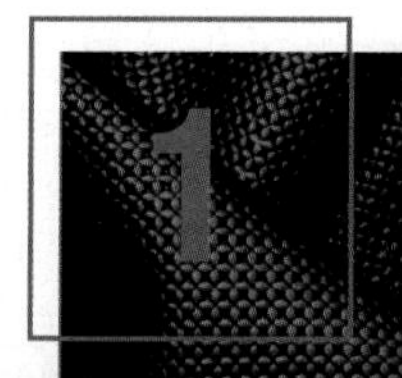

- Cosmetology instructor. Have you ever wondered how your instructor decided to start teaching? Many instructors had fantastic careers in the salon before they decided to dedicate themselves to teaching new professionals the tricks of the trade. If this career path interests you, spend some time with your school's instructors and ask them why they felt the call to go into education. Educating new cosmetologists can be very trying, but it can also be some of the most rewarding work a person can do.

These are but a few opportunities for career paths that await you on the road to a life-long cosmetology career. The wonderful thing about the professional beauty industry is that there are truly no limits to what you can do if you have a sincere interest in learning and giving back to your industry. Keep developing your skills in whatever way that interests you and soon you'll be coupling your skills and building a most creative and unique career.

SALON MANAGEMENT

If business is your calling, you will find that management opportunities in the salon and spa environment are quite diverse. They include being an inventory manager, department head, educator, special events manager (promotions), assistant manager and general manager. With experience, you can also add "salon owner" to this list of career possibilities. To ensure your success, it is wise to enroll in business classes to learn more about managing products, departments, and, above all, people.

Beyond defining your area of expertise, you must also decide whether you want to work in a:

- Specialty salon
- Full-service salon (hair, skin and nail services)
- Day spa (skin, body, nail, and hair services that emphasize beauty and wellness) (Figure 1-6)

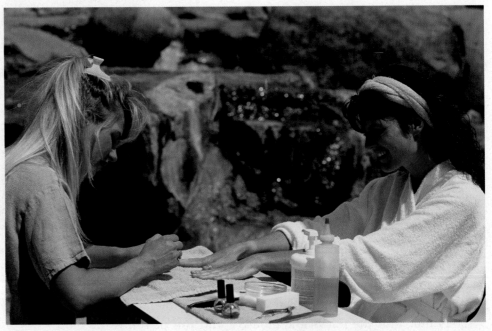

Figure 1-6 A day spa may offer nail, hair, body, and skin services.

To learn more about the various types of salon business models, see Chapter 32. There you will find a wealth of choices including national and regional chains, and low- and high-end salon opportunities.

A BRIGHT FUTURE

Clearly the field of cosmetology has broadened to encompass areas of specialization including esthetics and nail technology. As the cosmetology industry continues to grow, opportunities for professionals also increase. To make each day in school positively impact your future, focus on your studies, read trade publications cover to cover, become a member of relevant trade associations, and attend workshops outside of school. Remember, your license will unlock countless doors, but it is your personal dedication and passion that will fuel your career.

REVIEW QUESTIONS

1. What are the origins of appearance enhancement?
2. Name the advancements made in cosmetology during the 19th, 20th, and earlier centuries.
3. List some of the career opportunities available to licensed beauty practitioners.

CHAPTER GLOSSARY

cosmetology	The art and science of beautifying and improving the skin, nails, and hair, and the study of cosmetics and their applications.

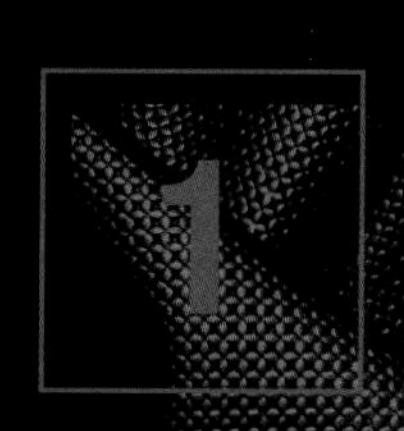

CHAPTER 2 LIFE SKILLS

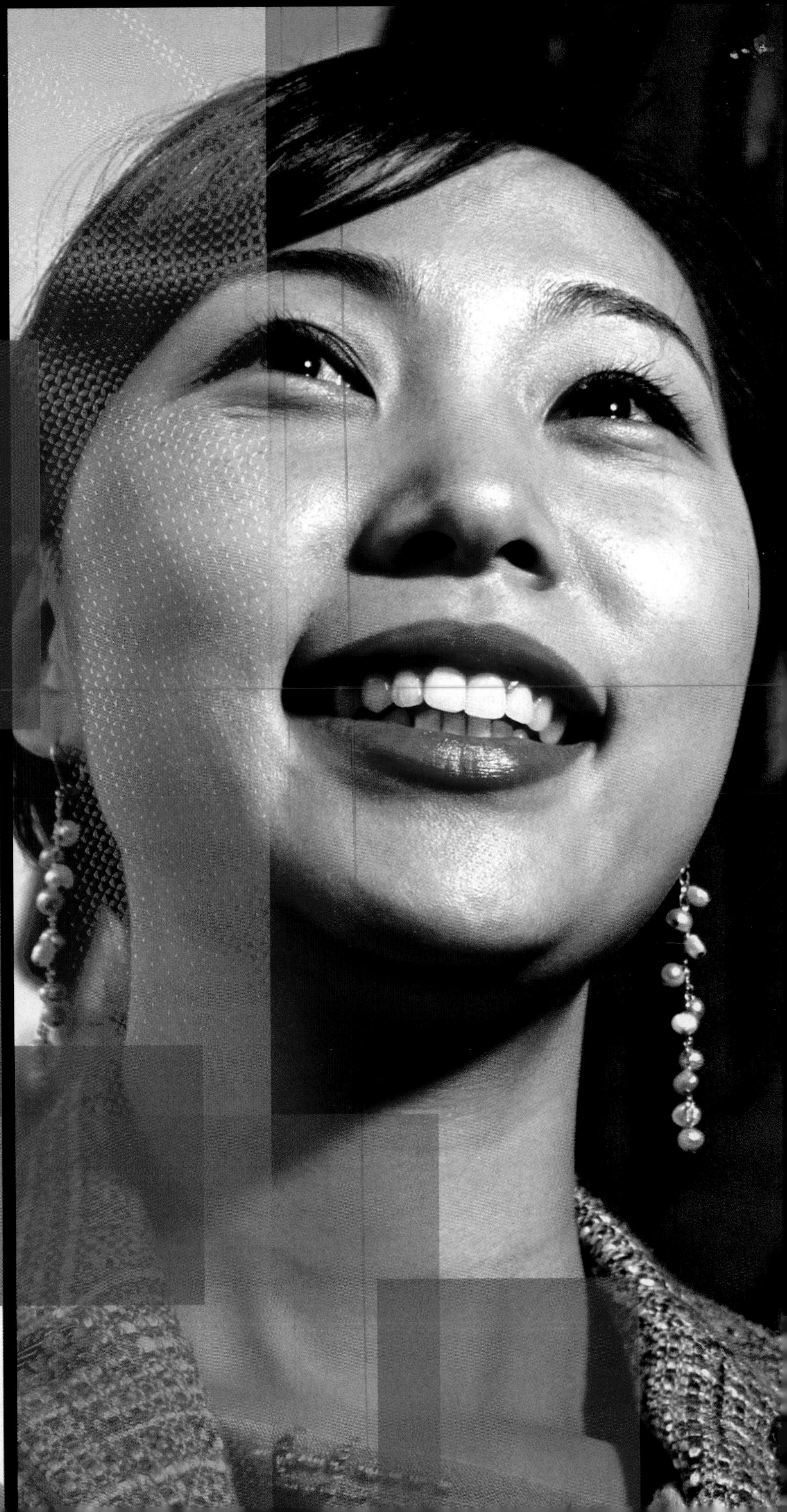

chapter outline

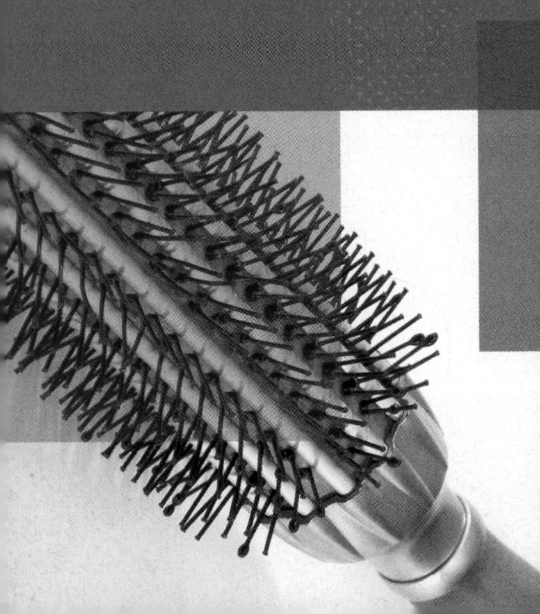

Learning Objectives

After completing this chapter, you will be able to:

- **List the principles that contribute to personal and professional success.**
- **Explain the concept of self-management.**
- **Create a mission statement.**
- **Explain how to set long- and short-term goals.**
- **Discuss the most effective ways to manage time.**
- **Describe good study habits.**
- **Define ethics.**
- **List the characteristics of a healthy, positive attitude.**

Key Terms

Page number indicates where in the chapter the term is used.

ethics
pg. 21

game plan
pg. 17

goal setting
pg. 18

mission statement
pg. 18

perfectionism
pg. 16

prioritize
pg. 19

procrastination
pg. 16

While going through cosmetology school has its own set of challenges, staying on course for your entire career can be difficult without having great life skills. This is particularly true of cosmetology since the hard-and-fast rules that apply to more structured industries are frequently absent in the salon business. By its nature, the salon is a creative workplace where you are expected to exercise your artistic talent. It is also a highly social atmosphere that requires strong self-discipline and excellent people skills. Besides making a solid connection with each client, you must always stay focused, and feel both competent and enthusiastic about taking care of every client's needs—no matter how you feel, or how many hours you have already worked. Your livelihood, as well as your own personal feelings of success, depend on how well you do this.

There are a great many life skills that can lead to a more satisfying and productive beauty career. Some of the most important life skills include:

- Being genuinely caring and helpful to others.
- Successfully adapting to different situations.
- Sticking to a goal and seeing a job to completion.
- Being consistent in your work.
- Developing a deep reservoir of common sense.
- Making good friends.
- Feeling good about yourself.
- Maintaining a cooperative attitude.
- Defining your own code of ethics, and living within your definition.
- Approaching all your work with a strong sense of responsibility.
- Mastering techniques that will help you become more organized.
- Having a sense of humor to bring you through difficult situations.
- Acquiring one of the greatest virtues: patience.
- Always striving for excellence.

RULES FOR SUCCESS

To be successful, you must take ownership of your education. While your instructors can create motivational circumstances and an environment to assist you in the learning process, the ultimate responsibility for learning is *yours.* To get the greatest benefits from your education, commit yourself to the following "rules" that will take you a long way down the road of success:

- Attend all classes.
- Arrive for class early.
- Have all necessary materials ready.
- Listen attentively to your instructor.
- Highlight important points.
- Take notes for later review.
- Pay close attention during summary and review sessions.
- When something is not clear, ask, ask, ask.

Continually seek further education. Never stop learning. The cosmetology industry is always changing. There are always new trends, techniques, products, and information. Read industry magazines, books, and attend trade shows and advanced educational classes throughout your career.

THE PSYCHOLOGY OF SUCCESS

Are you passionate about studying? Do you see yourself sustaining this passion 1 year, 5 years, or even 10 years from now? While cosmetology school is definitely challenging, it becomes much easier when you put that extra amount of effort, enthusiasm, and excitement into your studies. If your talent is not fueled by the passion necessary to sustain you over the course of your career, you can have all the talent in the world and still not be successful (Figure 2-1).

GUIDELINES FOR SUCCESS

Defining success is a very personal thing. There are some basic principles, however, that form the foundation of all personal and business success. You can begin your path to success right now by examining and putting these principles into practice.

Build self-esteem. Self-esteem is based on inner strength and begins with trusting your ability to reach your goals. It is essential that you begin working on improving your self-esteem while you are still a student.

Visualize. Imagine yourself working in your dream salon, competently handling clients, and feeling at ease and happy with your situation. The more you practice visualization, the easier you can turn the possibilities in your life into realities.

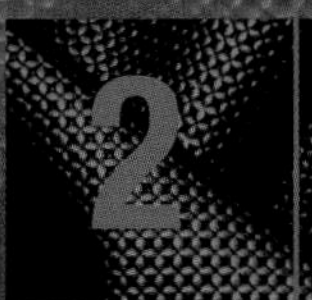

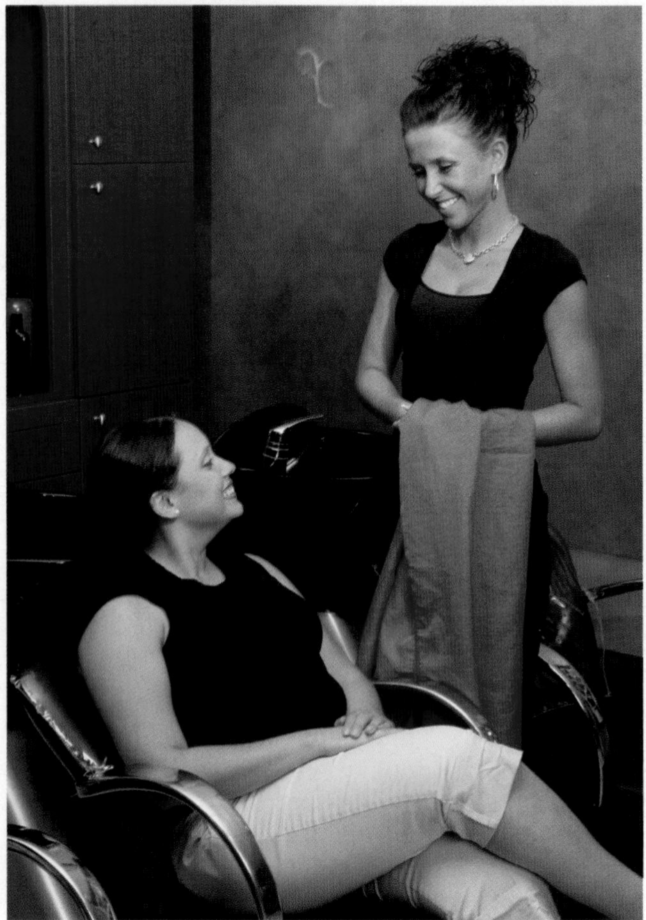

Figure 2-1 Loving your work is critical to your success.

Build on your strengths. Practice doing whatever it is that helps you maintain a positive self-image. If you are good at doing something (e.g., playing the guitar, running, cooking, gardening, or singing), the time you invest in this activity will allow you to feel good about yourself (Figure 2-2). Also remember that there may be things you are good at that you cannot see. You could be a good listener, for instance, or a caring and considerate friend.

Be kind to yourself. Put a stop to self-critical or negative thoughts that can work against you. If you make a mistake, tell yourself that it is okay and you will do your best next time.

Define success for yourself. Do not depend on other people's definitions of success; be a success in your own eyes. What is right for your father or sister, for instance, may not be right for you.

Practice new behaviors. Because creating success is a skill, you can help develop it by practicing positive new behaviors such as speaking with confidence, standing tall, or using good grammar.

Keep your personal life separate from your work. Talking about yourself and others at work is personally counterproductive, and causes the whole salon to suffer.

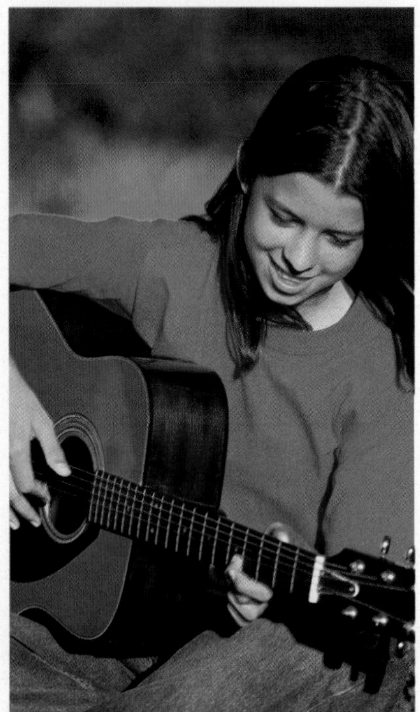

Figure 2-2 Spend time on the things you do well.

Keep your energy up. Successful cosmetologists do not run themselves ragged, nor do they eat, sleep, and drink beauty. They take care of their personal needs by spending time with family and friends, having hobbies, enjoying recreational activities, and so on.

Respect others. Make a point of relating to everyone you know with a conscious feeling of respect. Exercise good manners with others by using words like "please," "thank you," and "excuse me." Do not interrupt people and practice being a good listener.

Stay productive. There are three bad habits that can keep you from maintaining peak performance: (1) procrastination, (2) perfectionism, and (3) lack of a game plan. You will see an almost instant improvement when you work on eliminating these troublesome habits.

Procrastination is putting off until tomorrow what you can do today. This destructive, yet common habit is a characteristic of poor study habits ("I'll study tomorrow"). It may also be a symptom of taking on too much, which, in turn, is a symptom of faulty organization.

Perfectionism is the unhealthy compulsion to do things perfectly. Success is not measured by always doing things right. In fact, someone who never makes a mistake may not be trying hard enough. A better definition of success is to not give up, even when things get really tough.

short-term goal would be your graduation from cosmetology school. Short-term goals are usually those you wish to accomplish in a year or less.

Long-term goals are measured in larger sections of time such as 5 years, 10 years, or even longer. An example of a long-term goal is telling yourself that in 5 years you will own your own salon.

Once you have organized your thinking around your goals and written them down in "short-term" and "long-term" columns, divide each set of goals into workable segments. In this way, reaching your goals will not seem out of sight or overwhelming. For example, one of your biggest goals at the moment should be getting your license to practice your chosen career path. At first, the prospect of getting this license might seem to require a huge amount of time and effort. When you separate this goal into short-term goals (such as going to class on time, completing homework assignments, and mastering techniques), you begin to see how you can accomplish each one without too much difficulty.

The important thing to remember about goal setting is to have a plan and re-examine it often to make sure that you are staying on track. Even after successful people have accumulated fame, fortune, and respect, they still set goals for themselves. While they may adjust their goals and action plans as they go along, they never lose sight of the fact that their goals are what keep them going.

TIME MANAGEMENT

Many experts have researched how to make time more manageable. One thing they all agree on is that each of us has an "inner organizer." When we pay attention to our natural rhythms, we can learn how to manage our time most efficiently and reach our goals faster and with less frustration. Here are some tips from the experts.

- Learn to **prioritize** by making a list of tasks that need to be done in the order of most-to-least important.
- When designing your own time management system, make sure it will work for you. For example, if you are a person who needs a fair amount of flexibility, schedule in some blocks of unstructured time.
- Never take on more than you can handle. Learn to say "no" firmly but kindly, and mean it. You will find it easier to complete your tasks if you limit your activities, and do not spread yourself too thin.
- Learn problem-solving techniques that will save you time and needless frustration.
- Give yourself some down time whenever you are frustrated, overwhelmed, worried, or feeling guilty about something. You lose valuable time and energy when you are in a negative state of mind. Unfortunately, there may be situations—like being in the classroom—when you cannot get

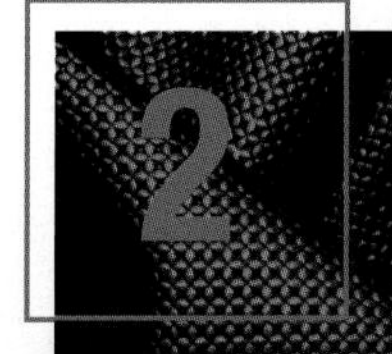

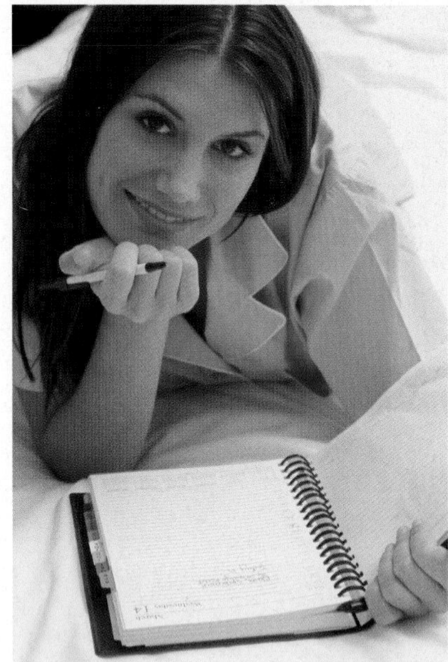

Figure 2-5 Keep a schedule for yourself and be sure to refer to it on a frequent basis.

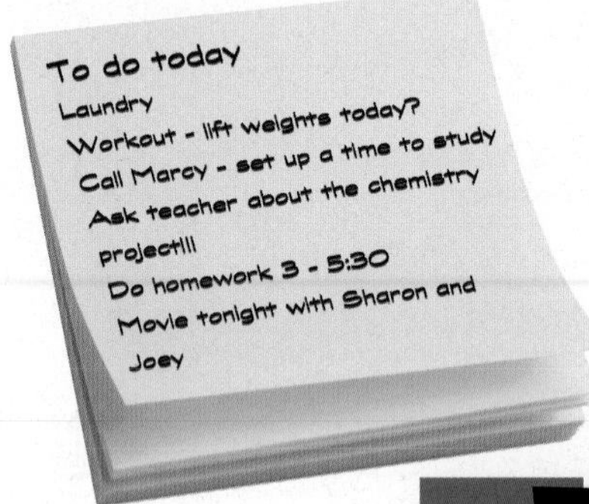

To do today
Laundry
Workout - lift weights today?
Call Marcy - set up a time to study
Ask teacher about the chemistry project!!!
Do homework 3 - 5:30
Movie tonight with Sharon and Joey

Figure 2-6 An example of a to-do list.

up and walk away. To handle these difficult times, try practicing the technique of deep breathing. Just fill your lungs as much as you can and exhale slowly. After about 5 to 10 breaths, you will find that you have calmed down, and your inner balance has been restored.

- Carry a notepad or an organizer with you at all times. You never know when a good idea might strike. Write it down before it slips your mind!
- Make daily, weekly, and monthly schedules for study and exam times, and any other regular commitments. Plan your leisure time around these commitments, and not the other way around (Figure 2-5).
- Identify the times of day when you are highly energetic, and when you just want to relax. Plan your schedule accordingly.
- Reward yourself with a special treat or activity for work well done and time managed efficiently.
- Do not neglect physical activity. Remember that exercise and recreation stimulate clear thinking and planning.
- Schedule at least one additional block of free time each day. This will be your hedge against events that come up unexpectedly like car trouble, baby-sitting problems, a friend in need, and so on.
- Understand the value of to-do lists for the day and week. They can help you prioritize your tasks and activities, which is key to organizing your time efficiently (Figure 2-6).
- Make time management a habit.

STUDY SKILLS

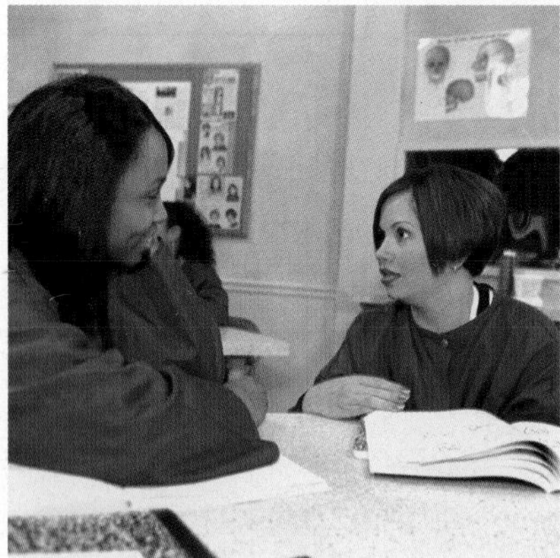

Figure 2-7 Studying with a friend can be effective and fun.

If you find studying overwhelming, focus on small tasks at a time. For example, instead of trying to study for 3 hours at a stretch and suffering a personal defeat when you fold after 40 minutes, set the bar lower by studying in smaller chunks of time. If your mind tends to wander in class, try writing down key words or phrases as your instructor discusses them. Any time you lose your focus, you can stay after class and ask questions based on your notes.

Another way to get a better handle on studying is to find other students who are open to being helpful and supportive. The more you discuss new material with others, the more comfortable you will become with it, and the more successful you will be. If possible, study together (Figure 2-7).

ESTABLISHING GOOD STUDY HABITS

Part of developing consistently good study habits is knowing where, when, and how to study.

WHERE

Establish a comfortable, quiet spot where you can study uninterrupted.

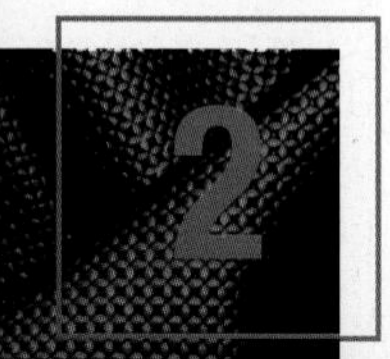

Have everything you need—books, pens, paper, proper lighting, and so on—before you begin studying.

Remain as alert as possible by sitting upright. Reclining will make you sleepy!

WHEN

- Start out by estimating how much study time you need.
- Study when you feel most energetic and motivated.
- Make good use of your time by planning to study while you are waiting in the doctor's office, taking a bus across town, and so on.

HOW

- Study a section of a chapter at a time, instead of the entire chapter at once.
- Make a note of key words and phrases as you go along.
- Test yourself on each section to ensure that you understand and remember the key points of each chapter.

Remember that every effort you make to follow through on your education is an investment in your future. The progress you make with your learning will increase your confidence and self-esteem across the board. In fact, when you have mastered a range of information and techniques, your self-esteem will soar right along with your grades.

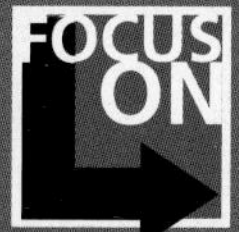

Focus on . . . The Goal

Determine whether your goal-setting plan is a good one by asking yourself these key questions:

- Are there specific skills I will need to learn in order to meet my goals?
- Is the information I need to reach my goals readily available?
- Would I be willing to seek out a mentor or a coach to enhance my learning?
- What is the best method or approach that will allow me to accomplish my goals?
- Am I always open to finding better ways of putting my plan into practice?

ETHICS

Ethics are the moral principles by which we live and work. In cosmetology, each state board sets the ethical standards for sanitation and safety that all professionals working in that state must follow. In the salon setting, ethics also entail the role you assume with your clients and fellow employees. When your actions show that you are respectful, courteous, and helpful, you are behaving in an ethical manner.

Here are five ways to show that you are an ethical person:

1. Provide skilled and competent services.
2. Be honest, courteous, and sincere.
3. Never share what clients have told you privately with others—even your closest friend.
4. Participate in ongoing education and stay on track with new information, techniques, and skills.
5. Always give correct information to clients about treatments and any products that they may want to purchase.

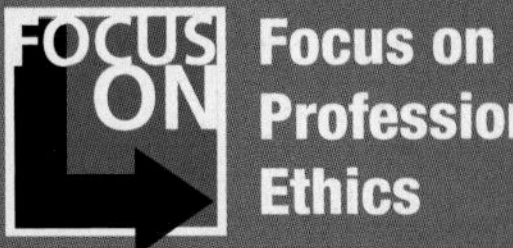

Focus on . . . Professional Ethics

Ethical people often embody the following qualities:

Self-care. Many service providers suffer from stress and eventual burnout because they focus most of their energy and time on other people and very little on themselves. If you are to be truly helpful to others, it is essential to take care of yourself. Try the self-care test to see how you rate (Figure 2-8).

Integrity. Maintain your integrity by making sure that your behavior and actions match your values. For example, if you believe that it is unethical to sell products just to make money, then do not do so. On the other hand, if you feel that a client needs products and additional services, it would be unethical *not* to give the client that information.

Discretion. Do not share your personal problems with clients. Likewise, never *breach confidentiality* by repeating personal information that clients have shared with you.

Communication. Your responsibility and ethical behavior extend to your communication with your customers and the other people with whom you work.

The Self-Care Test

Some people know intuitively when they need to stop, take a break, or even take a day off. Other people forget when to eat. You can judge how well you take care of yourself by noting how you feel physically, emotionally, and mentally. Here are some questions to ask yourself to see how you rate on the self-care scale.

1. Do you wait until you are exhausted before you stop working?
2. Do you forget to eat nutritious food and substitute junk food on the fly?
3. Do you say you will exercise and then put off starting a program?
4. Do you have poor sleep habits?
5. Are you constantly nagging yourself about not being good enough?
6. Are your relationships with people filled with conflict?
7. When you think about the future are you unclear about the direction you will take?
8. Do you spend most of your spare time watching TV?
9. Have you been told you are too stressed and yet you ignore these concerns?
10. Do you waste time and then get angry with yourself?

Score 5 points for each yes. A score of 0-15 says that you take pretty good care of yourself, but you would be wise to examine those questions you answered yes to. A score of 15-30 indicates that you need to rethink your priorities. A score of 30-50 is a strong statement that you are neglecting yourself and may be headed for high stress and burnout. Reviewing the suggestions in these chapters will help you get back on track.

Figure 2-8 Self-care test.

PERSONALITY DEVELOPMENT AND ATTITUDE

Some occupations require less interaction with people than others. For example, if you are a computer programmer, you may not be exposed to all different sorts of people every day. As a cosmetologist however, dealing with people from all walks of life is a major aspect of your work. It is useful, therefore, to have some sense of how different personalities and attitudes can affect your performance.

Refer often to the following ingredients of a healthy, well-developed attitude to see if they match your recipe.

Diplomacy. Being assertive is a good thing because it helps people know where you are coming from. However, it is a short step from being assertive to becoming aggressive, and even bullying. Take your attitude temperature to see how well you practice the art of tact. Being tactful means being straightforward, not critical. This is called "diplomacy."

Tone of voice. Here is a good example of an inborn personality trait that you can modify by softening the sound of your voice and speaking clearly. Also, if you have a positive attitude, you can deliver your words more pleasantly.

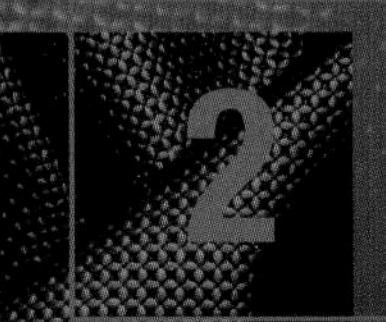

Emotional stability. Our emotions are important. Some people, though, have no control over their feelings, and may express themselves excessively or inappropriately. When they are happy, they get almost frantic; when they are angry, they fly into a rage. Learning how to handle a confrontation, as well as sharing how you feel without going overboard, are important indicators of maturity.

Sensitivity. Sensitivity is a combination of understanding, empathy, and acceptance. Being sensitive means being compassionate and responsive to other people.

Values and goals. Neither values nor goals are inborn characteristics; we acquire them as we move through life. They show us how to behave, and what to aim toward.

Receptivity. To be receptive means to be interested in other people, and to be responsive to their opinions, feelings, and ideas. Receptivity involves taking the time to really listen, instead of pretending to do so (Figure 2-9).

Communication skills. People with a warm, caring personality have an easy time talking about themselves and listening to what others have to say. When they want something, they can ask for it clearly and directly.

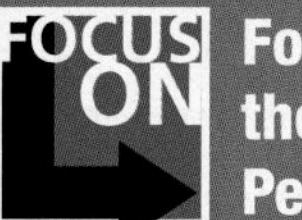

Focus on . . . the Whole Person

An individual's personality is the sum total of her or his inborn characteristics, attitudes, and behavioral traits. While you may not be able to alter most of your inborn characteristics, you certainly can work on your attitude. This is a process that continues throughout your life. In both your business and personal life, a pleasing attitude gains more associates, clients, and friends.

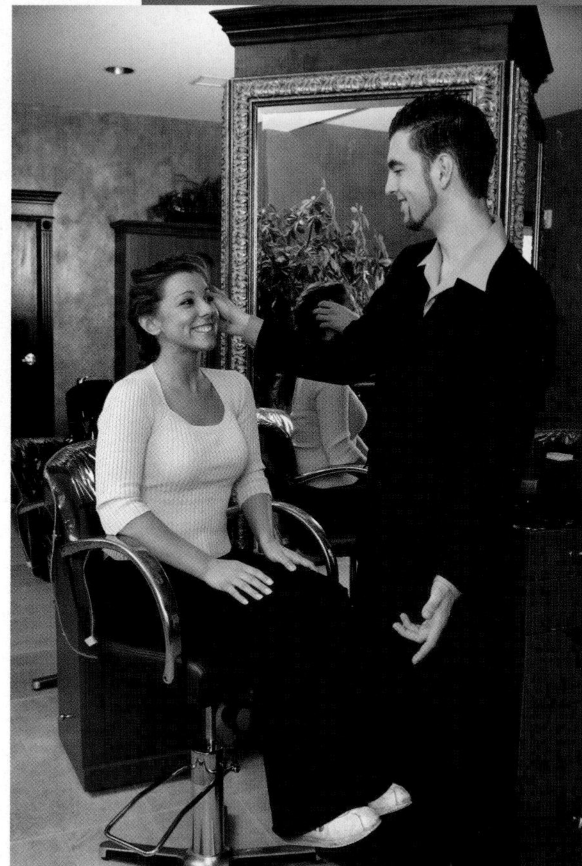

Figure 2-9 Being receptive is an important personal skill.

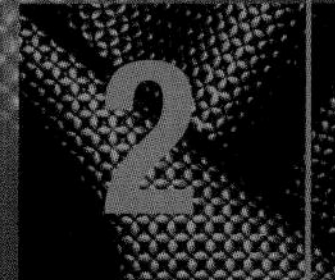

REVIEW QUESTIONS

1. How do you personally define success?
2. List and explain 10 basic guidelines for personal and professional success.
3. What are three common habits that can prevent people from being productive?
4. List at least three steps that you can take to enhance your creativity.
5. In one to five sentences, write a mission statement for yourself.
6. List three short-term and three long-term goals you have set for yourself.
7. Define "game plan" and how it can keep your career on target.
8. Why is it so important to learn how to manage your time?
9. List seven characteristics of a healthy, well-developed attitude.
10. List the qualities and characteristics of professional ethics.

CHAPTER GLOSSARY

ethics	Principles of good character, proper conduct, and moral judgment, expressed through personality, human relations skills, and professional image.
game plan	The conscious act of planning your life rather than just letting things happen.
goal setting	The identification of long- and short-term goals.
mission statement	A statement that sets forth the values that an individual or institution lives by and that establishes future goals.
perfectionism	A compulsion to do things perfectly.
prioritize	To make a list of tasks that need to be done in the order of most to least important.
procrastination	Putting off until tomorrow what you can do today.

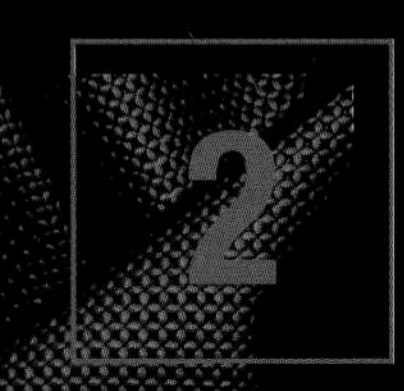

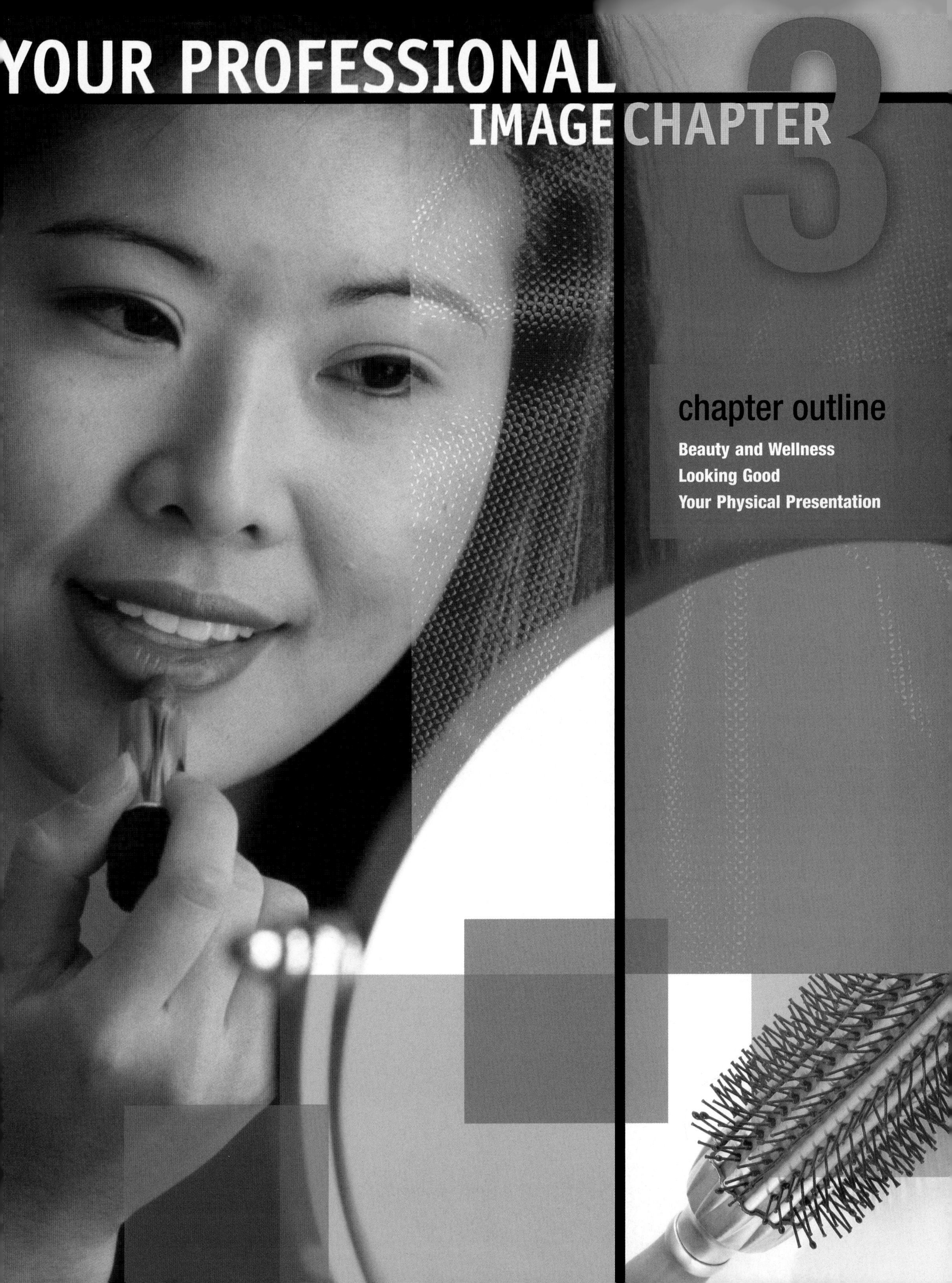

YOUR PROFESSIONAL IMAGE CHAPTER 3

chapter outline

Beauty and Wellness
Looking Good
Your Physical Presentation

Learning Objectives

After completing this chapter, you will be able to:

- **Understand professional hygiene.**
- **Explain the concept of dressing for success.**
- **Use appropriate methods to ensure personal health and well-being.**
- **Demonstrate an understanding of ergonomic principles and ergonomically correct postures and movement.**

Key Terms

Page number indicates where in the chapter the term is used.

ergonomics
pg. 30

personal hygiene
pg. 27

physical presentation
pg. 29

professional image
pg. 28

stress
pg. 29

Because you are in the image business, how you look and present yourself has a big influence on whether you will be successful working in your chosen career path within the field of cosmetology. If you are talking style, then you need to look stylish; if you are advising your clients about makeup, then your makeup must be current and beautifully applied. If you are recommending hand care services, it is critical that your hands and nails are well manicured. When your appearance and the way that you conduct yourself are in harmony with the beauty business, your chances of being successful in any area of cosmetology increase by as much as 100 percent! After all, when you look great, your clients will assume that you can make them look great, too (Figure 3-1).

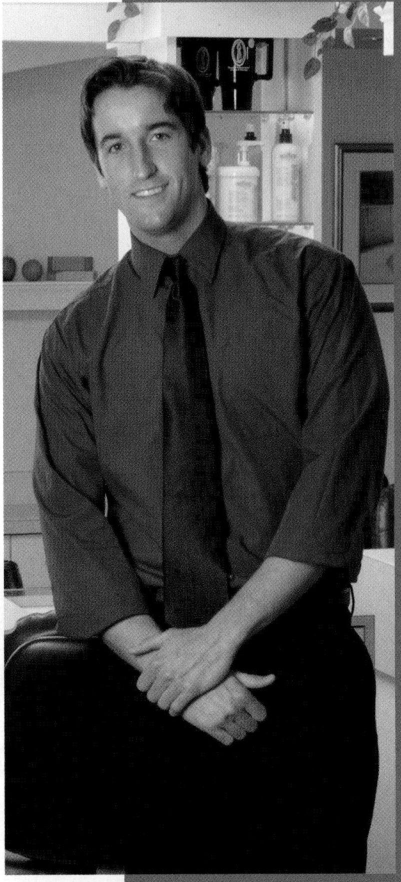
Figure 3-1 Project a professional image.

BEAUTY AND WELLNESS

PERSONAL HYGIENE

Being well groomed begins with looking and smelling fresh. This is especially important in the beauty business where practitioners are frequently only inches away from their clients during services. It is a given that you should shower or bathe every day, use deodorant before going to work, and generally be neat and clean. Beyond that, though, there are special considerations when working in a salon.

One weak moment of drinking coffee right before performing a service, for instance, or wearing something that needs laundering because you did not plan ahead, could spell disaster. Rather than telling you that you smell offensive, most clients will simply not return for another service. Equally distressing, they will typically tell three of their friends about the bad experience they had while sitting in your chair.

Personal hygiene is the daily maintenance of cleanliness by practicing good sanitary habits (Figure 3-2). Working as a stylist behind the chair, or doing makeup, nail care, or skin care means that you must be extremely meticulous about your hygiene.

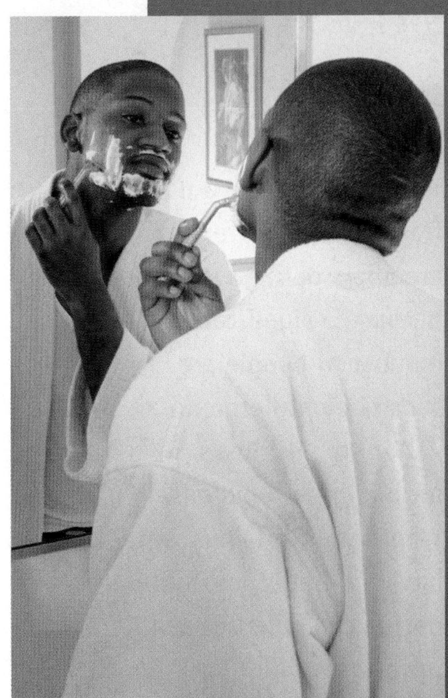
Figure 3-2 Practice meticulous personal hygiene every day.

One of the best ways to ensure that you always smell fresh and clean is to create a hygiene pack to keep in your station or locker. Your hygiene pack should include:

- Toothbrush and toothpaste
- Mouthwash
- Sanitizing hand wipes or liquid to freshen your hands between clients
- Floss
- Deodorant or antiperspirant

Your hygiene pack will be useful in following these guidelines:

- Wash your hands throughout the day as required, including at the beginning of each service.
- Use deodorant or antiperspirant.
- Brush and floss your teeth, and use mouthwash or breath mints throughout the day as needed.
- Do self-checks periodically to ensure that you smell and look fresh.
- If you smoke cigarettes, *do not* smoke during work hours. If you cannot wait until after work, make sure to smoke in a well-ventilated area at least 30 minutes before seeing your next client. Always brush your teeth, use mouthwash, and wash your hands after smoking if you are still servicing clients!

LOOKING GOOD

Naturally, in the line of work that you have chosen, an extremely important element of your image is having well-groomed hair, skin, and nails that serve as an advertisement for your commitment to professional beauty. Make sure that you:

- Put thought into your appearance every day.
- Keep your haircut and color in tip-top shape.
- Keep your skin well groomed.
- Determine the best length and grooming for your nails and meticulously maintain their appearance.
- Change your style frequently, or as often as you feel comfortable, to keep up with trends.

CAUTION

PERFUME

Many salons have a no-fragrance policy for staff members during work hours because a significant number of people are sensitive or allergic to a variety of chemicals, including perfume oils. Whether or not your salon has a no-fragrance policy, perfume should be saved for after work.

PERSONAL GROOMING

Many salon owners and managers view appearance, personality, and poise as being just as important as technical knowledge and skills. One of the most vital aspects of good personal grooming is the careful maintenance of your wardrobe. First and foremost, your clothes must be clean—not simply free of the dirt that you can see, but stain free, a feat that is sometimes difficult to achieve in a salon environment. Because you are constantly coming into contact with products and chemicals that can stain fabric in a nanosecond, it is a good idea to invest in an apron or smock to wear while handling such products. Be mindful about spills and drips when using chemicals, and avoid leaning on counters in the work area—particularly in the dispensary.

DRESS FOR SUCCESS

If you want to go out on the weekend and wear something wild and crazy, this is your choice. But while you are at your place of employment, you will need to consider whether your wardrobe selection expresses a **professional image** that is consistent with the image of the salon.

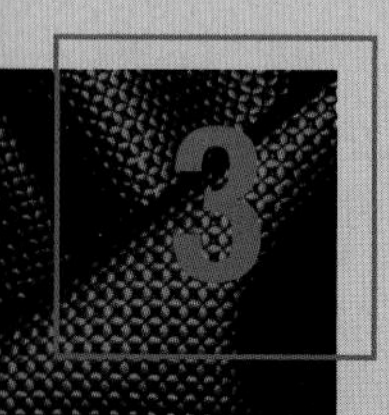

Common sense as well should rule when it comes to choosing clothes to wear at work. When shopping for work clothes, you should always visualize how you would look in them while performing professional client services. Is the image you present one that is acceptable to your clients?

To a large degree, your clothing should reflect the fashions of the season by embodying current styles, colors, textures, and so forth. Depending on where you work, you may be encouraged to wear stylish torn jeans and faded tees, or they may be expressly forbidden. Just remember to "tune in" to your salon's energy and clientele so that you can make the best clothing choices that promote your career as a promising stylist.

You should always be guided by your salon's dress code with regard to these matters, but the following guidelines are generally appropriate (Figure 3-3).

- Make sure that your clothing is clean, fresh, and in step with fashion.
- Choose clothing that is functional, as well as stylish.
- Accessorize your outfits, but make sure that your jewelry does not clank and jingle while working. This can be irritating to fellow professionals and drive clients to distraction.

Wear shoes that are comfortable, have a low heel, and good support. Ill-fitting shoes, and any type with high heels, are not the best choices to wear when performing services within the salon (Figure 3-4).

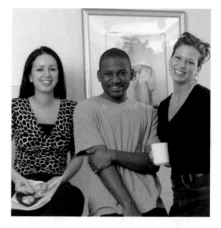

Figure 3-3 Be guided by your salon's dress code.

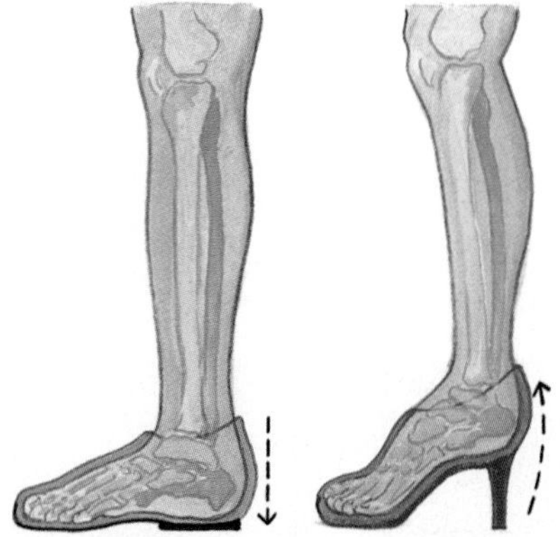

Figure 3-4 Working in high heels can throw off the body's balance.

THE ART OF MAKEUP

Makeup is an exciting category for beauty professionals. It helps promote your professional image, and is an area where some of your most lucrative sales can be made. You should always use makeup to accentuate your best features, and mask your less flattering ones. With that said, it is vital to always wear makeup at work. A freshly scrubbed face may look great for a leisurely day at the beach, but it does nothing to promote your image as a beauty professional while at work. Likewise, unless you are working in a trendy urban salon, things like heavily blackened eyes are generally best left to the club scene. Let the salon's image be your guide on the right makeup choices to wear for work (Figure 3-5).

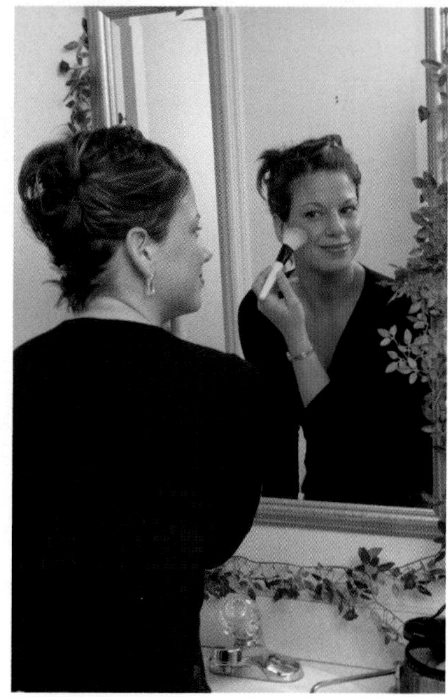

Figure 3-5 Expertly applied makeup is part of having a professional image.

YOUR PHYSICAL PRESENTATION

POSTURE

Good posture is a very important part of your **physical presentation.** It shows off your figure to its best advantage, and conveys an image of confidence. From a health standpoint, it can also prevent fatigue and many other physical problems. When you work within the field of cosmetology, sitting improperly can put a great deal of **stress** on your neck, shoulders,

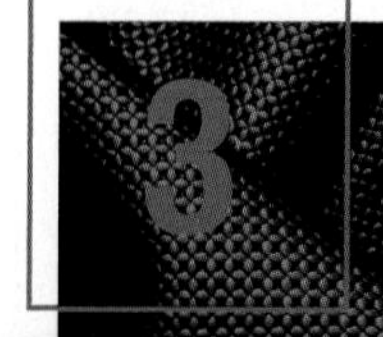

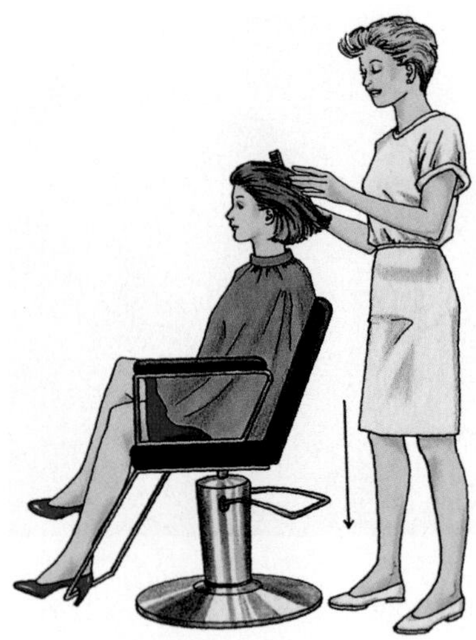

Figure 3-6 Good physical presentation.

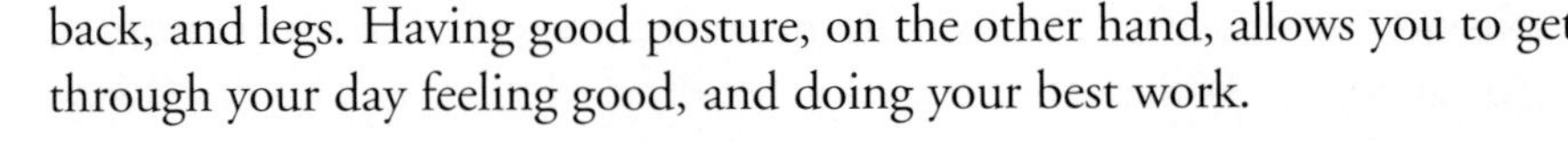

back, and legs. Having good posture, on the other hand, allows you to get through your day feeling good, and doing your best work.

Some guidelines for achieving and maintaining good work posture follow:

- Keep the neck elongated and balanced directly above the shoulders.
- Lift your upper body so that your chest is out and up (do not slouch).
- Hold your shoulders level and relaxed, not scrunched up.
- Sit with your back straight.
- Pull your abdomen in so that it is flat (Figure 3-6).

ERGONOMICS

Each year, hundreds of cosmetology professionals report musculoskeletal disorders, including carpal tunnel syndrome and back injuries. Beauty professionals expose their bodies to potential injury on a daily basis. Many have to stand or sit all day and hold their bodies in unnatural positions for long periods of time. They are susceptible to problems of the hands, wrists, shoulders, neck, back, feet, and legs. If not attended to, these problems can become career threatening.

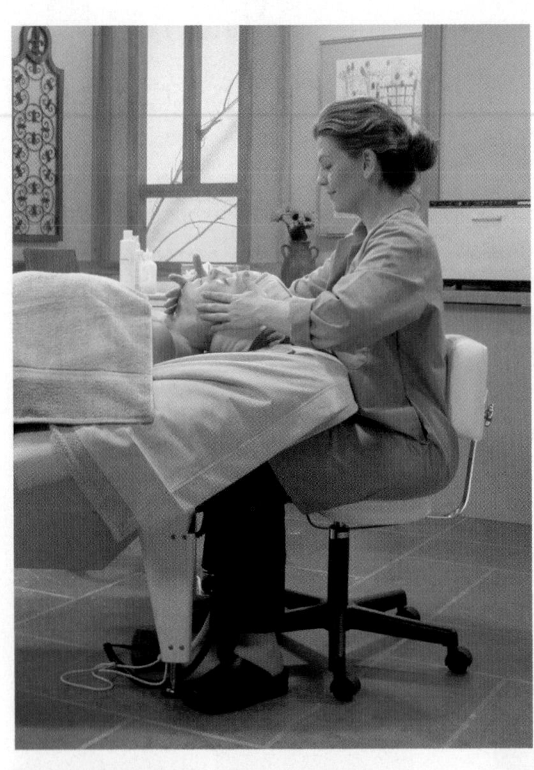

Figure 3-7 Proper positioning of the client on the facial bed.

Prevention is the key to alleviating these problems. An awareness of your body posture and movements, coupled with better work habits and proper tools and equipment, will enhance your health and comfort (Figure 3-7). An understanding of ergonomics is useful as well. **Ergonomics** is the study of how a workplace can best be designed for comfort, safety, efficiency, and productivity. It attempts to fit the job to the person, rather than the other way around. One example is a hydraulic chair that can be raised or lowered to accommodate different heights. Another is having ergonomically designed cutting shears and blow-dryers.

Stressful repetitive motions have a cumulative effect on the muscles and joints. Monitor yourself as you work to see if you are:

- Gripping or squeezing implements too tightly.
- Bending the wrist up or down constantly when using the tools of your profession.
- Holding your arms away from your body as you work.
- Holding your elbows more than a 60-degree angle away from your body for extended periods of time.
- Bending forward and/or twisting your body to get closer to your client.

Try the following measures to avoid some of the problems discussed above (Figure 3-8).

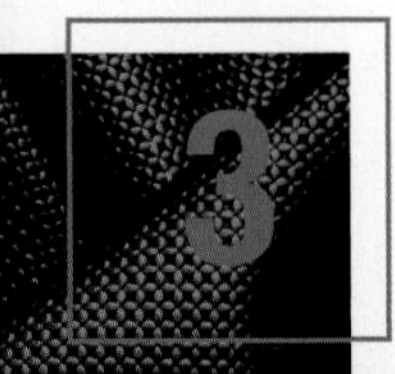

- Keep your wrists in a straight or neutral position as much as possible (Figure 3-9).
- When giving a manicure, do not reach across the table; have the client extend her hand across the table to you (Figure 3-10).
- Use ergonomically designed implements.
- Keep your back and neck straight.

If you work in an environment that has any physical discomfort built into it, as most places do, try to counter the problem by including regular stretching intervals to break up the repetitiveness of the motions you use. And, in every aspect of your work, always put your health first and then the task at hand. It will serve you well in the beauty business, and ensure a long, injury-free career.

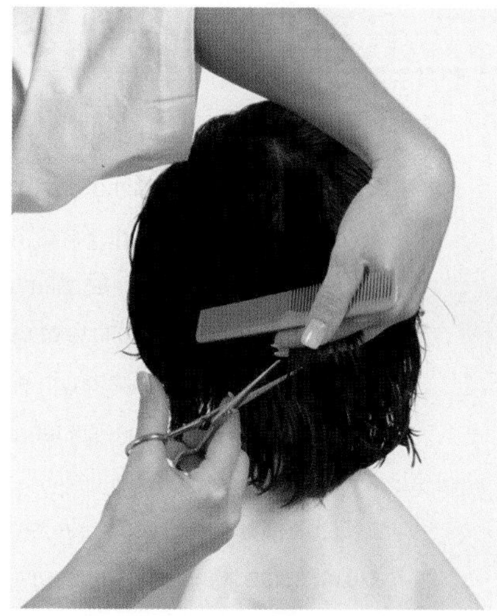

Figure 3-8 Improper haircutting position.

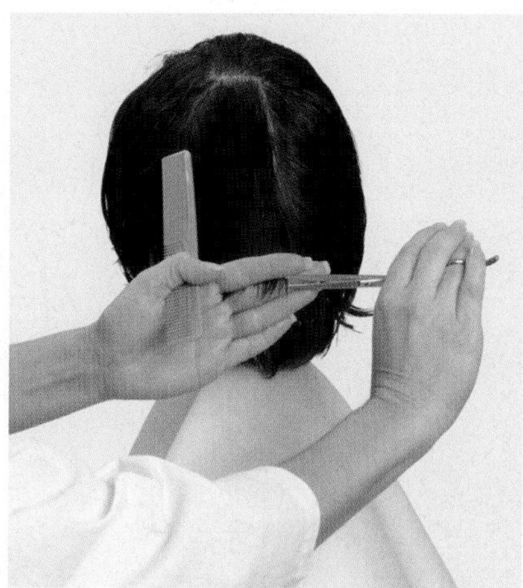

Figure 3-9 Correct wrist and hand position for haircutting.

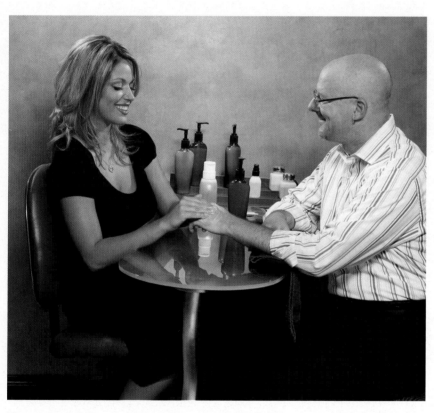

Figure 3-10 Follow proper ergonomic techniques when giving nail services.

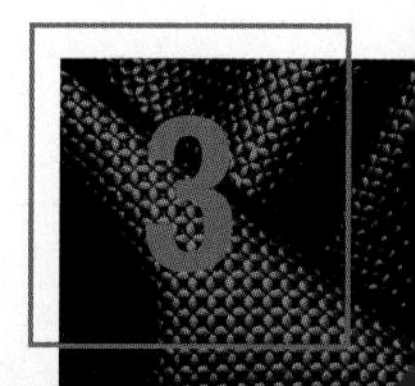

REVIEW QUESTIONS

1. List the elements of professional image.
2. List three basic habits of personal hygiene.
3. Identify what is included in a "hygiene pack." Where is it kept?
4. How often should you freshen up throughout the day?
5. List the general guidelines of dressing for success.
6. What is the role of posture in good health?
7. Assess your own work posture. How can it be improved?
8. Define the term "ergonomics."
9. List equipment or tools with ergonomic features.
10. List steps you can take to prevent potential injury to yourself with regard to ergonomics.

CHAPTER GLOSSARY

ergonomics	Study of how a workplace can best be designed for comfort, safety, efficiency, and productivity.
personal hygiene	Daily maintenance of cleanliness by practicing good sanitary habits.
physical presentation	Person's physical posture, walk, and movements.
professional image	Impression projected by a person engaged in any profession, consisting of outward appearance and conduct exhibited in the workplace.
stress	Inability to cope with a threat, real or imagined, to our well-being, which results in a series of responses and adaptations by our minds and bodies; tension caused by a situation.

COMMUNICATING FOR SUCCESS CHAPTER 4

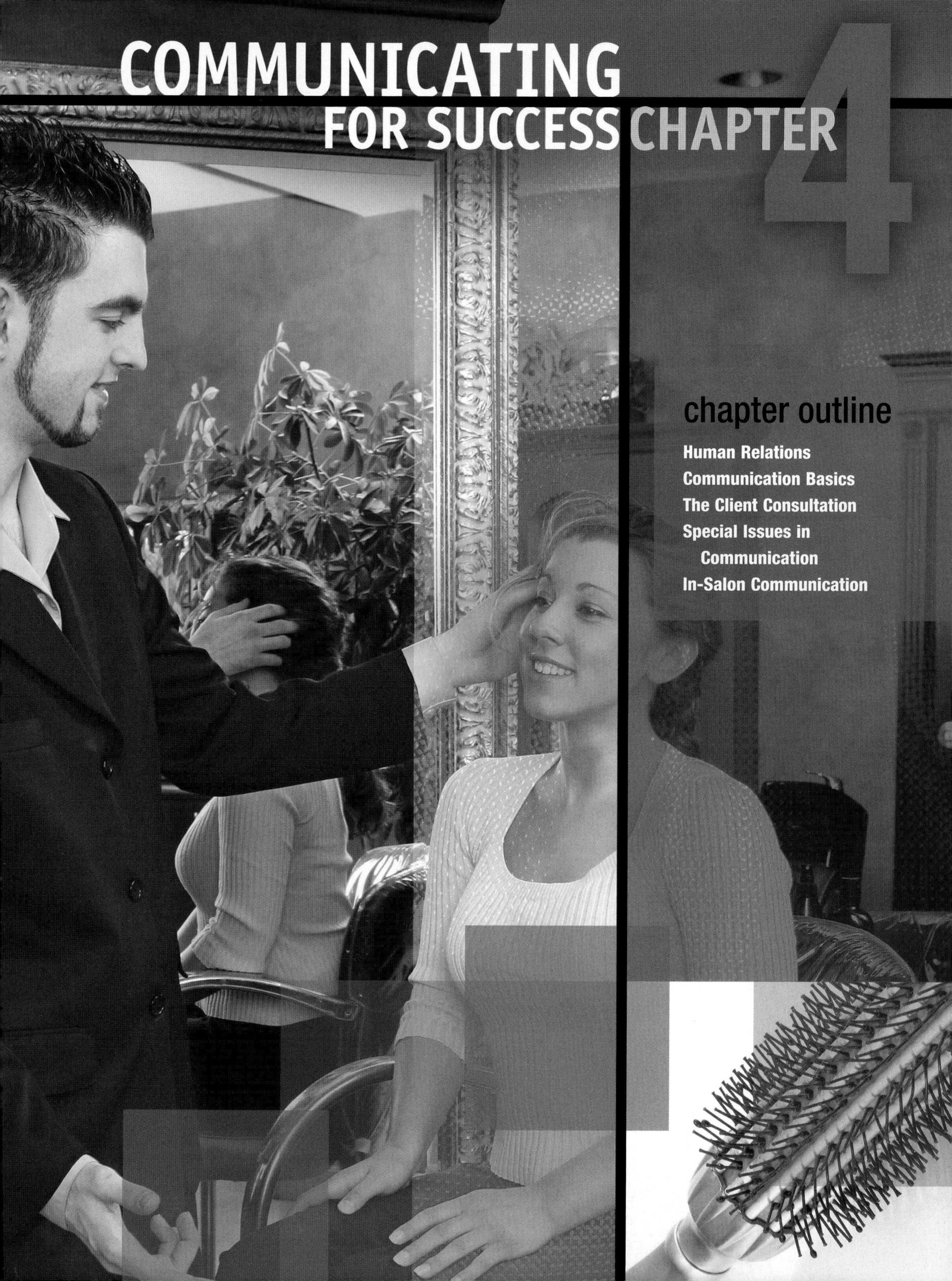

chapter outline

Learning Objectives

After completing this chapter, you will be able to:

- **List the golden rules of human relations.**
- **Explain the importance of effective communication.**
- **Conduct a successful client consultation.**
- **Handle delicate communications with your clients.**
- **Build open lines of communication with co-workers and salon managers.**

Key Terms

Page number indicates where in the chapter the term is used.

client consultation
pg. 40

communication
pg. 37

reflective listening
pg. 43

Do you have outstanding technical skills? Artistic talents? If you do, you are definitely on your way to becoming successful in your chosen career path within the field of cosmetology. It is important to realize, though, that technical and artistic skills can only take you so far. In order to have a thriving clientele, you must also master the art of communication (Figure 4-1). Effective human relations and communication skills build lasting client relationships, aid in your growth as a salon practitioner, and help prevent misunderstandings and unnecessary tension in the workplace.

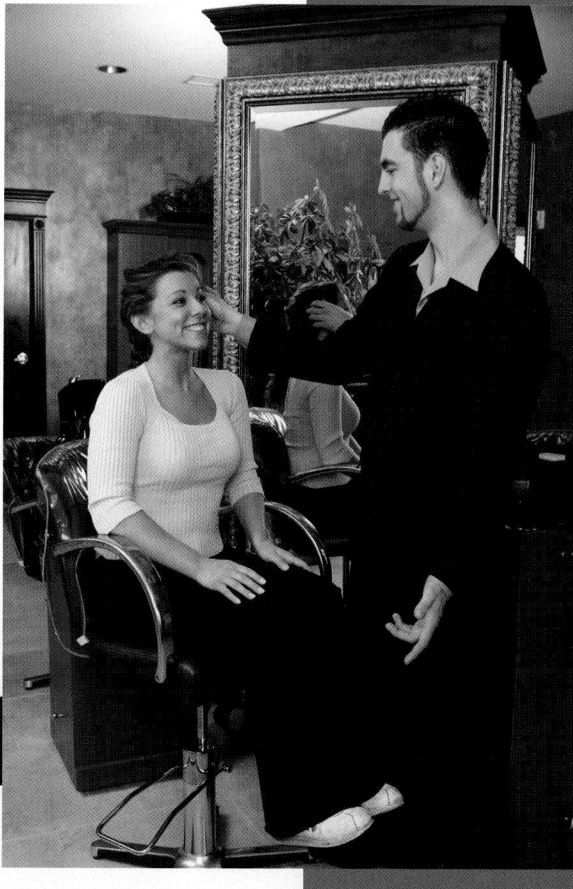

Figure 4–1 Communication is part of building lasting practitioner/client relationships.

HUMAN RELATIONS

No matter where you work, you will not always get along with everyone. It is not possible to always understand what people need, even when you know them well. Even if you do think you understand what people want, you cannot always be sure that you will satisfy them. This can lead to tension and misunderstanding.

The ability to understand people is the key to operating effectively in many professions. It is especially important in cosmetology where customer service is central to success. Most of your interactions will depend on your ability to communicate successfully with a wide range of people: your boss, co-workers, clients, and the different vendors who come into the salon to sell products. When you clearly understand the motives and needs of others, you are in a better position to do your job professionally and easily.

The best way to understand others is to begin with a firm understanding of yourself. When you know what makes you tick, it is easier to appreciate others and to help them get what they need. Basically, we all have the same needs. When we are treated with respect and people listen to us, we feel good about them and ourselves. When we create an atmosphere where customers and staff have confidence in us, we will get the respect we deserve. Good relationships are built on mutual respect and understanding. Here is a brief look at the basics of human relations along with some practical tips for dealing with situations that you are likely to encounter.

- A fundamental factor in human relations has to do with how secure we are feeling. When we feel secure, we are happy, calm, and confident, and we act in a cooperative and trusting manner. When we feel insecure, we become worried, anxious, overwhelmed, perhaps angry and suspicious, and usually we do not behave very well. We might be uncooperative, hostile, or withdrawn.

- Human beings are social animals. When we feel secure, we like to interact with other people. We enjoy giving our opinions, we take pleasure from having people help us, and we take pride in our ability to help others. When people feel secure with us, they are a joy to be with. You can help people feel secure around you by being respectful, trustworthy, and honest.
- No matter how secure you are, there will be times when you will be faced with people and situations that are difficult to handle. You may already have had such experiences. There are always some people who create conflict wherever they go. They can be rude, insensitive, or so full of themselves that being considerate just does not enter their minds. Even though you may wonder how anyone could be so unfeeling, just try to remember that this person at this particular time feels insecure or he/she wouldn't be acting this way.

To become skilled in human relations, learn to make the best of situations that could otherwise drain both your time and your energy. Here are some good ways to handle the ups and downs of human relations.

Respond instead of reacting. A fellow was asked why he did not get angry when a driver cut him off. "Why should I let someone else dictate my emotions?" he replied. A wise fellow, don't you think? He might have even saved his own life by not reacting with "an eye for an eye" mentality.

Believe in yourself. When you do, you trust your judgment, uphold your own values, and stick to what you believe is right. It is easy to believe in yourself when you have a strong sense of self-worth. It comes with the knowledge that you are a good person and you deserve to be successful. Believing in yourself makes you feel strong enough to handle almost any situation in a calm, helpful manner.

Talk less, listen more. There is an old saying that we were given two ears and one mouth for a reason. You get a gold star in human relations when you listen more than you talk. When you are a good listener, you are fully attentive to what the other person is saying. If there is something you do not understand, ask a question to gain understanding.

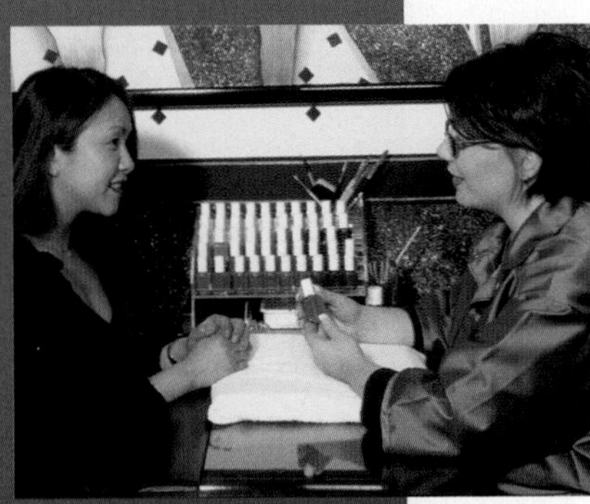

Figure 4-2 Be attentive to your client's needs.

Be attentive. Each client is different. Some are clear about what they want, others are aggressively demanding, while others may be hesitant. If you have an aggressive client, instead of trying to handle it by yourself, ask your manager for advice. You will likely be told that what usually calms difficult clients down is agreeing with them and then asking what you can do to make the service more to their liking. This approach is virtually guaranteed to work (Figure 4-2).

Take your own temperature. If you are tired or upset about a personal problem, or have had an argument with a fellow student, you may be feeling down about yourself and wish you were anywhere but in school. If this feeling lasts a short time, you will be able to get back on track easily enough and there is no cause for alarm. If, however, you begin to notice certain chronic behaviors about yourself once you are in a job, pay careful attention to what is happening. An important part of being in a service profession is taking care of yourself first and resolving whatever conflicts are going on so that you can take care of your clients. Trust can be lost in a second without even knowing it—and, once lost, trust is almost impossible to regain.

To conclude, human relations can be rewarding or demoralizing. It all depends on how willing you are to give.

THE GOLDEN RULES OF HUMAN RELATIONS

Keep the following guidelines in mind for a crash course in human relations that will always keep you in line and where you should be:

- Communicate from your heart; problem solve from your head.
- A smile is worth a million times more than a sneer.
- It is easy to make an enemy; it is harder to keep a friend.
- See what happens when you ask for help instead of just reacting.
- Show people you care by listening to them and trying to understand their point of view.
- Tell people how great they are (even when they are not acting so great).
- Being right is different from acting righteous.
- For every service you do for others, do not forget to do something for yourself.
- Laugh often.
- Show patience with other people's flaws.
- Build shared goals; be a team player and a partner to your clients.
- Always remember that listening is the best relationship builder.

COMMUNICATION BASICS

Communication is the act of successfully sharing information between two people, or groups of people so that it is effectively understood. You can communicate through words, voice inflections, facial expressions, body language, and visual tools (e.g., a portfolio of your work). When you and your client are both communicating clearly about an upcoming service, your chances of pleasing that person soar.

MEETING AND GREETING NEW CLIENTS

One of the most important communications you will have with a client is the first time you meet that person. Be polite, genuinely friendly and inviting (which you will continue to be in all your encounters), and remember that your clients are coming to you for services for which they are paying hard-earned cash (Figure 4-3). This means you need to court

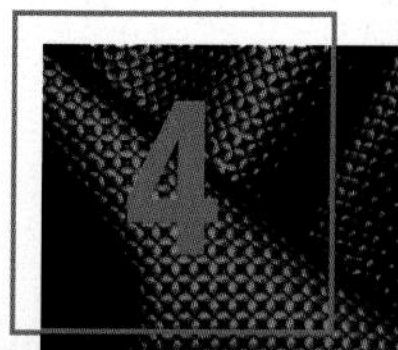

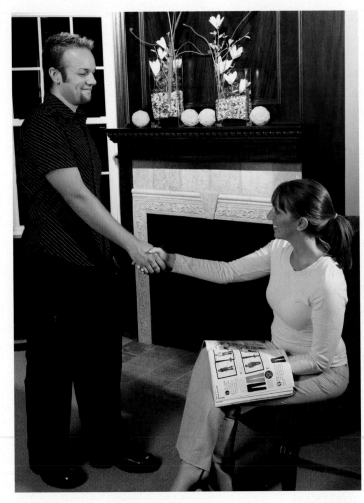

Figure 4-3 Welcome your client to the salon.

them every time they come to see you; otherwise, you may lose them to another stylist or salon.

To earn clients' trust and loyalty, you need to:

- Always approach a new client with a smile on your face. If you are having a difficult day or have a problem of some sort, keep it to yourself. The time you are with your client is for her needs, not yours.
- Always introduce yourself. Names are powerful and they are meant to be used. Many clients have had the experience of being greeted by the receptionist, ushered back to the service area, and when the service has been performed and the appointment is over, they have not learned the name of a single person.
- Set aside a few minutes to take new clients on a quick tour of the salon.
- Introduce them to people they may have interactions with while in the salon, including potential service providers for other services such as skin care or nail services.
- Be yourself. Do not try to trick your clients into thinking you are someone or something that you are not. Just be who you are. You will be surprised at how well this will work for you.

INTAKE FORM

An intake form—also called a "client questionnaire" or "consultation card"—should be filled out by every new client prior to sitting at your station. Whether in the salon or in school, this form can prove to be extremely useful (Figure 4-4).

Some salon intake forms ask for a lot of detailed information, and some do not. In cosmetology school, the consultation form may be accompanied by a release statement in which the client acknowledges that the service is being provided by a student who is still learning. This helps protect the school and the student from any legal action by a client who may be unhappy with the service.

How to Use the Client Intake Form

The client intake form can be used from the moment a new client calls the salon to make an appointment. When scheduling the appointment, let her know that you and the salon will require some information before you can begin the service, and that it is important for her to arrive 15 minutes prior to her appointment time to fill out a brief form. You will also have to allow time in your schedule to do a 5 minute to 15 minute client consultation, depending on the type of service you will be performing and the needs of the client.

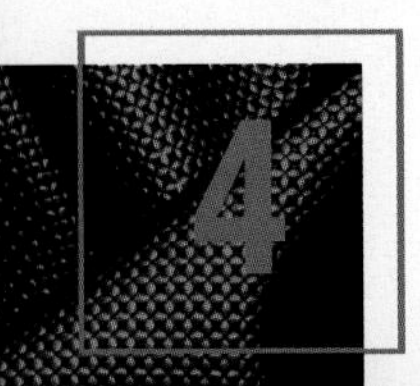

Client Intake Form

Dear Client,

Our sincerest hope is to serve you with the best hair care services you've ever received! We not only want you to be happy with today's visit, we also want to build a long-lasting relationship with you, the client.
In order for us to do so, we would like to learn more about you, your hair care needs and your preferences. Please take a moment now to answer the questions below as completely and as accurately as possible.

Thank you, and we look forward to building a "beautiful" relationship!

Name: ______________________________

Address: ______________________________

Phone Number: (day)__________ (evening)__________ (cell)__________

Email address: __________

Sex: _____ Male _____ Female Age:_____

How did you hear about our salon?______________________________

If you were referred, who referred you?______________________________

Please answer the following questions in the space provided. Thanks!

1. Approximately when was your last salon visit?______________________________
2. In the past year have you had any of the following services either in or out of a salon?

   ____ Haircut
   ____ Haircolor
   ____ Permanent Wave or Texturizing Treatment
   ____ Chemical Relaxing or Straightening Treatment
   ____ Highlighting or Lowlighting
   ____ Full head lightening
   ____ Manicure
   ____ Artificial nail services (please describe)
   ____ Pedicure
   ____ Facial/Skin Treatment
   ____ Other (please list any other services you've enjoyed at a salon that may not be listed here).
3. What are your expectations for your hair service(s) today?
4. Are you now, or have you ever been, allergic to any of the products, treatments, or chemicals you've received during any salon service—hair, nails, or skin? (Please explain)

   ____
5. Are you currently taking any medications? (Please list)

   ____
6. Please list all of the products that you use on your hair on a regular basis.
7. What tools do you use at home to style your hair?
8. What is the one thing that you want your stylist to know about you/your hair?
9. Are you interested in receiving a skin care, nail care or makeup consultation?
10. Would you like to be contacted via email aboout upcoming promotions and special events?

    Yes _____ No _____

Figure 4-4 The client intake form gives you an opportunity to build an excellent relationship with your clients. *Continued*

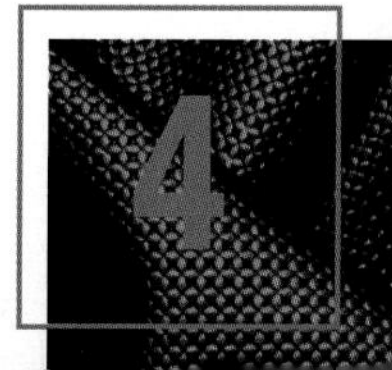

NOTE: If this card were used in a cosmetology school setting, it would include a release form at the bottom such as the one below.

Statement of Release: I hereby understand that supervised cosmetology students render these services for the sole purpose of practice and learning, and that by signing this form, I recognize and agree not to hold the school, its employees or the student liable for my satisfaction or the service outcome.

Client signature ______________________________ Date ______________________

Service Notes

Today's Date:

Today's Services:

Notes:

Today's Date:

Today's Services:

Notes:

Today's Date:

Today's Services:

Notes:

Today's Date:

Today's Services:

Notes:

Today's Date:

Today's Services:

Notes:

Figure 4–4 *(continued)*

THE CLIENT CONSULTATION

The **client consultation** is the verbal communication that determines the desired results. It is the single most important part of any service and should always be done *before* beginning any part of the service. Some professionals skip the client consultation altogether, or they make time for it only on a client's first visit to the salon. These professionals are making a serious mistake. A consultation should be performed, to some degree, as part of every single service and salon visit. It keeps good communication going, and allows you to keep your clients looking current and feeling satisfied with your services.

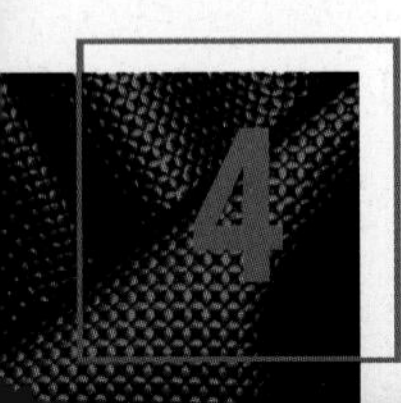

PREPARING FOR THE CLIENT CONSULTATION

In order for your time to be well spent during the client consultation, it is important to be prepared. To facilitate the consultation process, you should have certain important items on hand. These include styling books and hair swatches.

Have a variety of styling books that your clients can look through. There should be at least one that depicts short hair, one for medium-length hair, and one with longer styles, as well as an assortment of photos representing all hair color possibilities, such as blonds, reds, and darker colors.

In addition, it is always a good idea to have a portfolio of your own work on hand. Keep a camera at your station (a disposable or digital camera is fine) and take photos of whatever cuts, colors, perms, and other types of chemical or styling work you perform. A portfolio will help put new clients at ease about your abilities, and will help them decide what they want to have done. As you show the photos, explain why you performed the various services the way you did. This will help new clients understand why certain things can or cannot be achieved, and will also reassure them that you are knowledgeable and serious about their needs.

A handy tool, great for discussing haircolor, is a swatch book or ring. These are provided by the companies that manufacture hair color, and are generally packaged in a ring, book, or paper chart. Swatches are bundles of hair dyed to match a particular haircolor shade offered by the manufacturer. Usually made from a synthetic material, swatches are very durable and easy to use in consultations. If the swatch is long enough, it can be held up to the client's face or integrated into her own hair to see how it looks. Swatches are perfect "symbols" to help the stylist and client

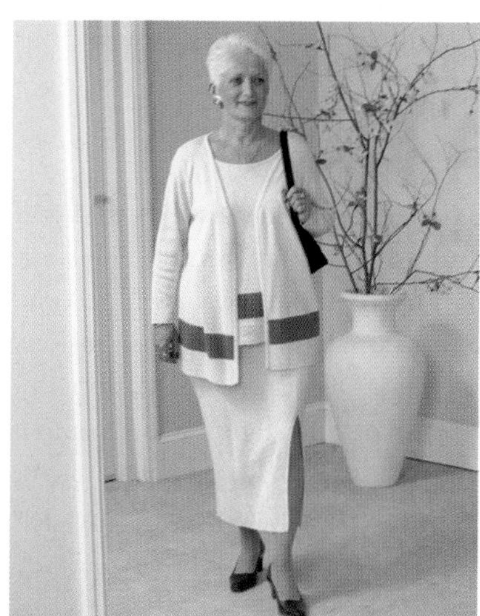

Figure 4-5 A "classic" look.

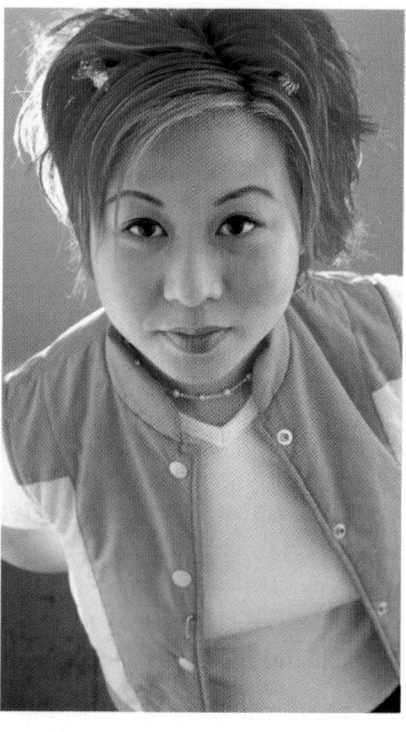

Figure 4-6 A "dramatic" look.

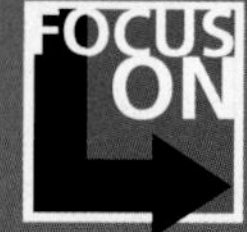

Focus on . . . Understanding the Total Look Concept

While the enhancement of your client's image should always be your primary concern, it is important to remember that the nails, skin, and hair adorn the body and are reflective of an entire lifestyle. How can you help a client make choices that reflect a personal sense of style? Start the process by doing a little research. Look for books or articles that describe different fashion styles, and become familiar with them. This exercise is useful for developing a profile of the broad fashion categories that you can refer to when consulting with clients.

For example, a person may be categorized as having a "classic" style if simple and sophisticated clothing, monochromatic colors, and no bright patterns are preferred. A person who prefers classic styling in her clothing would likely want a simple, elegant, and sophisticated look with respect to her nails, makeup, and hair .

Someone who prefers a more dramatic look, on the other hand, will choose nail designs, hairstyles, clothing and accessories that demand greater attention and allow for more options. These clients are likely to be more willing to try a variety of new products and spend more time having additional services that will help achieve the desired look (Figures 4-5 and 4-6).

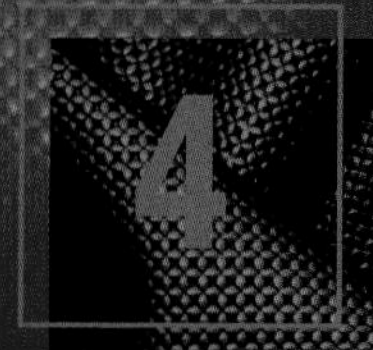

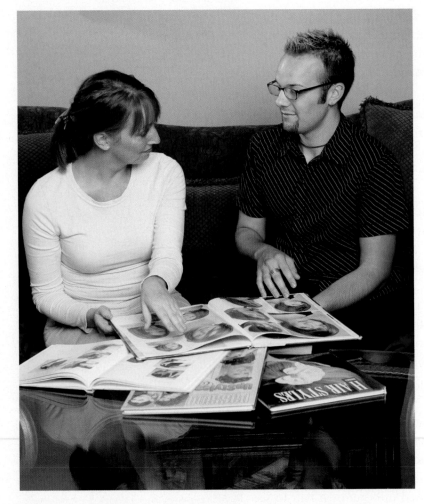

Figure 4-7 Use a photo collection to help confirm your client's choice.

reach a working level of communication on the subject of haircolor (Figure 4-7).

Many times, you will find yourself consulting with a client who asks for a specific cutting technique or color that she may have heard about from a friend or a previous stylist. You know that not every technique or color will work for everyone, and just because her friend was happy with the results does not mean that she will be. (Guess who will catch the blame?) In this situation, it may be the time to take her step-by-step through the process, explaining why a certain color is either right or wrong for her hair color, skin type, and lifestyle factors.

THE CONSULTATION AREA

Presentation counts for a lot in a business that is concerned with style and appearance. Once you have brought the client to your station to begin the consultation process, make sure she is comfortable. You and she are about to begin an important conversation that will clue you in to her needs and preferences. Your work area needs to be freshly cleaned and uncluttered. Have your photos, magazine clippings, and all other appropriate aids for the desired service available. You should read the intake form carefully, and refer to it often during the consultation process. Throughout the consultation, and especially once a course of action is decided on, make notes on the intake form. Record any formulations or products that you use and include any specific techniques you follow, or goals you are working toward, so that you can remember them for future visits.

10-STEP CONSULTATION METHOD

Every complete consultation needs to be structured in such a way that you cover all the key points that consistently lead to a successful conclusion. While this may seem like a lot of information to memorize, it will become second nature as you become more experienced and have many consultations under your belt. Depending on the service requested, the consultation will vary to some degree. For example, a full-head of high-lights will require a more detailed consultation than a haircut. To ensure that you always cover your bases, keep a list of the following 10 key points at your station for referral, and modify it as needed for the actual service.

1. **Review** the intake form that your client has filled out and feel free to make comments to break the ice and get the consultation going.

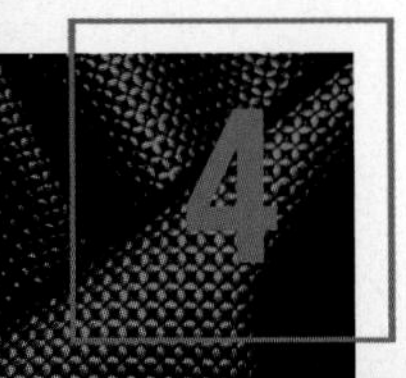

2. **Assess** your client's current style. Is it soft and unstructured? Carefully styled? Classic? Avant-garde? Is it in synch with her style of clothing and personal image?
3. **Preference.** Ask your client what she likes least and most about her current style. Is it too conservative? Does she love the fact that she only has to spend 10 minutes a day styling her hair? Was she happy with the style when it was first cut?
4. **Analyze.** Assess your client's thickness, texture, manageability, and condition. Is she particularly thin on top or at the temples? Check for strong hair growth patterns, including unruly cowlicks.
5. **Lifestyle.** Ask your client about her career and personal lifestyle.
   - Does she spend a great deal of time outdoors? Does she swim every day?
   - Is she a businesswoman? An artist? A stay-at-home mom?
   - Does she have a strong personal style that she wishes to project?
   - What are her styling habits? How often does she shampoo her hair?
   - How much time does she want to spend on her hair each day?
6. **Show and tell.** Encourage her to flip through your style books and point out styles, or even parts of styles, that she likes and why. This is a good time to get a real grasp on whether she not only understands, but accepts the limitations of her hair. Does she consistently point out thick, full hairstyles, for instance, when her own hair is quite thin? Is her hair curly, yet she consistently chooses smooth styles?

   In addition, listen to how she describes hair length. If she says she wants her hair short, for instance, does she mean up to her shoulders? Her ears? One-inch all over her head? When her bangs are dry, does she want them to still touch her eyebrows? Reiterating what she tells you using specific terms like "chin length" or "resting on the shoulders"—as opposed to short or long—and reinforcing your words both with pictures and your hands by pointing to where the hair would fall, are critical to having a clear understanding of what both of you are really saying.

   Listening to the client and then repeating, in your own words, what you think the client is telling you is known as **reflective listening.** Mastering this listening skill will help you to always be on target with your services, and to build a deep trust with your clients.
7. **Suggest.** Once you have enough information to make valid style suggestions, narrow your selections based on the following:
   - Lifestyle. The styles you choose must fit her styling parameters (time and effort), and meet her needs for business, personal, or both.
   - Hair type. You must base your recommendations on whether your client has (a) thick, medium, or thin hair; (b) fine, medium, or coarse hair; and (b) straight, wavy, curly, or extremely curly hair.
   - Face and body. Point out hairstyles that would look good with her face shape. Is she narrow across the temple area? If she is, you

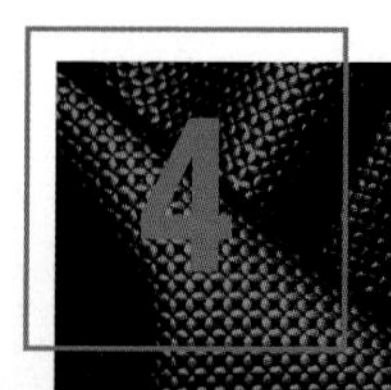

should suggest styles that add a little fullness in this area. If she has a noticeably small head, then a hairstyle that closely hugs her scalp would not be the best choice.

When making suggestions, qualify them by referencing the above parameters. For example: "I think this hairstyle would work well with the texture of your hair." Tactfully discuss any unreasonable expectations that she may have shared with you by picking out photos that are unrealistic based on her hair and personal needs. If her hair is damaged, you need to address intensive hair treatments, better home-care products, lifestyle changes, and the need to trim off damaged ends.

Never hesitate to suggest additional services to make her new haircut complete or better in some way. In addition to color, this could be a texture service for added movement or body, a relaxing to tame her curls, a makeup lesson to complement her new style, and so on.

8. **Color.** Unless she absolutely does not want to talk about color, color recommendations should be part of every consultation service. Everyone can use a glossing treatment, have their hair color enriched, or add some highlights or low lights to make their hair (and your work) even more attractive.

   Ask if she has colored her hair in the past. If she already has haircolor, find out how long it has been since it was last applied. Has she had color challenges in the past? Does she color her hair at home? Would she like to make a subtle or dramatic hair color change?

   When talking about color, be very careful to make sure you are both speaking the same language. Hairstylists are accustomed to the technical side of color and tend to use terms like "multidimensional highlighting," or "no-ammonia semi-permanent tint." This can be very confusing and misleading to clients. Make sure you explain yourself every step of the way, and use pictures whenever possible.

   Another thing you have to be very careful about is not taking clients literally when they say things like, "I want to be blond," or "I want to have red hair." Blond to a stylist may be Gwen Stefani platinum, while blond to a client may mean a few thin streaks of medium blond around the hair line. Red is also a sensitive subject. You may be dreaming of turning her conservative brown hair into a screaming blue-red work of art, and she may be envisioning brown with just a hint of red. Be careful and let pictures be your guide. Take hair swatches and twist them with the client's own hair strands so she can see the contrast.

9. **Upkeep.** Counsel every client on the salon maintenance, lifestyle limitations (blond hair and chlorine, for instance, are not a good match), and home maintenance that she will need to commit to in order to look her best.

10. **Repeat.** Reiterate everything that you have agreed upon. Make sure to speak in measured precise terms, and use visual tools to demonstrate

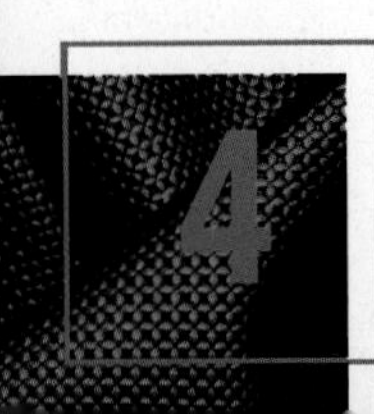

the end result. This is the most critical step of the consultation process because it determines the ultimate service(s). Take your time and be thorough.

CONCLUDING THE SERVICE

Once the service is finished and the client has let you know whether she is satisfied, take a few more minutes to record the results on the record card. Ask for her reactions and record them. Note anything you did that you might want to do again, as well as anything that does not bear repeating. Also, make note of the final results and any retail products that you recommended. Be sure to date your notes and file them in the proper place.

SPECIAL ISSUES IN COMMUNICATION

Although you may do everything in your power to communicate effectively, you will sometimes encounter situations that are beyond your control. The solution is not to try to control the circumstances, but to communicate past the issue. Your reactions to situations, and your ability to communicate in the face of problems, are critical to being successful in a "people" profession such as the beauty industry.

HANDLING TARDY CLIENTS

Tardy clients are a fact of life in every service industry. Because beauty professionals are so dependent on appointments and scheduling to maximize working hours, a client who is very late for an appointment, or one who is habitually late, can cause problems. One tardy client can make you late for every other client you service that day, and the pressure involved in making up for lost time can take its toll. You also risk inconveniencing the rest of your clients who are prompt for their appointments.

Here are a few guidelines for handling late clients.

- Know and abide by the salon's tardy or late policy. Many salons set a limited amount of time they allow a client to be late before they require them to reschedule. Generally, if clients are more than 15 minutes late, they should be asked to reschedule. Most will accept responsibility and be understanding about the rule, but you may come across a few clients who insist on being serviced immediately. Explain that you have other appointments and are responsible to those clients as well. Also explain that rushing through the service is unacceptable to both of you.
- If your tardy client arrives and you have the time to take her without jeopardizing other clients' appointments, let your client know why you are taking her even though she is late. You can deliver this information and still remain pleasant and upbeat. Say, "Oh, Ms. Lee, we're in luck!

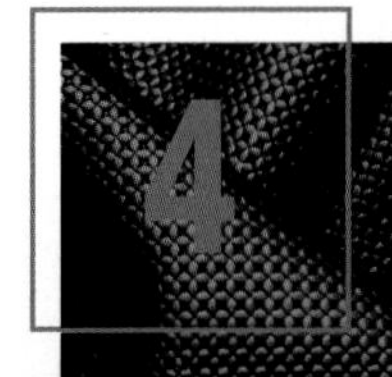

Even though you're a bit late, I can still take you because my next appointment isn't for two hours. Isn't it great that it worked out?" This lets her know that being late is not acceptable under normal circumstances, but that if you can accommodate her, you will.

- As you get to know your clients, you will learn who is habitually late. You may want to schedule such clients for the last appointment of the day or ask them to arrive earlier than their actual appointments. In other words, if a client is always 30 minutes late, schedule her for 2:30 but tell her to arrive at 2:00!

Imagine this scenario. In spite of your best efforts, you are running late. You realize that no matter what has happened in the salon that day, your clients want and deserve your promptness. If you have your clients' telephone numbers, call them and let them know about the delays. Give them the opportunity to reschedule, or to come a little later than their scheduled appointments. If you cannot reach them beforehand, be sure to approach them when they come into the salon and let them know that you are delayed. Tell them how long you think the wait will be, and give them the option of changing their appointment. Apologize for the inconvenience and show a little extra attention by personally offering them a beverage. Even if these clients are not happy about the delay, or they need to change their appointment, at least they will feel informed and respected.

HANDLING SCHEDULING MIX-UPS

We are all human, and we all make mistakes. Chances are you have gone to an appointment on a certain day, at a certain time, only to discover that you are in the wrong place, at the wrong time. The way you are treated at that moment will determine if you ever patronize that business again. The number-one thing to remember when you, as a professional, get involved with a scheduling mix-up is to be polite and never argue about who is correct. Being right may sound good, but this kind of situation is not about being right; it is about preserving your relationship with your client. If you handle the matter poorly, you run the risk of never seeing that client again.

Even if you know for sure that she is mistaken, tell yourself that the client is always right. Assume the blame if it helps keep her happy. *Do not, under any circumstances, argue the point with the client.*

Once you have the chance to consult your appointment book, you can say, "Oh, Mrs. Montez, I have you in my appointment book for 10:00, and unfortunately I have already scheduled other clients for 11:00 and 12:00. I'm so sorry about the mix-up. Can I reschedule you for tomorrow at 10:00?" Even though the client may be fuming, you need to stay disengaged. Your focus is to move the conversation away from who is at fault, and squarely in the direction of resolving the confusion. Make another appointment for the client and be sure to get her telephone number so that you can call and confirm the details of the appointment in advance (Figure 4-8).

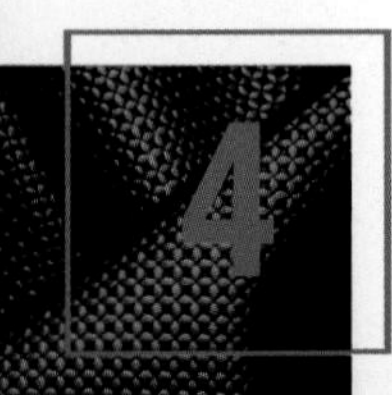

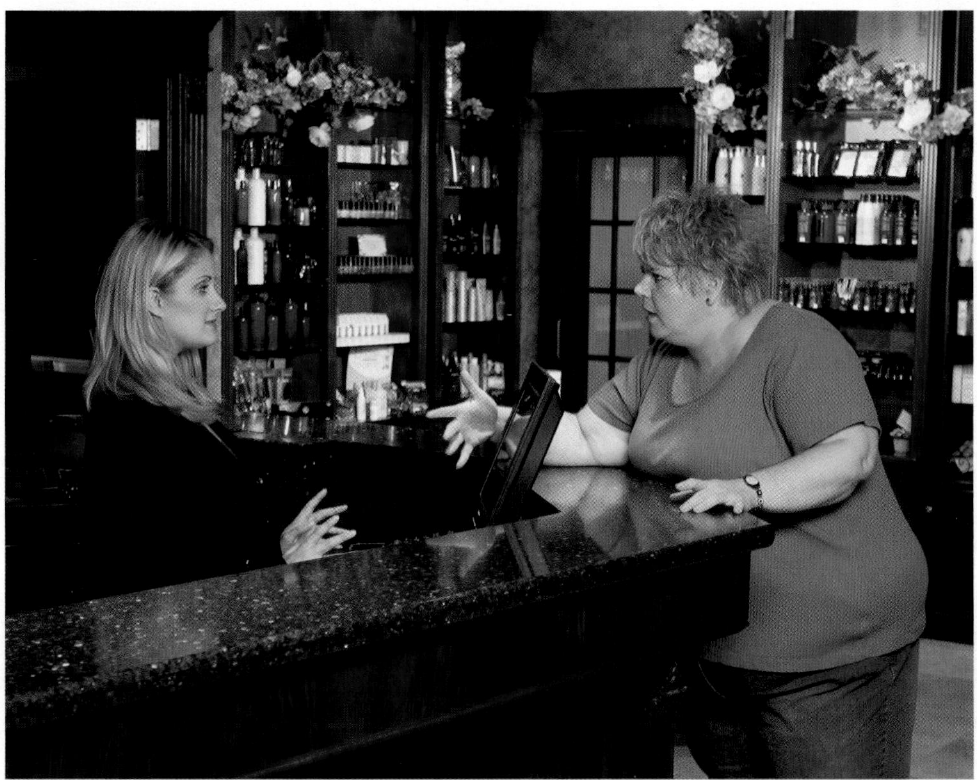

Figure 4–8 Accommodate an unhappy client promptly and calmly.

HANDLING UNHAPPY CLIENTS

No matter how hard you try to provide excellent service to your clients, once in a while you will encounter a client who is dissatisfied with the service. The way you and the salon handle this difficult situation will have lasting effects on you, the client, and the salon, so you need to know how best to proceed.

Once again, it is important to remember the ultimate goal: make the client happy enough to pay for the service and return for more of the same.

Here are some guidelines to follow.

- Try to find out why the client is unhappy. Ask for specifics. If she has a difficult time expressing herself, break the service down for her piece by piece until you determine exactly what has caused the dissatisfaction.
- If it is possible to change what she dislikes, do so immediately. If that is not possible, look at your schedule to see how soon you can do it. You may need to enlist the help of the receptionist in rescheduling your other appointments. If the client seems open to the suggestion, ask her to return to the salon at a time when you are free. If this is not possible, explain that you will begin her service, but will need to take your next client and will be relying on help from another practitioner. Do whatever you have to do to make her happy, and explain along the way who will be working with her and what the other practitioner will be doing.

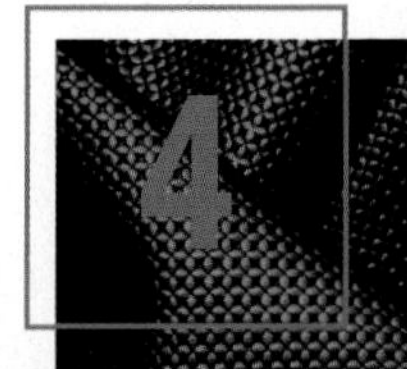

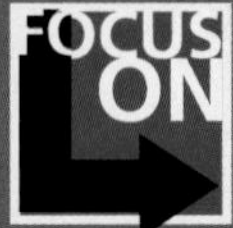

Focus on . . . Communication

At some point in your career you will no doubt have a disgruntled client who is unhappy about something that was done either during the service or in scheduling. No matter how well you communicate, handling a situation like this can be difficult. The best way to prepare is to practice. Role-play with a classmate, taking turns being the client and the practitioner. Role playing both sides of the issue will give you a better understanding of the entire situation.

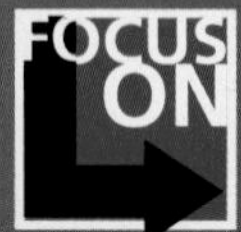

Focus on . . . Professionalism

A long-time client reveals to you one day that she and her husband are going through a messy divorce. You care for her and try to be understanding as she reveals increasingly personal details. Other practitioners and their clients are soon listening to every word of this conversation. You want to be helpful and supportive, but this is not the right time or place. What can you do?

Try this: Tell her you understand the situation is very difficult, but while she is in the salon, you want to do everything in your power to give her a break from it. Let her know that while she is in your care, you should both concentrate on her enjoyment of the services and not on the things that are stressing her.

She will appreciate the suggestion, and you will have put her back on the track of her real reason for coming to see you.

- If you cannot change what the client does not like, or it is simply impossible to change, you must honestly and tactfully explain the reason why you cannot make any changes. The client will not be happy, but you can offer any options that may be available.
- Again, never argue with the client or try to force your opinion. Unless you can change what has caused the dissatisfaction, this will just fuel the fire.
- Do not hesitate to call on a more experienced stylist or your salon manager for help. They have encountered a similar situation at some point in their careers and have insights that can help you.
- If, after you have tried everything, you are unable to satisfy the client, defer to your manager's advice on how to proceed. The client may be too upset to handle the situation maturely, and it may be easier for her to deal with someone else. This does not mean that you have failed; it simply means that another approach is needed.
- Confer with your salon manager after the experience. A good manager will not hold the event against you, but view it instead as an inevitable fact of life from which you can learn. Follow your manager's advice and move on to your next client. Use whatever you may have learned from the experience to perform future client consultations and services better.

GETTING TOO PERSONAL

Sometimes when a client forms a bond of trust with her stylist she may have a hard time differentiating between a professional and a personal relationship. That will be *her* problem, but you must not make it *your* problem. Your job is to handle your client relationships tactfully and sensitively. You cannot become your clients' counselor, career guide, parental sounding board, or motivational coach. Your job and your relationship with your clients are very specific: the goal is to advise and service clients with their beauty needs, and nothing more.

IN-SALON COMMUNICATION

Behaving in a professional manner is the first step in making this meaningful communication possible. Unfortunately, many beauty professionals act immaturely and get overly involved in the salon rumor mill.

The salon community is usually a close-knit one in which people spend long hours working side by side. For this reason, it is important to maintain boundaries around what you will and will not do or say at the salon. Remember, the salon is your place of business and, as such, must be treated respectfully and carefully.

COMMUNICATING WITH CO-WORKERS

As with all communication, there are basic principles that must guide your interactions. In a work environment, you will not have the opportunity to handpick your colleagues. There will always be people you like or relate to better than others, and people whose behaviors or opinions you find yourself in conflict with. These people can try your patience and your nerves, but they are your colleagues and are deserving of your respect.

Here are some guidelines to keep in mind as you interact and communicate with fellow staffers.

Treat everyone with respect. Regardless of whether you like someone, your colleagues are professionals who service clients who bring revenue into the salon. And, as practicing professionals, they have information they can offer you. Look at these people as having something to teach you, and hone in on their talents and their techniques.

Remain objective. Different types of personalities working side by side over long and intense hours are likely to breed some degree of dissension and disagreement. In order to learn and grow, you must make every effort to remain objective and resist being pulled into spats and cliques. When one or two people in the salon behave disrespectfully toward one another, the entire team suffers because the atmosphere changes. Not only will this be unpleasant for you, but it will also be felt by the clients who may decide to take their business elsewhere if they find the atmosphere in your salon too tense.

Be honest and be sensitive. Many people use the excuse of being honest as a license to say anything to anyone. While honesty is always the best policy, using unkind words or actions with regard to your colleagues is never a good idea. Be sensitive. Put yourself in the other person's place and think through what you want to say before you say it. That way, any negative or hurtful words can be suppressed.

Remain neutral. Undoubtedly, there will come a time when you are called on to make a statement or to "pick a side." Do whatever you can to avoid getting drawn into the conflict. If you have a problem with a colleague, the best way to resolve it is to speak with her or him directly and privately.

Speaking to, or gossiping with, others about someone never resolves a problem. It only makes it worse, and is often as damaging to you as it is to the object of your gossip.

Seek help from someone you respect. If you find yourself in a position where you are at odds with a co-worker, you may want to seek out a third party—someone who is not involved and who can remain objective—such as the manager or a more experienced practitioner. Ask for advice about how to proceed and really listen to what this mentor has to say. Since this person is not involved, he or she is more likely to see the situation as it truly is and can offer you valuable insights.

Do not take things personally. This is often easier said than done. How many times have you had a bad day, or been thinking about something totally unrelated, when a person asks you what's wrong, or wonders if you are mad at them? Just because someone is behaving in a certain

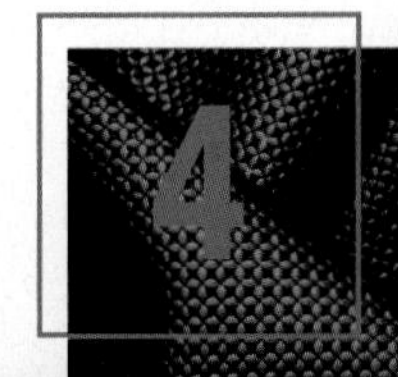

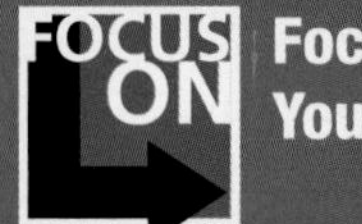

Focus on . . . Your Skills

Too much time spent on your personal life means time away from the task of perfecting your skills and artistry, and building up the business for yourself and the salon.

manner and you happen to be there, do not interpret the words or behaviors as being meant for you. If you are confused or concerned by someone's actions, find a quiet and private place to ask the person about it. The person may not even realize she was giving off any signals.

Keep your private life private. There is a time and a place for everything, but the salon is never the place to discuss your personal life and relationships. It may be tempting to engage in that kind of conversation, especially if others in the salon are doing so, and to solicit advice and opinions, but that is why you have friends. Co-workers can become friends, but those whom you selectively turn into friends are different from the ones whose chairs happen to be next to yours.

COMMUNICATING WITH MANAGERS

Another very important relationship for you within the salon is the one you will build with your manager. The salon manager is generally the person who has the most responsibility for how the salon is run in terms of daily maintenance and operations and client service. The manager's job is a very demanding one. Often, in addition to running a hectic salon, she also has a clientele that she personally services.

Your manager is likely to be the one who hired you and is responsible for your training and for how well you move into the salon culture. Therefore, your manager has a vested interest in your success. As a salon employee, you will see the manager as a powerful and influential person, but it is also important to remember that she is a human being. She isn't perfect, and she will not be able to do everything you think should be done in every instance. Whether she personally likes you or not, her job is to look beyond her personal feelings and make decisions that are best for the salon as a whole. The best thing you can do is to try to understand the decisions and rules that she makes whether you agree with them or not.

Many salon professionals utilize their salon managers in inappropriate ways by asking them to solve personal issues between staff members.

Inexperienced managers, hoping to keep everything flowing smoothly, may make the mistake of getting involved in petty issues. You and your manager must both understand that her job is to make sure the business is running smoothly, not to baby-sit temperamental practitioners.

Here are some guidelines for interacting and communicating with your salon manager.

Be a problem solver. When you need to speak with your manager about some issue or problem, think of some possible solutions beforehand. This will indicate that you are working in the salon's best interest and are trying to help, not make things worse.

Get your facts straight. Make sure that all your facts and information are accurate before you speak to your salon manager. This way you will avoid wasting time solving a "problem" that really does not exist.

Be open and honest. When you find yourself in a situation you do not understand or do not have the experience to deal with, tell your salon manager immediately and be willing to learn.

Do not gossip or complain about colleagues. Going to your manager with gossip or to "tattle" on a co-worker tells your manager that you are a troublemaker. If you are having a legitimate problem with someone and have tried everything in your power to handle the problem yourself, then it is appropriate to go to your manager. But you must approach her with a true desire to solve the problem, not just to vent.

Check your attitude. The salon environment, although fun and friendly, can also be stressful, so it is important to take a moment between clients to "take your temperature." Ask yourself how you are feeling. Do you need an attitude adjustment? Be honest with yourself.

Be open to constructive criticism. It is never easy to hear that you need improvement in any area, but keep in mind that part of your manager's job is to help you achieve your professional goals. She is supposed to evaluate your skills and offer suggestions on how to increase them. Keep an open mind and do not take her criticism personally.

COMMUNICATING DURING AN EMPLOYEE EVALUATION

Salons that are well run will make it a priority to conduct frequent and thorough employee evaluations. Sometime in the course of your first few days of work, your salon manager will tell you when you can expect your first evaluation. If she does not mention it, you might ask her about it and request a copy of the form she will use or the criteria on which you will be evaluated.

Take some time to look over this document. Be mindful that the behaviors and/or activities most important to the salon are likely to be the ones on which you will be evaluated. This is very useful information. You can begin to watch and rate yourself in the weeks and months ahead so you can assess how you are doing. Remember, everything you are being evaluated on is there for the purpose of helping you improve. Make the decision to approach these communications positively. As the time draws near for the evaluation, try filling out the form yourself. In other words, give yourself an evaluation, even if the salon has not asked you to do so. Be objective, and carefully think out your comments. Then, when you meet with the manager, show her your evaluation and tell her you are serious about your improvement and growth. She will appreciate your input and your desire. And, if you are being honest with yourself, there should be no surprises (Figure 4-9).

Before your evaluation meeting, write down any thoughts or questions you may have so you can share them with your manager. Do not be shy. If you want to know when you can take on more services, when your pay scale will be increased, or when you might be considered for promotion, this meeting is the appropriate time and place to ask. Many beauty professionals never take advantage of this crucial communication opportunity to discuss their future because they are too nervous, intimidated, or unprepared. Do not let that happen to you. Participate proactively in your career and in your success by communicating your desires and interests.

At the end of the meeting, thank your manager for taking the time to do an evaluation and for the feedback and guidance she has given you.

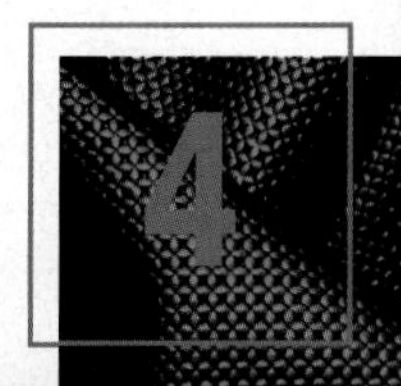

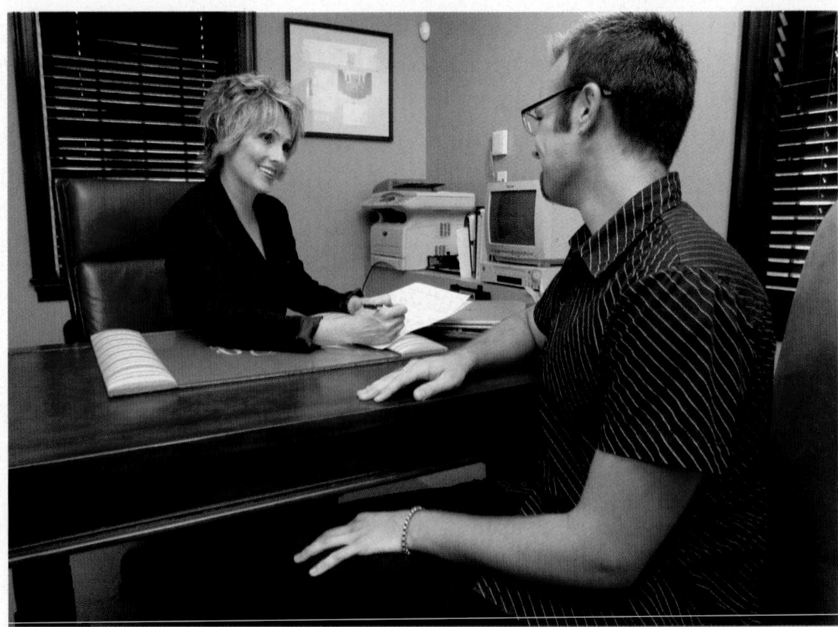

Figure 4–9 Your employee evaluation is a good time to discuss your progress with your manager.

REVIEW QUESTIONS

1. List the golden rules of human relations.
2. Define "communication."
3. How should you prepare for a client consultation?
4. What is the "total look" concept?
5. List and describe the 10 elements of a successful client consultation.
6. Name some types of information that should go on a client consultation card.
7. How should you handle tardy clients?
8. How should you handle a scheduling mix-up?
9. How should you handle an unhappy client?
10. List at least five things to remember when communicating with your co-workers.
11. List at least four guidelines for communicating with salon managers.

CHAPTER GLOSSARY

client consultation	Verbal communication with a client to determine desired results.
communication	The act of accurately sharing information between two people, or groups of people.
reflective listening	Listening to the client and then repeating, in your own words, what you think the client is telling you.

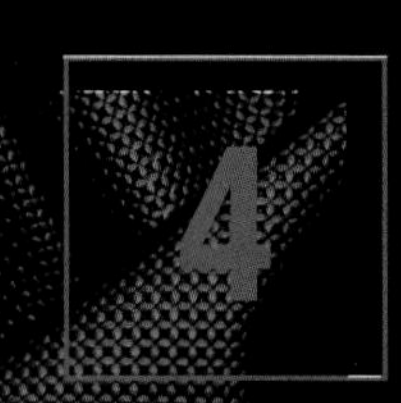

GENERAL SCIENCES

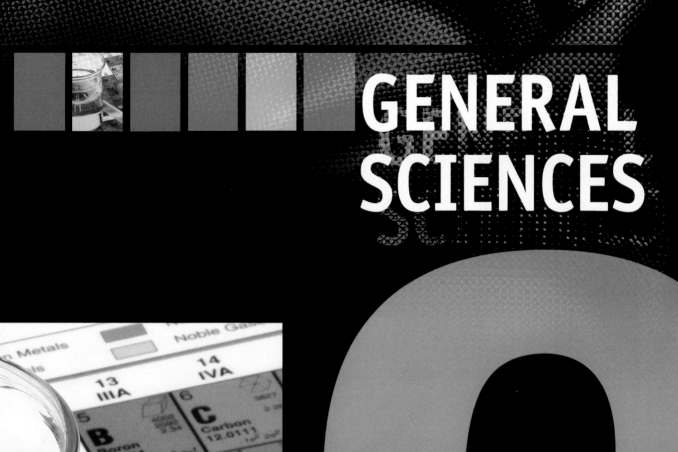

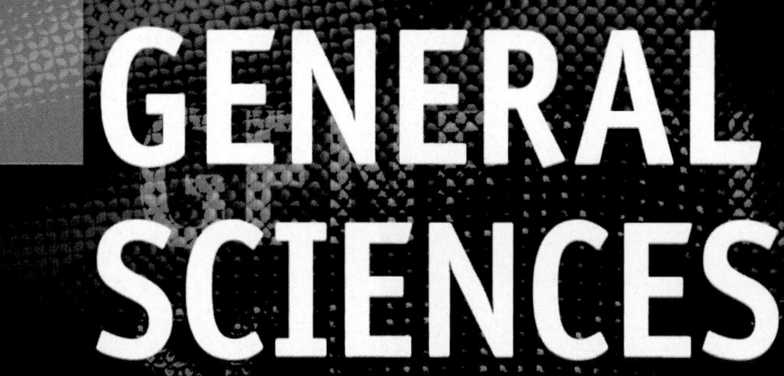

PART 2

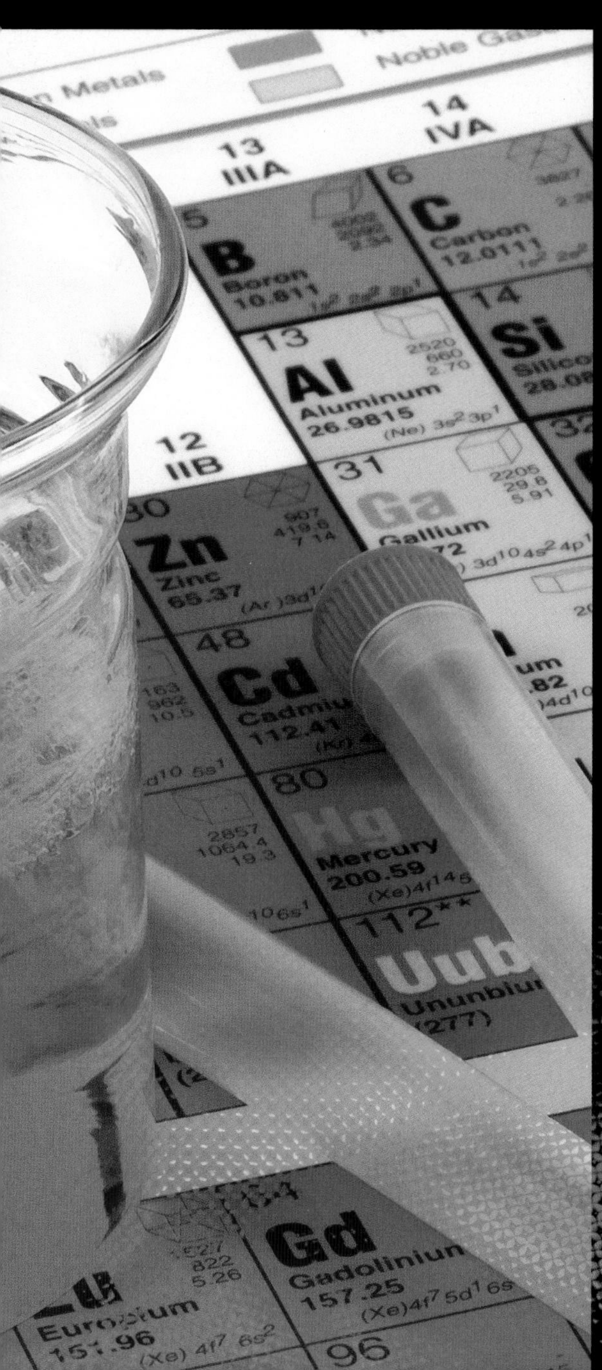

5 CHAPTER INFECTION CONTROL PRINCIPLES & PRACTICES

chapter outline

- Regulation
- Principles of Infection
- Principles of Prevention
- Disinfection Procedures
- Universal Precautions
- The Professional Salon Image

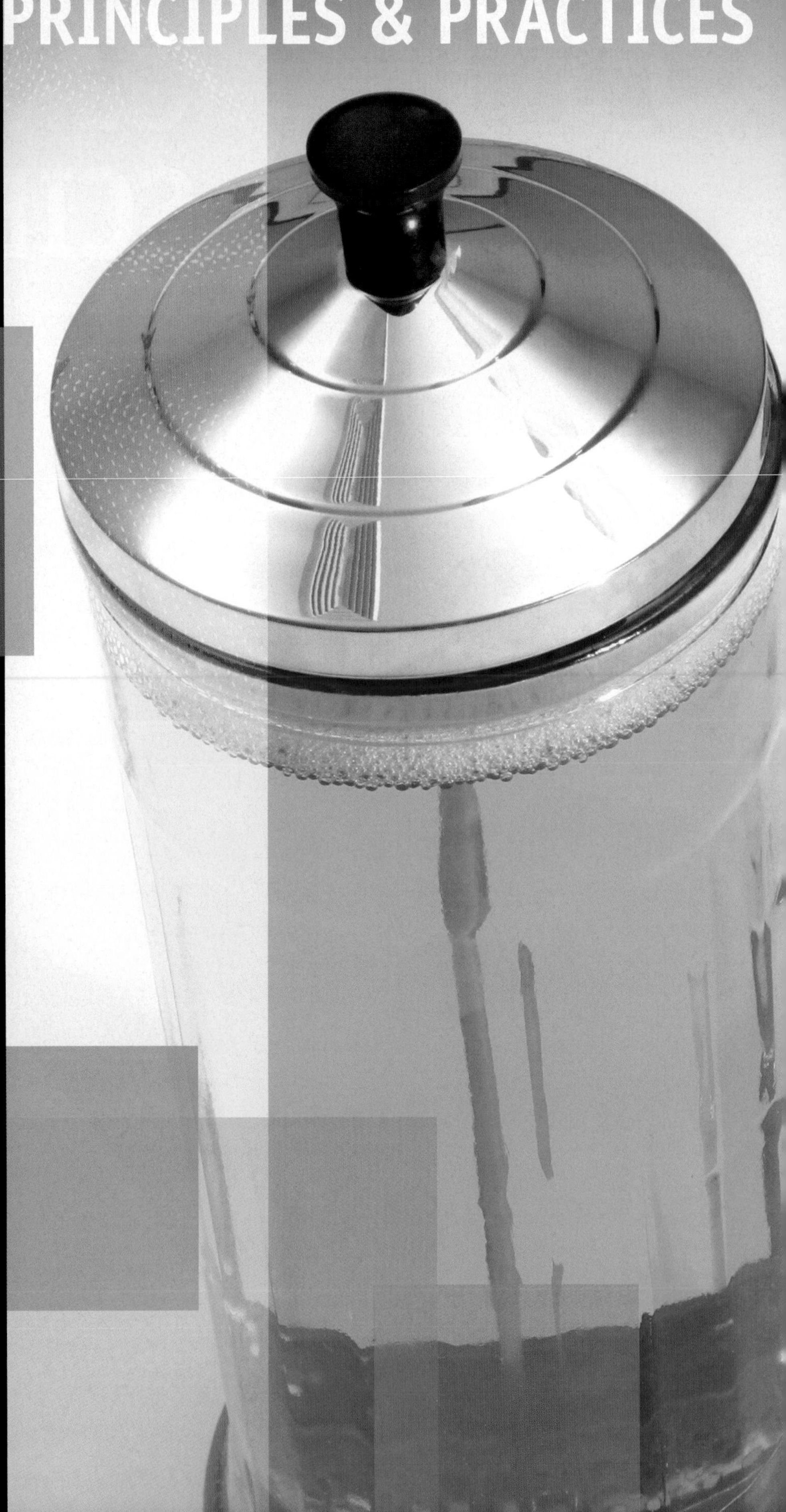

Learning Objectives

After completing this chapter, you will be able to:

- **Understand state laws and rules.**
- **List the types and classifications of bacteria.**
- **List the types of disinfectants and how they are used.**
- **Define hepatitis and HIV, and explain how they are transmitted.**
- **Describe how to safely clean and disinfect salon tools and equipment.**
- **Explain the differences between cleaning, disinfection and sterilization.**
- **Discuss Universal Precautions and your responsibilities as a salon professional.**

Key Terms

Page number indicates where in the chapter the term is used.

AIDS **pg. 65**
allergy **pg. 63**
antiseptics **pg. 77**
bacilli (singular: bacillus) **pg. 61**
bacteria **pg. 60**
bactericidal **pg. 60**
bloodborne pathogens **pg. 65**
cilia **pg. 61**
cocci **pg. 61**
contagious **pg. 64**
diagnosis **pg. 63**
diplococci **pg. 61**
disease **pg. 63**
disinfectable **pg. 71**
disinfectants **pg. 67**
disinfection **pg. 67**
efficacy **pg. 68**
exposure incident **pg. 79**
flagella (singular: flagellum) **pg. 61**
fungi **pg. 66**
fungicidal **pg. 60**
hepatitis **pg. 64**
HIV **pg. 65**
immunity **pg. 66**
infection **pg. 63**
infectious **pg. 62**
inflammation **pg. 63**
microorganism **pg. 62**
mildews **pg. 66**
motility **pg. 61**
Material Data Safety Sheet (MSDS) **pg. 56**
multi-use **pg. 71**
nonpathogenic **pg. 60**
occupational disease **pg. 63**
parasites **pg. 66**
pathogenic **pg. 60**
pediculosis capitis **pg. 66**
phenolics **pg. 69**
porous **pg. 71**
quaternary ammonium compounds (quats) **pg. 69**
sanitation or sanitizing **pg. 67**
scabies **pg. 66**
single-use or disposable **pg. 71**
sodium hypochlorite **pg. 70**
spirilla **pg. 61**
staphylococci **pg. 61**
sterilization **pg. 67**
streptococci **pg. 61**
tuberculocidal **pg. 59**
Universal Precautions **pg. 79**
virucidal **pg. 60**
virus **pg. 64**

EDITOR'S NOTE: Please notice that the words sanitation or sanitizing simply mean cleaning and that they may be used interchangeably throughout the chapter.

When reading this chapter, you may wonder if you are required to be part scientist or chemist to be a professional in the field of cosmetology. It is not important that you know the chemistry of the products that you use, or that you memorize medical terms, or that you know how to pronounce germs disinfectants will kill—what is important is that you know what to do and when to do it to keep clients safe. Understanding the basics of cleaning and disinfecting and following state rules will ensure that you have a long and successful career in the field of cosmetology.

REGULATION

Many different state and federal agencies regulate the practice of cosmetology. Federal agencies set guidelines for the manufacturing, sale, and use of equipment and chemical ingredients, and for safety in the workplace. State agencies regulate licensing, enforcement, and conduct when working in the salon.

FEDERAL AGENCIES

OSHA

The Occupational Safety and Health Administration (OSHA) was created as part of the U.S. Department of Labor to regulate and enforce safety and health standards to protect employees in the workplace. Regulating employee exposure to potentially toxic substances and informing employees about possible hazards of materials used in the workplace are key points of the Occupational Safety and Health Act of 1970. This regulation created the Hazard Communication Act, which requires that chemical manufacturers and importers assess the hazards associated with their products. Material Safety Data Sheets (MSDSs) are a result of this law.

The standards set by OSHA are important to the cosmetology industry because of the products used in salons. These standards address issues relating to handling, mixing, storing, and disposing of products, general safety in the workplace, and, most importantly, your right to know the hazardous ingredients in the products you use.

MATERIAL SAFETY DATA SHEET

Federal laws require that manufacturers supply a **Material Safety Data Sheet (MSDS)** for all products sold (Figure 5-1). MSDS sheets include information about hazardous ingredients, safe use and handling procedures, precautions to reduce the risk of harm and overexposure, flammability and data in case of a fire, proper disposal guidelines, and

Material Safety Data Sheet
May be used to comply with
OSHA's Hazard Communication Standard,
29 CFR 1910.1200. Standard must be
consulted for specific requirements.

U.S. Department of Labor
Occupational Safety and Health Administration
(Non-Mandatory Form)
Form Approved
OMB No. 1218-0072

IDENTITY *(As Used on Label and List)*	*Note: Blank spaces are not permitted. If any item is not applicable or no information is available, the space must be marked to indicate that.*

Section I

Manufacturer's Name	Emergency Telephone Number
Address *(Number, Street, City, State, and ZIP Code)*	Telephone Number for information
	Date Prepared
	Signature of Preparer *(optional)*

Section II — Hazardous Ingredients/Identity Information

Hazardous Components (Specific Chemical Identity; Common Names(s))	OSHA PEL	ACGIH TLV	Other Limits Recommended	% *(optional)*

Section III — Physical/Chemical Characteristics

Boiling Point		Specific Gravity (H_2O - 1)	
Vapor Pressure (mm Hg.)		Melting Point	
Vapor Density (Air - 1))		Evaporation Rate (Butyl Acetate - 1)	
Solubility in Water			
Appearance and Odor			

Section IV — Fire and Explosion Hazard Data

Flash Point (Method Used)	Flammable Limits	LEL	UEL
Extinguishing Media			
Special Fire Fighting Procedures			
Unusual Fire and Explosion Hazards			

(Reproduce locally) OSHA 174, Sept. 1985

Figure 5–1 Sample MSDS.

Continued

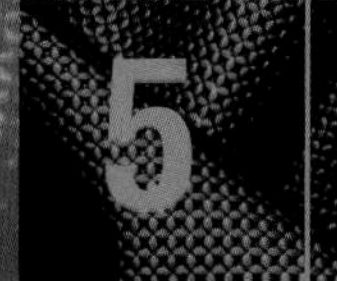

Material Safety Data Sheet (MSDS)

Section V — Reactivity Data

Stability	Unstable		Conditions to Avoid
	Stable		

Incompatibility (Materials to Avoid)

Hazardous Decomposition or Byproducts

Hazardous Polymerization	May Occur		Conditions to Avoid
	Will Not Occur		

Section VI — Health Hazard Data

Route(s) of Entry:	Inhalation?	Skin?	Ingestion?

Health Hazards *(Acute and Chronic)*

Carcenogenicity:	NTP?	IARC Monographs	OSHA Regulated?

Signs and Symptoms of Exposure

Medical Conditions
Generally Aggravated by Exposure

Emergency and First Aid Program

Section VII — Precautions for Safe Handling and Use

Steps to Be Taken in Case Material is Released or Spilled

Waste Disposal Method

Precautions to Be Taken in Handling and Storing

Other Precautions

Section VIII — Control Measures

Respiratory Protection (Specify Type)

Ventilation	Local Exhaust	Special
	Mechanical (General)	Other

Protective Gloves	Eye Protection

Other Protective Clothing or Equipment

Work/Hygienic Practices

Page 2

Figure 5-1 *(continued)*

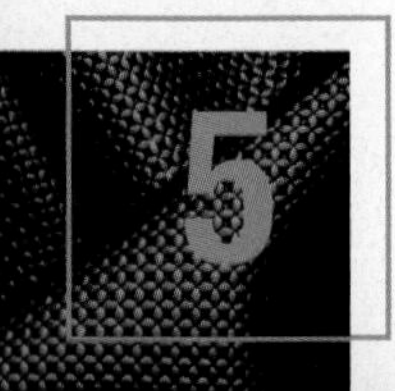

medical information should anyone have a reaction to the product. When necessary, the MSDS can be sent to a doctor, so that any reaction can be properly treated. OSHA and some state regulatory agencies require that MSDSs be kept available in the salon for all products that can cause harm. State inspectors can issue fines for the salon not having these available.

You can get MSDSs from the products' manufacturers, download them from the product manufacturer or distributor's website, or from distributors. Not having an MSDS poses a health risk to anyone in a salon who is exposed to hazardous materials and is a violation of federal regulations. Take the time to read all of this information to be certain that you are protecting yourself and your clients to the best of your ability.

ENVIRONMENTAL PROTECTION AGENCY (EPA)

The EPA licenses different types of disinfectants. The two types that are used in salons are hospital and tuberculocidal. Hospital products are safe for cleaning blood and body fluids in hospitals.

Tuberculocidal disinfectants are proven to kill the bacteria that causes tuberculosis, which is more difficult to kill (these products are also hospital products). This does not mean that you should use a tuberculocide; in fact, these products can be harmful to salon tools and equipment and they require special methods of disposal. Check the rules in your state to be sure that the product you choose complies with requirements.

It is against Federal Law to use any disinfecting product contrary to its labeling. This means that if you do not follow the instructions for mixing, contact time and the type of surface the disinfecting product can be used on, you have broken federal Law.

STATE REGULATORY AGENCIES

State regulatory agencies exist to protect the consumers' health, safety, and welfare while receiving services in the salon. These include licensing agencies, state boards of cosmetology, commissions, and health departments. They do this by requiring that everyone working in a salon or spa follow specific procedures. Enforcement of the rules through inspections and investigations of consumer complaints is also part of the agency's responsibility. The agency can issue penalties against both the salon owner and the operator's license ranging from warnings to fines, probation, and suspension or revocation of licenses. It is vital that you understand and follow the laws and rules in your state at all times – your license and your client's safety depend on it.

LAWS AND RULES—WHAT IS THE DIFFERENCE?

Laws are written by the legislature to determine the scope of practice (what each license allows the holder to do) and establish guidelines for regulatory agencies to make rules. *Laws* are also called *statutes. Rules* (also called *regulations*) are more specific than laws. Rules are written by the regulatory agency or board and determine how the law will be applied. Rules establish specific standards of conduct, and can be changed and updated.

Did You Know

A single practitioner can put many of her clients at risk if she does not practice stringent cleaning and disinfection guidelines. A case in point was the spread of a bacterium called *Mycobacterium fortuitum furunculosis* (MY-koh-bak-TIR-ee-um for-TOO-i-tum fur-UNK-yoo-LOH-sis), a microorganism that normally exists in tap water, and in small numbers is completely harmless. In 2000, over 100 clients of a California salon developed serious skin infections on their legs after receiving pedicures. The infection caused stubborn ugly sores that lingered for months, required the use of strong antibiotics, and, in some cases, caused scarring. The source of the infection was traced to the salon's whirlpool foot spas. Salon staff did not clean the foot spas properly, resulting in a build-up of hair and debris in the spas, which in turn created the perfect breeding ground for bacteria.

The outbreak was a catalyst for change in the industry. For instance, the California state government issued specific requirements for pedicure equipment aimed at preventing future outbreaks. In spite of these efforts in California and elsewhere, other outbreaks affecting hundreds of women have occurred since 2000; in 2006 alone, several deaths (and several lengthy hospital stays) resulting from pedicures were documented. Such developments have led to increased oversight measures by state agencies (and salon owners) as well as more stringent cleaning instructions and warnings by pedicure equipment manufacturers.

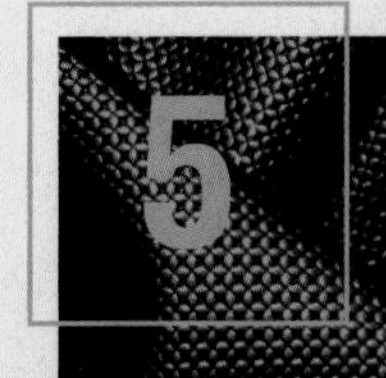

PRINCIPLES OF INFECTION

Being a salon professional is fun and rewarding, but it is also a great responsibility. One careless action could cause injury or infection, and you can lose your license to practice. Fortunately, preventing the spread of infections is easy if you know what to do and you practice what you have learned at all times. Safety begins and ends with YOU (Figure 5-2).

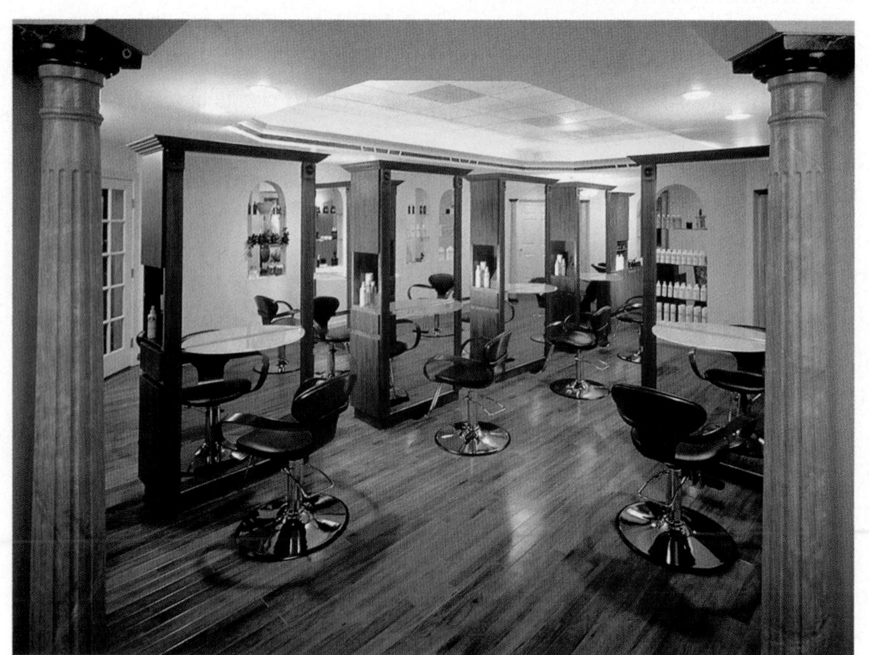

Figure 5-2 A sparkling clean salon gains your clients' confidence.

INFECTION CONTROL

There are three types of potentially infectious microorganisms that are important in the practice of cosmetology. These are bacteria, fungus, and virus. Remember, we are not seeking to treat any disease or condition, we are taking steps so that the tools and equipment we use are safe to use on clients. These steps are designed to prevent infection or disease. Disinfectants used in salons must be **bactericidal** (back-teer-uh-SYD-ul), **fungicidal** (fun-jih-SYD-ul), and **virucidal** (vy-rus-SYD-ul), meaning that when these are mixed and used according to the instructions on the label, these will kill potentially infectious bacteria, fungi and viruses.

Dirty salon tools and equipment may spread infections from client to client. You have an obligation to provide safe services and prevent consumers from harm by practicing safely. If they are infected or harmed because you did not correctly perform the services, you may be found legally responsible for their injury, infection, etc.

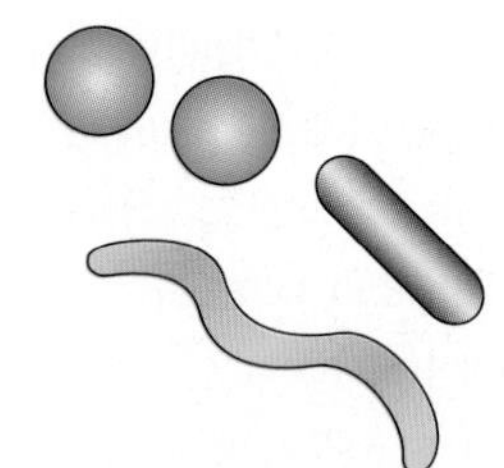

Figure 5-3 Some general forms of bacteria.

BACTERIA

Bacteria are one-celled microorganisms (my-kroh-OR-gah-niz-ums) with both plant and animal characteristics. Bacteria can exist almost anywhere: skin, water, air, decayed matter, body secretions, clothing, and under the free edge of fingernails. Bacteria are so small they can only be seen with a microscope. In fact, 1,500 rod-shaped bacteria will fit comfortably on the head of a pin!

TYPES OF BACTERIA

There are of thousands of (Figure 5-3) different kinds of bacteria that fall into two primary types—pathogenic and nonpathogenic. Most bacteria are **nonpathogenic** (completely harmless; do not cause disease). They can perform many useful functions. In the human body, nonpathogenic bacteria help the body break down food, protect against infection, and stimulate the immune system. **Pathogenic** (path-uh-JEN-ik) bacteria are

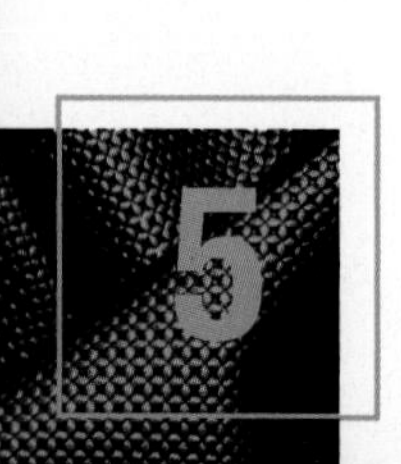

considered harmful because they may cause disease or infection when they invade the body. Preventing the spread of pathogenic microorganisms is why salons and schools must maintain sanitary standards. Tables 5-1 and 5-2 presents terms and definitions related to pathogens.

Classifications of Pathogenic Bacteria

Bacteria have distinct shapes that help to identify them. Pathogenic bacteria are classified as follows:

1. **Cocci** (KOK-sy) are round-shaped bacteria that appear singly (alone) or in the following groups (Figure 5-4).
   - **Staphylococci** (staf-uh-loh-KOK-sy)—Pus-forming bacteria that grow in clusters like a bunch of grapes. They cause abscesses, pustules, and boils (Figure 5-5).
   - **Streptococci** (strep-toh-KOK-eye)—Pus-forming bacteria arranged in curved lines resembling a string of beads. They cause infections such as strep throat and blood poisoning (Figure 5-6).
   - **Diplococci** (dip-lo-KOK-sy)—Spherical bacteria that grow in pairs and cause diseases such as pneumonia (Figure 5-7).
2. **Bacilli** (bah-SIL-ee) are short rod-shaped bacteria. They are the most common bacteria and produce diseases such as tetanus (lock-jaw), typhoid fever, tuberculosis, and diphtheria (Figure 5-8).
3. **Spirilla** (spy-RIL-ah) are spiral or corkscrew-shaped bacteria. They are subdivided into subgroups, such as *Treponema papillida,* which causes syphilis, a sexually transmitted disease (STD) or *Borrelia burgdorferi,* which causes Lyme disease (Figure 5-9).

MOVEMENT OF BACTERIA

Different bacteria move in different ways. Cocci rarely show active **motility** (self-movement). They are transmitted in the air, in dust, or within the substance in which they settle. Bacilli and spirilla are both motile and use slender, hairlike extensions, known as **flagella** (flu-JEL-uh; singular: flagellum) or **cilia** (SIL-ee-uh), for locomotion (moving about). A whiplike motion of these hairs moves the bacteria in liquid (Figure 5-10).

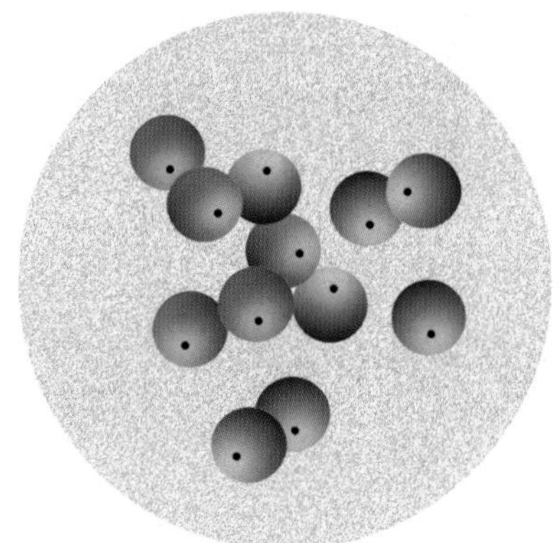

Figure 5-4 Cocci.

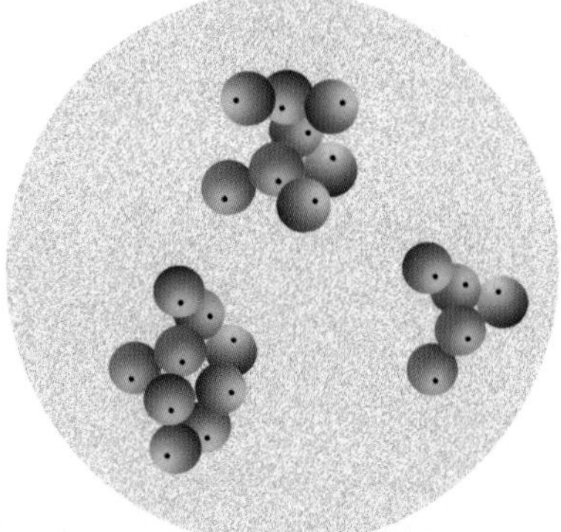

Figure 5-5 Staphylococci.

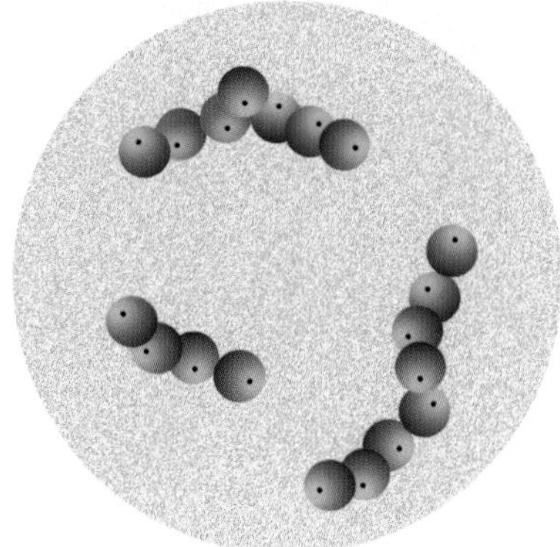

Figure 5-6 Streptococci.

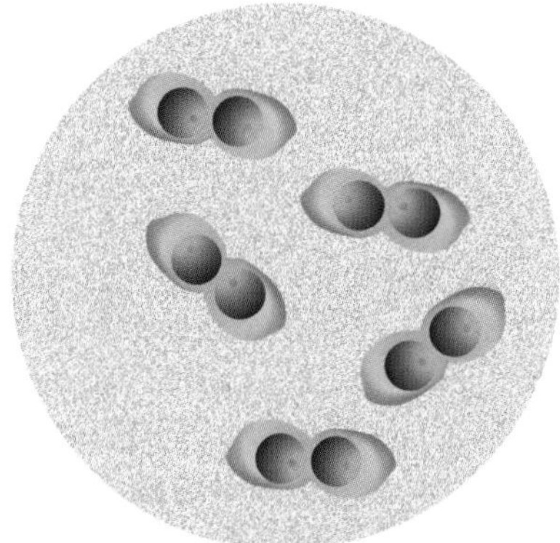

Figure 5-7 Diplococci.

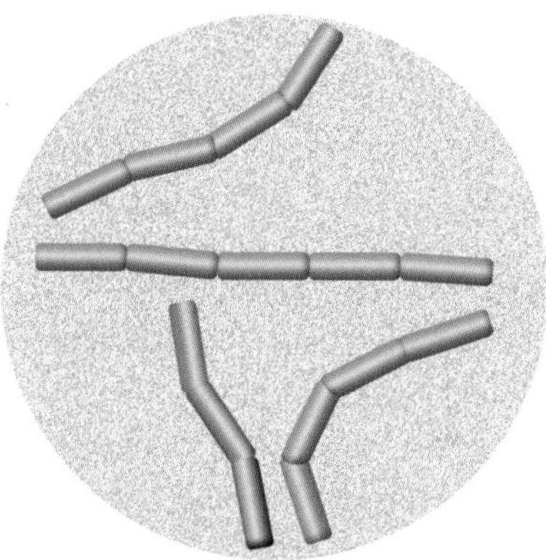

Figure 5-8 Bacilli.

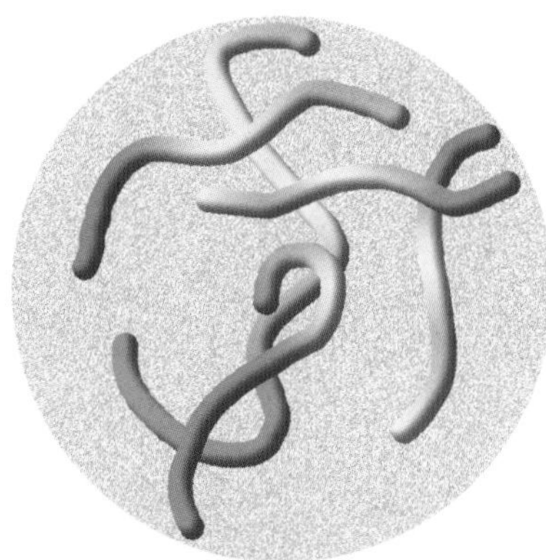

Figure 5-9 Spirilla.

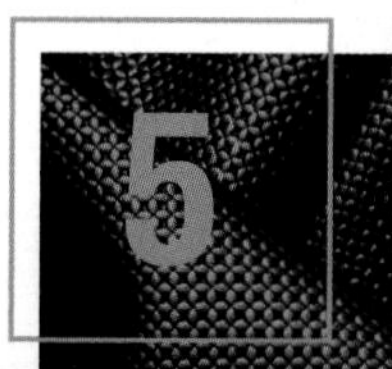

TERM	CAUSES OF DISEASE Definition
Bacteria (singular: bacterium)	One-celled microorganisms with both plant and animal characteristics. Some are harmful, some are harmless. Also known as microbes or germs.
Infectious	Communicable by infection from one person to another person or from one infected body part to another.
Microbes/germs	Nonscientific synonyms for disease-producing bacteria.
Microorganism	Any organism of microscopic to submicroscopic size.
-ology	Suffix meaning "study of" (e.g., microbiology).
Parasite	An organism that grows, feeds, and shelters on or in another organism, while contributing nothing to the survival of that organism.
Toxin	Any of various poisonous substances produced by some microorganisms.
Virus (plural: viruses)	A parasitic submicroscopic particle that infects cells of biological organisms. A virus is capable of replication only through taking over the host cell's reproduction machinery.

Table 5-1 Definitions Relating to Causes of Disease

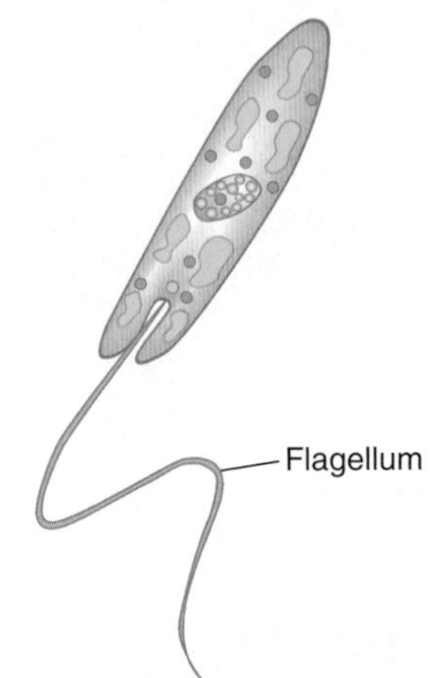

Figure 5-10 Bacteria with flagellum.

BACTERIAL GROWTH AND REPRODUCTION

Bacteria generally consist of an outer cell wall containing liquid called protoplasm. Cells manufacture their own food from what they can absorb from the surrounding environment. They give off waste products, grow, and reproduce. The life cycle of bacteria consists of two distinct phases: the active stage, and the inactive or spore-forming stage.

Active Stage

During the active stage, bacteria grow and reproduce. Bacteria multiply best in warm, dark, damp, or dirty places where food is available. When conditions are favorable, bacteria grow and reproduce. When they reach their largest size, they divide into two new cells. This division is called *mitosis* (my-TOH-sis). The cells that are formed are called daughter cells. When conditions become unfavorable and difficult for them to thrive, the bacteria either die or become inactive.

Inactive or Spore-Forming Stage

Certain bacteria, such as the anthrax and tetanus bacilli, coat themselves with waxy outer shells that are able to withstand long periods of famine, dryness, and unsuitable temperatures. In this stage, spores can be blown about and are not harmed by disinfectants, heat, or cold. When favorable conditions are restored, the spores change into the active form and begin to grow and reproduce. Although spores are dangerous if they enter the

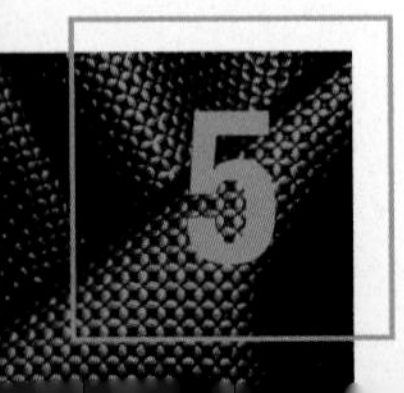

TERMS RELATED TO DISEASE	
TERM	**Definition**
Allergy	Reaction due to extreme sensitivity to certain foods, chemicals, or other normally harmless substances.
Contagious Disease	Disease that is communicable or transmittable by contact.
Contamination	The presence, or the reasonably anticipated presence, of blood or other potentially infectious materials on an item surface or visible debris/residues such as dust, hair, skin, etc.
Diagnosis	Determination of the nature of a disease from its symptoms.
Disease	Abnormal condition of all or part of the body, organ, or mind that makes it incapable of carrying on normal function.
Exposure Incident	Contact with non-intact skin, blood, body fluid or other potentially infectious materials that results from performance of an employees duties (previously called Blood Spill).
Infectious Disease	Disease caused by pathogenic microorganisms that are easily spread.
Inflammation	Condition in which a part of the body reacts to protect itself from injury, irritation, or infection, characterized by redness, heat, pain, and swelling.
Occupational Disease	Illnesses resulting from conditions associated with employment, such as prolonged and repeated overexposure to certain products or ingredients.
Parasitic Disease	Disease is caused by parasites, such as lice and ringworm.
Pathogenic Disease	Disease produced by disease-causing organisms, including bacteria, virus, and fungi.
Systemic Disease	Disease that affects the body generally, often due to under- or over-functioning of internal glands/organs.

Table 5-2 General Terms Relating to Disease

body during a surgical procedure and become active, they pose little to no risk to clients in a salon.

BACTERIAL INFECTIONS

An **infection** occurs when body tissues are invaded by disease-causing or pathogenic bacteria. There can be no bacterial infection without the presence of pathogenic bacteria. *Pus* is a fluid created by tissue inflammation, and contains white blood cells (see Chapter 6), bacteria, and dead cells. So if they are eliminated, clients cannot become infected. The presence of pus is a sign of a bacterial infection.

Staphylococci ("staph") are among the most common human bacteria, and are normally carried by about a third of the population. Staph can be picked up on doorknobs, countertops, and other surfaces, but is more

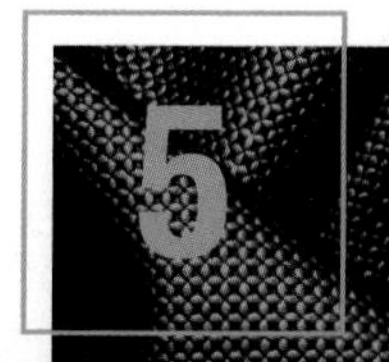

Did You Know?

The term Hospital Grade is a myth. The EPA does not 'grade' disinfectants; a product is approved for use in a hospital or it is not.

frequently spread through skin-to-skin contact, such as shaking hands or using unclean implements. If these bacteria get into the wrong place they can be very dangerous.

Staph is responsible for food poisoning and a wide range of diseases like toxic shock syndrome. Some bacteria are resistant to certain antibiotics. Staph infections occur most frequently among persons who have weakened immune systems, but can occur in otherwise healthy people. The symptoms usually appear as skin infections, such as pimples and boils that can be very difficult to cure and have resulted in death. Because of these highly resistant strains, it is important to clean and disinfect all tools and equipment used in the salon. You owe it to yourself and your clients!

A *local infection,* such as a pimple or abscess, is one that is confined to a particular part of the body and is indicated by a lesion containing pus. A *general infection* results when the bloodstream carries the bacteria or virus and their toxins (poisons) to all parts of the body. Syphilis is an example. When a disease spreads from one person to another by contact, it is said to be **contagious** (kon-TAY-jus) or communicable (kuh-MYOO-nih-kuhbul). Some of the more common contagious diseases that will prevent a salon professional from servicing a client are the common cold, ringworm, conjunctivitis (pinkeye), and viral infections. The chief sources of spreading these infections are dirty hands and implements; open sores, pus, mouth and nose discharges; and shared drinking cups, telephone receivers, and towels. Uncovered coughing or sneezing and spitting in public also spread germs.

VIRUSES

A **virus** (VY-rus) is a microorganism capable of infecting almost all plants and animals, including bacteria. They are so small that they can only be seen under the most sophisticated and powerful microscopes available. They cause common colds and other respiratory and gastrointestinal (digestive tract) infections. Other viruses that plague humans are measles, mumps, chicken pox, smallpox, rabies, yellow fever, hepatitis, polio, influenza, and HIV, which causes AIDS.

One difference between viruses and bacteria is that a virus can live and reproduce only by penetrating other cells and becoming part of them, while bacteria can live and reproduce on their own. Bacterial infections can usually be treated with specific antibiotics, while viruses are hard to kill without harming the body in the process. Viruses are not affected by antibiotics. Vaccination prevents viruses from growing in the body, but are not available for all viruses.

HEPATITIS

A bloodborne virus causes **hepatitis,** a disease that damages the liver. It is easier to contract hepatitis than HIV since it is present in all body fluids of infected individuals. Unlike HIV, hepatitis can live on a surface outside the body for long periods of time. It is vital that all surfaces that contact a client are thoroughly cleaned, especially if someone sneezes or coughs on them. Be sure to clean hands after coughing or sneezing.

There are three types of Hepatitis that are of concern within the salon—Hepatitis A, B, and C. Hepatitis B is the most difficult to kill on

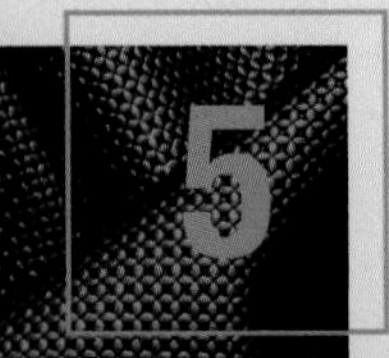

a surface, so check the label of the disinfectant you use to be sure that the product is effective against it. Those who work closely with the public can be vaccinated against Hepatitis. You may want to check with your doctor to see if this is an option for you.

HIV/AIDS

HIV (Human Immunodeficiency Virus) is the virus that causes **AIDS** (Acquired Immune Deficiency Syndrome). AIDS is a disease that breaks down the body's immune system. HIV is spread from person to person through blood and through other body fluids, such as semen and vaginal secretions. A person can be infected with HIV for many years without having symptoms, but testing can determine if a person is infected within 6 months after exposure to the virus according to the Centers for Disease Control and Prevention.

Sometimes people who are HIV-positive have never been tested and do not know they are infecting other people. The HIV virus is spread mainly through the sharing of needles by intravenous (IV) drug users, and less often by unprotected sexual contact or accidents with needles in healthcare settings. The virus is less likely to enter the bloodstream through cuts and sores. It is *not spread* by holding hands, hugging, kissing, sharing food or household items like the telephone, or even toilet seats. There are no documented cases of the virus being spread by food handlers, insects, or casual contact, or hair, skin and nail salon services.

BLOODBORNE PATHOGENS

Disease-causing bacteria or viruses that are carried through the body in the blood or body fluids, such as hepatitis and HIV, are called **bloodborne pathogens.** If you accidentally cut a client who is HIV-positive or is infected with hepatitis, and you continue to use the implement without cleaning and disinfecting it, you risk puncturing your skin or cutting another client with a contaminated tool. The spread of bloodborne pathogens is possible through shaving, nipping, clipping, facial treatments, waxing, or tweezing any time the skin is broken. Use great care to avoid damaging clients' skin during any type of service.

HOW PATHOGENS ENTER THE BODY

Pathogenic bacteria or viruses or fungi can enter the body through:

- broken skin, such as a cut or scratch—intact skin is an effective barrier to infection
- the mouth (contaminated water, food or fingers)
- the nose (inhaling dusts)
- the eyes or ears (less likely, but possible)
- unprotected sex

The body prevents and controls infections with:

- healthy, unbroken skin - the body's first line of defense
- body secretions, such as perspiration and digestive juices
- white blood cells within the blood that destroy bacteria
- antitoxins that counteract the toxins produced by bacteria and viruses

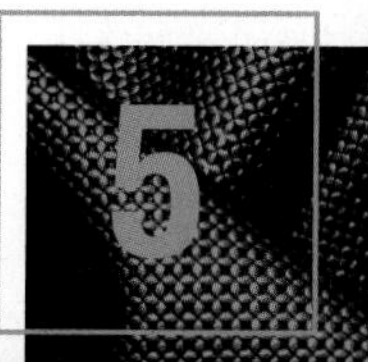

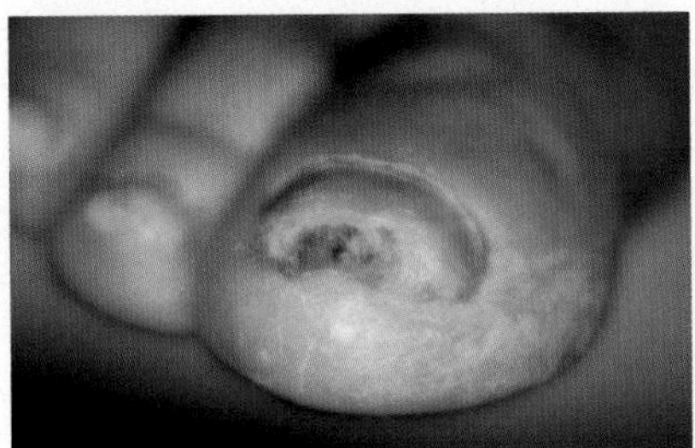

Figure 5-11 Nail fungus.

PARASITES

Parasites are plant or animal organisms that live in, or on, another living organism and draw their nourishment from that organism (referred to as a host). They must have a host to survive.

Fungi (FUN-jI), which include molds, **mildews,** and yeasts, can produce contagious diseases, such as ringworm. Hair stylists must clean and disinfect clipper blades to avoid spreading scalp and skin infections. *Tinea barbae* (Barber's Itch) is the most frequently encountered infection resulting from hair services, but others can occur. This infection affects the coarse hairs in the mustache and beard area, or around the neck and scalp, usually in men. Cleaning clippers of all visible hair, then disinfecting properly reduces the risk of spreading skin and scalp infections. Using compressed air to clean clipper blades is very effective and saves time.

Nail fungus can be spread by using dirty implements or by not properly preparing the surface of the natural nail before enhancement products are applied. Although they are not as common on the hands, nail fungus is usually a chronic condition that is localized to one or two fingers or toes, but can be spread to other nails or from client to client if implements are not properly cleaned and disinfected. The FDA has determined that topical treatments applied directly to the fingernails, skin, and toenails are not effective in eliminating fungal infections. The FDA prohibits sale of antifungal products for finger and toenails without a medical prescription. If the client is concerned about an infection of the nails, they should seek the advice of a doctor (Figure 5-11).

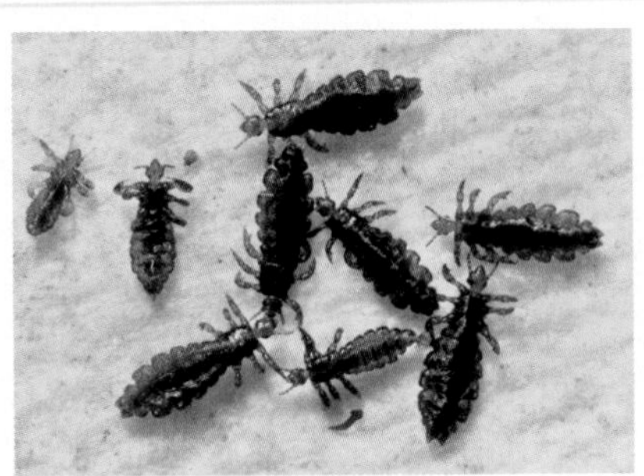

Figure 5-12 Head lice.

Head lice are another type of parasite responsible for contagious diseases and conditions (Figure 5-12). A skin disease caused by an infestation of head lice is called **pediculosis capitis (puh-dik-yuh-LOH-sis). Scabies (SKAY-beez)** is another contagious skin disease that is caused by the itch mite, which burrows under the skin. Contagious diseases and conditions caused by parasites should only be treated by a doctor. Contaminated countertops, tools and equipment should be thoroughly cleaned and then disinfected for 10 minutes with an EPA registered disinfectant or bleach solution.

IMMUNITY

Immunity is the ability of the body to destroy and resist infection. Immunity against disease can be either natural or acquired, and is a sign of good health. *Natural immunity* is partly inherited and partly developed through healthy living. *Acquired immunity* is immunity that the body develops after overcoming a disease, or through inoculation (such as flu vaccinations).

PRINCIPLES OF PREVENTION

There are three steps to decontamination. These are sanitation, disinfection, and sterilization. Because of the low risk of infection compared to medical facilities, salons are only concerned with the first two.

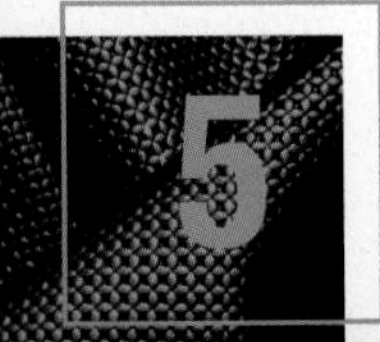

SANITATION

Sanitation or **sanitizing** is simply **cleaning.** Removing all visible dirt and debris is sanitizing. When a surface is properly cleaned, the number of germs on the surface is greatly reduced, as is the risk of infection. The vast majority of contaminants and pathogens can be washed from the surface through proper cleaning. This is why cleaning is the most important part of processing salon tools and equipment. A surface must be properly cleaned, or it cannot be properly disinfected. Using a disinfectant without cleaning first is like using mouthwash without brushing your teeth – it just does not work properly!

Cleaned surfaces can still harbor pathogens, but they are much less likely to spread infections.

Putting antiseptics on your skin or washing your hands is another example of sanitation. Your hands may appear clean when you are finished but there are still germs on them. Do not underestimate the importance of cleaning. It the most powerful and important way to prevent the spread of infection.

METHODS OF CLEANING

- Scrubbing with a brush
- Using an ultrasonic unit
- Using a solvent (i.e. on metal bits for electric files)

DISINFECTION

The second step of decontamination is **disinfection.** Disinfection is the process that kills most, but not necessarily all, microorganisms on non-living surfaces. In the salon setting, disinfection is extremely effective in controlling microorganisms on surfaces such as shears, nippers, and other multi-use tools and equipment.

Disinfectants are chemical agents that destroy all bacteria, fungi, and viruses, but not spores, on surfaces. *Disinfectants are not for use on human skin, hair, or nails.* Never use disinfectants as hand cleaners. All disinfectants clearly state on the label to avoid skin contact. This means your skin as well as the client's. Do not put your fingers directly into any disinfecting solution—these are pesticides and can be harmful to the skin if absorbed through the skin. If you mix a disinfectant in a container that is not labeled by the manufacturer, it must be labeled with the contents and the date mixed.

STERILIZATION

The word "sterilize" is often used incorrectly. **Sterilization** is the complete elimination of all microbial life, including spores, and is necessary only when surgical instruments cut into the vascular layers of the body (this does not mean an accidental cut). Methods of sterilization include high-pressure steam or dry heat autoclaves, and some chemicals. Simply exposing instruments to "steam", is not enough. To be effective against disease-causing pathogens, the steam must be pressurized, (i.e., an autoclave). Dry heat forms of sterilization are less efficient and require longer times at

Did You Know

Some state regulatory agencies prohibit the use of needles, lancets, and probes for salon services. Check with your state regulatory agency before offering any invasive services.

CAUTION

Manufacturers take great care to develop safe and highly effective systems. However, just because something is safe does not mean that it cannot be dangerous if used improperly. Any professional salon product can be dangerous if used incorrectly. Like all chemicals, disinfectants must always be used exactly as the label instructs. Disinfectants must be registered with the Environmental Protection Agency (EPA). Look for an EPA reg. number on the label.

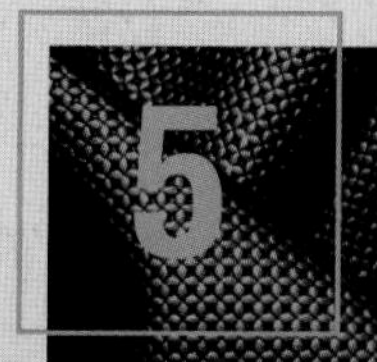

higher temperatures. Estheticians must sterilize reusable needles and probes that lance the skin, but it is best to use pre-sterilized disposable items for these procedures. Most people without medical training do not realize that the proper use of any autoclave requires cleaning, sterile rinse, *and* disinfection for 10 minutes in an EPA-registered Hospital germicide before sterilizing. Since surgical procedures are not performed in salons, sterilization of salon tools and equipment is not necessary.

CAUTION

Improperly mixing disinfectants, weaker or more concentrated than manufacturer's instructions, can dramatically reduce their effectiveness. Always add the disinfectant concentrate to the water when mixing. Quats contain detergents that will foam if you add water to the concentrate, which can result in an incorrect mixing ratio. The use of safety glasses and gloves is recommended.

CHOOSING A DISINFECTANT

To use a disinfectant properly, you must read and follow the manufacturer's instructions. Mixing ratios (dilution) and contact time is very important. Not all disinfectants have the same concentration, so be sure to mix the correct amount according to the instructions on the label. If the label does not have the word "concentrate" on it, the product is already mixed and must be used as is. All EPA disinfectants, even aerosol spray products for clippers, require 10-minute contact on precleaned, hard, nonporous surfaces. Alcohol (70% or higher) is also used to disinfect abrasive nail files and buffers used on healthy nails.

Disinfectants must have **efficacy** claims, on the label. This is a list of the specific germs the product is proven to kill when used according to the label instructions. Salons pose a very low infection risk when compared to hospitals. In hospitals, cleaning and disinfection standards are much stricter than in salons and for good reason.

Some types of disinfectants are much too dangerous (e.g., glutaraldehyde) for use in the salon environment, especially since the risk of causing serious infection is extremely low. There is some risk of spreading certain types of infections to salon clients; therefore, it is important to clean and disinfect correctly. Fortunately, any EPA-registered, liquid hospital disinfectant will be more than enough for salons. Hospital infection control guidelines now include the use of an EPA-registered *hospital* liquid disinfectant or bleach solution for clean-up of blood or body fluids. For this reason, when salon implements accidentally contact blood, body fluids, or unhealthy conditions, they should be cleaned and then completely immersed in an EPA-registered hospital disinfectant solution or 10% bleach solution.

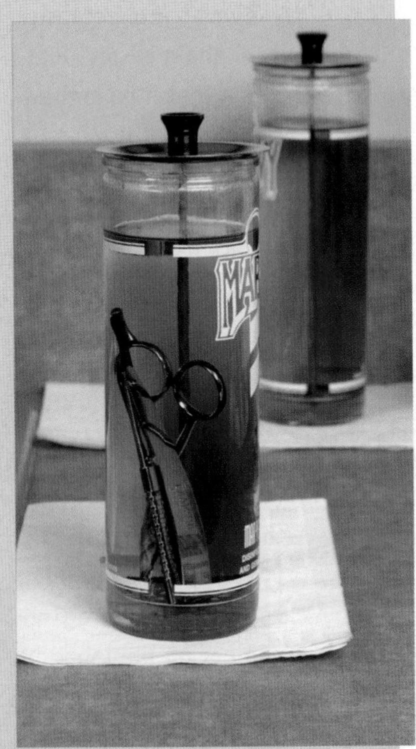

Figure 5-13 Completely immerse tools in disinfectant.

PROPER USE OF DISINFECTANTS

All implements must be thoroughly cleaned of all visible matter or residue before soaking in disinfectant solution because residue will interfere with the disinfectant and prevent them from being effective. Implements and tools must be completely immersed in disinfectant solution for the time specified on the product label. Complete immersion means enough liquid to cover all surfaces of the item, including the handles (Figure 5-13).

Disinfectant Tips

1. Use only on pre-cleaned, hard non-porous surfaces—not abrasive files or buffers.
2. Dilute according to the label of the product.
3. Immerse and soak according to the label of the product.

4. If a solution is sprayed on a clean surface, the solution must remain there for the time required by the product label. (Merely spraying and wiping is cleaning - NOT considered proper disinfection.)
5. If the product label states "complete immersion," this product cannot be used to disinfect by spraying.
6. Any use other than that on the label is a violation of Federal law.
7. If using an EPA-registered disinfectant in a whirlpool pedicure spa, the solution MUST be circulated for the time required by the label (the solution must go where the water was and remain there for the specified time), especially if the label states to disinfect by complete immersion.

Note: Absorbent nail files must be disposed of if they accidentally break the client's skin or contact unhealthy skin or nails.

TYPES OF DISINFECTANTS

QUATS

Quaternary ammonium compounds (KWAT-ur-nayr-ree uh-MOH-neeum), commonly called "**quats,**" are very safe and useful disinfectants. The most advanced type of these formulations are called "dual quats" because they contain sophisticated blends of quats that work together to dramatically increase the effectiveness of these disinfectants. Quat solutions disinfect implements usually in 10 minutes. These formulas contain anti-rust ingredients, but leaving tools in the solution for longer can cause damage. Complete immersion means enough liquid to cover all surfaces of the item being disinfected. Spraying is not adequate disinfection unless the solution saturates the surface and remains wet for the time specified by the product label.

PHENOLICS

Phenolics (fi-NOH-lik) are powerful tuberculocidal disinfectants. Phenolics have a very high pH and can cause damage to the skin and eyes; and some can be harmful to the environment. Phenolics have been used reliably over the years to disinfect salon tools, however, they do have some drawbacks. Phenol can damage plastic and rubber (phenolics should never be used to disinfect pedicure equipment) and can cause certain metals to rust. Extra care should be taken to avoid skin contact with phenolics.

ALCOHOL AND BLEACH

The word "alcohol" is often misunderstood. There are many different chemical compounds that are classified as alcohols. Two types of alcohol are used as disinfectants in the salon: ethyl (ETH-ul) alcohol (ethanol or grain alcohol) and isopropyl (eye-soh-PROH-pul) alcohol (isopropanol or rubbing alcohol). When used properly, both of these alcohols are considered to be useful and powerful disinfectants. Alcohol can be used to disinfect some items used in the salon, especially porous and absorbent items. To be effective, the concentration of ethyl and isopropyl alcohol must be 70 percent or higher. Since alcohol was used as a disinfectant

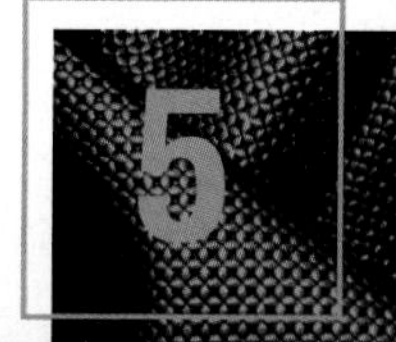

long before there was an EPA, it does not need an EPA registration number.

Household bleach (**sodium hypochlorite**) (SOH-dee-um hy-puh-KLOR-ite) is an effective disinfectant for all uses in the salon. Bleach has been used extensively as a disinfectant, long before the EPA existed, so it is not required to have an EPA registration number. Using too much bleach can damage some metals and plastics, so be sure to read the label for safe use. Bleach can be corrosive to metals and plastics, can cause skin irritation. To mix bleach solution, add a cup of household bleach to 1 gallon of water (128 oz). Store this solution away from heat and light.

CAUTION

Alcohol should never be used to clean up blood, or to disinfect any item that has contact with blood, body fluids, or unhealthy condition.

FUMIGANTS

Years ago formalin tablets were used as fumigants in dry cabinet "sanitizers." This was before EPA disinfectants came to market and before it was known that formaldehyde vapors may cause cancer in high concentrations. But the greater risk of using these tablets is the potential for developing allergic sensitivity in professionals who constantly breathe these vapors. Fumigants are no longer necessary in the salon for several reasons. First, the label clearly requires that these be kept in an airtight container, and it takes 24 hours to kill one fungus (remember that liquid disinfectants kill all fungi in 10 minutes). Second, the vapors are poisonous, and are extremely irritating to the eyes, nose, throat, and lungs, and can cause skin allergies, irritation, dryness, and rash. Third, using the product without following the label instructions is against federal law; and lastly, long-term exposure to formaldehyde vapors can aggravate existing lung problems, and may create other symptoms similar to those seen in people with chronic bronchitis or asthma.

CAUTION

Bleach is not magic! Like all disinfectants, bleach is inactivated (less effective) in the presence of materials such as oils, lotions, creams, and biological residue. If bleach is used to disinfect pedicure equipment, it is critical to use a detergent first to remove any residue from pedicure products.

Glutaraldehyde is a dangerous chemical used to sterilize surgical instruments in hospitals. It is not safe for salon use.

DISINFECTANT SAFETY

Disinfectants may cause serious skin and eye damage. Some disinfectants appear clear, while others are a little cloudy, especially phenolics. A good rule to remember is always *use caution* when handling these products and avoid skin contact!

SAFETY TIPS FOR DISINFECTANTS

- always wear gloves and safety glasses when mixing disinfectants (Figure 5-14).
- always add disinfectant to water, not water to disinfectant. Disinfectants contain detergents and will foam when water is added to them; this can result in an incorrect mixing ratio.
- use tongs, gloves, or a draining basket to remove implements from disinfectants.
- always keep disinfectants out of reach of children.
- never pour quats, phenols, alcohol, or any other disinfectant over your hands. If you get disinfectants on your skin, immediately wash your hands with soap and warm water and dry them thoroughly.

CAUTION

Fumigant tablets should never be left open in drawers or cabinets in the salon.

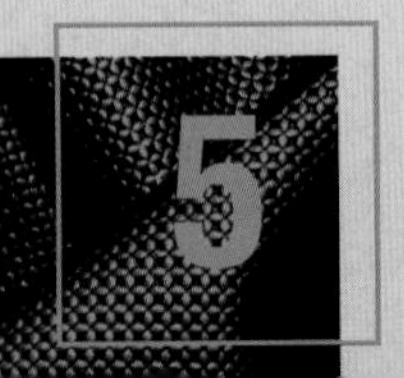

- carefully weigh and measure all products according to label instructions.
- never place any disinfectant or other product in an unmarked container (Figure 5-15).
- always follow the manufacturer's instructions for mixing, using, and disposal of disinfectants.
- change disinfectants every day, or more often if the solution becomes soiled or contaminated.

Jars or containers used to disinfect implements are often incorrectly called wet sanitizers. The purpose of these containers is to disinfect. Disinfectant containers must be covered but not airtight. Remember to clean the container every day as well. Always follow manufacturer's label instructions for disinfecting products.

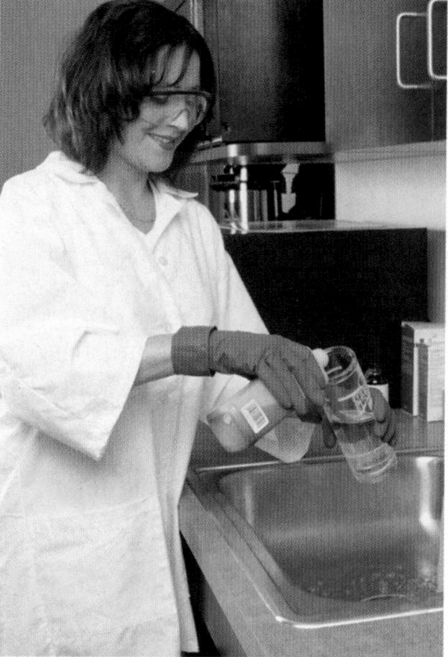

Figure 5-14 Wear gloves and safety goggles while handling disinfectants.

DISINFECT OR DISPOSE

How can you tell which items in the salon can be disinfected and used more than once? If the process of cleaning and disinfecting damages the item or changes its condition, it is a single-use item. There are two types of items used in salons - these are **multi-use** or reusable and **single-use** or **disposable** items.

Multi-use items can be cleaned, disinfected, and used on more than one person, even if the item is exposed to blood or body fluid. Examples of this are nippers, shears, combs, pushers, some nail files and buffers. Another word for these items is "**disinfectable,**" meaning these items can be disinfected.

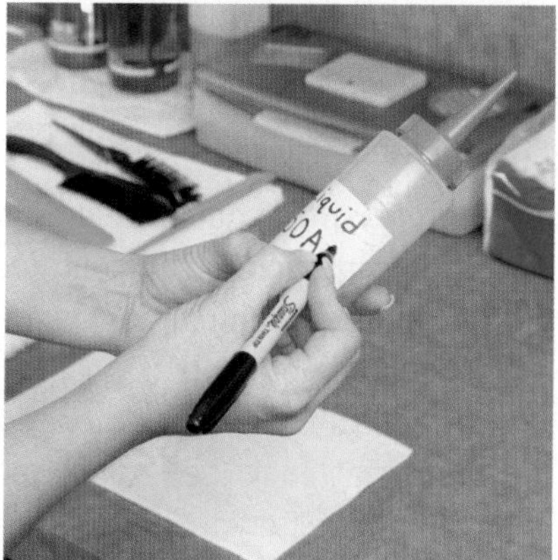

Figure 5-15 All containers should be labeled.

Porous means made or constructed of an absorbent material. Some porous items can be safely cleaned, disinfected, and used on more than one client. Examples of these are towels, chamois, and some nail files and buffers.

NOTE: If a porous item contacts broken skin, blood, body fluid or any unhealthy conditions, it must be discarded immediately—do not try to disinfect it. If you are not sure if an item can be safely cleaned, disinfected and used again—throw it out. Remember, **when in doubt, throw it out!**

Single-use disposable items cannot be used more than once, either because these cannot be cleaned of all visible residue (such as pumice stones used for pedicures), or because cleaning and disinfecting damages them. Examples of disposable items are orangewood sticks, cotton balls, gauze, tissues, paper towels, and some nail files and buffers.

DISINFECTION PROCEDURES

TOOLS AND EQUIPMENT

Tools and equipment must be cleaned and disinfected after each use and before they may be used on another client. Be certain to dilute and mix disinfectants according the label of the product that you choose. Mix disinfectants according to manufacturer's directions, always adding disinfectant to the water (Figure 5-16).

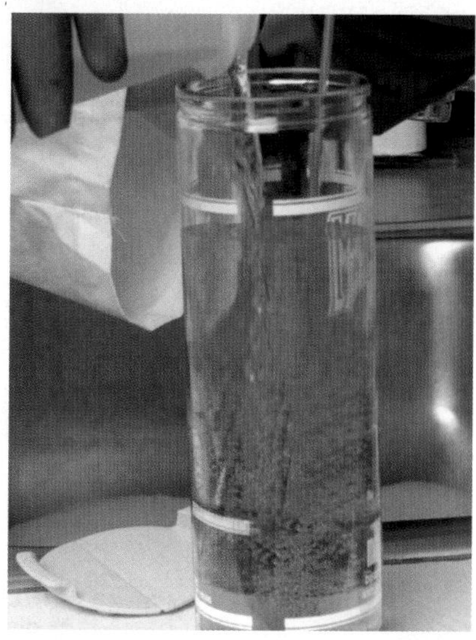

Figure 5-16 Carefully pour disinfectant into the water when preparing disinfectant solution.

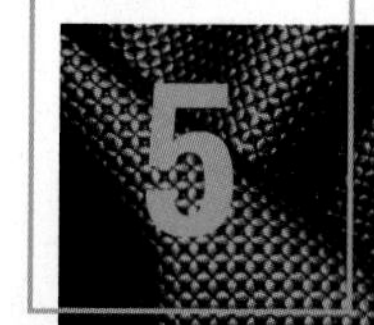

PROCEDURE 5-1

DISINFECTING NONELECTRICAL TOOLS AND EQUIPMENT

These include combs, brushes, rollers, picks, styling tools, scissors, tweezers, nail clippers, and multi-use abrasive nail files.

1. Clean tools and equipment to remove all visible matter and residue (Figure 5-17).
2. Rinse thoroughly and pat dry with a clean towel.
3. Completely immerse implements in a properly mixed disinfecting solution for 10 minutes (Figure 5-18) or per the manufacturer's directions.
4. Remove implements with tongs, basket, or gloves to avoid skin contact (Figure 5-19).
5. Rinse and dry tools thoroughly.
6. **Store disinfected implements.** Store disinfected implements in a clean container and in a sanitary manner between uses. A clean drawer can be used for storage of tools if only clean items are in it. Never seal tools inside a closed airtight container; they may not be completely dry, which can promote bacterial growth.

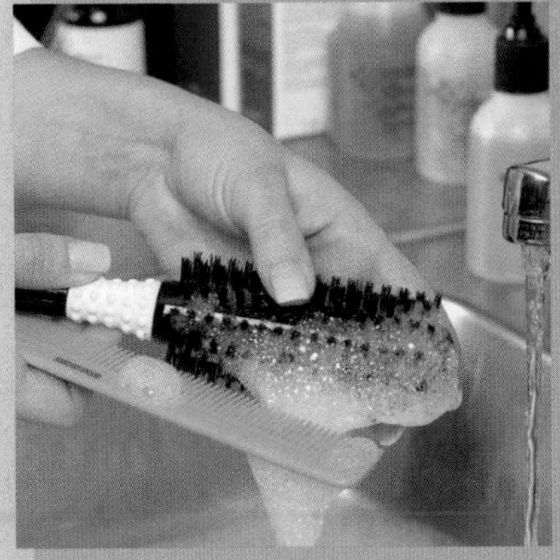

Figure 5–17 Remove all visible debris and residue from tools and implements.

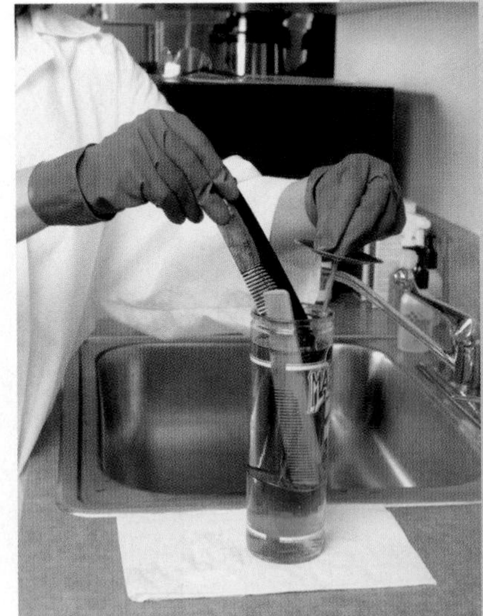

Figure 5–18 Submerge combs and brushes in disinfectant solution for 10 minutes.

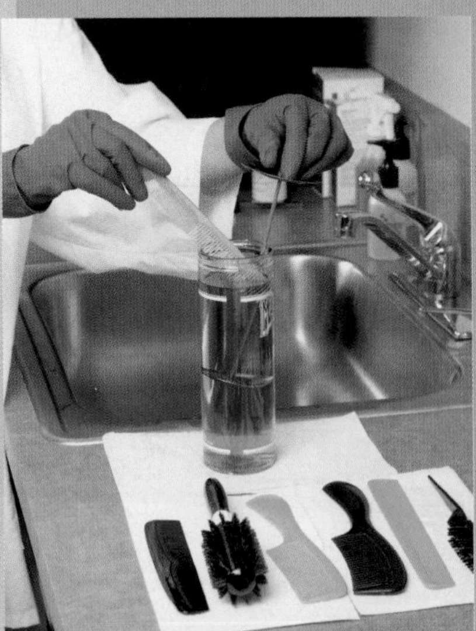

Figure 5–19 Remove implements with tongs, gloves, or a draining basket.

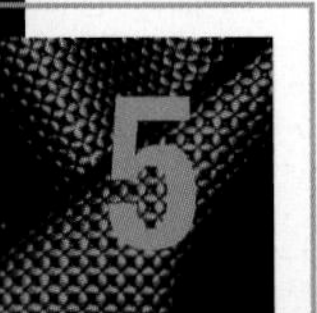

TOWELS, LINENS, AND CAPES

Clean towels and linens must be used for each client. Once a towel or linen has been used on a client, it must not be used again until it has been properly laundered. Store soiled linens and towels separate from clean linens and towels. It is not necessary to store clean towels in a closed container unless your regulatory agency requires it. Whenever possible, use disposable towels, especially in restrooms. Use disposable neck strips or towels to keep capes for cutting, shampooing, and chemical services from touching the client's skin. If a cape touches skin, do not use it again until it has been cleaned.

DISINFECTING ELECTRICAL EQUIPMENT

The contact points of equipment that cannot be immersed in liquid, such as hair clippers, electrotherapy tools, and nail drills, should be cleaned and disinfected using a regulatory oversight agency approved disinfectant designed for use on such devices. Follow the procedures recommended by the disinfectant product manufacture.

WORK SURFACES

Before beginning service for each client, all work surfaces (manicure tables, workstations, facial chairs, etc.) must be cleaned by wiping with a clean disposable towel. It is not necessary to disinfect tables and chairs unless the customer touches them with their skin, but they certainly need to be cleaned regularly (Figure 5-20). Clean doorknobs and handles daily to reduce germs on hands.

INDIVIDUAL CLIENT PACKS

You may save client packs with items like nail files and buffers as long as each item in the pack is cleaned, disinfected, and dried before being placed in the pack. Do not put single-use items in client packs stored between services. Never use bags or containers with an airtight seal to store tools or implements. Saving client tools to avoid cleaning and disinfecting is NOT safe and violates state rules. Remember, state rules require ALL tools and equipment be cleaned and disinfected before each use—even if used on the same person! This also applies to clients that bring their tools with them to the salon—before you use it, you must clean and then disinfect each item for 10 minutes! Remember, it is *your* license that is at risk if there is a problem, even if your client brings her tools with her. This practice should be vehemently discouraged.

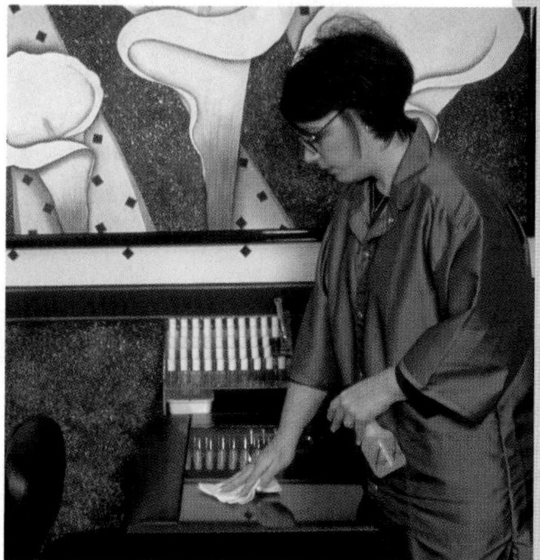

Figure 5-20 Clean manicure tables.

DISINFECTING FOOT SPAS AND PEDICURE EQUIPMENT

All equipment that holds water for pedicures, including whirlpool spas, "pipeless" units, foot baths, basins, tubs, sinks, and bowls, must be cleaned and disinfected after every

CAUTION

Ultraviolet (UV) sanitizers are useful storage containers, but they do not disinfect or sterilize.

CAUTION

Electric or bead "sterilizers" do not disinfect or sterilize implements. In fact, these devices can spread potentially infectious diseases and should never be used in salons. Remember: state rules require the use of liquid disinfecting solutions!

CAUTION

Remember that products and equipment that have the word "sanitizer" on the label are merely cleaners. Items must be both cleaned and disinfected after each and every use and before using them on another client.

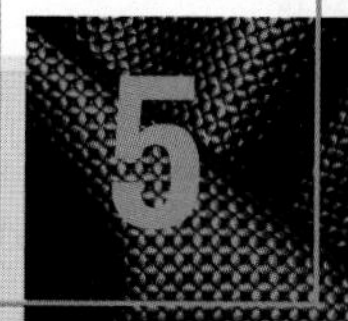

PROCEDURE 5-2

DISINFECTING FOOT SPAS AFTER EACH CLIENT

1. **Drain and remove debris.** Drain all water and remove all visible debris from the foot spa or basin; if there is a footplate or impeller, remove it and clean the areas behind and underneath.
2. **Thoroughly clean.** Clean the surfaces and walls of the foot spas or basin with chelating detergent and a brush to remove all visible debris, and rinse with clean, clear water. Although modern detergents aren't affected by hard water, soaps cause the minerals in hard water to buildup inside foot spas. Chelating detergents remove that mineral buildup and are an important first step in proper sanitation. Ethylene Diamine Tetra Acetic Acid (EDTA) is a very effective chelating agent commonly used in chelating detergents. Remember to clean and disinfect the brush.
3. **Disinfect basin.** Disinfect the foot basin with an EPA-registered, liquid hospital disinfectant for 10 minutes. If it is a whirlpool unit, the solution must be circulated. The solution must go every place the water was and must stay there for 10 minutes (or as indicated on the product label).
4. **Dry basin.** Wipe dry with a disposable towel. Cloth towels can transmit pathogens if they are not properly laundered between each client.
5. Record the time and date these procedures were performed in the pedicure logbook, if required by your state regulatory agency.

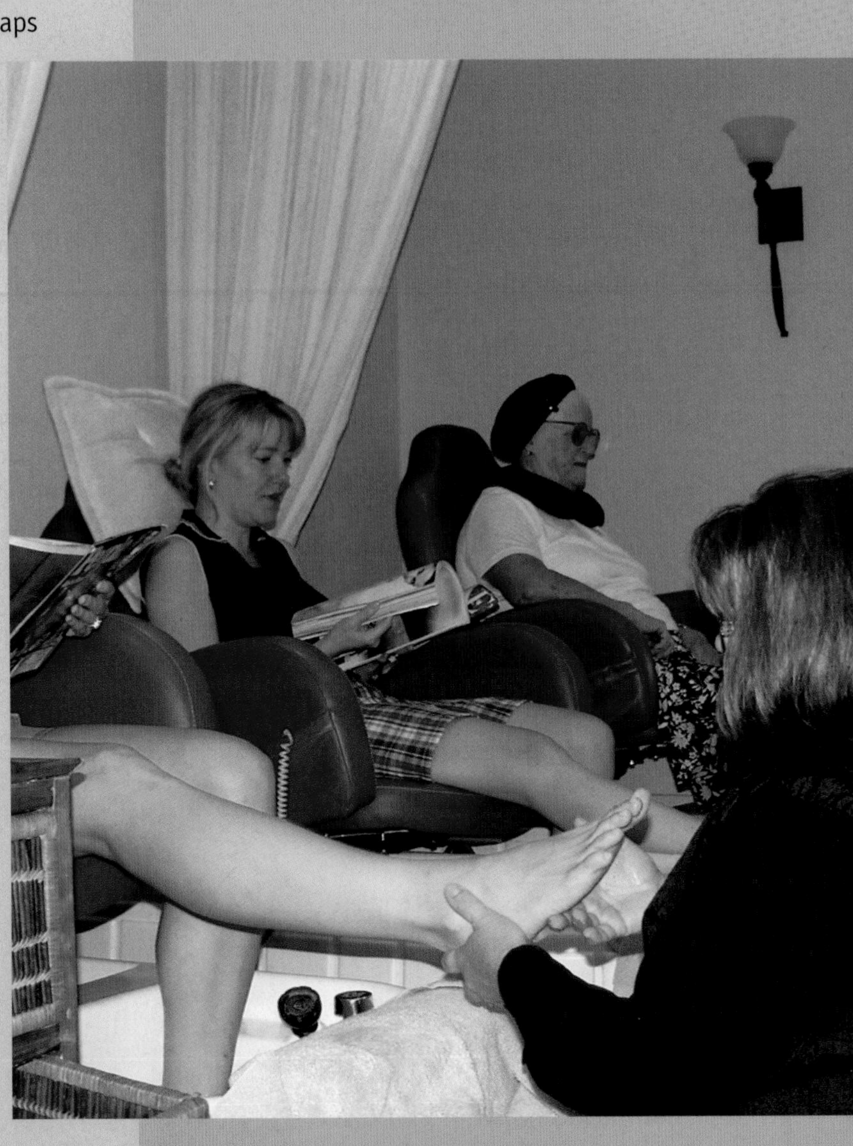

PROCEDURE 5-3

DISINFECTING FOOT SPAS AT THE END OF DAY

1. Remove the screen. Clean the screen and the area behind the screen of all visible residue and trapped materials with a brush and liquid soap and water. Replace the screen.
2. Fill the basin with warm water and chelating liquid soap. Flush the spa system for 5 minutes, and then rinse and drain.
3. Fill the basin with water and the correct amount of an EPA-registered, liquid hospital disinfectant. Circulate this solution through the basin for 10 minutes, and then drain and rinse.
4. Allow the unit to completely dry overnight.
5. Make a record of the date and time of this cleaning and disinfecting in the salon pedicure logbook if required by your state regulatory agency.

Foaming: If the disinfectant *foams* while it circulates, run the unit for about 90 seconds and turn off the jets. Leave the solution in the basin for the remainder of 10 minutes then drain.

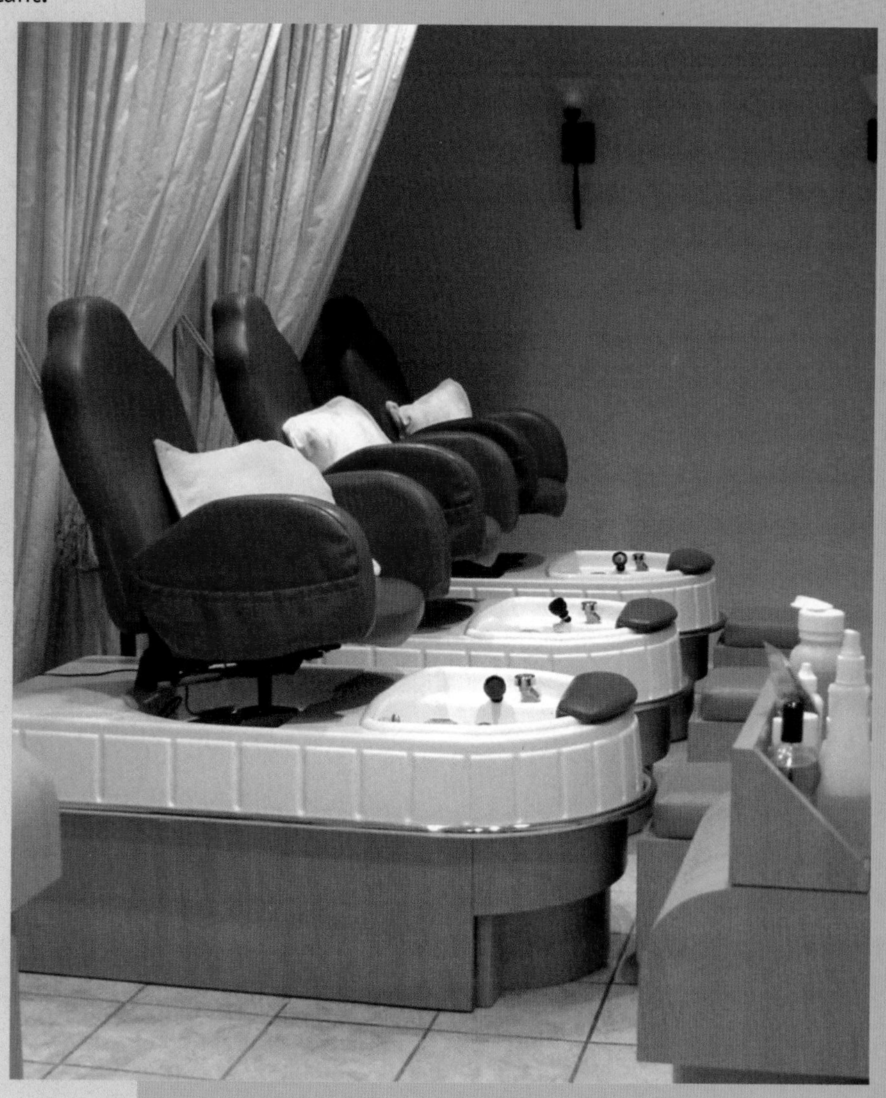

PROCEDURE 5-4

DISINFECTING FOOT SPAS AT LEAST ONCE EACH WEEK

1. Drain all water and remove all debris from the foot spa or basin. If there is a footplate or impeller, remove it and clean the areas behind and underneath.
2. Clean the surfaces and walls of the foot spas or basin with liquid soap and a brush to remove all visible debris, and rinse with clean, clear water; remember to clean and disinfect the brush.
3. Disinfect the foot basin with an EPA-registered, liquid Hospital disinfectant for 10 minutes. If it is a whirlpool unit, the solution must be circulated to ensure proper disinfection.
4. Do not drain the disinfectant solution. Turn off the unit and leave the solution in the unit overnight (6 to 10 hours).
5. In the morning, drain and rinse.
6. Record this procedure in the salon pedicure logbook if required by your state regulatory agency.

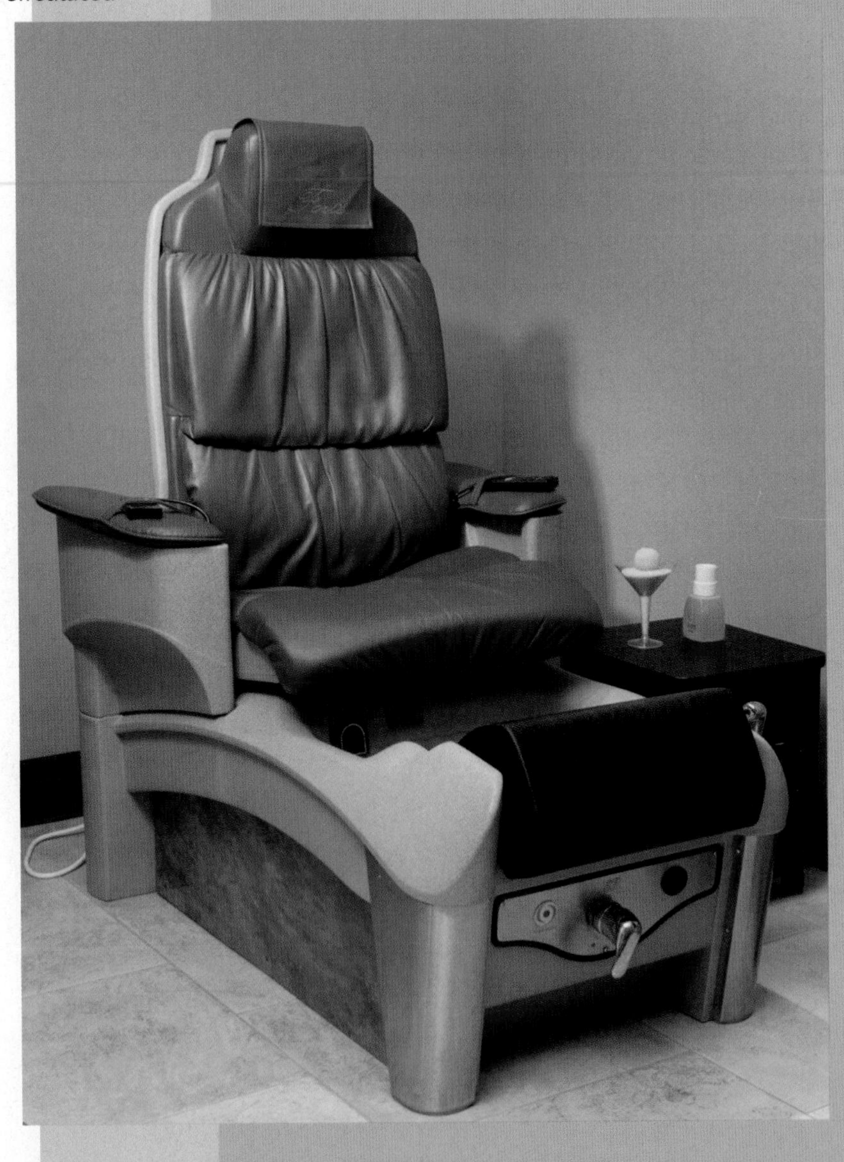

pedicure. Inspectors may issue fines if there is no logbook. Most pedicure spas hold 5 gallons of water—check with the manufacturer so that you use the correct amount of disinfectant. Remember: 128 ounces = 1 gallon.

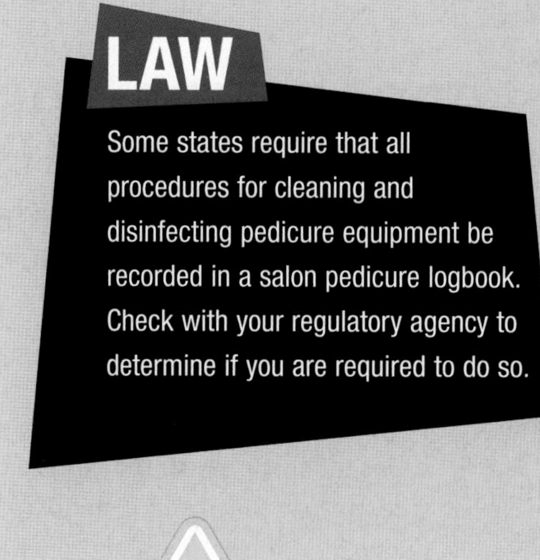

Some states require that all procedures for cleaning and disinfecting pedicure equipment be recorded in a salon pedicure logbook. Check with your regulatory agency to determine if you are required to do so.

DETERGENTS AND SOAPS

Using *chelating surfactant* soaps or detergents, which work to sequester debris, is very important for removing the residue from pedicure products like scrubs, salts, and masques. These detergents work in all types of water, are low-sudsing, and are especially formulated to work in the areas where hard water is prevalent. Check with your local distributor for pedicure cleaners that contain chelating detergents.

ADDITIVES, POWDERS, AND TABLETS

There is no additive, powder, or tablet that eliminates the need for you to clean and disinfect. You cannot replace proper cleaning and disinfection with a shortcut. These products cannot be used instead of EPA-registered, liquid disinfectant solutions. For example, be wary of products containing Chloramine-T because this chemical is not recognized as an effective disinfectant for use in the United States.

CAUTION

Never place client's feet in water that contains a disinfectant.

DISPENSARY

The dispensary must be kept clean and orderly, with the contents of all containers clearly marked. Store products according to manufacturers' instructions and away from heat. Keep MSDSs for all chemicals used in the salon.

HANDLING DISPOSABLE SUPPLIES

All items designed to be disposed of after a single use, such as orangewood sticks, cotton, gauze, neck strips, nail wipes, and paper towels, should be thrown away after one use. Anything exposed to blood, including skincare treatment debris, must be double-bagged and marked with a biohazard sticker or disposed of according to OSHA standards (separated from other waste and disposed of according to federal, state, and local regulations). Puncture-proof containers should be used for disposal of all sharps.

Remember: Disinfect or Discard.

CAUTION

Use liquid soaps in pump containers—bar soaps can grow bacteria.

WASHING HANDS

Hand washing is one of the most important actions to prevent spreading germs from one person to another. Hand washing removes germs from the folds and grooves of the skin and from under the free edge of the nail plate by lifting and rinsing them from the surface. In the salon, hands-both yours and the client's—should be thoroughly washed with soap and water before and after each service. Medical studies suggest that antimicrobial and antibacterial soaps are no more effective than regular soaps or detergents, and may actually promote the growth of resistant strains.

The use of a moisturizing hand lotion can help prevent dry skin, which can be caused by repeated hand washing.

WATERLESS HAND SANITIZERS

Antiseptics (ant-ih-SEP-tiks) are agents formulated for use on skin. Antiseptics can contain either alcohol or benzalkonium chloride (less

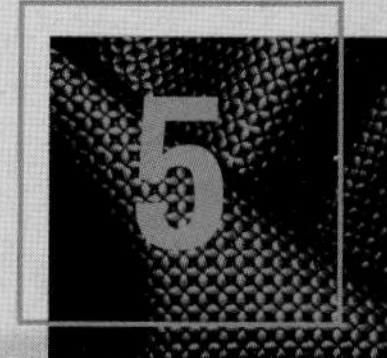

PROCEDURE 5-5

PROCEDURE FOR WASHING HANDS

1. Wet your hands with warm water.
2. Using liquid soap and a clean, disinfected soft-bristle nail brush, scrub your hands together and work up a good lather for at least 20 seconds. Give particular attention to the areas between the fingers, the nails, both sides of the hands, and the exposed portions of the arms (Figure 5-21). Be sure to use the nail brush to carefully scrub the underside of the nail plate where bacteria can hide.
3. Thoroughly rinse soap residue from your hands with warm water.
4. Dry your hands using a disposable paper towel, air blower, or clean cloth towel.

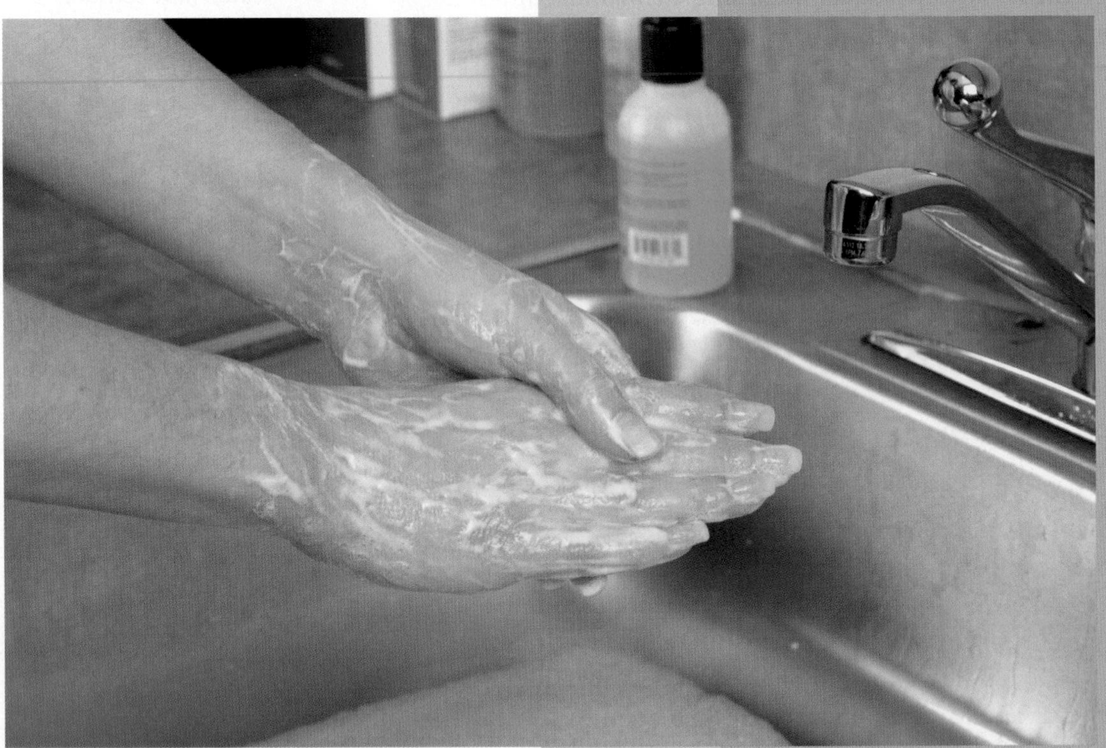

Figure 5-21 Proper hand-washing technique.

drying to the skin than alcohol). Both types of antiseptics are effective for cleaning (sanitizing) hands if soap and water are not available, but should not replace washing with soap, soft-bristle brush, and water. These agents are not the same as surface or implement disinfectants, so never use an antiseptic to disinfectant instruments or other surfaces.

UNIVERSAL PRECAUTIONS

The **Universal Precautions** are a set of guidelines published by OSHA that require the employer and the employee to assume that all human blood and body fluids are infectious for bloodborne pathogens. Because it is impossible to identify clients with infectious diseases, the same infection control practices should be used with all clients. In most instances, clients who are infected with Hepatitis B Virus or other bloodborne pathogens are *asymptomatic,* which means that they show no symptoms or signs of infection. Bloodborne pathogens are more difficult to kill than germs that live outside the body.

OSHA sets safety standards and precautions that protect employees when they are potentially exposed to bloodborne pathogens. Precautions include hand washing, wearing gloves, and proper handling and disposal of sharp instruments and items that have been contaminated by blood or other body fluids. It is important that specific procedures are followed if blood or body fluid is present.

CONTACT WITH BLOOD OR BODY FLUID

Accidents happen. If a client's skin is cut during a salon service, blood or body fluid can be present—this is called an **exposure incident.** If this should occur, follow these steps for the safety of both you and the client:

1. If a cut occurs during service, stop the service.
2. Wear gloves to protect yourself against contact with the client's blood.
3. Clean the injured area with an antiseptic—each salon must have a first aid kit.
4. Bandage the cut with an adhesive bandage.
5. Clean workstation as necessary.
6. Discard contaminated objects. Discard all disposable contaminated objects such as wipes or cotton balls by double-bagging (place the waste in a plastic bag and then in a trash bag). Use a biohazard sticker (red or orange) or a container for contaminated waste. Deposit sharp disposables in a sharps box (Figure 5-22).
7. Disinfect tools and implements. Remember, before removing your gloves, all tools and implements that have come into contact with blood or other body fluids must be thoroughly cleaned and completely immersed in an EPA-registered, hospital disinfectant solution or 10% bleach solution for 10 minutes. Because blood can carry pathogens, you should never touch an open sore or wound.

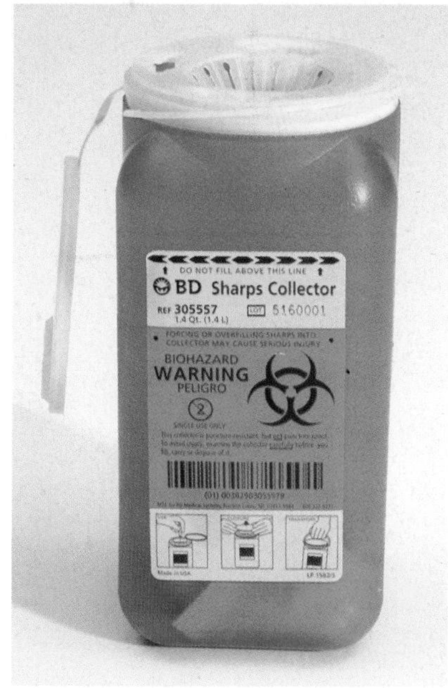

Figure 5-22 Sharps box.

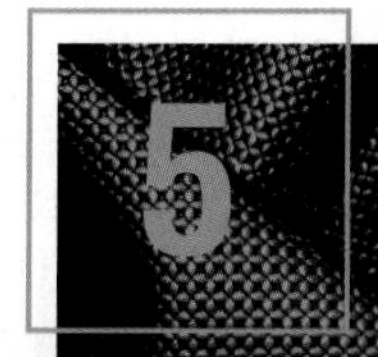

8. Remove your gloves. Wash your hands with soap and warm water before returning to the service.

THE PROFESSIONAL SALON IMAGE

Cleanliness should be a part of your normal routine as well as those who work with you. This way, you and your coworkers can project a steadfast professional image. The following are some simple guidelines that will keep the salon looking its best:

1. Keep floors clean. Sweep hair after every client. Mop floors and vacuum carpets every day.
2. Keep trash in a waste receptacle; covered containers may be necessary by mandate of your state regulatory agency and to reduce chemical odors and to look more professional.
3. Control dust, hair, and other debris.
4. Clean fans, ventilation systems, and humidifiers at least once each week.
5. Keep all work areas well lit.
6. Keep restrooms clean, including door handles.
7. Provide toilet tissue, paper towels, and liquid soap, and clean, soft-bristle nail brushes in the restroom.
8. Do not allow the salon to be used for cooking or living quarters.
9. Never place food in refrigerators used to store salon products.
10. Prohibit eating, drinking, and smoking in areas where services are performed or where product mixing occurs, i.e. back bar area.
11. Empty waste receptacles regularly throughout the day. A waste receptacle with a self-closing lid works best.
12. Make sure all containers are properly marked and properly stored.
13. Never place any tools or implements in your mouth or pockets.
14. Properly clean and disinfect all tools after each use.
15. Store clean and disinfected tools in a clean container or sanitary manner. Clean drawers may be used for storage if only clean items are stored in it.
16. Avoid touching your face, mouth, or eye areas during services.
17. Clean all work surfaces after every client. This includes manicure tables, facial chairs and tables, workstations, and shampoo bowls.
18. Always use clean linens on clients, and use disposable towels and linens. Keep soiled linens separate from clean linens. Use neck strips or towels to avoid skin contact with shampoo capes and cutting or chemical protection gowns.

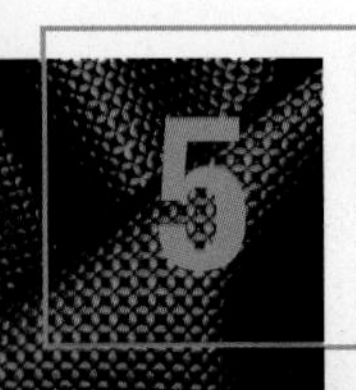

19. Use exhaust systems in the salon. Replacing the air in the salon with fresh air at least 4 times every hour is recommended to ensure proper air quality.

YOUR PROFESSIONAL RESPONSIBILITY

You have many responsibilities as a salon professional, but none is more important than protecting your clients' health and safety. Never take shortcuts for cleaning and disinfection—you cannot afford to skip steps or save money when it comes to safety.

Remember, it is *your* responsibility to follow state laws and rules. Keep your license current and notify the licensing agency if you move or change your name. Check the state website weekly for any changes to the rules.

REVIEW QUESTIONS

1. What are bacteria?
2. Name and describe the two main classifications of bacteria.
3. What are some of the beneficial functions performed by nonpathogenic bacteria?
4. Name and describe the three forms of pathogenic bacteria.
5. What is sanitation? Why is this important?
6. What is the primary purpose of regulatory agencies?
7. What is an exposure incident?
8. List the steps for cleaning and disinfecting electrical equipment.
9. List the three types of microorganisms that are important to cosmetology.
10. What is complete immersion?
11. Is HIV a risk in the salon? Why or why not?
12. What is a contagious or communicable disease?
13. How often should disinfectant solutions be changed?
14. Describe the procedure for taking care of blood or other body fluid in the salon.
15. How do you know if an item is disinfectable?
16. Can porous items be disinfected?
17. What is an MSDS? Where can you get an MSDS?
18. List the steps for cleaning and disinfecting pedicure equipment after each client.
19. Explain how to clean and disinfect the following: implements for haircutting and styling, nail implements, linens and capes, and electrical tools that cannot be immersed.
20. List at least six precautions to follow when using disinfectants.
21. What are Universal Precautions?

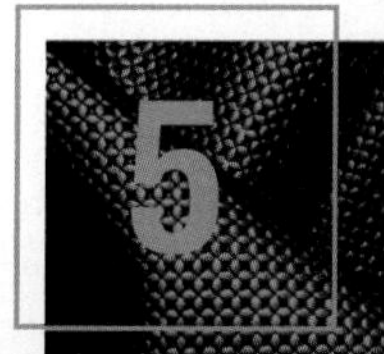

CHAPTER GLOSSARY

AIDS	Acquired immune deficiency syndrome, a disease caused by the HIV virus that breaks down the body's immune system.
allergy	Reaction due to extreme sensitivity to certain foods, chemicals, or other normally harmless substances.
antiseptics	Agents formulated for use on skin.
bacilli (singular: bacillus)	Short, rod-shaped bacteria; the most common bacteria; they produce diseases such as tetanus (lockjaw), typhoid fever, tuberculosis, and diphtheria.
bacteria	One-celled microorganisms. Some are harmful, some are harmless.
bactericidal	Capable of destroying bacteria.
bloodborne pathogens	Disease-causing microorganisms carried in the body by blood or body fluids.
cilia	Slender, hair-like extensions that permit locomotion in certain bacteria; their whip-like motion moves bacteria in liquid.
cocci	Round shaped bacteria that appear singly (alone) or in groups.
contagious disease	Disease that can be easily spread to others by contact.
diagnosis	Determining the nature of a disease or infection.
diplococci	Spherical bacteria that grow in pairs and cause diseases such as pneumonia.
disease	Abnormal condition of all or part of the body, organ, or mind that makes it incapable of carrying out normal function.
disinfectable	An item that can be disinfected.
disinfectants	Chemical agents that destroy most bacteria, fungi and viruses, but not spores, on surfaces.
disinfection	Process that eliminates most microorganisms, but is not effective against bacterial spores.
efficacy	Effectiveness with which a disinfecting solution kills germs, when used according to the label.
exposure incident	Contact with non-intact skin, blood, body fluid or other potentially infectious materials that results from performance of an employees duties.
flagella (singular: flagellum)	Slender, hair-like extensions that permit locomotion in certain bacteria; their whip-like motion moves bacteria in liquid.
fungi (singular: fungus)	Microscopic plant parasites, including molds, mildews, and yeasts.
fungicidal	Capable of destroying fungi.
hepatitis	Bloodborne virus that causes disease affecting the liver.
HIV	Human immunodeficiency virus; virus that can cause AIDS.
immunity	Ability of the body to destroy and resist infection.
infection	Invasion of body tissue by pathogenic bacteria.
infectious	Infection that can be spread from one person to another person or from one infected body part to another.
inflammation	Body's response to injury or infection with redness, heat, pain, and swelling.

CHAPTER GLOSSARY

microorganism	Any organism of microscopic to submicroscopic size.
mildews	Type of fungus that affects plants or grows on in animate objects but does not cause human infections in the salon setting.
motility	Self-movement.
Material Data Safety Sheet (MSDS)	Material Safety Data Sheet; safety information about products compiled by manufacturer.
multi-use	Items that can be cleaned, disinfected, and used on more than one person, even if the item is exposed to blood or body fluid.
nonpathogenic	Not harmful; organisms that may perform useful functions.
occupational disease	Illness resulting from conditions associated with employment.
parasites	Plant or animal organisms that derive nutrition from another organism.
pathogenic	Causing disease; may cause harmful conditions or illnesses in humans.
pediculosis capitis	Skin disease caused by infestation of head lice.
phenolics	Powerful tuberculocidal disinfectants.
porous	Absorbent, having pores or openings.
quaternary ammonium compounds	Type of disinfectant solution safe for all uses in the salon; commonly called quats.
sanitation or sanitizing	Cleaning to remove all visible residue and matter.
scabies	Contagious skin disease that is caused by the itch mite, which burrows under the skin.
single-use or disposable	Disposable items that cannot be used more than once, either because they cannot be cleaned of all visible residue (such as pumice stones used for pedicures), or because cleaning and disinfecting damages them.
sodium hypochlorite	Common household bleach; disinfectant for salon use.
spirilla	Spiral or corkscrew-shaped bacteria that can cause diseases such as syphilis and Lyme disease.
staphylococci	Pus-forming bacteria that grow in clusters like bunches of grapes, can cause abscesses, pustules and boils.
sterilization	Process that completely destroys all microbial life, including spores.
streptococci	Pus-forming bacteria arranged in curved lines resembling a string of beads; they can cause infections such as strep throat and blood poisoning.
tuberculocidal	Disinfectants that kill the bacteria that cause tuberculosis.
Universal Precautions	Set of guidelines published by the Occupational Safety and Health Administration that requires the employer and employee to assume that all human blood and body fluids contain pathogens and are thus infectious.
virucidal	Capable of destroying viruses.
virus	Microorganism that can invade plants and animals, including bacteria.

CHAPTER 6 GENERAL ANATOMY AND PHYSIOLOGY

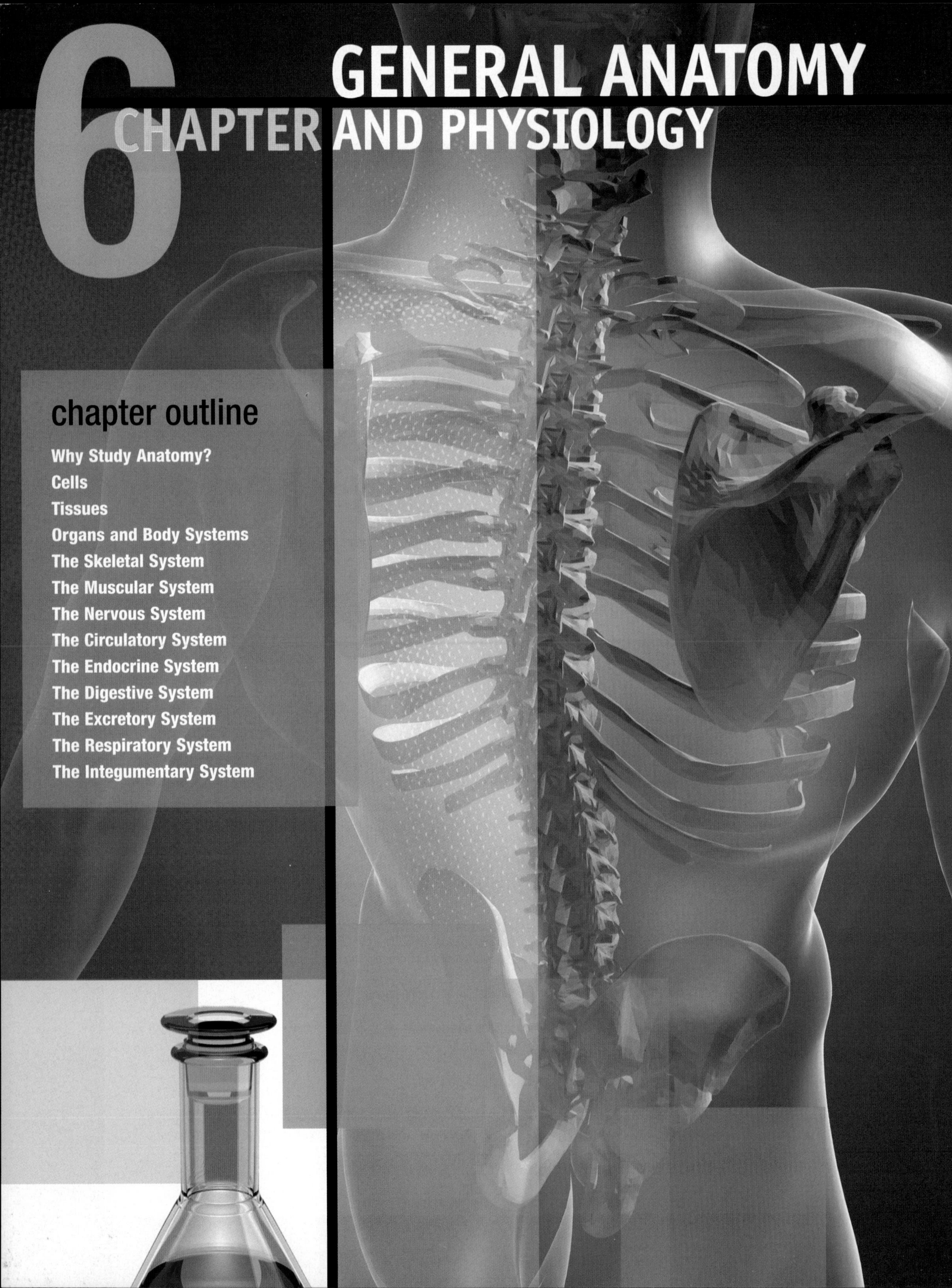

chapter outline

Learning Objectives

After completing this chapter, you will be able to:

- **Explain the importance of anatomy and physiology to the cosmetology profession.**
- **Describe cells, their structure, and their reproduction.**
- **Define tissue and identify the types of tissues found in the body.**
- **Name the 10 main body systems and explain their basic functions.**

Key Terms

Page number indicates where in the chapter the term is used.

abductors **pg. 98**
abductor hallucis **pg. 99**
adductors **pg. 98**
anabolism **pg. 88**
anatomy **pg. 87**
angular artery **pg. 106**
anterior auricular artery **pg. 107**
anterior tibial artery **pg. 107**
anterior tibial nerve **pg. 103**
arteries **pg. 105**
atrium **pg. 104**
auricularis anterior **pg. 96**
auricularis posterior **pg. 96**
auricularis superior **pg. 96**
auriculotemporal nerve **pg. 101**
autonomic nervous system **pg. 100**
axon **pg. 100**
belly (muscle) **pg. 95**
bicep **pg. 98**
blood **pg. 105**
blood vascular system **pg. 103**
body systems **pg. 89**
brain **pg. 100**
buccal nerve **pg. 102**
buccinator muscle **pg. 97**
capillaries **pg. 105**
cardiac muscle **pg. 94**
carpus **pg. 93**
catabolism **pg. 89**
cell membrane **pg. 88**
cells **pg. 87**
central nervous system **pg. 99**
cervical cutaneous nerve **pg. 102**
cervical nerves **pg. 102**
cervical verterbrae **pg. 92**
circulatory system **pg. 103**
clavicle **pg. 92**
common carotid artery **pg. 106**
common peroneal nerve **pg. 102**
connective tissue **pg. 89**
corrugator muscle **pg. 96**
cranium **pg. 91**
cytoplasm **pg. 88**
deep peroneal nerve **pg. 103**
deltoid **pg. 98**
dendrites **pg. 100**
depressor labii inferioris muscle **pg. 97**
diaphragm **pg. 109**
digestive system **pg. 108**
digits **pg. 93**
digital nerve **pg. 102**
dorsal **pg. 103**
dorsal cutaneous nerve **pg. 103**
dorsalis pedis artery **pg. 107**
endocrine (ductless) glands **pg. 108**
endocrine system **pg. 108**
epicranial aponeurosis **pg. 95**
epicranius **pg. 95**
epithelial tissue **pg. 89**
ethmoid bone **pg. 91**
excretory system **pg. 108**
exhalation **pg. 109**
exocrine (duct) glands **pg. 108**
extensors **pg. 98**
extensor digitorum brevis **pg. 99**
extensor digitorum longus **pg. 98**
external carotid artery **pg. 106**
external jugular vein **pg. 107**
facial artery **pg. 106**
femur **pg. 93**
fibula **pg. 93**
fifth cranial nerve **pg. 101**
flexors **pg. 98**
flexor digitorum brevis **pg. 99**
frontal artery **pg. 107**
frontal bone **pg. 91**
frontalis **pg. 95**
gastrocnemius **pg. 99**
glands **pg. 108**
greater auricular nerve **pg. 102**
greater occipital nerve **pg. 102**
heart **pg. 104**
hemoglobin **pg. 105**
histology **pg. 87**

Aside from medical practitioners, few professionals are licensed to actually touch people as part of their services. When performing cosmetology services, you are touching your clients in ways that few other people have ever done.

While understanding human anatomy overall is important, cosmetology is primarily restricted to the muscles, nerves, circulatory system, and bones of the head, face, neck, arms, hands, lower legs, and feet. Understanding these areas of anatomy will help you develop beneficial facial and massage techniques that can be used during facials or as part of a shampoo ritual at the shampoo station. Knowing the bones of the skull is important in the design of flattering hairstyles that gracefully drape the head, and for the skillful application of cosmetics.

WHY STUDY ANATOMY?

As a beauty professional, an overview of human anatomy and physiology will enable you to:

- Understand how the human body functions as an integrated whole.
- Recognize changes from the norm.
- Determine a scientific basis for the proper application of services and products such as scalp manipulations, facials, and hand and arm massages.

Anatomy is the study of the structures of the human body that can be seen with the naked eye, and what they are made up of. It is the science of the structure of organisms, or of their parts.

Physiology (fiz-ih-OL-oh-jee) is the study of the functions and activities performed by the body structures.

Histology (his-TAHL-uh-jee) is the study of the tiny structures found in living tissue, that is, microscopic anatomy.

CELLS

Cells are the basic units of all living things, from bacteria to plants and animals, and including human beings. Without cells, life does not exist. As a basic functional unit, the cell is responsible for carrying on all life

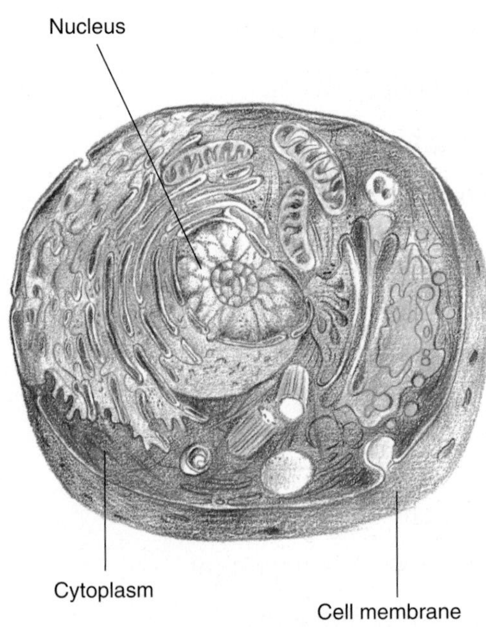

Figure 6–1 Anatomy of the cell.

processes. There are trillions of cells in the human body, and they vary widely in size, shape, and purpose.

BASIC CONSTRUCTION OF THE CELL

The cells of all living things are composed of a substance called **protoplasm** (PROH-toh-plaz-um), a colorless jelly-like substance in which food elements such as proteins, fats, carbohydrates, mineral salts, and water are present. You can visualize the protoplasm of a cell as being similar to the white of a raw egg. In addition to protoplasm, most cells also include the following (Figure 6-1):

The **nucleus** (NOO-klee-us) is the dense, active protoplasm found in the center of the cell. It plays an important part in cell reproduction and metabolism. You can visualize the nucleus as the yolk of a raw egg.

The **cytoplasm** (sy-toh-PLAZ-um) is all the protoplasm of a cell that surrounds the nucleus. It is the watery fluid that cells need for growth, reproduction, and self-repair.

The **cell membrane** acts like a balloon to contain the protoplasm, and allows certain types of substances to pass through its walls.

CELL REPRODUCTION AND DIVISION

Cells have the ability to reproduce, thus providing new cells for the growth and replacement of worn or injured ones. Most cells reproduce by dividing into two identical cells called daughter cells. This reproduction process is known as **mitosis** (my-TOH-sis). As long as conditions are favorable, the cell will grow and reproduce. This is true of human cells, plant cells, and single-cell creatures such as bacteria. Favorable conditions include an adequate supply of food, oxygen, and water; suitable temperatures; and the ability to eliminate waste products. If conditions become unfavorable, the cell will become impaired or may die. Unfavorable conditions include toxins (poison) and disease.

CELL METABOLISM

Metabolism (muh-TAB-uh-liz-um) is a chemical process that takes place in living organisms, whereby the cells are nourished and carry out their activities. Metabolism has two phases.

Anabolism (uh-NAB-uh-liz-um) is constructive metabolism, the process of building up larger molecules from smaller ones. During this process, the body stores water, food, and oxygen for the time when these substances will be needed for cell growth, reproduction, or repair.

Catabolism (kuh-TAB-uh-liz-um) is the phase of metabolism that involves the breaking down of complex compounds within the cells into smaller ones. This process releases energy that has been stored.

Anabolism and catabolism are carried out simultaneously and continually within the cells as part of their normal processes.

TISSUES

A **tissue** (TISH-oo) is a collection of similar cells that perform a particular function. Each tissue has a specific function and can be recognized by its characteristic appearance. Body tissues are composed of large amounts of water, along with various other substances. There are five types of tissue in the body.

- **Connective tissue** serves to support, protect, and bind together other tissues of the body. Examples of connective tissue are bone, cartilage, ligaments, tendons, fascia (which separates muscles), and fat or adipose tissue.
- **Epithelial tissue** (ep-ih-THEE-lee-ul) is a protective covering on body surfaces. Skin, mucous membranes, and the lining of the heart, digestive, respiratory organs, and glands are all examples of epithelial tissue.
- **Liquid tissue,** such as blood and lymph, carries food, waste products, and hormones through the body.
- **Muscular tissue** contracts and moves the various parts of the body.
- **Nerve tissue** carries messages to and from the brain and controls and coordinates all bodily functions. Nerve tissue is composed of special cells known as neurons, which make up the nerves, brain, and spinal cord.

ORGANS AND BODY SYSTEMS

Organs are groups of tissues designed to perform a specific function. Table 6-1 lists some of the most important organs of the body.

Body systems are groups of bodily organs acting together to perform one or more functions. The human body is composed of 10 major systems (Table 6-2).

ORGAN	Function
brain	controls the body
eyes	control vision
heart	circulates the blood
kidneys	excrete water and waste products
lungs	supply oxygen to the blood
liver	removes toxic products of digestion
skin	forms external protective covering of the body
stomach and intestines	digest food

Table 6-1 Some Major Body Organs and Their Functions

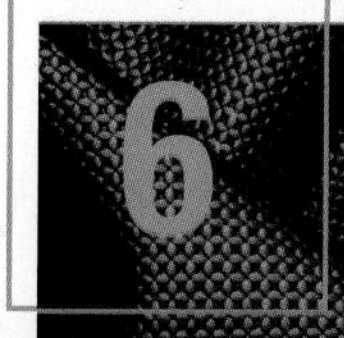

SYSTEM	Function
circulatory	controls the steady circulation of the blood through the body by means of the heart and blood vessels
digestive	changes food into nutrients and wastes; consists of mouth, stomach, intestines, salivary and gastric glands, and other organs
endocrine	affects the growth, development, sexual activities, and health of the entire body; consists of specialized glands
excretory	purifies the body by the elimination of waste matter; consists of kidneys, liver, skin, intestines, and lungs
integumentary	serves as a protective covering and helps in regulating the body's temperature; consists of skin, accessory organs such as oil and sweat glands, sensory receptors, hair, and nails
muscular	covers, shapes, and supports the skeleton tissue; also contracts and moves various parts of the body; consists of muscles
nervous	controls and coordinates all other systems and makes them work harmoniously and efficiently; consists of brain, spinal cord, and nerves
reproductive	responsible for processes by which plants and animals produce offspring
respiratory	enables breathing, supplying the body with oxygen, and eliminating carbon dioxide as a waste product; consists of lungs and air passages
skeletal	physical foundation of the body; consists of the bones and movable and immovable joints

Table 6-2 Body Systems and Their Functions

THE SKELETAL SYSTEM

The **skeletal system** is the physical foundation of the body. It is composed of 206 bones that vary in size and shape and are connected by movable and immovable joints. **Osteology** (ahs-tee-AHL-oh-jee) is the study of anatomy, structure, and function of the bones. **Os** means "bone," and is used as a prefix in many medical terms, such as osteoarthritis, a joint disease.

Except for the tissue that forms the major part of the teeth, bone is the hardest tissue in the body. It is composed of connective tissue consisting of about one-third organic matter, such as cells and blood, and two-thirds minerals, mainly calcium carbonate and calcium phosphate.

The primary functions of the skeletal system are to:

- Give shape and support to the body

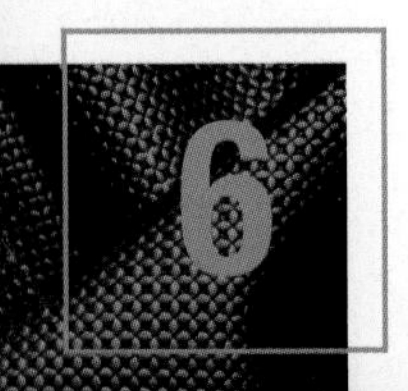

- Protect various internal structures and organs
- Serve as attachments for muscles and act as levers to produce body movement
- Help produce both white and red blood cells (one of the functions of bone marrow)
- Store most of the body's calcium supply as well as phosphorus, magnesium, and sodium

A **joint** is the connection between two or more bones of the skeleton. There are two types of joints: movable, such as elbows, knees, and hips; and immovable, such as the pelvis or skull, which allows little or no movement.

BONES OF THE SKULL

The skull is the skeleton of the head and is divided into two parts: the **cranium** (KRAY-nee-um), an oval, bony case that protects the brain; and the facial skeleton, which is made up of 14 bones (Figure 6-2).

BONES OF THE CRANIUM

The following are the cranium's eight bones:

- **Occipital bone** (ahk-SIP-ih-tul). Hindmost bone of the skull, below the parietal bones; forms the back of the skull above the nape.
- Two **parietal bones** (puh-RY-uh-tul). Form the sides and crown (top) of the cranium.
- **Frontal bone** (FRUNT-ul). Forms the forehead.
- Two **temporal bones** (TEM-puh-rul). Form the sides of the head in the ear region.
- **Ethmoid bone** (ETH-moyd). Light spongy bone between the eye sockets and forms part of the nasal cavities.
- **Sphenoid bone** (SFEEN-oyd). Joins all of the bones of the cranium together.

The ethmoid and sphenoid bones are not affected by massage.

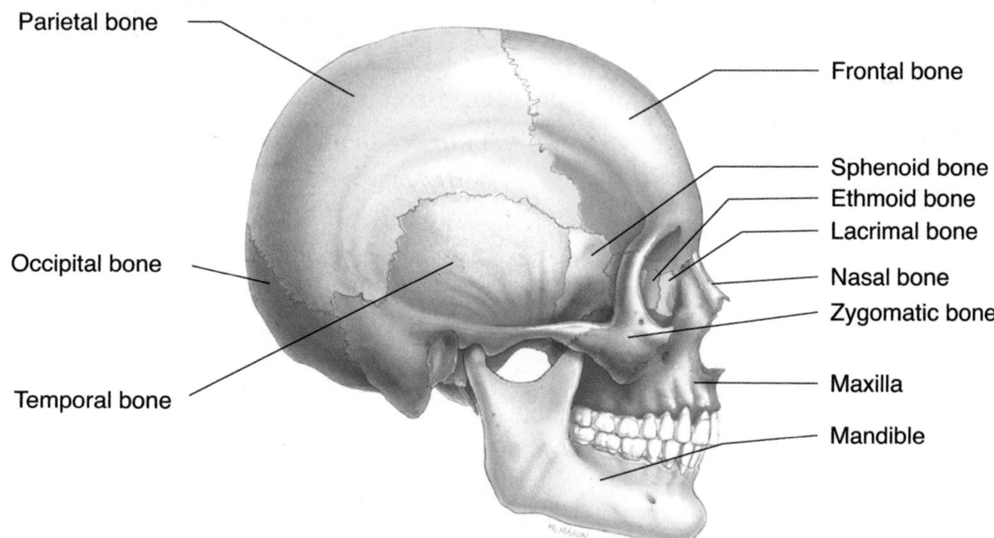

Figure 6-2 Bones of the cranium, face, and neck.

BONES OF THE FACE

Of the 14 bones of the face the bones involved in facial massage include:

- Two **nasal bones** (NAY-zul). They form the bridge of the nose.
- Two **lacrimal bones** (LAK-ruh-mul). Small, thin bones located at the front inner wall of the orbits (eye sockets).
- Two **zygomatic or malar bones** (zy-goh-MAT-ik). Form the prominence of the cheeks; cheekbones.
- Two **maxillae** (mak-SIL-ee). Bones of the upper jaw (singular: maxilla).
- **Mandible** (MAN-duh-bul). Lower jawbone; largest and strongest bone of the face.

The remaining facial bones are not recognized when performing services or massage and do not appear in Figure 6-2:

- Two **turbinal** (TUR-bih-nahl) **bones** (also referred to as turbinate bones). Thin layers of spongy bone on either of the outer walls of the nasal depression.
- **Vomer** (VO-mer) **bone**. Flat thin bone that forms part of the nasal septum.
- Two **palatine bones**. Forms the floor and outer wall of the nose, roof of the mouth, and floor of the orbits.

BONES OF THE NECK

The main bones of the neck follow:

- **Hyoid bone** (HY-oyd). U-shaped bone at the base of the tongue that supports the tongue and its muscles.
- **Cervical vertebrae** (SUR-vih-kul VURT-uh-bray). The seven bones of the top part of the vertebral column located in the neck region (Figure 6-3).

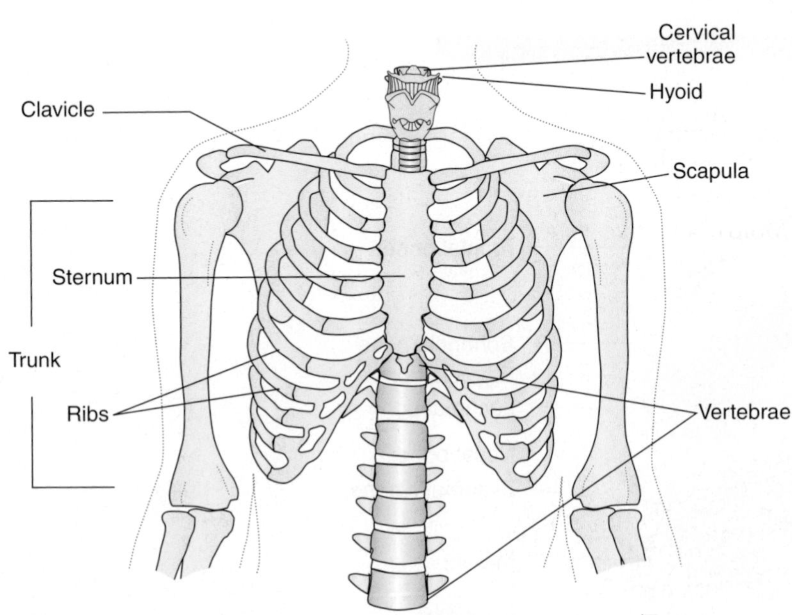

Figure 6-3 Bones of the neck, shoulder, and back.

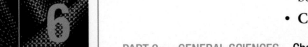

BONES OF THE CHEST, SHOULDER, AND BACK

The bones of the trunk or torso are comprised of:

- **Thorax** (THOR-aks). The chest; elastic, bony cage that serves as a protective framework for the heart, lungs, and other internal organs.
- **Ribs**. Twelve pairs of bones forming the wall of the thorax.
- **Scapula** (SKAP-yuh-luh). One of a pair of shoulder blades; a large, flat, triangular bone of the shoulder.
- **Sternum** (STUR-num). Breastbone; flat bone that forms the ventral (front) support of the ribs.
- **Clavicle**. Collarbone; bone that joins the sternum and scapula.

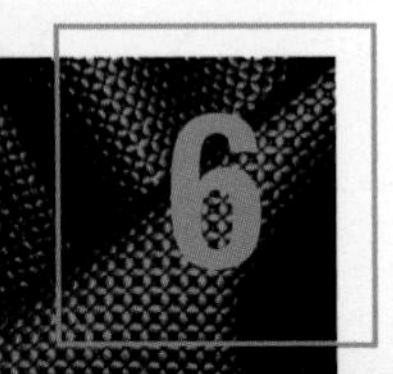

BONES OF THE ARMS AND HANDS

The important bones of the shoulder, arms, and hands that you should know about (Figures 6-4 and 6-5) include the following:

Humerus (HYOO-muh-rus). Uppermost and largest bone of the arm, extending from the elbow to the shoulder.

Ulna (UL-nuh). Inner and larger bone of the forearm (lower arm), attached to the wrist and located on the side of the little finger.

Radius (RAY-dee-us). Smaller bone in the forearm (lower arm) on the same side as the thumb.

Carpus (KAR-pus). The wrist; flexible joint composed of a group of eight small, irregular bones (carpals) held together by ligaments.

Metacarpus (met-uh-KAR-pus). Bones of the palm of the hand; parts of the hand containing five bones between the carpus and phalanges.

Phalanges (fuh-LAN-jeez). Bones in the fingers, or **digits** (also the toes), consisting of three bones in each finger and two in each thumb, totaling 14 bones.

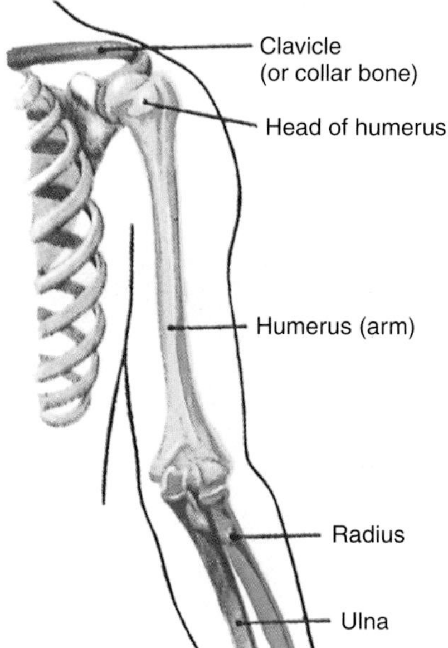

Figure 6–4 Bones of the arm.

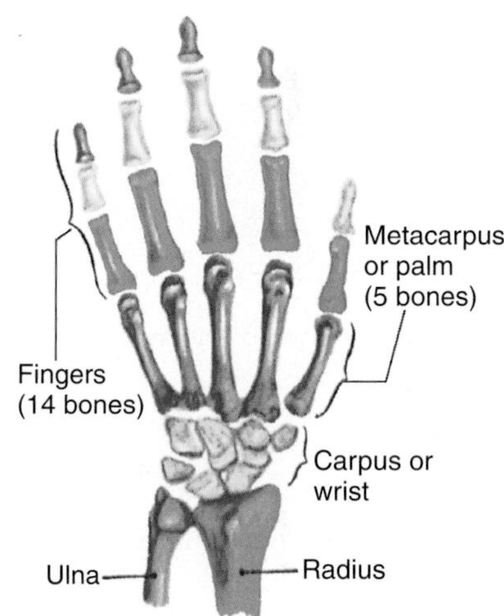

Figure 6–5 Bones of the hand.

BONES OF THE LEG AND FOOT

The **femur** (FEE-mur) is a heavy, long bone that forms the leg above the knee.

The **tibia** (TIB-ee-ah) is the larger of the two bones that form the leg below the knee. The tibia may be visualized as a "bump" on the big-toe side of the ankle.

The **fibula** (FIB-ya-lah) is the smaller of the two bones that form the leg below the knee. The fibula may be visualized as a "bump" on the little-toe side of the ankle.

The **patella** (pah-TEL-lah), also called the accessory bone, forms the knee cap joint (Figure 6-6).

The ankle joint is made up of three bones. The ankle joint is formed by the tibia, fibula, and the **talus** (TA-lus) or ankle bone of the foot.

The foot is made up of 26 bones. These can be subdivided into three general categories: seven **tarsal** (TAHR-sul) bones (talus, calcaneous, navicular, three cuneiform bones, and the cuboid), and five **metatarsal** (met-ah-TAHR-sul) bones, which are long and slender, like the metacarpal bones of the hand, and 14 bones called phalanges, which compose the toes.

The phalanges are similar to the finger bones. There are three phalanges in each toe, except for the big toe, which has only two (Figure 6-7).

THE MUSCULAR SYSTEM

The **muscular system** is the body system that covers, shapes, and supports the skeleton tissue. It contracts and moves various parts of the body.

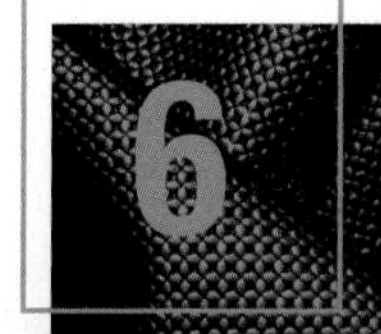

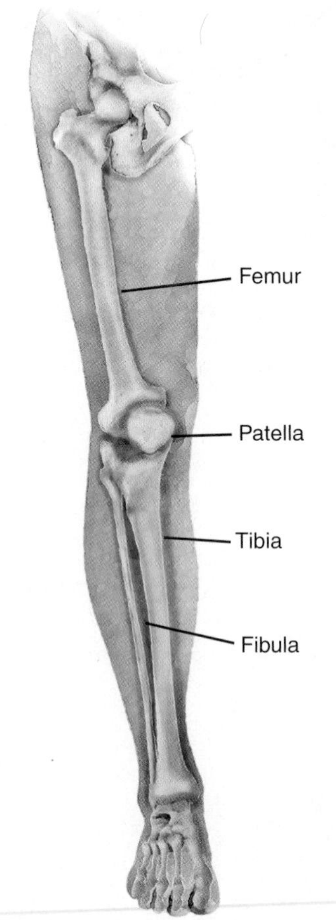

Figure 6-6 Bones of the leg.

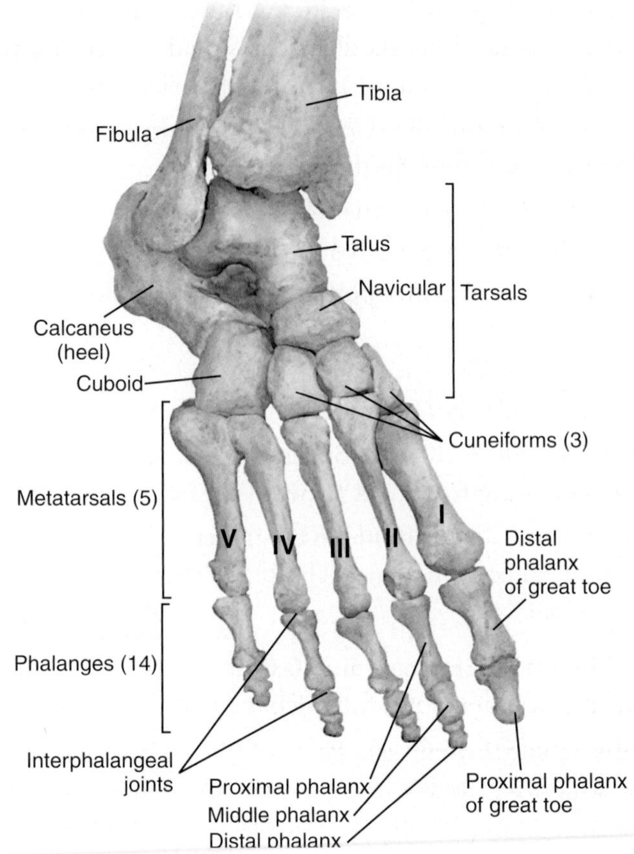

Figure 6-7 Bones of the foot and ankle.

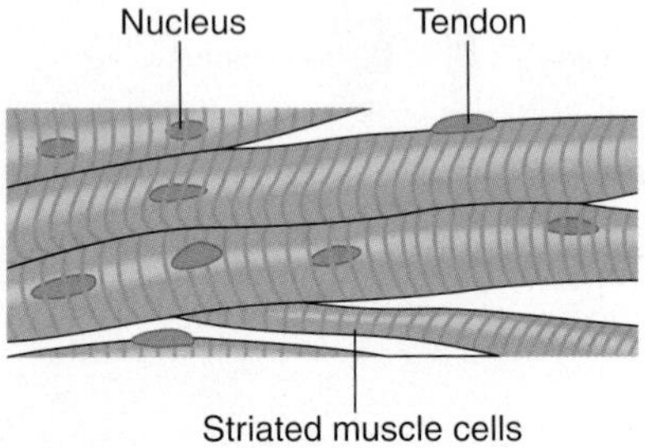

Figure 6-8 Striated muscles.

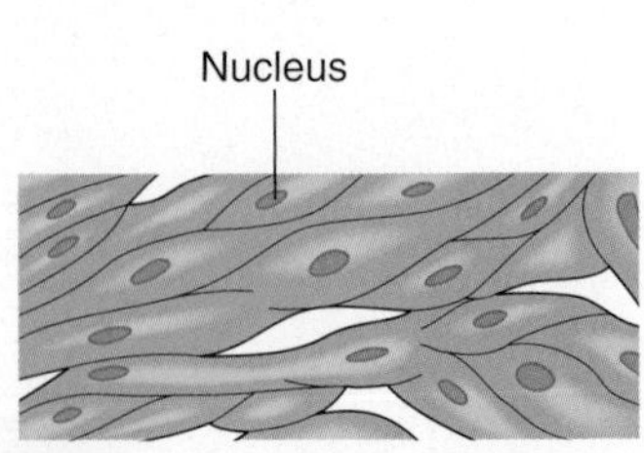
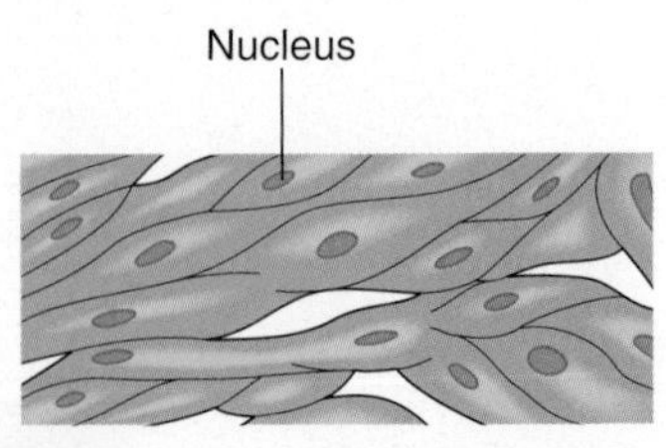

Figure 6-9 Nonstriated muscles.

The cosmetologist must be concerned with the voluntary muscles that control movements of the arms, hands, lower legs, and feet. It is important to know where these muscles are located and what they control.

Myology (my-AHL-uh-jee) is the study of the structure, function, and diseases of the muscles. The human body has over 600 muscles, which are responsible for approximately 40 percent of the body's weight. Muscles are fibrous tissues that have the ability to stretch and contract according to demands of the body's movements. There are three types of muscular tissue.

Striated muscles (STRY-ayt-ed), also called skeletal muscles, are attached to the bones and are voluntary or consciously controlled. Striated (skeletal) muscles assist in maintaining the body's posture, and protect some internal organs (Figure 6-8).

Nonstriated muscles, or smooth muscles, are involuntary and function automatically, without conscious will. These muscles are found in the internal organs of the body, such as the digestive or respiratory systems (Figure 6-9).

Cardiac muscle is the involuntary muscle that is the heart. This type of muscle is not found in any other part of the body (Figure 6-10).

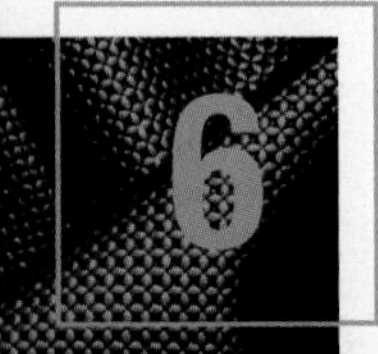

A muscle has three parts. The **origin** is the part that does not move; it is attached to the skeleton and is usually part of a skeletal muscle. The **insertion** is the part of the muscle at the more movable attachment to the skeleton. The **belly** is the middle part of the muscle. Pressure in massage is usually directed from the insertion to the origin.

Muscular tissue can be stimulated by:

- Massage (hand or electric vibrator)
- Electrical current (high frequency or faradic current)
- Light (infrared or ultraviolet)
- Dry heat (heating lamps or heating caps)
- Moist heat (steamers or moderately warm steam towels)
- Nerve impulses (through the nervous system)
- Chemicals (certain acids and salts)

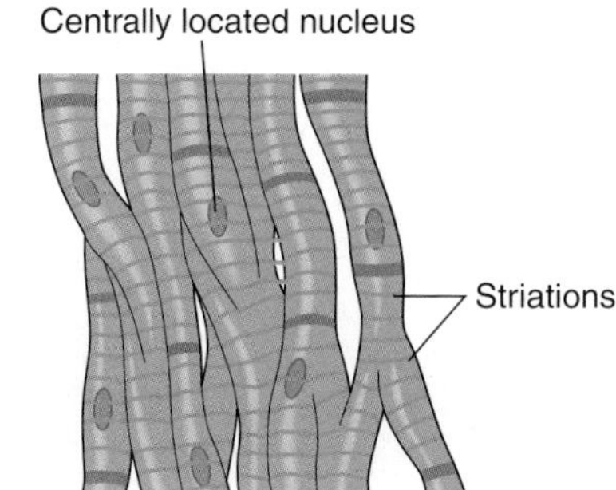

Figure 6–10 Cardiac muscle cells.

MUSCLES OF THE SCALP

- **Epicranius** (ep-ih-KRAY-nee-us) or occipito-frontalis (ahk-SIP-ih-tohfrun- TAY-lus). The broad muscle that covers the top of the skull consists of the occipitalis and frontalis.
- **Occipitalis** (ahk-SIP-i-tahl-is). Back of the epicranius; muscle that draws the scalp backward.
- **Frontalis** (frun-TAY-lus). Anterior (front) portion of the epicranius; muscle of the scalp that raises the eyebrows, draws the scalp forward, and causes wrinkles across the forehead.
- **Epicranial aponeurosis** (ep-ih-KRAY-nee-al ap-uh-noo-ROH-sus). Tendon that connects the occipitalis and frontalis (Figure 6-11).

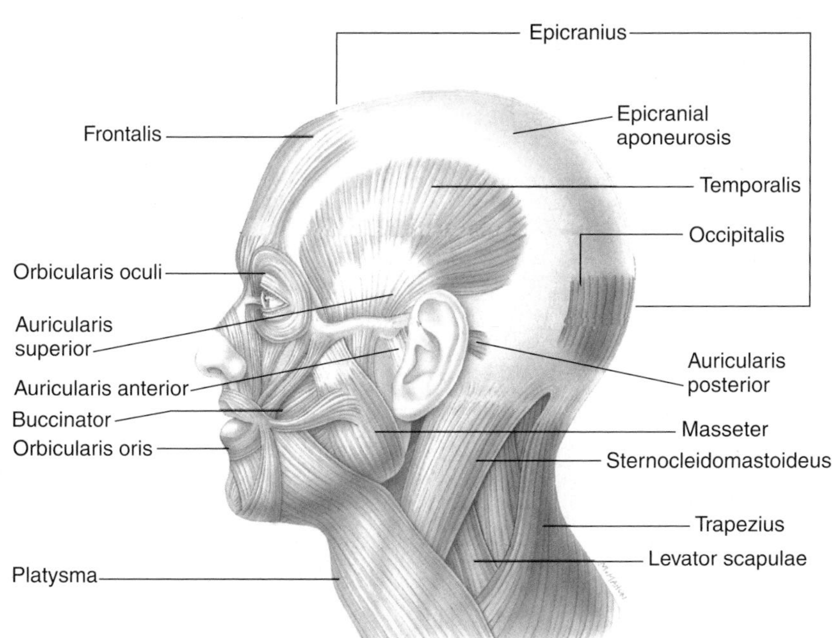

Figure 6–11 Muscles of the head, face, and neck.

MUSCLES OF THE EAR

Three muscles of the ear have no function (although some people can contract them to move the ears).

- **Auricularis superior** (aw-rik-yuh-LAIR-is). Muscle above the ear that draws the ear upward.
- **Auricularis anterior**. Muscle in front of the ear that draws the ear forward.
- **Auricularis posterior**. Muscle behind the ear that draws the ear backward.

MUSCLES OF MASTICATION (CHEWING)

The **masseter** (muh-SEE-tur) and the **temporalis** (tem-poh-RAY-lis) muscles coordinate in opening and closing the mouth, and are sometimes referred to as chewing muscles.

MUSCLES OF THE NECK

- **Platysma** (plah-TIZ-muh) **muscle**. Broad muscle extending from the chest and shoulder muscles to the side of the chin; responsible for lowering the lower jaw and lip.
- **Sternocleidomastoideus** (STUR-noh-KLEE-ih-doh-mas-TOYD-ee-us). Muscle of the neck that lowers and rotates the head.

MUSCLES OF THE EYEBROW

- **Corrugator muscle** (KOR-oo-gay-tohr). Muscle located beneath the frontalis and orbicularis oculi that draws the eyebrow down and wrinkles the forehead vertically (Figure 6-12).
- **Orbicularis oculi** (or-bik-yuh-LAIR-is AHK-yuh-lye) **muscle**. Ring muscle of the eye socket; enables you to close your eyes.

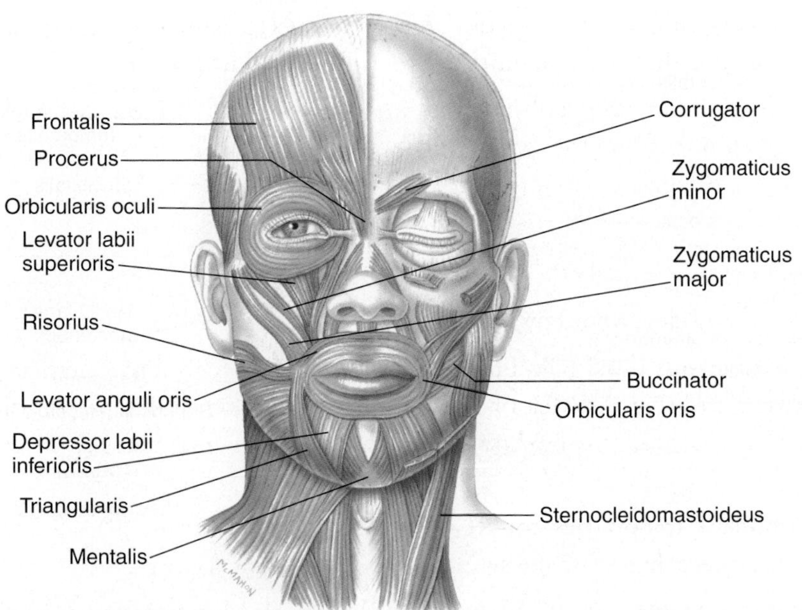

Figure 6-12 Muscles of the face.

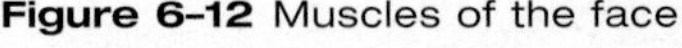

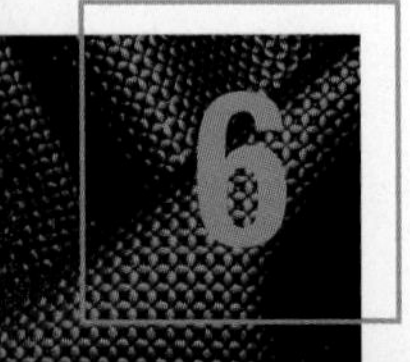

MUSCLES OF THE NOSE

- **Procerus** (proh-SEE-rus). Covers the bridge of the nose, lowers the eyebrows, and causes wrinkles across the bridge of the nose.
- Other nasal muscles that contract and expand the openings of the nostrils.

MUSCLES OF THE MOUTH

Important ones to know follow:

- **Buccinator** (BUK-sih-nay-tur) **muscle**. Thin, flat muscle of the cheek between the upper and lower jaw that compresses the cheeks and expels air between the lips.
- **Depressor labii inferioris** (dee-PRES-ur LAY-bee-eye in-FEER-ee-or-us) **muscle**. Also known as quadratus labii inferioris, a muscle surrounding the lower lip; lowers the lower lip and draws it to one side, as in expressing sarcasm.
- **Levator anguli oris** (lih-VAYT-ur ANG-yoo-ly OH-ris). Also known as caninus (kay-NY-nus), a muscle that raises the angle of the mouth and draws it inward.
- **Levator labii superioris** (lih-VAYT-ur LAY-bee-eye soo-peer-ee-OR-is). Also known as quadratus (kwah-DRA-tus) labii superioris, a muscle surrounding the upper lip; elevates the upper lip and dilates the nostrils, as in expressing distaste.
- **Mentalis** (men-TAY-lis). Muscle that elevates the lower lip and raises and wrinkles the skin of the chin.
- **Orbicularis oris** (or-bik-yuh-LAIR-is OH-ris) **muscle**. Flat band around the upper and lower lips that compresses, contracts, puckers, and wrinkles the lips.
- **Risorius** (rih-ZOR-ee-us). Muscle of the mouth that draws the corner of the mouth out and back, as in grinning.
- **Triangularis** (try-ang-gyuh-LAY-rus). Muscle extending alongside the chin that pulls down the corner of the mouth.
- **Zygomaticus** (zy-goh-MAT-ih-kus) major and minor. Muscles extending from the zygomatic bone to the angle of the mouth; elevate the lip, as in laughing.

MUSCLES THAT ATTACH THE ARMS TO THE BODY

These muscles are briefly summarized below.

Latissimus dorsi (lah-TIS-ih-mus DOR-see). Broad, flat superficial muscle covering the back of the neck and upper and middle region of the back, controlling the shoulder blade and the swinging movements of the arm (Figure 6-13).

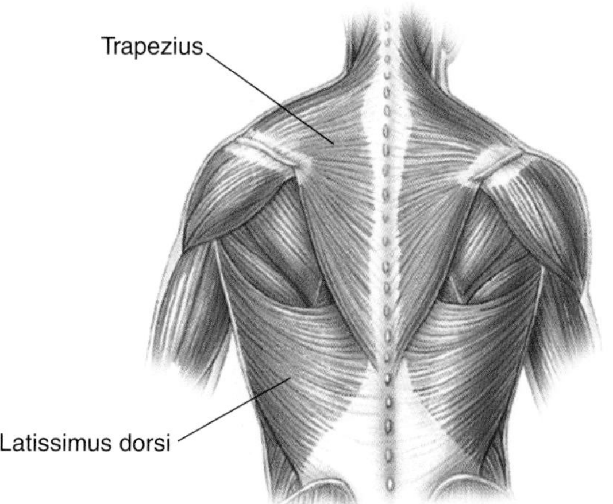

Figure 6-13 Muscles of the back and neck.

Pectoralis major (pek-tor-AL-is) and **pectoralis minor**. Muscles of the chest that assist the swinging movements of the arm.

Serratus anterior (ser-RAT-us an-TEER-ee-or). Muscle of the chest that assists in breathing and in raising the arm (Figure 6-14).

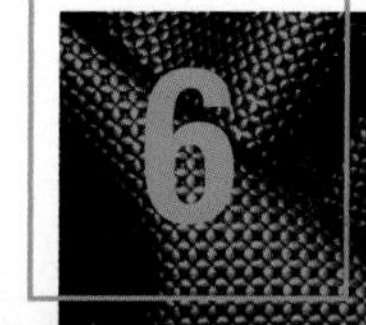

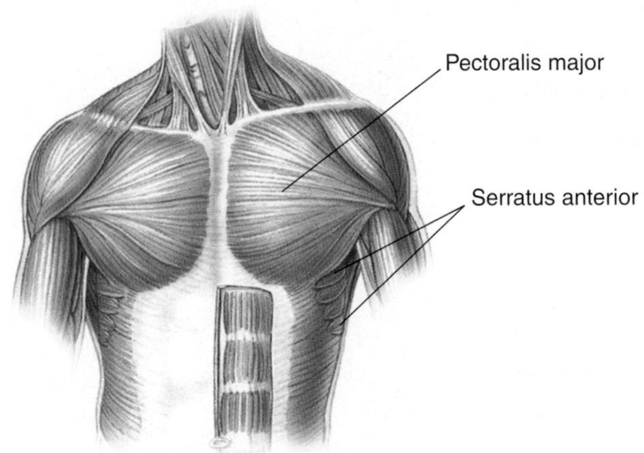

Figure 6-14 Muscles of the chest.

Trapezius (trah-PEE-zee-us). Muscle that covers the back of the neck and upper and middle region of the back; rotates and controls swinging movements of the arm.

MUSCLES OF THE SHOULDER AND ARM

There are three principal muscles of the shoulders and upper arms (Figure 6-15):

Bicep (BY-sep). Muscle producing the contour of the front and inner side of the upper arm; they lift the forearm and flex the elbow.

Deltoid (DEL-toyd). Large, triangular muscle covering the shoulder joint that allows the arm to extend outward and to the side of the body.

Tricep (TRY-sep). Large muscle that covers the entire back of the upper arm and extends the forearm.

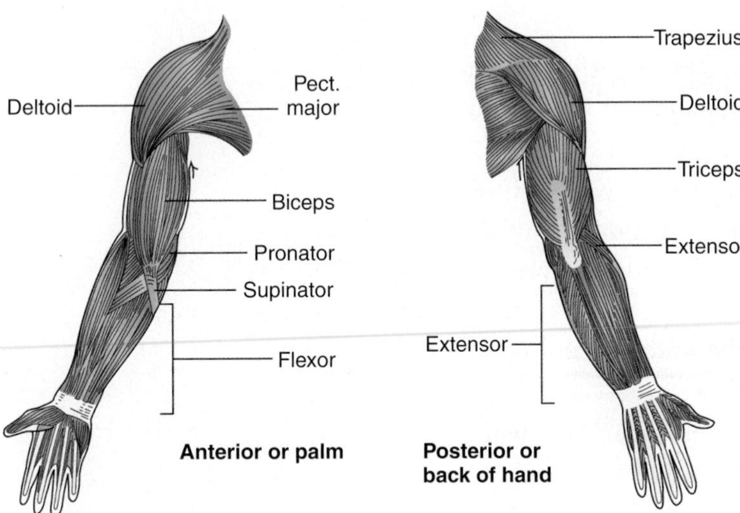

Figure 6-15 Muscles of the shoulder and arm.

The forearm is made up of a series of muscles and strong tendons. As a cosmetologist, you will be concerned with:

Extensors (ik-STEN-surs). Muscles that straighten the wrist, hand, and fingers to form a straight line.

Flexors (FLEK-surs). Extensor muscles of the wrist, involved in bending the wrist.

Pronators (proh-NAY-tohr). Muscles that turn the hand inward so that the palm faces downward.

Supinator (SOO-puh-nayt-ur). Muscle of the forearm that rotates the radius outward and the palm upward.

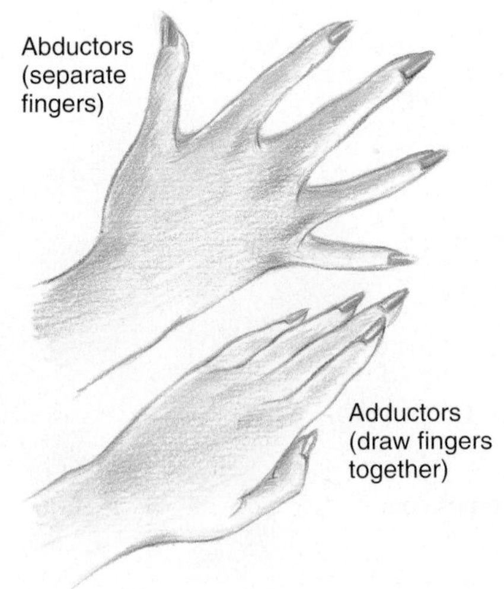

Figure 6-16 Muscles of the hand.

MUSCLES OF THE HAND

The hand is one of the most complex parts of the body, with many small muscles that overlap from joint to joint, providing flexibility and strength to open and close the hand and fingers. Important muscles to know include the:

Abductors (ab-DUK-turz). Muscles that separate the fingers (Figure 6-16).

Adductors (ah-DUK-turz). Muscles at the base of each finger that draw the fingers together.

MUSCLES OF THE LOWER LEG AND FOOT

As a practitioner, you will use your knowledge of the muscles of the foot and leg during a pedicure. The muscles of the foot are small and provide proper support and cushioning for the foot and leg (Figure 6-17).

The **extensor digitorum longus** (eck-STEN-sur-dij-it-TOHR-um LONG-us) bends the foot up and extends the toes.

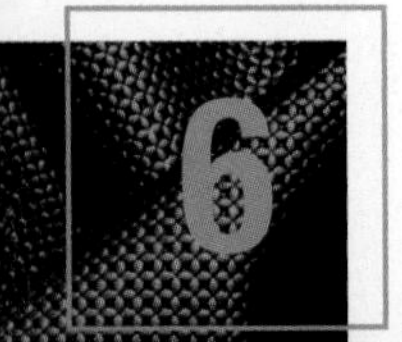

the hand from a hot object). Reflexes do not have to be learned; they are automatic.

NERVES OF THE HEAD, FACE, AND NECK

The largest of the cranial nerves is the **fifth cranial nerve,** also known as the *trifacial* (try-FAY-shul) or *trigeminal* (try-JEM-un-ul) nerve. It is the chief sensory nerve of the face, and serves as the motor nerve of the muscles that control chewing. It consists of three branches: **ophthalmic** (ahf-THALmik), **mandibular** (man-DIB-yuh-lur), and **maxillary** (MAK-suh-lair-ee) (Figure 6-21).

The following are the branches of the fifth cranial nerve that are affected by massage.

- **Auriculotemporal nerve** (aw-RIK-yuh-loh-TEM-puh-rul). Affects the external ear and skin above the temple, up to the top of the skull.
- **Infraorbital nerve** (in-fruh-OR-bih-tul). Affects the skin of the lower eyelid, side of the nose, upper lip, and mouth.
- **Infratrochlear nerve** (in-frah-TRAHK-lee-ur). Affects the membrane and skin of the nose.
- **Mental nerve**. Affects the skin of the lower lip and chin.
- **Nasal nerve** (NAY-zul). Affects the point and lower side of the nose.
- **Supraorbital nerve** (soo-pruh-OR-bih-tul). Affects the skin of the forehead, scalp, eyebrow, and upper eyelid.
- **Supratrochlear nerve** (soo-pruh-TRAHK-lee-ur). Affects the skin between the eyes and upper side of the nose.
- **Zygomatic nerve** (zy-goh-MAT-ik). Affects the muscles of the upper part of the cheek.

The seventh (facial) cranial nerve is the chief motor nerve of the face. It emerges near the lower part of the ear and extends to the muscles of the

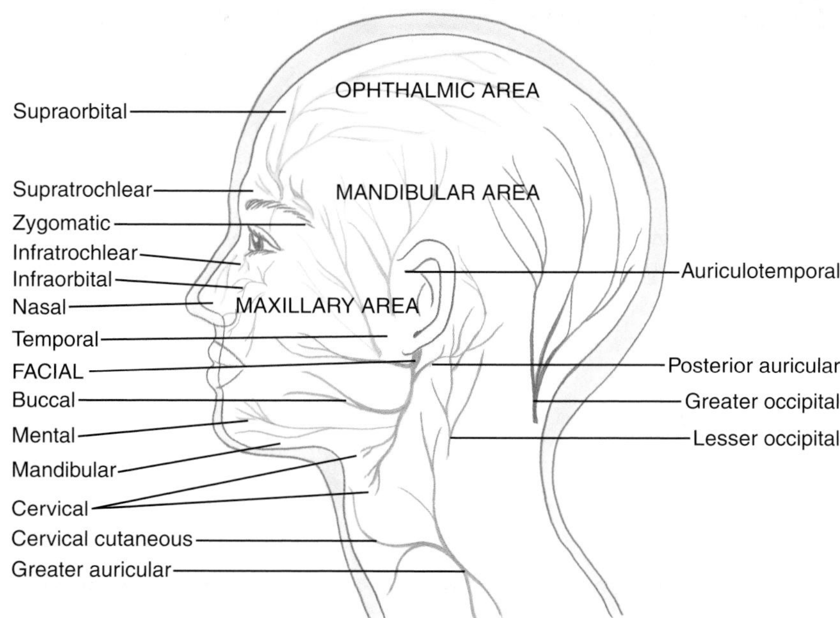

Figure 6-21 Nerves of the head, face and neck.

neck. Its divisions and their branches supply and control all the muscles of facial expression. The following are the most important branches of the facial nerve:

- **Posterior auricular nerve**. Affects the muscles behind the ear at the base of the skull.
- **Temporal nerve**. Affects the muscles of the temple, side of the forehead, eyebrow, eyelid, and upper part of the cheek.
- **Zygomatic nerve** (upper and lower). Affects the muscles of the upper part of the cheek.
- **Buccal nerve** (BUK-ul). Affects the muscles of the mouth.
- **Marginal mandibular nerve**. Affects the muscles of the chin and lower lip.
- **Cervical nerves** (SUR-vih-kul) (branches of the facial nerve). Affect the side of the neck and the platysma muscle.

Cervical nerves originate at the spinal cord, and their branches supply the muscles and scalp at the back of the head and neck, as follows:

- **Greater occipital nerve.** Located in the back of the head, affects the scalp as far up as the top of the head.
- **Smaller (lesser) occipital nerve.** Located at the base of the skull, affects the scalp and muscles behind the ear.
- **Greater auricular nerve.** Located at the side of the neck, affects the face, ears, neck, and parotid gland.
- **Cervical cutaneous nerve** (kyoo-TAY-nee-us). Located at the side of the neck, affects the front and sides of the neck as far down as the breastbone.

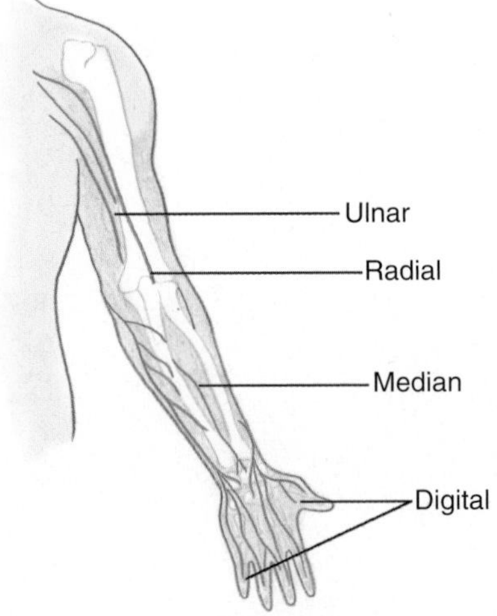

Figure 6-22 Nerves of the arm and hand.

NERVES OF THE ARM AND HAND

The principal nerves supplying the superficial parts of the arm and hand are as follows (Figure 6-22):

Digital nerve (DIJ-ut-tul) (sensory-motor), with its branches, supplies the fingers.

Radial nerve (RAY-dee-ul) (sensory-motor), with its branches, supplies the thumb side of the arm and back of the hand.

Median nerve (MEE-dee-un) (sensory-motor), smaller nerve than the ulnar and radial nerves that, with its branches, supplies the arm and hand.

Ulnar nerve (UL-nur) (sensory-motor), with its branches, affects the little finger side of the arm and palm of the hand.

NERVES OF THE LOWER LEG AND FOOT

The **tibial** (TIB-ee-al) **nerve,** a division of the sciatic nerve, passes behind the knee. It subdivides and supplies impulses to the knee, the muscles of the calf, the skin of the leg, and the sole, heel, and underside of the toes.

The **common peroneal** (per-oh-NEE-al) **nerve,** also a division of the sciatic nerve, extends from behind the knee to wind around the head of the fibula to the front of the leg where it divides into two branches. The

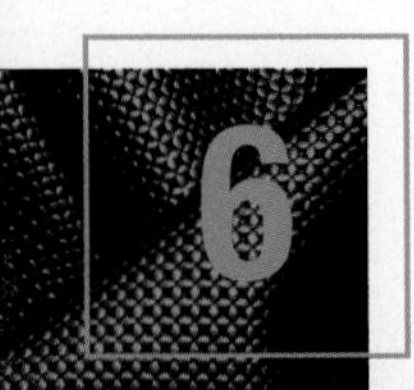

deep peroneal nerve, also known as the **anterior tibial nerve,** extends down to the front of the leg, behind the muscles. It supplies impulses to these muscles and also to the muscles and skin on the top of the foot and adjacent sides of the first and second toes. The **superficial peroneal nerve,** also known as the **musculocutaneous nerve,** extends down the leg, just under the skin, supplying impulses to the muscles and the skin of the leg, as well as to the skin and toes on the top of the foot, where it is called the dorsal (DOOR-sal) or **dorsal cutaneous nerve.**

The **saphenous** (sa-FEEN-us) **nerve** supplies impulses to the skin of the inner side of the leg and foot.

The **sural nerve** supplies impulses to the skin on the outer side and back of the foot and leg.

The **dorsal** (DOOR-sal) nerve supplies impulses to the skin on top of the foot (Figure 6-23).

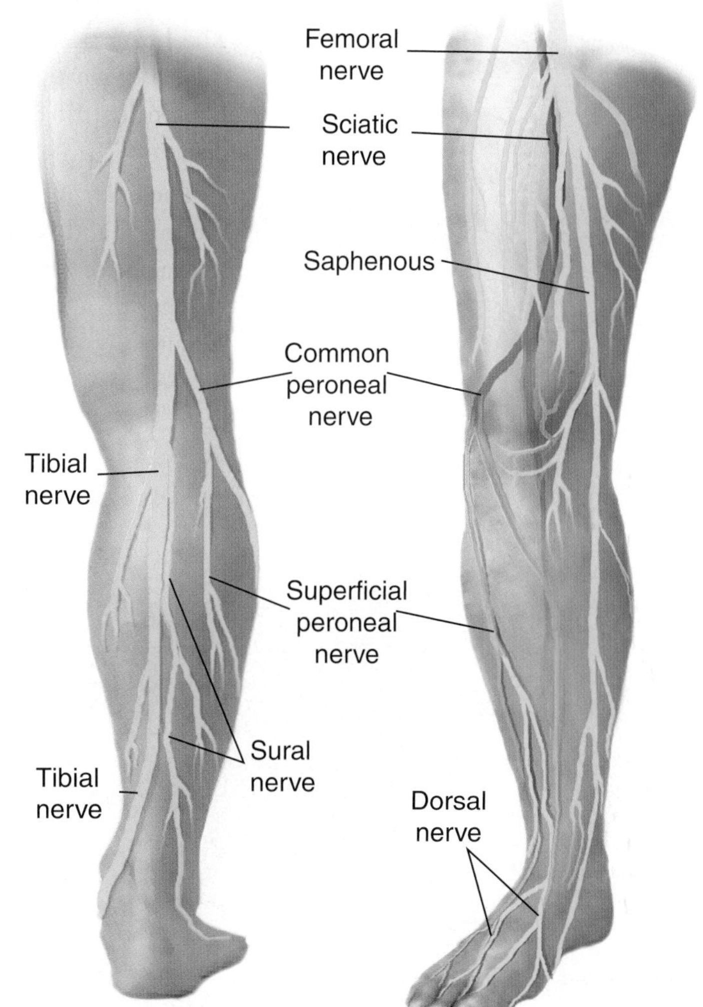

Figure 6-23 Nerves of the lower leg and foot.

THE CIRCULATORY SYSTEM

The **circulatory system**, also referred to as the cardiovascular or vascular system, controls the steady circulation of the blood through the body by means of the heart and blood vessels. The circulatory system is made up of two divisions:

The **blood vascular system**, which consists of the heart, arteries, veins, and capillaries for the distribution of blood throughout the body.

The **lymph vascular system** (LIMF VAS-kyoo-lur) or lymphatic system, which acts as an aid to the blood system and consists of the lymph, lymphatics (lymph vessels), lymph nodes, and other structures. **Lymph** is a clear yellowish fluid that circulates in the lymphatics of the body. It carries waste and impurities away from the cells.

THE HEART

The **heart** is often referred to as the body's pump. It is a muscular cone-shaped organ that keeps the blood moving within the circulatory system. It is enclosed by a membrane known as the **pericardium** (payr-ih-KAR-deeum).

The heart is the approximate size of a closed fist, weighs approximately 9 ounces, and is located in the chest cavity. The heartbeat is regulated by the vagus (tenth cranial) nerve and other nerves in the autonomic nervous system. In a normal resting state, the heart beats 72 to 80 times per minute.

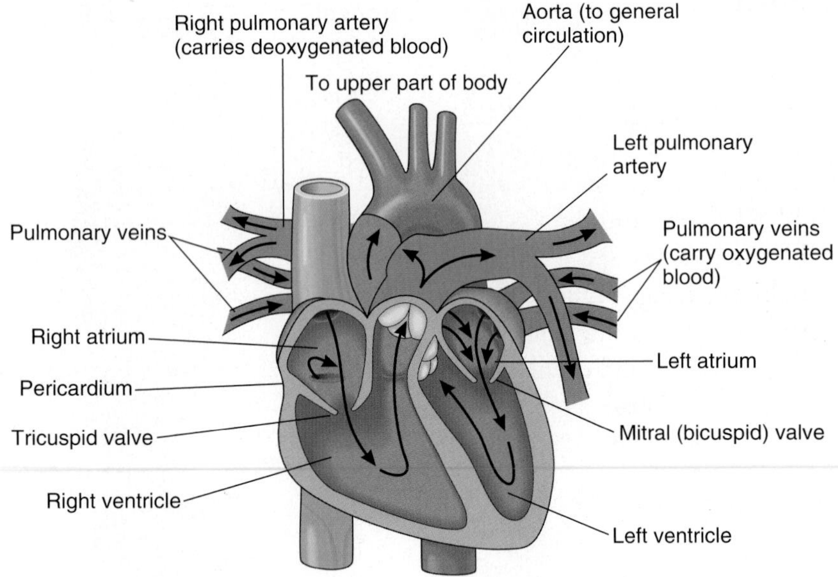

Figure 6-24 Anatomy of the heart.

The interior of the heart contains four chambers and four valves. The upper, thin-walled chambers are the right **atrium** (AY-tree-um) and left atrium. The lower, thick-walled chambers are the right **ventricle** (VENtruh-kul) and left ventricle. **Valves** between the chambers allow the blood to flow in only one direction. With each contraction and relaxation of the heart, the blood flows in, travels from the atria (plural of atrium) to the ventricles, and is then driven out, to be distributed all over the body (Figure 6-24).

The blood is in constant and continuous circulation from the time that it leaves the heart until it returns to the heart. Two systems attend to this circulation. **Pulmonary circulation** sends the blood from the heart to the lungs to be purified. **Systemic circulation** or general circulation carries the blood from the heart throughout the body and back to the heart. The following is an overview of how these systems work.

1. Blood flows from the body into the right atrium.
2. From the right atrium, it flows through the tricuspid valve into the right ventricle.
3. The right ventricle pumps the blood to the lungs, where it releases waste gases and receives oxygen. The blood is then considered to be oxygen rich.
4. The oxygen-rich blood returns to the heart, entering the left atrium.
5. From the left atrium, the blood flows through the mitral valve into the left ventricle.
6. The blood then leaves the left ventricle and travels to all parts of the body.

BLOOD VESSELS

The blood vessels are tube-like structures that include the arteries, capillaries, and veins. The function of these vessels is to transport blood to and from the heart, and then on to various tissues of the body.

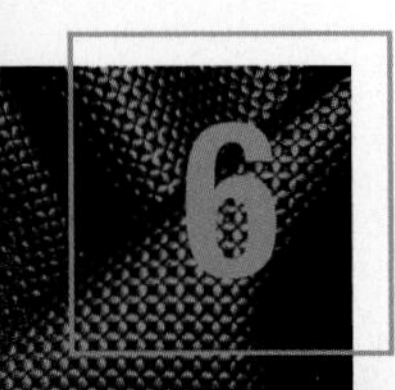

Arteries are thick-walled, muscular, flexible tubes that carry oxygenated blood away from the heart to the capillaries. The largest artery in the body is the aorta.

Capillaries are tiny, thin-walled blood vessels that connect the smaller arteries to the veins. They bring nutrients to the cells and carry away waste materials.

Veins are thin-walled blood vessels that are less elastic than arteries. They contain cup-like valves that prevent backflow and carry blood containing waste products from the various capillaries back toward the heart for cleaning and to pick up oxygen. Veins are located closer to the outer skin surface of the body than arteries (Figure 6-25).

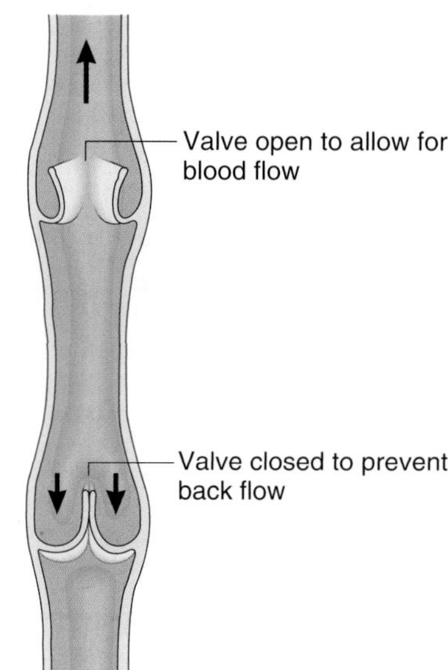

Figure 6-25 Valves in the veins.

THE BLOOD

Blood is a nutritive fluid circulating through the circulatory system. There are approximately 8 to 10 pints of blood in the human body, which contribute about 1/20th of the body's weight. Blood is approximately 80-percent water. It is sticky and salty, with a normal temperature of 98.6 Fahrenheit (36 Celsius). It is bright red in the arteries (except for the pulmonary artery) and dark red in the veins. The color change occurs with the exchange of carbon dioxide for oxygen as the blood passes through the lungs and the exchange of oxygen for carbon dioxide as the blood circulates throughout the body. Red blood is oxygen rich; blue blood is oxygen poor.

COMPOSITION OF THE BLOOD

Blood is composed of red and white cells, platelets, plasma, and hemoglobin.

Red blood cells are produced in the red bone marrow. They contain **hemoglobin** (HEE-muh-gloh-bun), a complex iron protein that binds to oxygen, which is the function of red blood cells, to carry oxygen to the body cells.

White blood cells, also called white corpuscles or leukocytes (LOO-kohsyts), perform the function of destroying disease-causing microorganisms.

Platelets are much smaller than red blood cells. They contribute to the blood-clotting process, which stops bleeding.

Plasma (PLAZ-muh) is the fluid part of the blood in which the red and white blood cells and platelets flow. It is about 90-percent water and contains proteins and sugars. The main function of plasma is to carry food and other useful substances to the cells and to take carbon dioxide away from the cells.

CHIEF FUNCTIONS OF THE BLOOD

Blood performs the following critical functions:

- Carries water, oxygen, food, to all cells of the body.
- Carries away carbon dioxide and waste products to be eliminated through the lungs, skin, kidneys, and large intestines.
- Helps to equalize the body's temperature, thus protecting the body from extreme heat and cold.

- Works with the immune system to protect the body from harmful microorganisms.
- Seals leaks found in injured blood vessels by forming clots, thus preventing further blood loss.

THE LYMPH VASCULAR SYSTEM

The lymph vascular system, also known as the lymphatic system, acts as an aid to the blood system. Lymph is circulated through the lymphatic vessels and filtered by the **lymph nodes**, which are found inside the lymphatic vessels. They filter the blood and help to fight infections.

The primary functions of the lymph vascular system are to:

- Carry nourishment from the blood to the body cells
- Act as a defense against invading microorganisms and toxins
- Remove waste material from the body cells to the blood
- Provide a suitable fluid environment for the cells

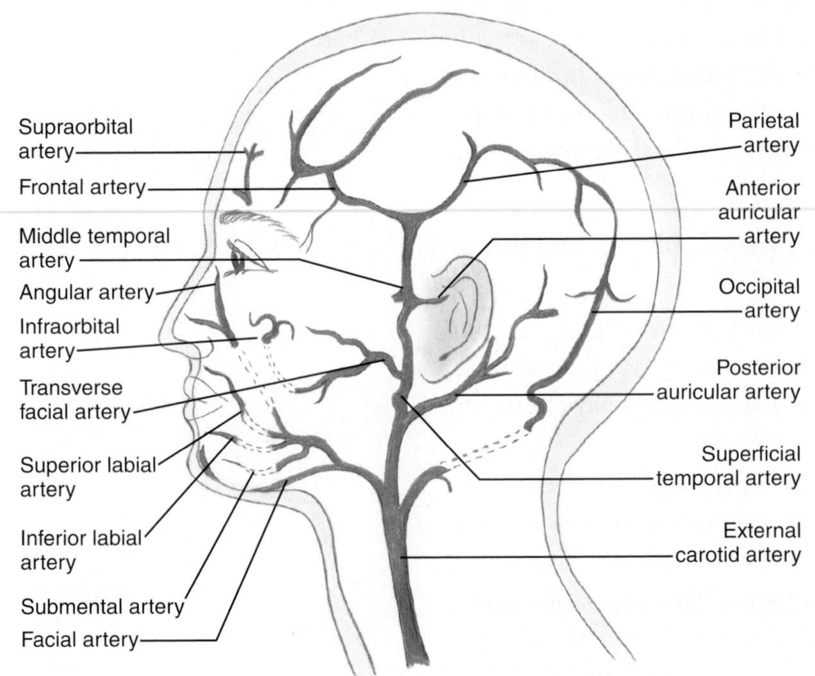

Figure 6-26 Arteries of the head, face, and neck.

ARTERIES OF THE HEAD, FACE, AND NECK

The **common carotid arteries** (kuh-RAHT-ud) are the main sources of blood supply to the head, face, and neck. They are located on both sides of the neck, and each is divided into an internal and external branch.

The **internal carotid artery** supplies blood to the brain, eyes, eyelids, forehead, nose, and internal ear. The **external carotid artery** supplies blood to the anterior (front) parts of the scalp, ear, face, neck, and side of the head (Figure 6-26).

The external carotid artery subdivides into a number of branches.

The **facial artery** or external maxillary artery supplies blood to the lower region of the face, mouth, and nose. Some of its branches include:

- **Submental artery** (sub-MEN-tul). Supplies blood to the chin and lower lip.
- **Inferior labial artery** (LAY-bee-ul). Supplies blood to the lower lip.
- **Angular artery** (ANG-gyoo-lur). Supplies blood to the side of the nose.
- **Superior labial artery**. Supplies blood to the upper lip and region of the nose.

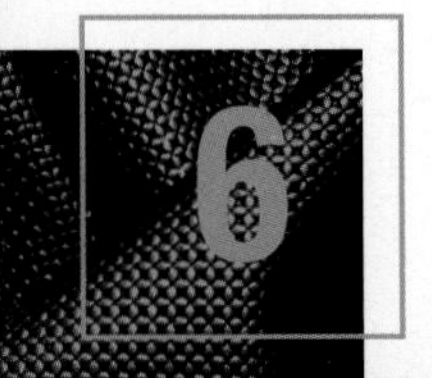

The **superficial temporal artery** is a continuation of the external carotid artery and supplies blood to the muscles of the front, side, and top of the head. Some of its important branches follow:

- **Frontal artery**. Supplies blood to the forehead and upper eyelids.
- **Parietal artery**. Supplies blood to the side and crown of the head.
- **Transverse facial artery** (tranz-VURS). Supplies blood to the skin and masseter.
- **Middle temporal artery**. Supplies blood to the temples.
- **Anterior auricular artery** Supplies blood to the front part of the ear.

Two other arteries that branch from the external carotid artery are the:

- **Occipital artery** Supplies blood to the skin and muscles of the scalp and back of the head up to the crown.
- **Posterior auricular artery**. Supplies blood to the scalp, the area behind and above the ear, and the skin behind the ear.

Two branches of the internal carotid artery that are important to know include the:

- **Supraorbital artery** (soo-pruh-OR-bih-tul). Supplies blood to the upper eyelid and forehead.
- **Infraorbital artery** (in-frah-OR-bih-tul). Supplies blood to the muscles of the eye.

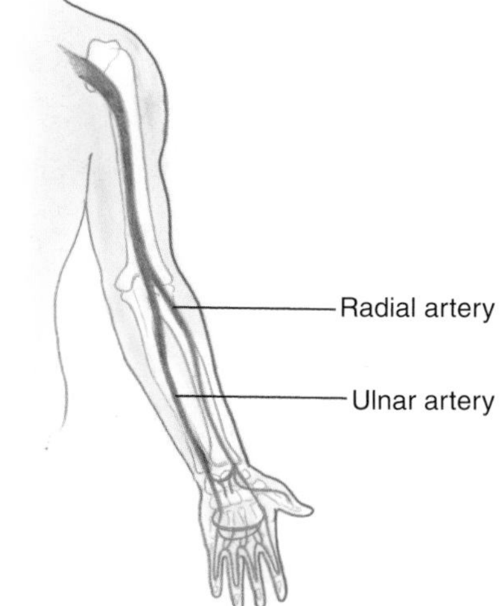

Figure 6–27 Arteries of the arm and hand.

VEINS OF THE HEAD, FACE, AND NECK

The blood returning to the heart from the head, face, and neck flows on each side of the neck in two principal veins: the **internal jugular** (JUG-yuh-lur) and **external jugular**. The most important veins of the face and neck are parallel to the arteries and take the same names as the arteries.

BLOOD SUPPLY OF THE ARM AND HAND

The ulnar and radial arteries are the main blood supply of the arms and hands (Figure 6-27). The **ulnar artery** and its numerous branches supply the little-finger side of the arm and palm of the hand. The **radial artery** and its branches supply the thumb side of the arm and the back of the hand.

While the arteries are found deep in the tissues, the veins lie nearer to the surface of the arms and hands.

BLOOD SUPPLY TO THE LOWER LEG AND FOOT

There are several major arteries that supply blood to the lower leg and foot.

The **popliteal** (pop-lih-TEE-ul) **artery** divides into two separate arteries known as the **anterior tibial** (TIB-ee-al) and the **posterior tibial.** The anterior tibial goes to the foot and becomes the **dorsalis pedis** which supplies the foot with the blood.

As in the arm and hand, the important veins of the lower leg and foot are almost parallel with the arteries and take the same names (Figure 6-28).

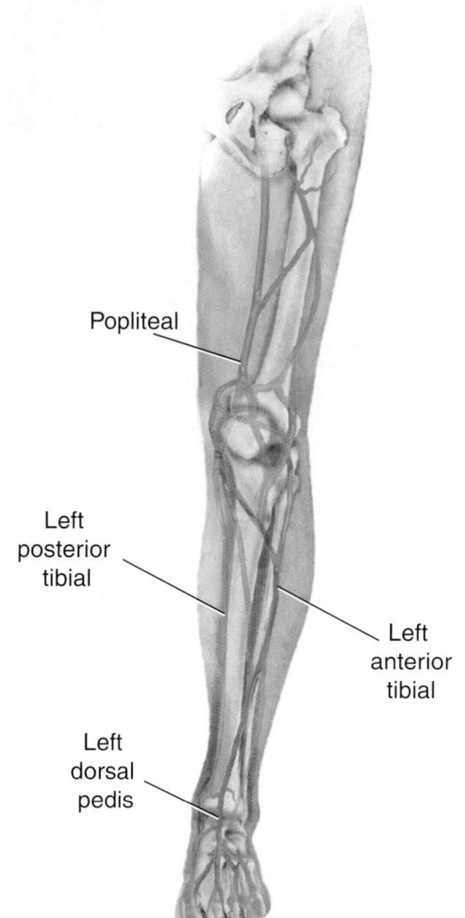

Figure 6–28 Arteries of the lower leg and foot.

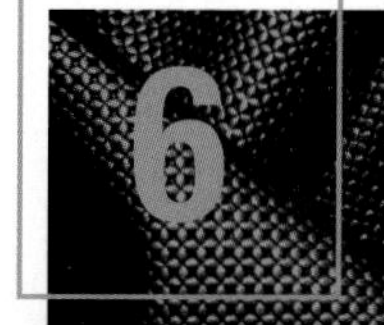

THE ENDOCRINE SYSTEM

The **endocrine system** (EN-duh-krin) is made up of a group of specialized glands that affect the growth, development, sexual activities, and health of the entire body. **Glands** are specialized organs that remove certain elements from the blood to convert them into new compounds.

There are two main types of glands:

Exocrine glands (EK-suh-krin) or duct glands produce a substance that travels through small tube-like ducts. Sweat and oil glands of the skin and intestinal glands belong to this group.

Endocrine glands or ductless glands release secretions called **hormones** directly into the bloodstream, which in turn influence the welfare of the entire body. Hormones, such as insulin, adrenaline, and estrogen, stimulate functional activity or secretion in other parts of the body. These hormones can also affect your moods, feelings, and emotions.

THE DIGESTIVE SYSTEM

The **digestive system**, also called the gastrointestinal (gas-troh-in-TES-tunul) system, is responsible for breaking down food into nutrients and waste.

Digestive enzymes (EN-zymz) are chemicals that change certain kinds of food into a form that can be used by the body. The food, now in soluble form, is transported by the bloodstream and used by the body's cells and tissues. The entire food digestion process takes about 9 hours to complete.

THE EXCRETORY SYSTEM

The **excretory system** (EK-skre-tor-ee) is responsible for purifying the body by eliminating waste matter. The metabolism of body cells forms various toxic substances that, if retained, could poison the body.

Each of the following organs plays a crucial role in the excretory system:

- The kidneys excrete waste containing urine.
- The liver discharges waste containing bile.
- The skin eliminates waste containing perspiration.
- The large intestine eliminates decomposed and undigested food.
- The lungs exhale carbon dioxide.

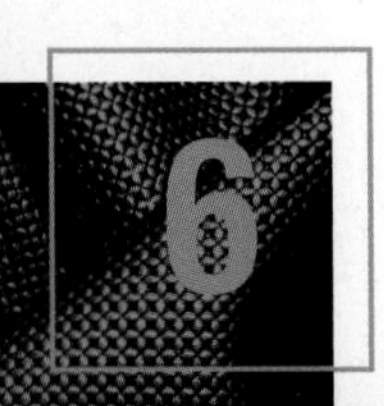

THE RESPIRATORY SYSTEM

The **respiratory system** enables breathing (**respiration**) and consists of the lungs and air passages. The **lungs** are spongy tissues composed of microscopic cells in which inhaled air is exchanged for carbon dioxide during one breathing cycle. The respiratory system is located within the chest cavity and is protected on both sides by the ribs. The **diaphragm** is a muscular wall that separates the thorax from the abdominal region and helps control breathing (Figure 6-29).

With each breathing cycle, an exchange of gases takes place. During **inhalation** (in-huh-LAY-shun), or breathing in, oxygen is passed into the blood. During **exhalation** (eks-huh-LAY-shun), or breathing outward, carbon dioxide (collected from the blood) is expelled from the lungs.

Oxygen is more essential than either food or water. Although people may survive for more than 60 days without food, and several days without water, if they are deprived of oxygen, they will die within a few minutes.

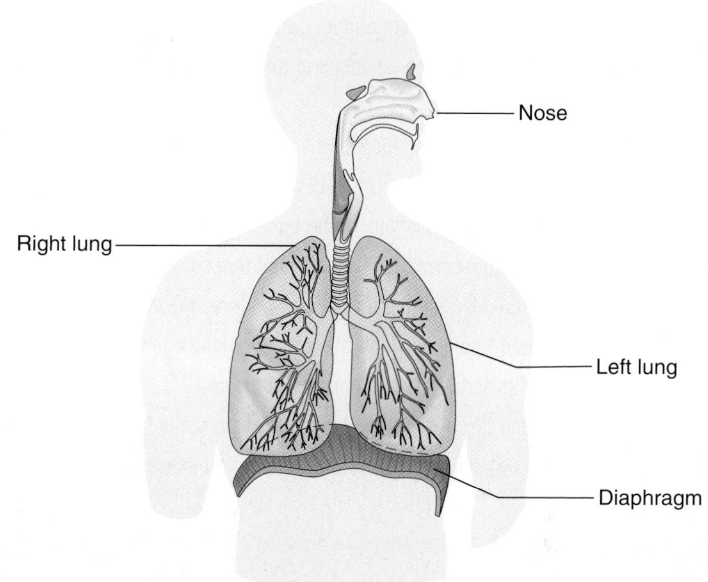

Figure 6-29 The respiratory system.

THE INTEGUMENTARY SYSTEM

The **integumentary system** is made up of the skin and its various accessory organs, such as the oil and sweat glands, sensory receptors, hair, and nails. (Skin anatomy and physiology are discussed in detail in Chapter 7.)

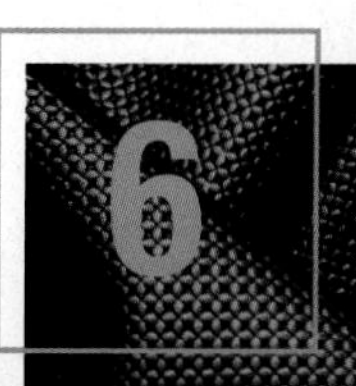

REVIEW QUESTIONS

1. Define anatomy, physiology, and histology.
2. Why is the study of anatomy, physiology, and histology important to the cosmetologist?
3. Name and describe the basic structures of a cell.
4. Explain cell metabolism and its purpose.
5. List and describe the functions of the five types of tissue found in the human body.
6. What are organs?
7. List and describe the functions of the main organs found in the body.
8. Name the 10 body systems and their main functions.
9. List the primary functions of the bones.
10. Name and describe the three types of muscular tissue found in the body.
11. Name and describe the three types of nerves found in the body.
12. Name and briefly describe the three type of blood vessels found in the body.
13. List and describe the components of blood.
14. Name and discuss the two types of glands found in the human body.
15. List the organs of the excretory system and their function.

CHAPTER GLOSSARY

abductors	Muscles that separate the fingers.
abductor hallucis	Muscle of the foot that moves the toes and help maintain balance while walking and standing.
adductors	Muscles at the base of each finger that draw the fingers together.
anabolism	Constructive metabolism; the process of building up larger molecules from smaller ones.
anatomy	Study of human body structure that can be seen with the naked eye, and what they are made up of; the science of the structure of organisms, or of their parts.
angular artery	Supplies blood to the side of the nose.
anterior auricular artery	Supplies blood to the front part of the ear.
anterior tibial artery	See "popliteal (pop-lih-TEE-ul) artery".
anterior tibial nerve	See "deep peroneal nerve".
arteries	Thick-walled, muscular, flexible tubes that carry oxygenated blood away from the heart to the capillaries.
atrium	The upper thin walled chambers of the heart.
auricularis anterior	Muscle in front of the ear that draws the ear forward.
auricularis posterior	Muscle behind the ear that draws the ear backward.

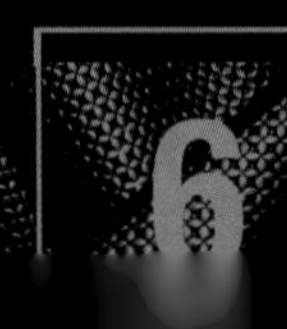

CHAPTER GLOSSARY

auricularis superior	Muscle above the ear that draws the ear upward.
auriculotemporal nerve	Affects the external ear and skin above the temple, up to the top of the skull.
autonomic nervous system	The part of the nervous system that controls the involuntary muscles; regulates the action of the smooth muscles, glands, blood vessels, and heart.
axon	The extension of a neuron by which impulses are sent away from the nerve cell.
belly (muscle)	Middle part of a muscle.
bicep	Muscle producing the contour of the front and inner side of the upper arm.
blood	Fluid circulating through the circulatory system (heart, veins, arteries, and capillaries).
blood vascular system	Group of structures (heart, arteries, veins, and capillaries) that distribute blood throughout the body.
body systems	Groups of bodily organs acting together to perform one or more functions. The human body is composed of 10 major systems.
brain	Part of the central nervous system contained in the cranium; largest and most complex nerve tissue; controls sensation, muscles, gland activity, and the power to think and feel emotions.
buccal nerve	Affects the muscles of the mouth
buccinator muscle	Thin, flat muscle of the cheek between the upper and lower jaw that compresses the cheeks and expels air between the lips.
capillaries	Thin-walled blood vessels that connect the smaller arteries to the veins.
cardiac muscle	The involuntary muscle that is the heart.
carpus	The wrist; flexible joint composed of a group of eight small, irregular bones held together by ligaments.
catabolism	The phase of metabolism that involves the breaking down of complex compounds within the cells into smaller ones resulting in the release of energy to perform functions such as muscular movement or digestion.
cell	Basic unit of all living things; minute mass of protoplasm capable of performing all the fundamental functions of life.
cell membrane	Part of the cell that encloses the protoplasm and permits soluble substances to enter and leave the cell.
central nervous system	Consists of the brain, spinal cord, spinal nerves, and cranial nerves.
cervical cutaneous nerve	Located at the side of the neck, affects the front and sides of the neck as far down as the breastbone.
cervical nerves	Affect the side of the neck and the platysma muscle.
cervical vertebrae	The seven bones of the top part of the vertebral column, located in the neck region.
circulatory system	System that controls the steady circulation of the blood through the body by means of the heart and blood vessels.
clavicle	Collarbone; bone joining the sternum and scapula.
common carotid artery	Artery that supplies blood to the face, head, and neck.
common peroneal nerve	A division of the sciatic nerve that extends from behind the knee to wind around the head of the fibula to the front of the leg where it divides into two branches.

CHAPTER GLOSSARY

connective tissue	Fibrous tissue that binds together, protects, and supports the various parts of the body such as bone, cartilage, and tendons.
corrugator muscle	Muscle located beneath the frontalis and orbicularis oculi that draws the eyebrow down and wrinkles the forehead vertically.
cranium	An oval, bony case that protects the brain.
cytoplasm	All the protoplasm of a cell except that which is in the nucleus; the watery fluid that contains food material necessary for growth, reproduction, and self-repair of the cell.
deep peroneal nerve	A nerve that extends down the front of the leg, behind the muscles. It supplies impulses to these muscles and also to the muscles and skin on the top of the foot and adjacent sides of the first and second toes.
deltoid	Large triangular muscle covering the shoulder joint that allows the arm to extend outward and to the side of the body.
dendrites	Tree-like branching of nerve fibers extending from a nerve cell; short nerve fibers that carry impulses toward the cell.
depressor labii inferioris muscle	Muscle surrounding the lower lip; depresses the lower lip and draws it to one side.
diaphragm	Muscular wall that separates the thorax from the abdominal region and helps control breathing.
digestive system	The mouth, stomach, intestines, and salivary and gastric glands that change food into nutrients and wastes.
digit	A finger or toe.
digital nerve	Nerve that, with its branches, supplies the fingers and toes.
dorsal	A nerve that extends up from the toes and foot, just under the skin, supplying impulses to toes and foot, as well as the muscles and skin of the leg, where it is called the superficial peroneal nerve or the musculo-cutaneous nerve.
dorsal cutaneous nerve	See "dorsal".
dorsalis pedis artery	See "popliteal".
endocrine (ductless) glands	Ductless glands that release hormonal secretions directly into the bloodstream.
endocrine system	Group of specialized glands that affect the growth, development, sexual activities, and health of the entire body.
epicranial aponeurosis	Tendon that connects the occipitalis and frontalis.
epicranius	The broad muscle that covers the top of the skull consists of the occipitalis and frontalis.
epithelial tissue	Protective covering on body surfaces, such as the skin, mucous membranes, and the lining of the heart, digestive and respiratory organs, and glands.
ethmoid bone	Light spongy bone between the eye sockets and forms part of the nasal cavities.
excretory system	Group of organs including the kidneys, liver, skin, intestines, and lungs that purify the body by the elimination of waste matter.
exhalation	The act of breathing outward, expelling carbon dioxide from the lungs.
exocrine (duct) glands	Duct glands that produce a substance that travels through small tube-like ducts, such as the sudoriferous (sweat) glands and the sebaceous (oil) glands.
extensors	Muscles that straighten the wrist, hand, and fingers to form a straight line.

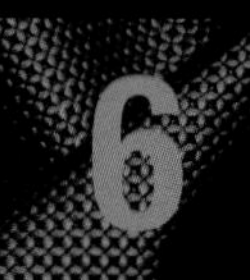

CHAPTER GLOSSARY

extensor digitorum brevis	Muscle of the foot that moves the toes and help maintain balance while walking and standing.
extensor digitorum longus	Muscle that bends the foot up and extends the toes.
external carotid artery	Supplies blood to the anterior (front) parts of the scalp, ear, face, neck, and side of the head.
external jugular vein	Vein located at the side of the neck that caries blood returning to the heart from the head, face, and neck.
facial artery	Supplies blood to the lower region of the face, mouth, and nose.
femur	A heavy, long bone that forms the leg above the knee.
fibula	The smaller of the two bones that form the leg below the knee. The fibula may be visualized as a "bump" on the little-toe side of the ankle.
fifth cranial nerve (also known as trifacial or trigeminal)	The chief sensory nerve of the face, and serves as the motor nerve of the muscles that control chewing.
flexors	Extensor muscles of the wrist involved in flexing the wrist.
flexor digitorum brevis	Muscle of the foot that moves the toes and help maintain balance while walking and standing.
frontal artery	Supplies blood to the forehead and upper eyelids.
frontal bone	Forms the forehead.
frontalis	Anterior (front) portion of the epicranius; muscle of the scalp that raises the eyebrows, draws the scalp forward, and causes wrinkles across the forehead.
gastrocnemius	Muscle that is attached to the lower rear surface of the heel and pulls the foot down.
glands	Specialized organs that remove certain constituents from the blood to convert them into new substances.
greater auricular nerve	Located at the side of the neck, affects the face, ears, neck, and parotid gland.
greater occipital nerve	Located in the back of the head, affects the scalp as far up as the top of the head.
heart	Muscular cone-shaped organ that keeps the blood moving within the circulatory system.
hemoglobin	Iron-containing protein in red blood cells that binds to oxygen.
histology	Science of the minute structures of organic tissues; microscopic anatomy.
hormones	Secretions produced by one of the endocrine glands and carried by the bloodstream or body fluid to another part of the body to stimulate a specific activity.
humerus	Uppermost and largest bone in the arm, extending from the elbow to the shoulder.
hyoid bone	U-shaped bone at the base of the tongue that supports the tongue and its muscles.
inferior labial artery	Supplies blood to the lower lip.
infraorbital artery	Supplies blood to the muscles of the eye.
infraorbital nerve	Affects the skin of the lower eyelid, side of the nose, upper lip, and mouth.
infratrochlear nerve	Nerve that affects the membrane and skin of the nose.

CHAPTER GLOSSARY

inhalation	The breathing in of air.
insertion	Part of the muscle at the more movable attachment to the skeleton.
integumentary system	The skin and its accessory organs, such as the oil and sweat glands, sensory receptors, hair, and nails.
internal carotid artery	Supplies blood to the brain, eyes, eyelids, forehead, nose, and internal ear.
internal jugular vein	Vein located at the side of the neck to collect blood from the brain and parts of the face and neck.
joint	Connection between two or more bones of the skeleton.
lacrimal bones	Small, thin bones located at the front inner wall of the orbits (eye sockets).
latissimus dorsi	Broad, flat superficial muscle covering the back of the neck and upper and middle region of the back, controlling the shoulder blade and the swinging movements of the arm.
levator anguli oris	Also known as caninus, a muscle that raises the angle of the mouth and draws it inward.
levator labii superioris	Also known as quadratus labii superioris, a muscle surrounding the upper lip; elevates the upper lip and dilates the nostrils, as in expressing distaste.
liquid tissue	Body tissue that carries food, waste products, and hormones (i.e., blood and lymph).
lungs	Spongy tissues composed of microscopic cells in which inhaled air is exchanged for carbon dioxide.
lymph	Clear yellowish fluid that circulates in the lymph spaces (lymphatic) of the body; carries waste and impurities away from the cells.
lymph nodes	Special structures found inside the lymphatic vessels that filter lymph.
lymph vascular system	Body system that acts as an aid to the blood system and consists of the lymph spaces, lymph vessels, and lymph glands.
mandible	Lower jawbone; largest and strongest bone of the face.
mandibular nerve	Affects the muscles of the chin and lower lip.
masseter	Muscles that coordinate with the temporalis muscles in opening and closing the mouth, and are sometimes referred to as chewing muscles.
maxillae (singular: maxilla)	Bones of the upper jaw.
maxillary nerve	Branch of the fifth cranial nerve that supplies the upper part of the face.
median nerve	Nerve that supplies the arm and hand.
mental nerve	Affects the skin of the lower lip and chin.
mentalis	Muscle that elevates the lower lip and raises and wrinkles the skin of the chin.
metabolism	Chemical process taking place in living organisms whereby the cells are nourished and carry out their activities.
metacarpus	Bones of the palm of the hand; parts of the hand containing five bones between the carpus and phalanges.
metatarsal	One of three subdivisions of the foot comprised of five bones, which are long and slender, like the metacarpal bones of the hand, help make-up the foot. All three subdivisions comprise 26 bones.

CHAPTER GLOSSARY

middle temporal artery	Supplies blood to the temples.
mitosis	Cells dividing into two new cells (daughter cells); the usual process of cell reproduction of human tissues.
motor nerves	Nerves that carry impulses from the brain to the muscles.
muscular system	Body system that covers, shapes, and supports the skeleton tissue; contracts and moves various parts of the body.
muscular tissue	Tissue that contracts and moves various parts of the body.
myology	Science of the nature, structure, function, and diseases of the muscles.
nasal bones	Bones that form the bridge of the nose.
nasal nerve	Affects the point and lower side of the nose.
nerves	Whitish cords made up of bundles of nerve fibers held together by connective tissue, through which impulses are transmitted.
nerve tissue	Tissue that controls and coordinates all body functions.
nervous system	Body system composed of the brain, spinal cord, and nerves; controls and coordinates all other systems and makes them work harmoniously and efficiently.
neuron	Nerve cell; basic unit of the nervous system, consisting of cell body, nucleus, dendrites, and axon.
neurology	Science of the structure, function, and pathology of the nervous system.
nonstriated muscle	Also called involuntary or smooth muscle; muscle that functions automatically without conscious will.
nucleus	Dense, active protoplasm found in the center of the cell; plays an important part in cell reproduction and metabolism.
occipital artery	Supplies blood to the skin and muscles of the scalp and back of the head up to the crown.
occipital bone	Hindmost bone of the skull, below the parietal bones; forms the back of the skull above the nape.
occipitalis	Back of the epicranius; muscle that draws the scalp backward.
ophthalmic nerve	Branch of the fifth cranial nerve that supplies the skin of the forehead, upper eyelids, and interior portion of the scalp, orbit, eyeball, and nasal passage.
orbicularis oculi muscle	Ring muscle of the eye socket; enables you to close your eyes.
orbicularis oris muscle	Flat band around the upper and lower lips that compresses, contracts, puckers, and wrinkles the lips.
organs	Structures composed of specialized tissues and performing specific functions.
origin	Part of the muscle that does not move; it is attached to the skeleton and is usually part of a skeletal muscle.
os	Bone.
osteology	The study of anatomy, structure, and function of the bones.
palatine bones	Form the floor and outer wall of the nose, roof of the mouth, and floor of the orbits.
parietal artery	Supplies blood to the side and crown of the head.
parietal bones	Form the sides and top of the cranium.

CHAPTER GLOSSARY

patella	Also called the accessory bone, forms the knee cap joint.
pectoralis major, pectoralis minor	Muscles of chest that assist the swinging movements of the arm.
pericardium	Double-layered membranous sac enclosing the heart.
peripheral nervous system	System of nerves and ganglia that connects the peripheral parts of the body to the central nervous system; it has both sensory and motor nerves.
peroneus brevis	Muscle that originates on the lower surface of the fibula. It bends the foot down and out.
peroneus longus	Muscle that covers the outer side of the calf and inverts the foot and turns it outward.
phalanges	Bones of the fingers or toes (singular: phalanx).
physiology	Study of the functions or activities performed by the body's structures.
plasma	Fluid part of the blood and lymph that carries food and secretions to the cells.
platelets	Blood cells that aid in the forming of clots.
platysma muscle	Broad muscle extending from the chest and shoulder muscles to the side of the chin; responsible for lowering the lower jaw and lip.
popliteal artery	Divides into two separate arteries known as the anterior tibial (TIB-ee-al) and the posterior tibial. The anterior tibial goes to the foot and becomes the dorsalis pedis which supplies the foot with blood.
posterior auricular artery	Supplies blood to the scalp, the area behind and above the ear, and the skin behind the ear.
posterior auricular nerve	Affects the muscles behind the ear at the base of the skull.
posterior tibial artery	See "popliteal artery".
procerus	Covers the bridge of the nose, lowers the eyebrows, and causes wrinkles across the bridge of the nose.
pronators	Muscles that turn the hand inward so that the palm faces downward.
protoplasm	Colorless jelly-like substance found inside cells in which food elements such as protein, fats, carbohydrates, mineral salts, and water are present.
pulmonary circulation	Blood circulation from heart to lungs to be purified.
radial artery	Artery that supplies blood to the thumb side of the arm and the back of the hand.
radial nerve	Supplies the thumb side of the arm and back of the hand.
radius	Smaller bone in the forearm on the same side as the thumb.
red blood cells	Blood cells that carry oxygen from the lungs to the body cells.
reflex	Automatic nerve reaction to a stimulus that involves the movement of specific muscles as a response to impulses carried along a motor neuron to a muscle, causing a spontaneous reaction.
reproductive system	Body system responsible for processes by which plants and animals produce offspring.
respiration	Act of breathing; the exchange of carbon dioxide and oxygen in the lungs and within each cell.

CHAPTER GLOSSARY

respiratory system	Body system consisting of the lungs and air passages; enables breathing, supplying the body with oxygen and eliminating carbon dioxide wastes.
ribs	Twelve pairs of bones forming the wall of the thorax.
risorius	Muscle of the mouth that draws the corner of the mouth out and back, as in grinning.
saphenous nerve	Supplies impulses to the skin of the inner side of the leg and foot.
scapula	One of a pair of shoulder blades; a large, flat, triangular bone of the shoulder.
sensory (afferent) nerves	Nerves that carry impulses or messages from the sense organs to the brain, where sensations of touch, cold, heat, sight, hearing, taste, smell, pain, and pressure are experienced.
serratus anterior	Muscle of the chest that assists in breathing and in raising the arm.
skeletal system	Physical foundation of the body, comprised of 206 bones that vary in size and shape and are connected by movable and immovable joints.
smaller occipital nerve	Located at the base of the skull, affects the scalp and muscles behind the ear.
soleus	Muscle that originates at the upper portion of the fibula and bends the foot down.
sphenoid bone	Joins all of the bones of the cranium together.
spinal cord	The portion of the central nervous system that originates in the brain, extends down to the lower extremity of the trunk, and is protected by the spinal column.
sternocleidomastoideus	Muscle of the neck that lowers and rotates the head.
sternum	Breastbone; flat bone that forms the ventral (front) support of the ribs.
striated muscle	Also called voluntary or skeletal muscle; muscle that is consciously controlled.
submental artery	Supplies blood to the chin and lower lip.
superficial peroneal nerve	A nerve that extends down the leg, just under the skin, supplying impulses to the muscles and the skin of the leg, as well as to the skin and toes on the top of the foot.
superficial temporal artery	Artery that supplies blood to the muscles of the front, side, and top of the head.
superior labial artery	Supplies blood to the upper lip and region of the nose.
supinator	Muscle of the forearm that rotates the radius outward and the palm upward.
supraorbital artery	Supplies blood to the upper eyelid and forehead.
supraorbital nerve	Affects the skin of the forehead, scalp, eyebrow, and upper eyelid.
supratrochlear nerve	Affects the skin between the eyes and upper side of the nose.
sural nerve	Supplies impulses to the skin on the outer side and back of the foot and leg.
systemic circulation	Circulation of blood from the heart throughout the body and back again to the heart; also called general

CHAPTER GLOSSARY

tarsal	One of the three subdivisions of the foot comprised of seven bones (talus, calcaneous, navicular, three cuneiform bones, and the cuboid). All three subdivisions comprise 26 bones.
temporal bone	Form the sides of the head in the ear region.
temporal nerve	Affects the muscles of the temple, side of the forehead, eyebrow, eyelid, and upper part of the cheek.
temporalis	Temporal muscle; one of the muscles involved in mastication (chewing).
thorax	The chest; elastic, bony cage that serves as a protective framework for the heart, lungs, and other internal organs.
tibia	The larger of the two bones that form the leg below the knee. The tibia may be visualized as a "bump" on the big-toe-side of the ankle.
tibial nerve	A division of the sciatic nerve that passes behind the knee. It subdivides and supplies impulses to the knee, the muscles of the calf, the skin of the leg, and the sole, heel, and underside of the toes.
tibialis anterior	Muscle that covers the front of the shin. It bends the foot upward and inward.
tissue	Collection of similar cells that perform a particular function.
transverse facial artery	Supplies blood to the skin and masseter.
trapezius	Muscle that covers the back of the neck and upper and middle region of the back; rotates and controls swinging movements of the arm.
triangularis	Muscle extending alongside the chin that pulls down the corner of the mouth.
tricep	Large muscle that covers the entire back of the upper arm and extends the forearm.
turbinal bones	Thin layers of spongy bone on either of the outer walls of the nasal depression.
ulna	Inner and larger bone of the forearm, attached to the wrist and located on the side of the little finger.
ulnar artery	Artery that supplies blood to the muscle of the little finger side of the arm and palm of the hand.
ulnar nerve	Nerve that affects the little finger side of the arm and palm of the hand.
valves	Structures that temporarily close a passage, or permit blood flow in one direction only.
veins	Thin-walled blood vessels that are less elastic than arteries; veins contain cup-like valves to prevent backflow and carry impure blood from the various capillaries back to the heart and lungs.
ventricle	The lower thick-walled chambers of the heart.
vomer bone	Flat thin bone that forms part of the nasal septum.
white blood cells	Blood cells that perform the function of destroying disease-causing microorganisms.
zygomatic/malar bones	Form the prominence of the cheeks; cheekbones.
zygomatic nerve	Affects the muscles of the upper part of the cheek.
zygomaticus	Muscles extending from the zygomatic bone to the angle of the mouth; elevate the lip, as in laughing.

SKIN STRUCTURE & GROWTH CHAPTER 7

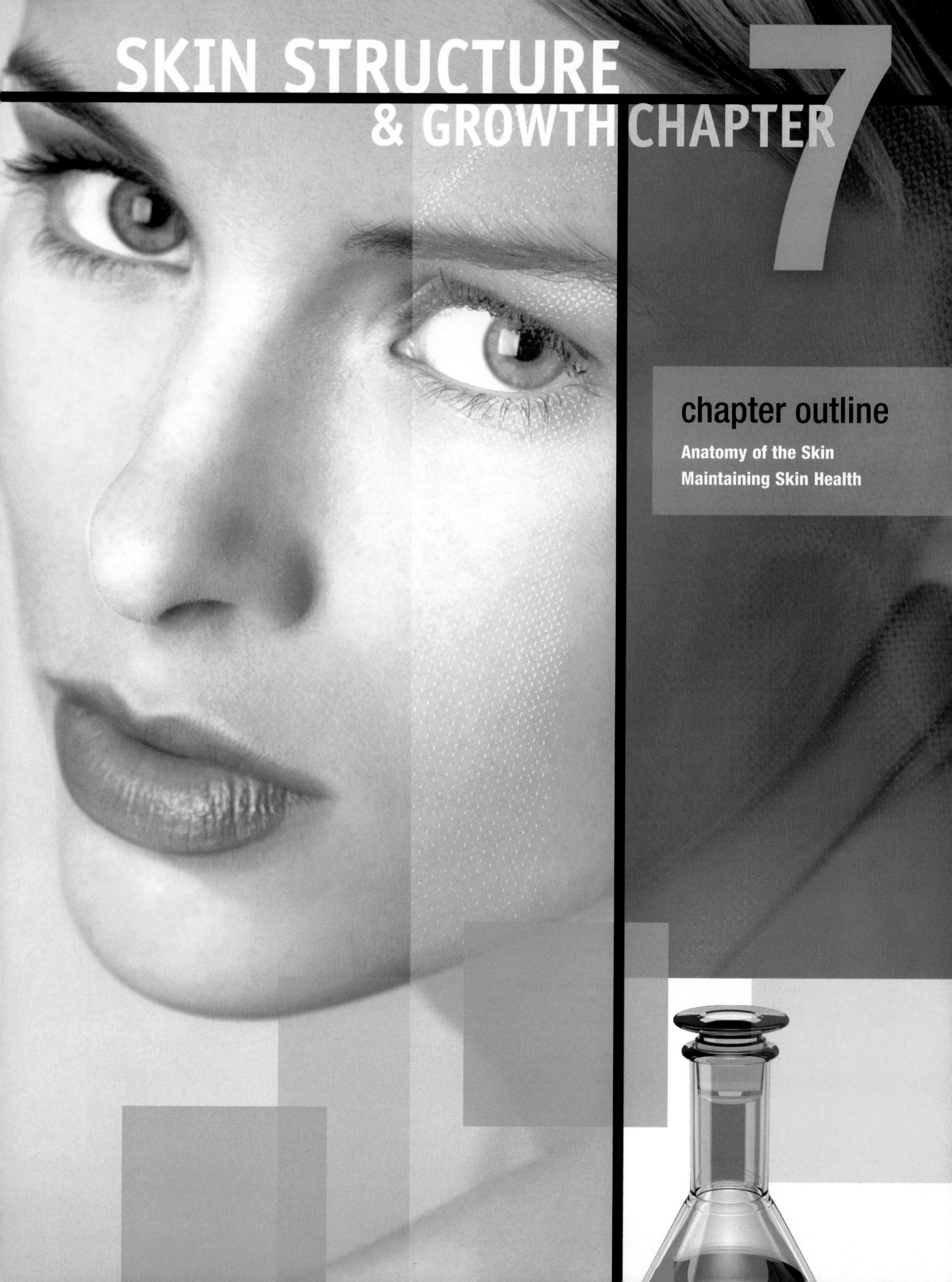

chapter outline

Learning Objectives

After completing this chapter, you will be able to:

- **Describe the structure and composition of the skin.**
- **List the functions of the skin.**

Key Terms

Page number indicates where in the chapter the term is used.

adipose **pg. 123**

basal cell layer **pg. 122**

blood **pg. 124**

collagen **pg. 125**

comedone **pg. 127**

dermatologist **pg. 121**

dermatology **pg. 121**

dermis **pg. 122**

elastin **pg. 126**

epidermal-dermal junction **pg. 123**

epidermis **pg. 122**

esthetician **pg. 121**

keratin **pg. 122**

melanin **pg. 124**

melanocytes **pg. 122**

motor nerve fibers **pg. 124**

papillary layer **pg. 123**

reticular layer **pg. 123**

retinoic acid **pg. 128**

sebaceous glands **pg. 126**

secretory coil **pg. 126**

secretory nerve fibers **pg. 124**

sensory nerve fibers **pg. 124**

stratum corneum **pg. 122**

stratum germinativum **pg. 122**

stratum granulosum **pg. 122**

stratum lucidum **pg. 122**

stratum spinosum **pg. 122**

subcutaneous tissue **pg. 123**

subcutis **pg. 123**

sudoriferous glands **pg. 126**

tactile corpuscles **pg. 123**

Vitamin A **pg. 128**

Vitamin C **pg. 128**

Vitamin D **pg. 128**

Vitamin E **pg. 129**

Clear glowing skin is one of today's most important hallmarks of beauty. With all the latest high-performance ingredients and state-of-the-art delivery systems, 21st-century skin care has entered the realm of high technology with products and services that truly help protect, nourish, and preserve the health and beauty of the skin.

No matter how advanced the latest skin-care technology may be, though, knowing how to care for skin begins with understanding its underlying structure and basic needs. As a licensed service provider, you also must recognize adverse conditions, including inflamed skin conditions, diseases, and infectious skin disorders.

ANATOMY OF THE SKIN

The medical branch of science that deals with the study of skin—its nature, structure, functions, diseases, and treatment—is called **dermatology.**

A **dermatologist** is a physician engaged in the science of treating the skin, its structures, functions, and diseases. An **esthetician** is a specialist in the cleansing, preservation of health, and beautification of the skin and body.

The skin is the largest organ of the body. If the skin of a typical 150-pound (68-kilogram) adult male were stretched out flat, it would cover about two square yards (1.7 square meters) and weigh about 9 pounds (4 kilograms). Our skin protects the network of muscles, bones, nerves, blood vessels, and everything else inside our bodies. It is our only barrier against the environment.

Healthy skin is slightly moist, soft, and flexible with a texture (feel and appearance) that ideally is smooth and fine-grained. The surface of healthy skin is slightly acidic, and its immune responses react quickly to organisms that touch or try to enter it. Appendages of the skin include hair, nails, and sweat and oil glands.

Our eyelids have the thinnest skin; the soles of our feet have the thickest skin.

Continued pressure on any part of the skin can cause it to thicken and develop into a callus. The skin of the scalp is constructed similarly to the skin elsewhere on the human body, but the scalp has larger and deeper hair follicles to accommodate the longer hair of the head.

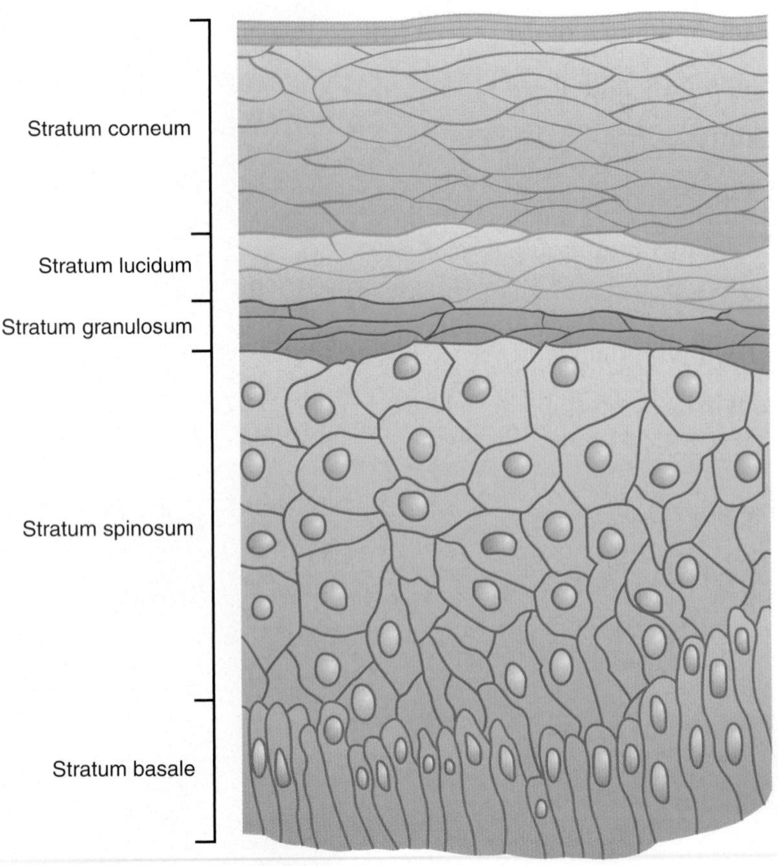

Figure 7-1 Layers of the skin.

The skin is composed of two main divisions: epidermis and dermis (Figure 7-1).

The **epidermis** (ep-uh-DUR-mis) is the outermost layer of the skin. This layer, also called the cuticle (KYOO-tih-kul), is the thinnest layer of skin and forms a protective covering for the body. It contains no blood vessels, but has many small nerve endings. The epidermis is made up of the layers discussed below.

The **basal cell layer,** also referred to as the **stratum germinativum** (jer-mih-nah-TIV-um), is the deepest layer of the epidermis. It is composed of several layers of differently shaped cells. It is the live layer of the epidermis, which produces new epidermal skin cells and is responsible for the growth of the epidermis. It also contains special cells called **melanocytes** (muh-LANuh-syts), which produce a dark skin pigment, called melanin, that protects the sensitive cells in the dermis below from the destructive effects of excessive ultraviolet rays of the sun or those from an ultraviolet lamp. The type of melanin produced also determines skin color.

The spiny layer, also referred to as the **stratum spinosum,** is just above the basal cell layer. It is in the spiny layer that the beginning of the process that causes skin cells to shed begins.

The **stratum granulosum** (gran-yoo-LOH-sum), or granular layer, consists of cells that look like distinct granules. These cells are almost dead and are pushed to the surface to replace cells that are shed from the skin surface layer.

The **stratum lucidum** (LOO-sih-dum) is the clear, transparent layer just under the skin surface; it consists of small cells through which light can pass.

The **stratum corneum** (STRAT-um KOR-nee-um), or horny layer, is the outer layer of the epidermis. The corneum is the layer we see when we look at the skin, and the layer treated by the practitioner. Its scale-like cells are continually being shed and replaced by cells coming to the surface from underneath. These cells are made up of **keratin,** a fiber protein that is also the principal component of hair and nails. The cells combine with lipids or fats produced by the skin to help make the stratum corneum a protective, waterproof layer.

The **dermis** (DUR-mis) is the underlying or inner layer of the skin. It is also called the derma, corium (KOH-ree-um), cutis (KYOO-tis), or true skin. This highly sensitive layer of connective tissue is about 25 times thicker than the epidermis. Within its structure, there are numerous blood vessels, lymph vessels, nerves, sweat glands, oil glands, and hair follicles, as well as arrector pili muscles (small muscles that work in connection with the hair follicles and cause "goose bumps") and papillae (small cone-shaped projections of elastic tissue that point upward into the epidermis). The dermis is comprised of two layers: the papillary or superficial layer, and the reticular or deeper layer (Figure 7-2).

The **papillary layer** (PAP-uh-lair-ee) is the outer layer of the dermis, directly beneath the epidermis. Here you will find the dermal papillae (puh-PIL-eye), which are small, cone-shaped elevations at the bottom of the hair follicles. Some papillae contain looped capillaries and others contain small structures called **tactile corpuscles** (TAK-tile KOR-pusuls), with nerve endings that are sensitive to touch and pressure. This layer also contains melanocytes, the pigment-producing cells. The top of the papillary layer where it joins the epidermis is called the **epidermal-dermal junction.**

The **reticular layer** (ruh-TIK-yuh-lur) is the deeper layer of the dermis that supplies the skin with oxygen and nutrients. It contains the following structures within its network:

- Fat cells
- Sweat glands
- Blood vessels
- Hair follicles
- Lymph vessels
- Arrector pili muscles
- Oil glands

Subcutaneous tissue (sub-kyoo-TAY-nee-us) is a fatty layer found below the dermis that some specialists regard as a continuation of the dermis. This fat tissue is also called **adipose** (AD-uh-pohs) or **subcutis** (sub-KYOO-tis) tissue, and varies in thickness according to the age, gender, and general health of the individual. It gives smoothness and contour to

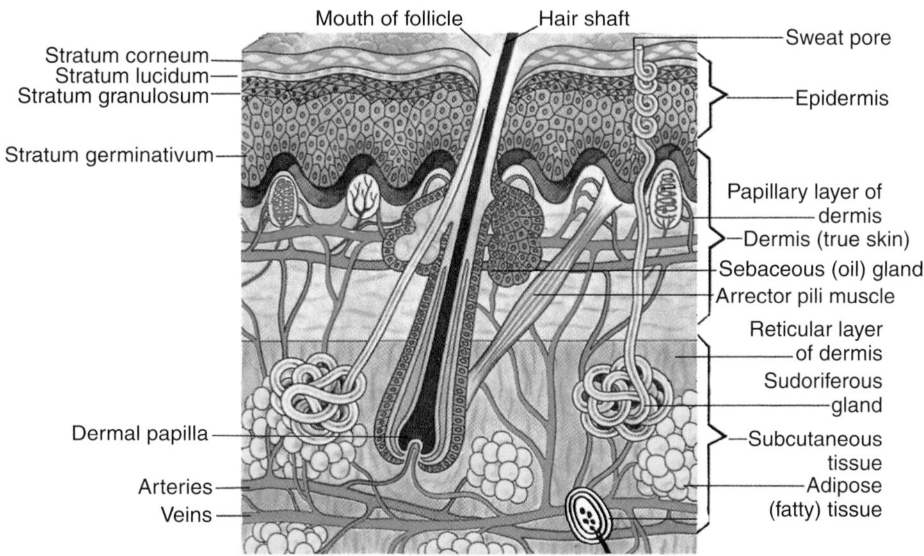

Figure 7-2 Structures of the skin.

the body, contains fats for use as energy, and also acts as a protective cushion for the outer skin.

HOW THE SKIN IS NOURISHED

Blood supplies nutrients and oxygen to the skin. Nutrients are molecules from food, such as protein, carbohydrates, and fats. These nutrients are necessary for cell life, repair, and growth.

Lymph, the clear fluids of the body that resemble blood plasma but contain only colorless corpuscles, bathe the skin cells, remove toxins and cellular waste, and have immune functions that help protect the skin and body against disease. Networks of arteries and lymph vessels in the subcutaneous tissue send their smaller branches to hair papillae, hair follicles, and skin glands.

NERVES OF THE SKIN

The skin contains the surface endings of the following nerve fibers:

Motor nerve fibers are distributed to the arrector pili muscles attached to the hair follicles. These muscles can cause goose bumps when a person is frightened or cold.

Sensory nerve fibers react to heat, cold, touch, pressure, and pain. These sensory receptors send messages to the brain.

Secretory nerve fibers are distributed to the sweat and oil glands of the skin. Secretory nerves, which are part of the autonomic nervous system, regulate the excretion of perspiration from the sweat glands and control the flow of sebum (a fatty or oily secretion of the sebaceous glands) to the surface of the skin.

SENSE OF TOUCH

The papillary layer of the dermis houses the nerve endings that provide the body with the sense of touch. These nerve endings register basic sensations such as touch, pain, heat, cold, and pressure. Nerve endings are most abundant in the fingertips. Complex sensations, such as vibrations, seem to depend on the sensitivity of a combination of these nerve endings.

SKIN COLOR

The color of the skin—whether fair, medium, or dark—depends primarily on **melanin,** the tiny grains of pigment (coloring matter) deposited into cells in the basal cell layer of the epidermis and the papillary layers of the dermis. The color of the skin is a hereditary trait and varies among races and nationalities. Genes determine the amount and type of pigment produced in an individual.

The body produces two types of melanin: pheomelanin, which is red to yellow in color, and eumelanin, which is dark brown to black. People with light-colored skin mostly produce pheomelanin, while those with dark-colored skin mostly produce eumelanin. In addition, individuals differ in the size of melanin particles (Figure 7-3).

Melanin protects sensitive cells against strong light rays. Daily use of a sunscreen with a sun protection factor (SPF) of 15 or higher can help the

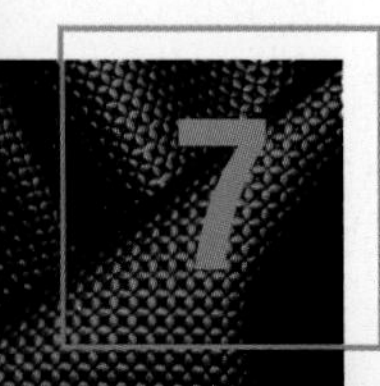

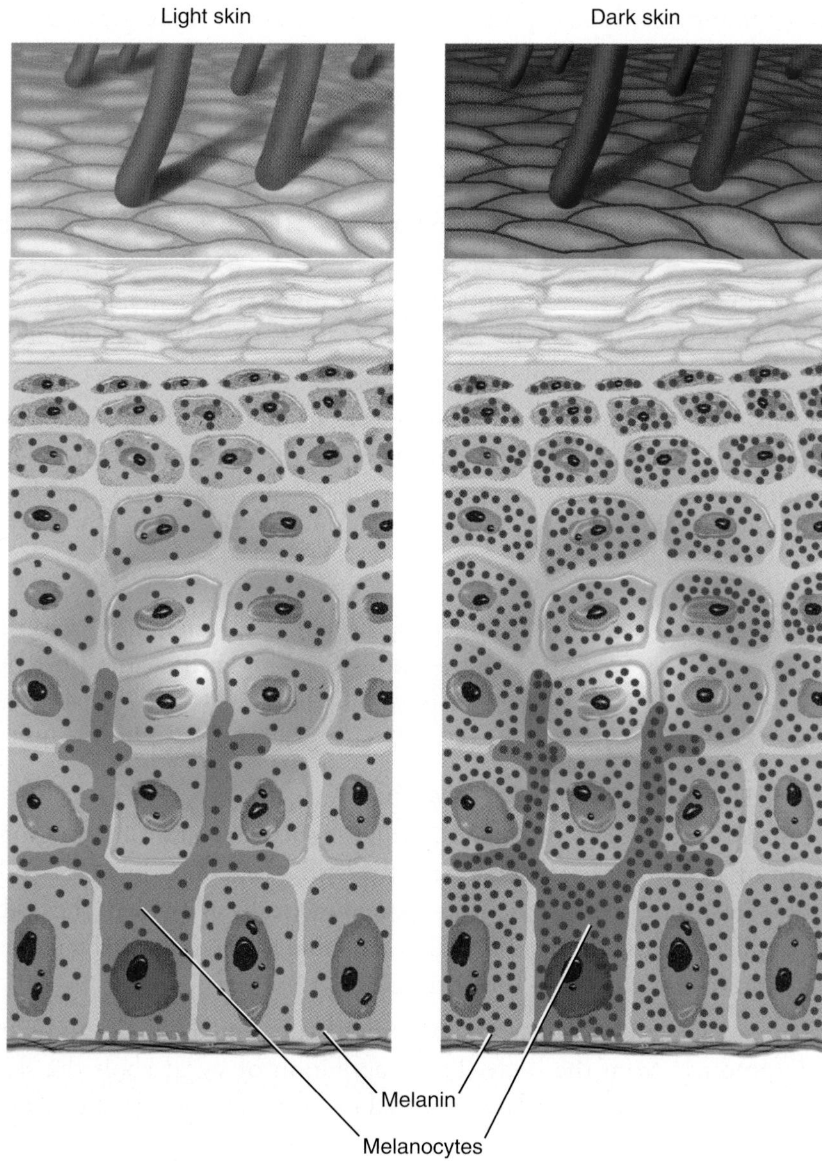

Figure 7-3 Melanocytes in the epidermis produce melanin.

melanin in the skin protect it from burning, and from receiving damage that can lead to skin cancer or premature aging.

STRENGTH AND FLEXIBILITY OF THE SKIN

The skin gets its strength, form, and flexibility from two specific structures composed of flexible protein fibers found within the dermis. These two structures, which make up 70 percent of the dermis, are called collagen and elastin.

Collagen is a fibrous protein that gives the skin form and strength. This fiber makes up a large portion of the dermis and helps give structural support to the skin by holding together all the structures found in this layer.

When collagen fibers are healthy, they allow the skin to stretch and contract as necessary. If collagen fibers become weakened due to a lack of moisture in the skin, environmental damage such as sun tanning or routine unprotected sun exposure, or frequent changes in weight, the skin will begin to lose its tone and suppleness. Wrinkles and sagging are often the result of collagen fibers losing their strength.

Collagen fibers are interwoven with **elastin,** a protein base similar to collagen that forms elastic tissue. This fiber gives the skin its flexibility and elasticity. Elastin helps the skin regain its shape, even after being repeatedly stretched or expanded.

Both of these fibers are important to the overall health and appearance of the skin. As we age, gravity causes these fibers to weaken, resulting in some degree of elasticity loss or skin sagging.

A majority of scientists now believe that most signs of skin aging are caused by sun exposure over a lifetime. Keeping the skin healthy, protected, moisturized, and free of disease will slow the weakening process and help keep the skin looking young longer.

GLANDS OF THE SKIN

The skin contains two types of duct glands that extract materials from the blood to form new substances: the **sudoriferous glands** (sood-uh-RIF-uhrus) or sweat glands, and the **sebaceous glands** (sih-BAY-shus) or oil glands (Figure 7-4).

SUDORIFEROUS (SWEAT) GLANDS

The sudoriferous or sweat glands, which excrete sweat from the skin, consist of a coiled base, or **secretory coil,** and a tube-like duct that ends at the skin surface to form the sweat pore. Practically all parts of the body are supplied with sweat glands, which are more numerous on the palms, soles, and forehead, and in the armpits.

The sweat glands regulate body temperature and help to eliminate waste products from the body. The evaporation of sweat cools the skin surface. Their activity is greatly increased by heat, exercise, emotions, and certain drugs.

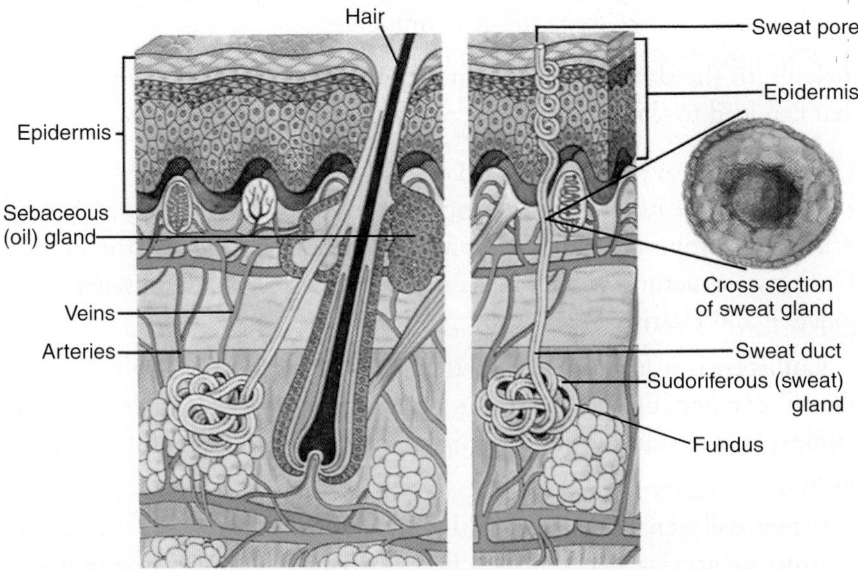

Figure 7-4 Sweat gland and oil gland.

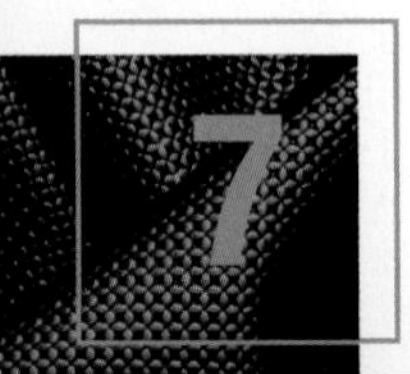

The excretion of sweat is controlled by the nervous system. Normally, one to two pints of liquids containing salts are eliminated daily through sweat pores in the skin.

SEBACEOUS (OIL) GLANDS

The sebaceous or oil glands of the skin are connected to the hair follicles. They consist of little sacs with ducts that open into the follicles. These glands secrete sebum, a fatty or oily secretion that lubricates the skin and preserves the softness of the hair. With the exception of the palms and soles, these glands are found in all parts of the body, particularly in the face and scalp, where they are larger.

Ordinarily, sebum flows through the oil ducts leading to the mouths of the hair follicles. However, when the sebum hardens and the duct becomes clogged, a pore impaction or **comedone** is formed, which may lead to an acne papule or pustule.

FUNCTIONS OF THE SKIN

The principal functions of the skin are protection, sensation, heat regulation, excretion, secretion, and absorption.

Protection. The skin protects the body from injury and bacterial invasion. The outermost layer of the epidermis is covered with a thin layer of sebum, and fatty lipids between the cells produced through the cell renewal process, which render it essentially waterproof. This outermost layer is resistant to wide variations in temperature, minor injuries, chemically active substances, and many forms of bacteria.

Sensation. By stimulating different sensory nerve endings, the skin responds to heat, cold, touch, pressure, and pain. When the nerve endings are stimulated, a message is sent to the brain. You respond by saying "ouch" if you feel pain, by scratching an itch, or by pulling away when you touch something hot. Sensory nerve endings are located near hair follicles (Figure 7-5).

Heat regulation. This means that the skin protects the body from the environment. A healthy body maintains a constant internal temperature of about 98.6 Fahrenheit (37 Celsius). As changes occur in the outside temperature, the blood and sweat glands of the skin make necessary adjustments to allow the body to be cooled by the evaporation of sweat.

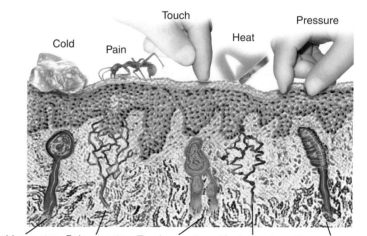

Figure 7-5 Sensory nerve endings in the skin.

Excretion. Perspiration from the sweat glands is excreted through the skin. Water lost through perspiration takes salt and other chemicals with it.

Secretion. Sebum, or oil, is secreted by the sebaceous glands. This oil lubricates the skin, keeping it soft and pliable. Oil also keeps hair soft. Emotional stress and hormone imbalances can increase the flow of sebum.

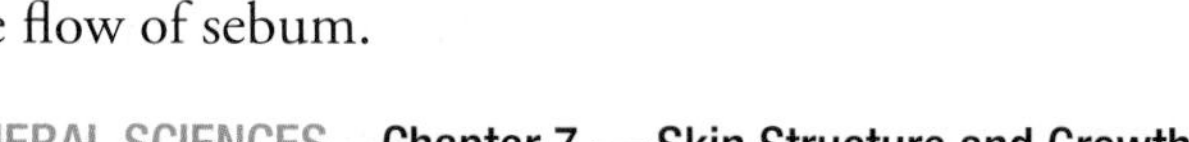

Absorption. Absorption is limited, but it does occur. Female hormones, when used as an ingredient of a face cream, can enter the body through the skin and influence it to a minor degree. Fatty materials, such as those used in many advanced skin care formulations, may be absorbed between the cells, and through the hair follicles and sebaceous gland openings.

MAINTAINING SKIN HEALTH

For your own benefit, as well as the benefit of your clients, you should have a basic understanding of how best to maintain healthy skin. In order to keep the skin and the body healthy, the old adage "you are what you eat" still holds true. Proper dietary choices help to regulate hydration (maintaining a healthy level of water in the body), oil production, and overall function of the cells. Eating foods found in all three basic food groups—fats, carbohydrates, and proteins—is the best way to support the health of the skin.

VITAMINS AND DIETARY SUPPLEMENTS

Vitamins play an important role in the skin's health, often aiding in healing, softening, and fighting diseases of the skin. Vitamins such as A, C, D, and E have all been shown to have positive effects on the skin's health when taken internally. Although experts agree that taking vitamins internally is still the best way to support the health of the skin, some external applications of vitamins have also been found to be useful in nourishing the skin. The following vitamins relate to the skin in particularly significant ways:

Vitamin A supports the overall health of the skin. This vitamin aids in the health, function, and repair of skin cells. Vitamin A is an antioxidant that can help prevent certain types of cancers, including skin cancer, and has been shown to improve the skin's elasticity and thickness. In its topical acid form as the prescription cream called **retinoic acid** or by its trade name, Retin-A®, vitamin A can be used to treat many different types of acne.

Vitamin C, also known as ascorbic acid or another topical form, magnesium ascorbyl phosphate, is an important element needed for proper repair of the skin and various tissues. This vitamin aids in, and even speeds up, the healing processes of the body. Vitamin C is also vitally important in fighting the aging process and promotes the production of collagen in the skin's dermal tissues, keeping the skin healthy and firm.

Vitamin D promotes the healthy and rapid healing of the skin. The best source of this vitamin is sunlight (in limited amounts). Vitamin D can also be obtained from fortified milk or orange juice. Because vitamin D helps to support the bone structure of the body, it has been made readily available in many fortified foods and dietary supplements.

Vitamin E, or tocopherol, used in conjunction with vitamin A, helps fight against, and protect the skin from, the harmful effects of the sun's rays. Vitamin E also helps to heal damage to the skin's tissues when used both internally and externally. When used externally in topical lotions or creams, vitamin E can help heal structural damage on the skin including severe burns and stretch marks.

Ideally, the nutrients the body needs for proper functioning and survival should come primarily from the foods we eat. If a person's daily food consumption is lacking in nutrients, an effective way to provide them is to take vitamins and mineral supplements (providing that the recommended daily allowance is not exceeded).

Clients will occasionally ask you about nutrition and their skin. While it is important that the professional know the basics of nutrition, cosmetologists are not registered dieticians, and should never give nutritional advice. Instead, refer the client to a registered dietician.

Did You Know

Research suggests that the benefits of water on human health and functioning are many:

Even mild dehydration will slow metabolism by as much as 3 percent.

Drinking lots of water can help stop hunger pangs for many dieters.

Lack of water is the principal cause of daytime fatigue.

A 2-percent drop in body water can trigger fuzzy short-term memory and trouble with basic math, and may cause difficulty focusing on a computer screen or printed page.

Pass the water, please!

WATER AND THE SKIN

There is one essential nutrient that no person can live without, and that is water. In order to function properly, the body and skin both rely heavily on the benefits of water. Water composes 50- to 70-percent of body weight.

Drinking pure water is essential to the health of the skin and body because it sustains the health of the cells, aids in the elimination of toxins and waste, helps regulate the body's temperature, and aids in proper digestion. All these functions, when performing properly, help keep the skin healthy, vital, and attractive.

The amount of water needed by an individual varies, depending on body weight and the level of daily physical activity. The following is an easy formula to help you determine how much water you need every day for maximum physical health: Take your body weight and divide by 16. The resulting number approximates how many 8-ounce glasses of water you should drink every day. For instance, if you weigh 160 pounds, you should drink 10 glasses of water a day. If intense physical activity is performed daily, add two extra glasses of water to the final number. This will help replace extra fluids lost while exercising (Figure 7-6).

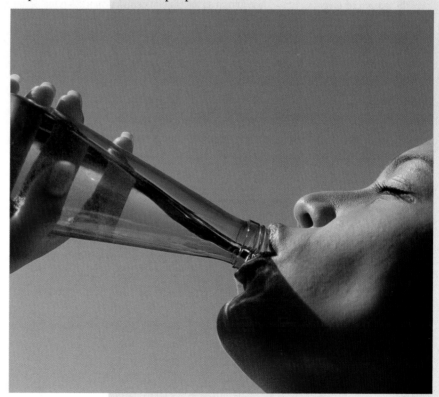

Figure 7-6 Water is essential for healthy skin.

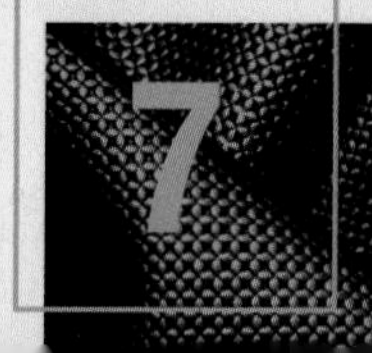

REVIEW QUESTIONS

1. Briefly describe healthy skin.
2. Name the main divisions of the skin and the layers within each division.
3. How is the skin nourished?
4. List the three types of nerve fibers found in the skin.
5. What is collagen?
6. Name the two types of glands contained within the skin and describe their functions.
7. What are the six important functions of the skin?
8. Define dermatology.

CHAPTER GLOSSARY

adipose	Tissue that gives smoothness and contour to the body, contains fats for use as energy, and also acts as a protective cushion for the outer skin.
basal cell layer	Also known as the stratum germinativum layer; the deepest, live layer of the epidermis that produces new epidermal skin cells and is responsible for growth.
blood	Nutritive fluid circulating through the circulatory system (heart, veins, arteries, and capillaries) to supply oxygen and nutrients to cells and tissues, and to remove carbon dioxide and waste from them.
collagen	Fibrous protein that gives the skin form and strength.
comedone	Pore impaction that could lead to an acne papule or pustule.
dermatologist	Physician engaged in the science of treating the skin, including its structures, functions, and diseases.
dermatology	Medical branch of science that deals with the study of skin and its nature, structure, functions, diseases, and treatment.
dermis	Underlying or inner layer of the skin; also called the derma, corium, cutis, or true skin.
elastin	Protein base similar to collagen that forms elastic tissue.
epidermal-dermal junction	The top of the papillary layer where it joins the epidermis.
epidermis	Outermost layer of the skin; also called cuticle.
esthetician	Specialist in the cleansing, preservation of health, and beautification of the skin and body.
keratin	Fiber protein that is the principal component of hair and nails.

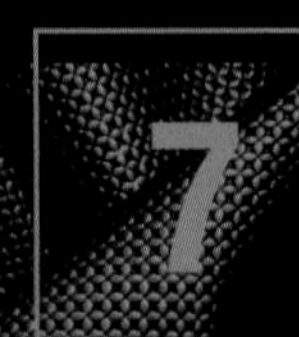

CHAPTER GLOSSARY

melanin	Tiny grains of pigment (coloring matter) deposited in the basal cell layer of the epidermis and papillary layers of the dermis.
melanocytes	Melanin-forming cells.
motor nerve fibers	Distributed to the arrector pili muscles attached to the hair follicles.
papillary layer	Outer layer of the dermis, directly beneath the epidermis.
reticular layer	Deeper layer of the dermis that supplies the skin with oxygen and nutrients; contains cells, vessels, glands, and follicles.
retinoic acid	Prescription cream for acne.
sebaceous glands	Oil glands of the skin connected to hair follicles.
secretory coil	Coiled base of sweat glands.
secretory nerve fibers	Distributed to the sweat and oil glands of the skin.
sensory nerve fibers	React to heat, cold, touch, pressure, and pain. These sensory receptors send messages to the brain.
stratum corneum	Outer layer of the epidermis.
stratum germinativum	Also known as the basal cell layer, the deepest live layer of the epidermis that produces new epidermal skin cells and is responsible for growth.
stratum granulosum	Granular layer of the epidermis.
stratum lucidum	Clear, transparent layer just under the skin surface.
stratum spinosum	Spiny layer of the epidermis.
subcutaneous tissue	Fatty layer found below the dermis that gives smoothness and contour to the body, contains fat for use as energy, and also acts as a protective cushion for the outer skin; also called adipose or subcutis tissue.
subcutis	See "adipose"
sudoriferous glands	Sweat glands of the skin.
tactile corpuscles	Small epidermal structures with nerve endings that are sensitive to touch and pressure.
Vitamin A	Aids in the health, function, and repair of skin cells.
Vitamin C	Is needed for proper repair of the skin and various tissues.
Vitamin D	Promotes the healthy and rapid healing of the skin.
Vitamin E	Helps fight against, and protect the skin from the harmful effects of the sun's rays.

CHAPTER 8 NAIL STRUCTURE & GROWTH

chapter outline

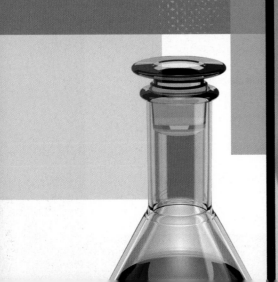

The Natural Nail
Nail Anatomy
Nail Growth
Know Your Nails

Learning Objectives

After completing this chapter, you will be able to:

- **Describe the structure and composition of nails.**
- **Discuss how nails grow.**

Key Terms

Page number indicates where in the chapter the term is used.

bed epithelium
pg. 135

cuticle
pg. 135

eponychium
pg. 135

free edge
pg. 135

hyponychium
pg. 135

ligament
pg. 135

lunula
pg. 135

matrix
pg. 135

nail bed
pg. 134

nail fold
pg. 136

nail groove
pg. 136

nail plate
pg. 135

nail unit
pg. 134

natural nail
pg. 134

onyx
pg. 134

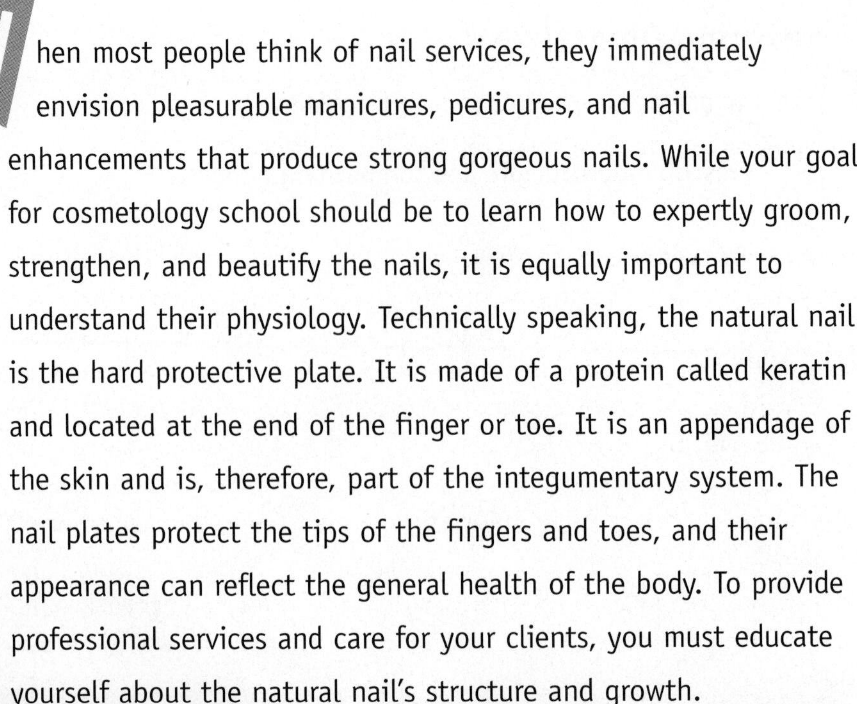

When most people think of nail services, they immediately envision pleasurable manicures, pedicures, and nail enhancements that produce strong gorgeous nails. While your goal for cosmetology school should be to learn how to expertly groom, strengthen, and beautify the nails, it is equally important to understand their physiology. Technically speaking, the natural nail is the hard protective plate. It is made of a protein called keratin and located at the end of the finger or toe. It is an appendage of the skin and is, therefore, part of the integumentary system. The nail plates protect the tips of the fingers and toes, and their appearance can reflect the general health of the body. To provide professional services and care for your clients, you must educate yourself about the natural nail's structure and growth.

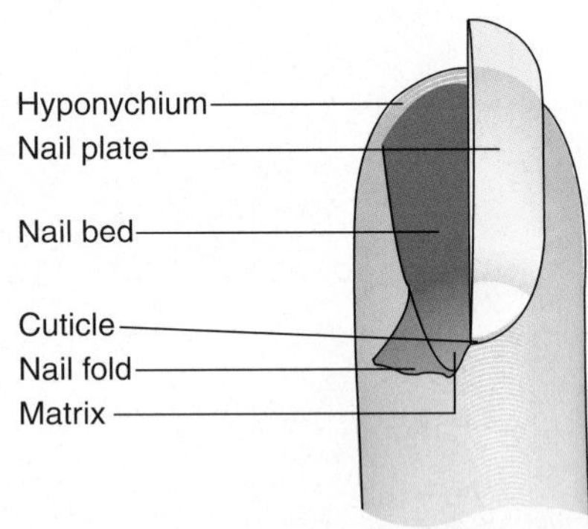

Figure 8-1 Structure of the natural nail.

THE NATURAL NAIL

The **natural nail,** which is technically referred to as **onyx** (AHN-iks), is composed mainly of keratin, the same protein found in skin and hair. The keratin in natural nails is harder than the keratin in hair or skin. A healthy nail should be whitish and translucent in appearance, with the pinkish color of the nail bed below showing through. The nail plate is relatively porous to water; allowing it to pass much more easily than it will pass through normal skin of equal thickness. The water content of the nail is related to the relative humidity of the surrounding environment. A healthy nail may look dry and hard, but it actually has a water content of between 15 and 25 percent. The water content directly affects the nail's flexibility. The lower the water content, the more rigid the nail becomes. Using an oil-based nail conditioner, or nail polish to coat the plate, can reduce water loss and improve flexibility.

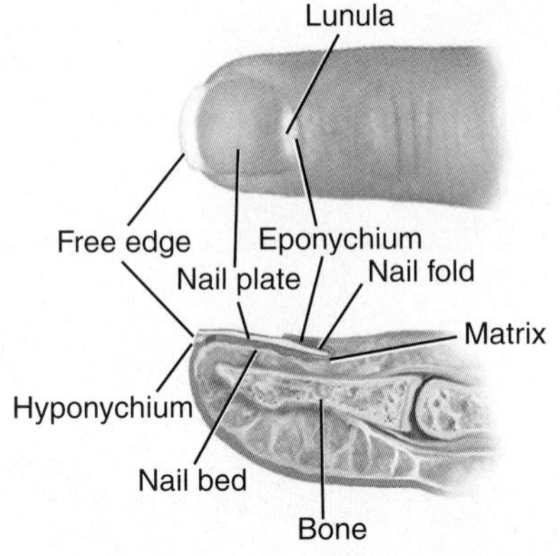

Figure 8-2 Cross-section of the nail.

NAIL ANATOMY

The natural **nail unit** consists of several anatomical parts necessary to produce the natural nail plate (Figures 8-1 and 8-2).

NAIL BED

The **nail bed** is the portion of living skin on which the nail plate sits. Because it is richly supplied with blood vessels, the area under the nail plate has a pinkish appearance in the area that extends from the lunula to

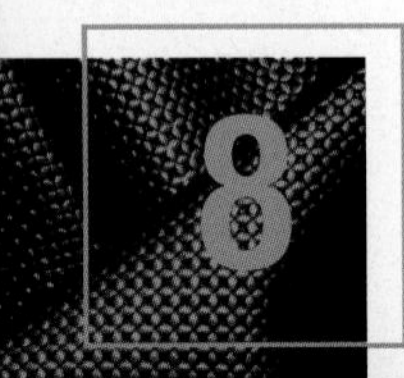

the area just before the free edge of the nail. The nail bed is supplied with many nerves, and is attached to the nail plate by a thin layer of tissue called the **bed epithelium** (ep-ih-THEE-lee-um). The bed epithelium helps guide the nail plate along the nail bed as it grows.

MATRIX

The **matrix** is where the natural nail is formed. The matrix is composed of matrix cells that produce other cells that become the nail plate. The matrix area contains nerves, lymph, and blood vessels to nourish the matrix cells. The matrix will continue to create new nail cells as long as it is nourished and kept in a healthy condition. The matrix extends from under the nail fold at the base of the nail plate. The visible part of the matrix that extends from underneath the living skin is called the **lunula** (LOO-nuh-luh). The lighter color of the lunula shows the true color of the matrix.

Growth of the nails can be affected if an individual is in poor health, a nail disorder or disease is present, or there has been an injury to the matrix.

NAIL PLATE

The **nail plate** is the most visible and functional part of the nail module. It is a hardened keratin plate that sits on and slides across the nail bed. It is formed by the matrix cells whose sole job is to create nail plate cells. The nail plate may appear to be one piece, but is actually constructed of about 100 layers of nail cells. The **free edge** is the part of the nail plate that extends over the tip of the finger or toe.

The **cuticle** (KYOO-tih-kul) is the dead colorless tissue attached to the nail plate. The cuticle comes from the underside of the skin that lies above the natural nail plate. This tissue is incredibly sticky and difficult to remove from the nail plate. Its job is to seal the space between the natural nail plate and living skin above to prevent entry of foreign material and microorganisms, thus helping to prevent injury and infection. The **eponychium** (ep-oh-NIK-eeum) is the living skin at the base of the nail plate covering the matrix area. The eponychium is sometimes confused with the cuticle. They are not the same. The cuticle is the dead tissue on the nail plate, where as the eponychium is living tissue. The cuticle comes from the underside of this area, where it becomes strongly attached to the new growth of nail plate and is pulled free to form a seal between the natural nail plate and the eponychium. The **hyponychium** (hy-poh-NIK-eeum) is the slightly thickened layer of skin that lies underneath the free edge of the nail plate. It creates a seal under the nail plate to prevent microorganisms from invading and infecting the nail bed.

SPECIALIZED LIGAMENTS

A **ligament** is a tough band of fibrous tissue that connects bones or holds an organ in place. Specialized ligaments attach the nail bed and matrix bed to the underlying bone. They are located at the base of the matrix and around the edges of the nail bed.

NAIL FOLDS

The **nail folds** are folds of normal skin that surround the nail plate. These folds form the **nail grooves,** which are the slits or furrows on the sides of the nail on which it moves as it grows.

NAIL GROWTH

The growth of the nail plate is affected by nutrition, exercise, and a person's general health. A normal nail grows forward from the matrix and extends over the tip of the finger. Normal, healthy nails can grow in a variety of shapes, depending on the shape of the matrix (Figure 8-3). The length, width, and curvature of the matrix determine the thickness, width, and curvature of the natural nail plate. For example, a longer matrix produces a thicker nail plate and a highly curved matrix creates a highly curved free edge.

The average rate of nail growth in the normal adult is about 1/10″ (3.7 mm) per month. Nails grow faster in the summer than they do in the winter. Children's nails grow more rapidly, whereas those of elderly persons grow at a slower rate. The nail of the middle finger grows fastest and the thumbnail grows the slowest. Nail growth rates increase dramatically during the last trimester of pregnancy due to hormonal changes in the body. The nail growth rate decreases dramatically after delivery and returns to normal, as do hormone levels in the body. It is a myth that this is due to taking prenatal care vitamins. Nail growth rates will accelerate whether or not a woman takes these vitamins. Although toenails grow slower than fingernails, they are thicker and harder.

NAIL MALFORMATION

If disease, injury, or infection occurs in the matrix, the shape or thickness of the nail plate can change. The natural nail will continue to grow as long as the matrix is healthy and undamaged. Ordinarily, replacement of the natural nail takes about 4 to 6 months. Toenails take 9 months to a year to be fully replaced. It should be noted that nails are not shed automatically or periodically, as is the case with hair.

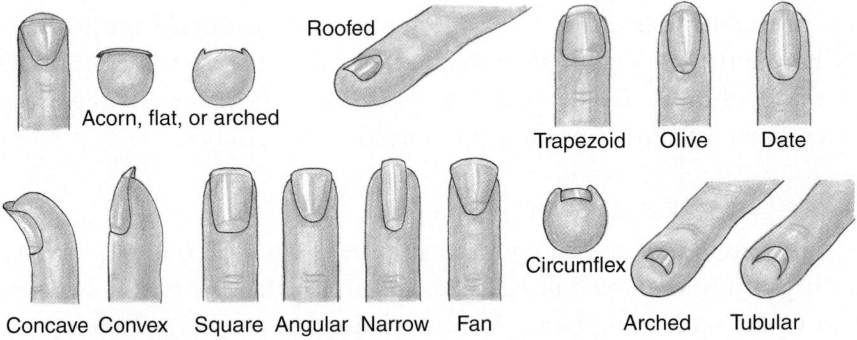

Figure 8-3 Various shapes of nails.

KNOW YOUR NAILS

Many nail care professionals are interested in nails because of the creative opportunities they present. As with every other area of cosmetology, this creativity must be grounded in a full awareness of the structure and physiology of the nails and the surrounding tissue. Working on good, strong, healthy nails can be a pleasure.

REVIEW QUESTIONS

1. Describe the appearance of a normal healthy nail.
2. What material is the nail plate made from?
3. Name six basic parts of the nail unit.
4. What part of the nail unit contains the nerve and blood supply?

CHAPTER GLOSSARY

bed epithelium	Thin layer of tissue between the nail plate and the nail bed.
cuticle	Dead tissue that tightly adheres to the nail plate.
eponychium	Living skin at the base of the nail plate covering the matrix area.
free edge	Part of the nail plate that extends over the tip of the finger or toe.
hyponychium	The slightly thickened layer of skin that lies beneath the free edge of the nail plate.
ligament	Tough bank of fibrous tissue that connects bones or holds an organ in place.
lunula	Whitish, half-moon shape at the base of the nail plate, caused by the reflection of light off the surface of the matrix.
matrix	Area where the natural nail is formed; this area is composed of matrix cells that make up the nail plate.
nail bed	Portion of the skin that the nail plate sits on.
nail fold	Fold of normal skin that surrounds the nail plate.
nail groove	Slit or furrow on the sides of the nail.
nail plate	Hardened keratin plate covering the nail bed.
nail unit	All the anatomical parts of the fingernail necessary to produce the natural nail plate.
natural nail	The hard protective plate of the nail, composed mailny of keratin.
onyx	The technical term for nail of the fingers or toes.

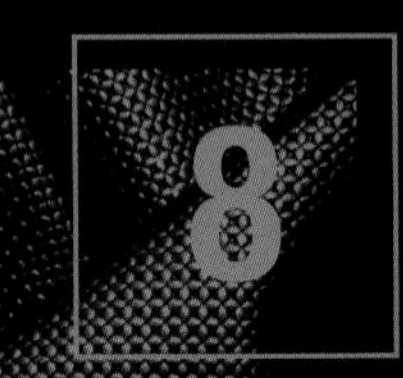

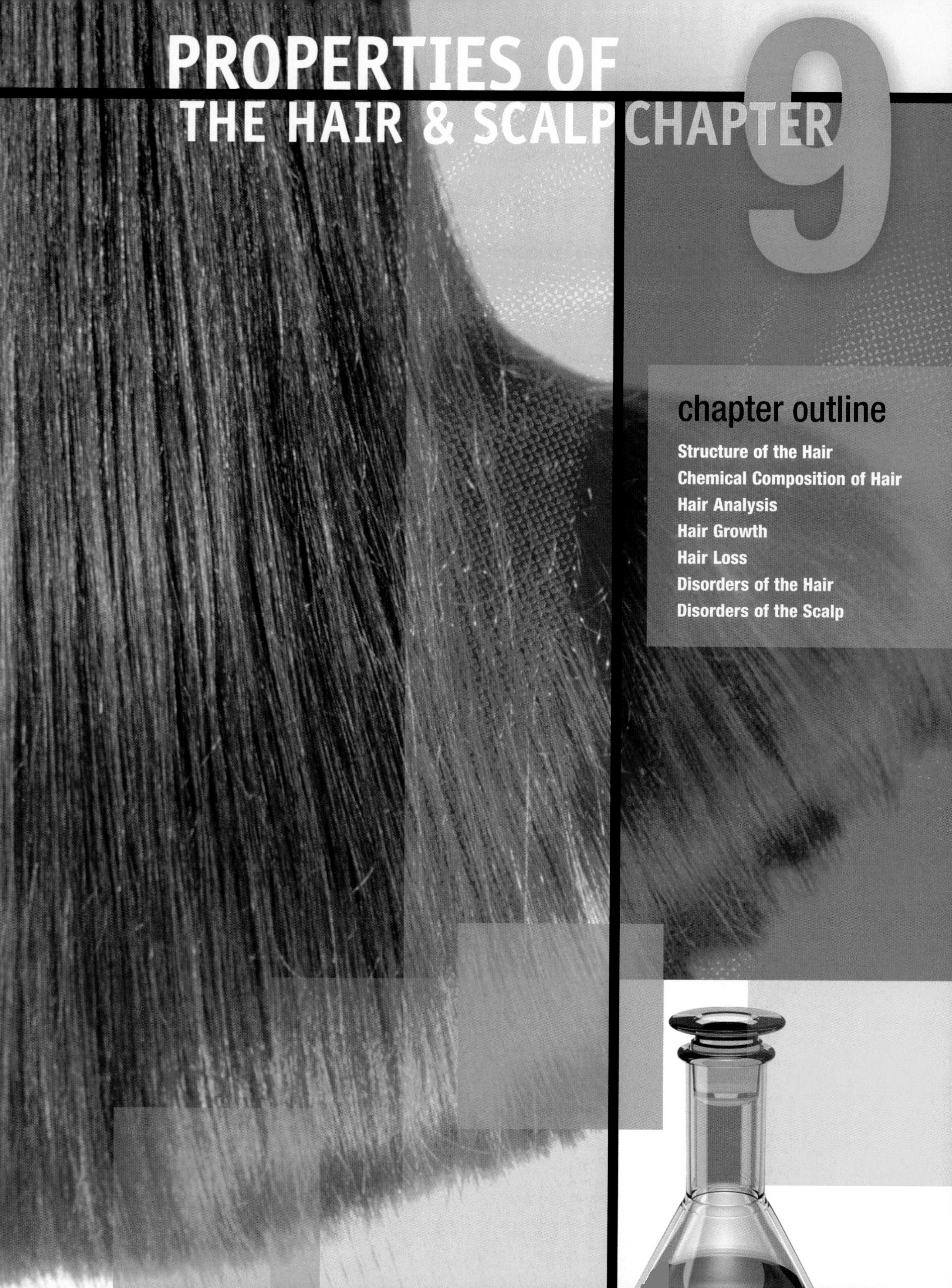

PROPERTIES OF THE HAIR & SCALP CHAPTER 9

chapter outline

Learning Objectives

After completing this chapter, you will be able to:

- **Name and describe the structures of the hair root.**
- **List and describe the three layers of the hair shaft.**
- **Describe the three types of side bonds in the cortex.**
- **List the factors that should be considered in a hair analysis.**
- **Describe the process of hair growth.**
- **Discuss the types of hair loss and their causes.**
- **Describe the options for hair loss treatment.**
- **Recognize hair and scalp disorders commonly seen in the salon and school, and know which can be treated by cosmetologists.**

Key Terms

Page number indicates where in the chapter the term is used.

alopecia pg. 154

alopecia areata pg. 155

amino acids pg. 144

anagen pg. 151

androgenic alopecia pg. 154

arrector pili pg. 143

canities pg. 156

carbuncle pg. 160

catagen pg. 151

COHNS elements pg. 144

cortex pg. 144

cowlick pg. 150

cuticle pg. 143

dermal papilla (plural: papillae) pg. 143

disulfide bond pg. 145

eumelanin pg. 146

follicle pg. 143

fragilitas crinium pg. 157

furuncle pg. 160

hair bulb pg. 143

hair density pg. 148

hair elasticity pg. 149

hair porosity pg. 149

hair root pg. 142

hair shaft pg. 142

hair stream pg. 150

hair texture pg. 147

helix pg. 145

hydrogen bond pg. 145

hypertrichosis pg. 156

integument pg. 142

keratinization pg. 144

malassezia pg. 158

medulla pg. 144

melanin pg. 145

monilethrix pg. 157

pediculosis capitis pg. 159

peptide bond (end bond) pg. 144

pheomelanin pg. 146

pityriasis pg. 158

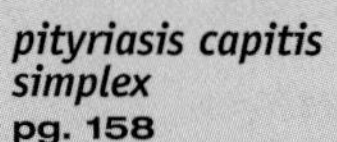

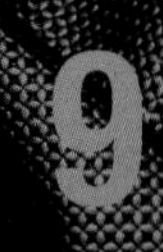

From Lady Godiva's infamous horseback ride, to all the sought-after celebrity styles that make headlines every day, hair has been one of humanity's most enduring obsessions. The term "crowning glory" aptly describes the importance placed on hair, such as how good we feel when our hair looks great, and just how distressing a "bad hair day" really can be. This is why hair stylists play such an important role in most people's lives.

As fascinating as hair styling may be, though, all professional hair services need to be based on a thorough understanding of the growth, structure, and composition of hair. It is the only way to know why hair grows and why it falls out, what creates natural color and texture, and how to spot an unhealthy scalp condition that could be harboring a communicable disease or even be causing permanent hair loss.

The scientific study of hair, and its diseases and care, is called **trichology** (trih-KAHL-uh-jee), which comes from the Greek words *trichos* (hair) and *ology* (the study of). As a cosmetologist, you will need to know as much as you can about the structure of hair, and how to keep it healthy. The more you learn, the more you will understand how salon services affect different hair types. That's the key to consistent results with your services and happy clients who recommend you to their friends.

The hair, skin, and nails are known collectively as the **integument** (in-TEG-yuh-ment), which is the largest and fastest growing organ of the human body. Although we no longer need hair for warmth and protection, hair still has an enormous impact on our psychology.

STRUCTURE OF THE HAIR

A mature strand of human hair is divided into two parts: hair root and hair shaft. The **hair root** is the part of the hair located below the surface of the scalp. The **hair shaft** is the portion of the hair that projects above the skin.

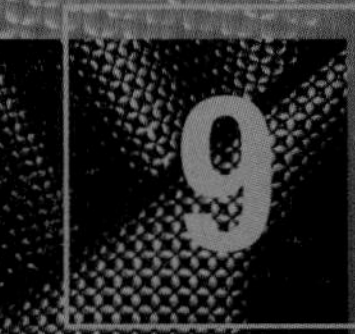

STRUCTURES OF THE HAIR ROOT

The main structures of the hair root include the follicle, bulb, papilla, arrector pili muscle, and sebaceous glands (Figure 9-1).

The **follicle** (FAWL-ih-kul) is the tube-like depression or pocket in the skin or scalp that contains the hair root. Hair follicles are distributed all over the body, with the exception of the palms of the hands and the soles of the feet. The follicle extends downward from the epidermis (the outer layer of skin) into the dermis (the inner layer of skin), where it surrounds the dermal papilla. It is not uncommon for more than one hair to grow from a single follicle.

The **hair bulb** is the lowest area or part of a hair strand. It is the thickened, club-shaped structure that forms the lower part of the hair root. The lower part of the hair bulb fits over and covers the dermal papilla.

The **dermal papilla** (puh-PIL-uh) (plural: papillae) is a small, cone-shaped area located at the base of the hair follicle that fits into the hair bulb. The dermal papilla contains the blood and nerve supply that provides the nutrients needed for hair growth.

The **arrector pili** (ah-REK-tohr PY-ly) is a tiny, involuntary muscle in the base of the hair follicle. Strong emotions or cold causes it to contract, which makes the hair stand up straight, resulting in "goose bumps."

Sebaceous glands (sih-BAY-shus) are the oil glands of the skin, connected to the hair follicles. The sebaceous glands secrete an oily substance called **sebum** (SEE-bum), which lubricates the hair and skin.

STRUCTURES OF THE HAIR SHAFT

The three main layers of the hair shaft are the cuticle, cortex, and medulla (Figure 9-2).

The **cuticle** (KYOO-ti-kul) is the outermost layer of hair. It consists of an overlapping layer of transparent, scale-like cells that look like shingles on a roof. The cuticle layer provides a barrier that protects the inner structure of hair as it lies tightly against the cortex. It is responsible for creating the shine and the smooth, silky feel of healthy hair.

To feel the cuticle, pinch a single healthy strand of hair between your fingers, starting near the scalp. Pull downward and feel the sleek, smooth feel of the hair. Next, pinch the end of the hair and move up the hair shaft. In this direction, the hair feels rougher because you are going against the natural growth of the cuticle layer. A healthy, compact cuticle layer is the hair's primary defense against damage. A lengthwise section of hair shows that although the cuticle scales overlap, each individual cuticle scale is attached to the cortex (Figure 9-3). These overlapping scales make up the

Did You Know

Although a healthy diet does not always guarantee a healthy hair and scalp, you are what you eat. Your body cannot produce healthy hair without the proper nutrients. The body can produce 11 of the 20 amino acids that make up hair, but the remaining nine must come from your daily diet. This is why crash dieting and anorexia can cause hair loss, lackluster hair and unhealthy scalp conditions. Proteins in meat, fish, eggs, and dairy products are good sources of these amino acids, as are food combinations such as peanut butter and bread, rice and beans, and beans and corn.

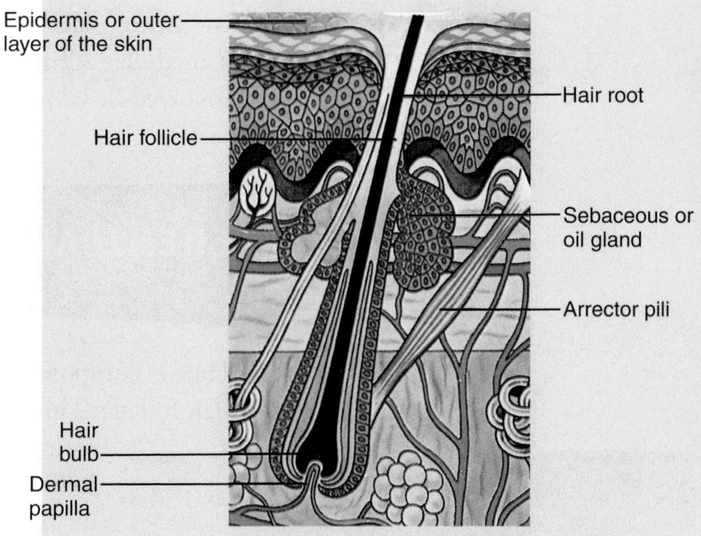

Figure 9-1 Structures of the hair.

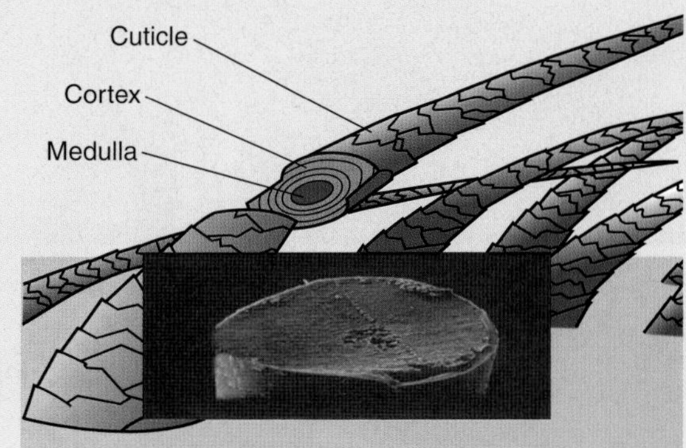

Figure 9-2 Cross-section of hair.

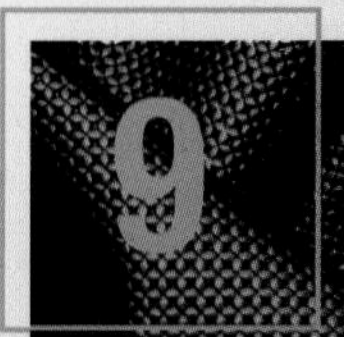

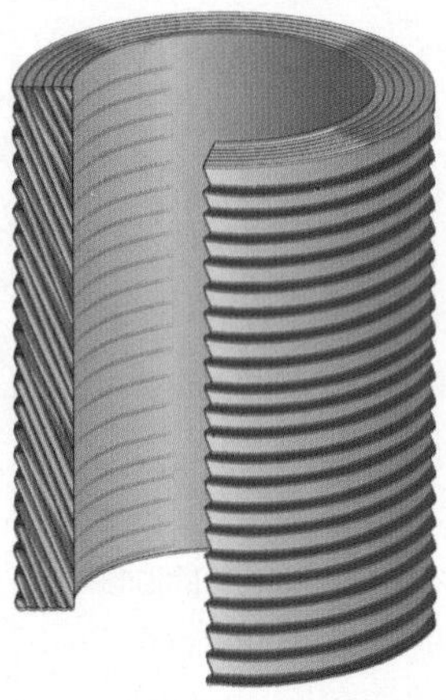

Figure 9-3 Cuticle layer.

cuticle layer. When viewed in cross-section, scales can be seen to overlap. Swelling the hair raises the cuticle layer and opens the space between the scales, which allows liquids to penetrate into the cortex.

A healthy cuticle layer protects the hair from penetration and prevents damage to hair fibers. Oxidation haircolors, permanent waving solutions, and chemical hair relaxers must have an alkaline pH in order to penetrate the cuticle layer, because a high pH swells the cuticle causing it to lift and expose the cortex.

The **cortex** is the middle layer of the hair. It is a fibrous protein core formed by elongated cells containing melanin pigment. About 90 percent of the total weight of hair comes from the cortex. The elasticity of the hair and its natural color are the result of the unique protein structures located within the cortex. The changes involved in oxidation haircoloring, wet setting, thermal styling, permanent waving, and chemical hair relaxing all take place within the cortex (Figure 9-4).

The **medulla** (muh-DUL-uh) is the innermost layer and is composed of round cells. It is quite common for very fine and naturally blond hair to entirely lack a medulla. Generally, only thick, coarse hair contains a medulla. All male beard hair contains a medulla. The medulla is not involved in salon services.

CHEMICAL COMPOSITION OF HAIR

Hair is composed of protein that grows from cells originating within the hair follicle. This is where the hair shaft begins. As soon as these living cells form, they begin their journey upward through the hair follicle. They mature in a process called **keratinization** (kair-uh-ti-ni-ZAY-shun). As these newly formed cells mature, they fill up with a fibrous protein called keratin, then move upward, lose their nucleus, and die. By the time the hair shaft emerges from the scalp, the cells of the hair are completely keratinized and are no longer living. The hair shaft that emerges from the scalp is a nonliving fiber composed of keratinized protein.

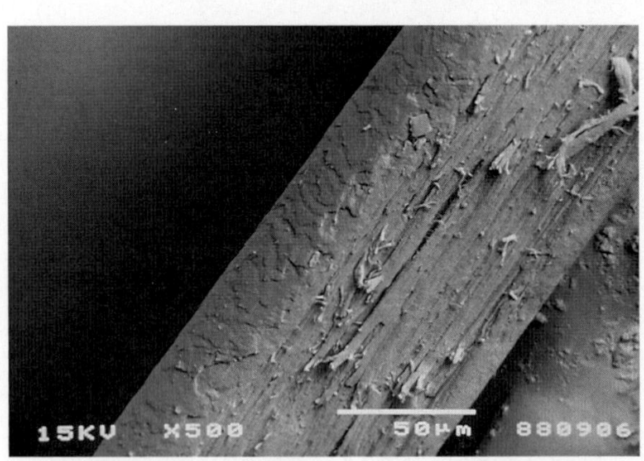

Figure 9-4 Hair shaft with part of cuticle stripped off, exposing the cortex.

Hair is approximately 90 percent protein. The protein is made up of long chains of amino acids, which, in turn, are made up of elements. The main elements that make up human hair are carbon, oxygen, hydrogen, nitrogen, and sulfur. These five elements are the major elements found in skin, hair, and nails, and are often referred to as the **COHNS elements.** Table 9-1 shows the percentages of each element in a typical strand of hair.

Proteins are made of long chains of **amino acids** (uh-MEE-noh AS-udz) that are linked together end to end like pop beads. The chemical bond that links amino acids is called a **peptide** (PEP-tyd) **bond or end bond.** A long chain of amino acids linked by peptide bonds is called a

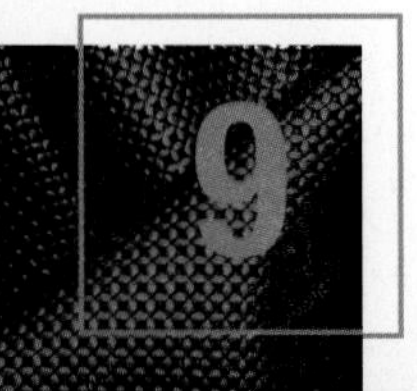

polypeptide (pahl-ee-PEP-tyd). Proteins are long, coiled, complex polypeptides made of amino acids. The spiral shape of a coiled protein is called a **helix** (HEE-licks) (Figure 9-5).

ELEMENT	Percentage in Normal Hair
Carbon	51%
Oxygen	21%
Hydrogen	6%
Nitrogen	17%
Sulfur	5%

Table 9-1 The COHNS Elements

SIDE BONDS OF THE CORTEX

The cortex is made up of millions of polypeptide chains. These **polypeptide chains** are cross-linked like the rungs on a ladder by three different types of side bonds. The three types of side bonds are called hydrogen, salt, and disulfide bonds (Figure 9-6). These side bonds hold the keratin fibers in place and account for the incredible strength and elasticity of human hair. They are essential to services such as wet sets, thermal styling, permanent waving, and chemical hair relaxing (see Chapter 18).

A **hydrogen bond** is a weak physical side bond that is easily broken by water or heat. Although individual hydrogen bonds are very weak, there are so many of them that they account for about one-third of the hair's overall strength.

A **salt bond** is also a weak, temporary side bond between adjacent polypeptide chains. Salt bonds are easily broken by strong alkaline or acidic solutions, and account for about one-third of the hair's overall strength.

A **disulfide** (dy-SUL-fyd) **bond** is a chemical side bond that is very different from the physical bonding of a hydrogen or salt bond. The disulfide bond joins the sulfur atoms of two neighboring cysteine (SIS-ti-een) amino acids to create cystine (SIS-teen). Although there are far fewer disulfide bonds than hydrogen or salt bonds, disulfide bonds are much stronger and account for about one-third of the hair's overall strength. Disulfide bonds are not broken by heat or water. Permanent waves, and chemical hair relaxers change the shape of hair by chemically changing the hair's disulfide bonds (Table 9-2).

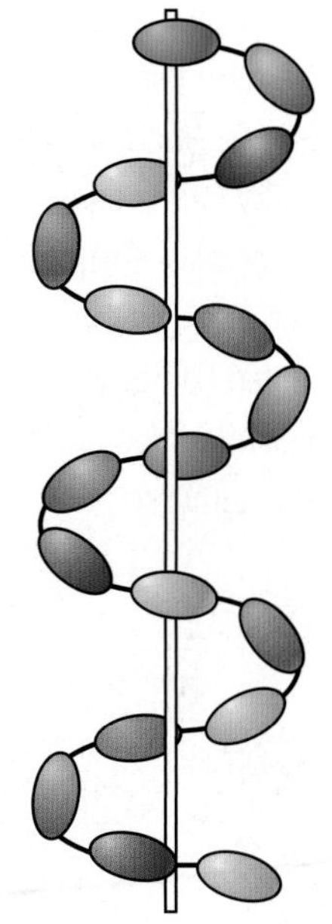

Figure 9-5 Polypeptide chains intertwine in a spiral shape called a helix.

Thio permanent waves break disulfide bonds, which are re-formed by thio neutralizers. Hydroxide chemical hair relaxers break disulfide bonds and then convert them to lanthionine bonds when the relaxer is rinsed from the hair. The disulfide bonds that are treated with hydroxide relaxers are broken permanently and can never be reformed (see Chapter 18).

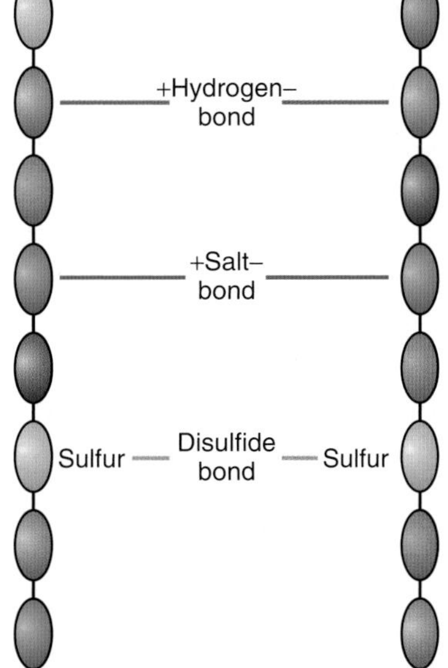

Figure 9-6 Side bonds between polypeptide chains.

HAIR PIGMENT

All natural hair color is the result of the pigment located within the cortex. **Melanin** (MEL-uh-nin) are the tiny grains of pigment

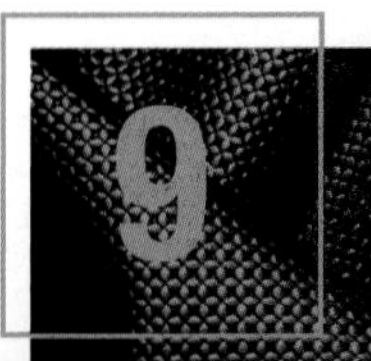

BOND	Type	Strength	Broken By	Re-formed By
hydrogen	side bond	weak physical	water or heat	drying or cooling
salt	side bond	weak physical	changes in pH	normalizing pH
disulfide	side bond	strong chemical	1. thio perms and thio relaxers 2. hydroxide relaxers	1. oxidation with neutralizer 2. converted to lanthionine bonds
peptide	end bond	strong chemical	chemical depilatories	not re-formed; hair dissolves

Table 9-2 Bonds of the Hair

Did You Know

The term "hair color" refers to the color of hair created by nature. "Haircolor" (one word) is the term used in the beauty industry to refer to artificial haircoloring products. Gray hair is caused by the absence of melanin. Gray hair grows from the hair bulb in exactly the same way that pigmented hair grows and has exactly the same structure, but without the melanin pigment.

in the cortex that give natural color to the hair. The two different types of melanin are eumelanin and pheomelanin.

1. **Eumelanin** (yoo-MEL-uh-nin) provides brown and black color to hair.
2. **Pheomelanin** (fee-oh-MEL-uh-nin) provides colors ranging from red and ginger to yellow/blond tones.

All natural hair color is the result of the ratio of eumelanin to pheomelanin, along with the total number and size of pigment granules.

WAVE PATTERN

The **wave pattern** of the hair refers to the shape of the hair strand, and is described as straight, wavy, curly, or extremely curly (Figure 9-7).

Natural wave patterns are the result of genetics. Although there are many exceptions, as a general rule, Asians tend to have extremely straight hair, Caucasians tend to have straight to wavy hair, and African Americans tend to have extremely curly hair. But straight, curly, and extremely curly hair occur in all races. This means that anyone of any race, or mixed race, can have hair with varying degrees of curliness from straight to extremely curly. Within a racial/ethnic group, individuals' hair varies according to degree of curliness.

The wave pattern may also vary from strand to strand on the same person's head. It is not uncommon for an individual to have different amounts of curl in different areas of the head. Individuals with curly hair often have straighter hair in the crown and curlier hair in other areas.

Several theories attempt to explain the cause of natural curly hair, but there is no single, definite answer that explains why some hair grows straight and other hair grows curly. The most popular theory claims that the shape of the hair's cross-section determines the amount of curl. This theory claims that hair with a round cross-section is straight, hair with an oval cross-section is wavy, and hair with a flat cross-section is curly. Although it is true that cross-sections of straight hair tend to be round and curlier hair tends to be more oval, modern microscopes have shown that a cross-section of hair can be almost any shape, including triangular, and that the shape of the cross-section does not always relate to the amount of curl.

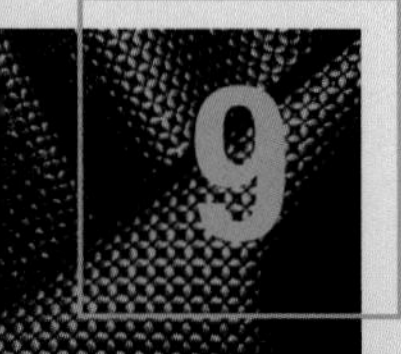

At present, natural curl is believed to be the result of one side of the hair strand growing faster than the other side. Since the side that grows faster will be slightly longer than the slower-growing side, tension within the strand causes the long side to curl around the short side. Hair that grows uniformly on both sides does not create tension and results in straight hair. However, this theory is still unproven.

EXTREMELY CURLY HAIR

Extremely curly hair grows in long twisted spirals. Cross-sections are highly oval and vary in shape and thickness along their length. Compared to straight or wavy hair, which tends to possess a fairly regular and uniform diameter along a single strand, extremely curly hair is fairly irregular, exhibiting varying diameters along a single strand. Some extremely curly hair has a natural tendency to form a coil like a telephone cord. Coiled hair usually has a fine texture, with many individual strands winding together to form the coiled locks that characterize this type of hair. Extremely curly hair often has low elasticity, breaks easily, and has a tendency to knot, especially on the ends. Gentle scalp manipulations, conditioning shampoo, and a detangling rinse help minimize tangles.

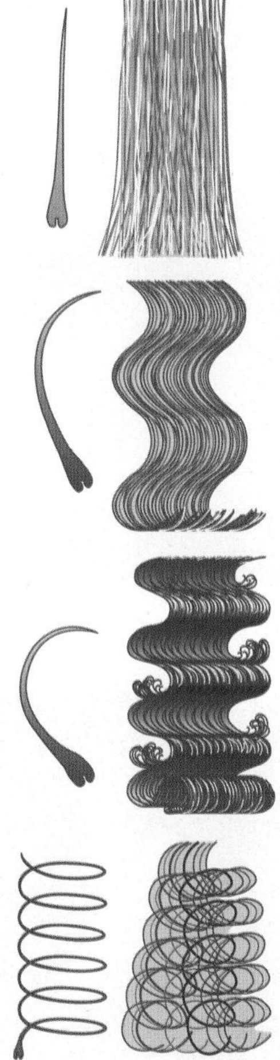

Figure 9-7 Straight, wavy, curly, and extremely curly hair strands.

HAIR ANALYSIS

All successful salon services must begin with a thorough analysis of the client's hair type and its present condition in order to determine the results that can reasonably be expected from the service. Because different types of hair react differently to the same service, it is essential that a thorough analysis be performed prior to all salon services. Hair analysis is performed by observation using the senses of sight, touch, hearing, and smell. The four most important factors to consider in hair analysis are texture, porosity, elasticity, and density. Other factors that you should also be aware of are growth pattern and dryness versus oiliness.

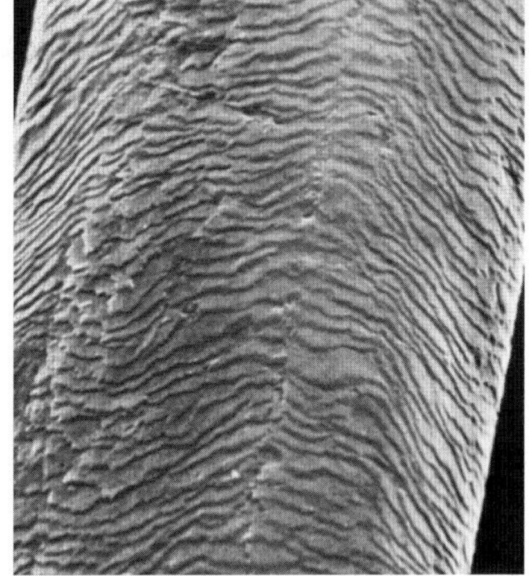

Figure 9-8 Coarse hair.

HAIR TEXTURE

Hair texture is the thickness or diameter of the individual hair strand. Hair texture can be classified as coarse, medium, or fine (Figures 9-8, 9-9, and 9-10). Hair texture can vary from strand to strand on the same person's head. It is not uncommon for hair from different areas of the head to have different textures. Hair from the nape (back of the neck), crown, temples, and front hairline of the same person may have different textures.

Coarse hair texture has the largest diameter. It is stronger than fine hair, for the same reason that a thick rope is stronger than a thin rope. It usually requires more processing than medium or fine hair, and is often more resistant to that processing. This is why it is more difficult for hair

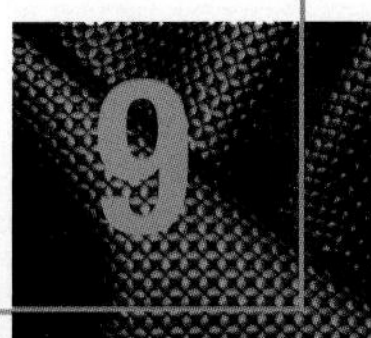

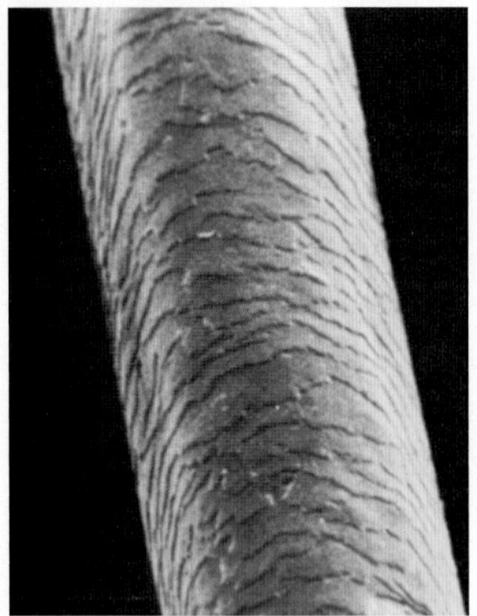
Figure 9-9 Medium hair.

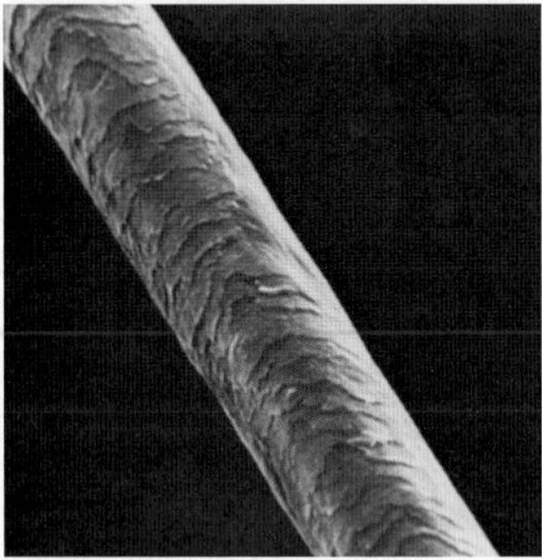
Figure 9-10 Fine hair.

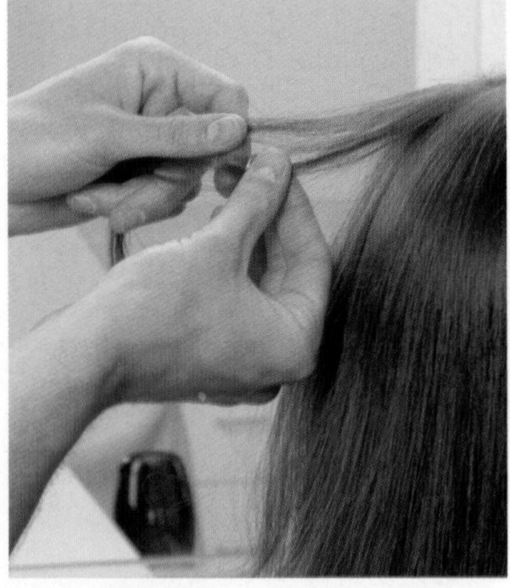
Figure 9-11 Testing for hair texture.

lighteners, haircolors, permanent waving solutions, and chemical hair relaxers to process on coarse hair.

Medium hair texture is the most common, and is the standard to which other hair is compared. Medium hair does not pose any special problems or concerns.

Fine hair has the smallest diameter and is more fragile, easier to process, and more susceptible to damage from chemical services than coarse or medium hair.

Hair texture can be determined by feeling a single dry strand between the fingers. Take an individual strand from four different areas of the head—front hairline, temple, crown, and nape—and hold the strand securely with one hand while feeling it with the thumb and forefinger of the other hand. With a little practice, you will be able to feel the difference between coarse, medium, and fine hair diameters (Figure 9-11).

HAIR DENSITY

Hair density measures the number of individual hair strands on 1 square inch (2.5 cm) of scalp. It indicates how many hairs there are on a person's head. Hair density can be classified as low, medium, or high (or thin, medium, or thick/dense). Hair density is different from hair texture in that individuals with the same hair texture can have different densities.

Some individuals may have coarse hair texture (each hair has a large diameter), but low hair density (a low number of hairs on the head). Others may have fine hair texture (each hair has a small diameter), but high hair density (a high number of hairs on the head).

The average hair density is about 2,200 hairs per square inch. Hair with high density (thick or dense hair) has more hairs per square inch, and hair with low density (thin hair) has fewer hairs per square inch. The average head of hair contains about 100,000 individual hair strands. The number of hairs on the head generally varies with the color of the hair. Blonds usually have the highest density, and people with red hair tend to have the lowest. Average hair density by hair color follows: blond, 140,000; brown, 110,000; black, 108,000; and red, 80,000 (Table 9-3).

HAIR COLOR	Average Number of Hairs on Head
Blond	140,000
Brown	110,000
Black	108,000
Red	80,000

Table 9-3 Average Number of Hairs on the Head by Hair Color

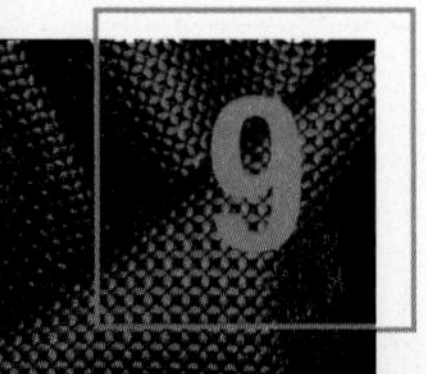

HAIR POROSITY

Hair porosity is the ability of the hair to absorb moisture. The degree of porosity is directly related to the condition of the cuticle layer. Healthy hair with a compact cuticle layer is naturally resistant to penetration. Porous hair has a raised cuticle layer that easily absorbs moisture.

Hair with low porosity is considered resistant (Figure 9-12). Chemical services performed on hair with low porosity require a more alkaline solution than those on hair with high porosity. Alkaline solutions raise the cuticle and permit uniform saturation and processing on resistant hair.

Hair with average porosity is considered to be normal hair (Figure 9-13). Chemical services performed on this type of hair will usually process as expected, according to the texture.

Hair with high porosity is considered overly porous hair and is often the result of previous overprocessing (Figure 9-14). Overly porous hair is damaged, dry, fragile, and brittle. Chemical services performed on overly porous hair require less alkaline solutions with a lower pH, which help prevent additional overprocessing and damage.

The texture of the hair can be an indication of its porosity, but it is only a general rule of thumb. Different degrees of porosity can be found in all hair textures. Although coarse hair normally has a low porosity and is resistant to chemical services, in some cases coarse hair will have high porosity, perhaps as the result of previous chemical services.

You can check porosity on dry hair by taking a strand of several hairs from four different areas of the head (front hairline, temple, crown, and nape). Hold the strand securely with one hand while sliding the thumb and forefinger of the other hand from the end to the scalp. If the hair feels smooth and the cuticle is compact, dense, and hard, it is considered resistant. If you can feel a slight roughness, it is considered porous. If the hair feels very rough, dry, or breaks, it is considered highly porous and may have been overprocessed (Figure 9-15).

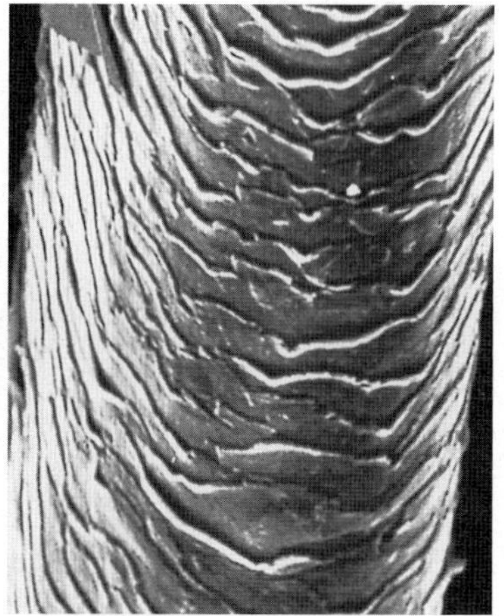

Figure 9-12 Low porosity (resistant hair).

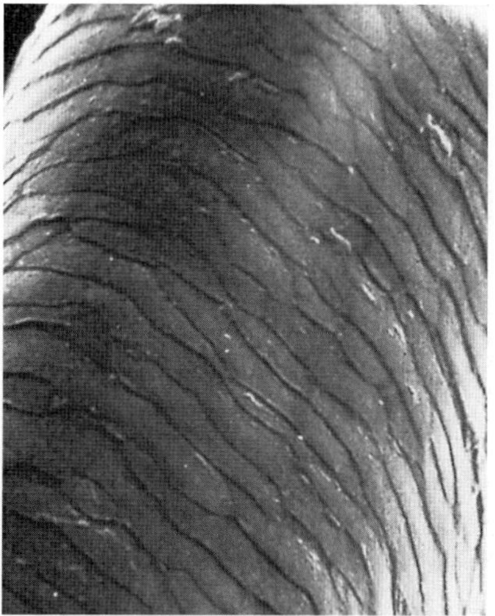

Figure 9-13 Average porosity (normal hair).

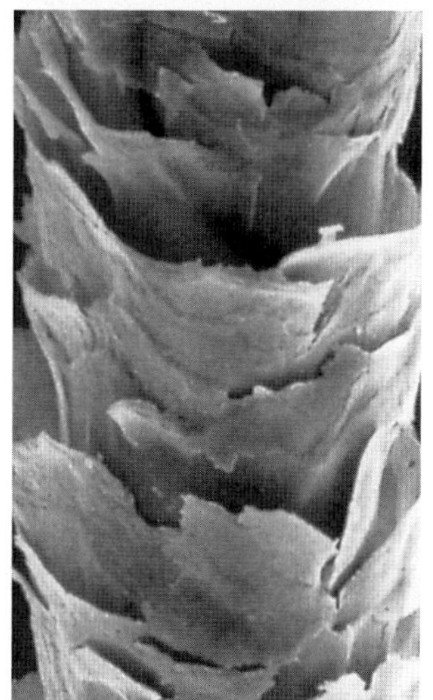

Figure 9-14 High porosity (overly porous).

HAIR ELASTICITY

Hair elasticity is the ability of the hair to stretch and return to its original length without breaking. Hair elasticity is an indication of the strength of the side bonds that hold the hair's individual fibers in place. Wet hair with normal elasticity will stretch up to 50% of its original length and return to that same length without breaking. Dry hair stretches about 20% of its length.

Hair with low elasticity is brittle and breaks easily. It may not be able to hold the curl from wet setting, thermal styling, or permanent waving. Hair with low elasticity is the result of weak side bonds that usually result from previous overprocessing. Chemical services performed on hair with low elasticity require a milder solution with a lower pH in order to minimize further damage and prevent additional overprocessing.

Check elasticity on wet hair by taking an individual strand from four different areas of the head (front hairline, temple, crown, and nape). Hold a single strand of wet hair securely and try to pull it apart (Figure 9-16).

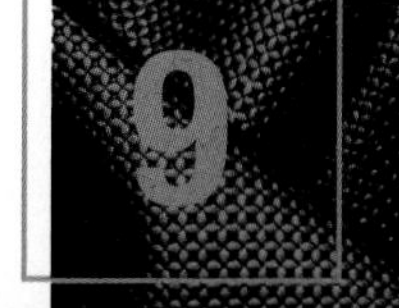

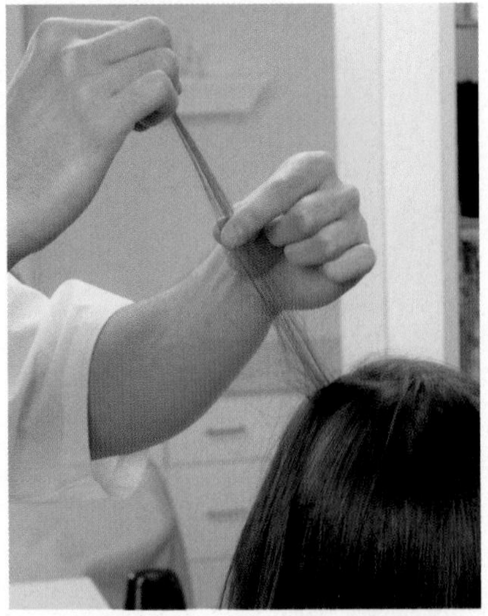

Figure 9-15 Testing for hair porosity.

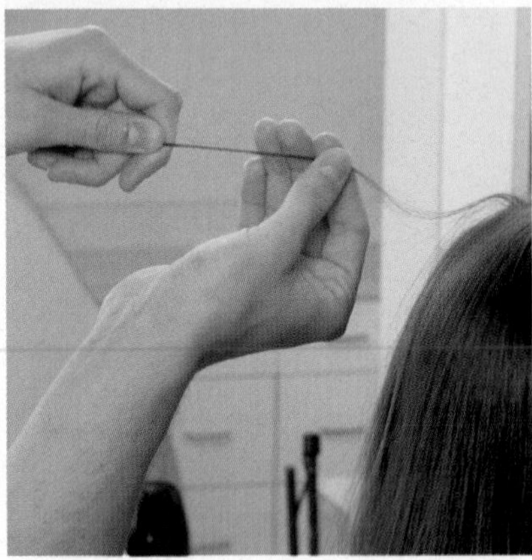

Figure 9-16 Testing for hair elasticity.

If the hair stretches and returns to its original length without breaking, it has normal elasticity. If the hair breaks easily or fails to return to its original length, it has low elasticity.

GROWTH PATTERNS

It is important when shaping and styling hair to consider the hair's growth patterns. Hair follicles do not usually grow perpendicular to the scalp. Most hair follicles grow at an angle other than 90 degrees, and most hair grows in a direction other than straight out from the head. These growth patterns result in hair streams, whorls, and cowlicks.

- A **hair stream** is hair flowing in the same direction, resulting from follicles sloping in the same direction. Two streams flowing in opposite directions form a natural part in the hair.
- A **whorl** is hair that forms in a circular pattern, as on the crown. A whorl normally forms in the crown with all the hair from that point growing down.
- A **cowlick** is a tuft of hair that stands straight up. Cowlicks are usually more noticeable at the front hairline, but they may be located anywhere.

DRY HAIR AND SCALP

Dry hair and scalp can be caused by inactive sebaceous glands, and is aggravated by excessive shampooing or dry air, such as during winter or in a desert climate. The lack of natural oils (sebum) leads to hair that appears dull, dry, and lifeless. Dry hair and scalp should be treated with products that contain moisturizers and emollients.

Frequent shampooing should be avoided, along with the use of strong soaps, detergents, or products with a high alcohol content because they could aggravate existing conditions. Dry hair should not be confused with overly porous hair that has been damaged by thermal styling, environmental effects (e.g., sunlight), or chemical services.

OILY HAIR AND SCALP

Oily hair and scalp is caused by improper shampooing or overactive sebaceous glands, and is characterized by a greasy buildup on the scalp and an oily coating on the hair. Oily hair and scalp can be treated by properly washing with a normalizing shampoo. A well-balanced diet, exercise, regular shampooing, and good personal hygiene are essential to controlling oily hair and scalp.

HAIR GROWTH

The two main types of hair found on the body are vellus and terminal hair (Figure 9-17).

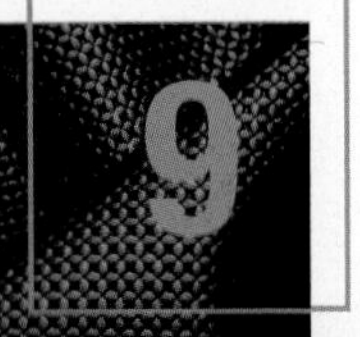

Vellus or lanugo hair is short, fine, and downy. Vellus hair is not pigmented and almost never has a medulla. It is commonly found on infants and can be present on children until puberty. On adults, vellus hair is usually found in places that are normally considered hairless (forehead, eyelids, and bald scalp), as well as nearly all other areas of the body, except the palms of the hands and the soles of the feet. Women normally retain 55 percent more vellus hair than men. Vellus hair helps in the efficient evaporation of perspiration.

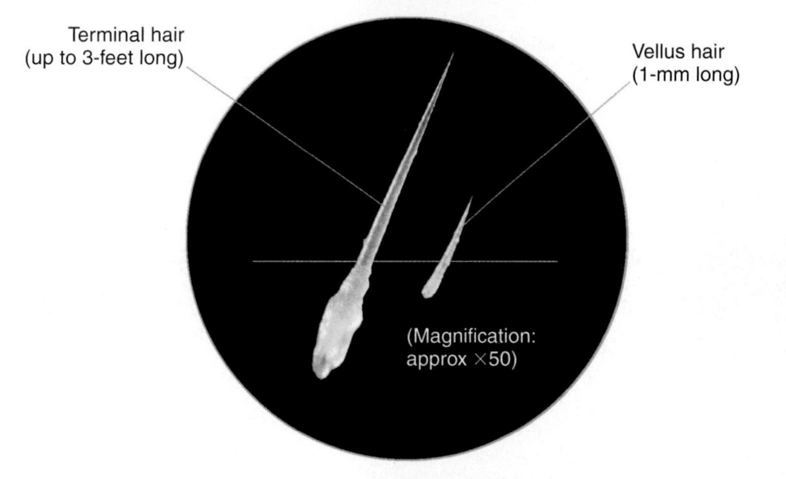

Figure 9-17 Terminal and vellus hair.

Terminal hair is the long hair found on the scalp, legs, arms, and bodies of males and females. Terminal hair is coarser than vellus hair and, with the exception of gray hair, it is pigmented. It usually has a medulla and is easily distinguished from vellus hair by its dark color and coarse texture.

Hormonal changes during puberty cause some areas of fine vellus hair to be replaced with thicker terminal hair. All hair follicles are capable of producing either vellus or terminal hair, depending on genetics, age, and hormones.

GROWTH CYCLES OF HAIR

Hair growth occurs in cycles. Each complete cycle has three phases that are repeated over and over again throughout life. The three phases are anagen, catagen, and telogen (Figure 9-18).

ANAGEN: THE GROWTH PHASE

During the **anagen** (AN-uh-jen) or growth phase, new hair is produced. New cells are actively manufactured in the hair follicle. During this phase, hair cells are produced faster than any other normal cell in the human body. The average growth of healthy scalp hair is about one half inch (1.25 centimeters) per month. The rate of growth varies on different parts of the body, between sexes, and with age. Scalp hair grows faster on women than on men. Scalp hair grows rapidly between the ages of 15 and 30, but slows down sharply after the age of 50.

About 90 percent of scalp hair is growing in the anagen phase at any one time. The anagen phase generally lasts from three to five years, but in some cases, it can last as long as ten years. The longer the anagen cycle is, the longer the hair is able to grow. This is why some people can only grow their hair down to their shoulders, while others can grow it down to the floor!

CATAGEN: THE TRANSITION PHASE

The **catagen** (KAT-uh-jen) phase is the brief transition period between the growth and resting phases of a hair follicle. It signals the end of the growth phase. During the catagen phase, the follicle canal shrinks and detaches from the dermal papilla. The hair bulb disappears and the

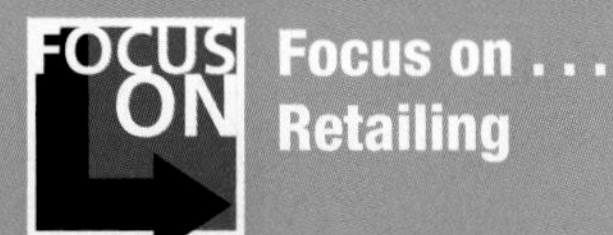

Focus on . . . Retailing

Did you know that selling retail products increases client retention? A client who takes home a retail product is more than twice as likely to return for services. Recommending products for home use is an important part of a successful career as a hairstylist. Your client needs to know which products to use and how to use them. A complete hair analysis will enable you to recommend the right products for your client with confidence. It is your job to know more about your client's specific needs than anyone else and to recommend the right products to satisfy those needs. Your clients do not want to make these decisions by themselves. They want your advice. Do not disappoint them.

ACTIVITY

Break up into groups of two or more in the classroom and analyze each other's hair. Hair analysis includes evaluating texture, density, porosity, and elasticity. Wave patterns, growth patterns, and the oiliness or dryness of the hair and scalp should also be noted. Follow the procedures in this textbook and use the same terminology. Write down results and present an oral report to the class. What is the most common texture among your classmates? The most common density?

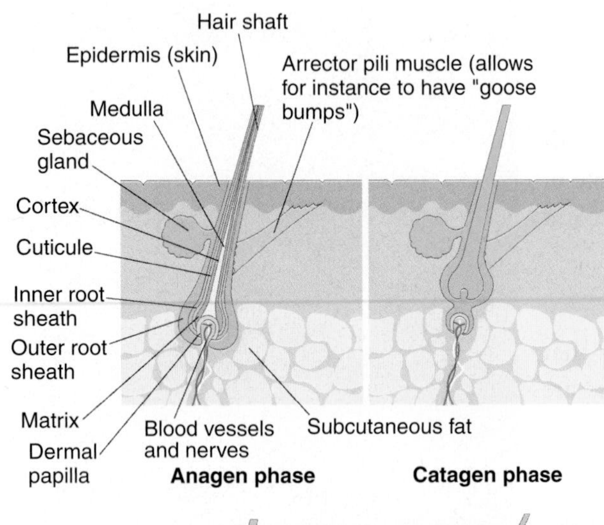

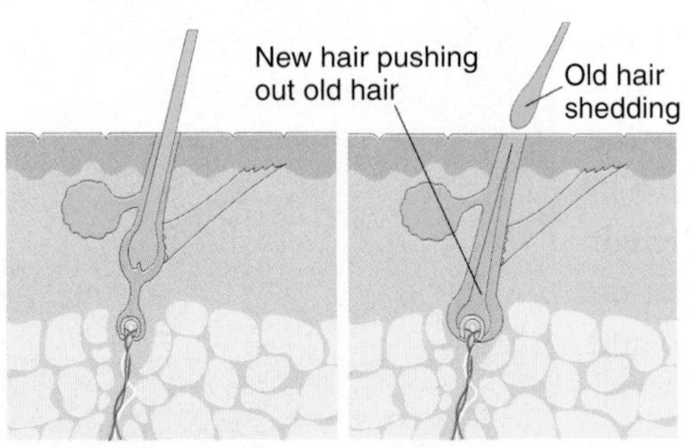

Figure 9-18 Cycles of hair growth.

shrunken root end forms a rounded club. Less than 1 percent of scalp hair is in the catagen phase at any one time. The catagen phase is very short and lasts from 1 to 2 weeks.

TELOGEN: THE RESTING PHASE

The **telogen** (TEL-uh-jen) or resting phase is the final phase in the hair cycle and lasts until the fully grown hair is shed. The hair is either shed during the telogen phase or remains in place until the next anagen phase, when the new hair growing in pushes it out. About 10 percent of scalp hair is in the telogen phase at any one time.

The telogen phase lasts for approximately 3 to 6 months. As soon as the telogen phase ends, the hair returns to the anagen phase and begins the entire cycle again. On average, the entire growth cycle repeats itself once every 4 to 5 years.

THE TRUTH ABOUT HAIR GROWTH

As a stylist, you may hear myths and opinions about hair growth from your clients or from other stylists. Here are some myths and facts about hair growth.

Myth: Shaving, clipping, and cutting the hair makes it grow back faster, darker, and coarser.

Fact: Shaving or cutting the hair has no effect on hair growth. When hair is blunt cut to the same length, it grows back more evenly. Although that may make it seem to grow back faster, darker, and coarser, shaving or cutting hair has no effect on hair growth.

Myth: Scalp massage increases hair growth.

Fact: There is no evidence that any type of stimulation or scalp massage increases hair growth. Minoxidil and finasteride are the only treatments that have been proven to increase hair growth and are approved for that purpose by the Food and Drug Administration (FDA). Products that claim to increase hair growth are regulated as "drugs," and are not "cosmetics."

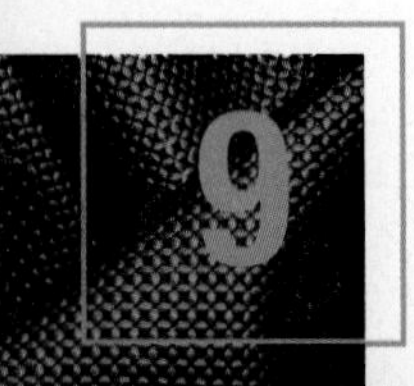

Myth: Gray hair is coarser and more resistant than pigmented hair.

Fact: Other than the lack of pigment, gray hair is exactly the same as pigmented hair. Although gray hair may be resistant, it is not resistant simply because it is gray. The pigmented hair on the same person's head is just as resistant as the gray hair. Gray hair is simply more noticeable than pigmented hair.

Myth: The amount of natural curl is always determined by racial background.

Fact: Anyone of any race, or mixed race, can have hair from straight to extremely curly. It is also true that within races, individuals have hair with different degrees of curliness.

Myth: Hair with a round cross-section is straight, hair with an oval cross-section is wavy, and hair with a flat cross-section is curly.

Fact: In general, cross-sections of straight hair are often round and curlier hair can be more oval, but cross-sections of hair can be almost any shape, including triangular. The shape of the cross-section does not always relate to the amount of curl or the shape of the follicle.

HAIR LOSS

Under normal circumstances, we all lose some hair every day. Normal daily hair loss is the natural result of the three phases of the hair's growth cycle.

The growth cycle provides for the continuous growth, fall, and replacement of individual hair strands. A hair that is shed in the telogen phase is replaced by a new hair, in that same follicle, in the next anagen phase. This natural shedding of hair accounts for normal daily hair loss. Although estimates of the rate of hair loss have long been quoted at 100 to 150 hairs per day, recent measurements indicate that the average rate of hair loss is closer to 35 to 40 hairs per day.

Over 63 million people in the United States suffer from abnormal hair loss. As a professional hair stylist, it is likely that you will be the first person that many of these people come to with questions about their hair loss. It is important that you have a basic understanding of the different types of hair loss and the products and services that are available.

THE EMOTIONAL IMPACT OF HAIR LOSS

Although the medical community does not always recognize hair loss as a medical condition, the anguish felt by many of those who suffer from abnormal hair loss is very real, and all too often overlooked. Results from a study that investigated perceptions of bald and balding men showed that compared to men who had hair, bald men were perceived as:

- less physically attractive (by both sexes)
- less assertive

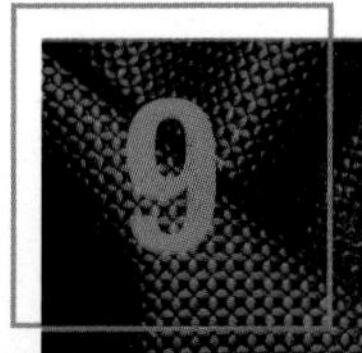

- less successful
- less personally likable
- older (by about 5 years)

Results of a study investigating how bald men perceive themselves showed that greater hair loss had a more significant impact than moderate hair loss. Men with more severe hair loss:

- experience significantly more negative social and emotional effects
- are more preoccupied with their baldness
- make some effort to conceal or compensate for their hair loss

For women, abnormal hair loss is particularly devastating. Women who experience hair loss sometimes try to disguise it from everyone, even their doctor (which is usually a mistake).

Women also tend to worry that their hair loss is a symptom of a serious illness. Studies indicate that women have a greater emotional investment in their appearance, and although abnormal hair loss is not as common in women as it is in men, it can be very traumatic. The large numbers of women with abnormal hair loss feel anxious, helpless, and less attractive. Many think that they are the only ones who have the problem.

TYPES OF ABNORMAL HAIR LOSS

Abnormal hair loss is called **alopecia** (al-oh-PEE-shah). The most common types of abnormal hair loss are androgenic alopecia, alopecia areata, and postpartum alopecia.

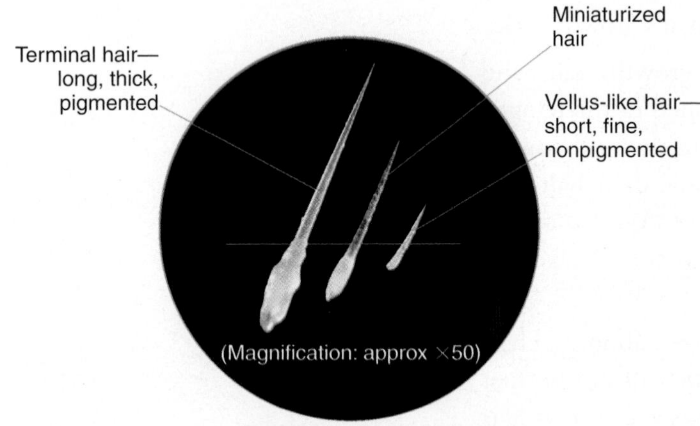

Figure 9-19 Miniaturization of the hair follicle.

ANDROGENIC ALOPECIA

Androgenic alopecia (an-druh-JEN-ik) or androgenetic (an-druh-je-NETik) alopecia is the result of genetics, age, and hormonal changes that cause miniaturization of terminal hair, converting it to vellus hair (Figure 9-19).

Androgenic alopecia can begin as early as the teens and is frequently seen by the age of 40. By age 35, almost 40 percent of both men and women show some degree of hair loss.

In men, androgenic alopecia is known as male pattern baldness and usually progresses to the familiar horseshoe-shaped fringe of hair. In women it shows up as generalized thinning over the entire crown area. Androgenic alopecia affects about 40 million men and 20 million women in the United States.

The mission of the National Alopecia Areata Foundation (NAAF) is to support research to find a cure or acceptable treatment for alopecia areata, to support those with the disease, and to educate the public. The NAAF can be contacted at P.O. Box 150760, San Rafael, CA 94915-0760, (415)472-3780, info@NAAF.org (www.alopeciaareata.com).

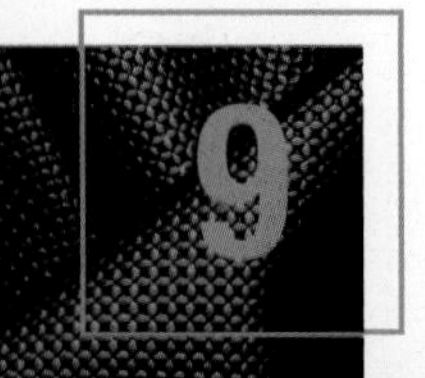

ALOPECIA AREATA

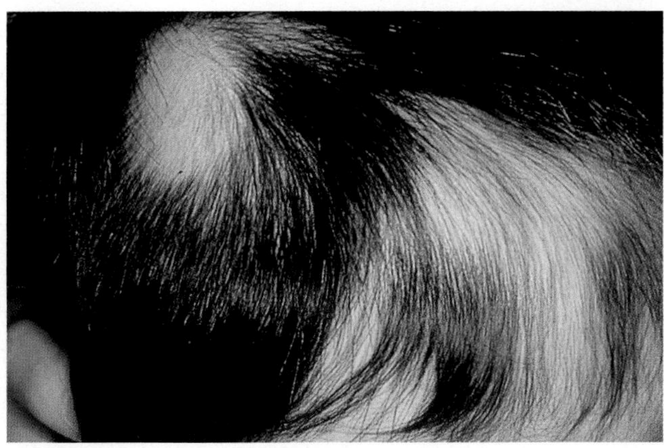

Figure 9-20 Alopecia areata.

Alopecia areata (air-ee-AH-tah) is characterized by the sudden falling out of hair in round patches or baldness in spots, and may occur on the scalp and elsewhere on the body. It is a highly unpredictable skin disease that affects almost 5 million people in the United States alone.

Alopecia areata is an autoimmune disorder that causes the affected hair follicles to be mistakenly attacked by a person's own immune system, with white blood cells stopping the hair growth (anagen) phase. Alopecia areata usually begins with one or more small, round, smooth bald patches on the scalp and can progress to total scalp hair loss (alopecia totalis), or complete body hair loss (alopecia universalis).

Alopecia areata occurs in males and females of all ages and race/ethnic backgrounds and most often begins in childhood. The scalp usually shows no signs of inflammation. Alopecia areata occurs in individuals who have no obvious skin disorder or disease (Figure 9-20).

POSTPARTUM ALOPECIA

Postpartum alopecia is temporary hair loss experienced at the conclusion of a pregnancy. For some women, pregnancy seems to disrupt the normal growth cycle of hair, with very little normal hair loss during pregnancy, but sudden and excessive shedding from 3 to 9 months after delivery. Although this is usually very traumatic to the new mother, the growth cycle generally returns to normal within 1 year after the baby is delivered.

HAIR LOSS TREATMENTS

Of all treatments that are said to counter hair loss, there are only two products—minoxidil and finasteride—that have been proven to stimulate hair growth and are approved by the FDA for sale in the United States.

Minoxidil is a topical (applied to the surface of the body) medication that is applied to the scalp twice a day, and has been proven to stimulate hair growth. It is sold over the counter (OTC) as a nonprescription drug. Minoxidil is available for both men and women and comes in two different strengths: 2% regular and 5% extra strength. It is not known to have any serious negative side effects.

Finasteride is an oral prescription medication for men only. Although finasteride is more effective and convenient than minoxidil, possible side effects include weight gain and loss of sexual function. Women may not use this treatment, and pregnant women or those who might become pregnant are cautioned not to even touch the drug because of the strong potential for birth defects.

In addition to the treatments described above, there are also several surgical options available. Transplants (hair plugs) are probably the most common permanent hair replacement technique. The process consists of removing small sections of hair, including the follicle, papilla, and bulb, from an area where there is a lot of hair (usually in the back) and transplanting

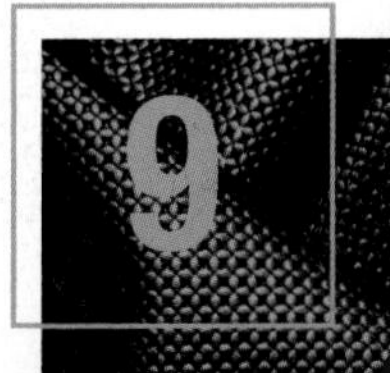

them into the bald area. These sections, or bulbs, grow normally in the new location. Only licensed surgeons may perform this procedure, and several surgeries are usually necessary to achieve the desired results. The cost of each surgery ranges from $8,000 to over $20,000.

Hair stylists can offer a number of nonmedical options to counter hair loss. Some salons specialize in nonsurgical hair replacement systems such as wigs, toupees, hair weavings, and hair extensions. With proper training, you can learn to fit, color, cut, and style wigs and toupees. Hair weavings and hair extensions allow you to enhance a client's natural hair and create a look that boosts self-esteem (see Chapter 17).

DISORDERS OF THE HAIR

The following disorders of the hair range from those that are commonplace and not particularly troublesome to those that are far more unusual or distressing.

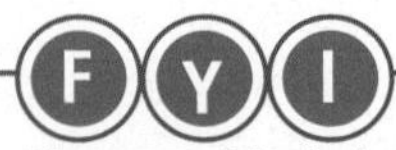

Abnormal hair loss is an unwanted side effect of chemotherapy or radiation cancer treatments. Look Good . . . Feel Better (LGFB) is a free, national public service program that teaches beauty techniques to women with cancer, helping them to boost their self-image and camouflage their hair loss. The program is open to all women cancer patients actively undergoing treatment for cancer. Each year, approximately 30,000 women participate in LGFB group sessions, and more than 200,000 women have been served by the organization since it was founded. Contact the LGFB program at 800-395-LOOK (800-395-5665) or through the web at www.lookgoodfeelbetter.org.

CANITIES

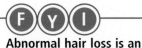

Canities (kah-NISH-ee-eez) is the technical term for gray hair. Canities results from the loss of the hair's natural melanin pigment. Other than the absence of pigment, gray hair is exactly the same as pigmented hair. The two types of canities are congenital and acquired.

1. Congenital canities exists at or before birth. It occurs in albinos, who are born without pigment in the skin, hair, and eyes, and occasionally in individuals with normal hair. A patchy type of congenital canities may develop either slowly or rapidly, depending on the cause of the condition.
2. Acquired canities develops with age and is the result of genetics. Although genetics is also responsible for premature canities, acquired canities may develop due to prolonged anxiety, or illness.

RINGED HAIR

Ringed hair is a variety of canities, characterized by alternating bands of gray and pigmented hair throughout the length of the hair strand.

HYPERTRICHOSIS

Hypertrichosis (hi-pur-trih-KOH-sis) or hirsuties (hur-SOO-shee-eez) is a condition of abnormal growth of hair. It is characterized by the growth of terminal hair in areas of the body that normally grow only vellus hair. A mustache or light beard on women are examples of hypertrichosis.

Treatments include electrolysis, photoepilation, laser hair removal, shaving, tweezing, electronic tweezers, depilatories, epilators, threading, and sugaring (see Chapter 21).

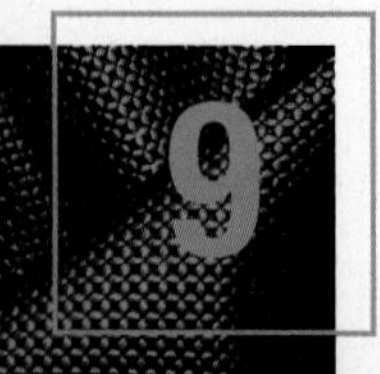

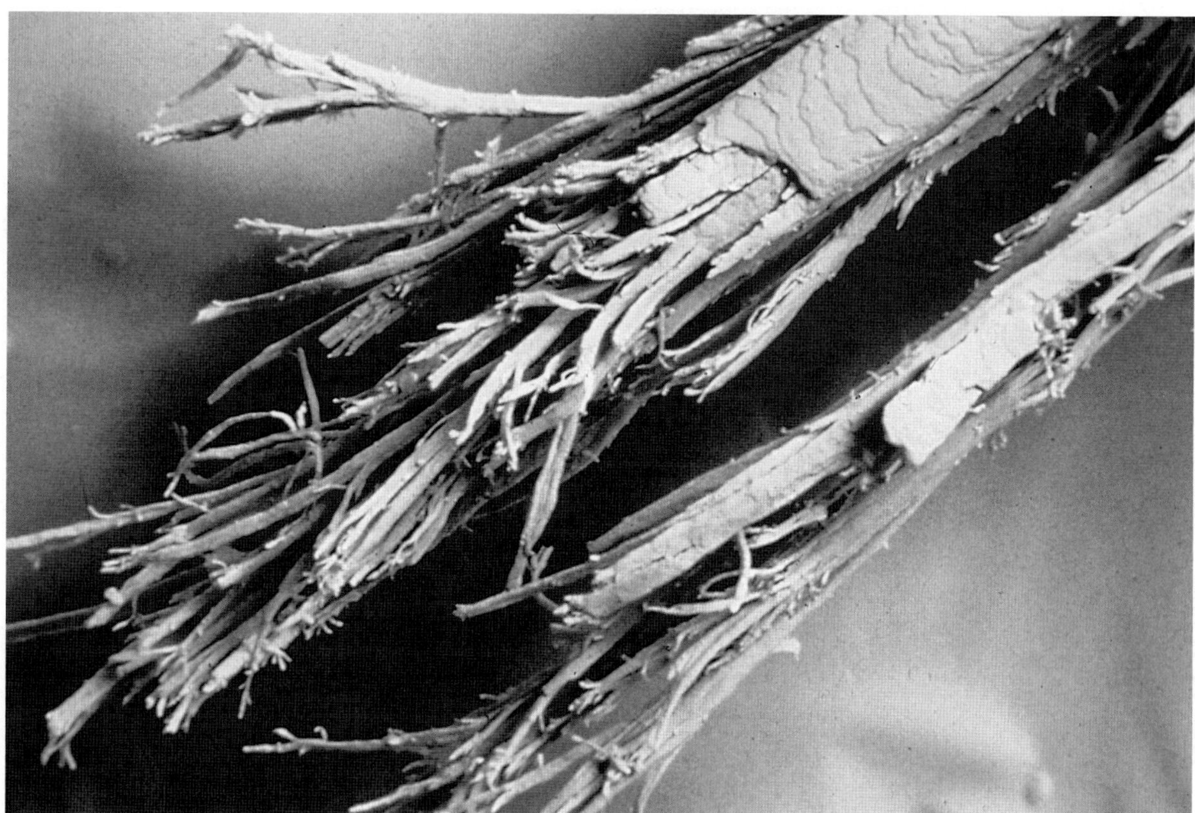

Figure 9-21 Trichoptilosis.

TRICHOPTILOSIS

Trichoptilosis (trih-kahp-tih-LOH-sus) is the technical term for split ends (Figure 9-21). Treatments include hair conditioning to soften and lubricate dry ends. The split ends may also be removed by cutting.

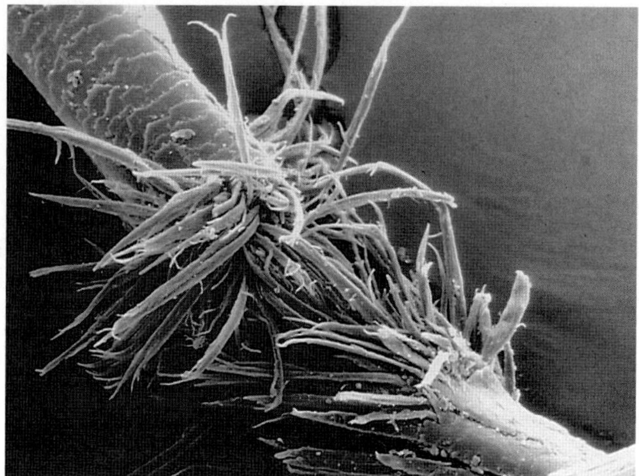

Figure 9-22 Trichorrhexis nodosa.

TRICHORRHEXIS NODOSA

Trichorrhexis nodosa (trik-uh-REK-sis nuh-DOH-suh) or knotted hair is characterized by brittleness and the formation of nodular swellings along the hair shaft (Figure 9-22). The hair breaks easily, and the broken fibers spread out like a brush along the hair shaft. Treatments include softening the hair with conditioners and moisturizers.

MONILETHRIX

Monilethrix (mah-NIL-ee-thriks) is the technical term for beaded hair (Figure 9-23). The hair breaks easily between the beads or nodes. Treatments include hair and scalp conditioning.

FRAGILITAS CRINIUM

Fragilitas crinium (fruh-JIL-ih-tus KRI-nee-um) is the technical term for brittle hair. The hairs may split at any part of their length. Treatments include hair and scalp conditioning.

DISORDERS OF THE SCALP

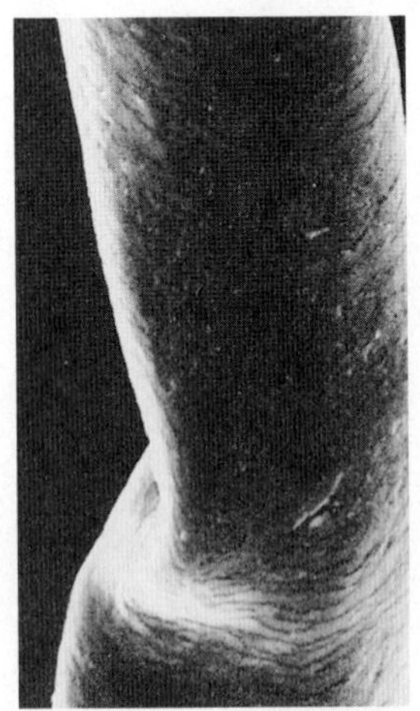

Figure 9-23 Monilethrix.

The skin is in a constant state of renewal. The outer layer of skin that covers your body is constantly being shed and replaced by new cells from below. The average person sheds about 9 pounds of "dead" skin each year. The skin cells of a normal, healthy scalp fall off naturally as small, dry flakes, without being noticed.

Dandruff can easily be mistaken for dry scalp because the symptoms of both conditions are a flaky, irritated scalp, but there is a difference. Dry scalp is dry, unlike the oily scalp that is common to dandruff. The flakes from a dry scalp are much smaller and less noticeable than the larger flakes seen with dandruff. Dry scalp can result from contact dermatitis, sunburn, or extreme age, and is usually made worse by a cold, dry climate.

DANDRUFF

Pityriasis (pit-ih-RY-uh-sus) is the medical term for dandruff, which is characterized by the excessive production and accumulation of skin cells. Instead of the normal shedding of tiny individual skin cells, one at a time, dandruff results from the accumulation of large visible clumps of cells.

Although the cause of dandruff has been debated over 150 years, current research confirms that dandruff is the result of a fungus called **malassezia** (mal-uh-SEEZ-ee-uh). Malassezia is a naturally occurring fungus that is present on all human skin but only develops the symptoms of dandruff when it grows out of control. Some individuals are also more susceptible to malassezia's irritating effects, and other factors such as stress, age, hormones, and poor hygiene can cause the fungus to multiply and dandruff symptoms to worsen.

Modern antidandruff shampoos contain the antifungal agents pyrithione zinc, selenium sulfide, or ketoconazole that control dandruff by suppressing the growth of malassezia. Antidandruff shampoos that contain pyrithione zinc are available in a variety of formulas for all hair types and are gentle enough to be used every day, even on color-treated hair. Frequent use of an antidandruff shampoo is essential for controlling dandruff. And although good personal hygiene and proper sanitation techniques are important, dandruff is not contagious.

The two principal types of dandruff are pityriasis capitis simplex and pityriasis steatoides.

Pityriasis capitis simplex (KAP-ih-tis SIM-pleks) is the technical term for classic dandruff that is characterized by scalp irritation, large flakes, and an itchy scalp. The scales may attach to the scalp in masses, scatter loosely in the hair, or fall to the shoulders. Regular use of antidandruff shampoos, conditioners, and topical lotions are the best treatment.

Pityriasis steatoides (stee-uh-TOY-deez) is a more severe case of dandruff characterized by an accumulation of greasy or waxy scalp scales, mixed with sebum, that stick to the scalp in crusts. When accompanied by redness and inflammation, the medical term is **"seborrheic dermatitis"** (seb-oh-REE-ik dur-muh-TY-tis). Occasionally, seborrheic dermatitis can also be found in the eyebrows or beard. A client with this condition should be referred to a physician.

FUNGAL INFECTIONS (TINEA)

Tinea (TIN-ee-uh) is the medical term for ringworm. It is characterized by itching, scales, and, sometimes, painful circular lesions. Several such patches may be present at one time. Tinea is caused by a fungal organism and not a parasite, as the old-fashioned term "ringworm" seems to suggest.

All forms of tinea are contagious and can be easily transmitted from one person to another. Infected skin scales or hairs that contain the fungi are known to spread the disease. Bathtubs, swimming pools, and unsanitary personal articles are also sources of transmission. Practicing approved sanitization and disinfection procedures will help prevent the spread of this disease. A client with this condition should be referred to a physician for medical treatment.

Tinea capitis (KAP-ih-tis) is another type of fungal infection characterized by red papules, or spots, at the opening of the hair follicles (Figure 9-24). The patches spread and the hair becomes brittle. Hair often breaks off, leaving only a stump, or may be shed from the enlarged open follicle.

Tinea favosa (fah-VOH-suh) is characterized by dry, sulfur-yellow, cup-like crusts on the scalp called **scutula** (SKUCH-ul-uh), which have a distinctive odor. Scars from tinea favosa are bald patches that may be pink or white and shiny.

PARASITIC INFECTIONS

Scabies is a highly contagious skin disease caused by a parasite called a "mite" that burrows under the skin. Vesicles (blisters) and pustules (inflamed pimples with pus) usually form on the scalp from the irritation caused by this parasite. Excessive itching results in scratching the infected areas and makes the condition worse. Practicing approved sanitization and disinfection procedures are very important to prevent the spread of this disease. A client with this condition must be referred to a physician for medical treatment.

Pediculosis capitis (puh-dik-yuh-LOH-sis KAP-ih-tis) is the infestation of the hair and scalp with head lice (Figures 9-25 and 9-26). As these parasites feed on the scalp, itching occurs and the scratching that usually results can cause an infection. Head lice are transmitted from one person to another by contact with infested hats, combs, brushes, and other personal articles. You can distinguish them from dandruff flakes by looking closely at the scalp with a magnifying glass.

Properly practicing state board—-approved sanitization and disinfection procedures will prevent the spread of this disease. Several nonprescription medications are available. A client with this condition should be referred to a physician or pharmacist.

Did You Know

Tinea barbae (Barber's Itch) is the most frequently encountered infection resulting from hair services that affects the coarse hairs in the mustache and beard area, or around the neck and scalp, usually in men (see chapter 5 for more details).

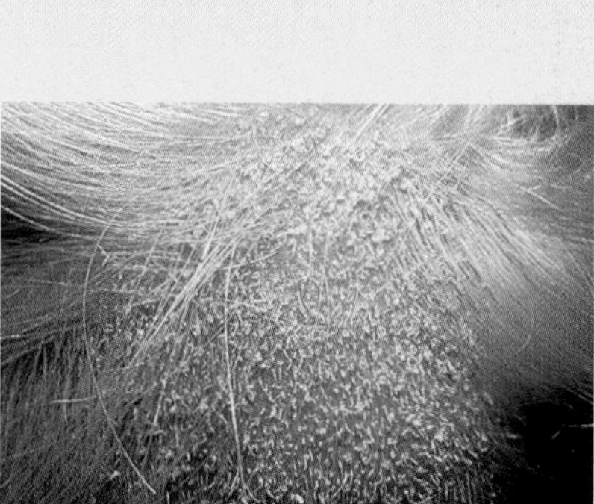

Figure 9-24 Tinea capitis.

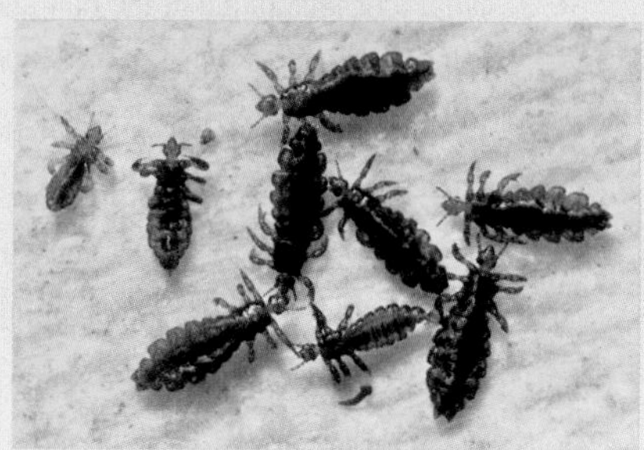

Figure 9-25 Head lice.

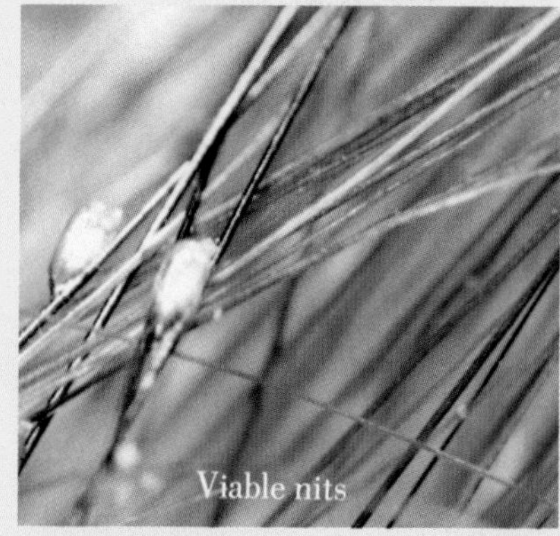

Figure 9-26 Nits (lice eggs).

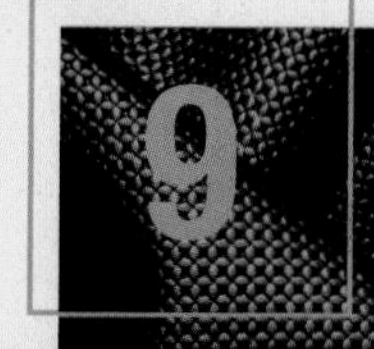

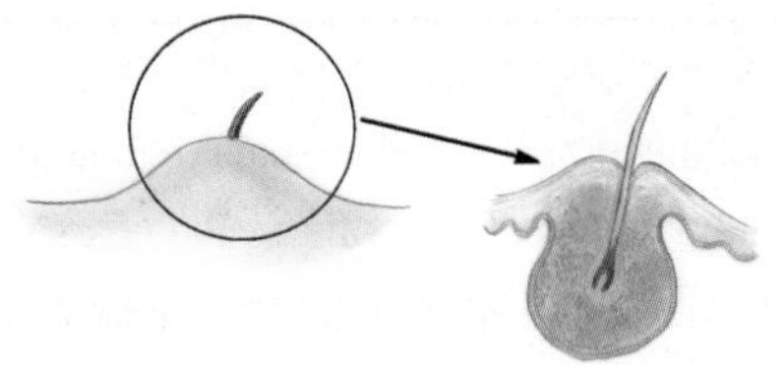

Figure 9-27 Furuncle (boil).

STAPHYLOCOCCI INFECTIONS

Staphylococci are bacteria that infect the skin or scalp. The two most common types of staphylococci infections are furuncles and carbuncles.

A **furuncle** (FYOO-rung-kul) or boil is an acute, localized bacterial infection of the hair follicle that produces constant pain (Figure 9-27). It is limited to a specific area and produces a pustule perforated by a hair.

A **carbuncle** (KAHR-bung-kul) is an inflammation of the subcutaneous tissue caused by staphylococci. It is similar to a furuncle but is larger.

Properly practicing regulatory agency—-approved sanitization and disinfection procedures will prevent the spread of these infections. A client with either condition must be referred to a physician for medical treatment.

REVIEW QUESTIONS

1. Name and describe the five main structures of the hair root.
2. Name and describe the three layers of the hair.
3. Explain the process of keratinization.
4. List and describe the three types of side bonds. Which are permanent and which are temporary? Which is strongest and why?
5. What are the differences between end bonds and side bonds?
6. Name and describe the two types of melanin responsible for natural hair color.
7. What four factors about the hair should be considered in a hair analysis?
8. Name and describe the different types of hair and their locations on the body.
9. What are the three phases of the hair growth cycle? What occurs during each phase ?
10. What is the reason for normal daily hair loss?
11. What are the most common types of abnormal hair loss?
12. What are the only two approved hair loss treatments?
13. Name the two main types of dandruff. Can either one be treated in the salon?
14. Which of the following scalp and hair disorders cannot be treated in the salon? Tinea capitis, trichoptilosis, trichorrhexis nodosa, ringed hair, tinea favosa, carbuncles, hypertrichosis, pediculosis capitis, scabies, monilethrix, fragilitas crinium, canities, and furuncles.

CHAPTER GLOSSARY

alopecia	Abnormal hair loss.
alopecia areata	The sudden falling out of hair in round patches or baldness in spots; may occur on the scalp and elsewhere on the body.
amino acids	Units that are joined together end to end by peptide bonds to form the polypeptide chains that comprise proteins.
anagen	Growth phase in the hair cycle in which a new hair shaft is created.
androgenic alopecia	Hair loss characterized by miniaturization of terminal hair which is converted to vellus hair; in men, it is known as male pattern baldness.
arrector pili	Minute, involuntary muscle in the base of the hair follicle that causes "goose bumps."
canities	Technical term for gray hair; results from the loss of the hair's natural melanin pigment.
carbuncle	Inflammation of the subcutaneous tissue caused by staphylococci; similar to a furuncle but larger.
catagen	The brief transition period between the growth and resting phases of a hair follicle.
COHNS elements	The five elements that make up human hair, skin, tissue and nails (carbon, oxygen, hydrogen, nitrogen, and sulfur).
cortex	Middle layer of the hair; a fibrous protein core formed by elongated cells containing melanin pigment.
cowlick	Tuft of hair that stands straight up.
cuticle	Outermost layer of hair, consisting of a single, overlapping layer of transparent, scale-like cells.
dermal papilla	Small, cone-shaped elevation located at the base of the hair follicle that fits into the hair bulb.
disulfide bond	Strong chemical side bonds that join the sulfur atoms of two neighboring cysteine amino acids to create cystine, which joins together two polypeptide strands like rungs on a ladder.
eumelanin	Melanin that gives brown and black color to hair.
follicle	Tube-like depression or pocket in the skin or scalp that contains the hair root.
fragilitas crinium	Technical term for brittle hair.
furuncle	Boil; acute, localized bacterial infection of the hair follicle.
hair bulb	Lowest part of a hair strand; the thickened, club-shaped structure that forms the lower part of the hair root.
hair density	The number of individual hair strands found on 1 square inch of scalp.
hair elasticity	Ability of the hair to stretch and return to its original length without breaking.

CHAPTER GLOSSARY

hair porosity	Ability of the hair to absorb moisture.
hair root	The part of the hair contained within the follicle, below the surface of the scalp.
hair shaft	The portion of hair that projects beyond the skin.
hair stream	Hair flowing in the same direction, resulting from follicles sloping in the same direction.
hair texture	Thickness or diameter of the individual hair strands.
helix	Spiral shape created by polypeptide chains that intertwine around each other.
hydrogen bond	Weak physical side bond that is easily broken by water or heat.
hypertrichosis (hirsuties)	Condition of abnormal growth of hair, characterized by the growth of terminal hair in areas of the body that normally grow only vellus hair.
integument	Largest and fastest growing organ of the body; composed of the hair, skin and nails.
keratinization	Process by which newly formed cells in the hair bulb mature, fill with keratin, move upward, lose their nucleus, and die.
malassezia	Naturally occurring fungus that is present on all human skin, and is responsible for dandruff.
medulla	Innermost layer of the hair, composed of round cells; often absent in fine hair.
melanin	Tiny grains of pigment in the cortex that give natural color to the hair.
monilethrix	Technical term for beaded hair.
pediculosis capitis	Infestation of the hair and scalp with head lice.
peptide bond or end bond	Chemical bond that joins amino acids to each other, end to end, to form a polypeptide chain.
pheomelanin	Melanin that provides natural hair colors from red and ginger to yellow/blond tones.
pityriasis	Dandruff; an inflammation of the skin characterized by the formation and flaking of fine, thin scales.
pityriasis capitis simplex	Technical term for classic dandruff; characterized by scalp irritation, large flakes, and itchy scalp.
pityriasis steatoides	Scalp inflammation marked by fatty (greasy or waxy) types of dandruff.
polypeptide chain	Long chain of amino acids linked by peptide bonds.

CHAPTER GLOSSARY

postpartum alopecia	Temporary hair loss experienced at the conclusion of a pregnancy.
ringed hair	Variety of canities characterized by alternating bands of gray and pigmented hair throughout the length of the hair strand.
salt bond	A weak, temporary side bond between adjacent polypeptide chains.
scabies	Highly contagious disease caused by mites that burrow under the skin.
scutula	Dry, sulfur-yellow, cup-like crusts on the scalp in tinea favosa or favus.
sebaceous glands	Oil glands of the skin connected to hair follicles.
seborrheic dermatitis	Medical term for pityriasis steatoides accompanied by redness and inflammation.
sebum	Oily secretion of the sebaceous glands, which lubricates the hair and skin.
telogen	Resting phase; the final phase in the hair cycle that lasts until the fully grown hair is shed.
terminal hair	Long hair found on the scalp, as well as on legs, arms, and body of both males and females.
tinea	Medical term for ringworm, a contagious condition caused by fungal infection.
tinea capitis	Fungal infection of the scalp characterized by red papules, or spots at the opening of hair follicles.
tinea favosa (tinea favus)	Fungal infection characterized by dry, sulfur-yellow, cup-like crusts on the scalp, called scutula.
trichology	Science dealing with the study of hair, its diseases, and care.
trichoptilosis	Technical term for split ends.
trichorrhexis nodosa	Knotted hair characterized by brittleness and the formation of nodular swellings along the hair shaft.
vellus or lanugo	Short, fine, unpigmented downy hair that appears on the body, with the exception of the palms of the hands and the soles of the feet.
wave pattern	Amount of "movement" in the hair strand; described as straight, wavy, curly, and extremely curly.
whorl	Hair that forms in a circular pattern, as on the crown.

CHAPTER 10 BASICS OF CHEMISTRY

chapter outline

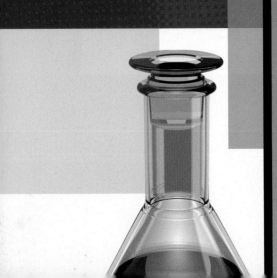

Learning Objectives

After completing this chapter, you will be able to:

- **Explain the difference between organic and inorganic chemistry.**
- **Discuss the different forms of matter—elements, compounds, and mixtures.**
- **Explain the difference between solutions, suspensions, and emulsions.**
- **Explain pH and the pH scale.**
- **Describe oxidation and reduction (redox) reactions.**

Key Terms

Page number indicates where in the chapter the term is used.

acids pg. 174
alkalis pg. 174
alkanolamines pg. 172
ammonia pg. 172
anion pg. 173
atom pg. 167
cation pg. 173
chemical change pg. 168
chemical properties pg. 168
chemistry pg. 166
combustion pg. 174
compounds pg. 167
element pg. 167
elemental molecules pg. 167
emulsion pg. 170
exothermic pg. 174
glycerin pg. 172
hydrophilic pg. 171
immiscible pg. 170
inorganic chemistry pg. 166
ion pg. 173
ionization pg. 173
lipophilic pg. 171
logarithm pg. 173
matter pg. 166
miscible pg. 170
molecule pg. 167
oil-in-water (O/W) emulsion pg. 171
organic chemistry pg. 166
oxidation pg. 174
oxidizing agent pg. 174
pH scale pg. 173
physical change pg. 168
physical mixture pg. 169
physical properties pg. 168
pure substance pg. 169
redox pg. 175
reduced pg. 174
reduction pg. 174
silicones pg. 172
solute pg. 169
solution pg. 169
solvent pg. 169
surfactants pg. 171
suspension pg. 170
volatile pg. 171
volatile organic compounds (VOC) pg. 172
water-in-oil (W/O) emulsion pg. 171

Cosmetology services in a modern salon would not be possible without the use of chemicals. To use professional products effectively and safely, all cosmetology professionals need to have a basic understanding of chemistry. This chapter will provide you with the overview you need.

CHEMISTRY

Chemistry is the science that deals with the composition, structures, and properties of matter, and how matter changes under different conditions.

Organic chemistry is the study of substances that contain carbon. Organic substances burn because they contain carbon. All living things, or things that were once alive, whether they are plants or animals, contain carbon. Although the term "organic" is often misused to mean "natural" because of its association with living things, all organic substances are not natural or healthy.

You may be surprised to learn that gasoline, motor oil, plastics, synthetic fabrics, pesticides, and fertilizers are all organic substances. All haircoloring products, chemical hair texturizers, shampoos, conditioners, and styling aids are organic. All artificial nail enhancements and nail polishes are organic. These products are manufactured from natural gas and oil, which are the remains of plants and animals that died millions of years ago. So, remember that "organic" does not mean "natural."

Inorganic chemistry is the study of substances that do not contain carbon. Inorganic substances do not burn because they do not contain carbon. Inorganic substances are not, and never were, alive. Metals, minerals, water, and air are inorganic substances. Hydrogen peroxide and hydroxide hair relaxers are examples of inorganic substances.

MATTER

Matter is any substance that occupies space and has mass (weight). All matter has physical and chemical properties, and exists in the form of a solid, liquid, or gas. Although matter has physical properties that we can touch, taste, smell, or see, not everything that we can see is matter. For instance, we can see visible light and electric sparks, but these are forms of energy, and energy is not matter. Energy does not occupy space or have physical properties, such as mass (weight). Energy is discussed in Chapter 11.

ELEMENTS

An **element** is the simplest form of matter and cannot be broken down into a simpler substance without a loss of identity. There are 90 naturally occurring elements, each with its own distinctive physical and chemical properties. All matter in the universe is made up of these 90 different elements.

Each element is identified by a single- or double-letter symbol, such as O for oxygen, C for carbon, H for hydrogen, N for nitrogen, and S for sulfur.

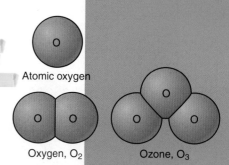

Atomic oxygen

Oxygen, O_2 Ozone, O_3

Figure 10-1 Elemental molecules contain atoms of the same element.

ATOMS

Atoms are the particles from which all matter is composed. Atoms are the structural units that make up the elements. Different elements are different from one another because the structure of their atoms is different. An **atom** is the smallest particle of an element that retains the properties of that element. Atoms cannot be divided into simpler substances by ordinary chemical means.

MOLECULES

Just as words are made by combining letters, molecules are made by combining atoms. A **molecule** is a chemical combination of two or more atoms. **Elemental molecules** are a chemical combination of atoms of the same element. Atmospheric oxygen in the air we breathe is an elemental molecule containing two atoms of the element oxygen and is written as O_2. Ozone, is a very dangerous form of oxygen and a major component of smog (Figure 10-1).

Compounds are chemical combinations of two or more atoms of different elements (Figure 10-2). Sodium chloride (NaCl), or common table salt, is a compound molecule that contains one atom of sodium (Na) and one atom of chlorine (Cl).

Sodium chloride, NaCl

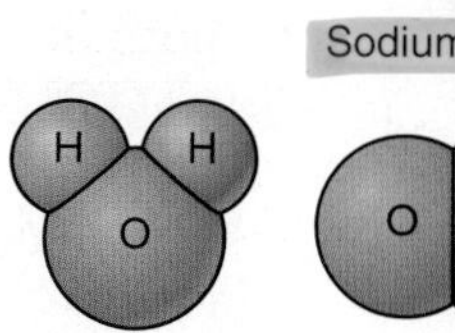

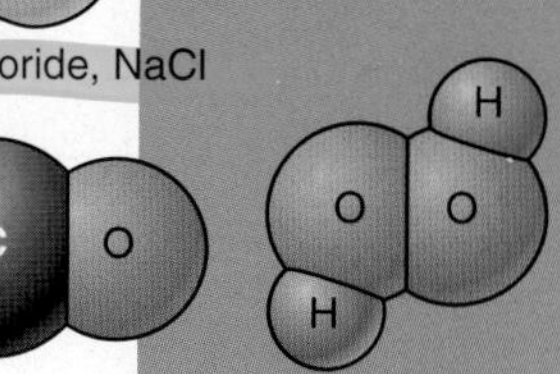

Water, H_2O Carbon dioxide, CO_2 Hydrogen peroxide, H_2O_2

Figure 10-2 Compound molecules contain atoms of different elements.

STATES OF MATTER

All matter exists in one of three physical forms: (1) solid, (2) liquid, or (3) gas.

These three forms are called the "states of matter" (Figure 10-3).

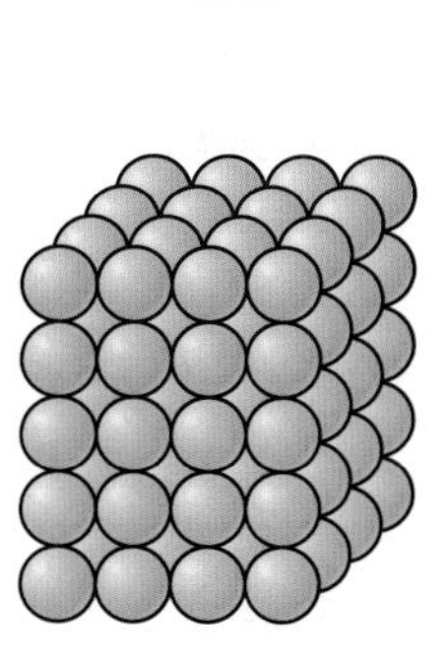

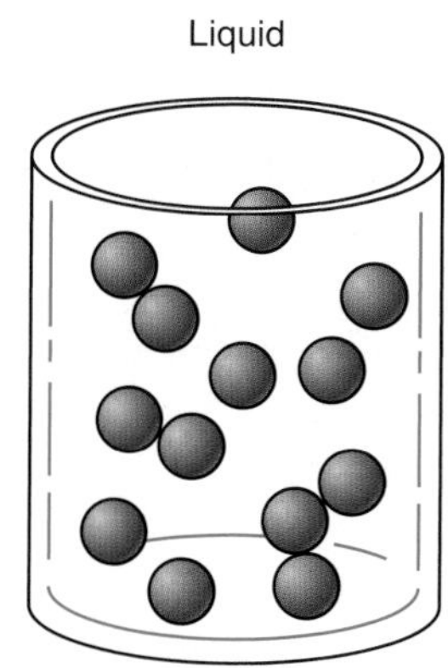

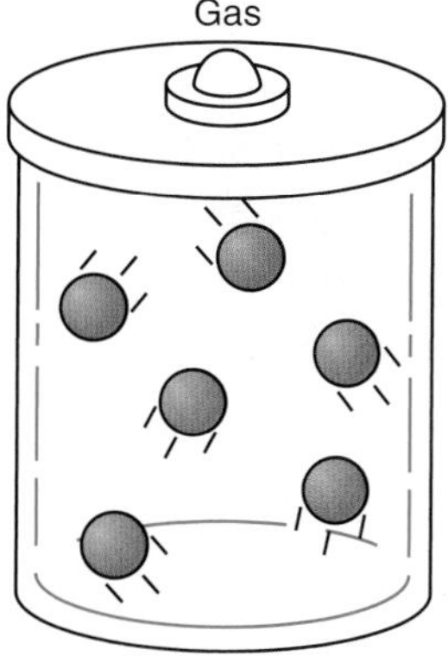

Figure 10-3 Solids, liquids, and gases.

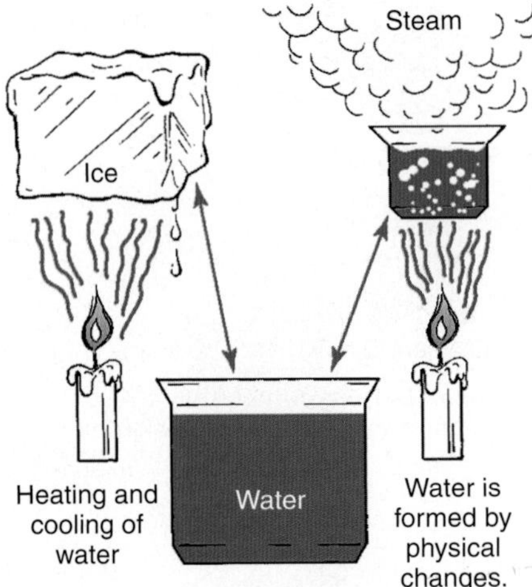

Figure 10-4 Physical changes.

Like many other substances, water (H_2O) can exist in all three states of matter, depending on its temperature. For instance, when water freezes, it turns to ice. When ice melts, it turns to water. When water boils, it turns to steam. When the steam cools, it turns back into water. The form of the water physically changes according to changes in the temperature, but it is still water (H_2O). It does not become a different chemical. It stays the same chemical, but in a different physical form. This is called a physical change.

The three different states of matter have the following distinct characteristics:

- Solids have a definite shape and volume. Ice is an example of a solid.
- Liquids have a definite volume, but not a definite shape. Water is an example of a liquid.
- Gases do not have a definite volume or shape. Steam is an example of a gas.

PHYSICAL AND CHEMICAL PROPERTIES

Every substance has unique properties that allow us to identify it. The two different types of properties are physical and chemical.

Physical properties are those characteristics that can be determined without a chemical reaction and do not involve a chemical change. Physical properties include color, size, weight, and hardness.

Chemical properties are those characteristics that can only be determined by a chemical reaction and a chemical change in the substance. Chemical properties include the ability of iron to rust and wood to burn. In both of these examples, oxidation is the chemical reaction that causes a chemical change in the substance.

PHYSICAL AND CHEMICAL CHANGES

Matter can be changed in two different ways. Physical forces cause physical changes and chemical reactions cause chemical changes.

A **physical change** is a change in the form, or physical properties, of a substance, without a chemical reaction or the creation of a new substance. A physical change is the result of physical forces that only change the physical properties of a substance, no chemical reaction is involved, and no new chemicals are formed. Solid ice undergoes a physical change when it melts into liquid water (Figure 10-4). A physical change occurs with the application of nonoxidation (temporary) haircolor or nail polish.

A **chemical change** is a change in the chemical and physical properties of a substance by a chemical reaction that creates a new substance or substances. A chemical change is the result of a chemical reaction that creates new chemicals that have new chemical and physical properties (Figure 10-5). Examples of a chemical change are the oxidation of haircolor and the polymerization of acrylic (methacrylate) nail enhancements.

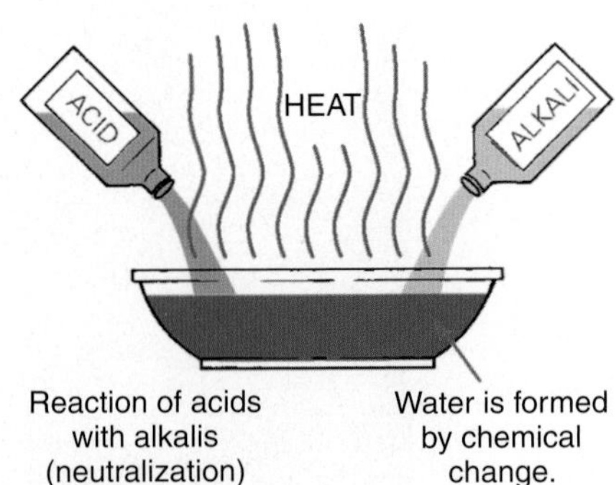

Figure 10-5 Chemical changes.

PURE SUBSTANCES AND PHYSICAL MIXTURES

All matter can be classified as either a pure substance or a physical mixture.

A **pure substance** is a chemical combination of matter, in definite proportions. Pure substances have unique properties. All atoms, elements, elemental molecules, and compound molecules are pure substances. Water is a pure substance that results from the chemical combination of two atoms of the element hydrogen and one atom of the element oxygen, in definite proportions. The properties of water (a liquid) are not the properties of hydrogen and oxygen (both gases). Pure substances include oxygen, ozone, water, and salt. Few of the products cosmetologists or manicurists use are pure substances.

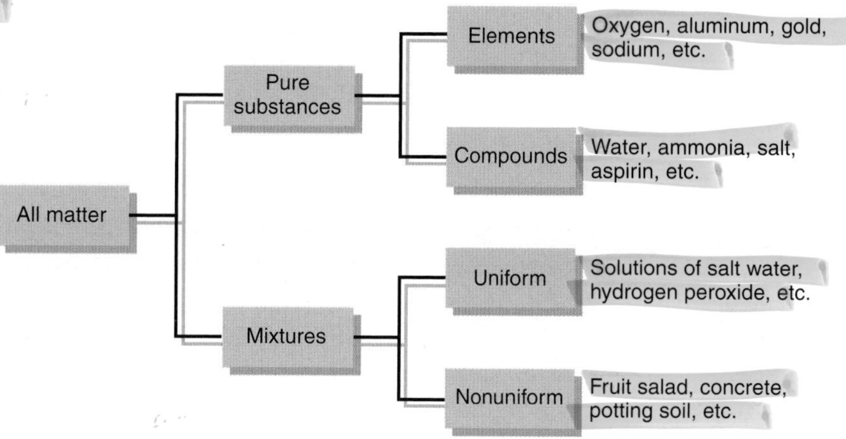

Figure 10-6 Pure substances and physical mixtures.

A **physical mixture** is a physical combination of matter in any proportion. The properties of a physical mixture are the combined properties of the substances in the mixture. Saltwater is a physical mixture of salt and water in any proportion. The properties of saltwater are the properties of salt and water. Saltwater is salty and wet. Most of the products a cosmetologist or manicurist uses are physical mixtures (Figure 10-6). See Table 10-1 for a summary of the differences between pure substances and physical mixtures.

SOLUTIONS, SUSPENSIONS, AND EMULSIONS

Solutions, suspensions, and emulsions are all physical mixtures. The difference between solutions, suspensions and emulsions is determined by the size of the particles and the solubility of the substances.

A **solution** is a stable mixture of two or more mixable substances. The **solute** is the substance that is dissolved in a solution. The **solvent** is the substance that dissolves the solute to form a solution.

Compounds	Physical Mixtures
Involve a chemical reaction	Do not involve a chemical reaction
Change the chemical properties	Change only the physical properties
Example: salt (NaCl)	Example: saltwater (blend of NaCl and H_2O)

Table 10-1 Chemical Compounds and Physical Mixtures

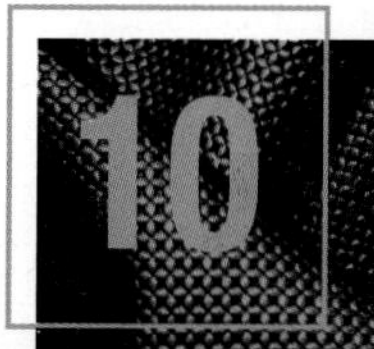

Miscible (MIS-uh-bul) liquids are mutually soluble, meaning that they can be mixed into stable solutions. Water and alcohol are examples of miscible liquids.

Immiscible liquids are not capable of being mixed into stable solutions. Water and oil are examples of immiscible liquids.

Solutions contain small particles that are invisible to the naked eye. Solutions are usually transparent, although they may be colored. They do not separate on standing. Saltwater is a solution of a solid dissolved in a liquid. Water is the solvent that dissolves the salt (solute) and holds it in solution.

A **suspension** is an unstable mixture of undissolved particles in a liquid. Suspensions contain larger and less miscible particles than solutions. The particles are generally visible to the naked eye but not large enough to settle quickly to the bottom. Suspensions are not usually transparent and may be colored. Suspensions are unstable and separate over time.

Oil and vinegar salad dressing is an example of a suspension, with tiny oil droplets suspended in the vinegar. The suspension will separate on standing and must be shaken well before using. Some lotions are suspensions and need to be shaken or mixed well before use. Calamine lotion and nail polish are examples of suspensions.

An **emulsion** is an unstable mixture of two or more immiscible substances united with the aid of an emulsifier. The term "emulsify" means "to form an emulsion." Although emulsions have a tendency to separate slowly over time, a properly formulated emulsion that is stored correctly should be stable for at least three years. Table 10-2 offers a summary of the differences among solutions, suspensions, and emulsions.

Solutions	Suspensions	Emulsions
Miscible	Slightly miscible	Immiscible
No surfactant	No surfactant	Surfactant
Small particles	Larger particles	Largest particles
Stable mixture	Unstable mixture	Limited stability
Usually clear	Usually cloudy	Usually a solid color
Salt water	Calamine lotion	Hair shampoos and conditioners

Table 10-2 Solutions, Suspensions, and Emulsions

Surfactants are substances that act as a bridge to allow oil and water to mix, or emulsify. The term "surfactant" (sur-FAK-tant) is a contraction for "surface active agent." A surfactant molecule has two distinct parts (Figure 10-7). The head of the surfactant molecule is **hydrophilic** (hy-drah-FIL-ik), meaning water-loving, and the tail is **lipophilic** (ly-puh-FIL-ik), meaning oil-loving. Since "like dissolves like," the hydrophilic head dissolves in water and the lipophilic tail dissolves in oil. So a surfactant molecule dissolves in both oil and water and temporarily joins them together to form an emulsion.

> **Did You Know**
>
> Soaps were the first surfactants. Soaps were made about 4,500 years ago by boiling oil or animal fat with wood ashes. Modern soaps are made from animal, vegetable, or synthetic fats or oils. Traditional soaps are highly alkaline and combine with the minerals in hard water to form an insoluble film that coats and dulls the hair. Modern synthetic surfactants have overcome these disadvantages and are superior to soaps.

In an **oil-in-water emulsion (O/W),** oil droplets are emulsified in water. The droplets of oil are surrounded by surfactants with their lipophilic tails pointing in. Tiny oil droplets form the internal portion of an O/W emulsion because the oil is completely surrounded by water (Figure 10-8). Oil-in-water emulsions do not feel as greasy as water-in-oil emulsions because the oil is "hidden," and water forms the external portion of the emulsion.

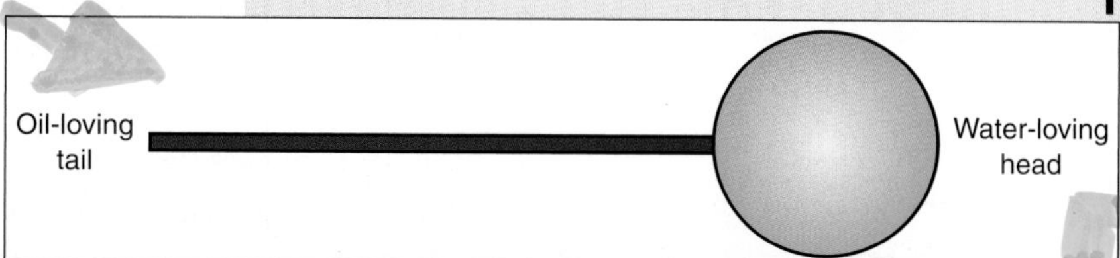

Figure 10-7 A surfactant molecule.

Mayonnaise is an example of an oil-in-water emulsion of two immiscible liquids. Although oil and water are immiscible, the egg yolk in mayonnaise emulsifies the oil droplets and distributes them uniformly in the water. Without the egg yolk as an emulsifying agent, the oil and water would separate. Most of the emulsions used in a salon are oil-in-water. Haircoloring, shampoos, conditioners, and hand creams are oil-in-water emulsions.

In a **water-in-oil emulsion (W/O),** water droplets are emulsified in oil. The droplets of water are surrounded by surfactants with their hydrophilic heads pointing in, (Figure 10-9). Tiny droplets of water form the internal portion of a W/O emulsion because the water is completely surrounded by oil. Water-in-oil emulsions feel more greasy than oil-in-water emulsions because the water is "hidden" and oil forms the external portion of the emulsion. Cold cream and styling creams are examples of water-in-oil emulsions.

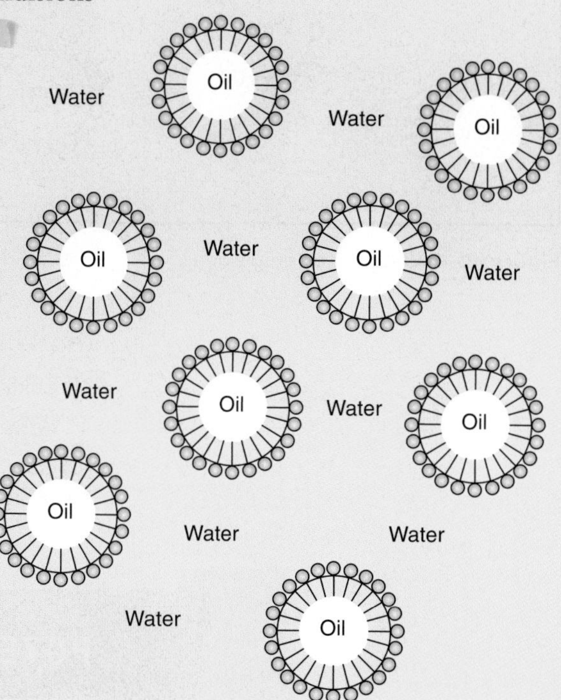

Figure 10-8 Oil-in-water emulsions.

OTHER PHYSICAL MIXTURES

Ointments, pastes, pomades, and styling waxes are semisolid mixtures made with any combination of petrolatum (petroleum jelly), oil, and wax.

Powders are a physical mixture of one or more types of solids. Off-the-scalp powdered hair lighteners are physical mixtures that may separate during shipping and storage, and should be thoroughly mixed before each use.

COMMON PRODUCT INGREDIENTS

Most people are familiar with **volatile** (VAHL-uh-tul) alcohols (those that evaporate easily) such as isopropyl alcohol (rubbing alcohol) and ethyl alcohol (alcoholic beverages). But there are many other types of

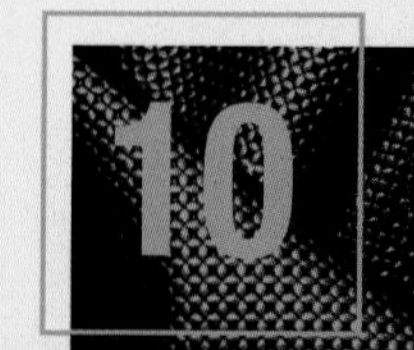

ACTIVITY

Have you ever heard the saying, "Oil and water don't mix"? Pour some water into a glass, and then add a little cooking oil (or other oil). What happens? Stir the water briskly with a spoon, and then observe for a minute or two. What does the oil do?

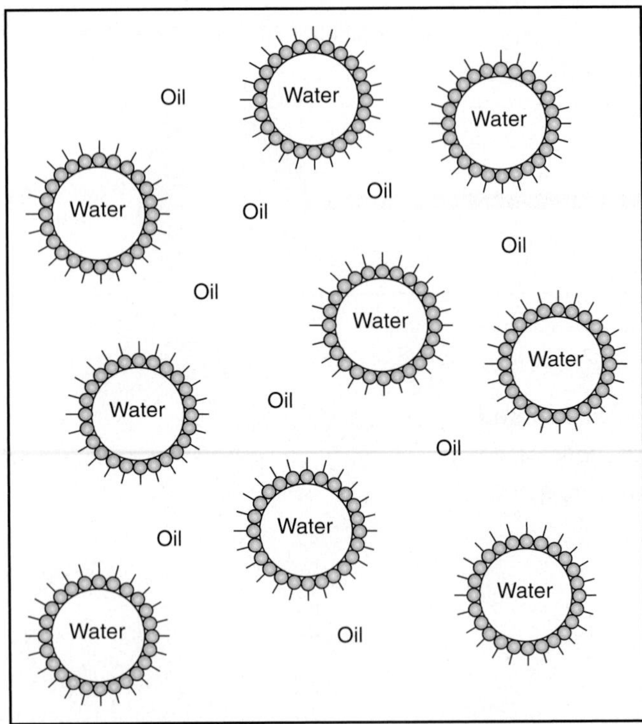

Figure 10-9 Water-in-oil emulsions.

alcohols, from free-flowing liquids to hard, waxy solids. Fatty alcohols, such as cetyl alcohol and cetearyl alcohol, are nonvolatile waxes that are used as hair conditioners.

Alkanolamines (al-kan-oh-LAH-mynz) are substances used to neutralize acids or raise the pH of many hair products. They are often used in place of ammonia because less odor is associated with their use.

Ammonia (uh-MOH-nee-uh) is a colorless gas with a pungent odor, composed of hydrogen and nitrogen. It is used to raise the pH in hair products to allow the solution to penetrate the hair shaft. Ammonium hydroxide and ammonium thioglycolate are examples of ammonia compounds that are used to raise the pH.

Glycerin (GLIS-ur-in) is a sweet, colorless, oily substance. It is used as a solvent and as a moisturizer in skin and body creams.

Silicones are a special type of oil used in hair conditioners and as water-resistant lubricants for the skin. Silicones are less greasy than other oils and form a "breathable" film that does not cause comedones (blackheads). Silicones also impart a silky smooth feel on the skin and great shine to hair.

Volatile organic compounds (VOCs) compounds contain carbon (organic) and evaporate very quickly (volatile). For example, a common VOC used in hairspray is SD alcohol (ethyl alcohol).

POTENTIAL HYDROGEN (pH)

Although pH is often discussed with regard to salon products, it is one of the least understood chemical properties. Understanding what pH is and how it affects the skin and hair is essential to understanding all salon services.

WATER AND pH

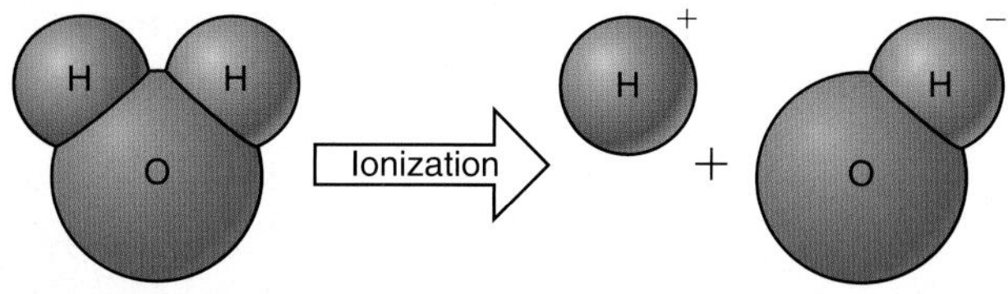

Figure 10-10 The ionization of water.

We cannot understand pH without first learning about ions. An **ion** (EYE-ahn) is an atom or molecule that carries an electrical charge. **Ionization** (eye-ahn-ih-ZAY-shun) causes an atom or molecule to split in two, creating a pair of ions with opposite electrical charges. An ion with a negative electrical charge is an **anion** (AN-eye-on). An ion with a positive electrical charge is a **cation** (KAT-eye-on).

In water, some of the water molecules (H_2O) naturally ionize into hydrogen ions and hydroxide ions. The pH scale measures these ions. The hydrogen ion (H^+) is acidic; the more hydrogen ions the substance has, the more acidic it will be. The hydroxide ion (OH) is alkaline; the more hydroxide ions the substance has, the more alkaline it will be. pH is only possible because of this ionization of water; only products that contain water can have a pH.

In pure water, each water molecule that ionizes produces one hydrogen ion and one hydroxide ion (Figure 10-10). Pure water has a neutral pH because it contains the same number of hydrogen ions as hydroxide ions. Pure water is neutral because it is an equal balance of acid and alkaline. Pure water is 50% acidic and 50% alkaline. The pH of any substance is always a balance of both acidity and alkalinity; as acidity increases, alkalinity decreases. The opposite is also true; as alkalinity increases, acidity decreases. Even the strongest acid also contains some alkalinity (Figure 10-11).

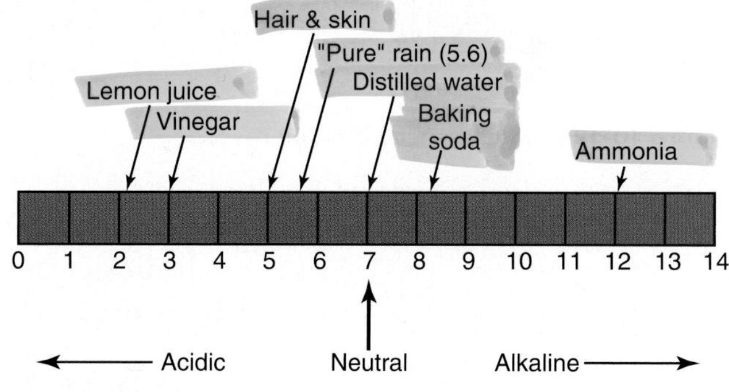

Figure 10-11 The pH scale.

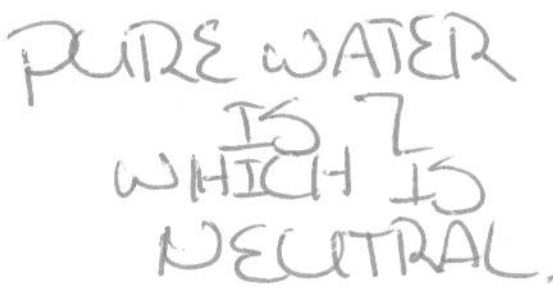

THE pH SCALE

The **pH scale** measures the acidity and alkalinity of a substance. Note that the term pH is written with a small *p* (which represents a quantity) and a capital *H* (which represents the hydrogen ion). The symbol pH represents the quantity of hydrogen ions.

The pH scale has a range from 0 to 14. A pH of 7 indicates a neutral solution, a pH below 7 indicates an acidic solution, and a pH above 7 indicates an alkaline solution.

The term **logarithm** (LOG-ah-rhythm) means multiples of ten. Because the pH scale is a logarithmic scale, a change of one whole number represents a ten-fold change in pH. That means that a pH of 8 is 10 times more alkaline than a pH of 7. A change of two whole numbers represents a change of 10 times 10, or a 100-fold change. That means that a pH of 9 is 100 times more alkaline than a pH of 7. A small change on the pH scale indicates a large change in pH.

pH is always a balance of both acidity and alkalinity. Pure water has a pH of 7 which is an equal balance of acid and alkaline. Although a pH of 7 is neutral on the pH scale, it is not neutral compared to the hair and skin, which have an average pH of 5. Pure water, with a pH of 7, is 100 times more alkaline than a pH of 5 (Figure10-11). Pure water is 100

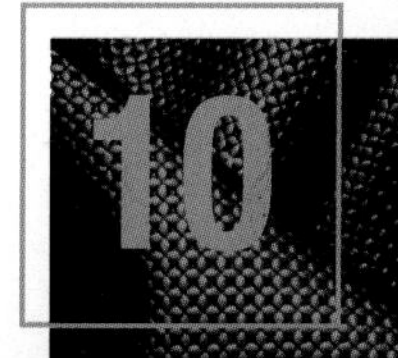

times more alkaline than your hair and skin. Pure water can cause the hair to swell as much as 20 percent, and is drying to the skin.

ACIDS AND ALKALIS

All **acids** owe their chemical reactivity to the hydrogen ion (H^+). Acids have a pH below 7.0, and turn litmus paper from blue to red. Acids contract and harden the hair. One such acid, thioglycolic acid, is used in permanent waving.

All **alkalis** (AL-kuh-lyz) owe their chemical reactivity to the hydroxide (OH-) ion. The terms "alkali" and "base" are interchangeable. Alkalis have a pH above 7.0, and turn litmus paper from red to blue. They feel slippery and soapy on the skin. Alkalis soften and swell the hair and skin. Sodium hydroxide, commonly known as lye, is a very strong alkali used in drain cleaners and chemical hair relaxers.

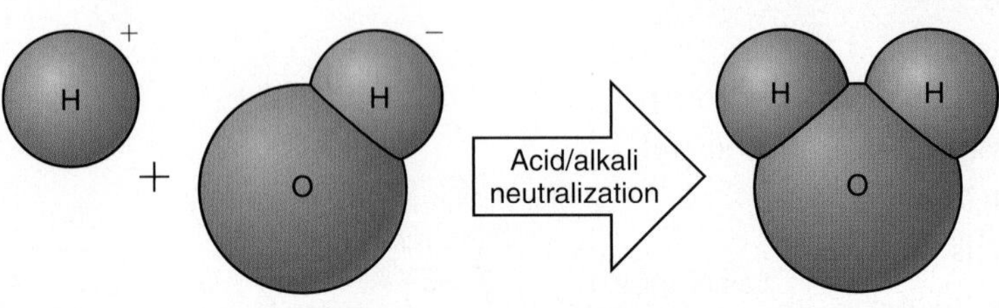

Figure 10-12 Acid/alkali neutralization reaction.

ACID-ALKALI NEUTRALIZATION REACTIONS

The same reaction that naturally ionizes water (H_2O) into hydrogen (H^+) ions and hydroxide ions (OH), also runs in reverse. When acids (H+) and alkalis (OH-) are mixed together in equal proportions, they neutralize each other to form water (H_2O) (Figure 10-12). The neutralizing shampoos and normalizing lotions used to neutralize hydroxide hair relaxers work by creating an acid-alkali neutralization reaction.

OXIDATION–REDUCTION (REDOX) REACTIONS

Oxidation–reduction (redox) reactions are responsible for the chemical changes created by hair colors, hair lighteners, permanent wave solutions, and neutralizers. The chemical services that we take for granted would not be possible without oxidation–reduction (redox) reactions.

OXIDATION REACTIONS

Oxidation is a chemical reaction that combines a substance with oxygen to produce an oxide. Chemical reactions that produce heat are called **exothermic** (ek-soh-THUR-mik). All oxidation reactions are exothermic.

Combustion (kum-BUS-chun) is the rapid oxidation of substance, accompanied by the production of heat and light. Lighting a match is an example of rapid oxidation. Since oxygen is needed, there cannot be a fire without air.

REDUCTION REACTIONS

When oxygen is added to a substance, the substance is oxidized. When oxygen is subtracted from a substance, the substance is **reduced,** and the chemical reaction is called **reduction.** An **oxidizing agent** is a substance that releases oxygen. Hydrogen peroxide (H_2O_2) is an example of an oxidizing agent. Hydrogen peroxide can be thought of as water (H_2O) with an "extra" atom of oxygen. When hydrogen peroxide is mixed with

ACTIVITY

Did you know that you can easily and safely test the pH of a solution? Litmus papers (pH test papers) can be used to indicate the pH of any salon product that contains water. You can test hair color, permanent waving solution, neutralizer, shampoo and conditioner, and skin care or nail care products.

You will need litmus papers (pH test papers), several small open containers, bottled drinking water, stirring sticks, and some white towels. Place the product you want to test in a small, open cup or bowl. If the product is a powder or is extremely thick, add a small amount of bottled water and stir thoroughly. Dip the litmus paper into the product.

Immediately place the paper on a white towel and compare the color obtained to the color on the package to determine the pH. Test anything you can think of, but it must contain water in order to have a pH. Be creative! What you discover may surprise you!

an oxidation hair color, oxygen is added to the hair color and the hair color is oxidized. At the same time, oxygen is subtracted from the hydrogen peroxide and the hydrogen peroxide is reduced. In this example, hair color is a reducing agent.

REDOX REACTIONS

Oxidation and reduction reactions always occur at the same time, and are referred to as redox reactions. **Redox** is a contraction for reduction-oxidation. Redox reactions involve a transfer between the oxidizing agent and the reducing agent. The oxidizing agent is reduced, and the reducing agent is oxidized.

Redox reactions can also take place without oxygen. Oxidation can also occur when hydrogen is subtracted from a substance. Thus, oxidation is the result of either the addition of oxygen, or the subtraction of hydrogen. Reduction can also occur when hydrogen is added to a substance. Consequently, reduction is the result of either the loss of oxygen or the addition of hydrogen (Figure 10-13).

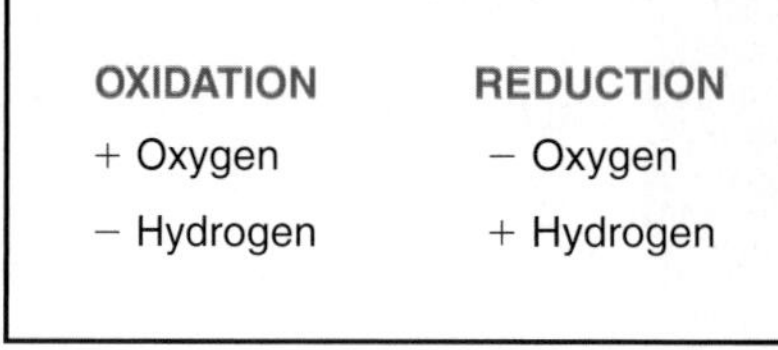

OXIDATION	REDUCTION
+ Oxygen	− Oxygen
− Hydrogen	+ Hydrogen

Figure 10-13 Chart for oxidation/reduction reactions.

YOU HAVE THE VALUE

There are many benefits for the client who takes advantage of the various salon services that use chemical products. While the use of chemical products has great benefits, always remember that there is a potential for injury as well. Your value as a salon professional depends on your ability to stay informed about new developments and products and how to use them effectively and safely.

REVIEW QUESTIONS

1. What is chemistry?
2. Why is a basic understanding of chemistry important?
3. What is the difference between organic and inorganic chemistry?
4. What are atoms?
5. What are elements?
6. What are the physical and chemical properties of matter? Give examples.
7. What is the difference between physical and chemical changes? Give examples.
8. Describe the three states of matter.
9. Explain elemental molecules, compound molecules, pure substances, and physical mixtures.
10. What is the difference between solutions, suspensions, and emulsions? Give examples.
11. Define pH and the pH scale.
12. Explain the difference between oxidation and reduction reactions.

CHAPTER GLOSSARY

acids	Solutions that have a pH below 7.0, and turn litmus paper from blue to red.
alkalis	Solutions that have a pH above 7.0, and turn litmus paper from red to blue.
alkanolamines	Substances used to neutralize acids or raise the pH of many hair products.
ammonia	Colorless gas with a pungent odor. Composed of hydrogen and nitrogen.
anion	An ion with a negative electrical charge.
atom	Smallest particle of an element that still retains the properties of that element.
cation	An ion with a positive electrical charge.
chemical change	Change in the chemical and physical properties of a substance due to a chemical reaction that creates a new substance or substances.
chemical properties	Characteristics that can only be determined by a chemical reaction and a chemical change in the substance.

CHAPTER GLOSSARY

chemistry	Science that deals with the composition, structures, and properties of matter, and how matter changes under various conditions.
combustion	Rapid oxidation of a substance, accompanied by the production of heat and light.
compounds	Combinations of two or more atoms of different elements chemically joined together.
element	The simplest form of matter; it cannot be broken down into a simpler substance without a loss of identity.
elemental molecules	A chemical combination of atoms of the same element.
emulsion	An unstable mixture of two or more immiscible substances united with the aid of an emulsifier.
exothermic	Chemical reactions that produce heat.
glycerin	Sweet, colorless, oily substance used as a solvent and moisturizer in skin and body creams.
hydrophilic	Water loving.
immiscible	Not capable of being mixed.
inorganic chemistry	Study of substances that do not contain carbon.
ion	An atom or molecule that carries an electrical charge.
ionization	Separation of an atom or molecule into positive and negative ions.
lipophilic	Oil loving.
logarithm	Multiples of ten.
matter	Any substance that occupies space and has mass (weight).
miscible	Capable of being mixed with another liquid in any proportion without separating.
molecule	A chemical combination of two or more atoms.
oil-in-water (O/W) emulsion	Oil droplets emulsified in water.
organic chemistry	Study of substances that contain carbon.
oxidation	A chemical reaction that combines a substance with oxygen to produce an oxide.
oxidizing agent	Substance that releases oxygen.

CHAPTER GLOSSARY

pH scale	Measures the acidity and alkalinity of a substance.
physical change	Change in the form or physical properties of a substance without the formation of a new substance.
physical mixture	Physical combination of matter, in any proportion.
physical properties	Characteristics that can be determined without a chemical reaction and that do not cause a chemical change in the substance.
pure substance	Chemical combination of matter in definite proportions.
redox	Contraction for reduction-oxidation; chemical reaction in which the oxidizing agent is reduced and the reducing agent is oxidized.
reduced	To subtract oxygen from or add hydrogen to a substance.
reduction	The chemical reaction of subtracting oxygen from, or adding hydrogen to, a substance.
silicones	Special type of oil used in hair conditioners and as water-resistant lubricants for the skin.
solute	Substance that is dissolved in a solution.
solution	Stable mixture of two or more mixable substances.
solvent	Substance that dissolves the solute to form a solution.
surfactants	Surface active agents; substances that act as a bridge to allow oil and water to mix, or emulsify.
suspension	Unstable mixture of undissolved particles in a liquid.
volatile	Easily evaporating.
volatile organic compounds (VOCs)	Substances containing carbon that evaporate quickly and easily.
water-in-oil (W/O) emulsion	Water droplets emulsified in oil.

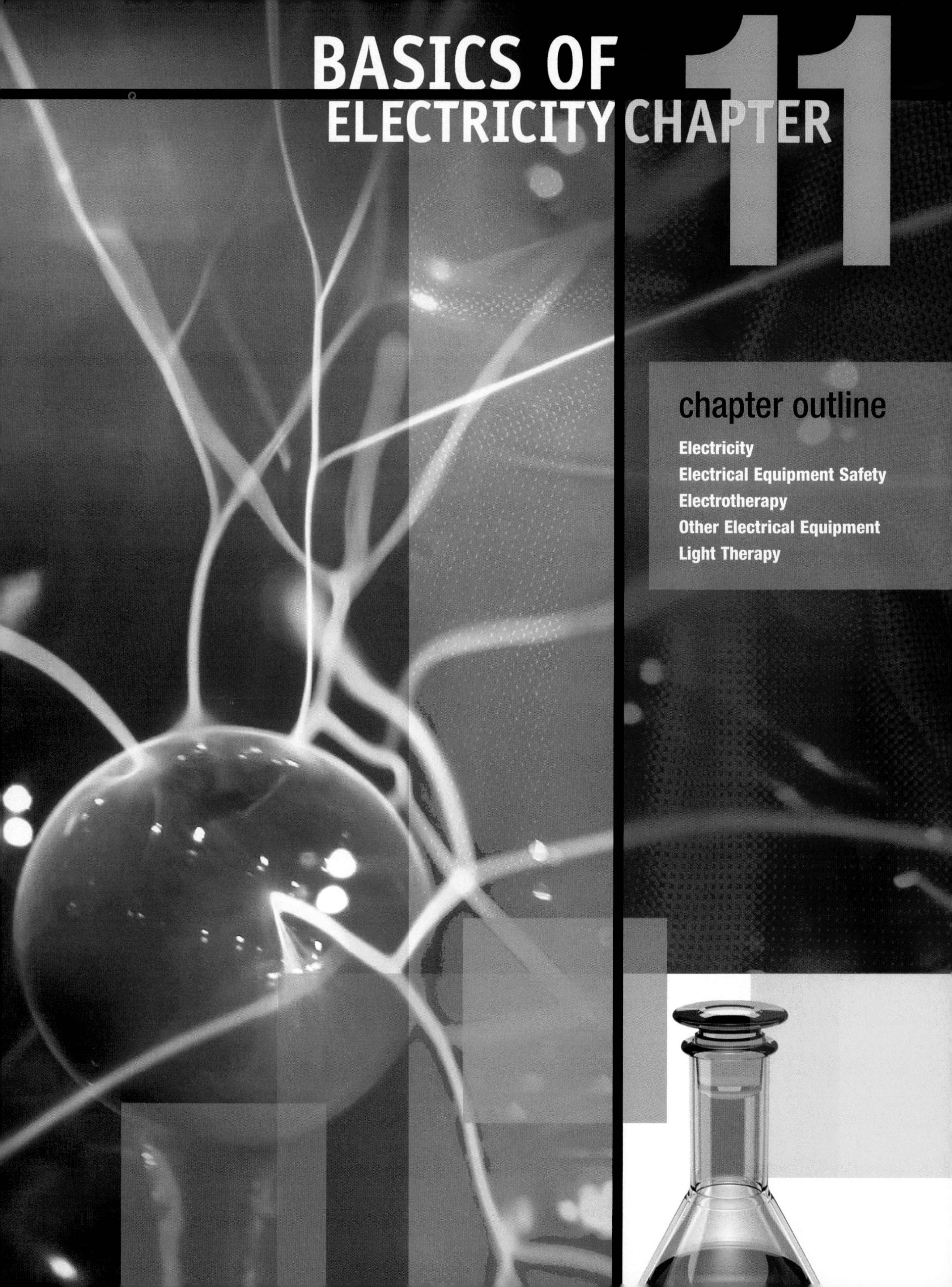

BASICS OF ELECTRICITY CHAPTER 11

chapter outline

- Electricity
- Electrical Equipment Safety
- Electrotherapy
- Other Electrical Equipment
- Light Therapy

Learning Objectives

After completing this chapter, you will be able to:

- Define the nature of electricity and the two types of electric current.
- Define electrical measurements.
- Understand the principles of electrical equipment safety.
- Define electric modalities used in cosmetology.
- Explain electromagnetic radiation and the visible spectrum of light.
- Describe the types of light therapy and their benefits.

Key Terms

Page number indicates where in the chapter the term is used.

Even if you have decided to join the professional cosmetology field because you love to style hair, your career will heavily rely on the use of electricity. To use your products and electricity effectively and safely, all cosmetology professionals need to have a basic working knowledge of their tools and how they are maintained.

ELECTRICITY

Just as we have provided you with a very general overview of chemistry, we will do the same with electricity since it, too, will play an important role in your work. Lightning on a stormy night is an effect of electricity. If you plug a poorly wired appliance into a socket and sparks fly out, you are also seeing the effects of electricity. You are not really "seeing" electricity, but instead its effects on the surrounding air. Electricity does not occupy space or have physical or chemical properties; therefore, it is not matter. If it is not matter, then what is it? **Electricity** is a form of energy that, when in motion exhibits magnetic, chemical, or thermal effects. It is a flow of electrons which are negatively charged particles that swirl around atoms like a swarm of bees.

An **electric current** is the flow of electricity along a conductor. All substances can be classified as conductors or insulators, depending on the ease with which an electric current can be transmitted through them.

A **conductor** is any substance that easily transmits electricity. Most metals are good conductors. Copper is a particularly good conductor, and is used in electric wiring and electric motors. The ionic compounds in ordinary water make it a good conductor. This explains why you should not swim in a lake during an electrical storm.

An **insulator** (IN-suh-layt-ur) or **nonconductor** is a substance that does not easily transmit electricity. Rubber, silk, wood, glass, and cement are good insulators. Electric wires are composed of twisted metal threads (conductor) covered with rubber (insulator). A **complete circuit** (SUR-kit) is the path of an electric current from the generating source through conductors and back to its original source (Figure 11-1).

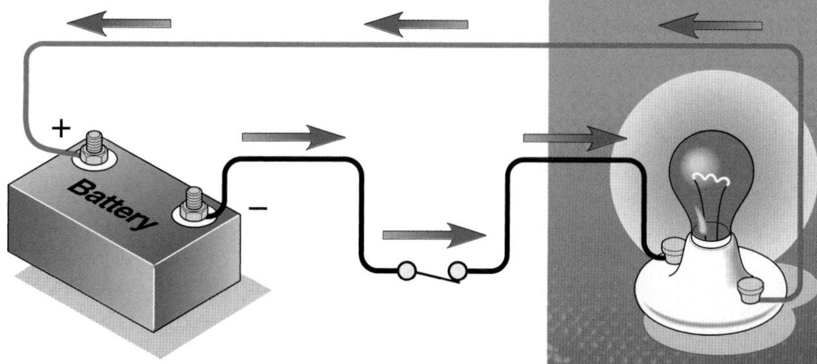

Figure 11-1 A complete electrical circuit.

TYPES OF ELECTRIC CURRENT

There are two kinds of electric current.

Direct current (DC) is a constant, even-flowing current that travels in one direction only. Flashlights, cellular telephones, and cordless electric drills use the direct current produced by batteries. The battery in your car stores electrical energy. Without it, your car would not start in the morning. A **converter** is an apparatus that changes direct current to alternating current. Some cars have converters that allow you to use appliances that would normally be plugged into an electrical wall outlet.

Alternating current (AC) is a rapid and interrupted current, flowing first in one direction and then in the opposite direction. This change in direction happens 60 times per second. Hair dryers and curling irons that plug into a wall outlet use alternating current produced by mechanical generators. A **rectifier** is an apparatus that changes alternating current to direct current. Cordless electric clippers and battery chargers use a rectifier to convert the AC current from an electrical wall outlet to the DC current needed to recharge their DC batteries.

ELECTRICAL MEASUREMENTS

The flow of an electric current can be compared to water flowing through a garden hose. Individual electrons flow through a wire in the same way that individual water molecules flow through a hose.

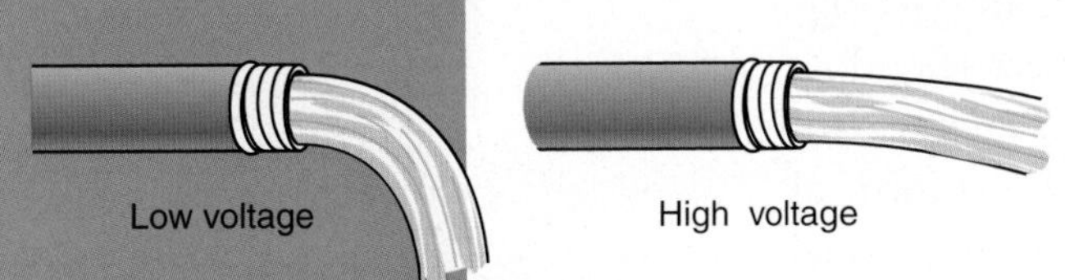

Figure 11-2 Volts measure the pressure or force that pushes electrons forward.

A **volt** (V), or voltage, is the unit that measures the pressure or force that pushes the flow of electrons forward through a conductor, much like the water pressure that pushes the water molecules through the hose (Figure 11-2). Without pressure, neither water nor electrons would flow. Car batteries are 12 volts, normal wall sockets that power your hair dryer and curling iron are 110 volts, and most air conditioners and clothes dryers run on 220 volts. A higher voltage indicates more pressure or force.

An **amp** (A), or ampere (AM-peer), is the unit that measures the amount of an electric current (the number of electrons flowing through a conductor). Just as a water hose must be able to expand as the amount of water flowing through it increases, so a wire must expand with an increase in the amount of electrons (amps). A hair dryer rated at 12 amps must have a cord that is twice as thick as one rated at 5 amps; otherwise, the cord might overheat and start a fire. A higher amp rating indicates a greater number of electrons and a stronger current (Figure 11-3).

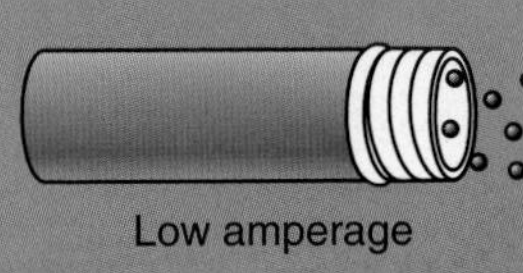

High amperage

Figure 11-3 Amps measure the number of electrons flowing through the wire.

A **milliampere** (mil-ee-AM-peer) is one-thousandth of an ampere. The current for facial and scalp treatments is measured in milliamperes; an ampere current would be much too strong and would damage the skin or body.

An **ohm** (O) is a unit that measures the resistance of an electric current. Current will not flow through a conductor unless the force (volts) is stronger than the resistance (ohms).

A **watt** (W) is a measurement of how much electric energy is being used in 1 second. A 40-watt light bulb uses 40 watts of energy per second.

A **kilowatt** (K) is 1,000 watts. The electricity in your house is measured in kilowatts per hour (kwh). A 1,000-watt (1-kilowatt) hair dryer uses 1,000 watts of energy per second.

ELECTRICAL EQUIPMENT SAFETY

When working with electricity, you must always be concerned with your own safety, as well as the safety of your clients. All electrical equipment should be inspected regularly to determine whether it is in safe working order. Sloppy electrical connections and overloaded circuits can result in an electrical shock, a burn, or even a serious fire.

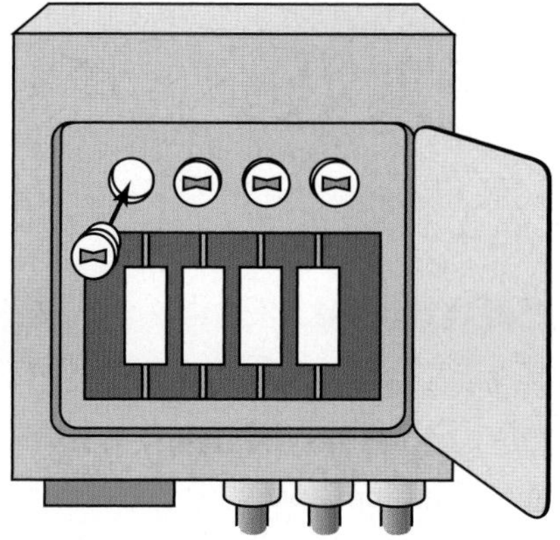

Figure 11-4 Fuse box.

SAFETY DEVICES

A **fuse** (FYOOZ) is a special device that prevents excessive current from passing through a circuit. It is designed to blow out or melt when the wire becomes too hot from overloading the circuit with too much current (i.e., too many appliances or faulty equipment). To re-establish the circuit, disconnect the appliance, check all connections and insulation, and insert a new fuse (Figure 11-4).

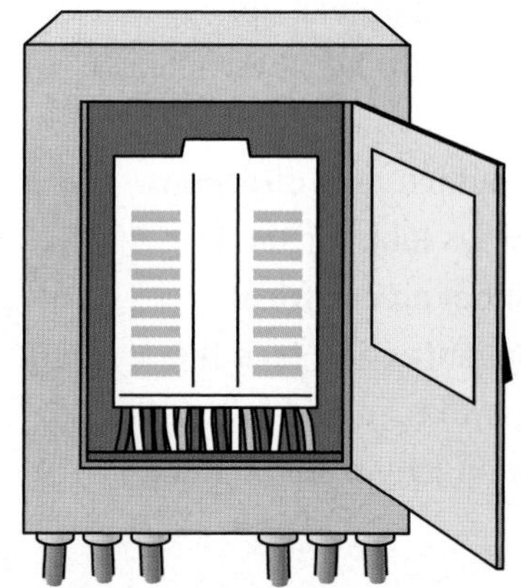

Figure 11-5 Circuit breakers.

A **circuit breaker** is a switch that automatically interrupts or shuts off an electric circuit at the first indication of overload. Circuit breakers have replaced fuses in modern electric circuits. They have all the safety features of fuses but do not require replacement, and can simply be reset. Your hair dryer has a circuit breaker located in the electric plug designed to protect you and your client in case of an overload or short circuit. When a circuit breaker shuts off, you should disconnect the appliance and check all connections and insulation before resetting (Figure 11-5).

The principle of "grounding" is another important way of promoting electrical safety. All electrical appliances must have at least two electrical connections. The "live" connection supplies current to the circuit. The ground connection completes the circuit and carries the current safely away to the ground. If you look closely at electrical plugs with two rectangular prongs, you will see that one is slightly larger than the other. This guarantees that the plug can only be inserted one way, and protects you and your client from electrical shock in the event of a short circuit.

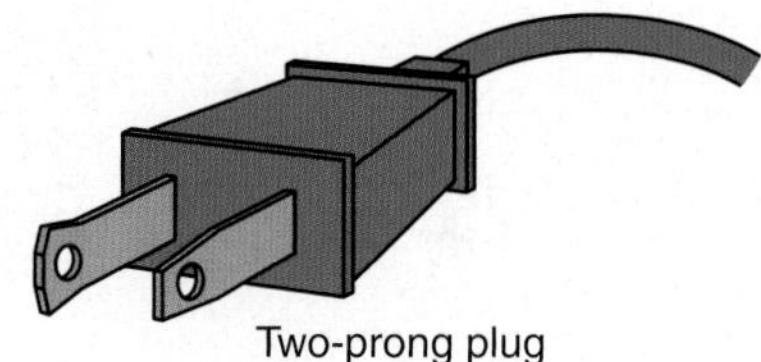

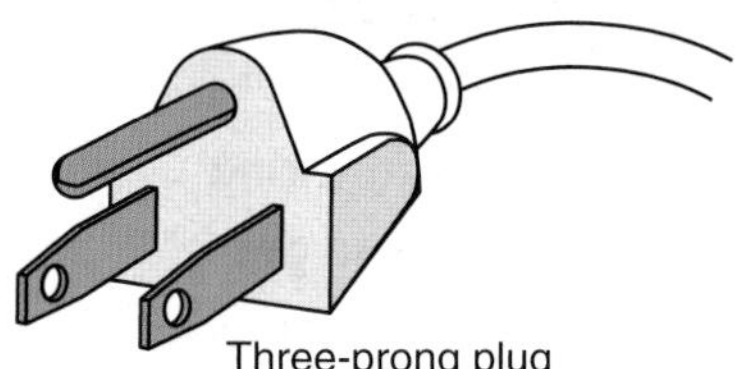

Figure 11-6 Two-prong and three-prong plugs.

For added protection, some appliances have a third, circular, electrical connection that provides an additional ground. This extra ground is designed to guarantee a safe path for electricity if the first ground fails or is improperly connected. Appliances with a third circular ground offer the most protection for you and your client (Figure 11-6).

GUIDELINES FOR SAFE USE OF ELECTRICAL EQUIPMENT

Careful attention to electrical safety helps to eliminate accidents and to ensure greater client satisfaction. The following reminders will help ensure the safe use of electricity.

- All the electrical appliances you use should be UL certified (Figure 11-7).
- Read all instructions carefully before using any piece of electrical equipment.
- Disconnect all appliances when not in use.

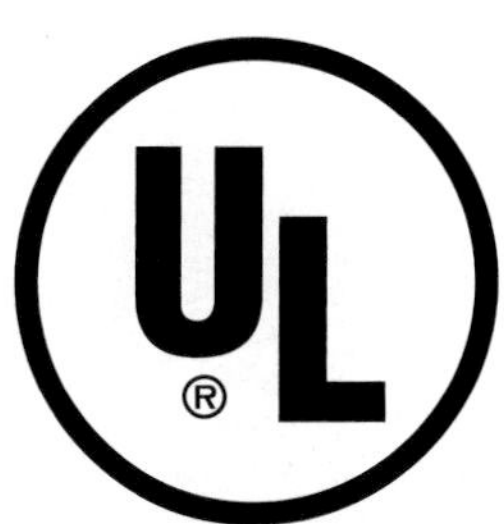

Figure 11-7 UL symbol as it appears on electrical devices.

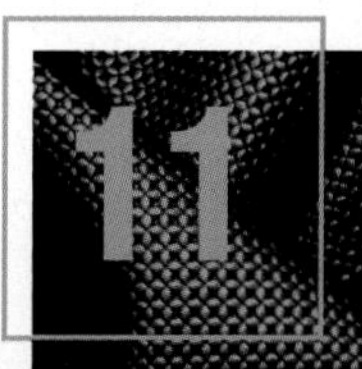

CAUTION

Underwriter's Laboratory (UL) certifies the safety of electrical appliances. Curling irons, hair dryers, and electric clippers that are UL approved are certified to be safe when used according to the manufacturer's directions. Always look for the UL symbol on electrical appliances and take the time to read and follow the manufacturer's directions.

CAUTION

Never tamper with wiring or electrical plugs to get them to fit into a receptacle that they were not designed for.

- Inspect all electrical equipment regularly.
- Keep all wires, plugs, and electrical equipment in good repair.
- Use only one plug to each outlet; overloading may cause the circuit breaker to pop (Figure 11-8).
- You and your client should avoid contact with water and metal surfaces when using electricity; do not handle electrical equipment with wet hands.
- Do not leave your client unattended while connected to an electrical device.
- Keep electrical cords off the floor and away from people's feet; getting tangled in a cord could cause you or your client to trip.
- Do not attempt to clean around electric outlets while equipment is plugged in.
- Do not touch two metal objects at the same time if either is connected to an electric current.
- Do not step on or place objects on electrical cords.
- Do not allow electrical cord to become twisted; it can cause a short circuit.
- Disconnect appliances by pulling on the plug, not the cord.
- Do not attempt to repair electrical appliances unless you are qualified.

ELECTROTHERAPY

Electronic facial treatments are commonly referred to as electrotherapy. A **wall plate** (facial stimulator) is an instrument that plugs into an ordinary wall outlet and produces different types of electric currents that are used for facial and scalp treatments. These currents are called **modalities.** Each modality produces a different effect on the skin.

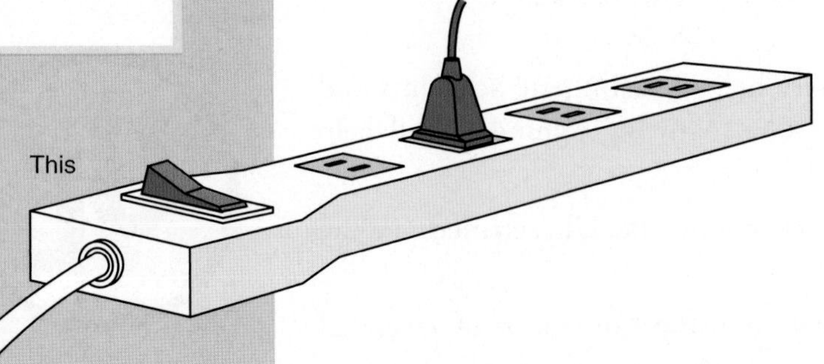

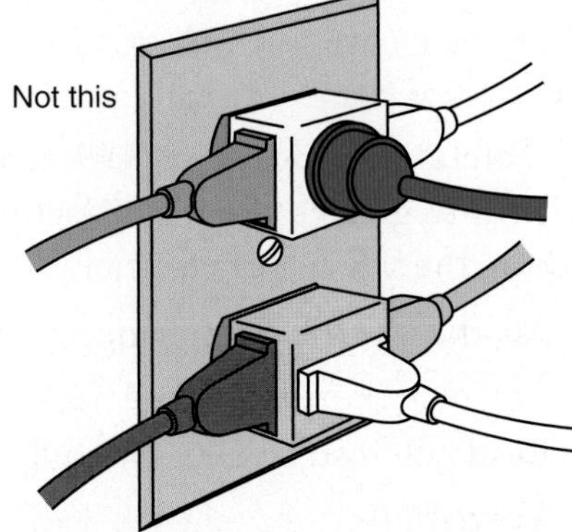

Figure 11-8 One plug per outlet.

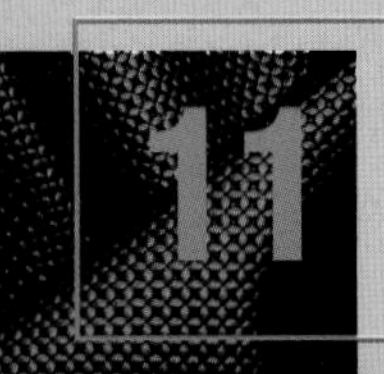

An **electrode** is an applicator for directing the electric current from the machine to the client's skin. It is usually made of carbon, glass, or metal. Each modality requires two electrodes—one negative and one positive—to conduct the flow of electricity through the body (except the Tesla high frequency).

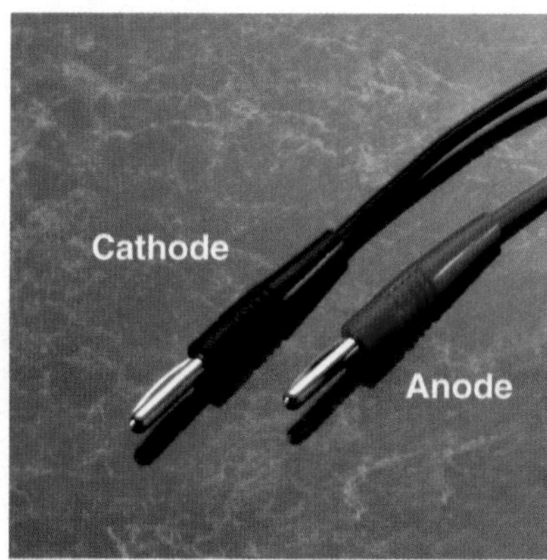

Figure 11-9 Anode and cathode.

POLARITY

Polarity indicates the negative or positive pole of an electric current. Electrotherapy devices always have one negatively charged pole and one positively-charged pole. The positive electrode is called an **anode** (AN-ohd). The anode is usually red and is marked with a "P" or a plus (+) sign. The negative electrode is called a **cathode** (KATH-ohd). It is usually black and is marked with an "N" or a minus (−) sign (Figure 11-9). If the electrodes are not marked, the following polarity tests will tell you which is which.

Separate the two tips of the conducting cords from each other and immerse them in a glass of salt water. Turn the selector switch of the appliance to galvanic current, and then turn up the intensity. More active bubbles will accumulate at the negative pole than at the positive pole.

Another test involves placing the tips of the conducting cords on two separate pieces of moist blue litmus paper. The paper under the positive pole will turn red, while the paper under the negative pole will stay blue. If you use red litmus paper, the paper under the positive pole will remain red and the paper under the negative pole will turn blue.

Do not let the tips of the cords touch or you will cause a short circuit. The polarity tests can be dangerous and should only be performed with your instructor's supervision.

MODALITIES

The two main modalities used in cosmetology are galvanic and Tesla high-frequency.

GALVANIC CURRENT

The most commonly used modality is **galvanic current.** It is a constant and direct current (DC), having a positive and negative pole, and produces chemical changes when it passes through the tissues and fluids of the body.

Two different chemical reactions are possible, depending on the polarity (negative or positive) that is used (see Table 11-1). The **active electrode** is the electrode used on the area to be treated. The **inactive electrode** is the opposite pole from the active electrode. Note that the effects produced by the positive pole are the exact opposite of those produced by the negative pole.

IONTOPHORESIS

Iontophoresis (eye-ahn-toh-foh-REE-sus) is the process of introducing water-soluble products into the skin with the use of electric current, such as the use of the positive and negative poles of a galvanic machine.

Cataphoresis (kat-uh-fuh-REE-sus) forces acidic substances into deeper tissues using galvanic current from the positive toward the negative pole.

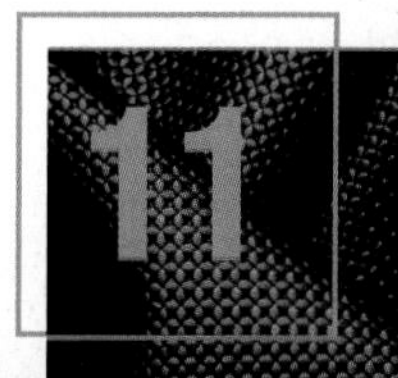

Positive Pole (Anode)	Negative Pole (Cathode)
Produces acidic reactions	Produces alkaline reactions
Closes the pores	Opens the pores
Soothes nerves	Stimulates and irritates the nerves
Decreases blood supply	Increases blood supply
Contracts blood vessels	Expands blood vessels
Hardens and firms tissues	Softens tissues

Table 11-1 Effects of Galvanic Current

CAUTION

Do not use negative galvanic current on skin with broken capillaries or pustular acne conditions, or on a client with high blood pressure or metal implants.

Anaphoresis (an-uh-for-EES-sus) is the process of forcing liquids into the tissues from the negative toward the positive pole. **Desincrustation** (des-inkrus-TAY-shun) is a process used to soften and emulsify grease deposits (oil) and blackheads in the hair follicles. This process is frequently used to treat acne, milia (small, white cyst-like pimples), and comedones (blackheads and whiteheads).

TESLA HIGH-FREQUENCY CURRENT

The **Tesla high-frequency current** is a thermal or heat-producing current with a high rate of oscillation or vibration. It is commonly called the violet ray and is used for both scalp and facial treatments. Tesla current does not produce muscle contractions, and its effects can be either stimulating or soothing, depending on the method of application. The electrodes are made from either glass or metal, and only one electrode is used to perform a service (Figure 11-10). Benefits from the use of Tesla high-frequency current are summarized below.

- Stimulates blood circulation
- Improves glandular activity
- Increases elimination and absorption
- Increased metabolism
- Improves germicidal action
- Relieves congestion

CAUTION

Tesla high-frequency current should not be used on clients who are pregnant, suffer from epilepsy (seizures) or asthma, or who have high blood pressure, a sinus blockage, a pacemaker, or metal implants.

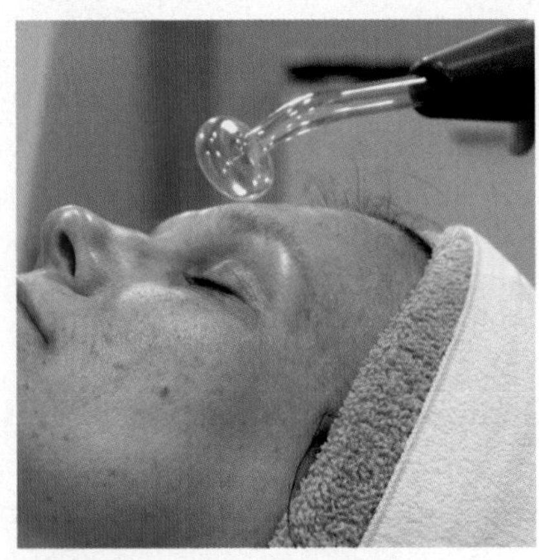

Figure 11-10 Applying high-frequency current with a facial electrode.

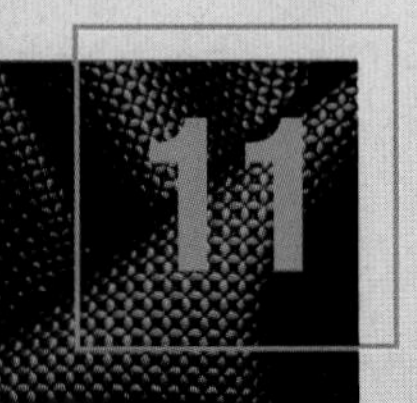

OTHER ELECTRICAL EQUIPMENT

Conventional hood hair dryers or heat lamps are sources of dry heat that can be used to shorten chemical processing time. Since dry heat causes evaporation, the hair must be covered with a plastic cap to avoid drying the hair during a chemical process. Several small holes should be placed in the cap to allow for the escape of excess heat and any gases that might form.

Electric curling and flat irons are available in many types and sizes. They have built-in heating elements and plug directly into a wall outlet.

Heating caps provide a uniform source of heat, and can be used with hair and scalp conditioning treatments.

Several different types of haircolor processing machines, or accelerating machines, shorten the time it takes to process chemical hair services. These processors usually look similar to a hood dryer and dispense a hot water vapor inside the hood. A haircolor service processed with a machine at 90°F (32°C) will process twice as fast as it would at a normal room temperature of 72°F (22°C).

A steamer or vaporizer produces moist, uniform heat that can be applied to the head or face. Steamers warm and cleanse the skin by increasing the flow of both oil and sweat. Some steamers may also be used for hair and scalp conditioning treatments. Estheticians often add essential oils to a facial steamer as part of a skin therapy, and to enhance general well-being.

As a salon professional, you may use equipment to perform light therapy treatments. Before we explore the specific types of equipment involved, it is important to have some basic understanding of what light is and how it works.

LIGHT THERAPY

Visible light is **electromagnetic radiation** that we can see. Electromagnetic radiation is also called "radiant energy" because it carries, or radiates, energy through space on waves. These waves are similar to the waves caused when a stone is dropped on the surface of the water. The distance between two successive peaks is called the **wavelength.** Long wavelengths have low frequency, meaning that the number of waves is less frequent (fewer waves) within a given length. Short wavelengths have higher frequency because the number of waves is more frequent (more waves) within a given length (Figure 11-11).

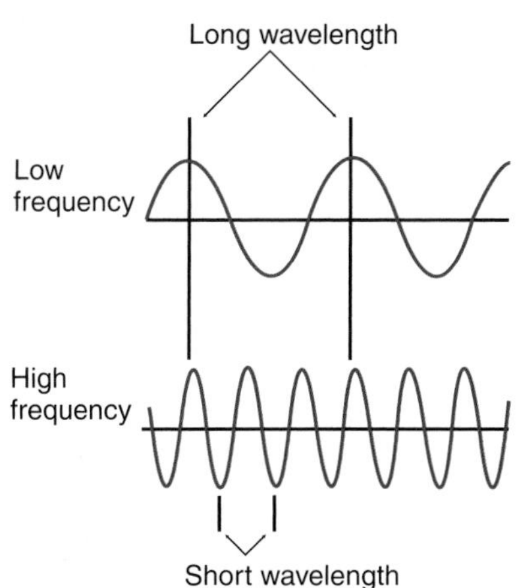

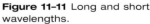

Figure 11-11 Long and short wavelengths.

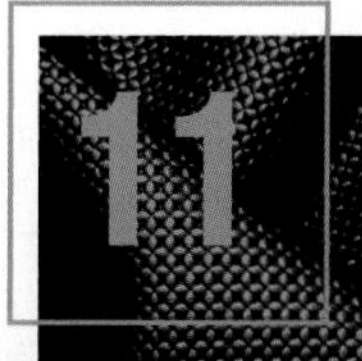

CAUTION

The vibrator should never be used when there is heart disease or when fever, abscesses, or inflammation are present.

CAUTION

The client's eyes should always be protected during any light therapy treatment. Use cotton pads saturated with boric acid solution, witch hazel, or distilled water. To avoid damage to the eyes, both cosmetologist and client should always wear safety goggles when working with ultraviolet rays.

The entire range of wavelengths of electromagnetic radiation (radiant energy) is called the "electromagnetic spectrum." Visible light is the part of the electromagnetic spectrum that we can see. Visible light makes up 35 percent of natural sunlight.

Ultraviolet rays and infrared rays are also forms of electromagnetic radiation, but they are invisible because their wavelengths are beyond the visible spectrum of light. Invisible rays make up 65 percent of natural sunlight (Figure 11-12).

Within the visible spectrum of light, violet has the shortest wavelength and red has the longest. The wavelength of infrared is just below red, and the wavelength of ultraviolet is just above violet. Infrared and ultraviolet rays are not really light at all. Again, they are the wavelengths of electromagnetic radiation that are just beyond the visible spectrum.

INFRARED

Infrared rays make up 60 percent of natural sunlight. Infrared rays have longer wavelengths, penetrate deeper, and produce more heat than visible light.

Infrared lamps are used mainly during hair treatments and to process hair color, and should be operated at a distance of at least 30 inches (76 centimeters), for an exposure time of about 5 minutes. Check the comfort of your client frequently during the service. Never leave the client unattended.

VISIBLE LIGHT

Visible light rays are the primary source of light used in facial and scalp treatments. The bulbs used for therapeutic visible light therapy are white, red, and blue.

White light is referred to as "combination light" because it is a combination of all visible rays of the spectrum. It also has the benefits

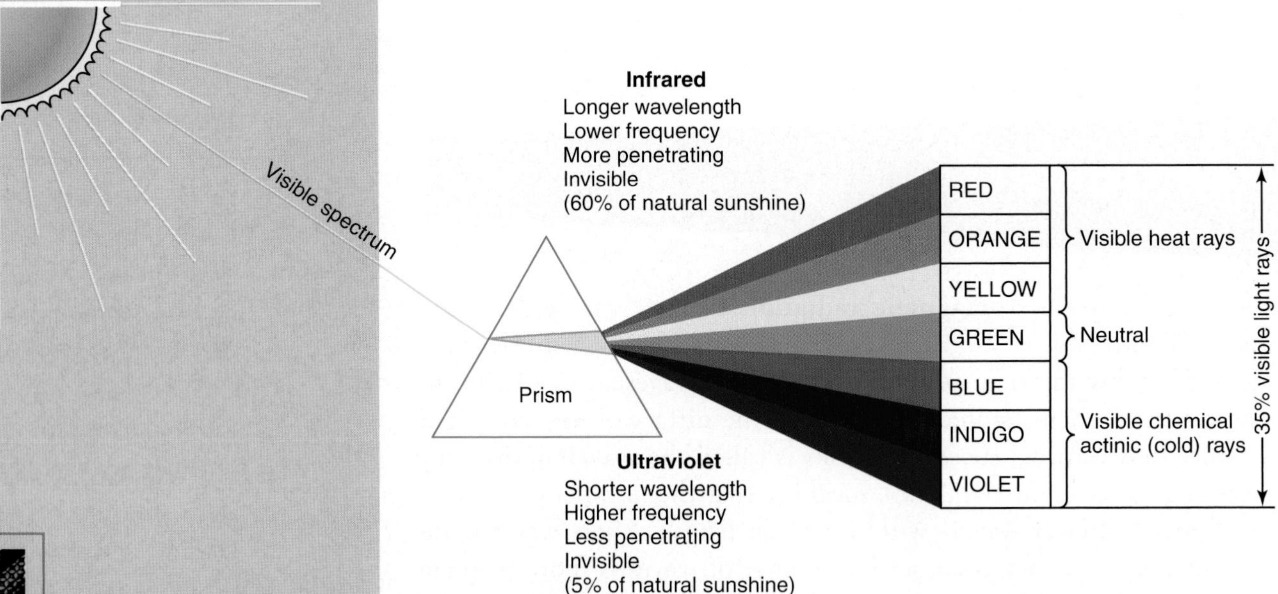

Figure 11-12 The visible spectrum.

of all rays of the visible spectrum. **Blue light** should only be used on bare oily skin. It contains few heat rays, is the least penetrating, and has some germicidal and chemical benefits. **Red light** is used on dry skin in combination with oils and creams. Red light penetrates the deepest and produces the most heat.

ULTRAVIOLET

Ultraviolet (UV) rays make up 5% of natural sunlight, and are also referred to as cold rays or actinic rays. Ultraviolet rays have shorter wavelengths, penetrate less, and produce less heat than visible light. UV rays also produce chemical effects and kill germs. UV also prompts the skin to produce Vitamin D, a fat-soluble vitamin that promotes mineralization of bones. Overexposure to UV rays, though, can cause premature aging of the skin and skin cancer. Incidents of skin cancer have reached a near-epidemic level, with over 1 million new cases being diagnosed each year. It is estimated that one in five Americans will develop skin cancer, and 90 percent of those cancers will be the result of exposure to UV radiation from the sun, sun lamps, and tanning beds.

APPLICATION OF ULTRAVIOLET RAYS

Although the application of ultraviolet rays can be beneficial, it must be done with the utmost care. UV rays are applied with a lamp at a distance of 30 to 36 inches (76 to 91 centimeters). The therapy should begin with exposure times of 2 to 3 minutes, with a gradual increase in exposure time to 7 or 8 minutes.

LIGHT VERSUS HEAT ENERGY

Catalysts are used to make reactions happen more quickly. Some catalysts use heat as an energy source while others use light. Whatever the source, catalysts absorb energy like a battery. At the appropriate time, they pass this energy to the initiator and the reaction begins. For example, light-cured nail enhancements use UV light. UV rays are invisible, have shorter wavelengths, and are less penetrating than visible lights. They also produce chemical effects and kill germs. All other nail products use heat energy.

You can see why it is important to protect UV-curing products from light. Sunlight and even artificial room lights can start polymerization in the container. The same can happen when heat-curing monomers are placed in a hot car trunk, a store window, or other warm area. The high heat may also cause polymerization in the container. Products that require normal "incandescent" light bulbs are *not* light-curing monomers. They are using the extra heat released from the light bulb to speed evaporation of solvents.

Did You Know

Although salon lighting is not a form of light therapy, the quality of this light can have an effect on your work and your client's satisfaction. Fluorescent light is produced by fluorescent lamps and is much cooler (green-blue) than natural sunlight. Incandescent light is produced by standard (tungsten) light bulbs and is warmer (yellow-gold) than either natural sunlight or fluorescent light. Your client's hair and skin will appear more green-blue when viewed with fluorescent lighting, and more golden when viewed with incandescent lighting.

Be careful when handling fluorescent light bulbs; they contain dangerous substances, including mercury. Avoid breaking fluorescent bulbs, and dispose of used bulbs properly.

CAUTION

Overexposure to UV rays can produce painful burns and blistering, increase the risk of skin cancer, and cause premature aging of the skin. Never leave your client unattended during the exposure time.

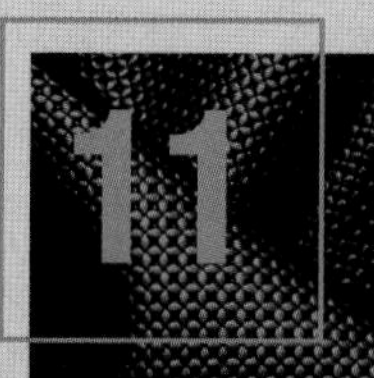

REVIEW QUESTIONS

1. Describe the two types of electric current and give examples of each.
2. List the four main types of electrical measurements. What do they measure?
3. List and describe the two main electric modalities or currents used in cosmetology.
4. List and describe the two main types of light therapy.
5. What is electromagnetic radiation? What is visible light? What is white light?
6. Name two important precautions to observe when using light therapy.

CHAPTER GLOSSARY

active electrode	Electrode used on the area to be treated.
alternating current (AC)	Rapid and interrupted current, flowing first in one direction and then in the opposite direction.
amp	Unit that measures the amount of an electric current (quantity of electrons flowing through a conductor).
anaphoresis	Process of forcing liquids into the tissues from the negative toward the positive pole.
anode	Positive electrode.
blue light	Therapeutic light that should only be used on bare oily skin; contains few heat rays, is the least penetrating, and has some germicidal and chemical benefits.
catalysts	Any substances having the power to increase the velocity (speed) of a chemical reaction.
cataphoresis	Process of forcing acidic substances into deeper tissues using galvanic current from the positive toward the negative pole.
cathode	Negative electrode.
circuit breaker	Switch that automatically interrupts or shuts off an electric circuit at the first indication of overload.
complete circuit	The path of an electric current from the generating source through conductors and back to its original source.
conductor	Any substance, material, or medium that easily transmits electricity.

CHAPTER GLOSSARY

converter	Apparatus that changes direct current to alternating current.
direct current (DC)	Constant, even-flowing current that travels in one direction only.
desincrustation	Process used to soften and emulsify grease deposits (oil) and blackheads in the hair follicles.
electric current	Flow of electricity along a conductor.
electricity	Form of energy that, when in motion, exhibits magnetic, chemical, or thermal effects; a flow of electrons.
electrode	Applicator for directing the electric current from machine to client's skin.
electromagnetic radiation	Also called radiant energy because it carries, or radiates, energy through space on waves.
fuse	Special device that prevents excessive current from passing through a circuit.
galvanic current	Constant and direct current (DC), having a positive and negative pole and producing chemical changes when it passes through the tissues and fluids of the body.
inactive electrode	Opposite pole from the active electrode.
infrared rays	Invisible rays that have longer wavelengths, penetrate deeper, and produce more heat than visible light.
insulator or nonconductor	Substance that does not easily transmit electricity.
iontophoresis	Process of introducing water-soluble products into the skin with the use of electric current, such as the use of the positive and negative poles of a galvanic machine.
kilowatt	1,000 watts.
milliampere	One-thousandth of an ampere.
modalities	Currents used in electrical facial and scalp treatments.
ohm	Unit that measures the resistance of an electric current.
polarity	Negative or positive pole of an electric current.
rectifier	Apparatus that converts alternating current to direct current.
red light	Therapeutic light used on dry skin in combination with oils and creams; penetrates the deepest and produces the most heat.

CHAPTER GLOSSARY

Tesla high-frequency current	Thermal or heat-producing current with a high rate of oscillation or vibration; also called violet ray.
ultraviolet (UV) rays	Invisible rays that have short wavelengths, are the least-penetrating rays, produce chemical effects, and kill germs; also called cold rays or actinic rays.
visible light	The primary source of light used in facial and scalp treatments.
volt	Unit that measures the pressure or force that pushes the flow of electrons forward through a conductor.
wall plate	Instrument that plugs into an ordinary wall outlet and produces various types of electric currents that are used for facial and scalp treatments.
watt	Measurement of how much electric energy is being used in one second.
wavelength	Distance between successive peaks of electromagnetic waves.
white light	Referred to as combination light because it is a combination of all visible rays of the spectrum.

HAIR CARE

PART 3

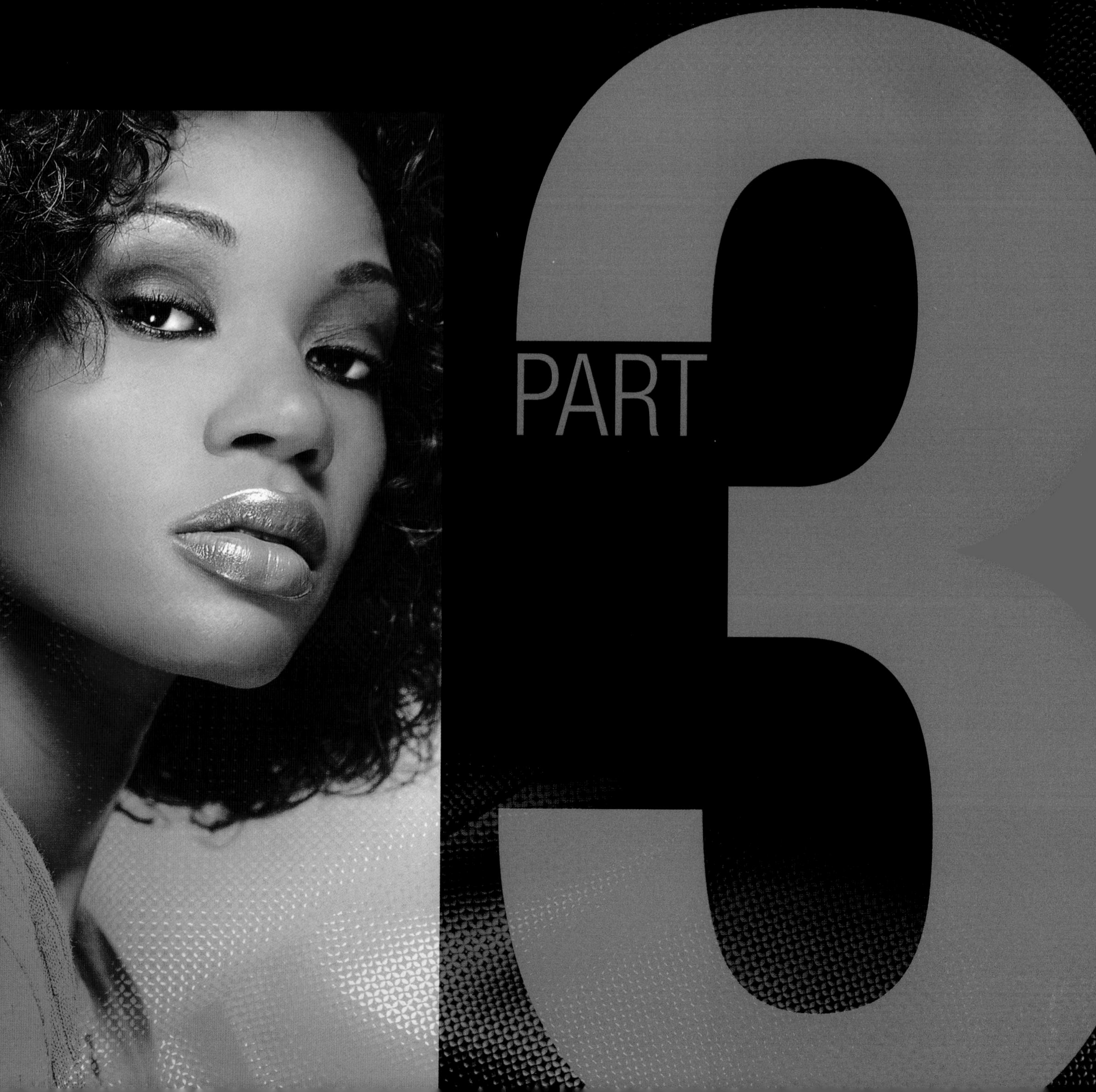

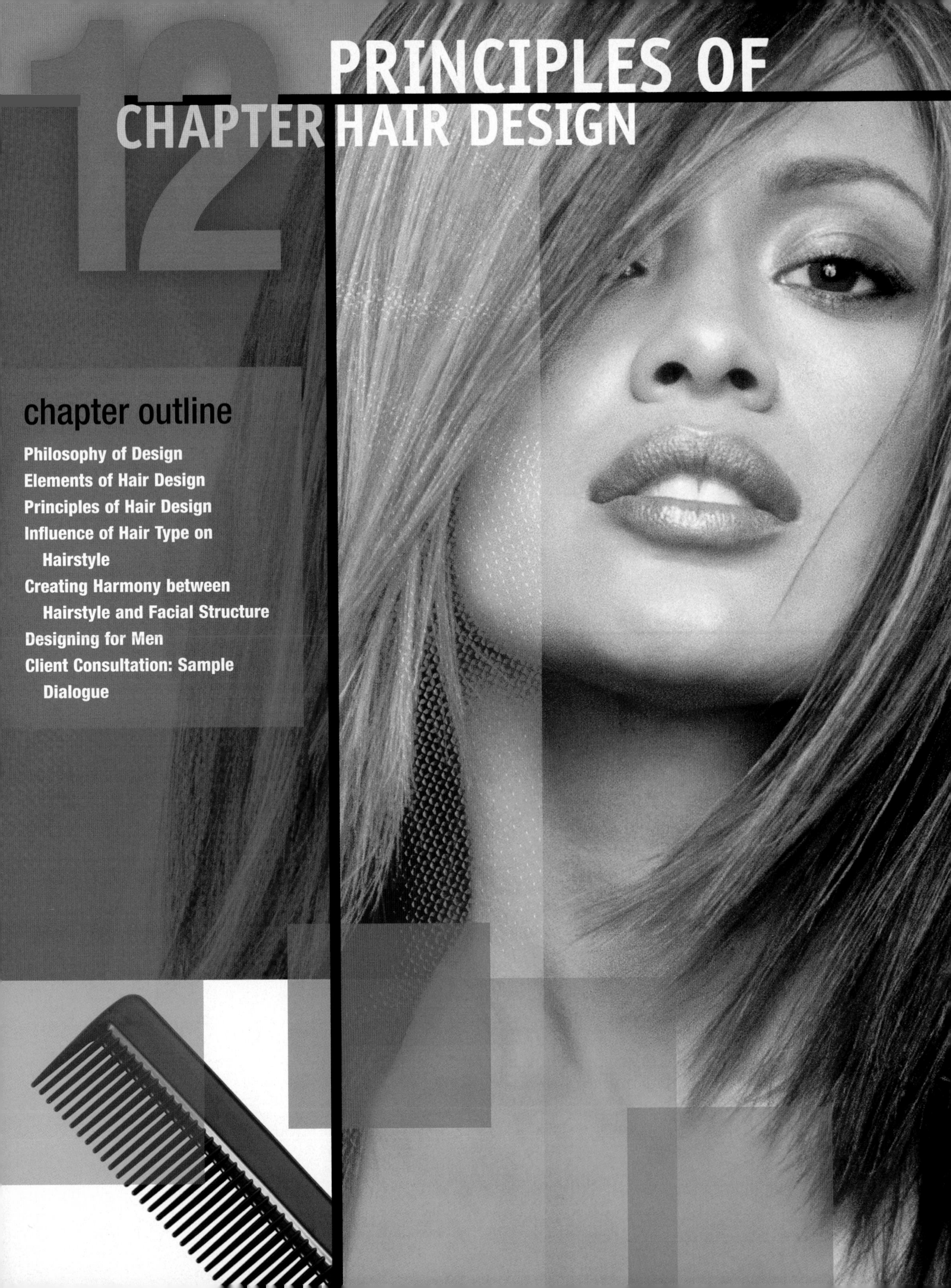

CHAPTER 12 PRINCIPLES OF HAIR DESIGN

chapter outline

Learning Objectives

After completing this chapter, you will be able to:

- **List the five elements of hair design.**
- **List the five principles of hair design.**
- **Identify different facial shapes.**
- **Demonstrate how to design hairstyles to enhance or camouflage facial features.**
- **Explain design considerations for men.**

Key Terms

Page number indicates where in the chapter the term is used.

asymmetrical balance pg. 203
balance pg. 202
bang area/fringe pg. 213
concave profile pg. 209
contrasting lines pg. 198
convex profile pg. 209
curved lines pg. 198
design texture pg. 199
diagonal lines pg. 197
emphasis or focus pg. 204
form pg. 199
harmony pg. 204
horizontal lines pg. 197
parallel lines pg. 198
proportion pg. 202
profile pg. 209
rhythm pg. 203
single lines pg. 198
space pg. 199
straight profile pg. 209
symmetrical balance pg. 203
transitional lines pg. 198
vertical lines pg. 197

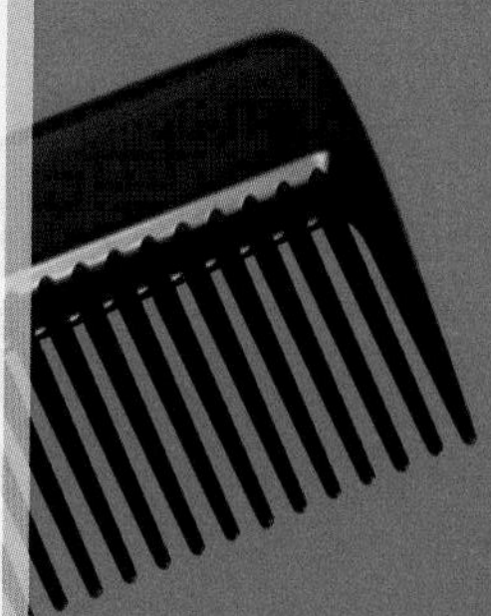

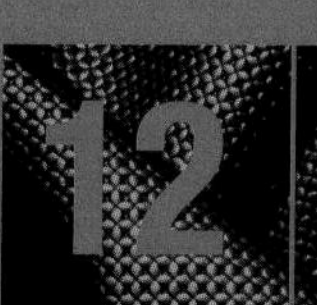

Design is the foundation of all artistic applications. All artists—architects, fashion designers, and interior designers, among many other designers—have a strong visual eye. So do you, since you have chosen to pursue a career in the beauty industry.

Do you want to be known as a good stylist or a great one? As a stylist, your goal is to learn how to design the best hairstyle for your client. That process begins with analyzing the entire person by using the elements and principles of design to enhance positive features and minimize the negative ones. An understanding of design and art principles will help you develop the artistic skill and judgment needed to create the best possible design for your client.

PHILOSOPHY OF DESIGN

A good designer always sees the end result before beginning. A good example is when an architect designs a building; he first visualizes it completed in drawings, and then takes the necessary steps to create the design in a model.

Inspiration can come from almost anywhere, at any time. Movies, TV, magazines, videos, a person on the street, and so on can often spark the creative process. One of the best sources of inspiration can be found in nature. The rhythm and movement of ocean waves have inspired painters, poets, composers, and hairstylists. The shapes, colors, patterns, and textures of plants, animals, and minerals are also a great source of visual ideas. At times, you may find yourself looking to the past for inspiration. A hairstyle from an earlier time might inspire you, as you reinvent it in a way that works for today (Figures 12-1 and 12-2). Modern inspiration for fashion often starts on the streets and in the clubs. Hair design usually follows fashion trends to create the total look.

Once inspired, you will then need to decide which tools and techniques—such as cutting shears, flat irons, permanent wave, hair color, and so forth—are needed to achieve your design. It is always a good idea when working out a design to first practice on a mannequin head. As you develop or practice a technique, there is always the chance that your original concept will turn into something entirely different. There are no failures if the experience is a lesson learned. Be open to change, and the creative process will be exciting and satisfying.

As a designer, you will need to develop a visual understanding of which hairstyles work best on which face shapes and body types. It takes time to train your eye to recognize the best design decision. You cannot achieve a trained eye simply through book learning. It may help you to review these pages over and over, but please do not get frustrated if it takes a while to understand this chapter. Sometimes the best teacher is time and the trial-and-error process that comes with experience. All good stylists have made a significant number of "design mistakes" in the past—-a great stylist will learn from the experience and grow. Having a strong design foundation will help make you a great stylist. Once you have these skills, your creative juices will kick in and you can move beyond the basics.

Having a strong foundation in technique and skills will allow you to take calculated risks. It is important in this field to take those risks. Too many stylists confine themselves to the basics where they feel safe. But "safe" can translate into "dull." If you are looking for a satisfying career in the long term do not allow yourself to become what is known in the beauty industry as a "cookie cutter" hairdresser who learns a new haircut and then gives it to everyone who sits in her chair for the next month. Always be exploring new possibilities, customizing your design to each client's individual needs and lifestyle. *Think out of the box!* Great hairstylists find inspiration everywhere by keeping an eye out for what is new in the beauty industry and by dedicating themselves to their continuing education. You can keep growing by having your eyes and mind always open to learning.

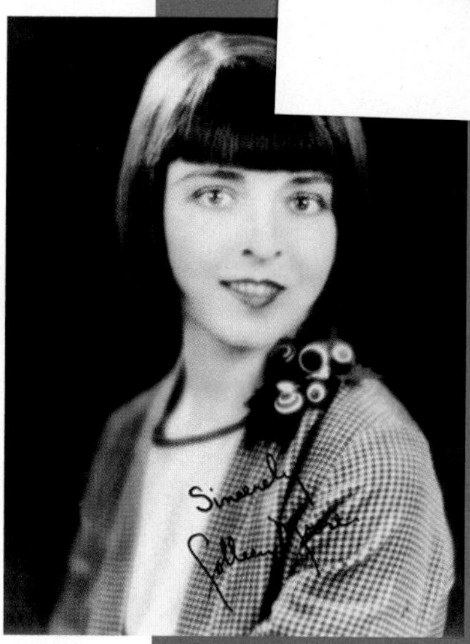

Figure 12-1 Colleen Moore, 1920s film star—the original flapper introduces the bob.

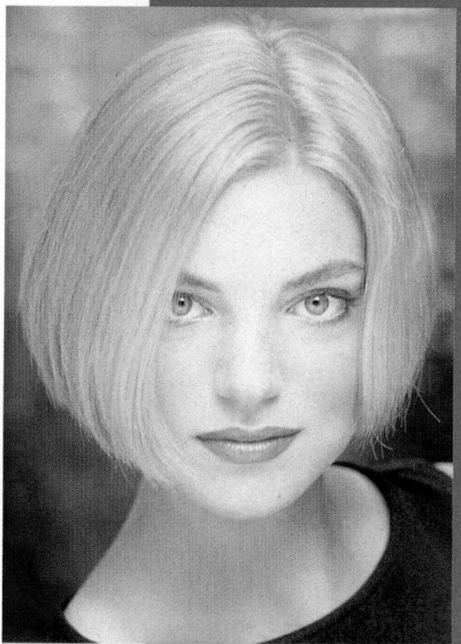

Figure 12-2 Contemporary bob.

ELEMENTS OF HAIR DESIGN

To begin to understand the creative process involved in hairstyling, it is critical to learn the five basic elements of three dimensional design. These elements are line, form, space, texture, and color.

LINE

Line defines form and space. The presence of one nearly always means that the other two are involved. Lines create the shape, design, and movement of a hairstyle. The eye follows the lines in a design. They can be straight or curved. There are four basic types of lines.

1. **Horizontal lines** create width in hair design. They extend in the same direction and maintain a constant distance apart—from the floor or horizon (Figure 12-3).
2. **Vertical lines** create length and height in hair design. They make a hairstyle appear longer and narrower as the eye follows the lines up and down (Figure 12-4).
3. **Diagonal lines** are positioned between horizontal and vertical lines. They are often used to emphasize or minimize facial features. Diagonal lines are also used to create interest in hair design (Figure 12-5).

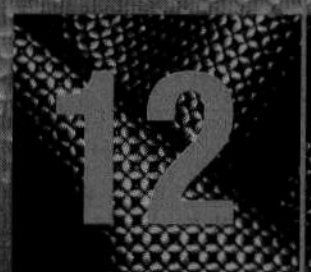

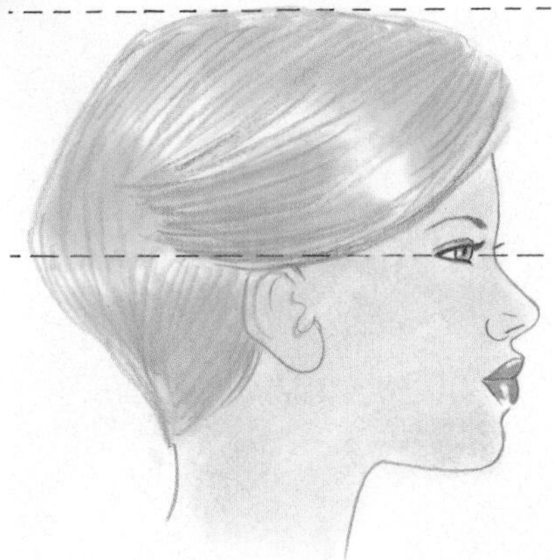

Figure 12-3 Horizontal lines in a hairstyle.

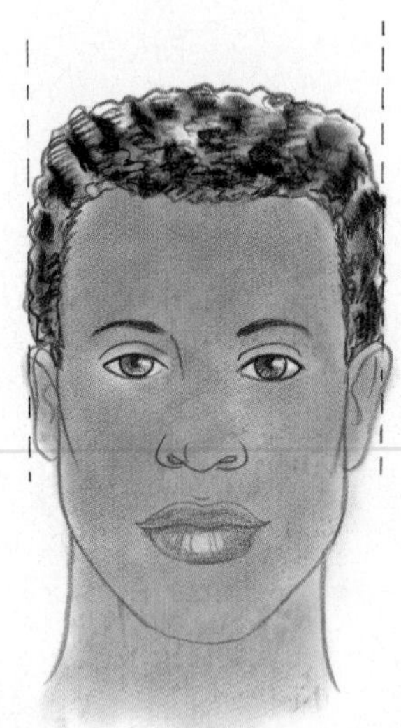

Figure 12-4 Vertical lines in a hairstyle.

4. **Curved lines** soften a design. They can be large or small, a full circle, or just part of a circle (Figure 12-6). They can be placed horizontally, vertically, or diagonally. Curved lines repeating in opposite directions create a wave (Figure 12-7).

DESIGNING WITH LINES

Hairstyles are created by the type of line or combination you choose.

1. **Single lines.** An example of this is the one-length hairstyle. These hairstyles are best worn on clients requiring the lowest maintenance when styling their hair (Figure 12-8).
2. **Parallel lines** are repeating lines in a hairstyle. They can be straight or curved. The repetition of lines creates more interest in the design. A finger wave is an example of a style using curved, parallel lines (Figure 12-9).
3. **Contrasting lines** are horizontal and vertical lines that meet at a 90-degree angle. These lines create a hard edge. Contrasting lines in a design are usually for clients able to carry off a strong look (Figure 12-10).
4. **Transitional lines** are usually curved lines that are used to blend and soften horizontal or vertical lines (Figure 12-11).

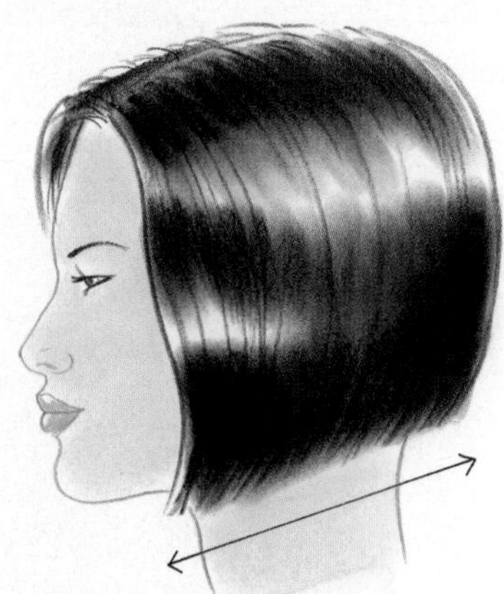

Figure 12-5 Diagonal lines in a hairstyle.

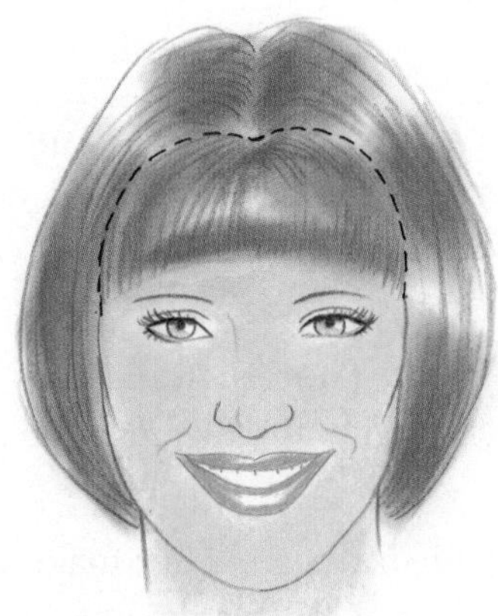

Figure 12-6 Curved lines in a hairstyle.

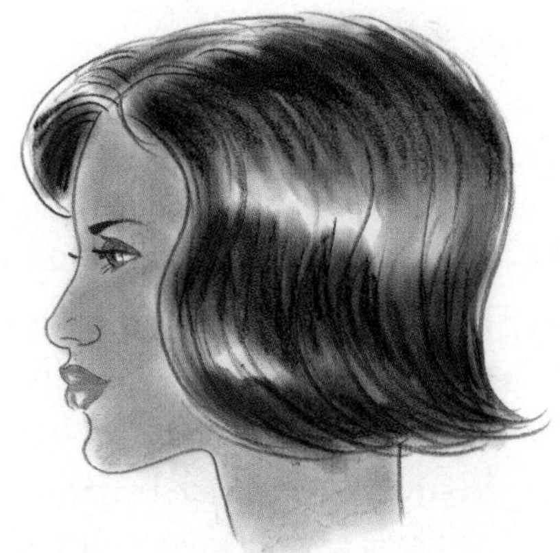

Figure 12-7 Wave.

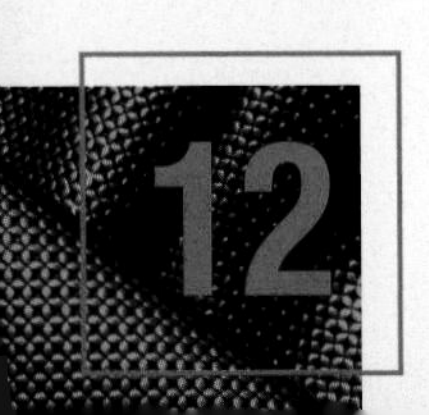

FORM

Form is the mass or general outline of a hairstyle. It is three-dimensional and has length, width, and depth. Form or mass may also be called volume. The silhouette is usually the part of the overall design that a client will respond to first. Generally, simple forms are best to use and are more pleasing to the eye. The hair form should be in proportion to the shape of the head and face, the length and width of the neck, and the shoulder line (Figure 12-12).

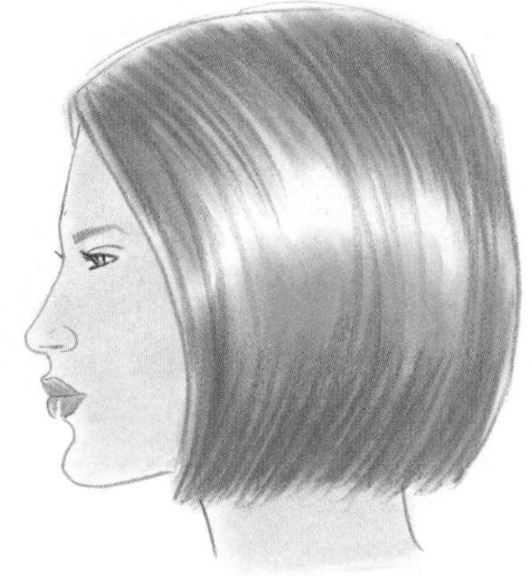

Figure 12-8 Single-line hairstyle.

SPACE

Space is the area surrounding the form or the area the hairstyle occupies. We are more aware of the (positive) form than the (negative) spaces. In hair design, with every movement the relationship of the form and space change. From every angle a hairstylist must keep in mind not only the forms being created, but the spaces as well. The space may contain curls, curves, waves, straight hair, or any combination.

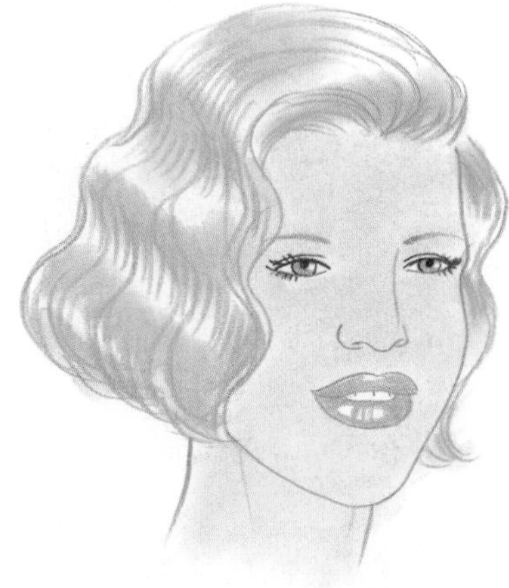

Figure 12-9 Repeating lines in a hairstyle.

DESIGN TEXTURE

Design texture refers to wave patterns that must be taken into consideration when designing a style for your client. All hair has a natural wave pattern, which is described as straight, wavy, curly, or extremely curly. For example, straight hair reflects light better than other wave patterns, so it reflects the most light when it is cut to a single length (Figure 12-13). Wavy hair can be combed into waves that create horizontal lines (Figure 12-14). Curly hair and extremely curly hair do not reflect much light and could be coarse to the touch. Curly hair creates a larger form than straight or wavy hair (Figures 12-15 and 12-16).

CREATING DESIGN TEXTURE WITH STYLING TOOLS

Texture can be created temporarily with the use of heat and/or wet styling techniques. Curling irons or hot rollers can be used to create a wave or curl.

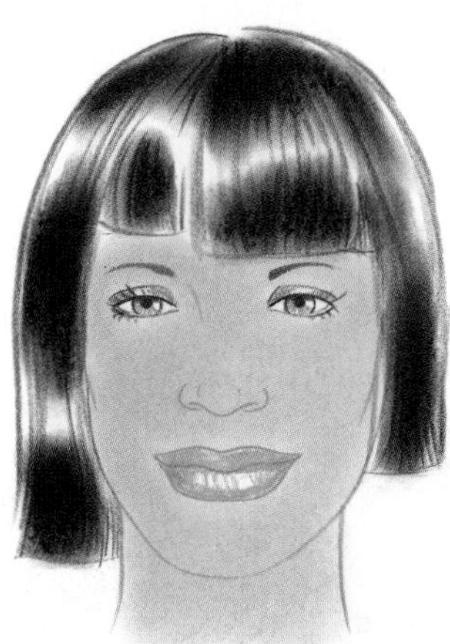

Figure 12-10 Contrasting lines.

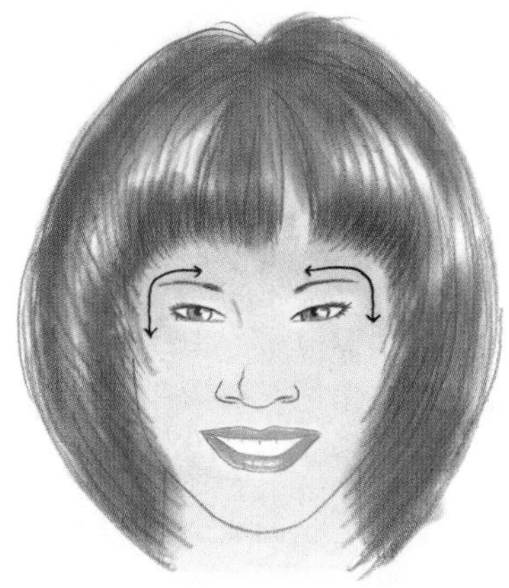

Figure 12-11 Transitional lines.

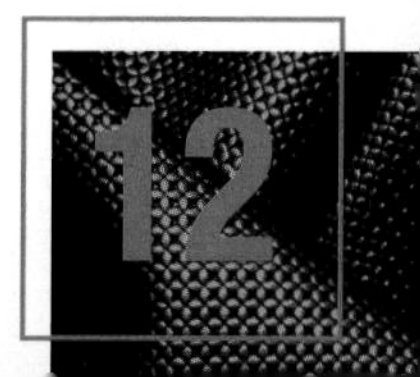

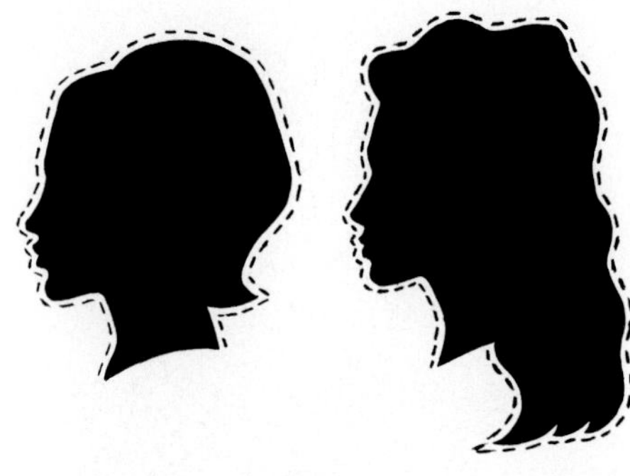

Figure 12-12 The outline of the hairstyle is the form.

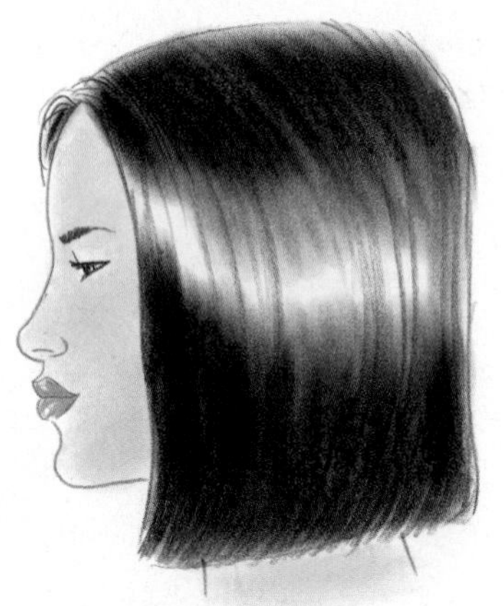

Figure 12-13 Straight hair.

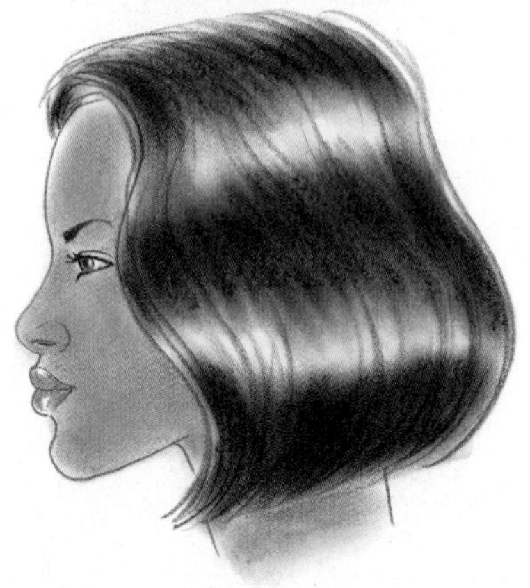

Figure 12-14 Wavy hair.

Curly hair can be straightened with a blow-dryer or flat iron (Figure 12-17).

Crimping irons are used to create interesting and unusual wave patterns like zigzags. Hair can also be wet-set with rollers or pin curls to create curls and waves. Finger waves are another way of creating temporary wave pattern changes (Figures 12-18 to 12-20). You will learn more about styling techniques in subsequent chapters.

CHANGING DESIGN TEXTURE WITH CHEMICALS

Chemical wave pattern changes are considered permanent (Figure 12-21). They last until the new growth is long enough to alter the design. Curly hair can be straightened with relaxers, while straight hair can be curled with permanent waves. These techniques are covered in detail in Chapter 18.

TIPS FOR DESIGNING WITH WAVE PATTERNS

1. When using many wave pattern combinations together you create a look that is very busy. This is fine for the client who wants to achieve a multitextured look, but may be less appropriate for a more conservative professional client.
2. Smooth wave patterns accent the face and are particularly useful when you wish to narrow a round head shape (Figure 12-22).

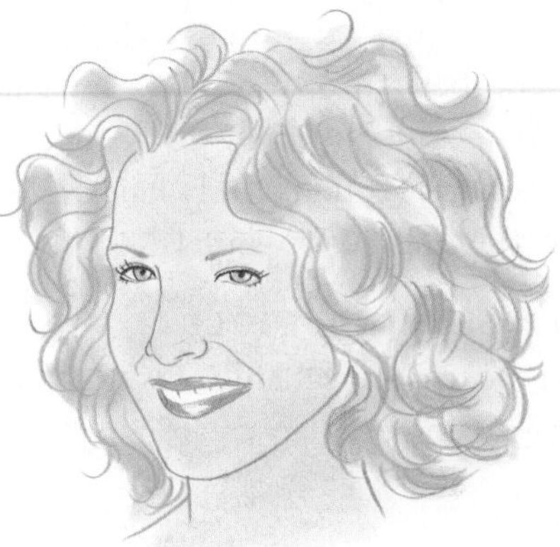

Figure 12-15 Curly hair.

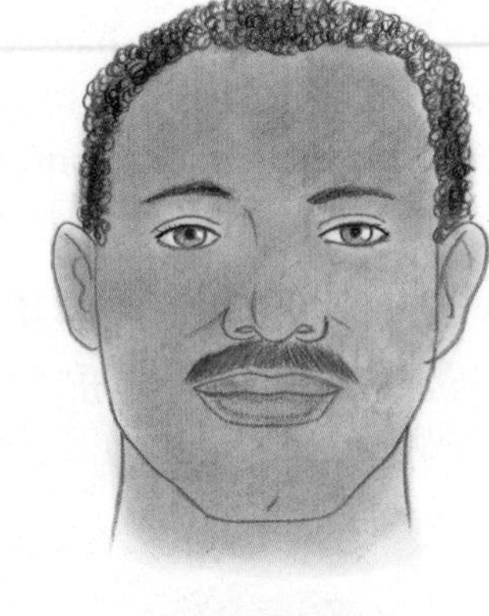

Figure 12-16 Very curly hair.

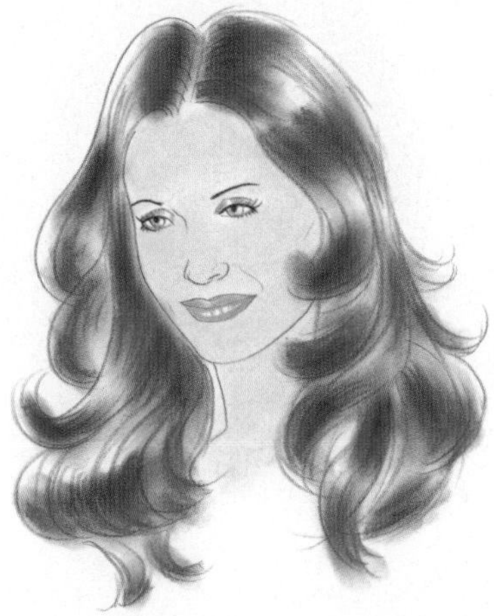

Figure 12-17 Wave patterns can be altered temporarily.

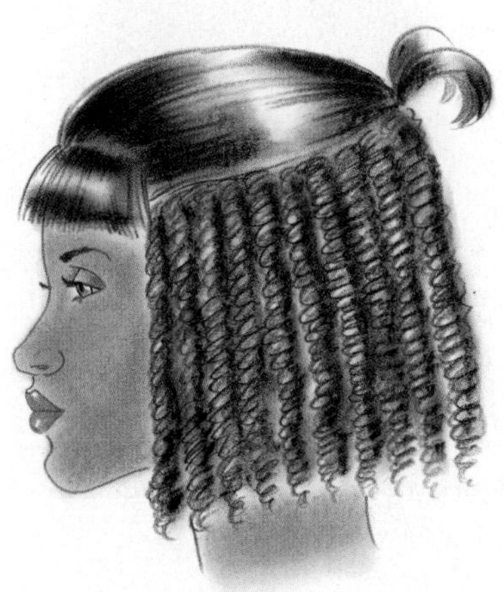

Figure 12-18 Combining wave patterns.

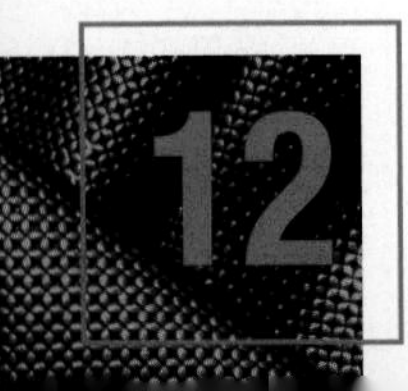

3. Curly wave patterns take attention away from the face and can be used to soften square or rectangular features (Figure 12-23).

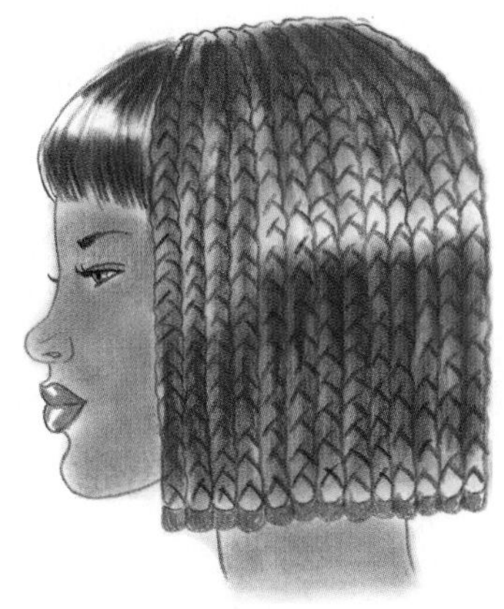

Figure 12–19 Fine braids create temporary waves.

COLOR

Color plays an important role in hair design, both visually and psychologically. It can be used to make all or part of the design appear larger or smaller. Color can help define texture and line, and tie design elements together. In Chapter 19, you will learn more about enhancing hair design using hair color as an important element.

DIMENSION WITH COLOR

Light colors and warm colors create the illusion of volume. Dark and cool colors recede or move in toward the head, creating the illusion of less volume. The illusion of dimension, or depth, is created when colors that are lighter and warmer alternate with those that are darker and cooler (Figures 12-24 and 12-25).

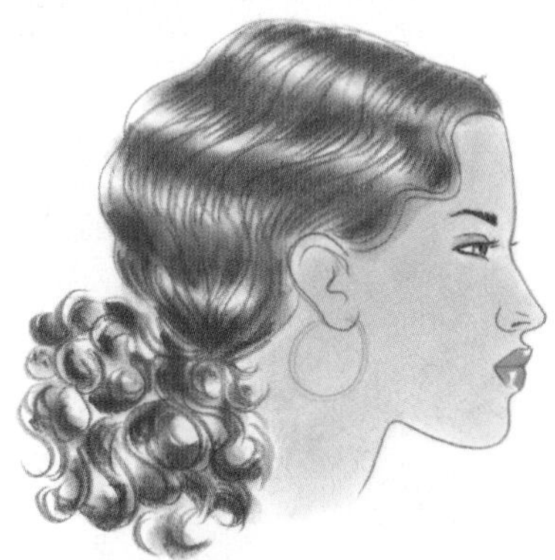

Figure 12–20 Finger waves and curls.

LINES WITH COLOR

Because the eye is drawn to the lightest color, you can use a light color to draw a line in the hairstyle in the direction you want the eye to travel. A single line of color, or a series of repeated lines, can create a bold, dramatic accent (Figure 12-26).

COLOR SELECTION

When choosing a color, be sure that the tone is compatible with the skin tone of the client. If a client has a gold tone to her skin, warm hair colors are more flattering than cool hair colors. For a more conservative or natural look when using two or more colors, choose colors with similar tones within two levels of each other. When using high-contrast colors in most salon situations, use one color sparingly. A strong contrast can create an attention-grabbing look and should only be used on clients who are trendy and can carry off a bold look (Figure 12-27).

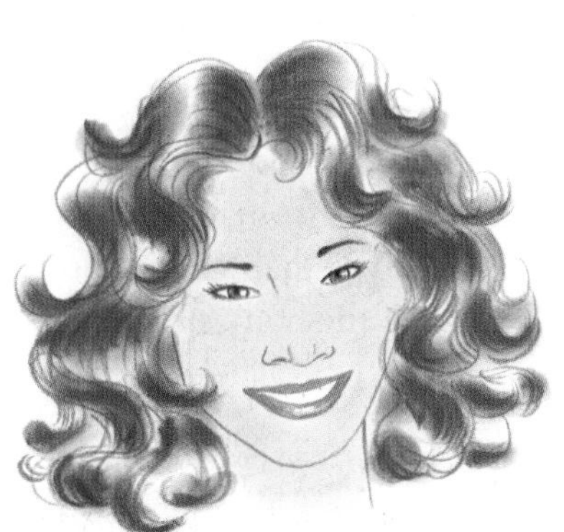

Figure 12–21 Chemically altered hairstyle.

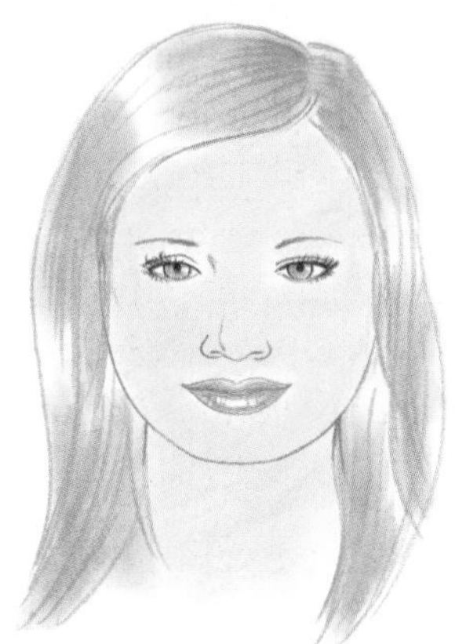

Figure 12–22 Straight wave patterns are flattering on round faces.

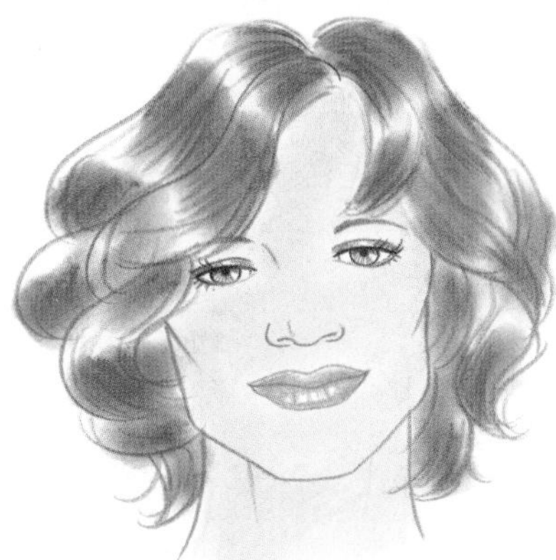

Figure 12–23 Curly wave patterns soften angular faces.

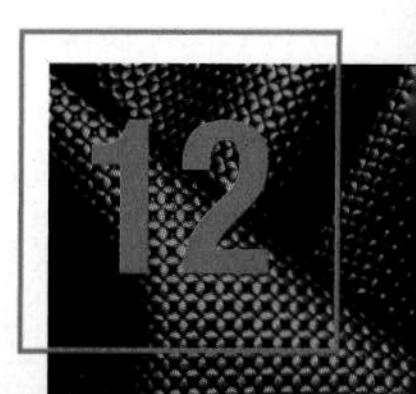

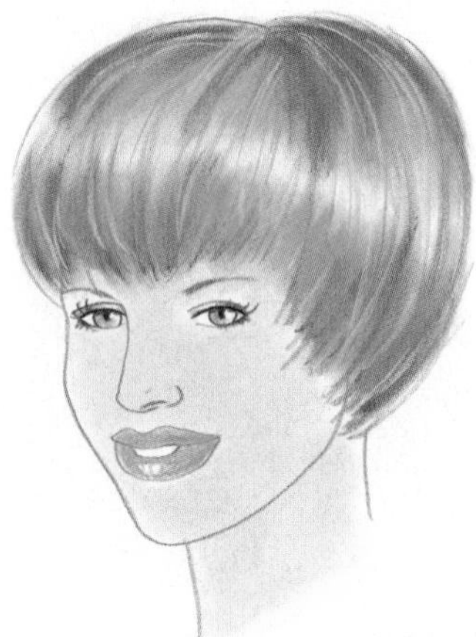

Figure 12-24 Light colors appear closer to the surface.

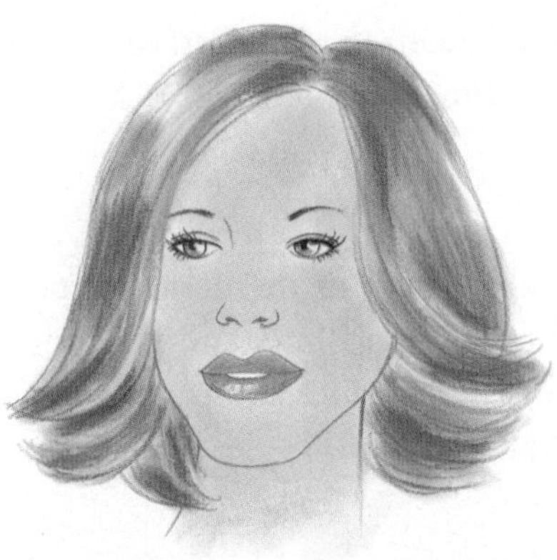

Figure 12-25 Creating dimension with color.

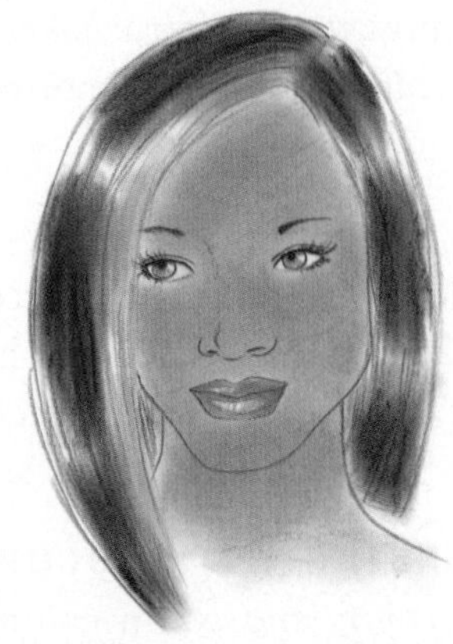

Figure 12-26 Contrasting color accents the line.

PRINCIPLES OF HAIR DESIGN

Five important principles in art and design—proportion, balance, rhythm, emphasis, and harmony—are also the basis of hair design. The better you understand these principles, the more confident you will feel about creating styles that are pleasing to the eye.

PROPORTION

Proportion is the comparative relationship of one thing to another. For example, a 60-inch TV set might be considered out of proportion or scale in a very small bedroom. A person with a very small chin and a very wide forehead might be said to have a head shape that is not in proportion. A well-chosen hairstyle could create the illusion of better proportion (Figures 12-28 and 12-29).

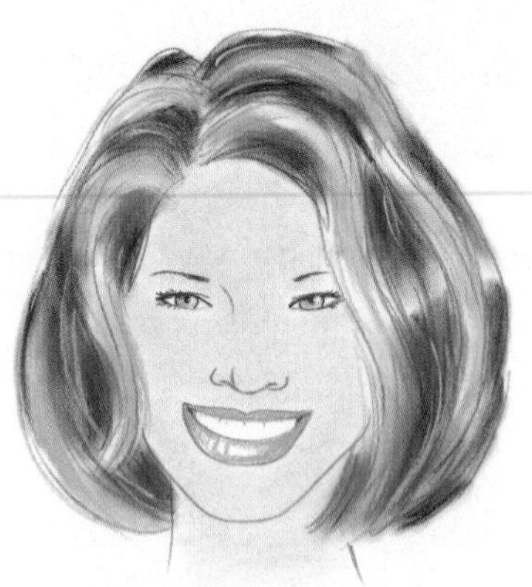

Figure 12-27 Strong color contrast.

BODY PROPORTION

It is essential when designing a hairstyle that you take into account the client's body shape and size. Challenges in body proportion become more obvious if the hair form is too small or too large. When choosing a style for a woman with large hips or broad shoulders, for instance, you would normally create a style with more volume (Figure 12-30). But the same large hair form would appear out of proportion on a petite woman (Figure 12-31). A general guide for "classic" proportion is that the hair should not be wider than the center of the shoulders, regardless of the body structure.

BALANCE

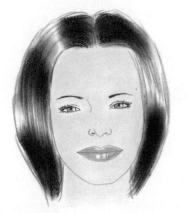

Balance is establishing equal or appropriate proportions to create symmetry. In hairstyling, it can be the proportion of height to width. Balance can be symmetrical or asymmetrical. Often when you are dissatisfied with a finished hair design, it is because the style is out of balance.

Figure 12-28 Facial features out of proportion.

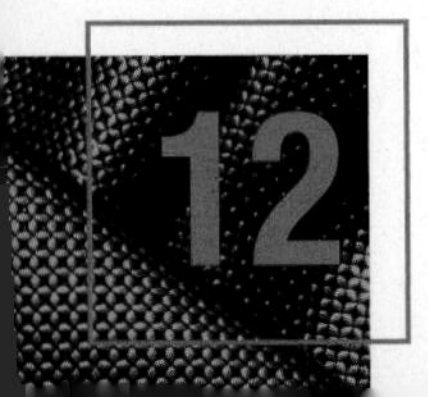

To measure symmetry, divide the face into four equal parts. The lines cross at the central axis, the reference point for judging the balance of the hair design. You can then decide if the hairstyle looks pleasing to the eye and is in correct balance (Figure 12-32).

Symmetrical balance occurs when an imaginary line drawn through the center of the face and two resulting halves form a mirror image of one another. Both sides of the hairstyle are the same distance from the center, the same length, and have the same volume when viewed from the front (Figures 12-33 to 12-35).

Asymmetrical balance has the two imaginary halves, having equal visual weight, or appear equal but the form may be positioned unevenly. Opposite sides of the hairstyle are different lengths or have a different volume. Asymmetry can be horizontal or diagonal (Figures 12-36 and 12-37).

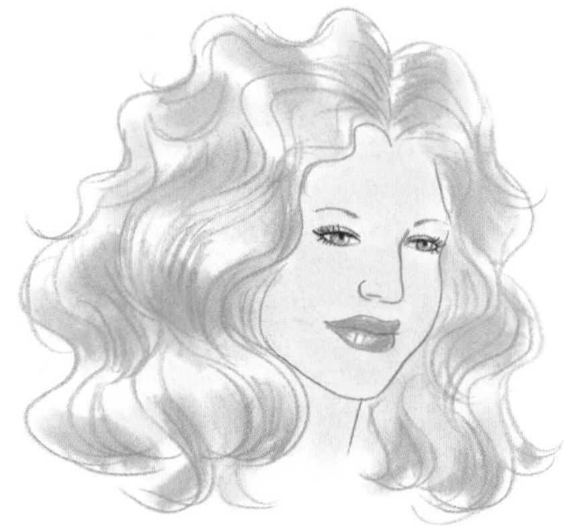

Figure 12-29 Hair out of proportion to face.

RHYTHM

Rhythm is a regular pulsation or recurrent pattern of movement in a design. In music or dance it can be fast or slow. A fast rhythm moves quickly in hair design; tight curls are an example. A slow rhythm can be seen in larger shapings or long waves (Figures 12-38 and 12-39).

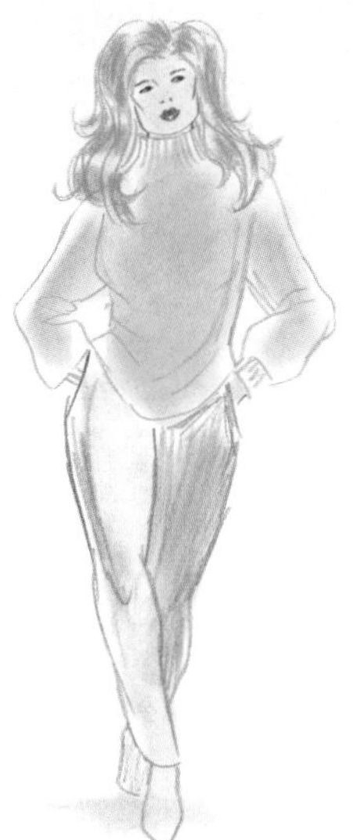

Figure 12-30 A large hairstyle balances a large body structure.

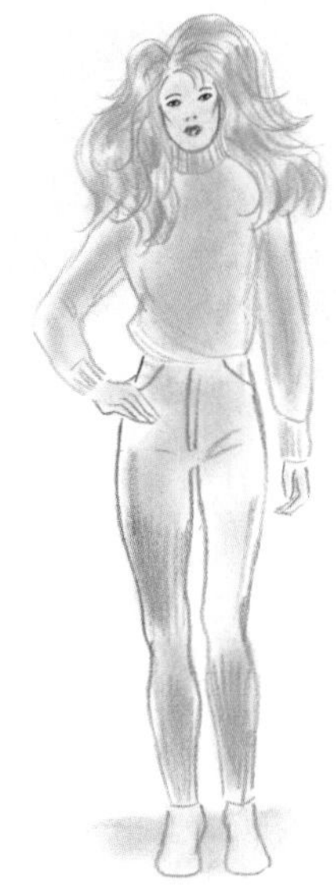

Figure 12-31 A large hairstyle makes a petite woman look smaller.

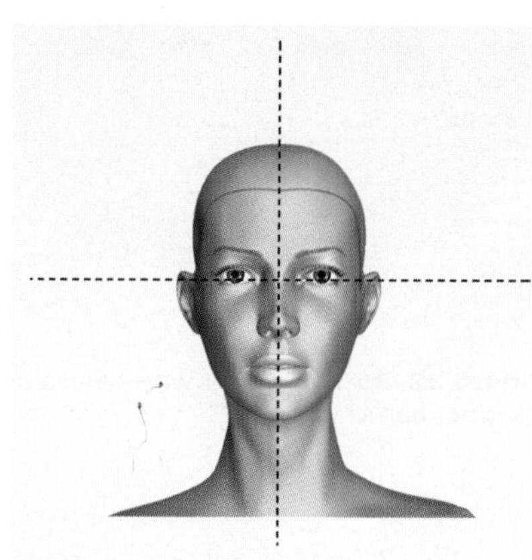

Figure 12-32 Measuring symmetry of the head.

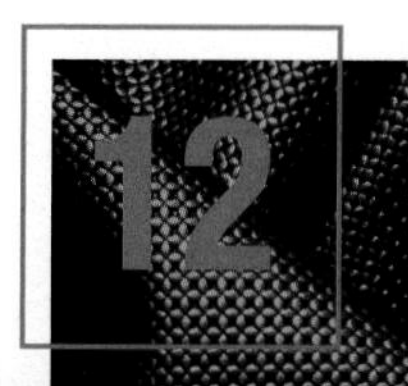

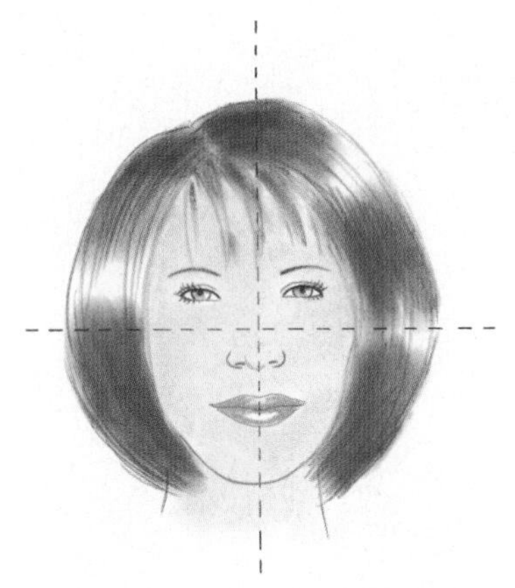

Figure 12-33 Both sides equidistant from center.

EMPHASIS

The **emphasis or focus** in a design is what draws the eye first before traveling to the rest of the design. A hairstyle may be well balanced, with good rhythm and harmony, and yet still be boring. Create interest with an area of focus or emphasis by using the following:

- Wave patterns (Figure 12-40)
- Color (Figure 12-41)
- Change in form (Figure 12-42)
- Ornamentation (Figure 12-43)

Choose an area of the head or face that you want to emphasize. Keep the design simple so that it is easy for the eye to follow from the point of emphasis through to the rest of the style. You can have multiple points of emphasis as long as they are decreasing in size and importance, and by not using too many. Remember, less is more.

HARMONY

Harmony is the creation of unity in a design and is the most important of the art principles. Harmony holds all the elements of the design together. When a hairstyle is harmonious, it has a form with interesting

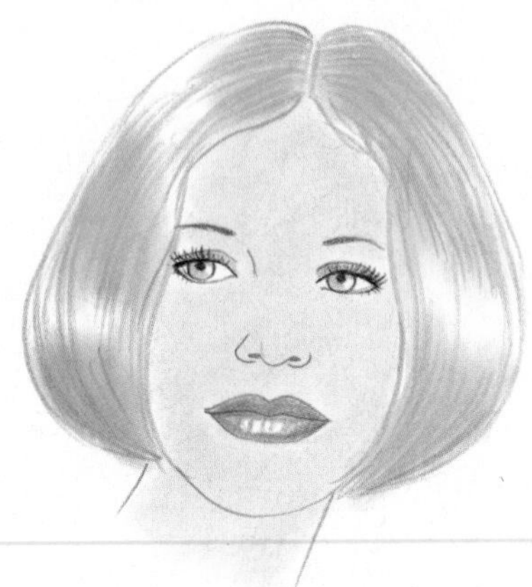

Figure 12-34 Perfect symmetry.

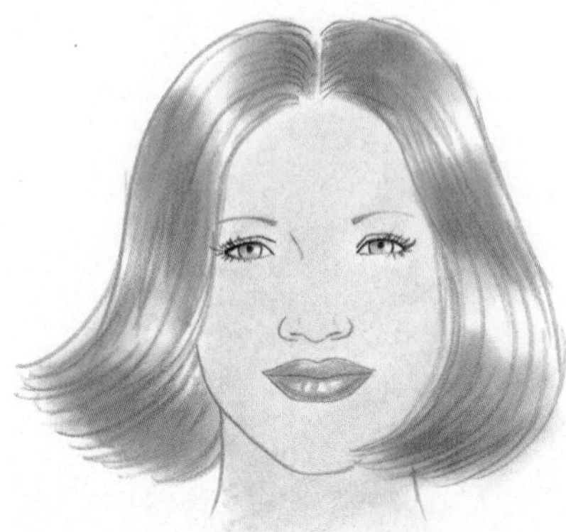

Figure 12-35 Symmetry with different shapes, same volume.

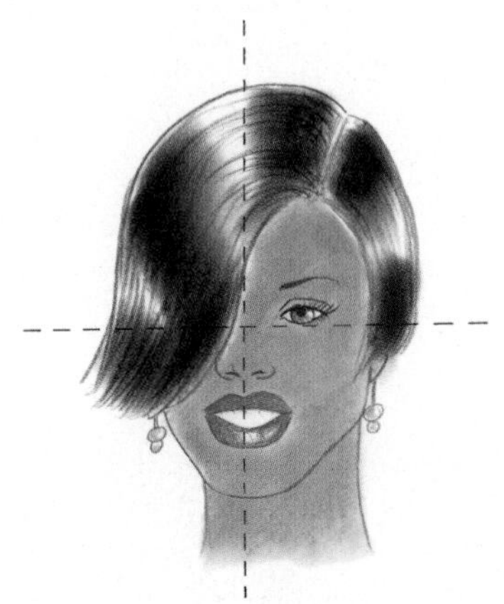

Figure 12-36 Horizontal asymmetry.

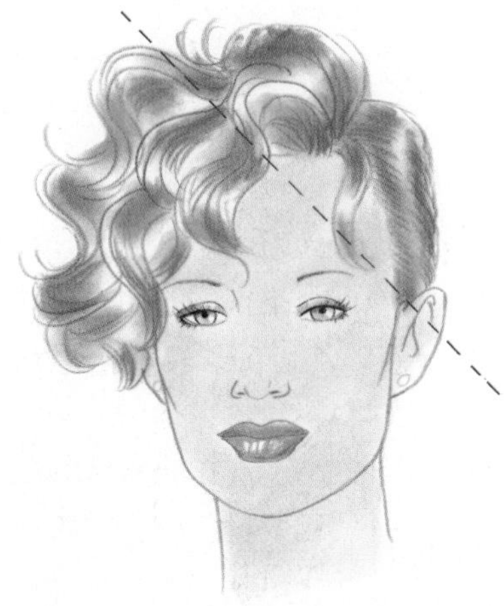

Figure 12-37 Diagonal asymmetry.

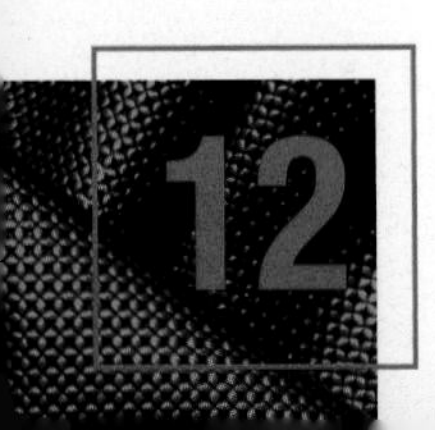

lines, a pleasing color or combination of colors and textures, and a balance and rhythm that together strengthen the design. A harmonious design is never too busy, and is in proportion to the client's facial and body structure, and includes an area of emphasis from which the eyes move to the rest of the style.

The principles of design may be used in modern hairstyling and makeup to guide you as you decide how best to achieve a beautiful appearance for your client. The best results are obtained when each of your client's facial features are properly analyzed for their strengths and weaknesses. Your job is to accentuate a client's best features and to downplay features that do not add to the person's appearance. Every hairstyle you create for every client should be properly proportioned to body type and correctly balanced to the person's head and facial features, and it should attractively frame their face. An artistic and suitable hairstyle will take into account physical characteristics of the client such as the following:

- Shape of the head, front view (face shape), profile, and back view
- Features (perfect as well as imperfect features)
- Body posture

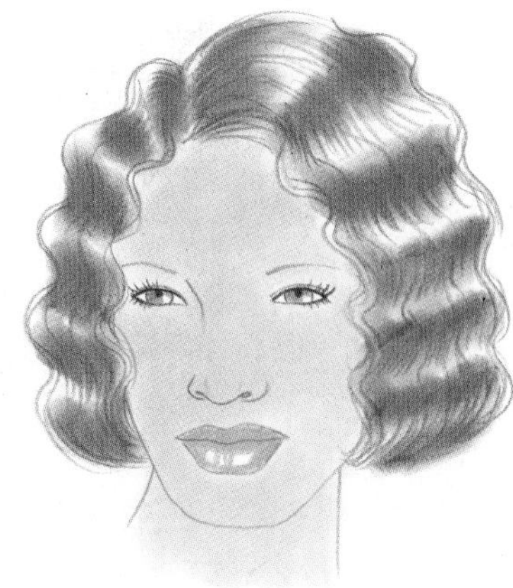

Figure 12-38 Fast rhythm.

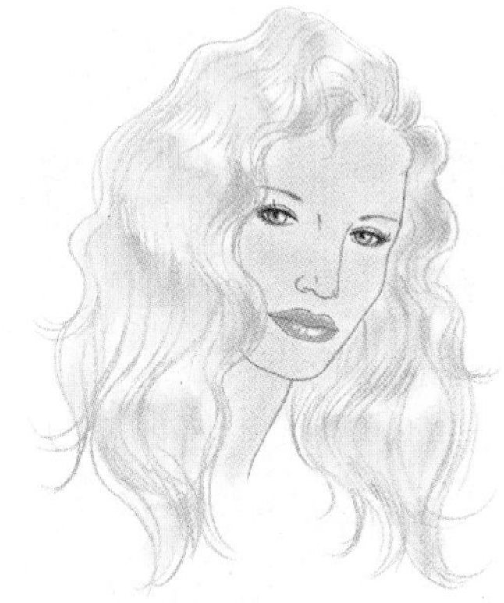

Figure 12-39 Slow rhythm.

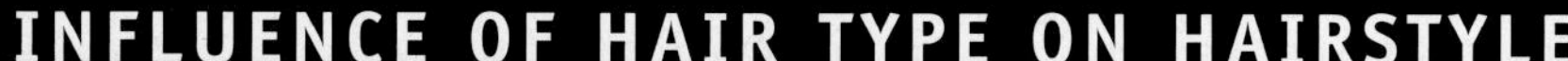

INFLUENCE OF HAIR TYPE ON HAIRSTYLE

Your client's hair type is a major consideration in the selection of a hairstyle. Hair type is categorized by two defining characteristics: wave patterns and hair texture.

All hair has natural wave patterns that must be taken into consideration when designing a style for your client. These wave patterns are straight, wavy, curly, and extremely curly. Hair texture and density are also important factors in choosing a style. The basic hair textures are fine, medium, and coarse. Hair density or hair per square inch ranges from thin to thicker.

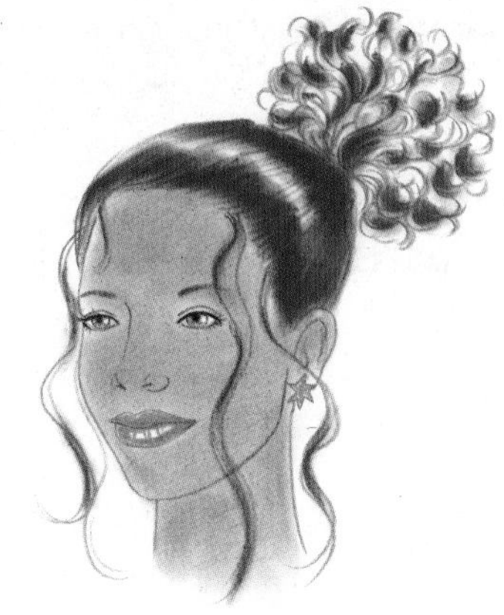

Figure 12-40 Creating emphasis with various wave patterns.

Keep in mind the following guidelines for different types of hair:

- *Fine, straight hair.* This combination usually hugs the head shape due to the fact that there is no body or volume. The silhouette is small and narrow. If this is not appropriate for the client based on the characteristics of her features or her body structure, think about what styling aids or chemical services can be recommended to achieve the most flattering style. Left natural, the hair may not offer enough support for options in styling.
- *Straight, medium hair.* This type of hair offers more versatility in styling. This hair type responds well to blow-drying with various sized brushes and has a good amount of movement. It will respond well to rollers and thermal styling.
- *Straight, coarse hair.* This hair is hard to curl and carries more volume than the previous two types. It casts a slightly wider silhouette and

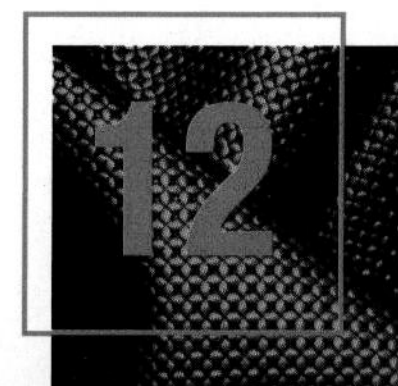

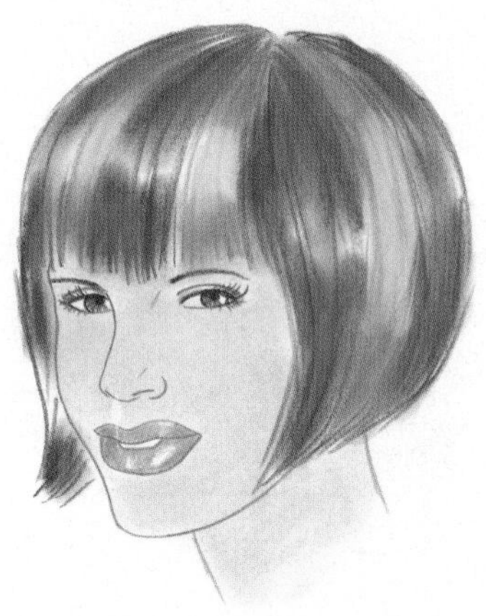

Figure 12-41 Creating emphasis with color.

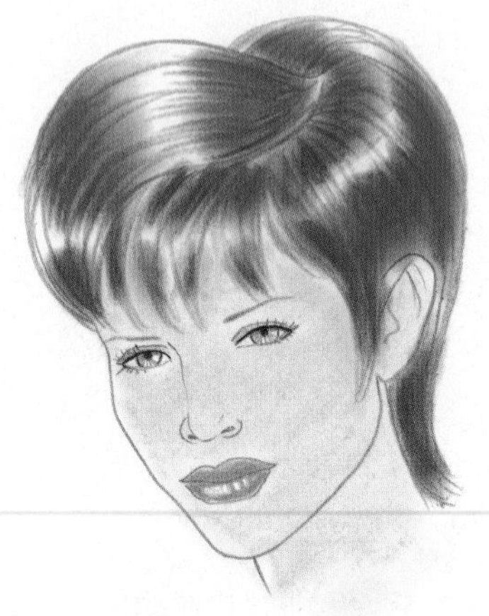

Figure 12-42 Creating emphasis with form changes.

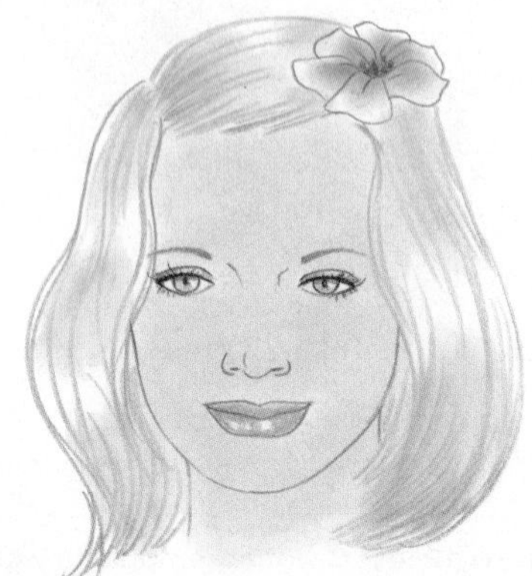

Figure 12-43 Ornament as focal point.

responds well to thermal styling. Flat brushes are better for this hair type because of a wide diameter in the hair shaft. Blow-drying with round brushes can make this hair type look too "poofy." Chemical services may also take a little longer to process.

- *Wavy, fine hair.* This type of hair can appear fuller with the appropriate haircut and style. With layering, it will look fuller, and it responds well to blow-drying and chemical services. This hair can be fragile so be careful not to overdo any of these services. If the desired result is straight hair, it will straighten easily by blow-drying, but you may sacrifice volume. If diffused, the hair will have a fuller appearance.
- *Wavy, medium hair.* This type of hair offers the most versatility in styling. This hair can be diffused to look curly, or be easily straightened by blow-drying.
- *Wavy, coarse hair.* This silhouette could get very wide, and the hair could appear unruly if it is not shaped properly. Blow-drying is often much easier for the stylist than for the client. If the client is not good at working with her own hair, try to work out a flattering shape that is easy to maintain. This client often feels that her hair leaves her trapped between being too wavy to be left in a straight style, but not curly enough for a curly style. A soft perm could easily bring her to a wash-and-wear curly style or another chemical service such as a mild relaxer may work very well if the client prefers a straighter look.
- *Curly, fine hair.* This hair when left long often separates revealing the client's scalp unless the hair is thick in density. It responds well to mild relaxers and to color services. Blow-drying straight may be difficult unless the hair is cut into short layers, and if the client is not going to be in a humid environment.
- *Curly, medium hair.* This type creates a wide silhouette, and when left natural gives a soft romantic look. The wide silhouette should be in proportion to the client's body shape, and not overwhelm it. When shaping the hair, keep in mind where the weight line of the haircut will fall. This hair responds well to relaxers and color.
- *Curly, coarse hair.* This hair needs heavy styling products to weight it down. It is easy for this type of hair to overwhelm any client. Keep in mind while cutting this combination that the hair will shrink considerably when dry, making it appear much shorter.
- *Very curly, fine hair.* The most flattering shape for the client must be determined first, and then second—for ease of styling—this hair type is generally best left short. If the hair is left long, the silhouette will be wide and extremely voluminous. Chemical services and hair pressing (temporary straightening) take well, but be careful because the hair may be fragile.
- *Extremely curly, medium hair.* This silhouette can get very wide, as the hair can look wider rather than longer as it grows. Chemical relaxers work very well to make the shape narrower, and hair pressing is also a good option. Thermal styling could follow the pressing. If the hair is

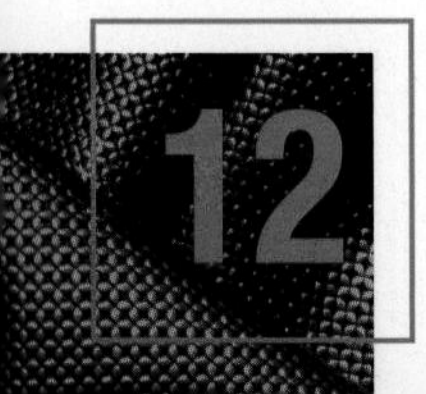

left in its natural state, cropping it close to the head in a flattering shape is great for ease of styling and low maintenance.

- *Extremely curly, coarse hair.* This silhouette will be extremely wide. Chemical relaxing is often recommended to make it easier to style with other thermal services. This hair type is often too thick to tie back in a ponytail, so if the client does not want any chemical services, and wants easy care, suggest short, cropped layers to make the silhouette narrower.

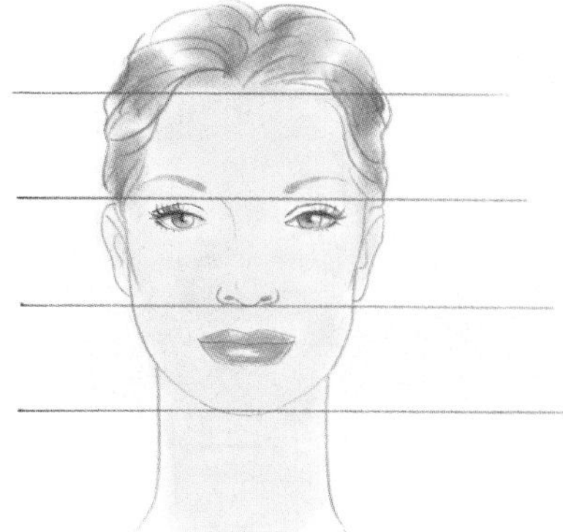

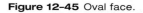

Figure 12-44 Ideal facial proportions.

CREATING HARMONY BETWEEN HAIRSTYLE AND FACIAL STRUCTURE

A client's facial shape is determined by the position and prominence of the facial bones. A good way to determine facial shape is to pull all the client's hair completely off the face using a towel or ponytail, so that you can better observe just the client's face. There are seven basic facial shapes: oval, round, square, triangle (pear shaped), oblong, diamond, and inverted triangle (heart shaped). To recognize each facial shape and to be able to style the hair in the most flattering design with that facial shape in mind, you should be acquainted with the characteristics of each. Remember, when designing a style for your client's facial type, you generally are trying to create the illusion of an oval-shaped face.

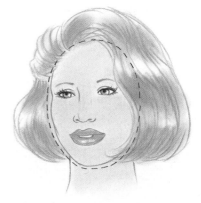

To determine a facial shape divide the face into three zones: forehead to eyebrow, eyebrows to end of nose, and end of nose to bottom of chin.

Figure 12-45 Oval face.

OVAL FACIAL TYPE

The contour and proportions of the oval face shape form the basis and ideals for modifying all other facial types (Figure 12-44).

Facial contour: The oval face is about one-and-a-half times longer than its width across the brow. The forehead is slightly wider than the chin (Figure 12-45). A person with an oval face can wear any hairstyle unless there are other considerations, such as eyeglasses, length and shape of nose, or profile (see the section on special considerations).

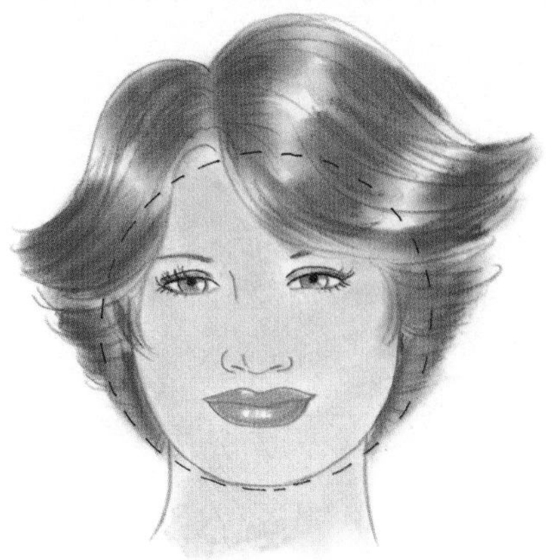

Figure 12-46 Round face.

ROUND FACIAL TYPE

Facial contour: Round hairline and round chin line; wide face.

Aim: To create the illusion of length to the face, this will make the face appear slimmer.

Styling choice: A hairstyle that has height or volume on top and closeness or no volume at the sides (Figure 12-46).

SQUARE FACIAL TYPE

Facial contour: Wide at the temples, narrow at the middle third of the face, and squared off at the jaw.

Aim: To offset or round out the square features.

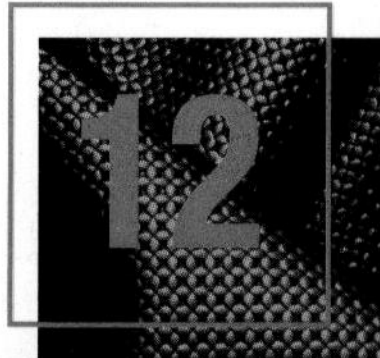

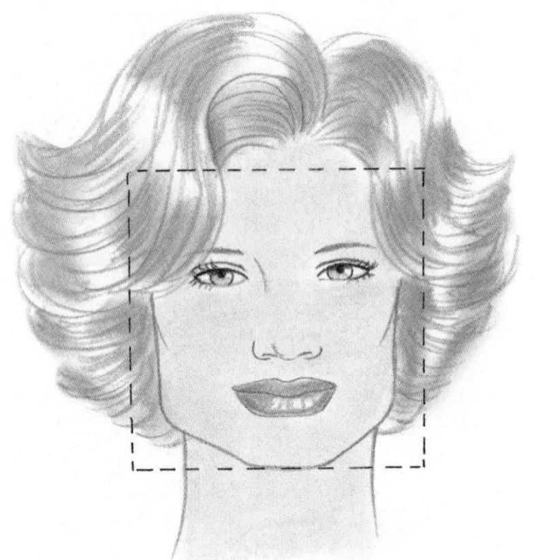

Figure 12-47 Square face.

Styling choice: Soften the hair around the temples and jaw, by bringing the shape or silhouette close to the head form. Create volume around the areas between the temples and jaw, by adding width around the ear area, for example (Figure 12-47).

TRIANGULAR (PEAR-SHAPED) FACIAL TYPE

Facial contour: Narrow forehead, wide jaw, and chin line.

Aim: To create the illusion of width in the forehead.

Styling choice: A hairstyle that has volume at the temples and some height at the top. You can disguise the narrowness of the forehead with a soft bang or fringe (Figure 12-48).

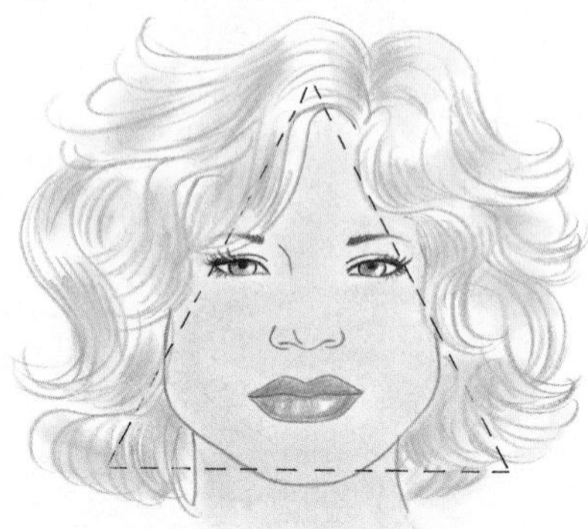

Figure 12-48 Triangular face.

OBLONG FACIAL TYPE

Facial contour: Long, narrow face with hollow cheeks.

Aim: To make the face appear shorter and wider.

Styling choice: Keep the hair fairly close to the top of the head. Add volume on the sides to create the illusion of width. The hair should not be too long, as this would elongate the oblong shape of the face. Chin length is the most effective (Figure 12-49).

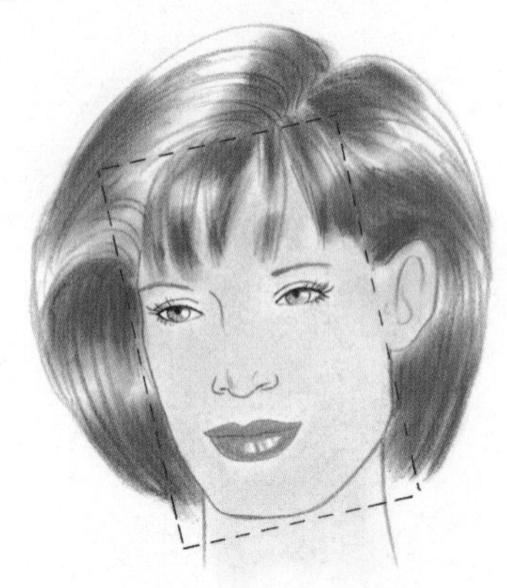

Figure 12-49 Oblong face.

DIAMOND FACIAL TYPE

Facial contour: Narrow forehead, extreme width through the cheekbones, and narrow chin.

Aim: To reduce the width across the cheekbone line.

Styling choice: Increasing the fullness across the jaw line and forehead while keeping the hair close to the head at the cheekbone line helps create an oval appearance. Avoid hairstyles that lift away from the cheeks or move back from the hairline on the sides near the ear area (Figure 12-50).

INVERTED TRIANGLE (HEART-SHAPED) FACIAL TYPE

Facial contour: Wide forehead and narrow chin line.

Aim: To decrease the width of the forehead and increase the width in the lower part of the face.

Styling choice: Style the hair close to the head with no volume. A bang or fringe is recommended. Gradually increase the width of the silhouette as you style the middle third of the shape in the cheekbone area and near the ears, and keep the silhouette at its widest at the jaw and neck area (Figure 12-51).

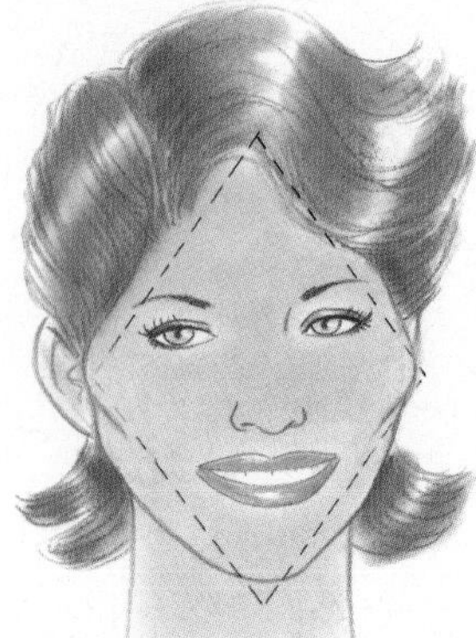

Figure 12-50 Diamond face.

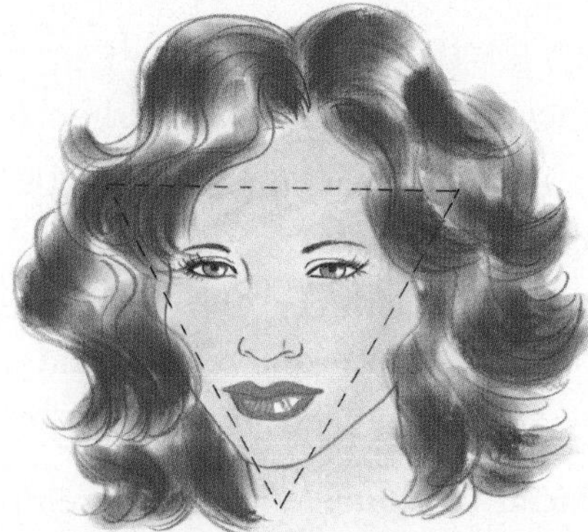

Figure 12-51 Inverted triangle-shaped face (heart-shaped face).

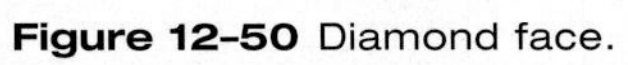

ACTIVITY

Bring to class pictures of models and celebrities from magazines, and look at them with your classmates to analyze facial shapes. What styles work or do not work? What hairstyle would you suggest if they were your clients? Why?

PROFILES

The **profile** is the outline of the face, head, or figure seen in a side view. There are three basic profiles: straight, convex, and concave.

The **straight** profile is considered the ideal. It is neither **convex** (curving outward) nor **concave** (curving inward), although even a straight profile has a very slight curvature. Generally, all hairstyles are flattering to the straight or ideal profile (Figure 12-52).

The **convex** profile has a receding forehead and chin. It calls for an arrangement of curls or bangs over the forehead. Keep the style close to the head at the nape and move hair forward in the chin area (Figures 12-53 and 12-54).

The **concave** profile has a prominent forehead and chin, with other features receded inward. It should be accommodated by softly styling the hair at the nape with an upward movement. Do not build hair onto the forehead (Figures 12-55 and 12-56).

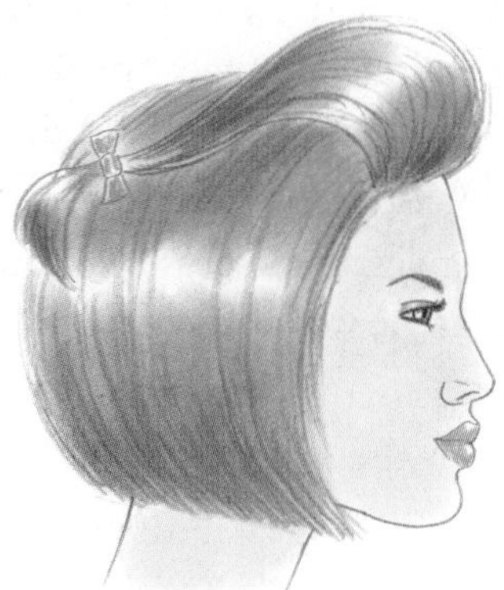

Figure 12-52 Straight profile.

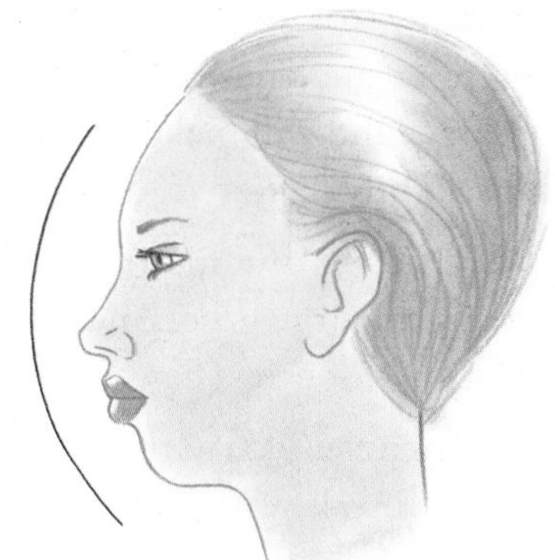

Figure 12-53 Convex profile.

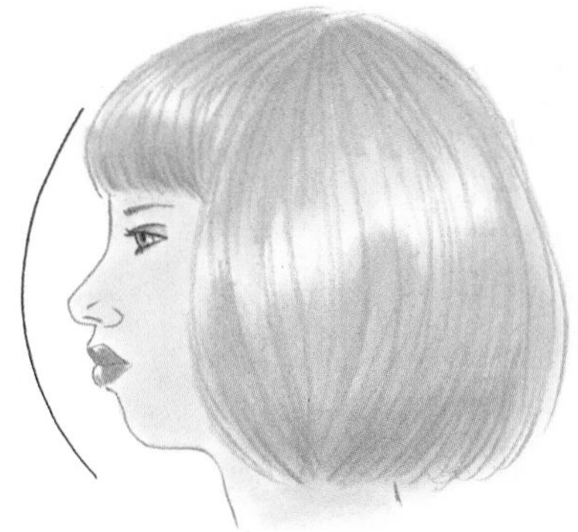

Figure 12-54 Styling for convex profile.

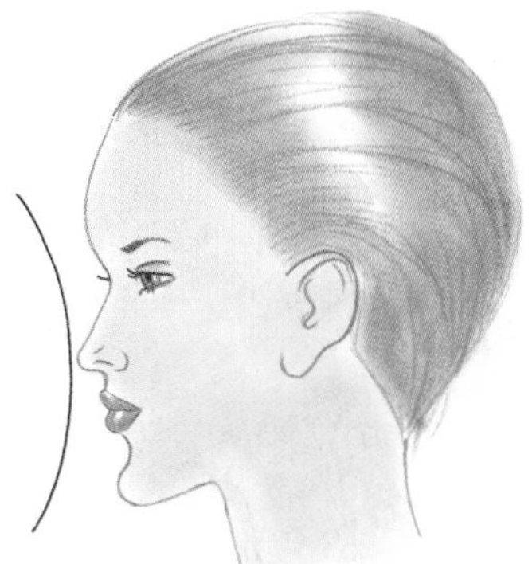

Figure 12-55 Concave profile.

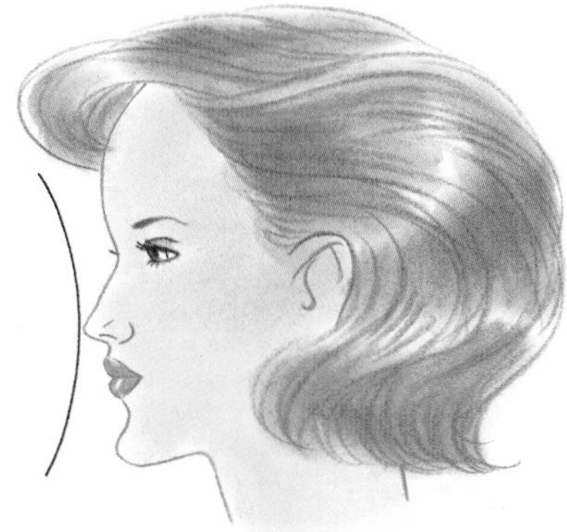

Figure 12-56 Styling for concave profile.

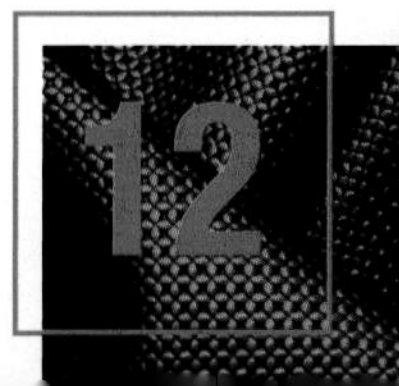

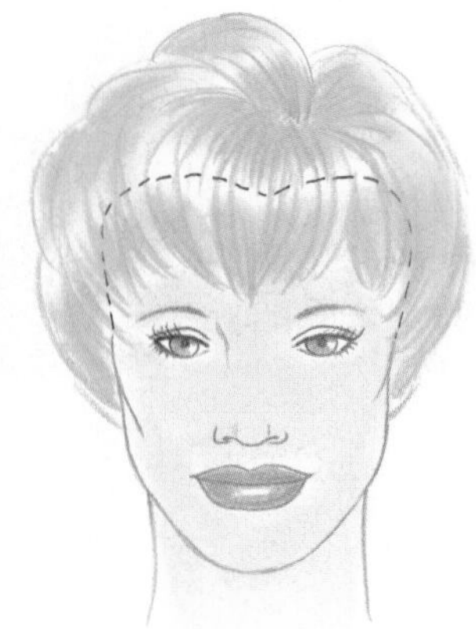

Figure 12-57 Wide forehead.

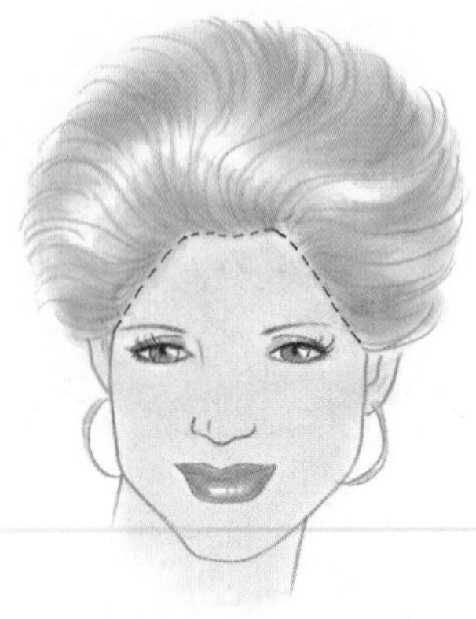

Figure 12-58 Narrow forehead.

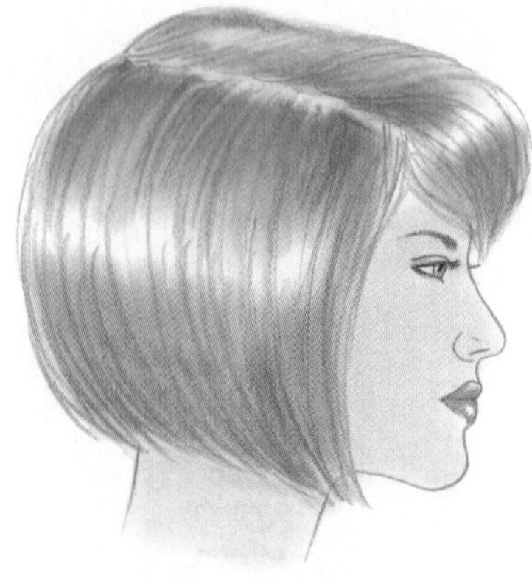

Figure 12-59 Receding forehead.

SPECIAL CONSIDERATIONS

An understanding of facial features and proportions will make it easier for you to analyze each client's face. You can then apply the design principles you have learned to help balance facial structural challenges. Dividing the face into three sections is one way to do this analysis (see Figure 12-32).

TOP THIRD OF THE FACE

Wide forehead: Direct hair forward over the sides of the forehead (Figure 12-57).

Narrow forehead: Direct hair away from the face at the forehead. Lighter highlights may be used at the temples to create the illusion of width (Figure 12-58).

Receding forehead: Direct the bangs over the forehead with an outwardly directed volume (Figure 12-59).

Large forehead: Use bangs with little or no volume to cover the forehead (Figure 12-60).

MIDDLE THIRD OF THE FACE

Close-set eyes: Usually found on long, narrow faces. Direct hair back and away from the face at the temples. A side movement from a diagonal back part with some height is advisable. A slight lightening of the hair at the corner of the eyes will give the illusion of width (Figure 12-61).

Wide-set eyes: Usually found on round or square faces. Use a higher half bang to create length in the face. This will give the face the illusion of being larger and will make the eyes appear more proportional. The hair should be slightly darker at the sides than the top (Figure 12-62).

Crooked nose: Asymmetrical, off-center styles are best, as they attract the eye away from the nose. An asymmetrical style will accentuate the fact that the face is not even (Figure 12-63).

Wide, flat nose: Draw the hair away from the face and use a center part to help elongate and narrow the nose (Figure 12-64).

Long, narrow nose: Stay away from styles that are tapered close to the head on the sides, and have height on top. Middle parts or too much hair

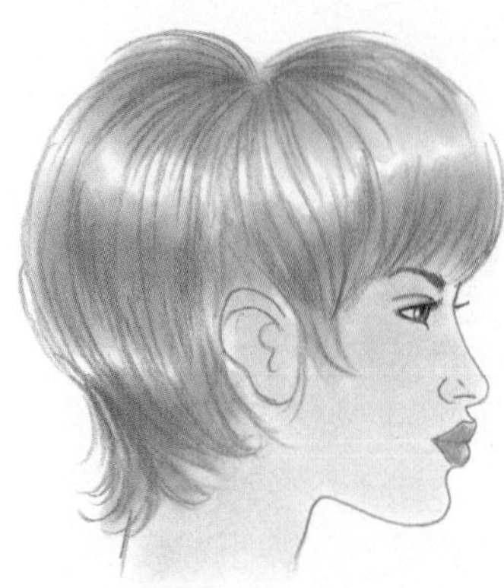

Figure 12-60 Large forehead.

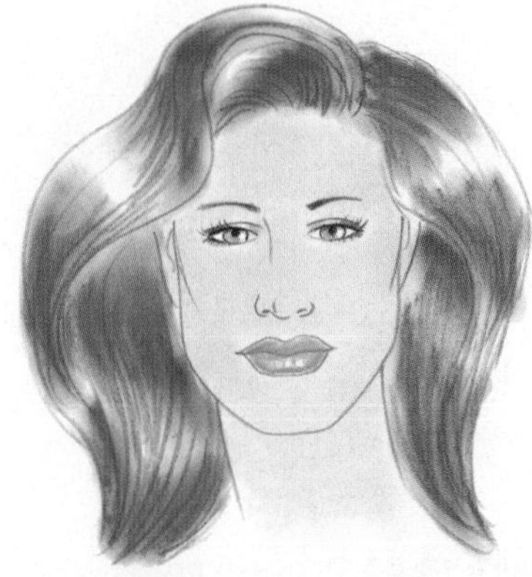

Figure 12-61 Close-set eyes.

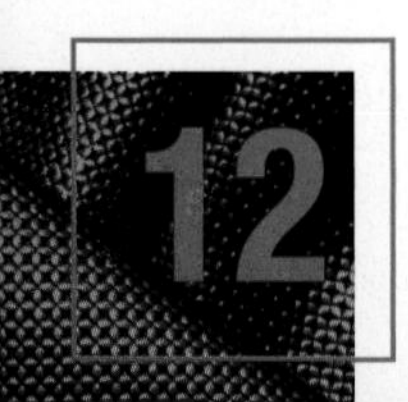

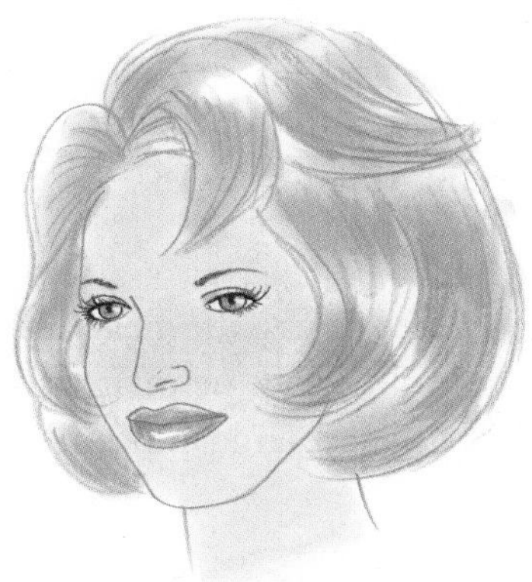

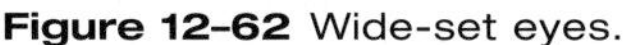

Figure 12-62 Wide-set eyes.

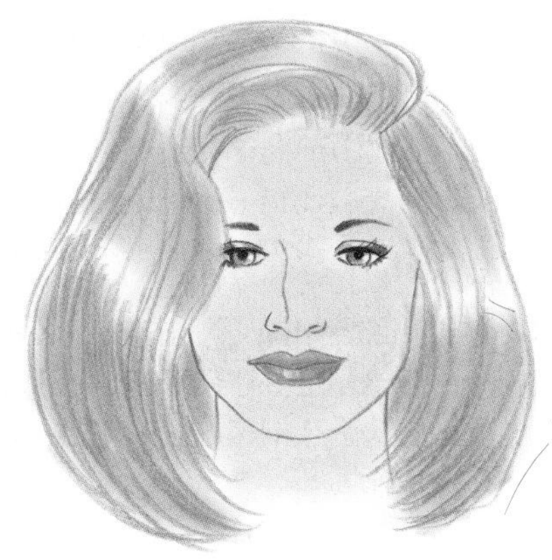

Figure 12-63 Crooked nose.

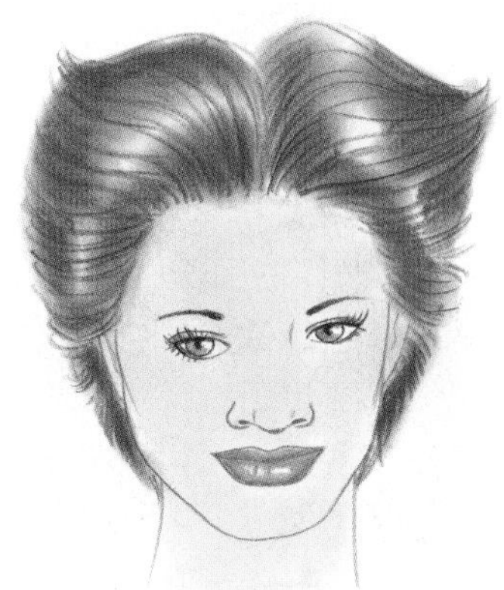

Figure 12-64 Wide nose.

directed toward the face are also poor choices. This will only accentuate any long, narrow features on the face. Instead, select a style where the hair moves away from the face, creating the illusion of wider facial features (Figure 12-65).

Small nose: A small nose often gives a child-like look; therefore it is best to design an age-appropriate hairstyle that would not be associated with children. Hair should be swept off the face, creating a line from nose to ear. The top hair should be moved off the forehead to give the illusion of length to the nose (Figure 12-66).

Prominent nose: To draw attention away from the nose, bring hair forward at the forehead with softness around the face (Figure 12-67).

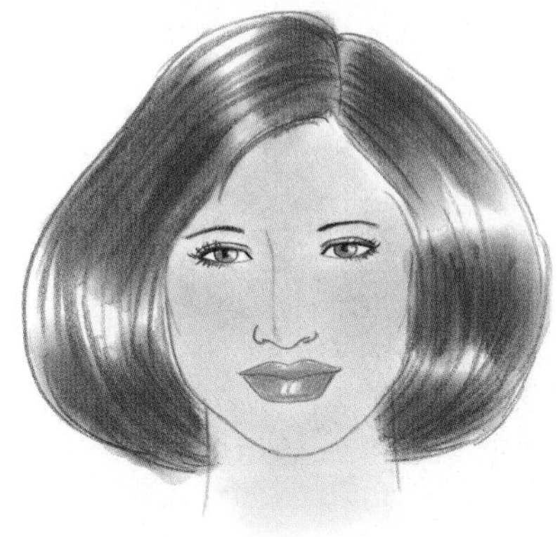

Figure 12-65 Long, narrow, nose.

LOWER THIRD OF THE FACE

Round jaw: Use straight lines at the jaw line (Figure 12-68).

Square jaw: Use curved lines at the jaw line (Figure 12-69).

Long jaw: Hair should be full and fall below the jaw to direct attention away from it (Figure 12-70).

Receding chin: Hair should be directed forward in the chin area (Figure 12-71).

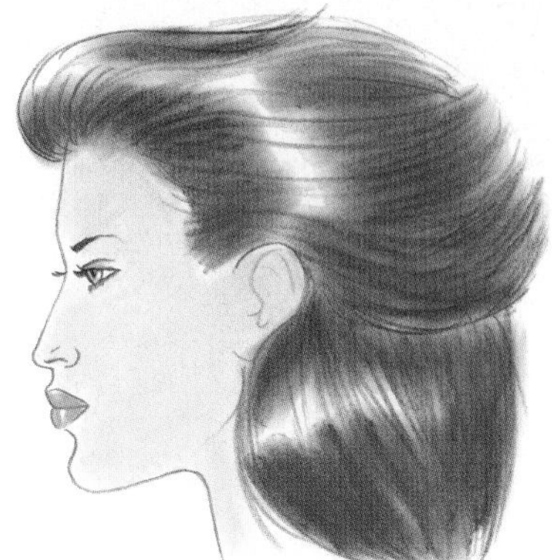

Figure 12-66 Small nose.

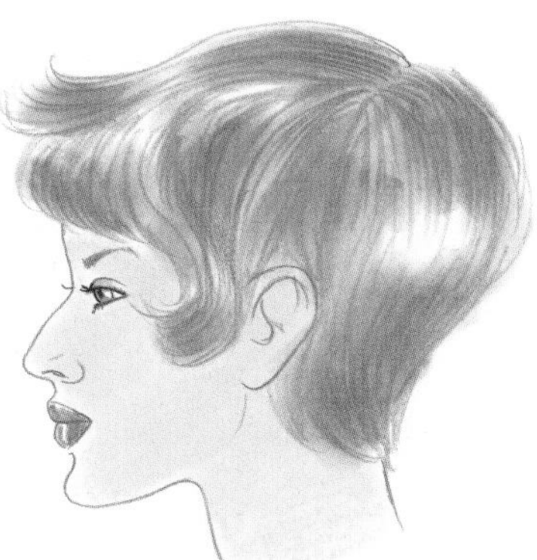

Figure 12-67 Prominent nose.

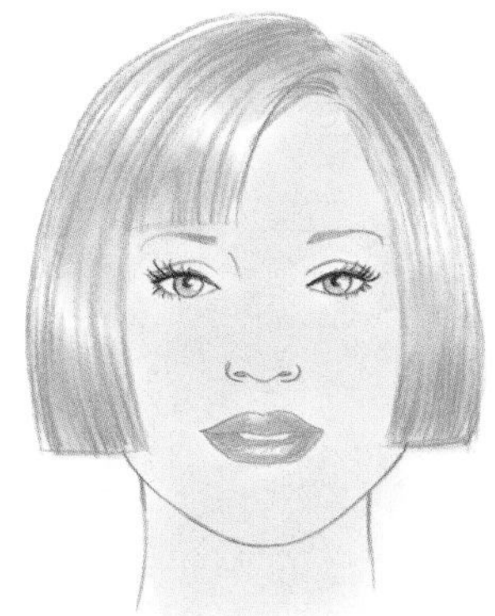

Figure 12-68 Round jaw.

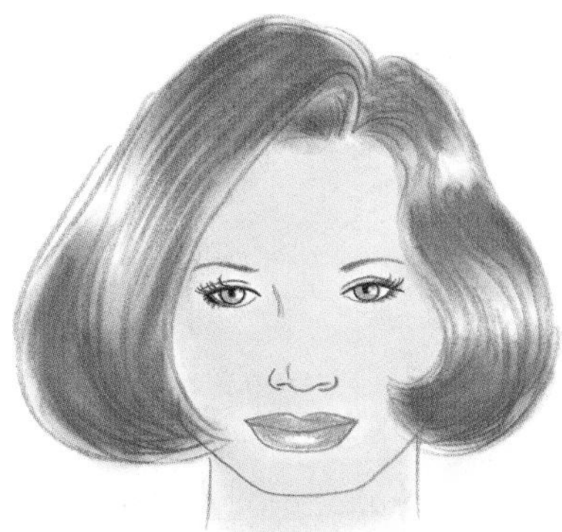

Figure 12-69 Square jaw.

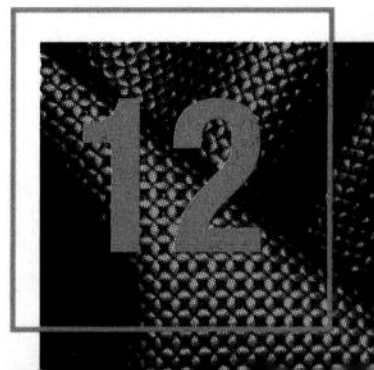

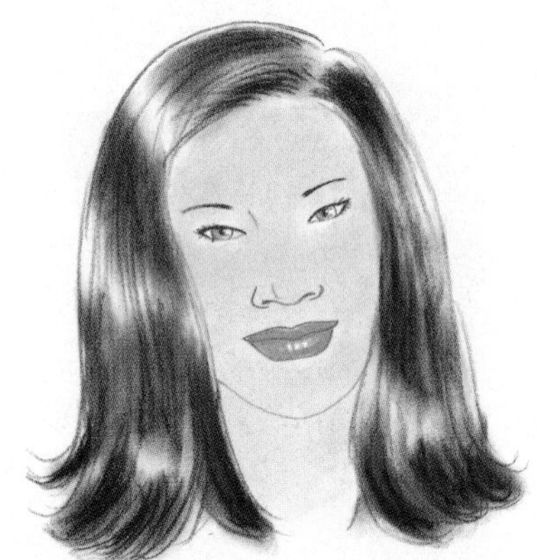

Figure 12-70 Long jaw.

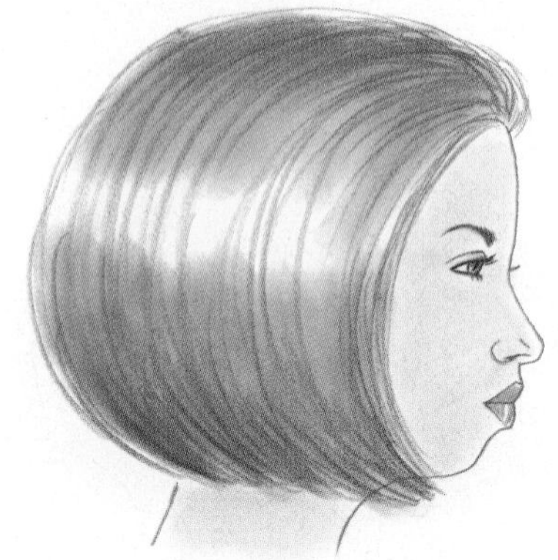

Figure 12-71 Receding chin.

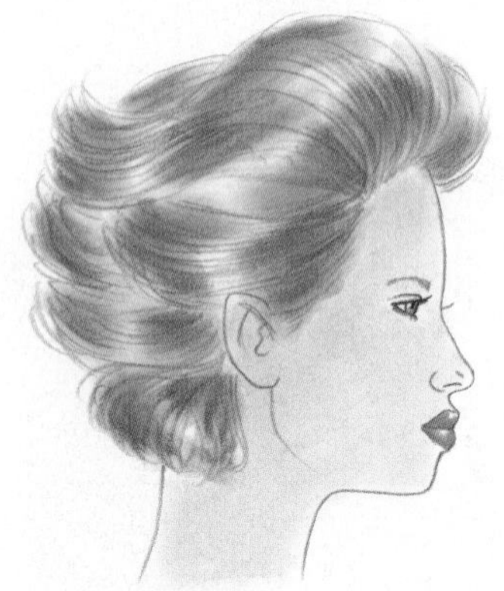

Figure 12-72 Small chin.

Small chin: Move the hair up and away from the face along the chin line (Figure 12-72).

Large chin: The hair should be either longer or shorter than the chin line so as to avoid drawing attention to the chin (Figure 12-73).

HEAD SHAPE

Not all head shapes are round. It is important to feel the head shape before deciding on a hairstyle. Design the style with volume in areas that are flat or small while reducing volume in areas that are large or prominent (Figure 12-74).

STYLING FOR PEOPLE WHO WEAR GLASSES

Eyeglasses have become a fashion accessory, and many people change their eyewear as often as their clothes. It is important for you to know whether your clients ever wear glasses so you can take that into account when designing the appropriate hairstyle. Keep in mind that when a client puts on her glasses, the arms of the glasses (the part that rests on the ear) can push the hair at the ear and cause it to stick out.

If you are choosing a short haircut, you may want to reconsider the length of the hair around the ear, opting to either leave it a little longer or cut the hair above and around the ear. For styling purposes, choose a style in which there is enough hair covering the ear (fine hair may "pop" out at the ear), or direct the hair away from the face, so that the arms of the glasses are not an issue.

HAIR PARTS

Hair parts can be the focal point of a hairstyle. Because the eye is drawn to a part, you must be careful in the placement. It is usually best to use a natural part, whenever possible. You may, however, want to create a part according to your client's head shape or facial features, or for a desired hairstyle. It is often challenging to create a hairstyle working against the natural crown part. For best results, you might try to incorporate the natural part into the finished style. The following are suggestions for hair parts that suit the various facial types.

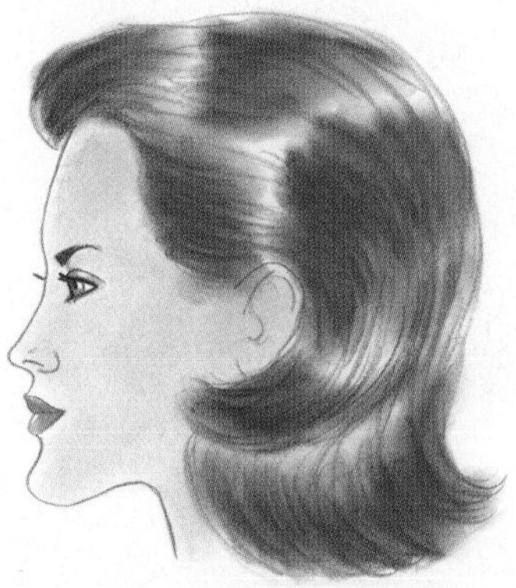

Figure 12-73 Large chin.

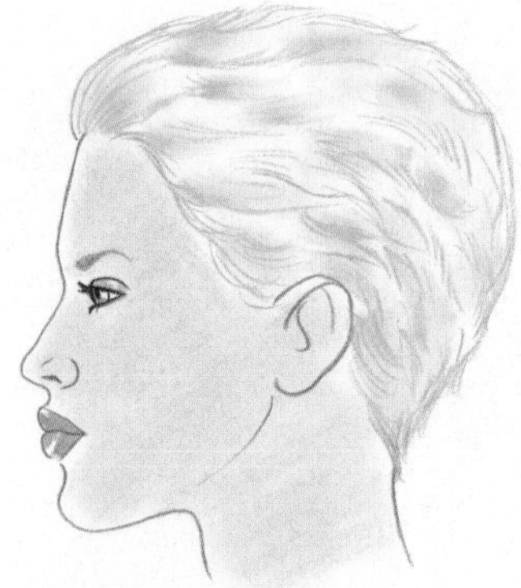

Figure 12-74 Perfect oval.

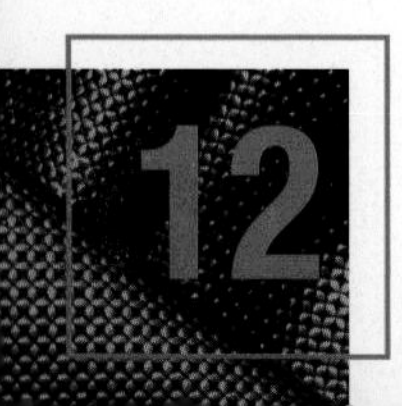

PARTS FOR THE BANG (FRINGE)

The **bang area,** or **fringe,** is the triangular section that begins at the apex, or high point of the head, and ends at the front corners. The bang is parted in three basic ways.

1. A triangular part is the basic parting for bang sections (Figure 12-75).
2. A diagonal part gives height to a round or square face and width to a long, thin face (Figure 12-76).
3. A curved part is used for a receding hairline or high forehead (Figure 12-77).

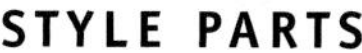

STYLE PARTS

There are four other parts that can be used to highlight facial features.

1. Center parts are classic. They are used for an oval face, but also give an oval illusion to wide and round faces. Remember to avoid using center parts on people with prominent noses (Figure 12-78).
2. Side parts are used to direct hair across the top of the head. They help develop height on top and make thin hair appear fuller (Figure 12-79).
3. Diagonal back parts are used to create the illusion of width or height in a hairstyle (Figure 12-80).
4. Zigzag parts create a dramatic effect (Figure 12-81).

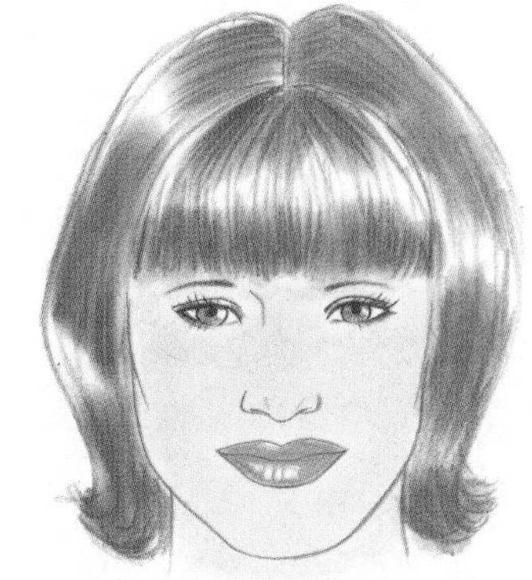

Figure 12-75 Triangular part.

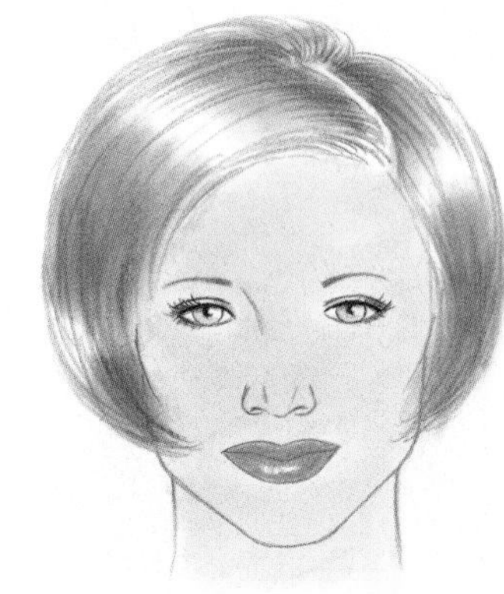

Figure 12-76 Diagonal part in fringe.

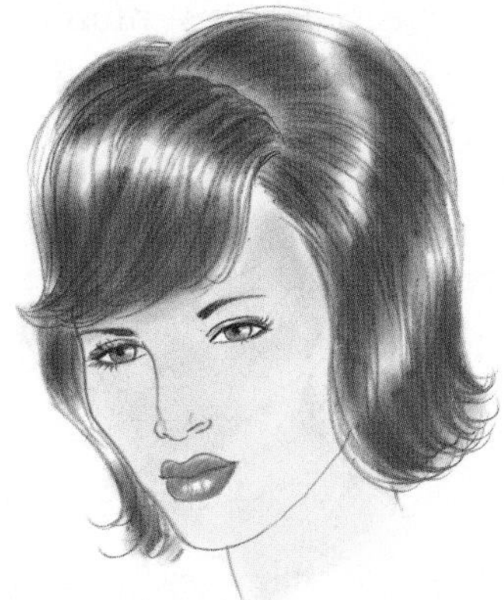

Figure 12-77 Curved part.

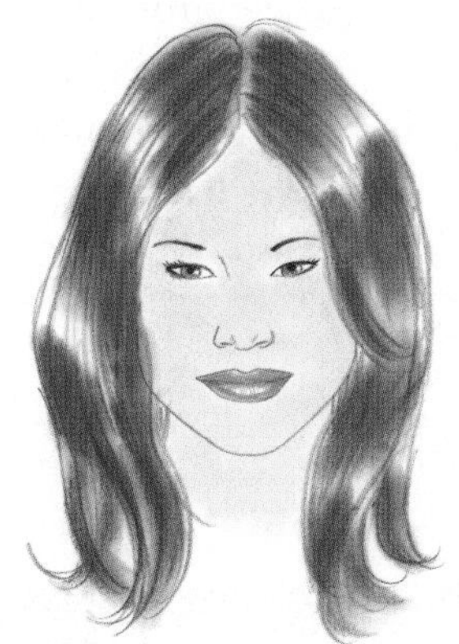

Figure 12-78 Center part.

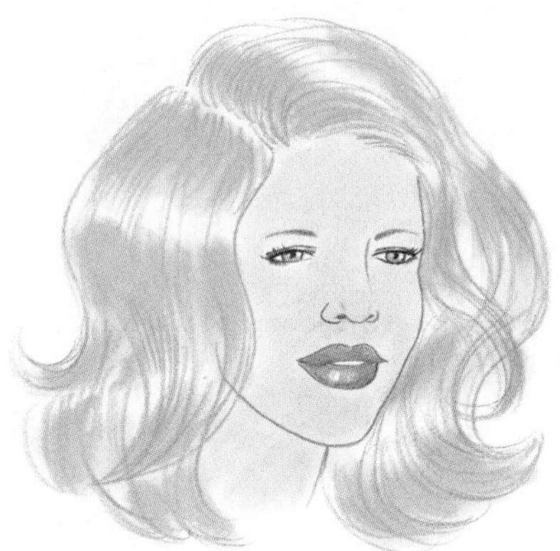

Figure 12-79 Side part.

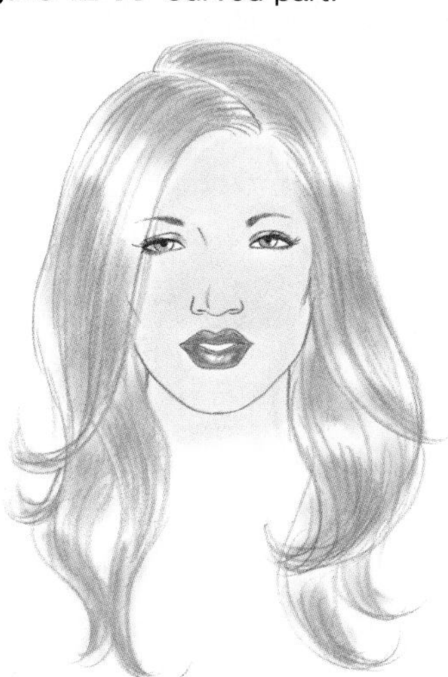

Figure 12-80 Diagonal part.

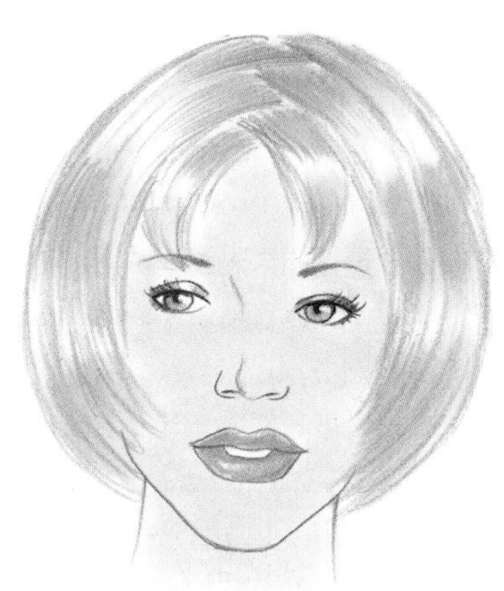

Figure 12-81 Zigzag part.

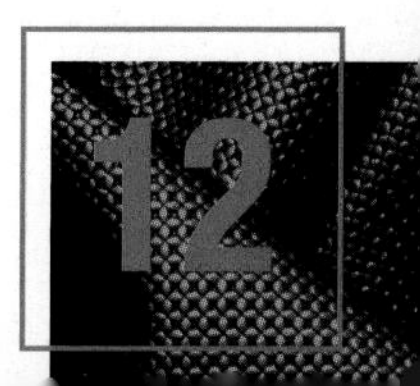

DESIGNING FOR MEN

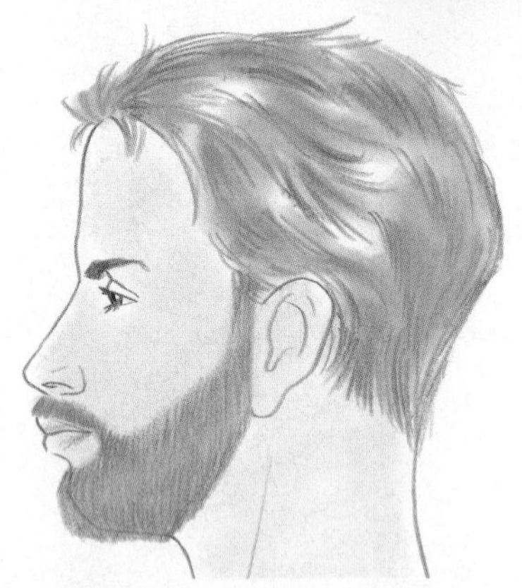

Figure 12-82 Full beard and mustache.

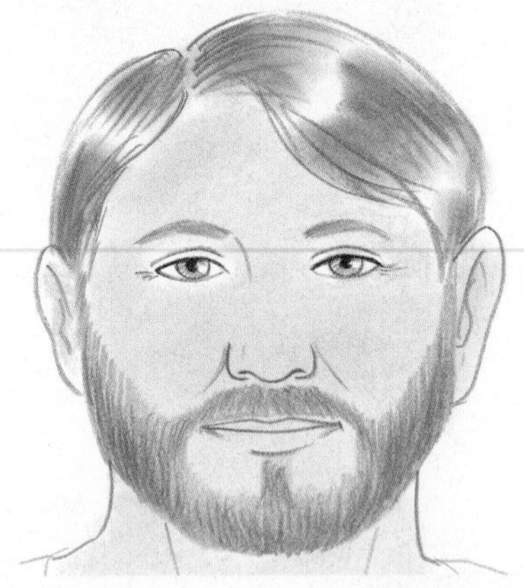

Figure 12-83 Closely trimmed beard and mustache.

All the design principles and elements you have just read about work for men's hairstyles, as well as for women's. Men's styles have become more individualized since the early 1960s, when the Beatles hit the music and fashion scene and greatly revolutionized men's hairstyling. Now all hair lengths are acceptable for men, giving them more choices than ever before. As a professional, you should be able to recommend styles that are both flattering and appropriate for the client's lifestyle, career, and hair type.

CHOOSING MUSTACHE AND BEARD SHAPES

Mustaches and beards can be great ways to camouflage facial flaws on male clients. For example, if a man does not have a prominent chin when you look at his profile, a neatly trimmed full beard and mustache may be a good solution (Figure 12-82). If a man has a wide face and full cheeks, a fairly close-trimmed beard and mustache would be very thinning (Figure 12-83).

A man who is balding with closely trimmed hair also could look very good in a closely groomed beard and mustache. Sideburns, mustaches, and beard shapes are largely dictated by current trends and fashions. No matter what the trend is, it is important that the shapes appear well groomed and are flattering to the client.

CLIENT CONSULTATION: SAMPLE DIALOGUE

The design process is a collaboration between stylist and client, beginning with the client consultation. Ellen, a new client at the salon, has just met Nicole, who is going to style her hair (Figure 12-84).

Nicole: Hi, Ellen. My name is Nicole and I'll be working with you today. Is there anything you would like to tell me or ask me about your hair?

Ellen: Well, I don't want it cut too short, and I like to keep my ears covered. I have a picture I tore out from a magazine that I want to show you.

(Nicole notices that the picture is of a model with a different kind of hair texture, and a cut about 3 inches shorter than what Ellen currently has.)

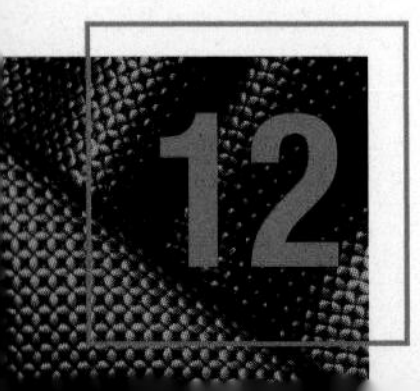

Nicole: This is a great look. I could achieve this for you with a permanent wave and a haircut. I would have to cut about three inches off the length and add some layers. How much time do you have in the morning to spend on your hair? Also, are you currently taking any medications, because they could have a negative effect on your perm.

Ellen: Well, let's keep it about an inch longer than this picture, and I am a little nervous about layering my hair. My mornings are very busy, getting my son off to school and getting myself ready to go to work. And no, I'm not taking any medications.

(Nicole realizes that Ellen is looking for a wash-and-wear style consistent with her lifestyle needs. She believes that the layering would help soften the lines of Ellen's square face.)

Nicole: Well, I can show you how you can easily style your hair with gel and cut your styling time in half by diffusing your curls. I think it would be fine to leave it an inch longer, but I really do feel that the layering would be most flattering to your features and would soften the whole look.

Ellen: Okay, that sounds great. Let's do it!

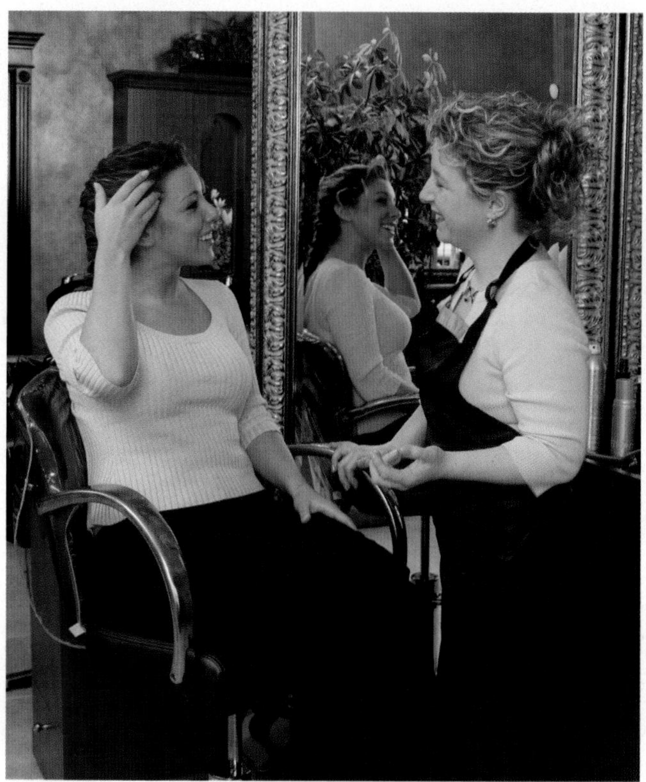

Figure 12-84 A client consultation.

REVIEW QUESTIONS

1. Name the five elements of design.
2. Name the five principles of hair design.
3. Why must the stylist consider the client's entire body when designing a hairstyle?
4. What are symmetrical and asymmetrical balances?
5. What is considered the most important art principle and why?
6. Explain how hair design can be used to highlight or camouflage facial features.
7. List and describe the seven facial shapes.
8. Name at least five facial features that must be considered when designing a hairstyle.
9. What is the difference between a convex and concave profile?
10. How do the elements and principles of hair design apply to men?

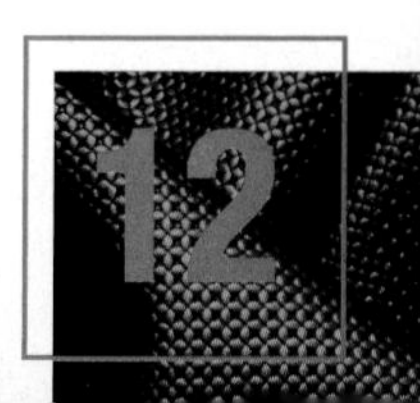

CHAPTER GLOSSARY

asymmetrical balance	Hairstyle design that features unequal proportions designed to balance facial features.
balance	Establishing equal or appropriate proportions to create symmetry. In hairstyling, it signifies the proper degree of height to width.
bang area/fringe	Triangular section that begins at the apex, or high point of the head, and ends at the front corners; fringe.
concave profile	Curving inward.
contrasting lines	Horizontal and vertical lines that meet at a 90-degree angle.
convex profile	Curving outward.
curved lines	Lines on an angle, used to soften a design.
design texture	Wave pattern.
diagonal lines	Lines positioned between horizontal and vertical lines.
emphasis or focus	The place in a hairstyle where the eye is drawn first before traveling to the rest of the design.
form	Outline of the overall hairstyle as seen from all angles.
harmony	Orderly and pleasing arrangement of shapes and lines.
horizontal lines	Lines parallel to the floor or horizon; creates width in design.
parallel lines	Repeating lines in a hairstyle; may be straight or curved.
proportion	Harmonious relationship among parts or things, or the comparative relation of one thing to another.
profile	Outline of the face, head, or figure seen in a side view.
rhythm	Regular, recurrent pattern of movement in a hairstyle.
single lines	A hairstyle with only one line such as the one-length hairstyle.
space	Area that the hairstyle occupies; also thought of as the area inside the form.
straight profile	Neither convex nor concave.
symmetrical balance	Hairstyle design that is similar on both sides of the face.
transitional lines	Usually curved lines that are used to blend and soften horizontal or vertical lines.
vertical lines	Lines that are straight up and down; creates length and height in hair design.

SHAMPOOING, RINSING, & CONDITIONING

CHAPTER 13

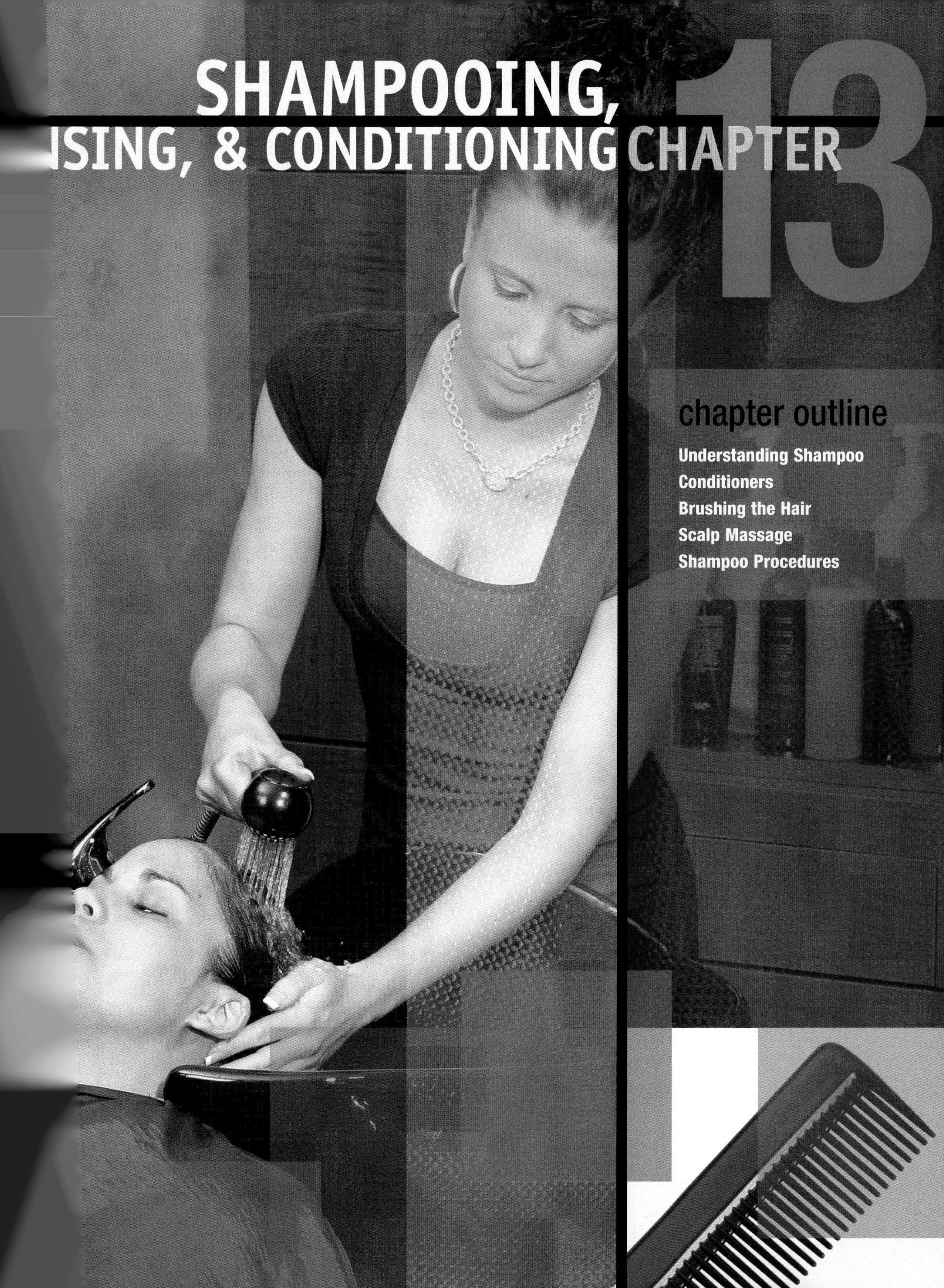

chapter outline

Learning Objectives

After completing this chapter, you will be able to:

- **Explain the importance of pH in shampoo selection.**
- **Explain the role of surfactants in shampoo.**
- **Discuss the uses and benefits of various types of shampoos and conditioners.**
- **Perform proper scalp manipulations as part of a shampoo service.**
- **Demonstrate proper shampooing and conditioning procedures.**

Key Terms

Page number indicates where in the chapter the term is used.

acid-balanced shampoo
pg. 223

balancing shampoos
pg. 224

clarifying shampoos
pg. 224

color-enhancing shampoos
pg. 224

conditioners
pg. 224

conditioning or moisturizing shampoos
pg. 223

deep-conditioning treatments
pg. 226

dry or powder shampoo
pg. 224

hard water
pg. 221

humectants
pg. 225

hydrophilic
pg. 222

instant conditioners
pg. 226

lipophilic
pg. 222

medicated scalp lotions
pg. 227

medicated shampoos
pg. 224

moisturizers
pg. 226

nonstripping
pg. 223

protein conditioners
pg. 226

scalp astringent lotions
pg. 227

scalp conditioners
pg. 227

soft water
pg. 221

spray-on thermal protectors
pg. 227

surfactants
pg. 222

When a client visits a salon for the first time, she immediately begins making judgments about her surroundings. How does the salon look? What kind of music is playing? Does the receptionist greet her with a smile and call her by name? While all of this is part of having a good experience, it is what happens next when she moves into the service area that can make or break you. One of the most important experiences that a stylist provides is the shampoo, which can be heavenly, forgettable, or even a nightmare.

While shampooing is an important preliminary step that prepares the hair for a variety of services, it can also be a soothing, pleasurable experience that sets the mood for the entire visit. The shampoo is an opportunity to provide the client with quality relaxation time in the salon that is free from the stresses of the day. It can be nurturing and, when done well, feel as good as an overall body massage. Remember: If a client is happy with her shampoo, she is far more likely to be happy with her entire service.

UNDERSTANDING SHAMPOO

The shampoo provides a good opportunity to analyze the client's hair and scalp. Always check for these conditions: (1) dry, dehydrated hair; (2) dry, tight scalp, (3) oily scalp, (4) abnormal flaking on the scalp, (5) open wounds or scalp irritations, (6) scalp disorders or diseases, (7) thinning, and (8) excessive hair left in the sink trap after shampooing.

In salons where shampoos are performed by salon assistants, the shampoo person should always alert the stylist about any hair or scalp conditions, including suspected diseases or disorders. A client with an infectious disease is never to be treated in the salon and should be referred to a physician.

Naturally, the primary purpose of a shampoo is to cleanse the hair and scalp prior to receiving a service. This is also the time you need to educate your client about the importance of home care and of using quality hair care products at home.

To be effective, a shampoo must remove all dirt, oils, cosmetics, and skin debris without adversely affecting either the scalp or hair. The scalp and hair need to be cleansed regularly to combat the accumulation of

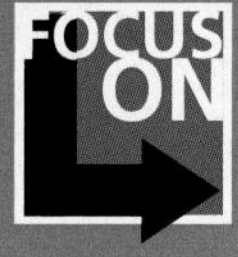

Focus on . . . Service: Eight Ways to Make a Good Shampoo Experience Great!

1. The scalp is always massaged according to the preference of the client. Some clients have a sensitive scalp and want a very light massage, while others lack sensitivity and want a firm massage. In order to service every client to the best of your ability, find out their preference before shampooing her or his hair.
2. Always ask the client if the water feels too warm, too cool, or just right, and adjust the temperature accordingly.
3. Do not allow the water or your hands to touch a woman's face while shampooing. This may remove part of her base makeup, and can turn an otherwise great shampoo into an unpleasant experience.
4. It is easy to miss the very nape of the neck when shampooing and rinsing, so be careful reaching it, and then check this area before escorting the client to your station.
5. Offer a cool rinse to your client. Explain how good it is for the hair (closes the cuticle). If the client objects, though, do not insist. Many people find even tepid water to be a chilling experience.

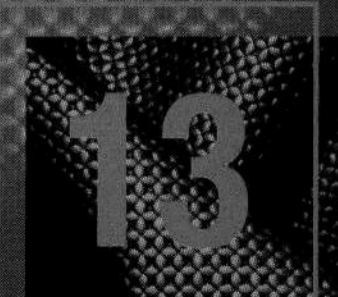

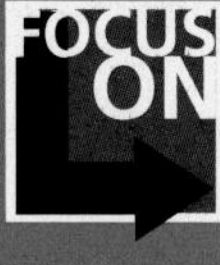

Focus on . . . Service: Eight Ways to Make a Good Shampoo Experience Great!—cont'd

6. Throughout the shampoo, be very careful not to drench the towel that is draped around the neck. If the towel becomes damp, replace it with a clean, dry towel before leaving the shampoo area.
7. When blotting the hair after the shampoo, be careful not to go beyond the hair line. If you do this, you may remove part of your client's makeup and she may feel self-conscious for her entire visit.
8. When learning to give a great shampoo, include a great massage. You may hear your clients say, "Don't stop, you can do that for hours," every time they come to you (Figure 13-1). Even though you may hear this five times a day, it is always satisfying to know that you are making your clients feel good!

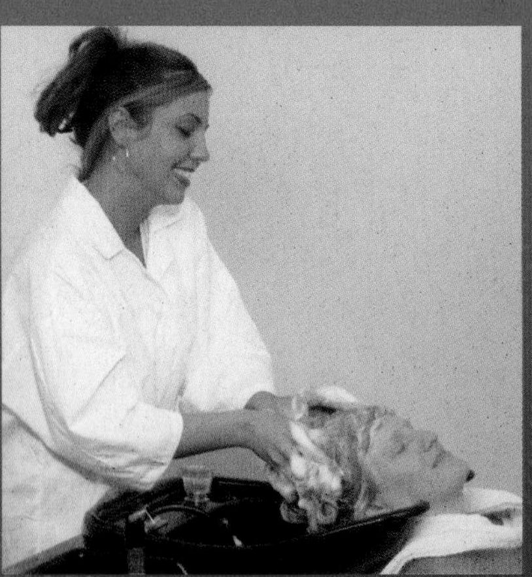

Figure 13-1 The shampoo is an enjoyable part of the salon experience.

oils and perspiration that mix with the natural scales and dirt to create a breeding ground for disease-producing bacteria. Hair should only be shampooed as often as necessary. Excessive shampooing strips the hair of its protective oil (sebum) that, in small amounts, seals and protects the hair's cuticle. As a general rule, oily hair needs to be shampooed more often than normal or dry hair.

TYPES OF SHAMPOO

There are many types of shampoo available on the market today. As a professional cosmetologist, you should become skilled at selecting shampoos that support the health of the hair, whether it is natural, color-treated, fine and limp, or coarse and wiry. Always read labels and accompanying literature carefully so that you can make informed decisions about the use of various shampoos. Careful attention to knowing your products will help you in recommending them as home-care items for purchase by your clients.

Select a shampoo according to the condition of the client's hair and scalp. Hair can usually be characterized as oily, dry, normal, or chemically treated. Your client might even have an oily scalp with dry hair, possibly due to overprocessing. Hair is not considered normal or virgin if it has been lightened, colored, permed, chemically relaxed, abused by the use of harsh shampoos, or damaged by improper care and exposure to the elements, such as wind, sun, cold, or heat.

Using the right hair-care products at home can make all the difference in how your clients' hair looks, feels, and behaves. It is your job to recommend and educate them about which products they should be using, as well as how and why. Otherwise, they will make their own uninformed decisions, and perhaps even buy inferior products at the drugstore or supermarket. The wrong product choice can make even a good haircut look bad, and can affect the outcome of a chemical service. Only professional products are guaranteed when purchased in the salon.

In the words of Vidal Sassoon: "If you don't look good, we don't look good!"

Remember: You want your clients to look their best so that they become good advertising for you.

THE pH SCALE

Chapter 10 of this book provides you with an overview of important chemistry basics, including pH and surfactants. Refer to that chapter as necessary. To save you some steps, though, the following is a review of pH as it applies to shampoo (Figure 13-2).

Understanding pH levels will help you select the proper shampoo for your client. The amount of hydrogen in a solution, which determines whether it is alkaline or acid, is measured on a pH scale that has a range from 0 to 14. A shampoo that is acidic can have a pH ranging from 0 to 6.9; a shampoo that is alkaline can have a pH rating of 7.1 or higher. The more alkaline the shampoo, the stronger and harsher the shampoo. A high-pH shampoo can leave the hair dry, brittle, and porous, and cause fading in color-treated hair. A slightly acidic shampoo more closely matches the ideal pH of hair.

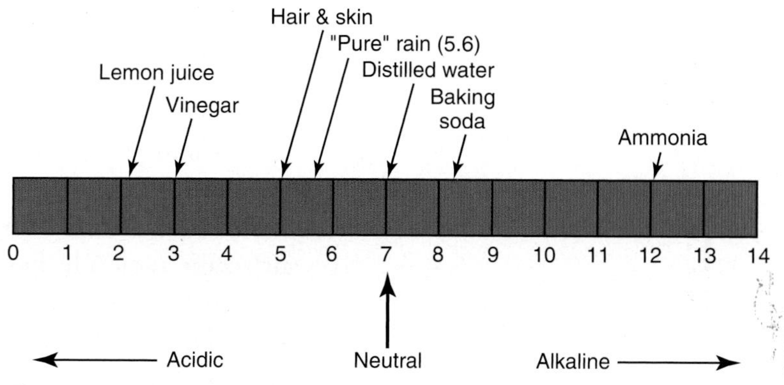

Figure 13-2 The pH scale.

THE CHEMISTRY OF WATER

Water is the most abundant and important element on Earth. It is classified as a "universal solvent" because it is capable of dissolving more substances than any other solvent known to science.

Fresh water from lakes and streams is purified by sedimentation (matter sinking to the bottom) and filtration (water passing through a porous substance, such as a filter paper or charcoal) to remove suspended clay, sand, and organic material. Small amounts of chlorine are then added to kill bacteria. Boiling water at a temperature of 212° F (100° C) will also destroy most microbes. Water can be further treated by distillation, a process of heating water so that it becomes a vapor, and then condensing the purified vapor so that it collects as a liquid. This process is often used in the manufacturing of cosmetics.

Water is of crucial importance in the cosmetology industry because it is used for shampooing, mixing solutions, and many other functions. Depending on the kinds and amounts of minerals present in water, water can be classified as either hard or soft. You will be able to make a more professional shampoo selection if you know whether the water in your salon and area is hard or soft. Most water softener companies can supply you with a water-testing kit to determine whether you have hard or soft water and even to what degree (soft, slightly hard, moderately hard, hard, or extremely hard).

Soft water is rain water or chemically softened water. It contains small amounts of minerals and, therefore, allows soap and shampoo to lather freely. For this reason, it is preferred for shampooing. **Hard water** is often in well water and contains minerals that reduce the ability of soap or shampoo to lather readily. It may also change the results of the haircoloring service. However, a water treatment process can soften hard water.

THE CHEMISTRY OF SHAMPOOS

To determine which shampoo will leave your client's hair in the best condition for the intended service, you need to understand the chemical and botanical ingredients regularly found in shampoos. Most shampoos have many of these ingredients in common. It is often the small differences in formulation that make one shampoo better than another for a particular hair texture or condition.

Water is the main ingredient in most shampoos. Generally it is not just plain water, but purified or deionized water. The water is deionized to remove impurities such as calcium and magnesium and other metal ions that would interfere with other ions and make the product unstable.

Water is usually the first ingredient listed, which indicates that the shampoo contains more water than anything else. From there on,

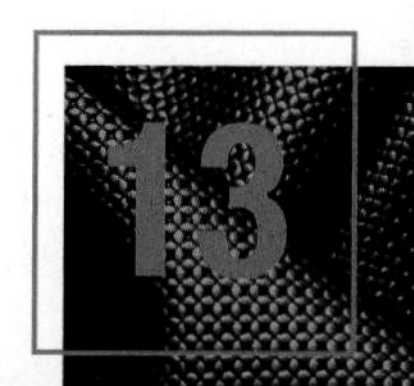

ingredients are listed in descending order, according to the percentage of each ingredient in the shampoo.

SURFACTANTS

The second ingredient that most shampoos have in common is the primary surfactant or base detergent. These two terms, **surfactant** and detergent, mean the same thing: cleansing or "surface active agent." A surfactant molecule has two ends: a **hydrophilic** (hy-drah-FIL-ik) or water-attracting "head," and a **lipophilic** (ly-puh-FIL-ik) or oil-attracting "tail." During the shampooing process, the hydrophilic head attracts water, and the lipophilic tail attracts oil. This creates a push-pull process that causes the oils, dirt, and deposits to roll up into little balls that can be lifted off in the water and rinsed from the hair (Figure 13-3, Figure 13-4, Figure 13-5, and Figure 13-6).

Other ingredients are added to the base surfactants to create a wide variety of shampoo formulas. Moisturizers, oils, proteins, preservatives, foam enhancers, and perfumes are all standard components of shampoo.

TYPES OF SHAMPOO

Shampoo products account for the most dollars spent in hair care products. Consumer studies show that the fastest growth items in the shampoo market are products that are retailed through professional

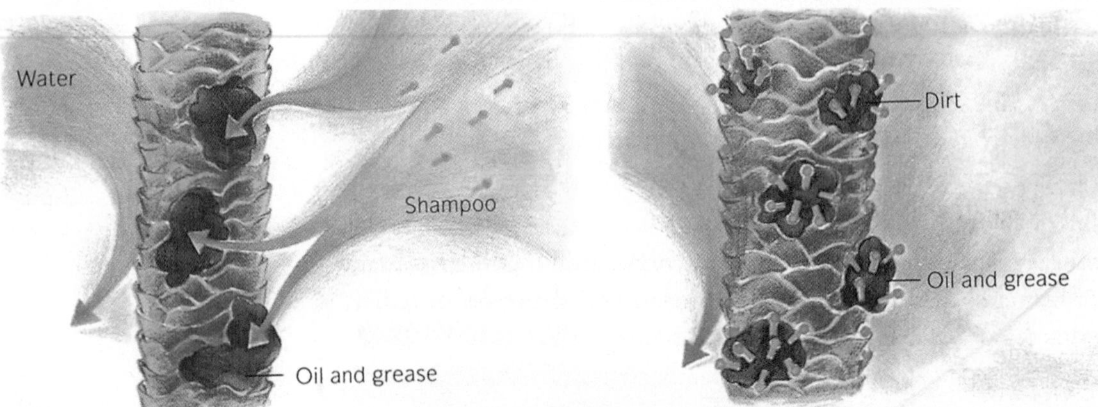

Figure 13-3 The tail of the shampoo molecule is attracted to oil and dirt.

Figure 13-4 Shampoo causes oils to roll up into small globules.

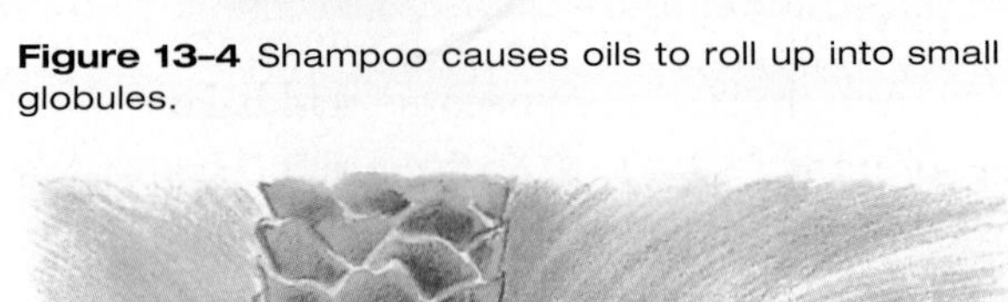

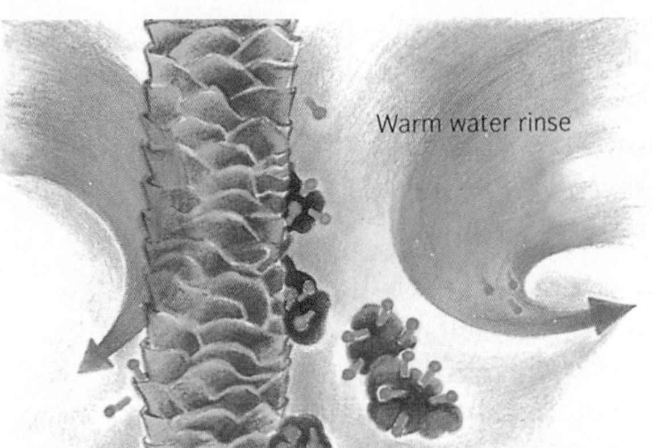

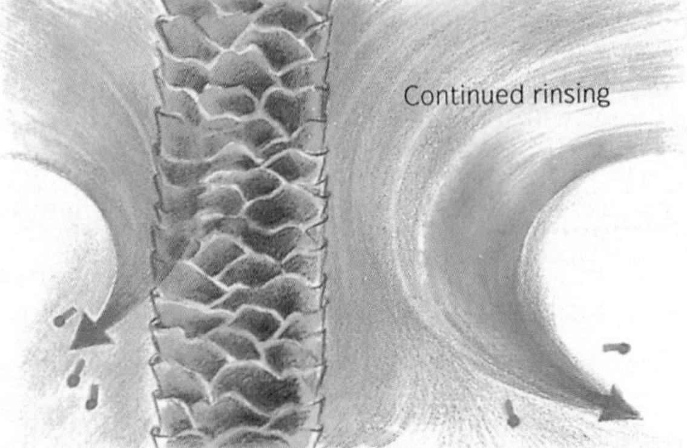

Figure 13-5 During rinsing, the heads of the shampoo molecules attach to water molecules and cause debris to roll off.

Figure 13-6 Thorough rinsing washes away debris and excess shampoo.

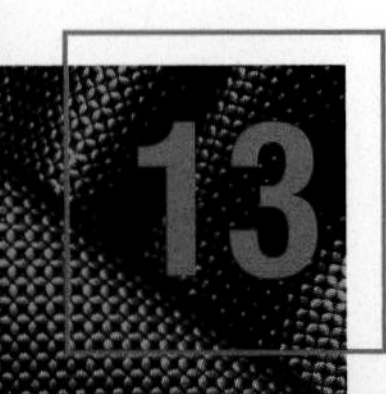

ACTIVITY

List all the hair products used in your school, along with what types of hair these products are best used on. Analyze the hair of one or two classmates and recommend a particular shampoo and conditioner. List the benefits of each product for that particular "client." With your instructor's guidance, you might even try using your recommended choices on your classmates. Keep a record of what products you use, how the hair feels and behaves afterward, and your classmates' own opinions about the products.

salons. This is good news for salon professionals, but never allow yourself to be overconfident if you want to succeed at sales. You will have to be as knowledgeable and sophisticated as possible about the products you are selling, and as skilled as you can be in demonstrating their use.

Clients are becoming increasingly informed about beauty products from reading about them in beauty magazines and other consumer reports. Your credibility as a professional will be in question if your client is better informed than you are.

Many good shampoos exist for every type of hair or scalp condition. There are shampoos for dry, oily, fine, coarse, limp, lightened, permed, relaxed, or color-treated and chemically treated hair. There are shampoos that add a slight amount of color to highlighted hair, and those that cleanse hair of styling product buildup, mineral deposits, and so forth. There are shampoos that deposit a coating on the hair, and shampoos that remove coatings from the hair.

The list of ingredients is your key to determining which shampoo will leave a client's hair shiny and manageable, which will treat a scalp or hair condition, and which will prepare the hair for a chemical treatment. Now that you are familiar with pH and the chemistry of water and shampoo, here are some of the different types of shampoos.

ACID BALANCED

An **acid-balanced shampoo** is balanced to the pH of skin and hair (4.5 to 5.5). Any shampoo can become acid balanced by the addition of citric, lactic, or phosphoric acid. Some experts believe that an acid pH of 4.5 to 5.5 is essential to prevent excessive dryness and hair damage during the cleansing process. Acid-balanced shampoos help to close the hair cuticle and are recommended for hair that has been color treated or lightened.

CONDITIONING OR MOISTURIZING SHAMPOOS

Conditioning or **moisturizing shampoos** are designed to make the hair smooth and shiny, avoid damage to chemically treated hair, and improve manageability of the hair. Protein and biotin are just two examples of conditioning agents that boost shampoos so that they can meet current grooming needs. These conditioning agents restore moisture and elasticity, strengthen the hair shaft, and add volume. They also are **nonstripping,** meaning that they do not remove artificial color from the hair.

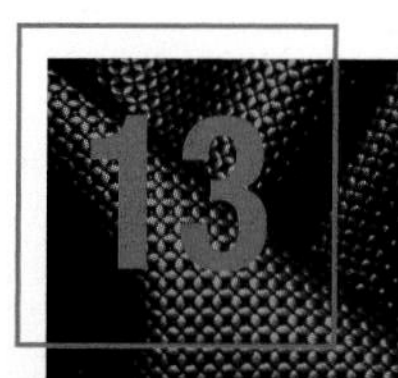

Did You Know

In the 1960s, beauty pioneer Jheri Redding revolutionized the salon industry by being the first to market pH-balanced shampoos. He went around the country staging demonstrations that showed how acidic shampoos (pH below 7) outperformed alkaline shampoos. When Redding dipped a piece of litmus paper into his shampoo, it would come up a glowing orange, pink, or gold. The litmus test on his competitors' products would come up a murky purple or black. Most cosmetic chemists today agree that a low pH is good for all hair, and especially chemically treated hair.

MEDICATED SHAMPOOS

Medicated shampoos contain special chemicals or drugs that are very effective in reducing excessive dandruff or relieving other scalp conditions. Some medicated shampoos have to be prescribed by a physician. They are generally quite strong and could affect the color of tinted or lightened hair. In some cases, the shampoo must remain on the scalp for a longer period of time than other shampoos in order for the active ingredient to work. Always read and follow the manufacturer's instructions carefully.

CLARIFYING SHAMPOOS

Clarifying shampoos contain an acidic ingredient such as apple cider vinegar to cut through product buildup that can flatten hair. They also increase shine. These shampoos should only be used when a buildup is evident, perhaps once a week to once every 2 weeks, depending on how much styling product a client tends to use.

BALANCING SHAMPOOS

For oily hair and scalp, **balancing shampoos** wash away excess oiliness, while preventing the hair from drying out.

DRY OR POWDER SHAMPOOS

Sometimes, the state of a client's health makes a wet shampoo uncomfortable or hard to manage. For instance, an elderly client may experience some discomfort at the shampoo bowl due to pressure on the back of the neck. In such a case, it is advisable to use a **dry** or **powder shampoo,** which cleanses the hair without the use of soap and water. The powder picks up dirt and oils as you brush or comb it through the hair. It also adds volume to the hair. Follow the manufacturer's instructions. Never give a dry shampoo before performing a chemical service.

COLOR-ENHANCING SHAMPOOS

Color-enhancing shampoos are created by combining the surfactant base with basic color pigments. They are similar to temporary color rinses because they are attracted to porous hair and result in only slight color changes that are removed with plain shampooing. Color shampoos are used to brighten, to add a slight hint of color, and to eliminate unwanted color tones such as gold or brassiness, and overly cool strands.

SHAMPOOS FOR HAIRPIECES AND WIGS

Prepared wig-cleaning solutions are available for these hair enhancements (see Chapter 17).

CONDITIONERS

Conditioners are special chemical agents applied to the hair to deposit protein or moisturizer, to help restore its strength and give it body, or to protect it against possible breakage. Conditioners are a temporary remedy

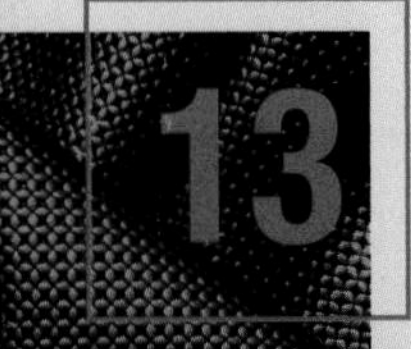

for hair that feels dry, appears damaged, or is damaged. They can only repair hair to a certain extent; they cannot "heal" damaged hair, and cannot improve the quality of new hair growth.

Heredity, health, and diet control the texture and structure of the hair. Conditioners are valuable because they can minimize the damage to hair during a cosmetology service. They can restore luster, shine, manageability, and strength while the damaged hair grows long enough to be cut off and replaced by new hair. Because of frequent shampooing, heavy use of thermal styling tools, generous use of hair color products, and the ever-present blow dryer being used at high heat, conditioning is a must for clients who care about their hair.

Conditioners can also be too much of a good thing. Habitual use can lead to a buildup on the hair, making it heavy and oily. The stylist should know when to choose between a cream rinse, which simply removes tangles, and a conditioning treatment, which repairs damaged hair. Always read the instructions on the bottle. If the manufacturer recommends that the product be used once a week, using it every day can lead to unsatisfactory results.

Conditioners, also known as "reconstructors" or even "hair masks," are available in the following three basic types:

- *Rinse-out.* Finishing rinses or cream rinses that are rinsed out after they are worked through the hair for detangling.
- *Treatment or repair.* Deep-penetrating conditioners that are left on the hair for 10 to 20 minutes, restoring protein and moisture. Sometimes it is necessary for the client to sit under a heated dryer for deeper penetration.
- *Leave-in.* Applied to the hair and not rinsed out.

Most conditioners contain silicone along with moisture-binding **humectants** (hew-MECK-tents), substances that absorb moisture or promote the retention of moisture. Silicone reflects light and makes the hair appear shiny. Other ingredients reduce frizz and bulk up the hair. Most treatments and leave-ins contain proteins, which penetrate the cortex and reinforce the hair shaft from within.

Even though a product may be formulated to improve the quality of the hair, it can cause damage over time if used incorrectly. Conditioners can build up on the hair shaft and make your hair heavy and oily, leading you to think that it is time to shampoo again. This constant shampooing strips the hair shaft of its protective oils, which prompts you to condition your hair more, creating a vicious cycle. If you use a gentle shampoo that is appropriate for your hair type with a little conditioner only when and where you need it, you can avoid this problem. Pass this on to your clients.

Conditioners affect the hair in different ways. The cuticle, or outermost layer, is made up of overlapping scales. A healthy cuticle lies down smoothly and reflects light, giving the appearance of shiny hair. Conditioners smooth the cuticle and coat the hair shaft to achieve the

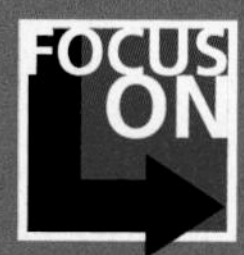

Focus on . . . Retailing

Some stylists view the shampoo as "down time," and use it to talk about what they did the night before. It is important to remember that your time, and your client's time, is valuable and can be better spent. You can begin to establish your professional relationship during the shampoo by giving the client information about what you are doing and why. Let the client know what shampoo you are using, and why you have selected it especially for their hair. Mention that these products are available for purchase, and emphasize their benefits.

There is no need to be pushy, or to see this as being pushy. Just be yourself and always be honest. When clients are concerned about the health and appearance of their hair, or they have been unhappy with what they have been using at home, they will often make a purchase based on your advice and will thank you for your professional recommendation. You will often find that the stylist with the highest client retention usually also has the highest retail/home-care sales in the salon. This stylist has gained the clients' trust and respect in them as a professional.

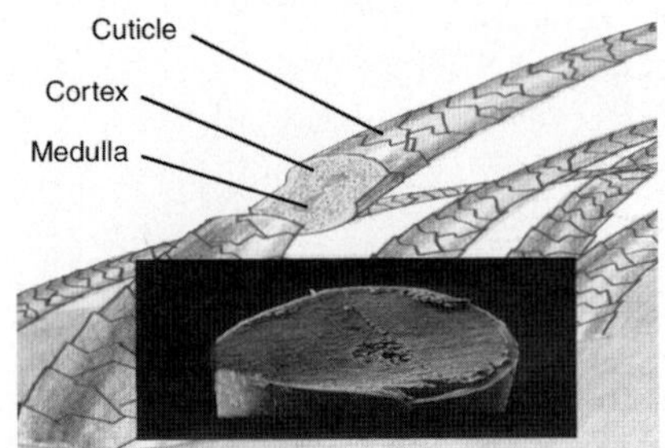

Figure 13-7 Cuticle, cortex, and medulla of the hair shaft.

same effect. So do detangling rinses or cream rinses, although they are not as heavy.

The cortex makes up 90 percent of the hair strand. It can be penetrated with protein conditioners to temporarily reconstruct the hair. Moisturizing conditioners also contain humectants that attract moisture from the air and are absorbed into the cortex (Figure 13-7).

INSTANT CONDITIONERS

Instant conditioners include products that either remain on the hair for a very short period (1 to 5 minutes), or are left in the hair during styling ("leave-in" conditioners). Instant conditioners contain humectants to improve the appearance of dry, brittle hair.

Most conditioners fall in the pH range of 3.5 to 6.0, and restore the pH balance after an alkaline chemical treatment. Those conditioners are designed primarily to balance pH. They are considered instant because of their short application time. They generally contain an acid that balances the alkalinity of a prior chemical service.

MOISTURIZERS

Heavier and creamier than instant conditioners, **moisturizers** also have a longer application time (10 to 20 minutes). They contain many of the same ingredients as instant conditioners, but are formulated to be more penetrating and to have longer staying power. Some moisturizers involve the application of heat. Quaternary ammonium compounds (quats) are included in the chemical formulation of moisturizers due to their ability to attach themselves steadfastly to hair fibers and to provide longer-lasting protection than instant conditioners.

PROTEIN CONDITIONERS

Protein conditioners are designed to slightly increase hair diameter with a coating action, thereby adding body to the hair. They are often referred to as protein treatments and facilitate the hairstyling process. Protein conditioners are available in several strengths. Choose the strength appropriate to the condition, texture, and quality of the hair you are treating.

Concentrated protein conditioners have traditionally had a brown liquid appearance. They are used to improve the strength of the hair and to temporarily close split ends. These conditioners are designed to pass through the cuticle, penetrate into the cortex, and replace the keratin that has been lost from the hair. They improve appearance, equalize porosity, and increase elasticity. The excess conditioner must be rinsed from the hair before setting. Concentrated protein treatments are generally not given immediately following a chemical treatment, as they can alter the desirable rearrangement of protein bonds formed by a permanent wave, relaxer, or hair coloring.

DEEP-CONDITIONING TREATMENTS

Deep-conditioning treatments, also known as hair masks or conditioning packs, are chemical mixtures of concentrated protein in the heavy cream base of a moisturizer. They penetrate the cuticle layer and are the chosen therapy when an equal degree of moisturizing and protein treatment is desired.

OTHER CONDITIONING AGENTS

Other conditioning agents that you need to be familiar with follow:

- **Spray-on thermal protectors** are applied to hair prior to any thermal service to protect the hair from the harmful effects of blow drying, thermal irons, or electric rollers.
- **Scalp conditioners,** usually found in a cream base, are used to soften and improve the health of the scalp. They contain moisturizing and emollient ingredients.
- **Medicated scalp lotions** are conditioners that promote healing of the scalp.
- **Scalp astringent lotions** remove oil accumulation from the scalp and are used after a scalp treatment and before styling.

Table 13-1 lists products suitable for various hair types.

BRUSHING THE HAIR

Correct hair brushing stimulates the blood circulation to the scalp; helps remove dust, dirt, and hair-spray buildup from the hair; and gives hair added shine. You should include a thorough hair brushing as part of every

Hair Type	Fine	Medium	Coarse
Straight	Volumizing shampoo Detangler, if necessary Protein treatments	Acid-balanced shampoo Finishing rinse Protein treatments	Moisturizing shampoo Leave-in conditioner Moisturizing treatments
Wave, Curly, Extremely Curly	Fine hair shampoo Light leave-in conditioner Protein treatments Spray-on thermal protectors	Acid-balanced shampoo Leave-in conditioner Moisturizing treatment	Moisturizing shampoo Leave-in conditioner Protein and moisturizing treatments
Dry & Damaged (Perms, Color, Relaxers, Blow-drying, Sun, Hot Irons)	Gentle cleansing shampoo Light leave-in conditioner Protein and moisturizing repair treatments Spray-on thermal protection	Shampoo for chemically treated hair Moisturizing conditioner Protein and moisturizing repair treatments	Deep-moisturizing shampoo for damaged hair Leave-in conditioner Deep conditioning treatments and hair masks

Table 13-1 Matching Products to Hair Types

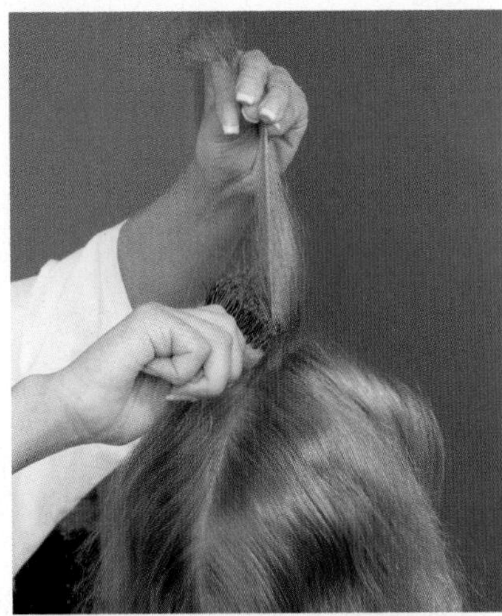

Figure 13-8 Begin the brushing stroke.

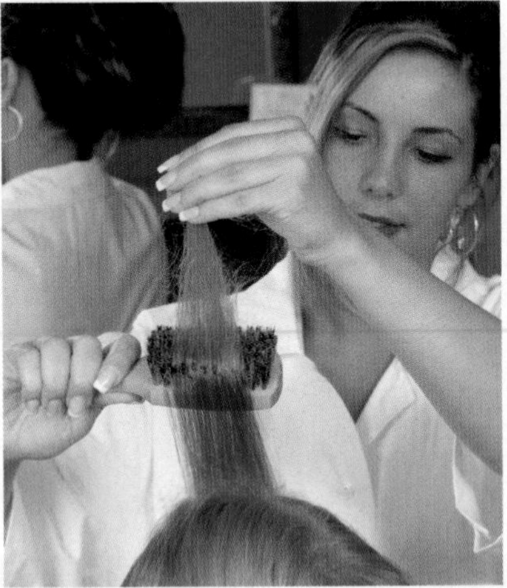

Figure 13-9 Brush the hair.

shampoo and scalp treatment, regardless of whether your client's hair and scalp are dry or oily. The three exceptions to hair brushing follow.

- Do not brush before giving a chemical service.
- Do not brush if the scalp is irritated.
- Never brush the scalp.

Hair services that you should not be brushing, shampooing, or massaging the scalp include:

- Single-process and double-process haircolor
- Highlighting
- Most chemical relaxers (follow manufacturer's directions)
- Some temporary and semipermanent haircolor (follow manufacturer's directions)

If shampooing is recommended, shampoo gently to avoid scalp irritation.

Also, never use a comb to loosen scales from the scalp. The most highly recommended hairbrushes are those made from natural bristles. Natural bristles have many tiny overlapping layers or scales, which clean and add luster to the hair. Hairbrushes with nylon bristles are shiny and smooth and are more suitable for hairstyling.

To brush the hair, first part it through the center from front to nape. Then part a section about an inch (1.25 cm) off the center parting to the crown of the head. Hold this section of hair in your left hand (Figure 13-8). Rotate the brush by turning the wrist slightly and sweep the bristles the full length of the hair shaft (Figure 13-9). Repeat three times. Then part the hair again an inch from the first parting and continue until the entire head has been brushed.

SCALP MASSAGE

The two basic requirements for a healthy scalp are cleanliness and stimulation. Since similar manipulations are given with all scalp treatments, you should learn to give them with a continuous, even motion that will stimulate the scalp and help to relax the client. Scalp massage is most effective when given as a series of treatments once a week for a normal scalp and more frequently when scalp disorders are present, in conjunction with treatment by a dermatologist. Do not massage or manipulate a client's scalp if abrasions are present.

Scalp massage is performed **prior** to the shampoo. It is this "extra" service that will keep your clients coming back to you. Knowing the muscles, the location of blood vessels, and the nerve points of the scalp and neck will help guide you to those areas most likely to benefit from massage movements. For this information, see Chapter 6.

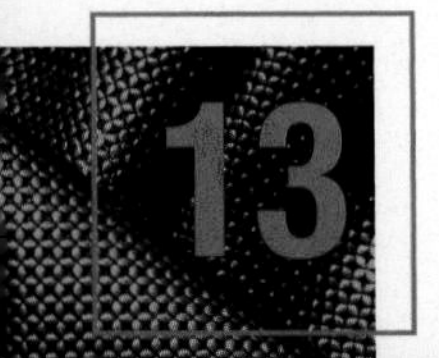

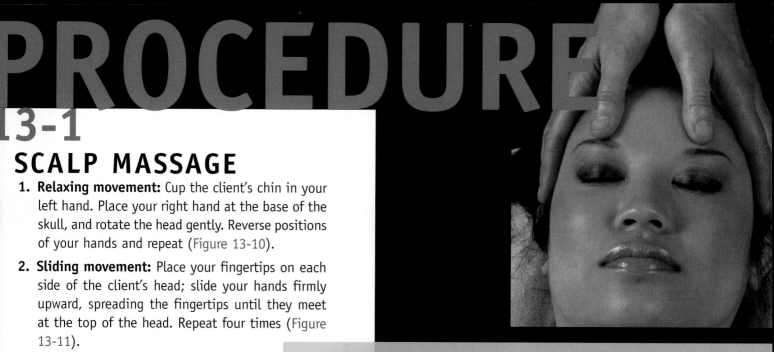

PROCEDURE 13-1

SCALP MASSAGE

1. **Relaxing movement:** Cup the client's chin in your left hand. Place your right hand at the base of the skull, and rotate the head gently. Reverse positions of your hands and repeat (Figure 13-10).
2. **Sliding movement:** Place your fingertips on each side of the client's head; slide your hands firmly upward, spreading the fingertips until they meet at the top of the head. Repeat four times (Figure 13-11).
3. **Sliding and rotating movement:** Same as (2), except that after sliding the fingertips 1 inch (2.5 cm), rotate and move the client's scalp. Repeat four times (Figure 13-12).
4. **Forehead movement:** Hold the back of the client's head with your left hand. Place your stretched thumb and the fingers of your right hand on the client's forehead. Move your hand slowly and firmly upward to 1 inch past the hairline. Repeat four times. (Figure 13-13).
5. **Scalp movement:** Place the palms of your hands firmly against the client's scalp. Lift the scalp in a rotary movement, first with your hands placed above her ears, and second with your hands placed at the front and back of her head (Figure 13-14).
6. **Hairline movement:** Place the fingers of both hands at the client's forehead. Massage around her hairline by lifting and rotating (Figure 13-15).

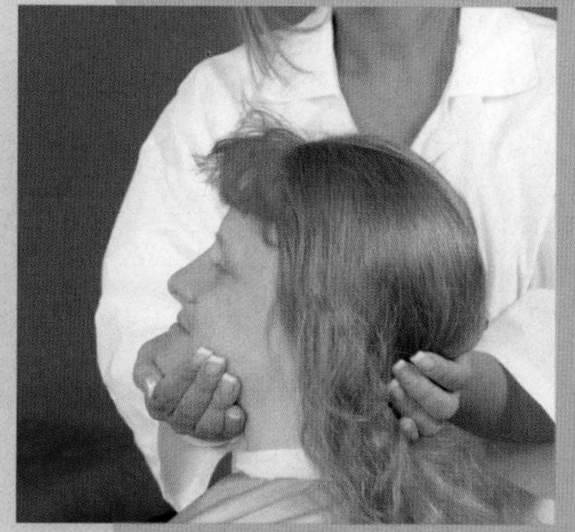

Figure 13–10 Relaxing movement.

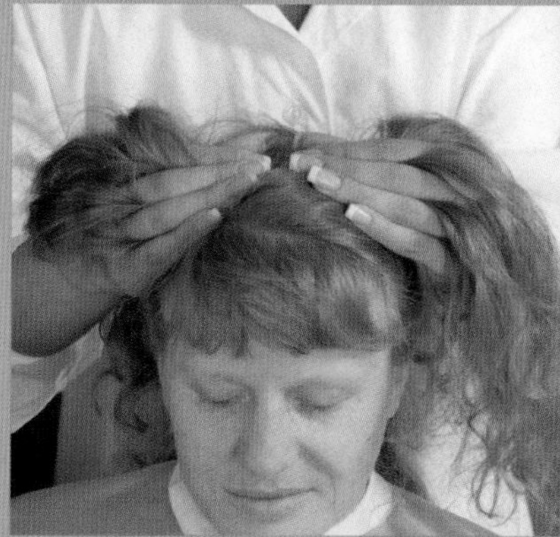

Figure 13–11 Sliding movement.

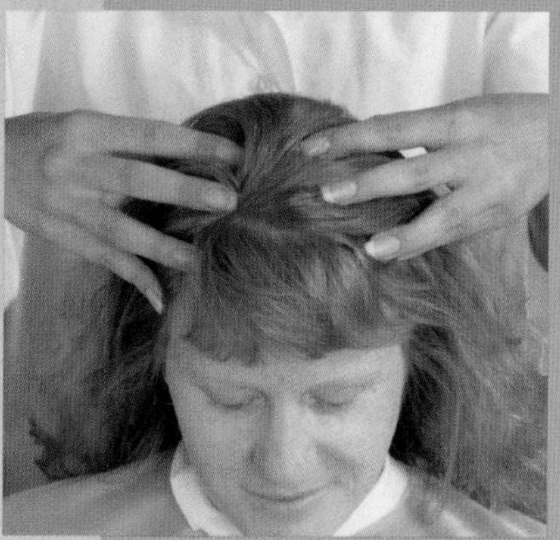

Figure 13–12 Sliding and rotating movement.

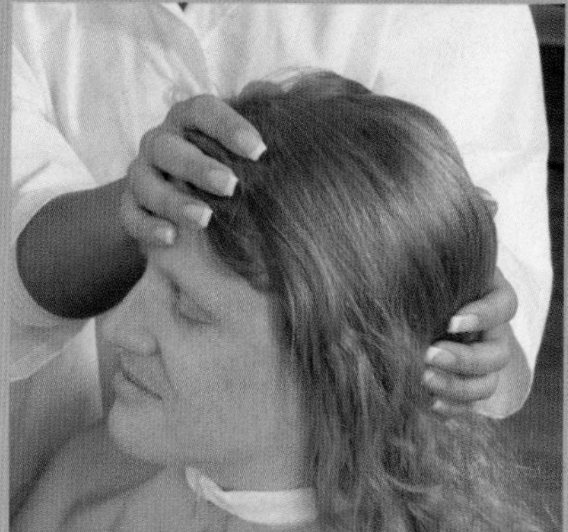

Figure 13–13 Forehead movement.

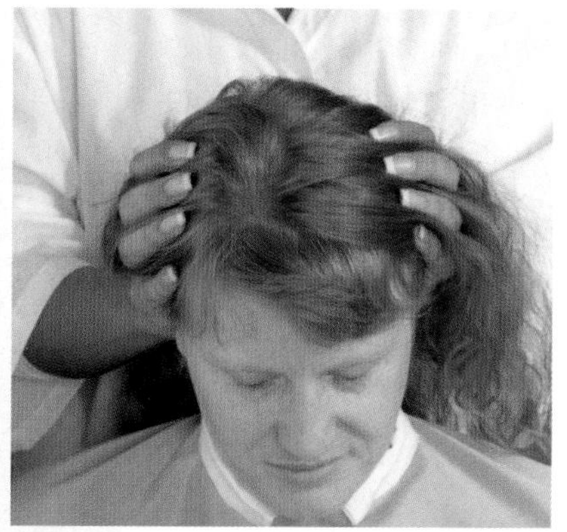

Figure 13–14 Scalp movement.

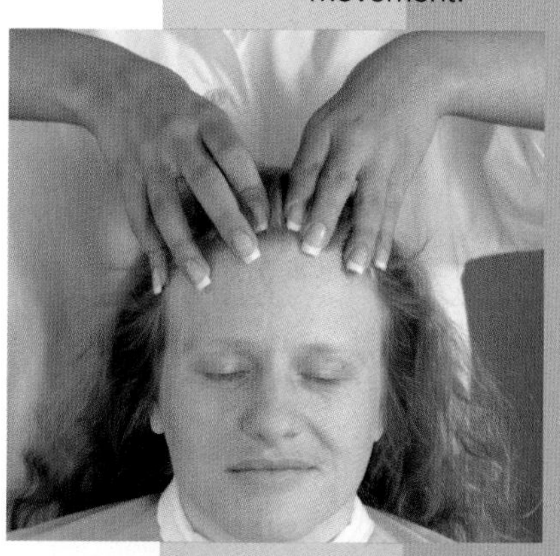

Figure 13–15 Hairline movement.

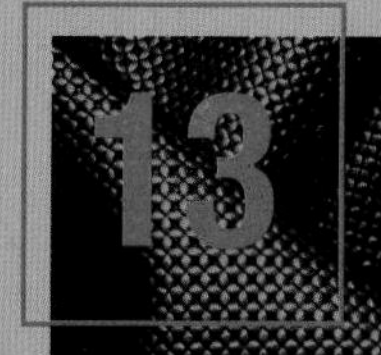

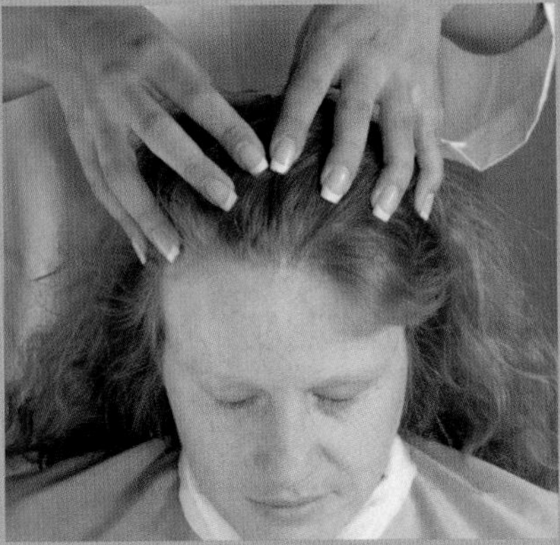
Figure 13-16 Front scalp movement.

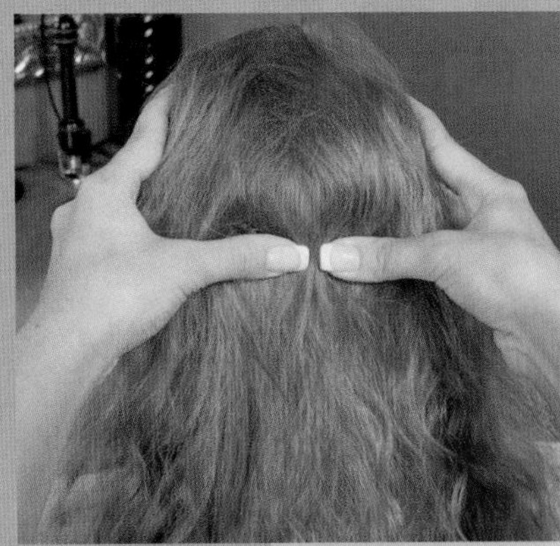
Figure 13-17 Back scalp movement.

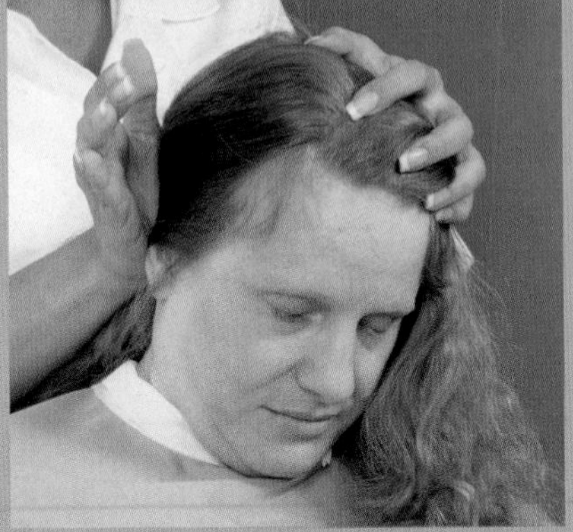
Figure 13-18 Ear-to-ear movement.

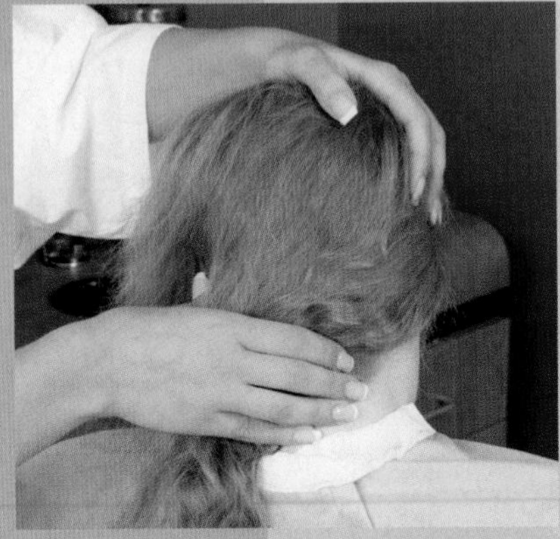
Figure 13-19 Back movement.

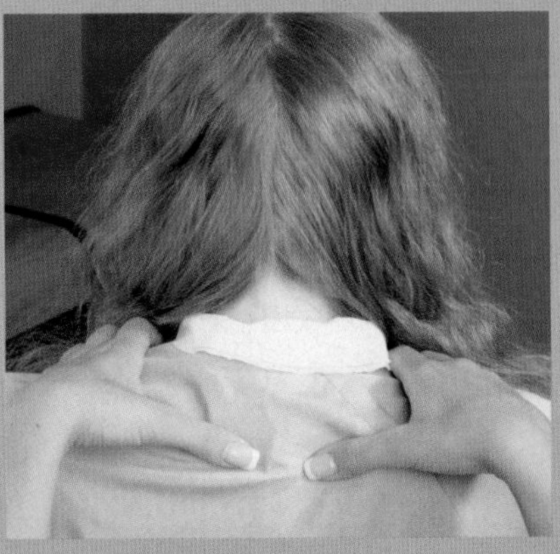
Figure 13-20 Shoulder movement.

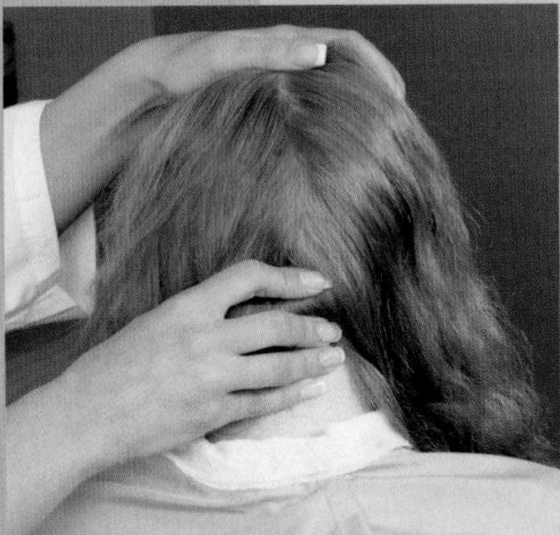
Figure 13-21 Spine movement.

7. **Front scalp movement:** Dropping back 1 inch, repeat the preceding movement over entire front and top of the scalp (Figure 13-16).
8. **Back scalp movement:** Place the fingers of each hand on the sides of the client's head. Starting below her ears, manipulate the scalp with your thumbs, working upward to the crown. Repeat four times. Repeat thumb manipulations, working toward the center back of the head (Figure 13-17).
9. **Ear-to-ear movement:** Place your left hand on the client's forehead. Massage from the right ear to the left ear along the base of the skull with the heel of your hand, using a rotary movement (Figure 13-18).
10. *Back movement:* Place your left hand on the client's forehead and stand to her left. Using your right hand, rotate from the base of the client's neck, along the shoulder, and back across the shoulder blade to the spine. Slide your hand up the client's spine to the base of her neck. Repeat on the opposite side (Figure 13-19).
11. *Shoulder movement:* Place both your palms together at the base of the client's neck. Using a rotary movement, catch the muscles in your palms and massage along the shoulder blades to the point of her shoulders, and then back again. Then massage from the shoulders to the spine and back again (Figure 13-20).
12. *Spine movement:* Massage from the base of the client's skull down the spine with a rotary movement. Using firm finger pressure, bring your hand slowly to the base of the client's skull (Figure 13-21).

SCALP MANIPULATION TECHNIQUE

There are several ways to effectively manipulate the scalp. The scalp manipulation procedure found on pages 229 and 230 may be adjusted in accordance with your instructor's recommendations.

With each massage movement, place the hands under the hair so that the length of the fingers, balls of the fingertips, and cushions of the palms can stimulate the muscles, nerves, and blood vessels of the scalp area.

SHAMPOO PROCEDURES

Before getting into the actual specifics of shampoo procedures, a few words about posture are in order. Maintaining good posture will protect you against the muscle aches, back strain, discomfort, fatigue, and other physical problems that can result from performing shampoos. Correct posture will also help you maintain an attractive image, an important consideration given your role as a model to your clients. The most important rule regarding posture is to always keep your shoulders back while performing the shampoo. This way, you will avoid slumping over the client. Remember, too, to hold your abdomen in, thereby lifting your upper body. Free-standing shampoo bowls allow for healthier body alignment and help reduce strain on the back and shoulders (Figure 13-22).

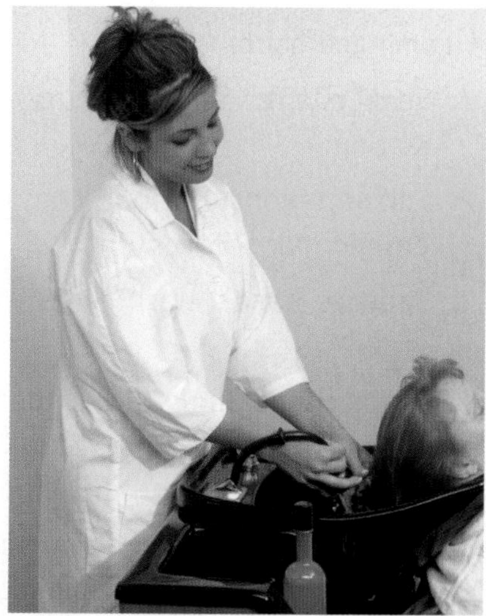

Figure 13-22 Correct posture at the shampoo bowl.

SHAMPOOING CHEMICALLY TREATED HAIR

Chemically treated hair tends to be drier and more fragile than natural hair. Therefore, a mild shampoo formulated especially for chemically treated hair is recommended. Chemically treated hair also tends to tangle. Use a wide-tooth comb to gently remove tangles, beginning at the nape, and work your way up to the frontal area. Do not force the comb through the hair. Use a conditioner, if necessary. Hair that has been relaxed or straightened tends to be less tangled, but it may mat if not moisturized properly before drying.

PROCEDURE 13-2

BASIC SHAMPOO

PREPARATION FOR SHAMPOOING NORMAL OR CHEMICALLY TREATED HAIR

The following implements and materials are routinely used when performing the shampoo service.

- Towels
- Shampoo cape
- Shampoo
- Conditioner (optional)
- Comb and hairbrush

1. **Seat client.** Seat client comfortably at workstation.
2. **Perform consultation.** Consult with client on desired hair services.
3. **Sanitize hands.** Wash hands with soap and warm water.
4. **Drape client.** Turn collar to the inside, if necessary. Place towel lengthwise across client's shoulders, crossing ends beneath the chin (Figure 13-23).
5. **Place cape.** Place cape over the towel and fasten in the back so that cape does not touch the client's skin.
6. **Place towel.** Place another towel over the cape and secure in the front (Figure 13-24).
7. **Remove objects.** Remove hair ornaments, hairpins, and so on.
8. **Remove jewelry.** Have client remove jewelry and glasses.
9. **Analyze scalp.** Examine condition of hair and scalp and select appropriate products.
10. **Brush.** Brush hair thoroughly, if applicable.
11. **Massage scalp,** if applicable.

BRUSHING

1. **Part hair.** Use half-head parting.
2. **Part subsection.** Take subsection inch from front hairline to crown.

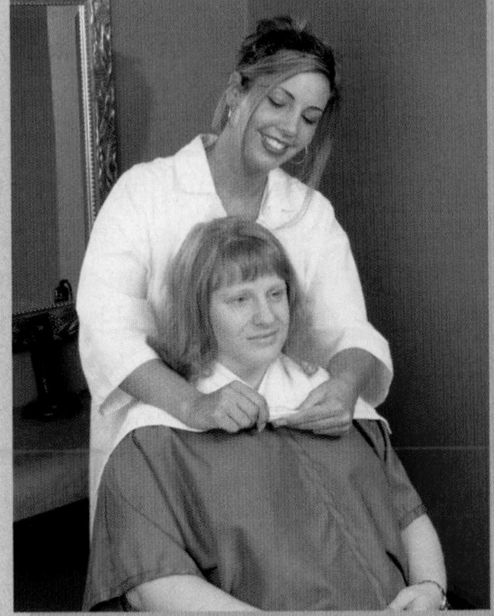

Figure 13-23 Cross ends of the towel under the chin.

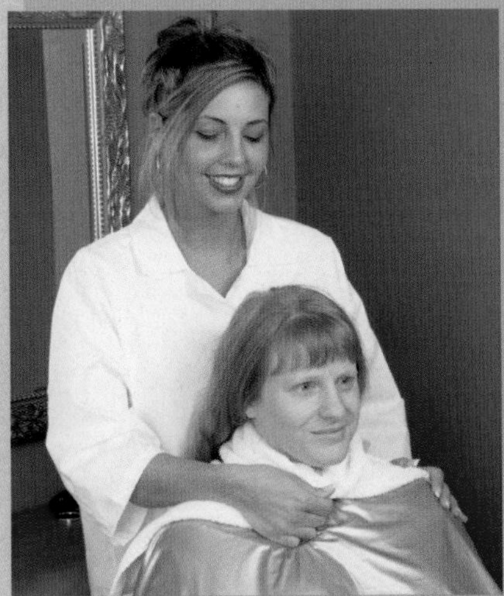

Figure 13-24 Place another towel over cape.

3. **Hold strand.** Hold hair in nondominant hand between thumb and fingers.
4. **Position brush.** Lay brush (held in dominant hand) with bristles down on hair close to scalp.
5. **Rotate brush.** Turn wrist slightly and sweep bristles full length of hair shaft.
6. **Repeat.** Repeat brushing three times on each strand.
7. **Complete brushing.** Continue brushing until entire head has been brushed.

SHAMPOO SERVICE

1. **Seat client.** Seat client comfortably at shampoo sink.
2. **Place cape.** Place cape over back of shampoo chair to prevent water from running down client's neck (Figure 13-25).
3. **Adjust water.** Adjust volume and temperature of water spray. (Test on inner wrist; monitor by keeping fingers under spray.)
4. **Saturate hair.** Wet hair with warm water. Lift hair and work it with free hand; protect client's face, ears, and neck from spray (Figure 13-26, Figure 13-27, Figure 13-28).
5. **Apply shampoo.** Apply small amounts of shampoo. Begin at the hairline, and work back and into lather using cushions of fingertips.

Reminder: Do *not* use firm pressure if following shampoo with a chemical service, if client's scalp is tender or sensitive, or if the client requests less pressure.

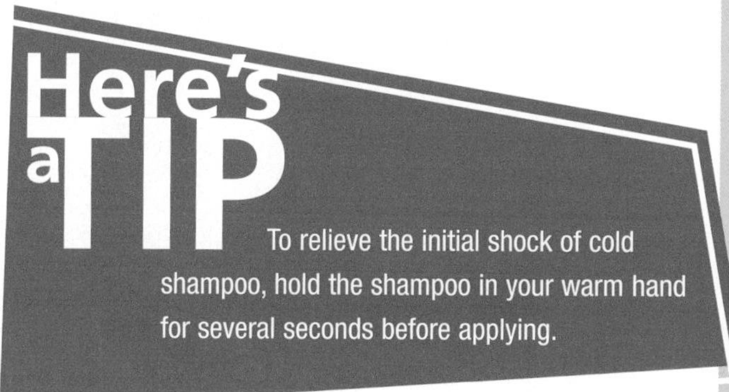

To relieve the initial shock of cold shampoo, hold the shampoo in your warm hand for several seconds before applying.

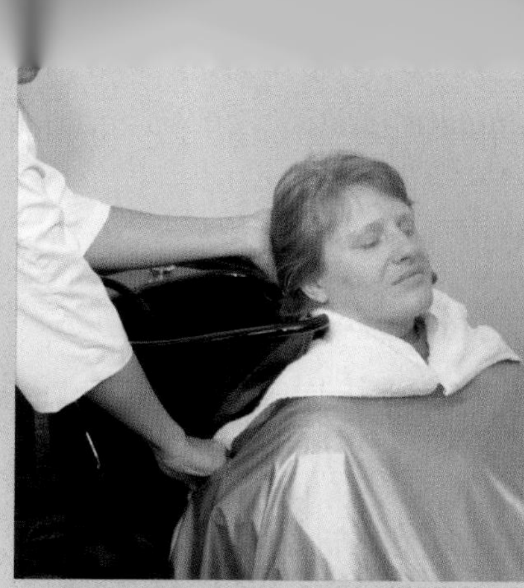
Figure 13-25 Adjust cape over back of shampoo chair.

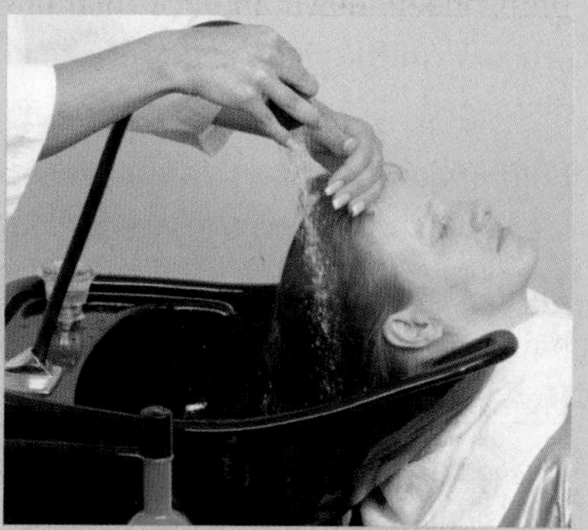
Figure 13-26 Protect the face.

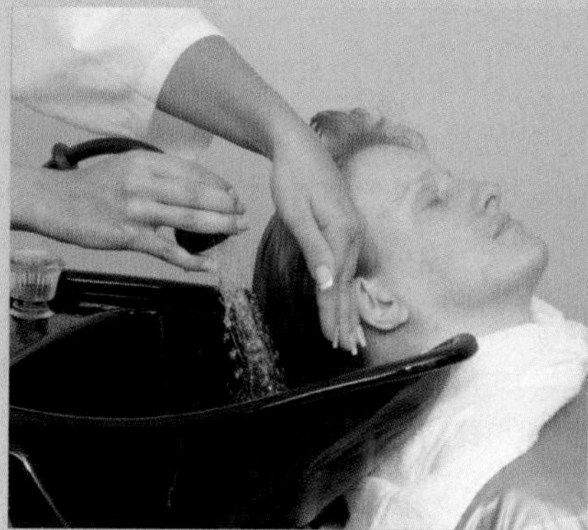
Figure 13-27 Protect the ears.

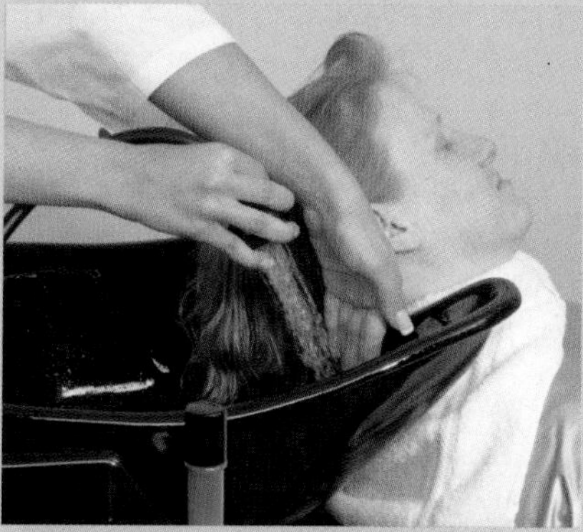
Figure 13-28 Protect the neck.

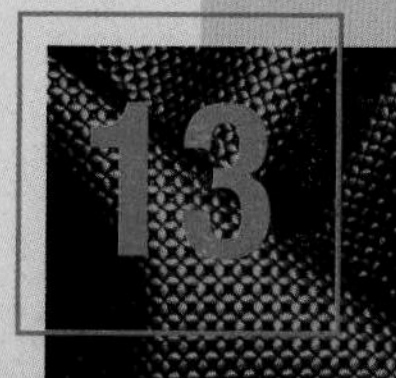

6. **Manipulate scalp.** Perform manipulations as follows:
   a. Begin at front hairline and work in back and forth movement until top of head is reached (Figure 13-29).
   b. Continue to back of head, shifting fingers back about 1 inch at a time.
   c. Lift head with left hand; with right hand start at top of right ear, using back and forth movement, and work to back of the head (Figure 13-30).
   d. Drop fingers down about 1 inch and repeat the process until right side of head has been massaged.
   e. Beginning at the left ear, repeat the prior two steps on the left side of head.
   f. Allow client's head to relax and work around hairline with thumbs in a rotary movement.
   g. Repeat all steps until scalp has been thoroughly massaged. Remove excess lather by squeezing hair gently.
7. **Rinse hair thoroughly.** Using strong spray:
   a. Lift hair at crown and back with fingers of left hand to permit spray to rinse hair thoroughly (Figure 13-31).
   b. Cup left hand along nape line and pat the hair, forcing spray against base scalp area.
8. **Shampoo again if needed.**
9. **Gently squeeze excess water from hair.** Apply conditioner avoiding base of hair near scalp. Gently comb conditioner through, distributing it with a wide-tooth comb (Figure 13-32).

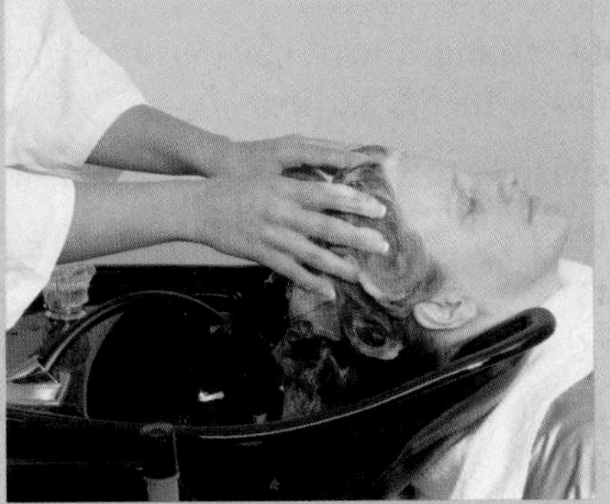
Figure 13-29 Manipulate the scalp.

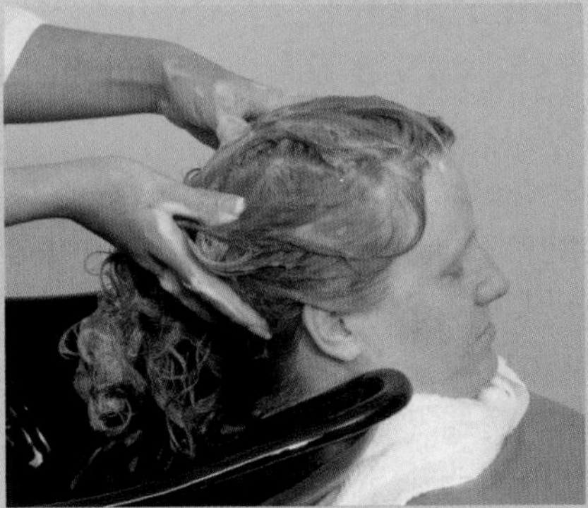
Figure 13-30 Lift the client's head

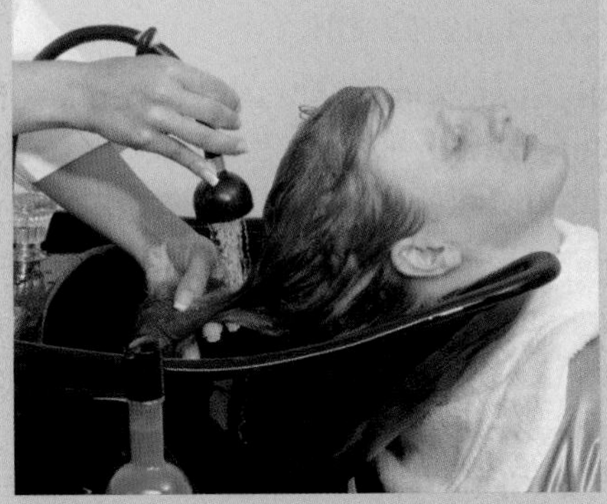
Figure 13-31 Rinse the client's hair.

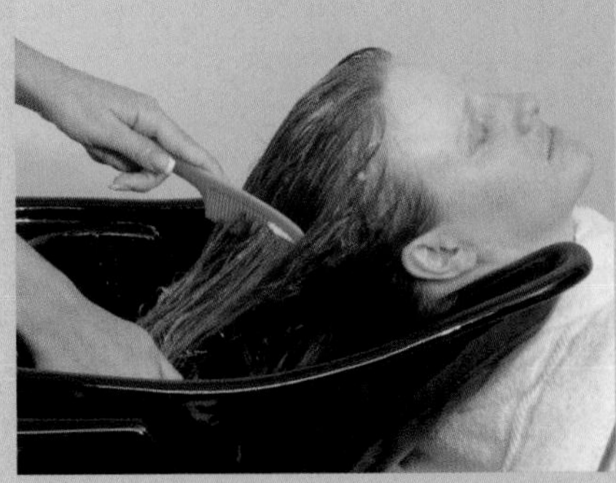
Figure 13-32 Comb conditioner through client's hair.

10. **Condition as recommended.** Rinse thoroughly and finish with a cool water rinse to seal cuticle.
11. **Place plastic cap on head.** If conditioner is to remain on hair more than 1 minute, place plastic cap on head and sit client upright for recommended time. If deep-conditioning treatment is applied, placing client under a heated dryer may be required; follow directions carefully (Figure 13-33).
12. **Partially towel dry hair.** While still at the shampoo bowl, partially towel dry hair as follows:
    a. Remove excess moisture from hair at shampoo bowl.
    b. Wipe excess moisture from around client's face and ears with ends of towel.
    c. Lift towel and drape over client's head.
    d. Place hands on top of towel and massage until hair is partially dry (Figure 13-34).
13. **Clean shampoo bowl.** Clean out shampoo bowl, removing any loose hair.
14. **Comb client's hair.** Comb client's hair, beginning with the end at the nape of the neck.
15. **Change drape.** Change the drape if necessary.

CLEAN-UP AND SANITATION

1. **Discard used materials.** Place unused supplies in proper place.
2. **Dispose of soiled towels.** Place soiled towels in hamper.
3. **Remove hair from combs and brushes.** Disinfect for the required time.
4. **Sanitize shampoo bowl.** Disinfect shampoo bowl after each client.
5. **Wash hands.** Wash your own hands with soap and warm water.

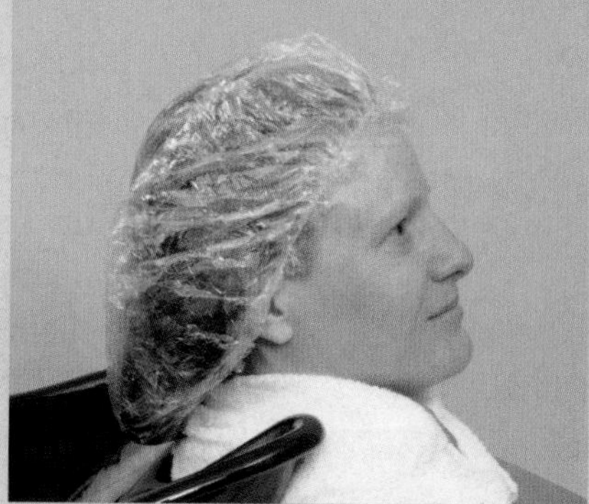

Figure 13-33 Some conditioners require a plastic cap.

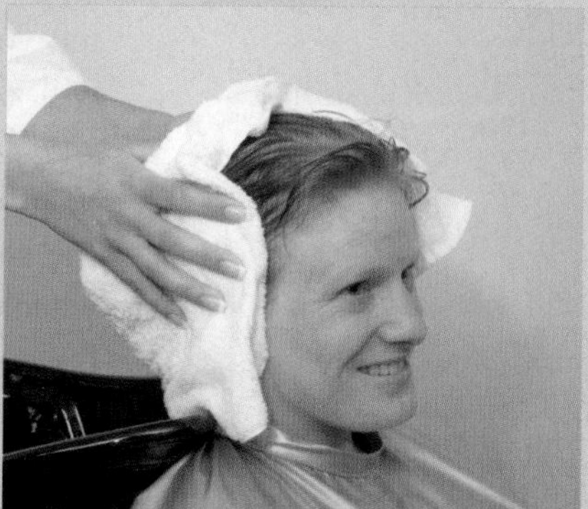

Figure 13-34 Towel-blot the client's hair.

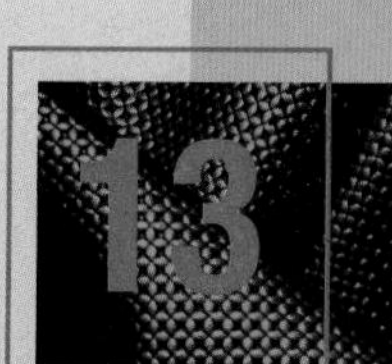

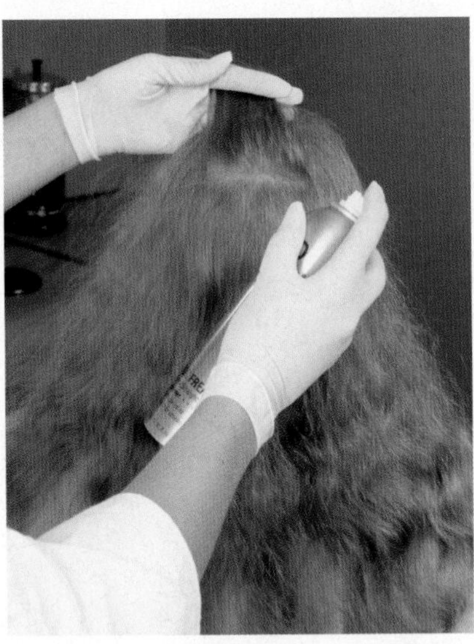

Figure 13-35 Applying powder or dry shampoo.

APPLYING DRY SHAMPOOS

Sometimes, as mentioned earlier, the state of a client's health makes a wet shampoo uncomfortable or hard to manage. For instance, an elderly client may experience some discomfort at the shampoo bowl due to pressure on the back of the neck. In such cases, it is advisable to use a dry or powder shampoo. A dry shampoo can be applied at the stylist's station, with the client draped as for a chemical service. Follow the manufacturer's directions, as they will vary. For the most part, you will be applying the powder directly to the hair from scalp to the ends, and then brushing through with a natural bristle brush to remove oil and dirt (Figure 13-35).

SHAMPOOING CLIENTS WITH SPECIAL NEEDS

Clients with disabilities or those who are wheelchair-bound will usually tell you how they prefer to be shampooed. Some clients in wheelchairs will allow you to shampoo their hair while they remain seated in their wheelchairs, facing the shampoo bowl and bending forward, with a towel to protect their face. If the wheelchair is the correct height in relation to the shampoo bowl, shampoo as normal while the client remains in the wheelchair. Sometimes, a client will arrive in the salon with her hair freshly shampooed from home, and sometimes a dry shampoo is appropriate. The same goes for clients with other special needs. Always ask about their preferences and make their comfort and safety a priority.

ACTIVITY

Role playing is a good way to practice recommending retail products to clients. Pair off with a classmate. One takes the role of the stylist and the other plays a client. Your "scene" might go like this:

Stylist: Have you encountered any problems with your scalp or hair since your last salon visit, Mrs. Benson? Any itchiness or flaking?

Mrs. Benson: No. I don't usually have scalp problems this time of year. But in the winter I do.

Stylist: Any dryness?

Mrs. Benson: Well, ever since I started having my hair highlighted, it does feel a little drier.

Stylist: Chemical services often dry the hair. I'm going to use this shampoo for color-treated hair and finish with this moisturizing conditioner. (Show and place shampoo and conditioner bottles in client's hands.)

Mrs. Benson: That sounds good. But won't the conditioner make my hair feel limp?

Stylist: I'll be using a light-weight conditioner only on your ends where you need it. It'll leave your hair silky and shiny and not weigh it down. If you like it, you can purchase some before you leave. You know, using the right shampoo and conditioner will help keep your hair healthy between visits to the salon.

Mrs. Benson: Great! Let's do it!

PROCEDURE 13-3

GENERAL HAIR AND SCALP TREATMENTS

NORMAL HAIR AND SCALP TREATMENTS

The purpose of a general scalp treatment is to keep the scalp and hair in a clean and healthy condition. A hair or scalp treatment should be recommended only after a hair and scalp examination. If the client does not have the time to sit for a treatment, recommend scheduling the treatment at a later, more convenient time. If the client does request a treatment at that time, it should be given either before or after the shampoo, depending on which treatment is given.

1. Drape the client.
2. Brush hair for 5 minutes.
3. Apply scalp conditioner.
4. Apply heat for about 5 minutes.
5. Manipulate scalp for 10 to 20 minutes.
6. Shampoo the hair.
7. Towel dry the hair.
8. Apply scalp lotion and/or styling aids.

DRY HAIR AND SCALP TREATMENTS

This treatment should be used when there is a deficiency of natural oil on the scalp and hair. Select scalp preparations containing moisturizing and emollient ingredients. Avoid the use of strong soaps, preparations containing a mineral oil or sulfonated oil base, greasy preparations, and lotions with high alcohol content. In this treatment, a scalp steamer, which resembles a hooded dryer, is used.

1. **Drape.** Drape the client.
2. **Brush hair.** Brush the client's hair for about 5 minutes.
3. **Apply preparation.** Apply the scalp preparation for this condition.
4. **Apply steamer.** Apply the scalp steamer for 7 to 10 minutes, or wrap the head in warm steam towels for 7 to 10 minutes.
5. **Shampoo hair.** Give a mild shampoo.
6. **Towel dry.** Towel dry the hair and scalp thoroughly.
7. **Apply scalp cream.** Apply moisturizing scalp cream sparingly with a rotary, frictional motion.
8. **Stimulate scalp.** Stimulate the scalp with direct high-frequency current, using the glass rake electrode, for about 5 minutes.
9. **Rinse hair.** Rinse the hair thoroughly.

CAUTION

Do not use high-frequency current on hair treated with tonics or lotions that contain alcohol.

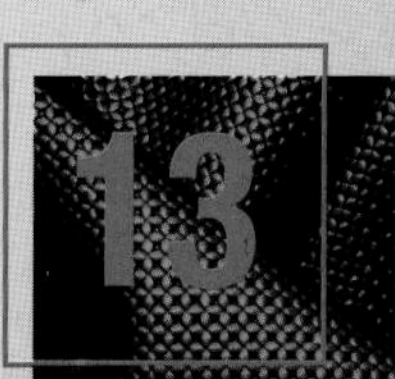

OILY HAIR AND SCALP TREATMENTS

Excessive oiliness is caused by overactive sebaceous (oil) glands. Manipulate the scalp and knead it to increase blood circulation to the surface. Any hardened sebum in the pores of the scalp will be removed with gentle pressing or squeezing. To normalize the function of these glands, excess sebum should be flushed out with each treatment.

1. **Drape.** Drape the client.
2. **Brush hair.** Brush the client's hair for about 5 minutes.
3. **Apply scalp lotion.** Using a cotton pledget (a tuft of cotton), apply a medicated scalp lotion to the scalp only (Figure 13-36).
4. **Apply lamp or heat.** Apply infrared lamp or heated dryer for about 5 minutes.
5. **Manipulate the scalp.**
6. **Shampoo hair.** Shampoo with a corrective shampoo for oily hair.
7. **Towel dry the hair.**
8. **Apply current.** Apply direct high-frequency current for 3 to 5 minutes (Figure 13-37).
9. **Apply astringent.** Apply a scalp astringent and/or suitable styling aids.

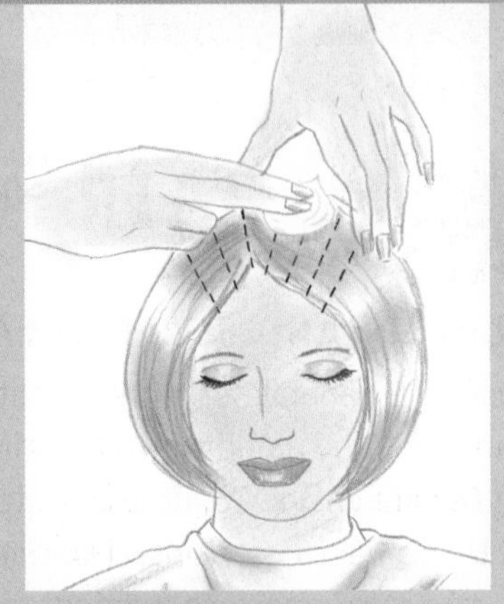

Figure 13-36 Apply scalp lotion with cotton pledget.

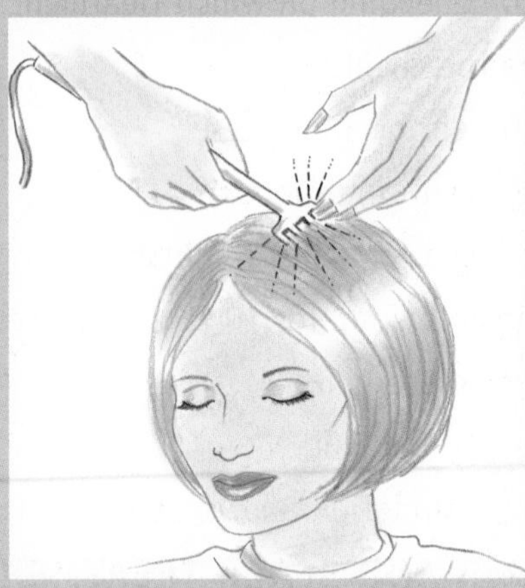

Figure 13-37 Apply high-frequency current.

ANTIDANDRUFF TREATMENTS

Dandruff is the result of a fungus called malassezia. Antidandruff shampoos, conditioners, and topical lotions contain antifungal agents that control dandruff by suppressing the growth of malassezia. Moisturizing salon treatments also soften and loosen scalp scales that stick to the scalp in crusts. You may treat a scalp with a dandruff condition with the following procedure.

1. **Drape.** Drape the client.
2. **Shampoo hair.** Shampoo with an antidandruff shampoo.
3. **Towel dry.** Towel dry the hair.
4. **Apply conditioner.** Apply an antidandruff conditioner or lotion.
5. **Apply heat or steamer.** Apply heat with an infrared lamp or scalp steamer for about five minutes (optional).
6. **Shampoo with an antidandruff shampoo.**

Because of the ability of fungus to resist treatment, additional salon treatments and the frequent use of antidandruff products at home should be recommended.

CAUTION

Some antidandruff lotions are alcohol based and should not be used in conjunction with infrared lamps.

REVIEW QUESTIONS

1. Why is pH an important factor in shampoo selection?
2. Name four ways in which water can be purified.
3. What is the chemical action of surfactants in shampoo?
4. What shampoo and/or conditioner is appropriate for use on dandruff? On product buildup? On damaged hair?
5. What is the action of conditioner on the hair?
6. What is the purpose of brushing the hair prior to shampooing?
7. Describe the draping procedure for a shampooing service.
8. What hair services should not be preceded by shampooing, brushing, or massage?
9. Describe the hair and scalp treatment for oily hair, dry hair, and dandruff.
10. When are scalp massages performed?

CHAPTER GLOSSARY

acid-balanced shampoo	Shampoos that are balanced to the pH of skin and hair (4.5 to 5.5).
balancing shampoos	Shampoos that wash away excess oiliness from oily hair and scalp, while preventing the hair from drying out.
clarifying shampoos	Shampoos containing an acidic ingredient such as cider vinegar to cut through product buildup that can flatten hair; also increase shine.
color-enhancing shampoos	Shampoos created by combining the surfactant base with basic color pigments.
conditioners	Special chemical agents applied to the hair to deposit protein or moisturizer, to help restore its strength and give it body, or to protect it against possible breakage.
conditioning or moisturizing shampoos	Shampoos designed to make the hair smooth and shiny, avoid damage to chemically treated hair, and improve manageability of the hair.
deep-conditioning treatments	Chemical mixtures of concentrated protein and the heavy cream base of a moisturizer; used to provide treatments when an equal degree of moisturizing and protein treatment is required.
dry or powder shampoo	Shampoos that cleanse the hair without the use of soap and water.

CHAPTER GLOSSARY

hard water	Water containing certain minerals that reduce the ability of soap or shampoo to lather.
humectants	Substances that absorb moisture or promote the retention of moisture.
hydrophilic	Capable of combining with or attracting water.
instant conditioners	Conditioners that either remain on the hair for a very short period (1 to 5 minutes) or are left in the hair during styling ("leave-in" conditioners).
lipophilic	Capable of attracting oil.
medicated scalp lotions	Conditioners that promote healing of the scalp.
medicated shampoos	Shampoos containing special chemicals or drugs for reducing excessive dandruff or relieving other scalp conditions.
moisturizers	Products formulated to add moisture to dry hair, with a heavier formulation than instant conditioners and a longer application time.
nonstripping	Description of products that do not remove artificial color from the hair.
protein conditioners	Products designed to slightly increase hair diameter with a coating action, thereby adding body to the hair.
scalp astringent lotions	Products used to remove oil accumulation from the scalp; used after a scalp treatment and before styling.
scalp conditioners	Products, usually in a cream base, used to soften and improve the health of the scalp.
soft water	Rain water or chemically softened water that lathers easily with soap or shampoo.
spray-on thermal protectors	Products applied to hair prior to any thermal service to protect it from the harmful effects of blow-drying, thermal irons, or electric rollers.
surfactants	Cleansing or surface active agent.

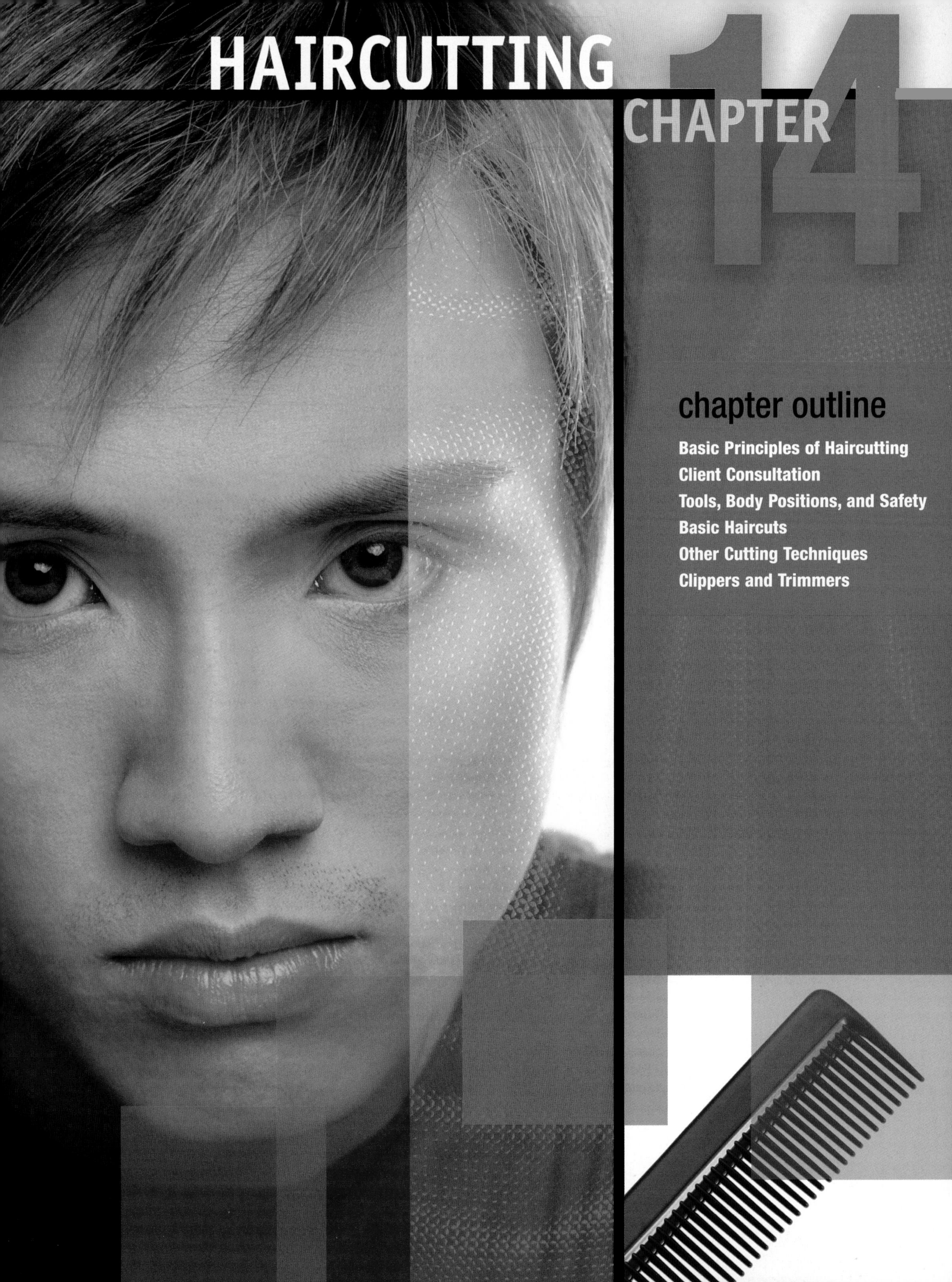

HAIRCUTTING

CHAPTER 14

chapter outline

Basic Principles of Haircutting
Client Consultation
Tools, Body Positions, and Safety
Basic Haircuts
Other Cutting Techniques
Clippers and Trimmers

Learning Objectives

After completing this chapter, you will be able to:

- **Identify reference points on the head form and understand their role in haircutting.**
- **Define angles, elevations, and guidelines.**
- **List the factors involved in a successful client consultation.**
- **Demonstrate the safe and proper use of the various tools of haircutting.**
- **Demonstrate mastery of the four basic haircuts.**
- **Demonstrate mastery of other haircutting techniques.**

Key Terms

Page number indicates where in the chapter the term is used.

angle **pg. 245**

apex **pg. 244**

bang (fringe) **pg. 245**

beveling **pg. 245**

blunt haircut **pg. 258**

carving **pg. 288**

clipper-over-comb **pg. 292**

cross-checking **pg. 260**

crown **pg. 245**

cutting line **pg. 246**

distribution **pg. 282**

elevation **pg. 246**

four corners **pg. 244**

free-hand notching **pg. 287**

free-hand slicing **pg. 289**

graduated haircut **pg. 258**

graduation **pg. 246**

growth pattern **pg. 251**

guideline **pg. 247**

hairline **pg. 251**

head form **pg. 243**

interior **pg. 247**

interior guideline **pg. 273**

layered haircut **pg. 258**

layers **pg. 258**

line **pg. 245**

long-layered haircut **pg. 259**

nape **pg. 245**

notching **pg. 287**

over-direction **pg. 248**

palm-to-palm **pg. 257**

parietal ridge **pg. 243**

part/parting **pg. 246**

perimeter **pg. 247**

point cutting **pg. 286**

razor-over-comb **pg. 290**

razor rotation **pg. 290**

reference points **pg. 243**

scissor-over-comb (shear-over-comb) **pg. 285**

sections **pg. 246**

slicing **pg. 288**

slide cutting **pg. 285**

slithering (effilating) **pg. 288**

stationary guideline **pg. 247**

subsections **pg. 246**

tapers **pg. 292**

tension **pg. 255**

texturizing **pg. 286**

traveling guideline **pg. 247**

uniform layers **pg. 273**

weight line **pg. 258**

Rapunzel, Samson, Joan of Arc, and the Beatles are just a few haircuts that have influenced many of us over the years. Haircuts through history have often demonstrated a change in the thinking of the time. Consider women bobbing their hair to express a newfound freedom in the 1920s or men and women who by not cutting their hair demonstrated protest during the 1960s. You will be able to give a great haircut once you have an understanding of the techniques and tools of cutting. And perhaps one day you will create the haircut that will rock the world.

BASIC PRINCIPLES OF HAIRCUTTING

Good haircuts begin with an understanding of the shape of the head, referred to as the **head form** or head shape. Hair responds differently on various areas of the head, depending on the length and the cutting technique used. Being aware of where the head form curves, turns, and changes will help you achieve the look that you and your client are seeking.

REFERENCE POINTS

Reference points on the head mark where the surface of the head changes, such as the ears, jaw line, occipital bone, or apex. These points are used to establish design lines (Figure 14-1).

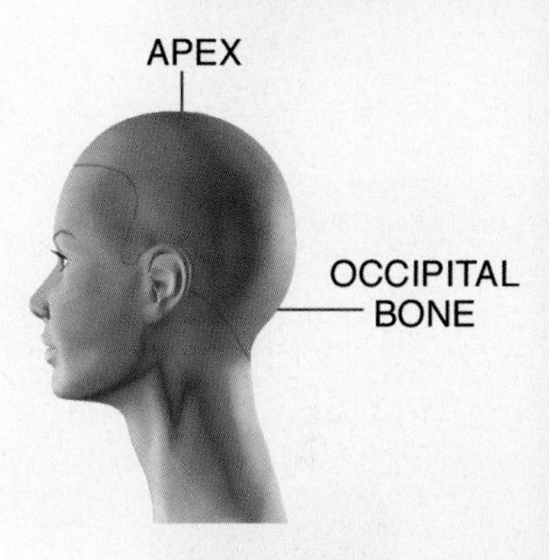

Figure 14-1 Reference points.

An understanding of head shape and reference points will help you in the following ways:

- Finding balance within the design, so that both sides of the haircut turn out the same
- Ability to recreate the same haircut
- Showing where and when it is necessary to change technique to make up for irregularities in the head form (e.g., if a client has a flat crown, you may choose to use a technique in that area to achieve more volume)

Standard reference points are defined below.

- **Parietal ridge.** The widest area of the head, starting at the temples and ending at the bottom of the crown. This area is easily found by placing a comb flat on the side of the head: the parietal ridge is found where the head starts to curve away from the comb. Also referred to as the crest area (Figure 14-2).

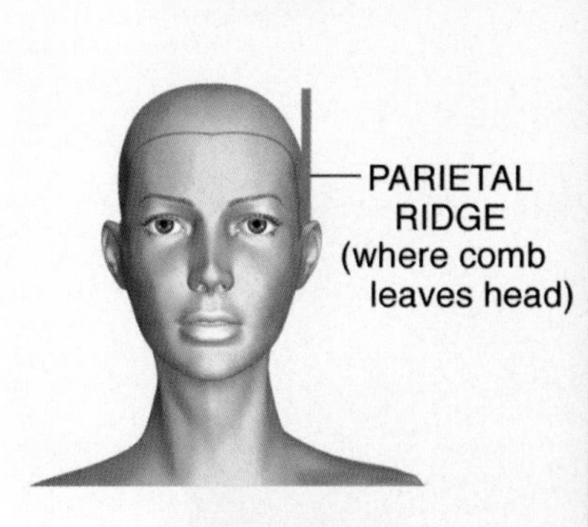

Figure 14-2 The parietal ridge.

- **Occipital bone.** The bone that protrudes at the base of the skull is the occipital bone. To find the occipital bone, simply feel the back of

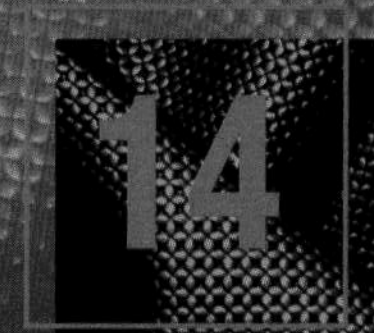

the skull, or place a comb flat against the nape and find where the comb leaves the head (Figure 14-3).

- **Apex.** Highest point on the top of the head. This area is easily located by placing a comb flat on the top of the head. The comb will rest on that highest point (Figure 14-4).
- **Four corners.** May be located in two different ways. First, place two combs flat against the side and back, locating the back corner at the point where the two combs meet (Figure 14-5). Second, make two diagonal lines crossing the apex of the head, pointing directly to the front and back corners (Figure 14-6).

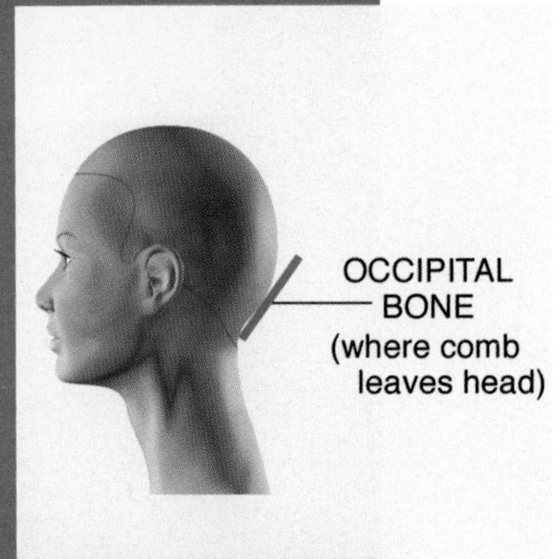

Figure 14-3 The occipital bone.

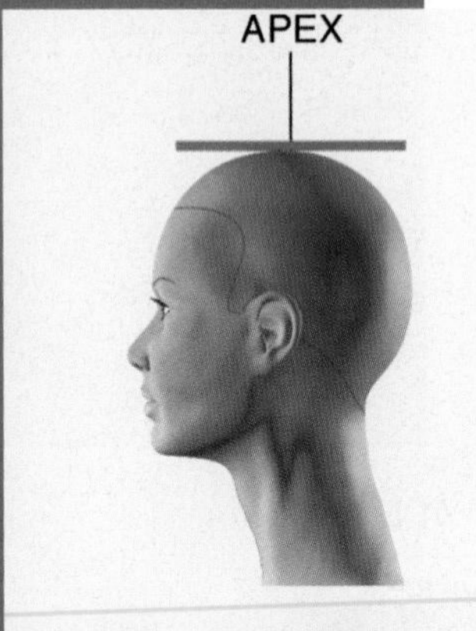

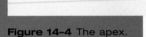

Figure 14-4 The apex.

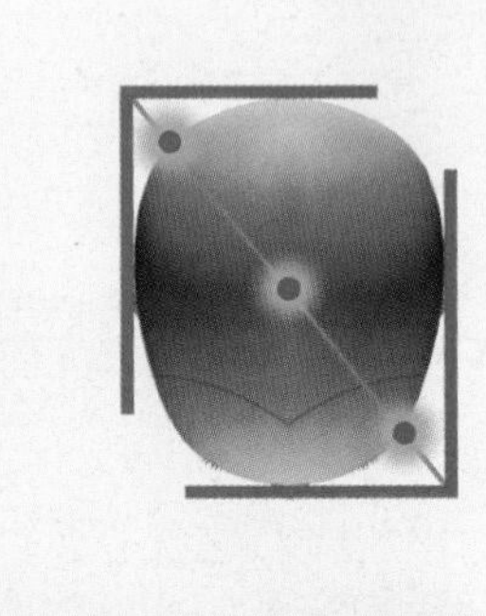

Figure 14-5 Locating the four corners.

You will not necessarily use every reference point for every haircut, but it is important to know where they are. The location of the four corners, for example, signals a change in the shape of the head from flat to round and vice versa. This change in the surface can have a significant effect on the outcome of the haircut. For example, the two front corners represent the widest points in the bang area. Cutting past these points can cause the bang to end up on the sides of the haircut once it is dry, creating an undesirable result.

AREAS OF THE HEAD

The areas of the head are described below (Figure 14-7).

- Top. By locating the parietal ridge, you can find the hair that grows on the top of the head. This hair "lies" on the head shape. Hair that grows below the parietal, or crest, "hangs" because of gravity. You can locate the top by parting the hair at the parietal ridge, and continuing all the way around the head.
- Front. By making a parting, or drawing a line from the apex to the back of the ear, you can separate the hair that naturally falls in front of the ear, from the hair behind the ear. Everything that falls in front of the ear is considered the front.
- Sides. The sides are easy to locate. They include all hair from the back of the ear forward, and below the parietal ridge.

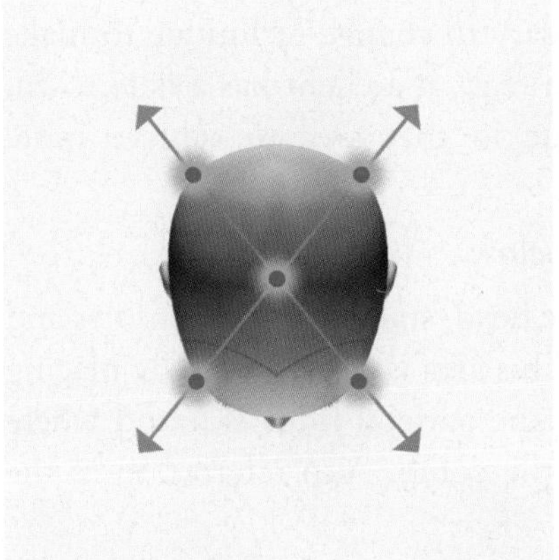

Figure 14-6 Another way to locate the four corners.

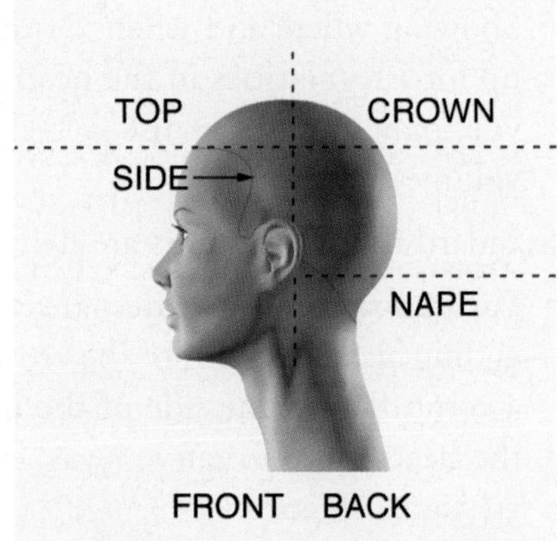

Figure 14-7 The areas of the head.

- **Crown.** The crown is the area between the apex and the back of the parietal ridge. On many people, the crown is often flat and the site of cowlicks or whorls. Because of this it is extremely important to pay special attention to this area when haircutting.
- **Nape.** The nape is the area at the back part of the neck and consists of the hair below the occipital bone. The nape can be located by taking a horizontal parting, or making a horizontal line across the back of the head at the occipital bone.
- Back. By making a parting or drawing a line from the apex to the back of the ear, you can locate the back of the head, which consists of all the hair that falls naturally behind the ear. When you have identified the front, you have also identified the back.
- **Bang (fringe) area.** The bang (fringe) area is a triangular section that begins at the apex and ends at the front corners (Figure 14-8). This area can be located by placing a comb on top of the head so that the middle of the comb is balanced on the apex. The spot where the comb leaves the head in front of the apex is where the bang area begins. Note how the bang area, when combed into a natural falling position, falls no farther than the outer corners of the eyes.

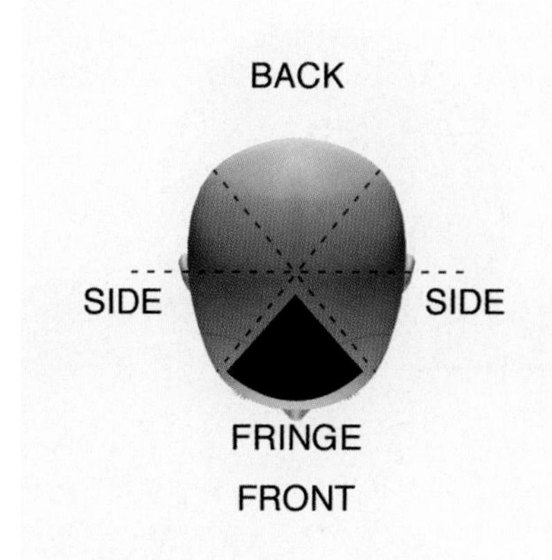

Figure 14-8 The bang area.

LINES AND ANGLES

Every haircut is made up of lines and angles. A **line** is a thin continuous mark used as a guide. An **angle** is the space between two lines or surfaces that intersect at a given point.

The two basic lines used in haircutting are straight and curved. The head itself is made up of curved and straight lines. By cutting lines into the hair, the hair will fall into a shape. (Figure 14-9). There are three types of straight lines in haircutting: horizontal, vertical, and diagonal (Figure 14-10).

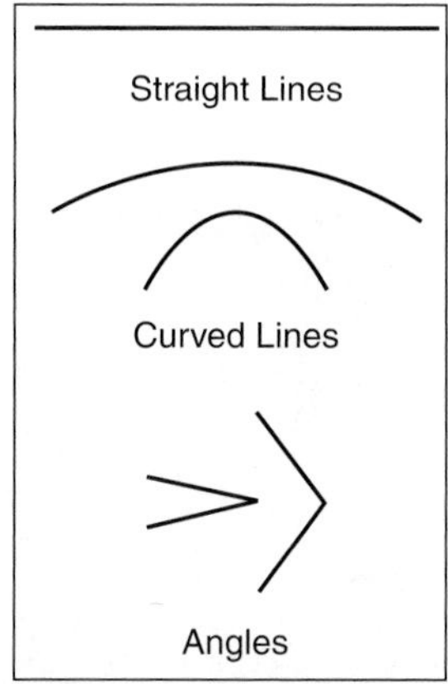

Figure 14-9 Lines and angles.

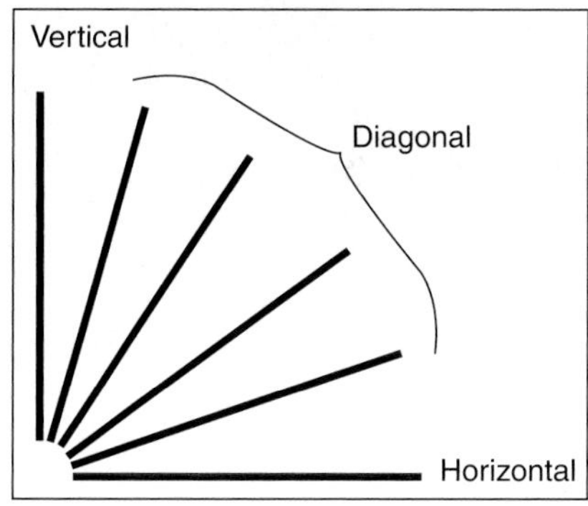

Figure 14-10 Horizontal, vertical, and diagonal lines.

- **Horizontal lines** are parallel to the horizon or the floor. Horizontal lines direct the eye from one side to the other. Horizontal lines build weight and are used to create one-length and low-elevation haircuts and weight (Figure 14-11).
- **Vertical lines** are usually described in terms of up and down and are perpendicular to the floor; they are the opposite of horizontal. Vertical lines remove weight to create graduated or layered haircuts, and are used with higher elevations (Figure 14-12).
- **Diagonal lines** are between horizontal and vertical. They have a slanting or sloping direction. Diagonal lines are used to create fullness in a haircut and to blend long layers into short layers (see Figure 14-13).

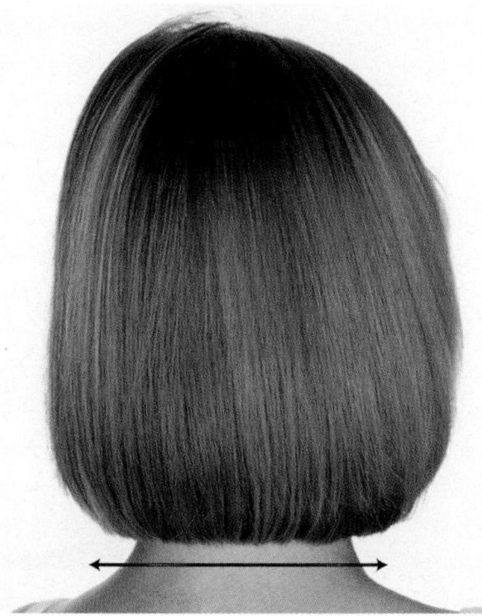

Figure 14-11 Horizontal line on a haircut.

Beveling and stacking are techniques using diagonal lines by cutting the ends

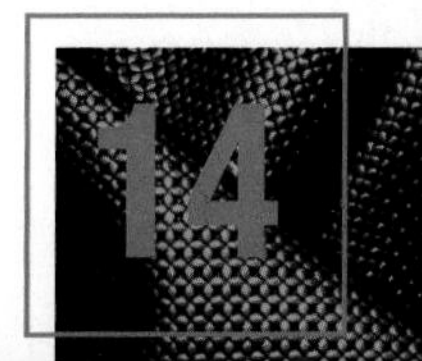

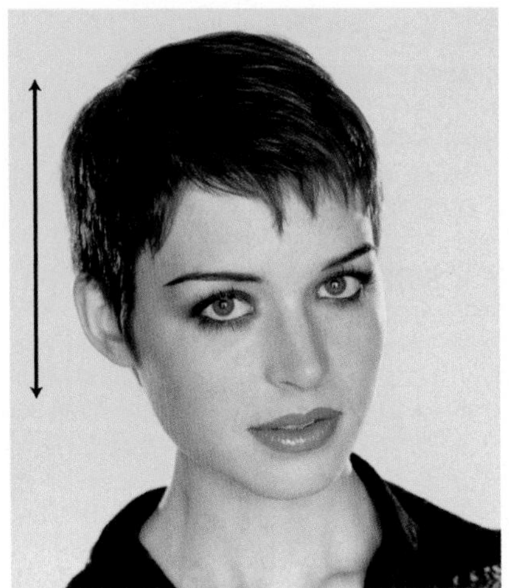
Figure 14-12 Vertical lines on a haircut.

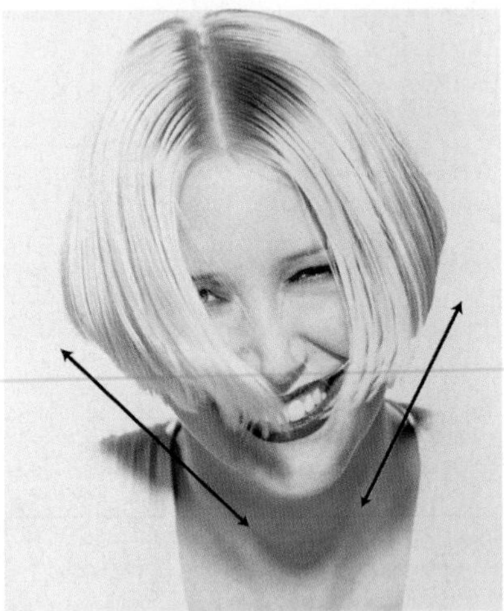
Figure 14-13 Diagonal lines on a haircut.

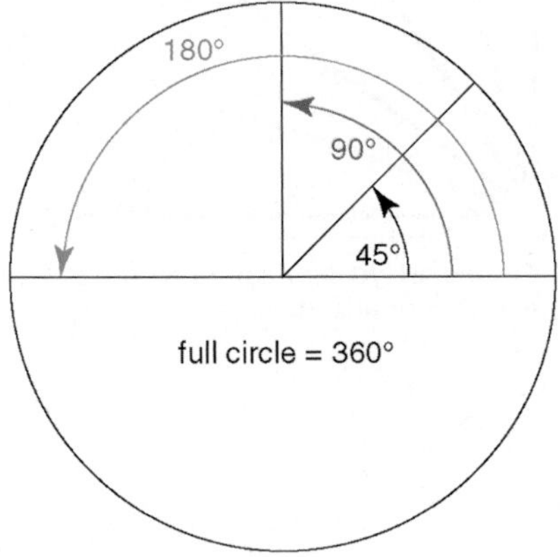

Figure 14-14 Angles.

of the hair with a slight increase or decrease in length. Angles are important elements in creating a strong foundation and consistency in haircutting (Figure 14-14) because this is how shapes are created.

ELEVATION

For control during haircutting, the hair is parted into uniform working areas, called **sections.** Each section may be divided into smaller partings called **subsections.** A **part** or **parting** is the line dividing the hair at the scalp, separating one section of hair from another, creating subsections. **Elevation** is the angle or degree at which a subsection of hair is held, or elevated, from the head when cutting. It is sometimes referred to as "projection" or simply "lifting" the hair. Elevation creates **graduation** and layers, and is usually described in degrees (Figure 14-15). In a blunt or one-length haircut, there is no elevation (0 degrees). Elevation occurs when you lift any section of hair above 0 degrees. If a haircut is not a single length, you can be sure that elevation was used.

When a client brings in a picture of a haircut she would like, you should be able to look at the picture and determine what elevations were used. Once you understand the effects of elevation, you can create any shape you desire. The most commonly used elevations are 45 and 90 degrees. *The more you elevate the hair, the more graduation you create.* When the hair is elevated below 90 degrees, you are building weight. When you elevate the hair at 90 degrees or higher, you are removing weight, or layering the hair. The length of the hair also affects the end result. The weight of longer hair often makes it appear heavier or less layered. You will usually need to use less elevation on curly hair than on straighter textures, or leave the hair a bit longer because of shrinkage when it dries.

CUTTING LINE

The **cutting line** is the angle at which the fingers are held when cutting the line that is cut creating the end shape. It is also known as cutting position, cutting angle, finger angle, and finger position. The cutting line can be described as horizontal, vertical, or diagonal, or by using degrees (Figures 14-16 to 14-18).

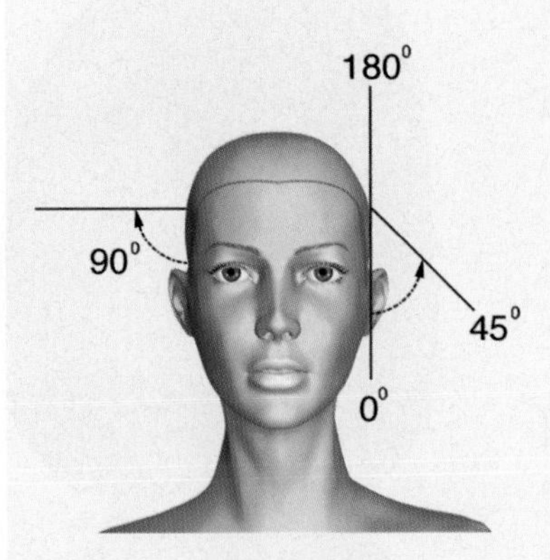

Figure 14-15 Angles relative to the head form.

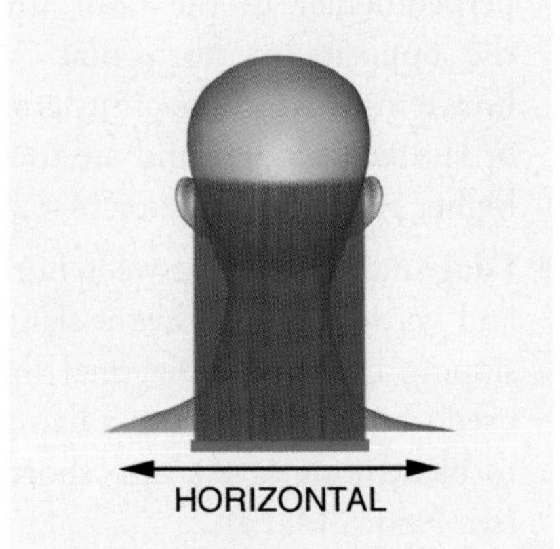

Figure 14-16 Horizontal cutting line.

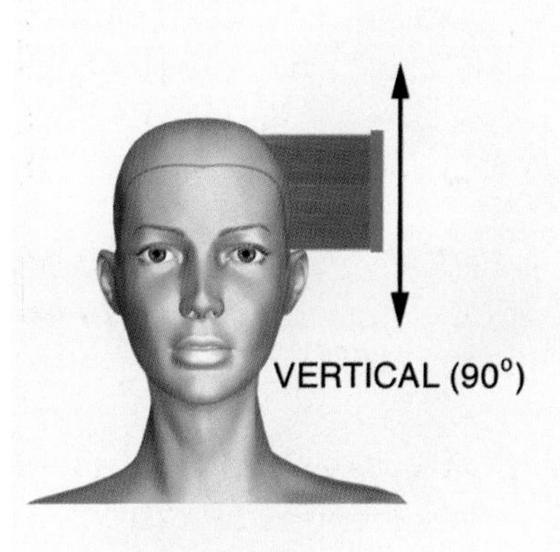

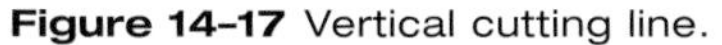

Figure 14-17 Vertical cutting line.

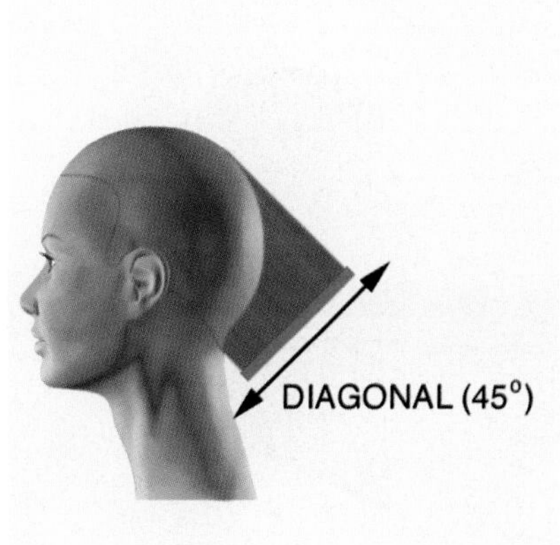

Figure 14-18 Diagonal cutting line.

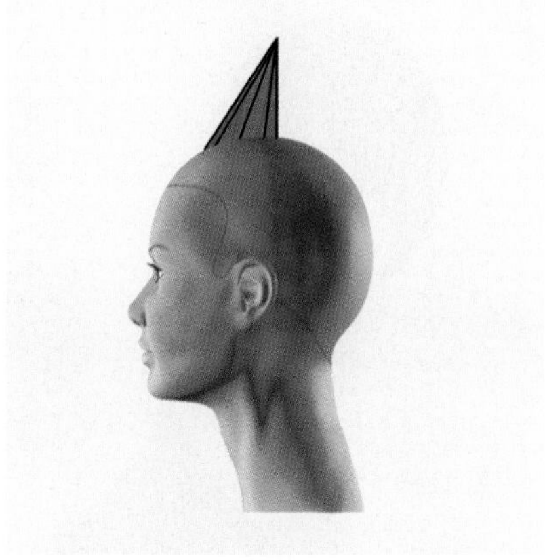

Figure 14-19 Stationary guideline.

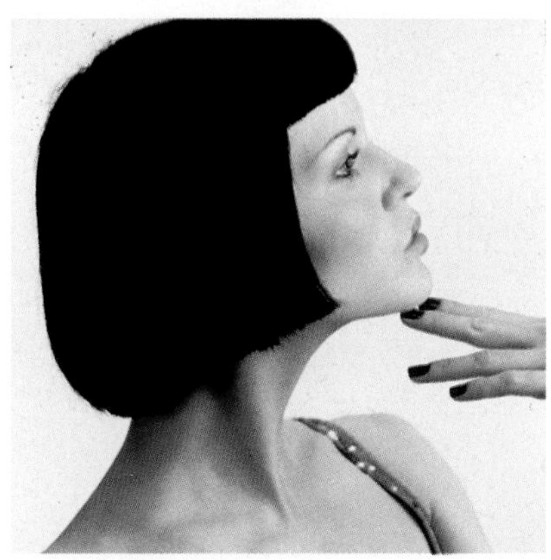

Figure 14-20 Blunt (one-length) haircut.

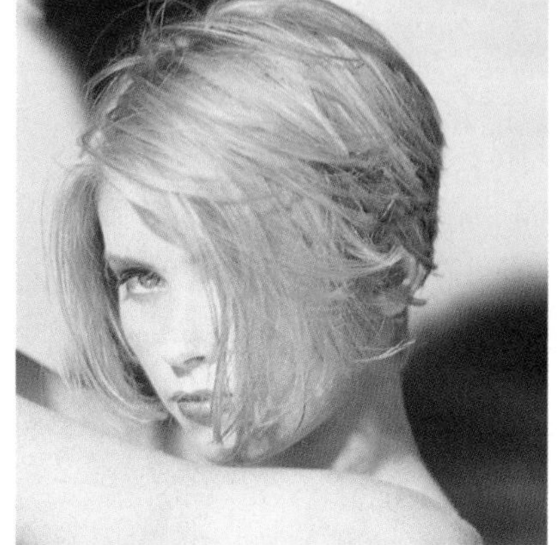

Figure 14-21 Graduated haircut.

GUIDELINES

A **guideline** (sometimes called a guide) is a section of hair that determines the length that the hair will be cut, located either at the **perimeter** (outer line) or the **interior** (inner or internal part) of the cut. It is usually the first section cut when creating a shape. The two basic guidelines in haircutting are stationary and traveling.

- A **stationary guidelin**e does not move (Figure 14-19). All other sections are combed to the stationary guideline and cut at the same angle and length. Stationary guidelines are used in blunt (single-length) haircuts (Figure 14-20), or if using over-direction to create a length or weight increase in a haircut (Figure 14-21).
- A **traveling guideline,** or movable guideline, moves as the haircut progresses. Traveling guidelines are used when creating layered or graduated haircuts (Figures 14-22 and 14-23). It travels with you as you work through the haircut (Figure 14-24). When you use a traveling guide, you take a small slice of the previous subsection and move it to the next position, or subsection, where it becomes your new guideline.

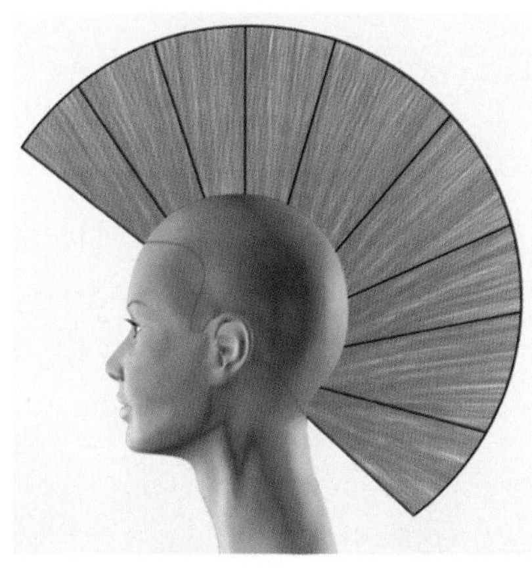

Figure 14-22 Traveling guideline.

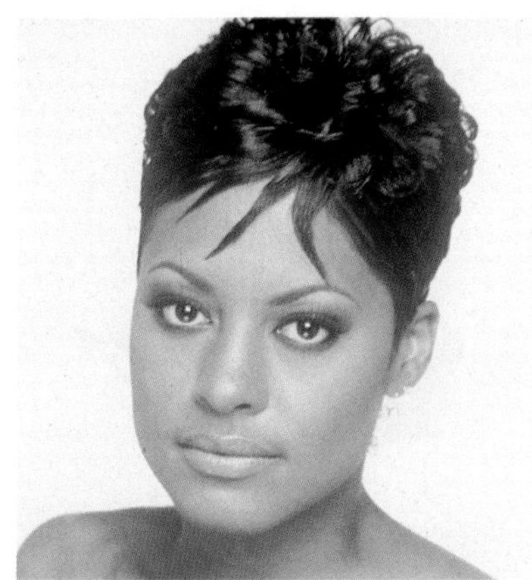

Figure 14-23 Uniform layered haircut.

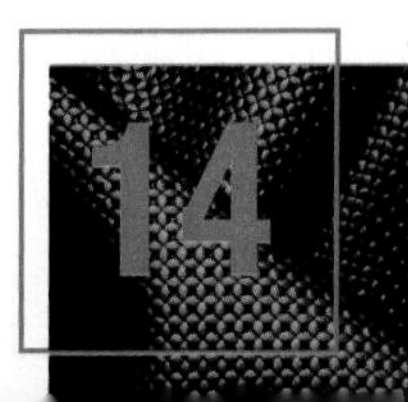

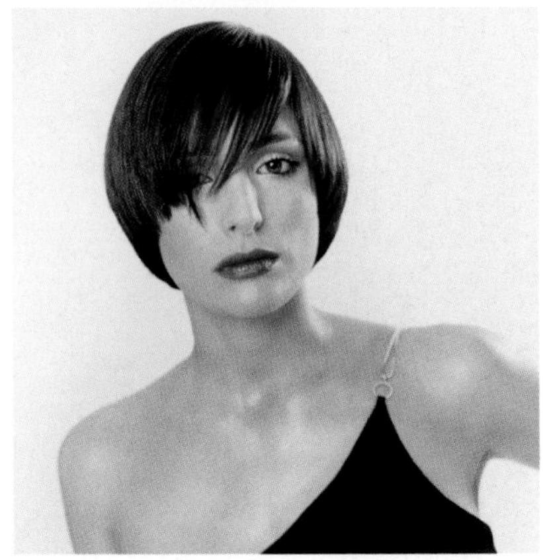

Figure 14-24 Graduated haircut.

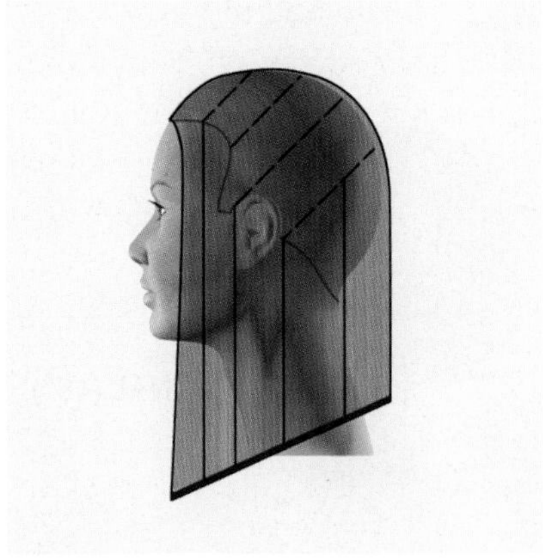

Figure 14-25 Blunt cut variation: design.

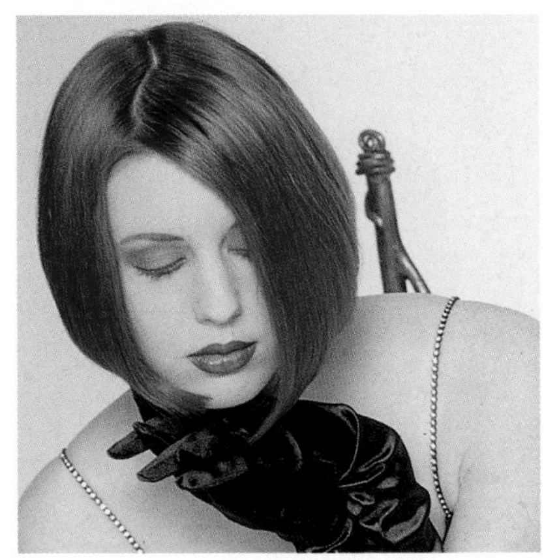

Figure 14-26 Finished blunt cut variation.

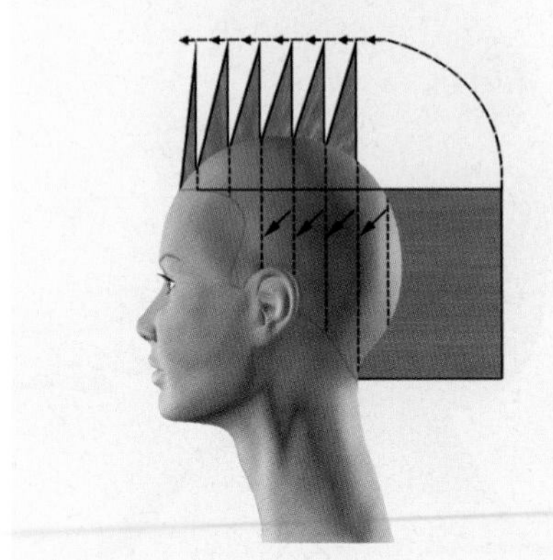

Figure 14-27 Layered cut variation: design.

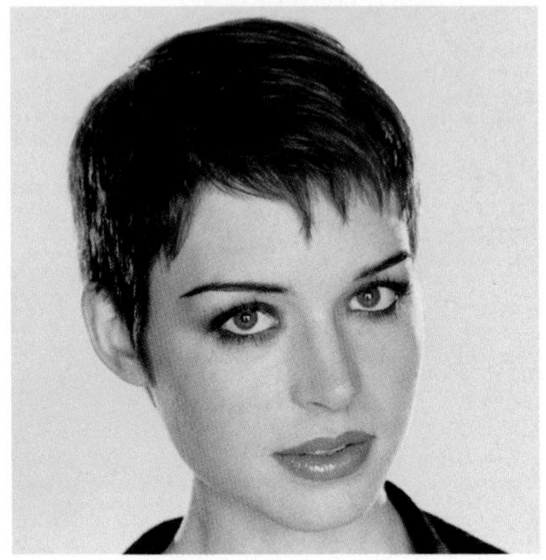

Figure 14-28 Finish layered cut variation.

The following are just a few of the shapes that can be created by using different elevations, cutting lines, and stationary and traveling guidelines. Keep in mind the varying amounts of weight that result from these combinations.

Figures 14-25 and 14-26 show a blunt (one-length haircut) cut with no elevation, a diagonal cutting line, and a stationary guideline. To achieve the layered shape in Figures 14-27 and 14-28, a 90-degree elevation was used, with a vertical cutting line and a traveling guideline. The next shape (Figures 14-29 and 14-30) was cut using a 45-degree elevation throughout the sides and back, creating a stacked effect with a diagonal (45-degree) cutting line. The top was cut using a 90-degree elevation (layered), and the entire shape was created using a traveling guideline.

OVER-DIRECTION

Over-direction is best understood by comparing it to elevation. Whereas elevation is simply the degree that you lift a section away from the head, over-direction occurs when you comb the hair away from its natural falling position, rather than straight out from the head, toward a guideline. Over-direction is used mostly in graduated and layered haircuts, and where you want to create a length increase in the design.

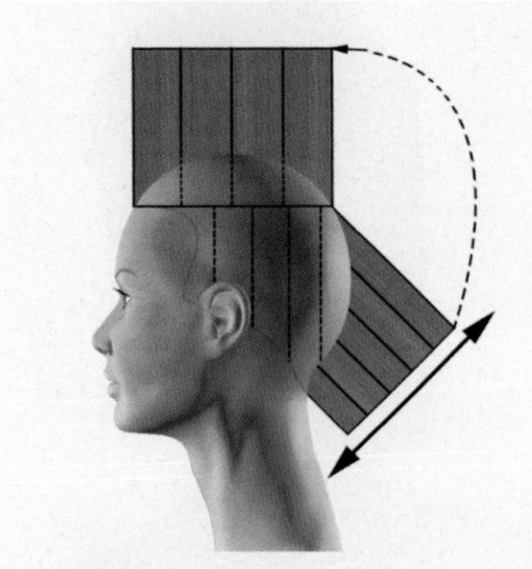

Figure 14-29 Graduated cut variation: design.

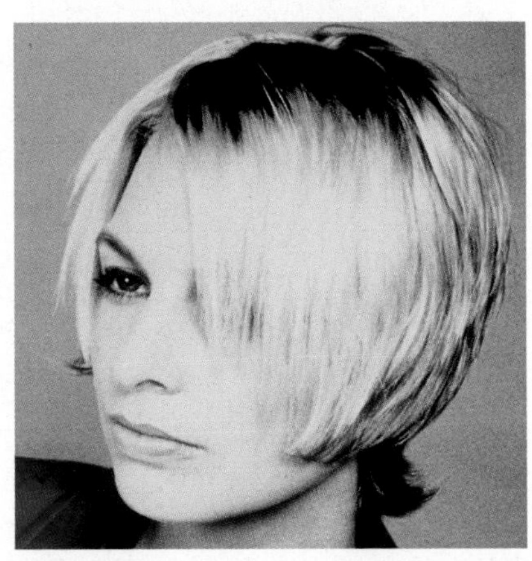

Figure 14-30 Finished graduated cut variation.

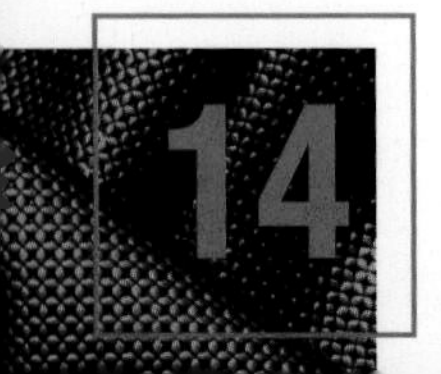

For example, you are working on a layered haircut and want the hair to be longer toward the front. You can over-direct the sections to a stationary guide at the back of the ear (Figures 14-31 and 14-32). Or, if you are creating a haircut with shorter layers around the face and longer layers in the back, you can over-direct sections to a stationary guide at the front (Figures 14-33 and 14-34).

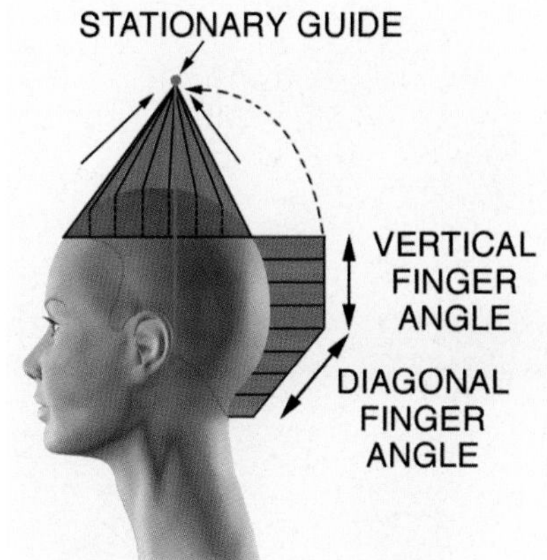

Figure 14-31 Over-direction in layered cut: design.

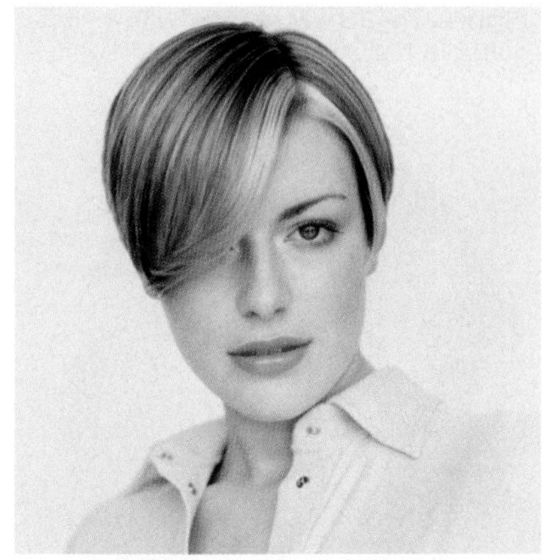

Figure 14-32 Finished layer cut.

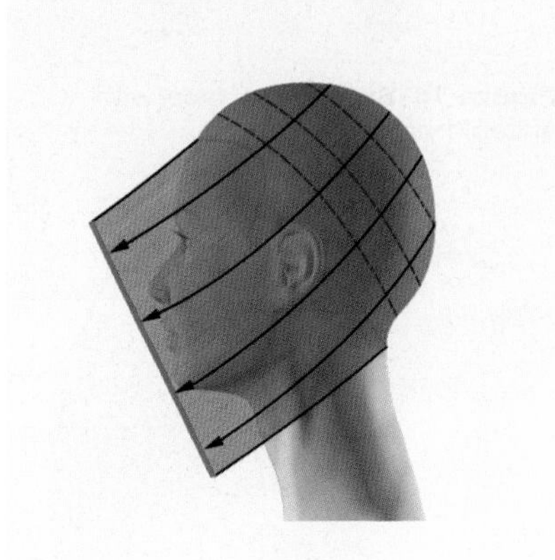

Figure 14-33 Over-direction in long layered cut: design.

CLIENT CONSULTATION

A great haircut always begins with a great consultation. A consultation is a conversation between you and your client where you find out what the client is looking for, offer suggestions and professional advice, and come to a joint decision about the most suitable haircut. If the client has a particular look in mind, you can discuss whether that look would be appropriate.

It can be difficult when a client asks for something that you know will not be the best look for her. This is when you will want to use gentle persuasion and positive reinforcement to offer alternative suggestions that will work with the client's hair texture, face shape, and lifestyle.

A great place to begin the consultation is to analyze the client's freshly cleansed and unstyled hair for its natural behavior and then ask the client if there is anything she would like to ask or tell you about her hair. Sometimes she may ask you for your suggestions. Before recommending anything, there are many factors to consider. How much time is the client willing to spend on her hair every day? What is her lifestyle? Does she want something that is classic or trendy? A good example is when a client with naturally curly thick hair is asking for a haircut that is really designed for straight hair, will she be willing to take the time to blow dry it straight every day? This is the time when you will need to analyze hair density and texture, growth patterns, and hairline, or if the client has hair that grows straight up at the nape and is requesting a short haircut that is soft and wispy at the nape. In cases like this, because her hairline will not lie down, you must suggest other haircuts that will work with her kind of hairline.

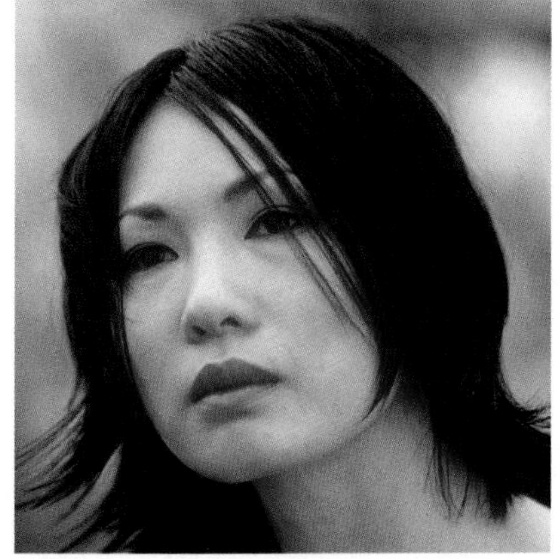

Figure 14-34 Finished long layered cut.

FACE SHAPE

Another part of the consultation is analyzing the face shape. To analyze the shape of a client's face, pull all the hair away with a clip or wrap the hair in a towel. Look for the widest areas, the narrowest areas, and the balance of the features. A quick way to analyze a face shape is to determine if it is wide or

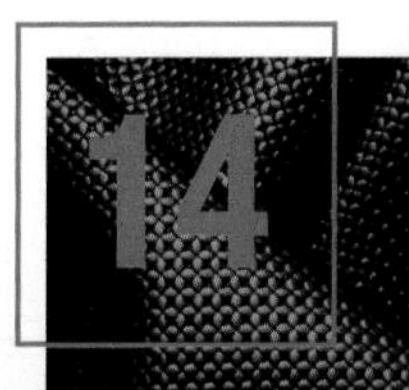

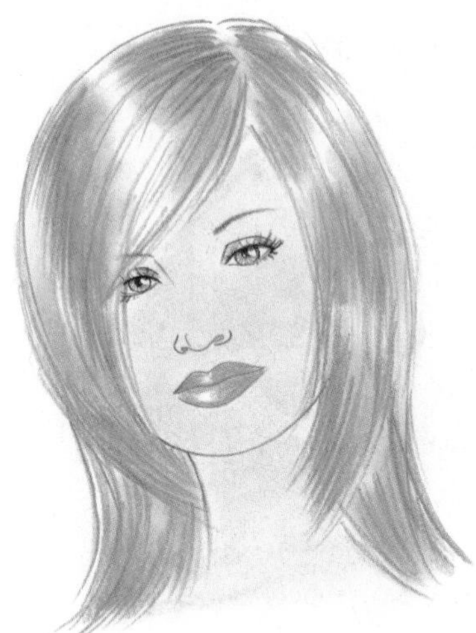

Figure 14-35 Wide face with suitable hairstyle.

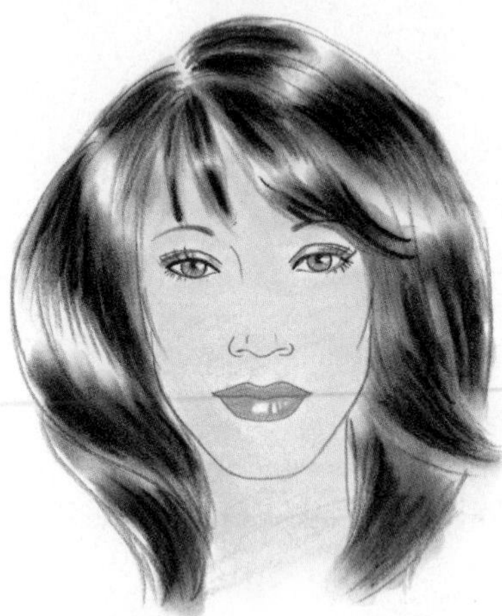

Figure 14-36 Narrow face with suitable hairstyle.

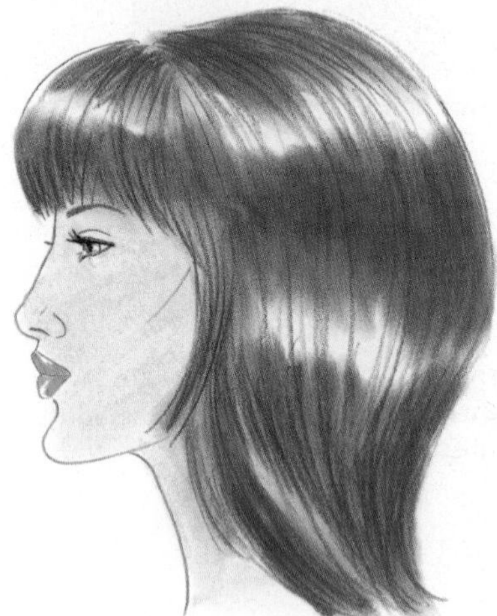

Figure 14-37 Flattering style for client with prominent chin.

long. Look for the features that you want to bring out, and those you might want to de-emphasize. See Chapter 12 for examples of face shapes.

By analyzing the face shape, you can begin to make decisions about the best haircut for the client. An important thing to remember is that weight and volume draw attention to an area. For example, if a client has a wide face, a hairstyle with fuller sides makes the face appear wider, whereas a narrower shape will give length to the face. If the client has a long face, a hairstyle with fullness on the sides will add width. If a client has a narrow forehead, on the other hand, you can add visual width by increasing volume or weight in that area. In order to balance out face shapes or draw the eye away from certain areas, you need to add or remove weight or volume in other areas. Figures 14-35 and 14-36 illustrate two face shapes and haircuts that help create balance.

Another important point to consider is the client's profile, or how she looks from the side. Turn the chair so you can see your client from the side. Pull the hair away from the face and up and away from the neck. What do you see? Look for features to emphasize, such as a nice jaw line or lovely neck. Look also for features to draw attention away from, such as a prominent or receding chin, a double chin, or an overly large nose. The haircut you choose should flatter the client by emphasizing good features and taking attention away from features that are not as flattering. For example, if a client has a prominent chin, you will want to balance the shape by adding volume or weight somewhere else (Figure 14-37). If the client has a prominent nose, you can balance the shape of the profile by adding weight in the appropriate place (Figure 14-38).

The consultation is also the time to decide on the type of part the client will wear. Will you be working with her natural part, a center part, or a side part?

During the consultation, it is helpful to use parts of the face and body as points of reference when describing the length of the haircut. For example, you could say, "Would you like your hair to be chin length or shoulder length?"

Hair shrinks when it dries. Once you and the client have decided on the length, keep in mind that the hair will shrink ¼ inch (0.6 centimeters) to ½ inch (1.25 centimeters) after it is dry. In other words, you need to cut the hair ¼ to ½ inch longer than the desired length. If the hair is curly, it will shrink ½ to 2 inches (5 centimeters) or more. Be sure to check with your instructor when deciding on the length for curly-haired clients.

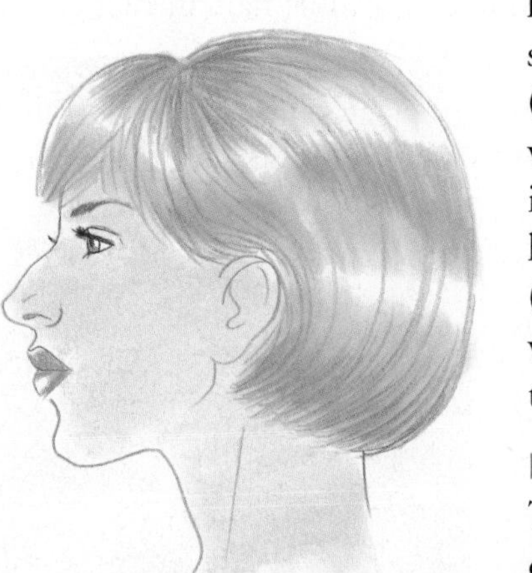

Figure 14-38 Flattering style for client with prominent nose.

HAIR ANALYSIS

There are five characteristics that determine the behavior of the hair (see Chapter 9 for a more thorough discussion):

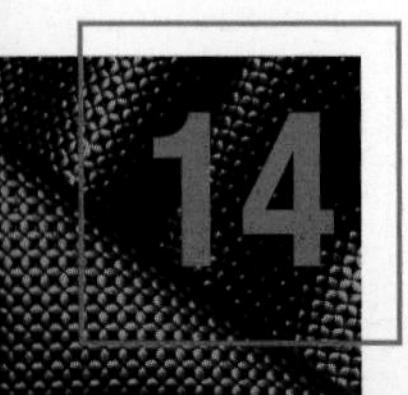

- Texture
- Density
- Porosity
- Elasticity
- Growth patterns

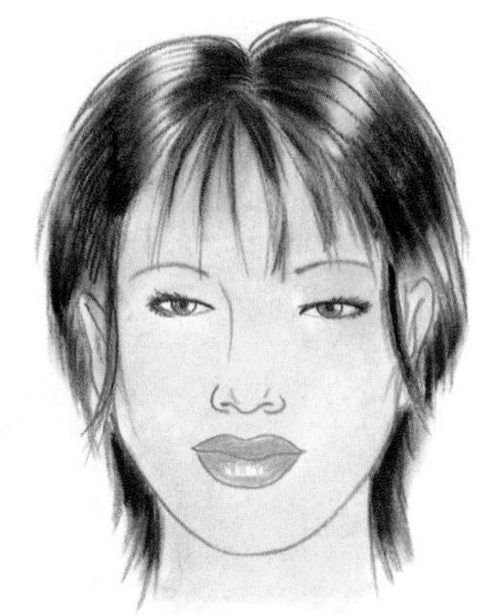

Figure 14-39 Uniform layered cut on fine, thin hair.

HAIRLINES AND GROWTH PATTERNS

Both the hairline and growth patterns are important to examine. The **hairline** is the hair that grows at the outermost perimeter along the face, around the ears, and on the neck. The **growth pattern** is the direction in which the hair grows from the scalp, also referred to as natural fall or natural falling position. Cowlicks, whorls, and other growth patterns affect where the hair ends up once it is dry (see Chapter 9). You may need to use less tension when cutting these areas to compensate for hair being pushed up when it dries, especially in the nape, or to avoid getting a "hole" around the ear in a one-length haircut. Another crucial area is the crown (there may be some wild things going on up there!).

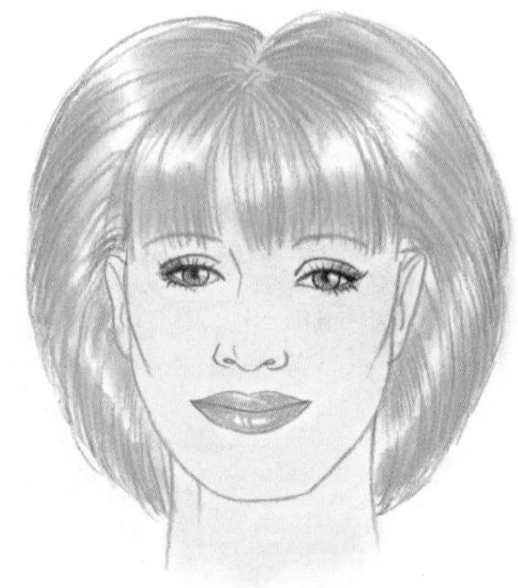

Figure 14-40 Uniform layered cut on thick, coarse hair.

HAIR DENSITY

Hair density is the number of individual hair strands on 1 square inch of scalp. It is usually described as thin, medium, or thick.

HAIR TEXTURE

Hair texture is based on the thickness or diameter of each hair strand, usually classified as coarse, medium, and fine. A fine hair strand is much "skinnier" than a coarse hair strand. A client may, in fact, have fine-textured hair with a thick density, meaning that the individual hairs are fine, but there are a lot of them. Or a client may have coarse texture but thin density, meaning the individual hairs are "fatter," but they are spaced farther apart.

Density and texture are important because the different hair types respond differently to various types of cutting. Some hair types need more layers, and some need more weight. For example, coarse hair tends to stick out more, especially if it is cut too short; fine hair can be cut to very short lengths and still lie flat. However, if a client has fine (texture) and thin (density) hair, cutting too short can result in the scalp showing through (Table 14-1).

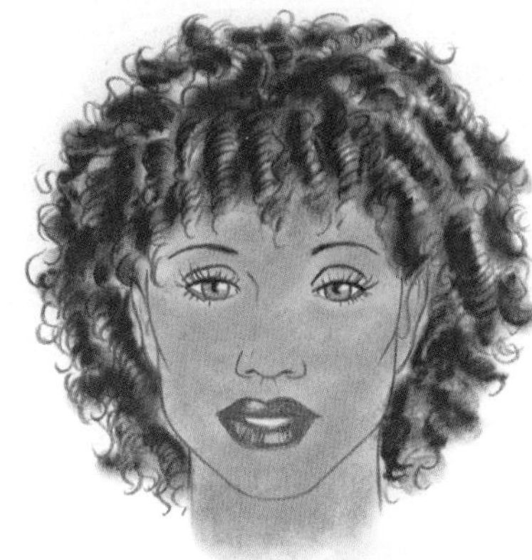

Figure 14-41 Uniform layered cut on medium curly hair.

WAVE PATTERN

The wave pattern, or the amount of movement in the hair strand, varies from client to client, as well as within the same head of hair. A client may have stick-straight hair (no wave), wavy hair, curly hair, extremely curly hair, or anything in between.

Imagine the same haircut cut at the same length on different types of hair: fine thin hair (Figure 14-39), thick coarse hair (Figure 14-40), and medium curly hair (Figure 14-41).

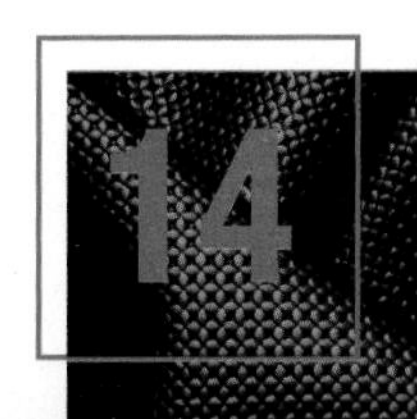

TEXTURE	DENSITY		
	Thin	**Medium**	**Thick**
Fine	Limp, needs weight	Great for many cuts, especially blunt and low elevation. Razor cuts are good.	Usually needs more texturizing. Suitable for many haircuts.
Medium	Needs weight. Graduated shapes work well.	Great for most cuts. Hair can handle texturizing.	Many shapes are suitable. Texturizing usually necessary.
Coarse	Maintain some weight. Razor cuts not recommended.	Great for many shapes. Razor cuts appropriate if hair is in good condition.	Very short cuts do not work. Razors may frizz and "expand" hair. Maintain some length to weigh hair down.

Table 14-1 Density and texture.

TOOLS, BODY POSITIONS, AND SAFETY

How do you choose and use the right tool for the job? To find the answer you will need to understand the function and characteristics of your tools, how to use them in a way that is safe for both yourself and your client, and how to position your body so that your energy and effectiveness are maximized and protected.

Figure 14-42 Haircutting shears and thinning shears.

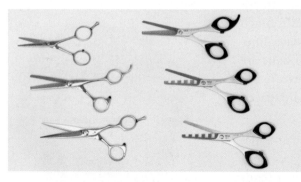

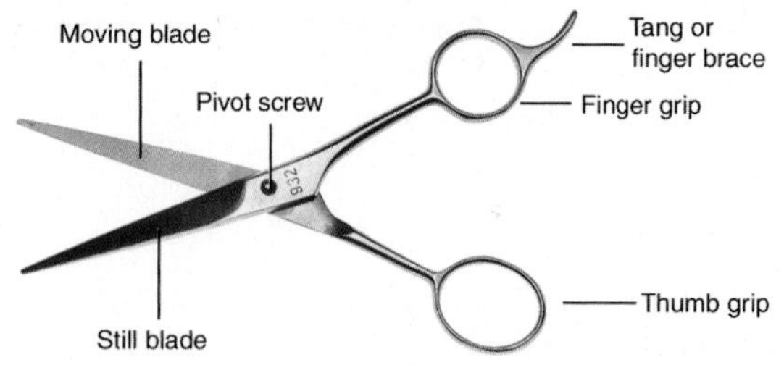

Figure 14-43 Parts of haircutting shears.

HAIRCUTTING TOOLS

There are several tools that you will need for haircutting. Understanding these implements, and the results you can achieve with them, is necessary for creating a great haircut. To do your best work, buy and use only high-quality professional implements from a reliable manufacturer, use them properly, and take good care of them. They can last a lifetime.

- **Haircutting shears.** Mainly used to cut blunt or straight lines in hair. May also be used to "slide cut," "point cut," and other texturizing techniques (discussed later in this chapter). The words *shears and scissors* are often used interchangeably (Figures 14-42 and 14-43).
- **Texturizing shears.** Mainly used to remove bulk from the hair. Sometimes referred to as thinning shears, tapering shears, or notching shears. Many types of thinning shears are used today, with varying amounts of teeth in the blades. A general rule of thumb is that the more teeth there are, the less

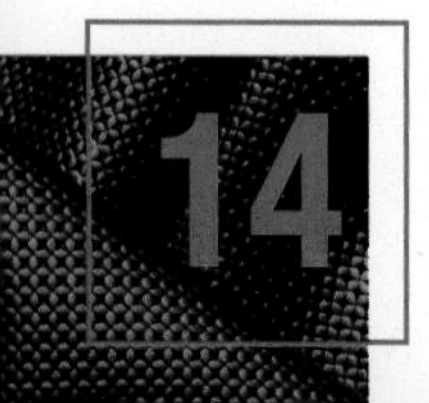

hair is removed. Notching shears are usually designed to remove more hair, with larger teeth set farther apart.

- **Straight razors or feather blades** are mainly used when a softer effect is desired on the ends of the hair. Razors can be used to create an entire haircut, to thin hair out, or to texturize in certain areas. They come in different shapes and sizes, with or without guards (Figure 14-44 and 14-45).
- **Clippers.** Mainly used when creating short haircuts, short tapers, fades, and flat tops. Clippers may be used without a guard to "shave" hair right to the scalp, with cutting guards at various lengths, or with the "clipper-over-comb" technique (Figure 14-46).
- **Trimmers** (also called edgers). A smaller version of clippers, mainly used to remove excess or unwanted hair at the neckline and around the ears, and create crisp outlines. Trimmers are mostly used on men's haircuts and very short haircuts for women.
- **Sectioning clips**. These come in a variety of shapes, styles, and sizes and can be made of plastic or metal. In general, two types are used: jaw or butterfly clips and duckbill clips. Both come in large and small sizes.
- **Wide-tooth comb.** Mainly used to detangle hair. Rarely to be used when performing a haircut.
- **Tail comb.** Mainly used to section and subsection the hair.
- **Barber comb.** Mainly used for close tapers on the nape and sides when using the scissor-over-comb technique. The narrow end of the comb allows the shears to get very close to the head.
- **Styling or cutting comb.** Also referred to as an all-purpose comb, it is used for most haircutting procedures. It can be 6 to 8 inches in length and has fine teeth at one end and wider teeth at the other (Figure 14-47).

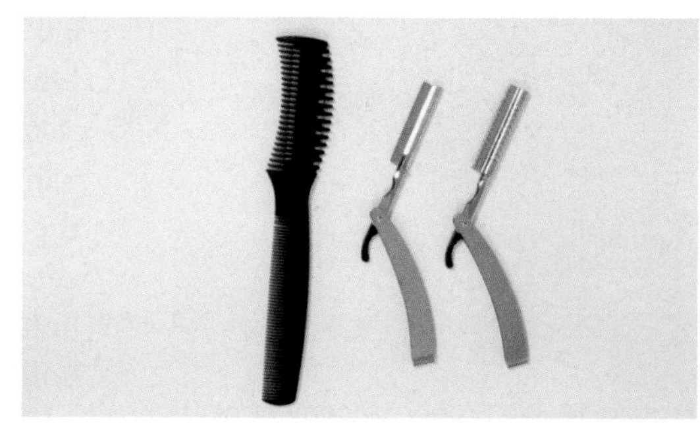

Figure 14-44 Razors.

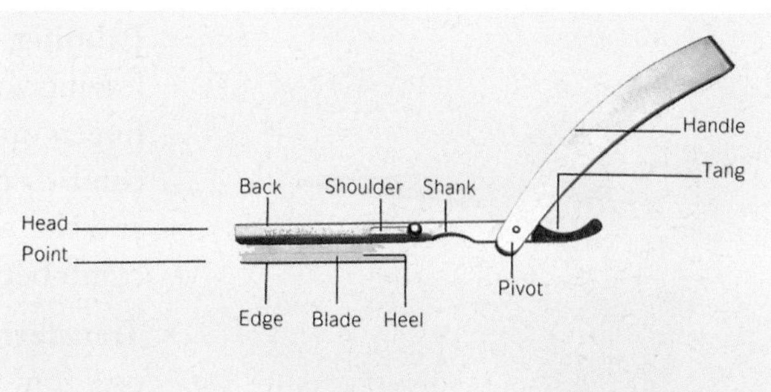

Figure 14-45 Parts of a razor.

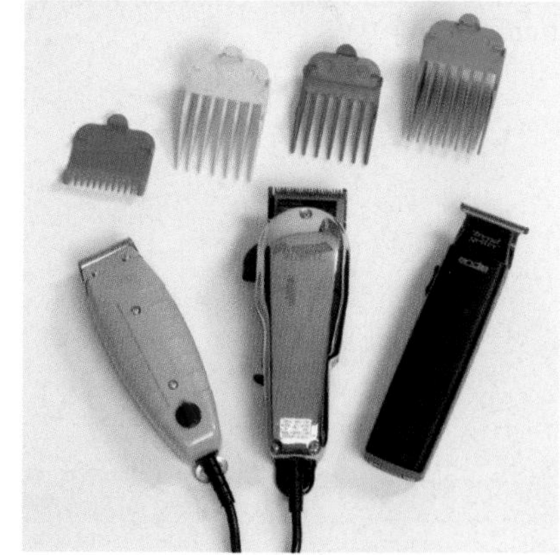

Figure 14-46 Clippers and trimmers.

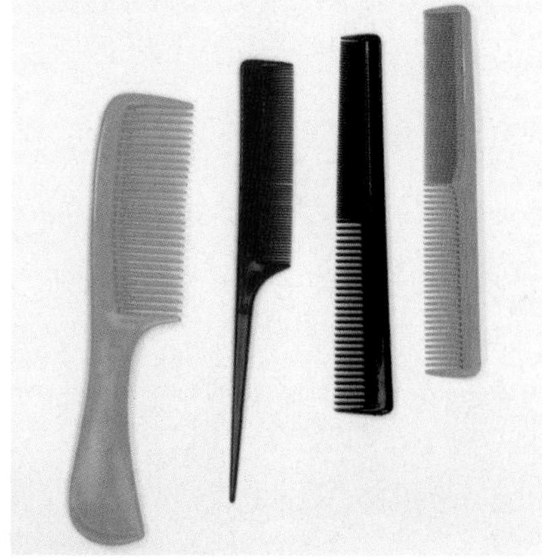

Figure 14-47 From left to right: wide-tooth comb, tail comb, barber comb, and styling comb.

HOLDING YOUR TOOLS

Two important reasons to properly hold your tools:

1. Gives you the most control, and the best results when cutting hair.
2. Can help you avoid muscle strain in your hands, arms, neck, and back.

HOLDING YOUR SHEARS

1. Open your right hand (left hand if you are left-handed), and place the ring finger in the finger grip of the still blade, and the little finger in the finger tang (brace) (Figure 14-48).
2. Place the thumb in the finger grip (thumb grip) of the moving blade (Figure 14-49).
3. Practice opening and closing the shears. Concentrate on moving only your thumb. A great way to get the feel of this is to lay the still blade against the palm or forefinger of your other hand, which holds it still while you move the other blade with your thumb (Figure 14-50).

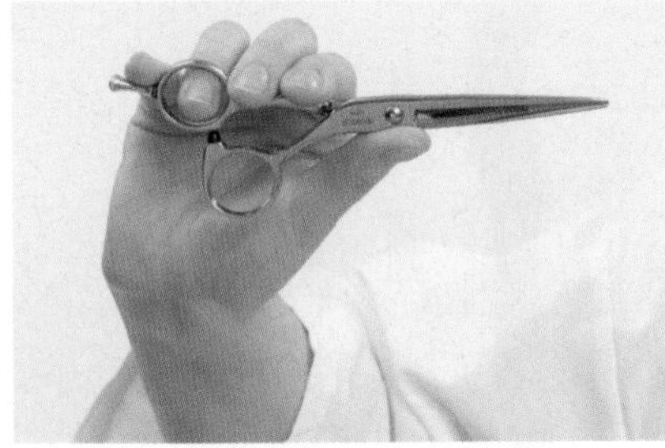

Figure 14-48 Proper placement of ring finger and little finger.

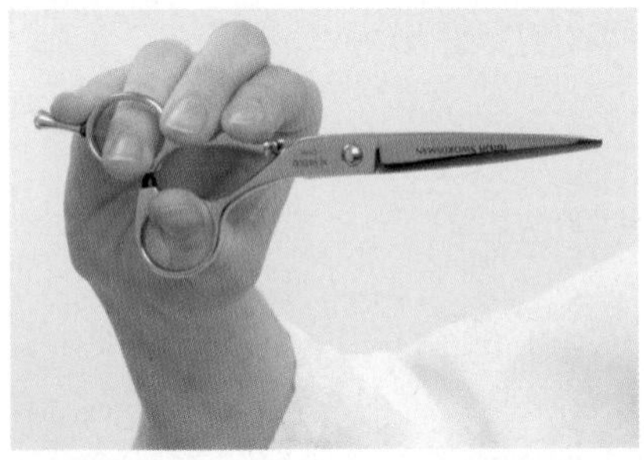

Figure 14-49 Proper placement of thumb.

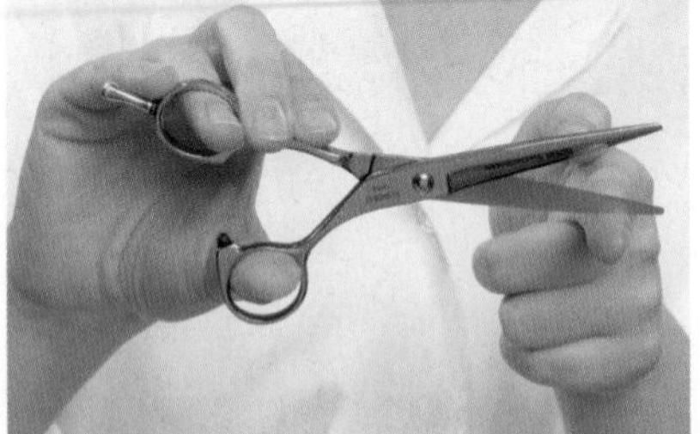

Figure 14-50 Still and moving blades.

HOLDING THE SHEARS AND COMB

During the haircutting process, you will be holding both the comb and shears at the same time. You may be tempted to put the comb down while cutting, but doing so will waste a lot of time. It is best to learn from the beginning how to hold both tools during the entire haircut. In general, your cutting hand (dominant hand) does most of the work. It holds the shears, parts the hair, combs the hair, and cuts the hair. Your holding hand does just that: it holds the sections of hair and the comb while cutting. The holding hand helps you maintain control while cutting.

- **Palming the shears.** Remove your thumb from the thumb grip, leaving your ring and little fingers in the grip and finger rest. Curl your fingers in to "palm" the shears, which keeps them closed while you comb or part the hair (Figure 14-51). This allows you to hold the comb and the shears at the same time. While palming the shears, hold the comb between thumb, index, and middle fingers (Figure 14-52).
- **Transferring the comb.** After you have combed a subsection into position, you will need to free up your cutting hand. Once your fingers are in place at the correct cutting position, transfer the comb by placing it between the thumb and index finger of your holding hand (the hand holding the subsection) (Figure 14-53). You are now ready to cut the subsection.

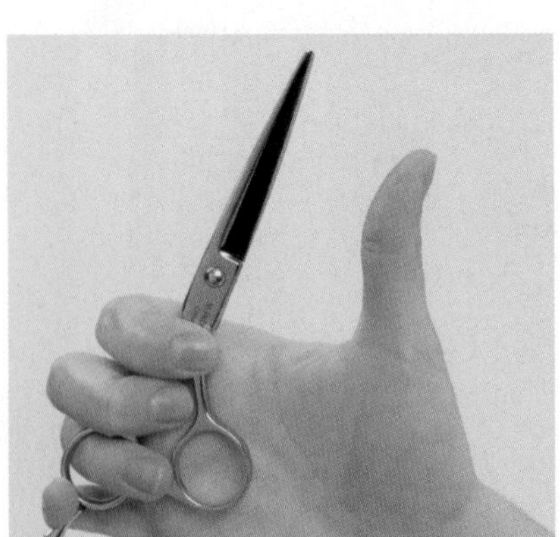

Figure 14-51 Palming the shears.

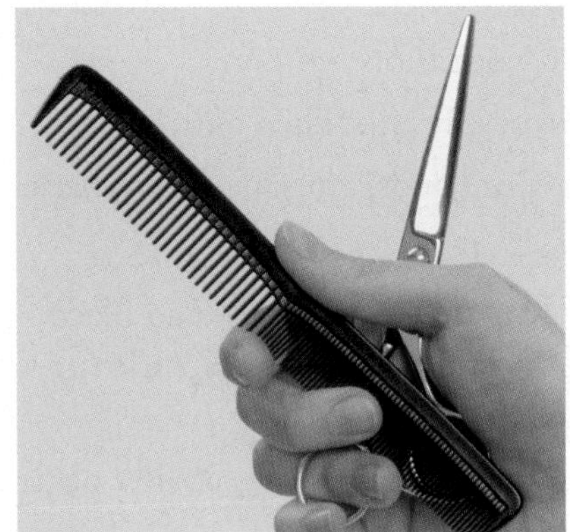

Figure 14-52 Holding comb and shears.

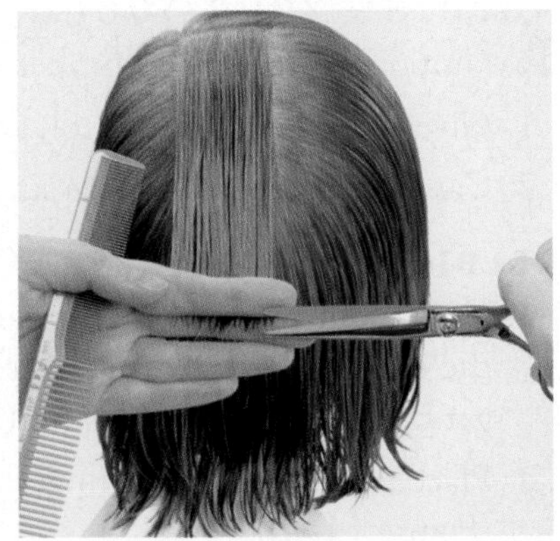

Figure 14-53 Transferring the comb.

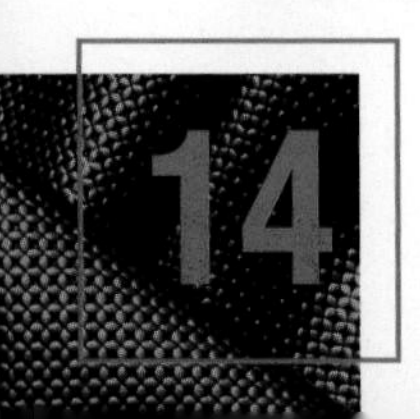

HOLDING THE RAZOR

The straight razor or feather blade is a versatile tool that can be used for an entire haircut, or for detailing and texturizing. Holding and working with a razor feels very different from holding and working with shears. The more you practice holding and palming the razor, the more comfortable you will become with this tool. There are two methods for holding the razor for cutting.

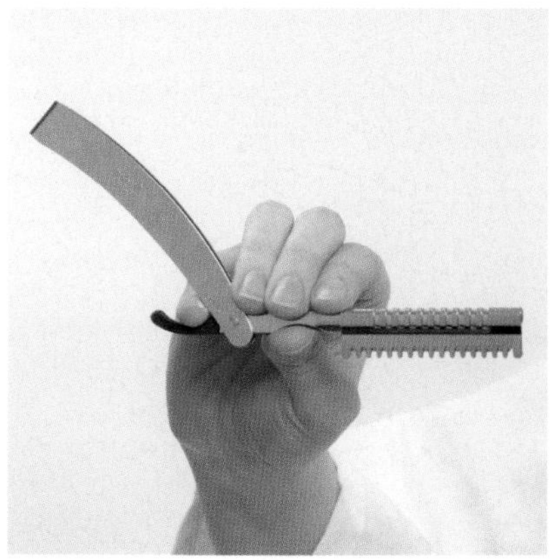

Figure 14-54 Holding razor properly.

Method A

1. **Open razor.** Open the razor so that the handle is higher than the shank. Place the thumb on the thumb grip, and the index, middle, and ring fingers on the shank.
2. **Place finger in tang.** Place the little finger in the tang, underneath the handle (Figure 14-54).
3. **Position razor.** When cutting a subsection, position the razor on top of the subsection, the part facing you, for maximum control (Figure 14-55).

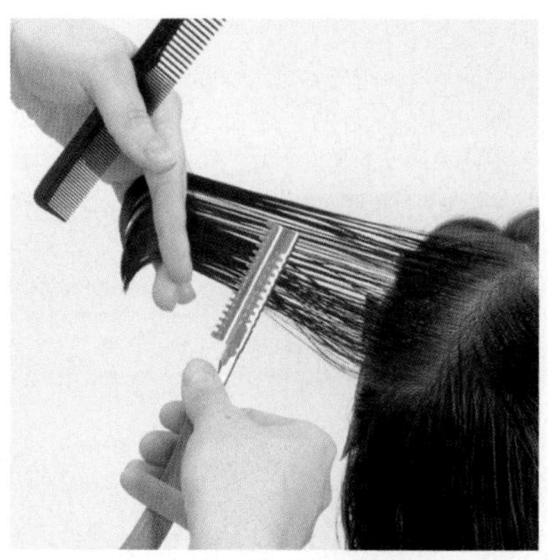

Figure 14-55 Holding razor for cutting.

Method B

1. **Open razor.** Open the razor until the handle and shank form a straight line.
2. **Wrap fingers.** Place the thumb on the grip and wrap the fingers around the handle (Figure 14-56).

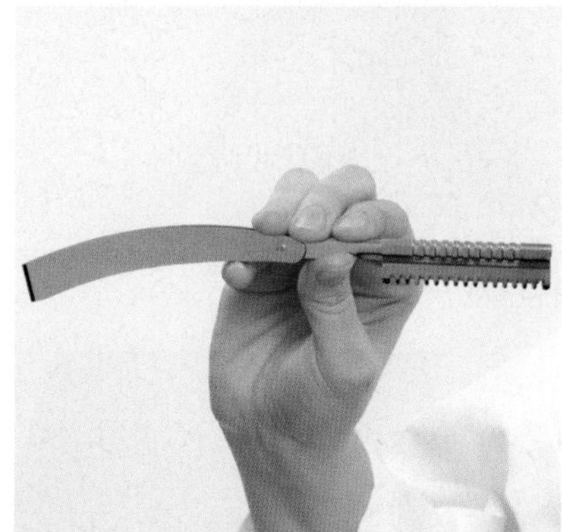

Figure 14-56 Alternate method of holding razor.

Just as you need to be able to hold the comb and the shears in your cutting hand while working, you also need to palm the razor so that you can comb and section hair during a haircut. Curl your ring finger and little finger to palm the razor. Hold the comb between your thumb and index and middle fingers (Figure 14-57). Most accidents with razors happen when combing the hair, not when cutting the hair, because of a loose grip when palming. Be sure to practice keeping a firm grip on the razor with the ring and little fingers, which keeps the open blade from sliding and cutting your hand while you comb the hair.

HANDLING THE COMB

Both the wide and fine teeth of the comb are regularly used when cutting hair. The wide teeth are used for combing and parting hair, while the finer teeth comb the section before cutting. The finer teeth provide more tension, and are useful when cutting around the ears, when dealing with difficult hairlines, and when cutting curly hair. Plan on spending some time practicing how to turn the comb in your hand while palming the shears.

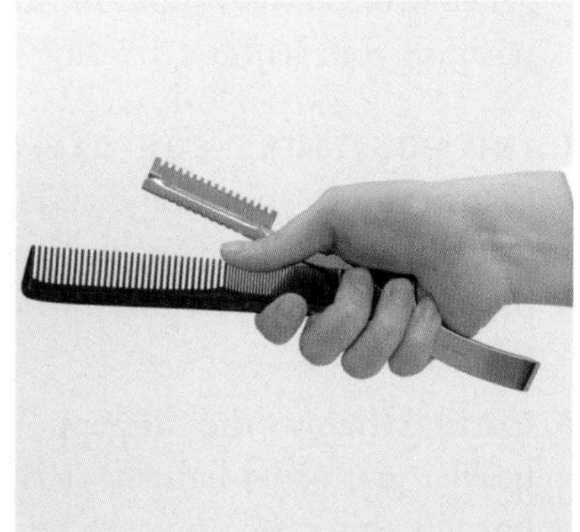

Figure 14-57 Palming the razor.

TENSION

Tension in haircutting is the amount of pressure applied when combing and holding a subsection, created by stretching or pulling the subsection.

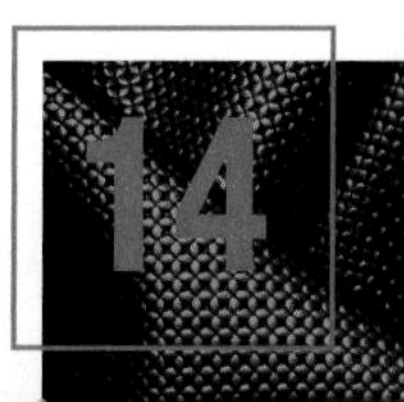

Tension ranges from minimum to maximum. You control tension with your fingers when you hold the subsection of hair between them. Consistent tension is important for constant, even results in a haircut. Use maximum tension on straight hair when you want precise lines. With curly or wavy hair, less tension is better because, a lot of tension will result in the hair shrinking even more than usual as it dries. Minimum tension should be used around the ears and on hairlines with strong growth patterns.

POSTURE AND BODY POSITION

Posture (how you stand and sit) and body position (how you hold your body when cutting hair) are important habits to be aware of. As a working cosmetologist, you will be spending many hours on your feet and you may want to consider using a cutting stool and wearing proper footwear as preventive measures. Good posture and body position will help you avoid future back problems and ensure better haircutting results. The correct body position will help you move more efficiently through the haircut, thereby maintaining more control over the process.

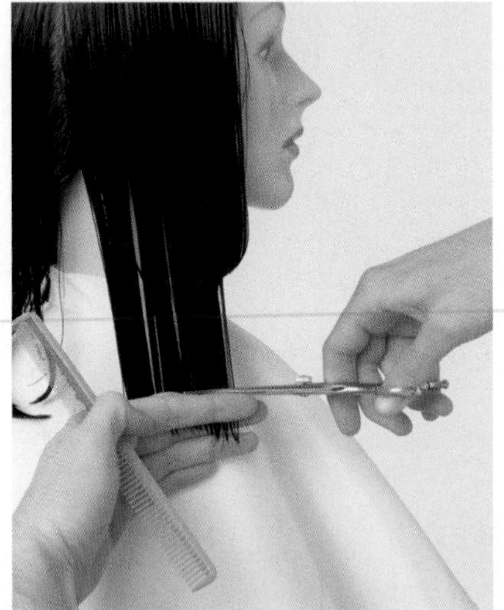

Figure 14-58 Cutting over the fingers.

- **Position the client.** Not only is your body position important, but so is your client's. Make sure that your client is sitting up straight and her legs are not crossed. Gentle reminders as the haircut progresses may be necessary. Remember, you can move the client by turning the chair, which gives you the option of keeping your body in the same place or angling the client's chair so you can see what you are doing in the mirror.
- **Center your weight.** When working, keep your body weight centered and firm. When standing keep your knees slightly bent, rather than locked. Instead of bending at the waist, try bending one knee if you need to lean slightly one way or the other. When sitting, keep both feet on the floor.
- **Work in front of your section.** When cutting hair, a general rule of thumb is to stand or sit directly in front of the area you are cutting. By doing this, you keep your body weight centered, and you will automatically find yourself moving around the head during a haircut. If you want to sit or stand in the same place, or be able to view what you are doing in the mirror, you need to move the client's chair. As a general rule, always stand in front of the area you are working on, and position your hands according to the cutting line.

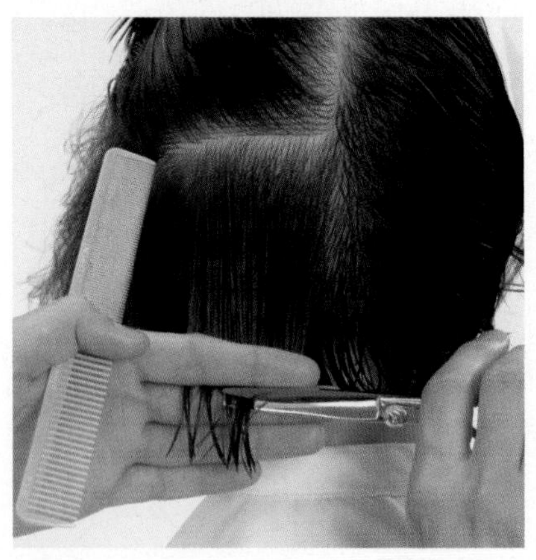

Figure 14-59 Cutting below the fingers.

HAND POSITIONS FOR DIFFERENT CUTTING ANGLES

- **Cutting over your fingers.** There are some situations in which you will be cutting over your fingers or on top of your knuckles. This hand position is used most often when cutting uniform or increasing layers (Figure 14-58).
- **Cutting below the fingers.** When cutting a one-length bob or a heavier graduated haircut, it is customary to use a horizontal cutting line. In this case, you will be cutting below your fingers, or on the inside of your knuckles (Figure 14-59).

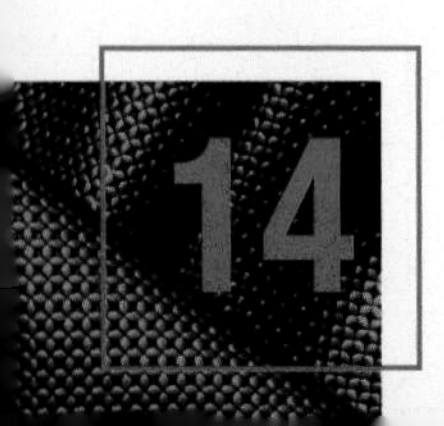

- **Cutting palm-to-palm.** When cutting with a vertical or diagonal cutting line, cutting palm-to-palm is the best way to maintain control of the subsection, especially with regard to elevation and overdirection. Cutting palm-to-palm means that the palms of both hands are facing each other while cutting. This is different from cutting on the top of your fingers or knuckles. Cutting palm-to-palm also helps to prevent strain on your back as you work (Figure 14-60 and Figure 14-61).

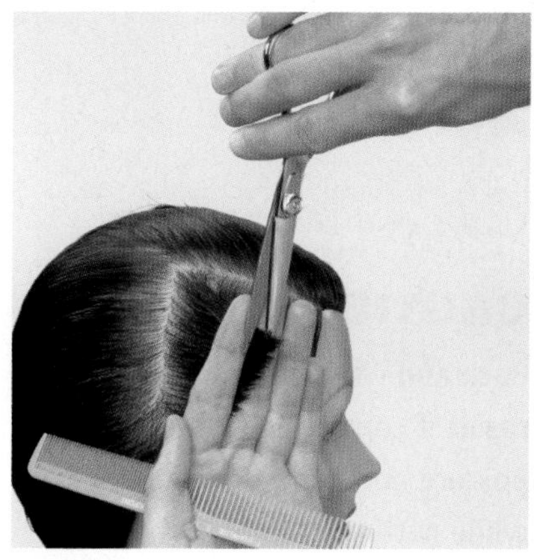

Figure 14-60 Cutting palm-to-palm, vertical cutting line.

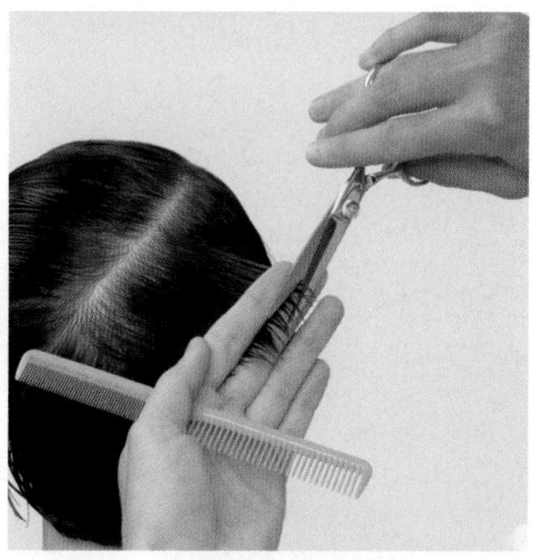

Figure 14-61 Cutting palm-to-palm, diagonal cutting line.

Learning how to control your shears is important because there are many techniques that can be difficult to learn if you are not holding the shears properly (e.g., scissor-over-comb and point cutting).

SAFETY IN HAIRCUTTING

It is absolutely essential for you to keep in mind that when you are cutting hair, accidents can happen. You will be handling sharp tools and instruments, and you must always protect yourself and your client by following the proper precautions.

Always palm the shears and the razor when combing or parting the hair. This keeps the points of the shears closed and pointed away from the client while combing, which prevents you from cutting yourself or the client. Palming the shears also reduces strain on the index finger and thumb while combing the hair.

- Do not cut past the second knuckle when cutting below your fingers, or when cutting palm-to-palm. The skin is soft and fleshy past the second knuckle, and is easy to cut.
- When cutting around the ears, or in the case of shorter haircuts, take extra care not to accidentally cut the ear. Cuts on the ears can produce large amounts of blood!
- When cutting the bangs (fringe), or any area close to the skin, balance the shears by placing the tip of the index finger of your left hand (right hand if you cut left-handed) on the pivot screw and the knuckles of your left hand against the skin (Figure 14-62). This helps prevent clients from being accidentally poked with the shears if they move suddenly. This also helps to balance your shears and cut a cleaner line.
- When working with a razor, learn with a guard. Never practice holding, palming, or cutting with the razor without a guard unless directed and supervised by your instructor.
- Take extra care when removing and disposing of the razor blade. Place the blade in its original sleeve, or wrap it in a paper towel to protect others from getting cut.

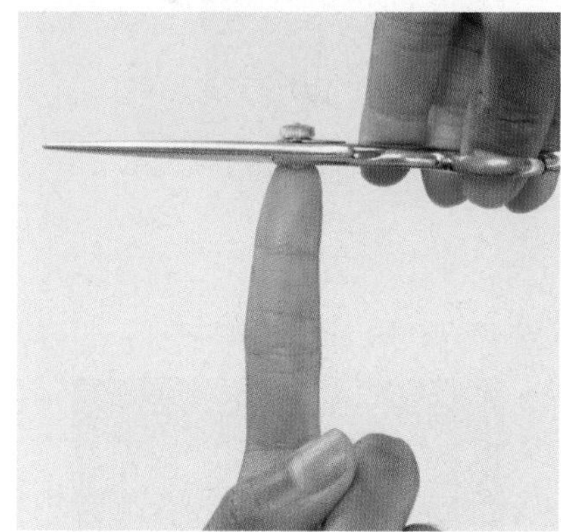

Figure 14-62 Balancing scissors.

SANITATION AND DISINFECTION GUIDELINES

1. **Wash hands.** Wash your hands with soap and warm water before and after each client.

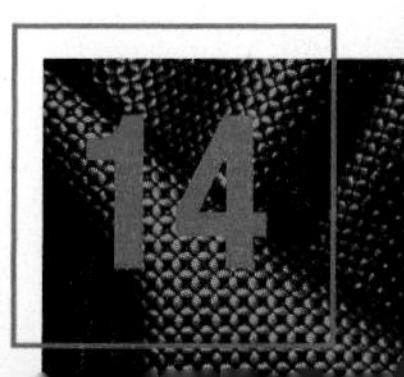

CAUTION

Back and wrist strain may result if correct body posture and hand position while cutting are not maintained.

2. **Sweep hair.** Before blow-drying your client, sweep up cut hair and dispose of it properly.
3. **Drape client.** Drape the client properly for the shampoo and the haircutting procedures.
4. **Sanitize implements and tools.** Always sanitize combs, brushes, shears, clips, and other implements after each haircut by washing thoroughly and placing in a disinfectant solution or by another method approved by your state board. See Chapter 5 for disinfection and storage procedures.
5. **Replace blade.** Replace the blade in your razor before each new client. Discard used blades in a puncture-proof container.
6. **Maintain shears.** Keep your shears in good working order by lubricating with a few drops of oil and wiping with a chamois (or dry cloth).
7. **Sanitize your workstation after each client.**

BASIC HAIRCUTS

The art of haircutting is made up of variations on four basic haircuts: blunt, graduated, layers, and long layers. An understanding of these basic haircuts is essential before you can begin experimenting with other cuts and effects.

In a **blunt haircut,** also known as a one-length haircut, all the hair comes to a single hanging level, forming a weight line. The **weight line** is a visual "line" in the haircut, where the ends of the hair hang together. The blunt cut is also referred to as a zero-elevation cut or no-elevation cut, because it has no elevation or overdirection. It is cut with a stationary guide. The cutting line can be horizontal, diagonal, or rounded. Blunt haircuts are excellent for finer and thinner hair types, because all the hair is cut to one length, therefore making it appear thicker (Figure 14-63).

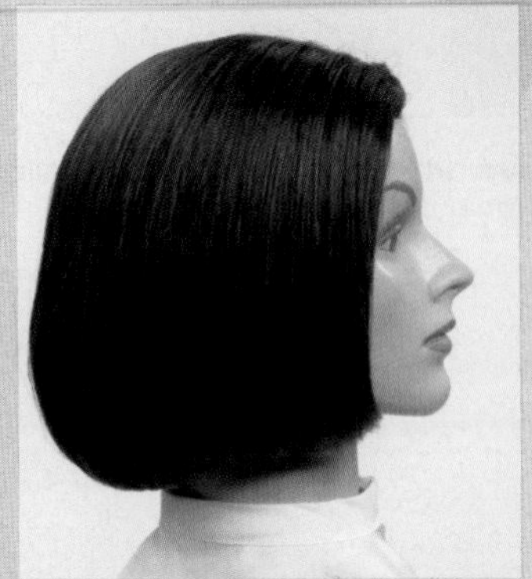

Figure 14-63 Blunt haircut.

A **graduated haircut** is a graduated shape or wedge, having an effect that results from cutting the hair with tension, low-to-medium elevation, or over-direction. The most common elevation is 45 degrees. In a graduated haircut, there is a visual buildup of weight in a given area. The ends of the hair appear to be "stacked." There are many variations and effects you can create with graduation simply by adjusting the degree of elevation, the amount of over-direction, or your cutting line (Figure 14-64).

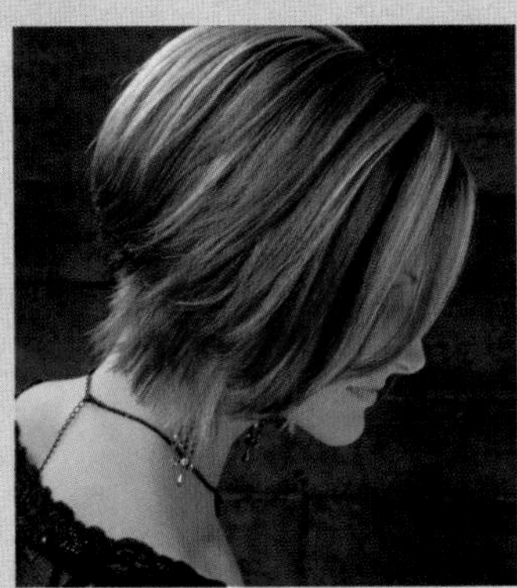

Figure 14-64 Graduated haircut.

A **layered haircut** is a graduated effect achieved by cutting the hair with elevation or over-direction. The hair is cut at higher elevations, usually 90 degrees and above. Layered haircuts generally have less weight than graduated haircuts. In a graduated haircut, the ends of the hair appear closer together. In a layered haircut, the ends appear farther apart. **Layers** create movement and volume in the hair by releasing weight. A layered haircut can be created with a traveling guide, a stationary guide, or both (Figure 14-65).

Another basic haircut is the **long-layered haircut.** The hair is cut at a 180-degree angle. This technique gives more volume to hairstyles and can be combined with other basic haircuts. The resulting shape will have shorter layers at the top and increasingly longer layers toward the perimeter (Figure 14-66).

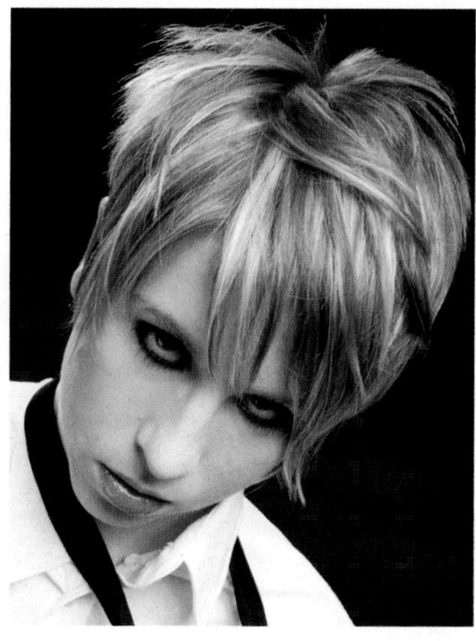

Figure 14-65 Layered haircut.

By using these four basic concepts, you are able to create any haircut you want. Every haircut is made up of one, two, or three of these basic techniques. Add a little texturizing, slide cutting, or scissor-over-comb, and you have advanced haircutting. Advanced haircutting is simply learning the basics and then applying them in any combination to create unlimited shapes and effects.

GENERAL HAIRCUTTING TIPS

- *Always take consistent and clean partings,* which will give an even amount of hair in each subsection and produce more precise results.
- *Take extra care* when working in the crown and neckline, which sometimes have very strong growth patterns. These areas are potential "danger zones."
- *Another danger zone* is the hair that grows around the ear or hangs over the ear in a finished haircut. Allow for the ear sticking out by either keeping more weight in this area, or cutting with minimal tension.
- *Always use consistent tension.* Tension may range from maximum to minimum. You can maintain light tension by using the wide teeth of the comb, and by not "pulling" the subsection too tightly. Be consistent with the tension you are using in the area on which you are working.
- *Pay attention to head position.* If the head is not upright, it may alter the amount of elevation and over-direction.

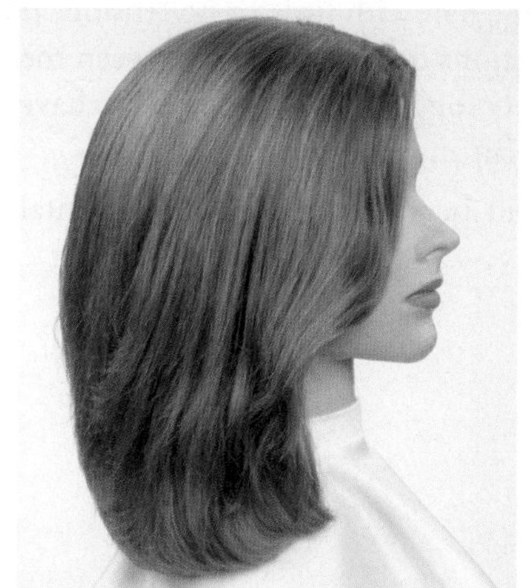

Figure 14-66 Long layered haircut.

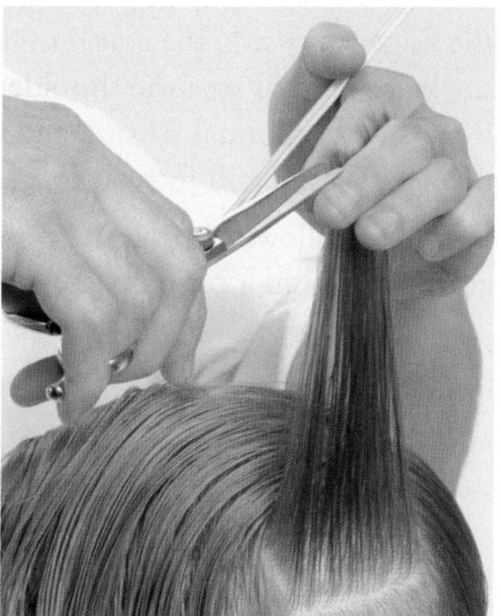

Figure 14-67 Cross-checking.

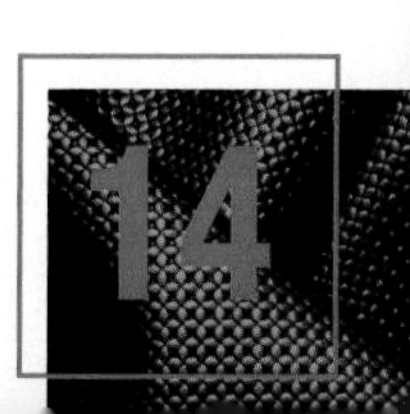

- *Maintain an even amount of moisture in the hair.* Dry hair responds to cutting differently than wet hair, and may give you uneven results in the finished haircut.
- *Always work with your guideline.* If you cannot see the guide, your subsection is too thick. Go back and take a smaller subsection before cutting. Taking too big of subsection can result in a big mistake. By using smaller sections, if a mistake is made, it is smaller and therefore easier to correct.
- *Always cross-check the haircut.* **Cross-checking** is parting the haircut in the opposite way that you cut it to check for precision of line and shape. For example, if you use vertical partings in a haircut, cross-check the lengths with horizontal partings (Figure 14-67).
- *Use the mirror to see your elevation.* You can also turn the client sideways so that you can see one side in the mirror while working on the opposite side. This helps create even lines and maintains visual balance while working.
- *Check both sides.* Always check that both sides are even by standing in front of your client as well.
- *Cutting curly hair.* Remember that curly hair shrinks more than straight hair, anywhere from ½ to 2 inches or more (1.25 to 5 centimeters). Always leave the length longer than the desired end result.

THE BLUNT HAIRCUT

The client's head should be upright and straight for this cut. If you tilt the head forward, the hair will not fall into its natural position. If you cut a blunt haircut with the head forward, you will make two discoveries: (1) the line will not fall as you cut it, and (2) you will have created some graduation where you did not intend to.

Blunt haircuts may be performed by either holding the sections between the fingers or using the comb to hold the hair with little or no tension. If the hair length is past the shoulders, sections need to be held between the fingers with minimal tension and for very long hair it may be best to have the client stand and for you to sit on a cutting stool to cut.

In the following procedure, you will be working with a horizontal cutting line and a center part.

PROCEDURE 14-1

BLUNT HAIRCUT

IMPLEMENTS AND MATERIALS

- Towels
- Shampoo cape
- Shampoo and conditioner
- Cutting cape
- Wide-tooth comb
- Cutting or styling comb
- Four sectioning clips
- Haircutting shears
- Spray water bottle
- Neck strip

PREPARATION

1. **Perform consultation.** Perform the client consultation and hair analysis.
2. **Drape client.** Drape the client for shampooing, using two towels.
3. **Shampoo.** Shampoo and condition the hair as necessary.
4. **Towel dry.** Towel dry the hair. Remove the towel around the neck and dispose of properly, leaving the second towel in place to prevent excess water from dripping on the client.
5. **Escort client to station.** Escort the client back to the styling chair. Secure a neck strip around the client's neck (Figure 14-68). Place a cape over the neck strip and fasten in the back. Fold the neck strip down over the cape so that no part of the cape touches the client's skin (Figure 14-69).

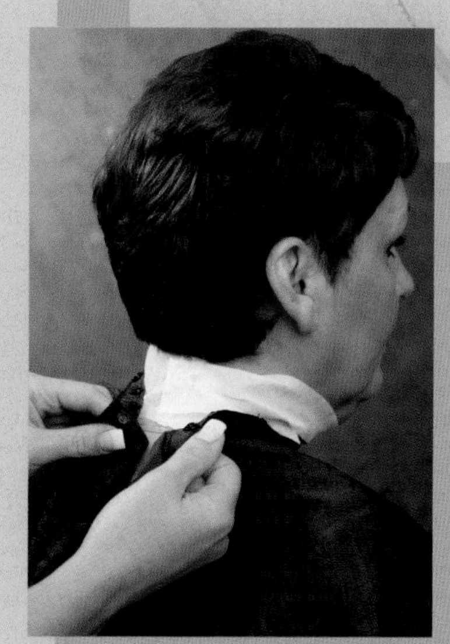

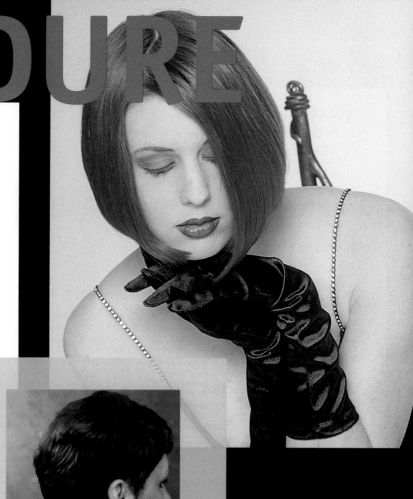

Figure 14-68 Place a neck strip around the client's neck.

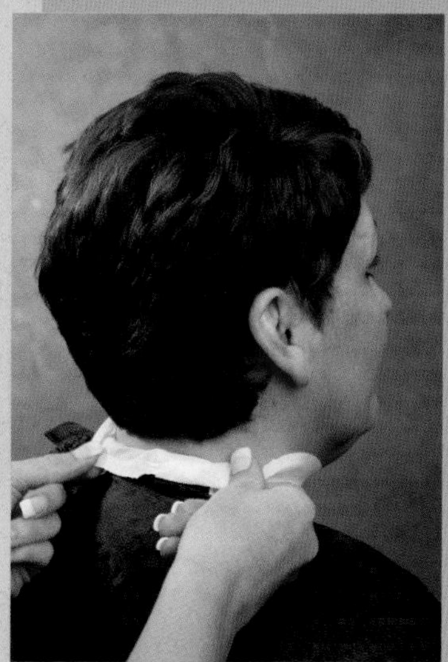

Figure 14-69 Fold the neck strip down.

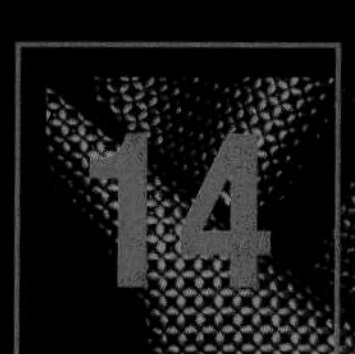

PROCEDURE

1. **Detangle and part hair.** Detangle the hair with the wide-tooth comb. Then comb the hair back from the hairline and push the hair gently forward with the palm of the hand. Use the comb and other hand to separate the hair where it parts, or part it the way the client will be wearing it.
2. **Divide hair in two parts.** Take a center part that runs from the front hairline to the nape, dividing the head in two (Figure 14-70).
3. **Find apex of head.** Find the apex of the head. Take a parting that runs from the apex to the back of the ear on both sides and clip. You have now divided the head into four sections (Figure 14-71).
4. **Create first subsection.** Beginning at the nape, on the left side, take a horizontal parting ¼ to ½ inch (0.6 to 1.25 centimeters) from the hairline, depending on the density of the hair. This creates the first subsection (Figure 14-72 and Figure 14-73).
5. **Comb subsection.** With the client's head upright, comb the subsection in a natural fall from scalp to ends. With your dominant hand, comb the subsection again, stopping just above the cutting line. Make sure the comb is horizontal and just above the cutting line (desired length). Cut the subsection straight across against the comb, remembering to keep your shears horizontal and parallel to the floor (Figure 14-74). Repeat on the right-hand side, using the length of your first subsection as a guide (Figure 14-75). Check to make sure your cutting line is straight before moving on. You have now created your guideline for the entire haircut.

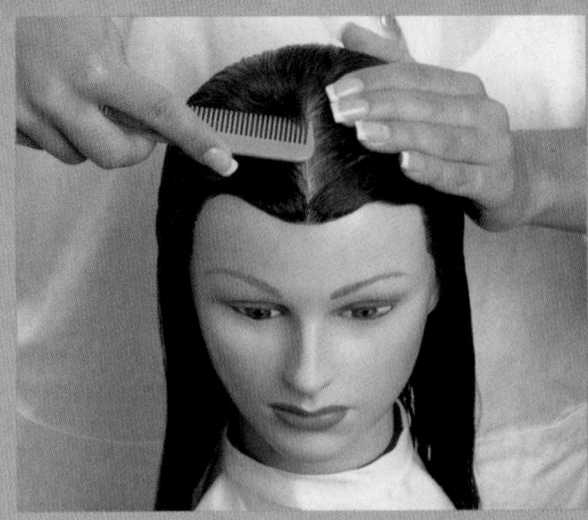

Figure 14-70 Center part.

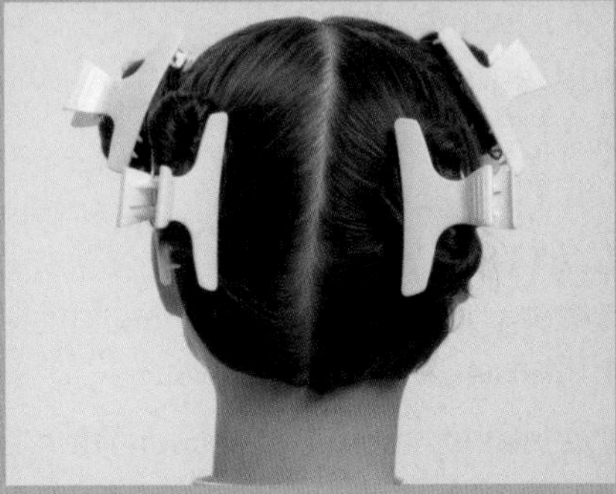

Figure 14-71 Hair parted into four sections.

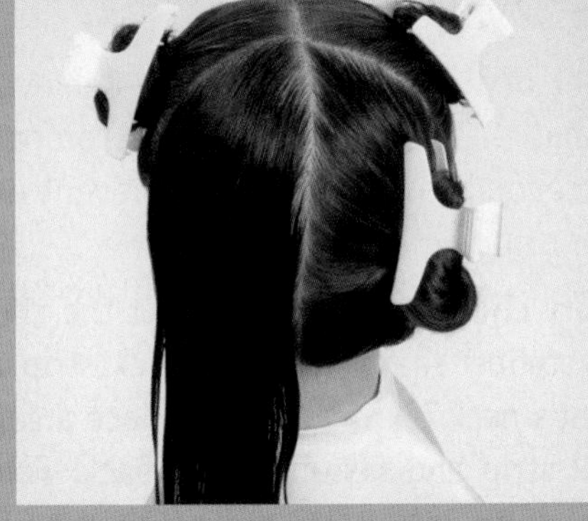

Figure 14-72 One section prepared for parting.

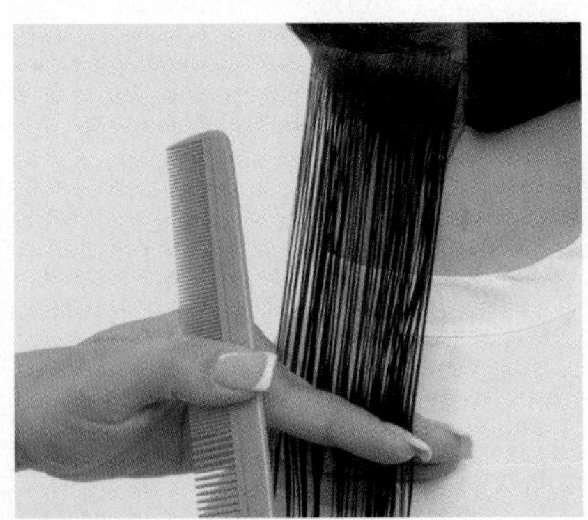

Figure 14-73 First subsection.

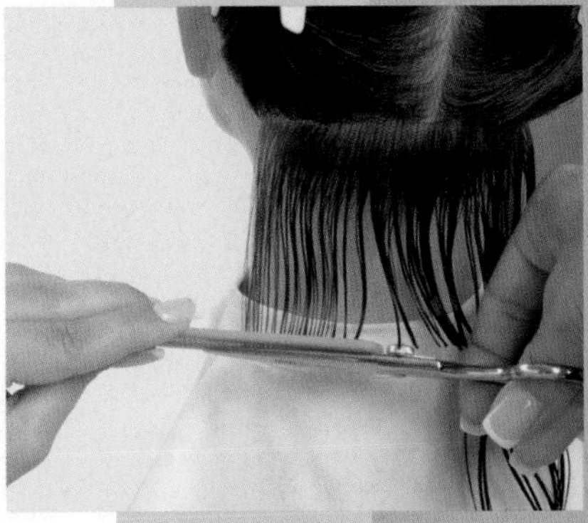

Figure 14-74 Cut first subsection on left.

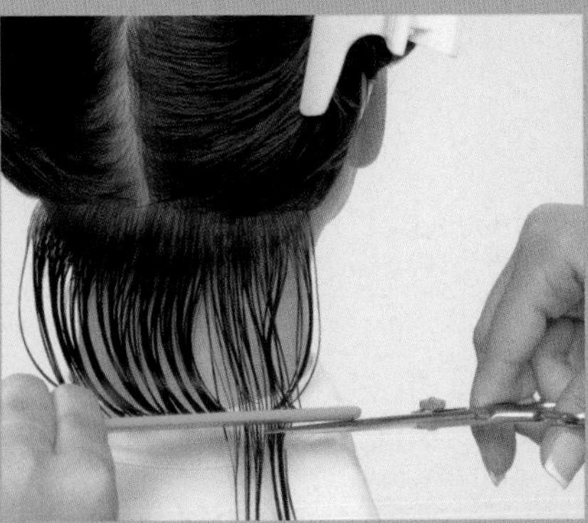

Figure 14-75 Cut first subsection on right.

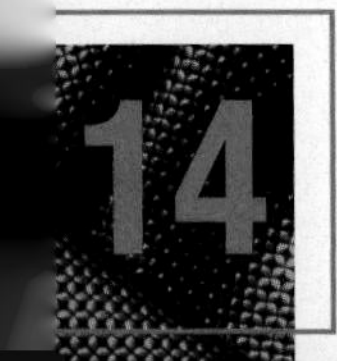

Here's a TIP

The density (thickness) of the hair will determine the size of the subsection. The thicker the hair, the narrower the subsection; the thinner the hair, the wider the subsection. In other words, to create narrower subsections, your partings need to be closer together. To create wider subsections, your partings should be farther apart. If there is too much hair in one subsection, it becomes difficult to see your guideline and to control the hair, because the hair is "pushed" away as you close the shears, producing an uneven line.

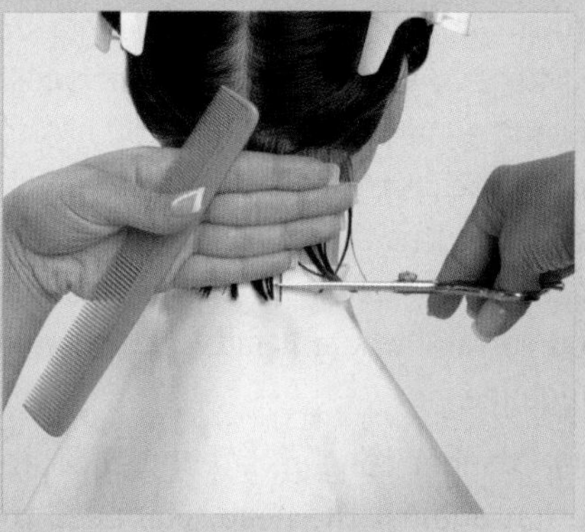

Figure 14-76 Hold the hair against the skin.

6. **Alternative method.** If the hairline lies down nicely, an alternate way of cutting a blunt line in the nape is to comb down the subsection and hold the hair against the skin with the edge of your nondominant hand. Cut the guideline below your hand, making sure that your shears are horizontal and parallel to the floor (Figure 14-76).
7. **Continue cutting.** Returning to the left side, take another horizontal parting, creating a subsection the same size as your previous subsection. As a rule, you should be able to see the guideline through the new subsection. If you cannot see the guide, take a smaller subsection. Comb the hair down in a natural fall, and cut the length to match the guide (Figure 14-77). Repeat on the right side (Figure 14-78).
8. **Continue cutting back.** Continue working up the back of the head, alternating from the left section to the right section, using ½-inch subsections.
9. **Cut crown area.** When you reach the crown area (danger zone), pay close attention to the natural fall of the hair. Comb the hair into its natural falling position, and cut with little or no tension to match the guide (Figure 14-79). You have now completed the back of the haircut.

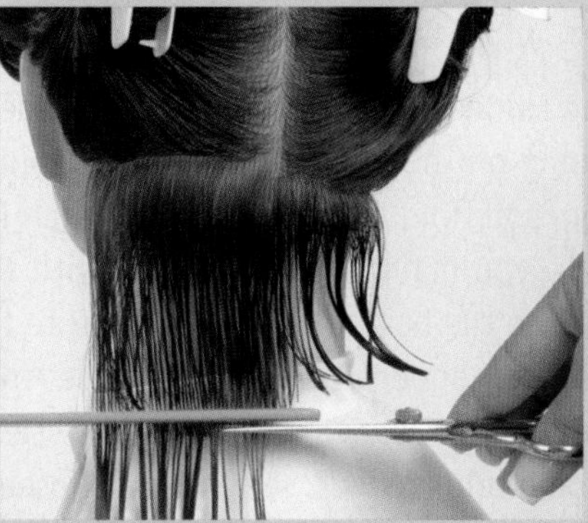

Figure 14-77 Second subsection on left.

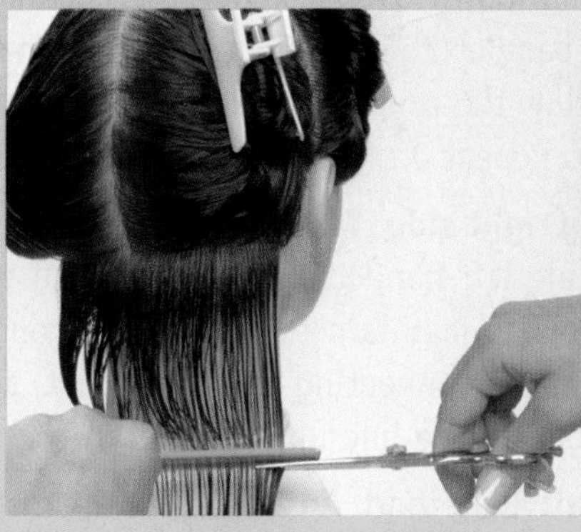

Figure 14-78 Second subsection on right.

Here's a TIP

Using the comb to control the hair allows you to cut with very little tension. This allows the hair to do what it naturally wants to do, and still maintain a clean line.

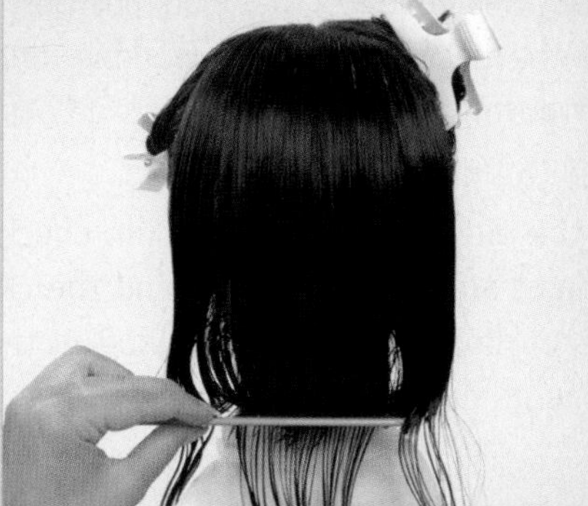

Figure 14-79 Comb the crown into natural fall.

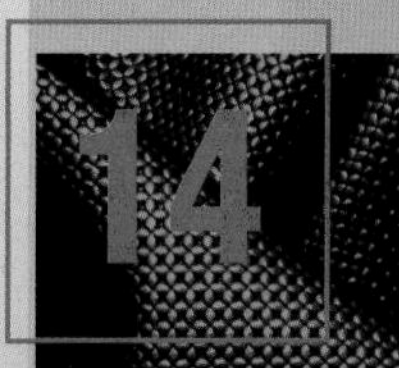

The crown area is called the "danger zone" because it is where irregular growth patterns are most often found. The crown can be challenging when you are doing blunt haircuts. Look at the scalp to see the natural growth pattern. You may want to leave this area out until the very end of the haircut, or cut it slightly longer than the guideline. Once the hair is dry, you can see where it falls, and then match the length to the guideline.

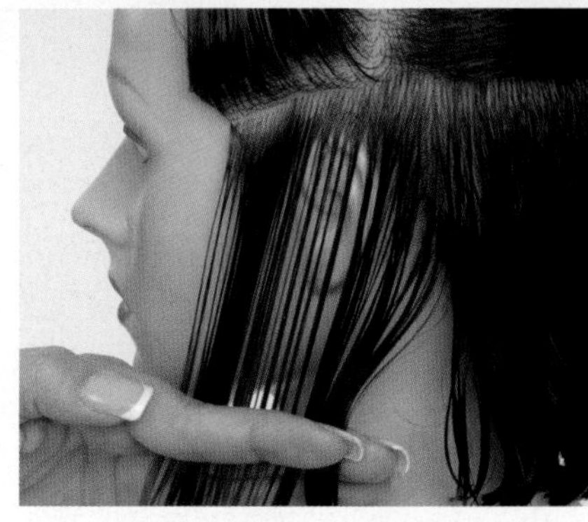

Figure 14-80 Take a horizontal parting on the left side.

Another "danger zone" is around the ears. Because ears do not lie flat against the head, you need to take special steps to keep an even cutting line. Always work with very little tension or no tension around the ears, unless you are working with shorter layers.

10. **Cutting sides.** Now move to the sides of the haircut. Beginning on the left side, take a horizontal parting and part off a portion from the back area to match (Figure 14-80). This will help you maintain consistency with the blunt line when connecting the back to the sides. Be sure to take a subsection that is large enough to give you an even amount of hair at the cutting line, allowing for the ears sticking out. Comb the hair from scalp to ends, release the subsection, and allow the hair to hang in a natural fall. Using the wide teeth, place the comb back into the subsection just below the ear. Slide the comb down to just above the cutting line. Holding the comb parallel to the floor, cut the hair straight across just below the comb, connecting the line to the back (Figure 14-81). Repeat on the right-hand side (Figure 14-82).

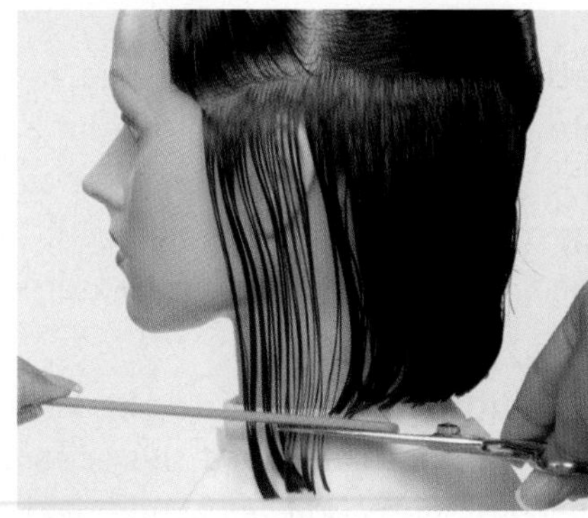

Figure 14-81 Cut the first subsection.

11. **Cutting right side.** When working on the right side (left side if you are left-handed), your shears will be pointing toward the back. To maintain consistency in your line, take smaller subsections, connecting at the ear first, and gradually move forward with the line until you reach the face.

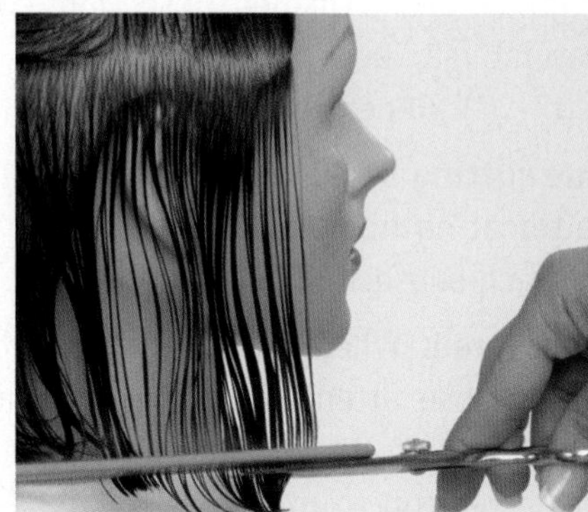

Figure 14-82 Repeat on the right.

12. **Alternative method.** An alternative approach to the right side (left side if you are left-handed) is to turn your wrist so that your palm is facing upward and your shears are pointed toward the face. This requires that you position your body slightly behind the section you are working on, with your elbow straight down. Either method gives a consistent result in your line (Figure 14-83).
13. **Check the sides.** Before moving on, check that both sides of the haircut are even. Stand behind the client and check the lengths on both sides while looking in the mirror. Make any adjustments needed (Figure 14-84).

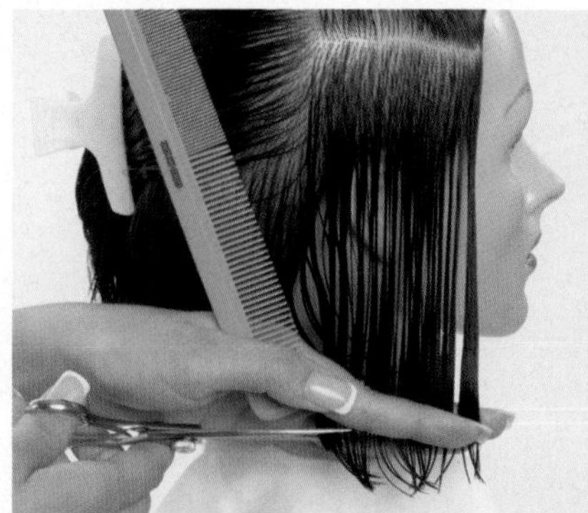

Figure 14-83 Cutting on the right side.

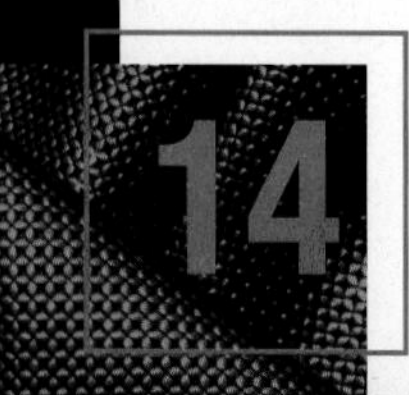

14. **Continue on left side.** Continue working up the left side with horizontal partings, until all the hair has been cut to match the guide. When cutting the hair that falls along the face, make sure to comb the hair so it lies on the side, not the front, of the face. Repeat on the right side.

15. **Cross-check haircut.** Cross-check the haircut using vertical sections, making sure that you do not over-direct the hair. Elevate the hair slightly and cut off any excess hair, removing only minimal amounts (Figure 14-85).

16. **Sweep hair.** Sweep up cut hair from the floor and dispose of properly.

17. **Blow-dry the haircut.** In order to get a true reading of the haircut, it is best to perform a smooth blow-dry, with very little lift at the scalp.

18. **Check the line.** Once the haircut is dry, have the client stand. Check the line in the mirror. You should see an even, horizontal line all the way around the head. This is the time to clean up any hair at the neckline and check where the hair falls when dry (Figure 14-86). Use the wide teeth of the comb to connect the crown area. If this section was left longer during the haircut, now is the time to connect it into the line (Figure 11-87).

19. **Remove drape.** Remove the drape and neck strip from the client and dispose of properly.

20. **Clean neck and face.** Brush loose hair from the client's neck and face. Escort the client to the reception area.

CLEANUP AND SANITATION

1. **Disinfect tools and implements.** Disinfect all shears, combs, and brushes used during the haircut by immersing in a hospital-level disinfectant.
2. **Sanitize workstation.** Sanitize your workstation, making sure that it is clean and neat for your next client.
3. **Wash hands.** Wash your hands with soap and warm water.

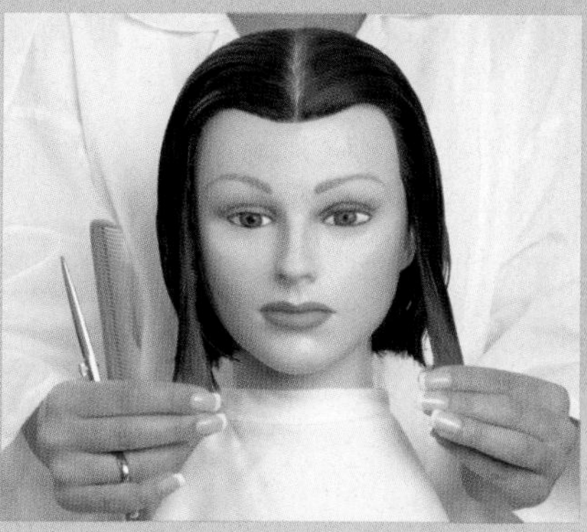

Figure 14-84 Check both sides.

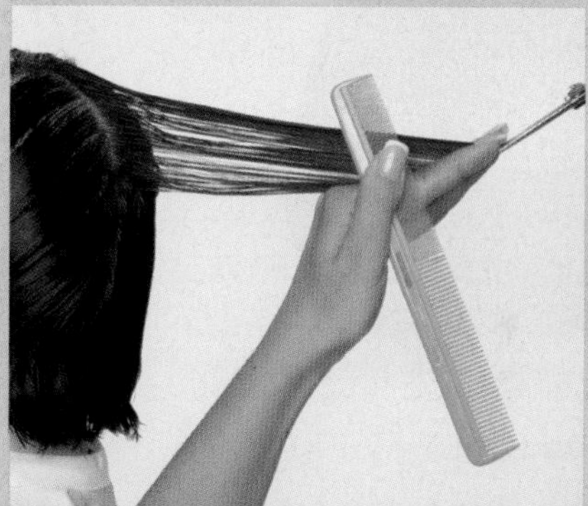

Figure 14-85 Cross-check with vertical subsections.

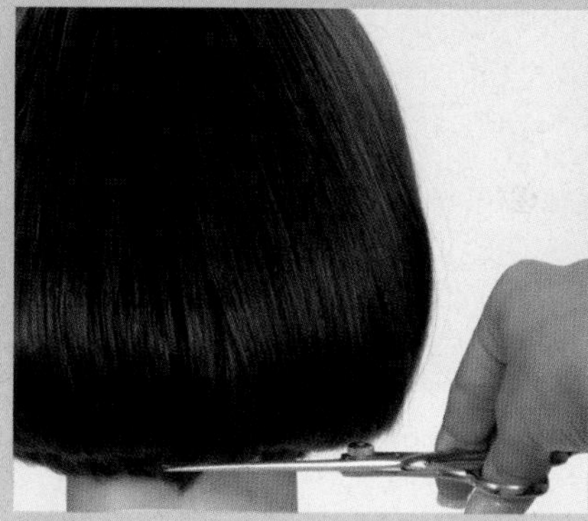

Figure 14-86 Clean up the neckline.

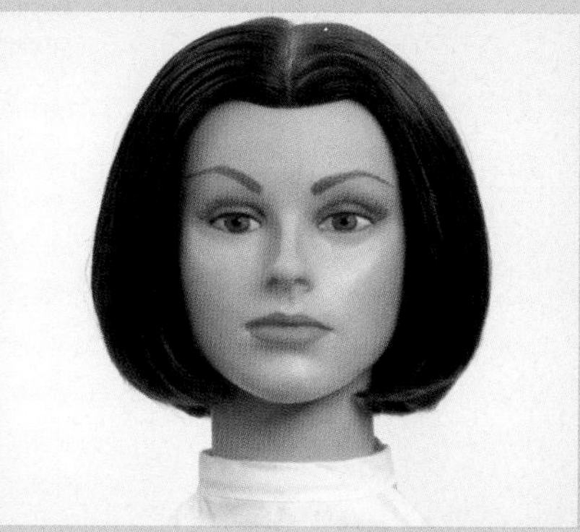

Figure 14-87 Finished blunt haircut.

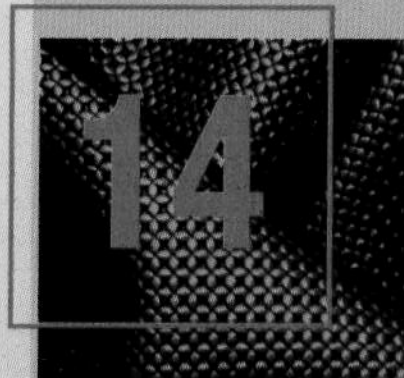

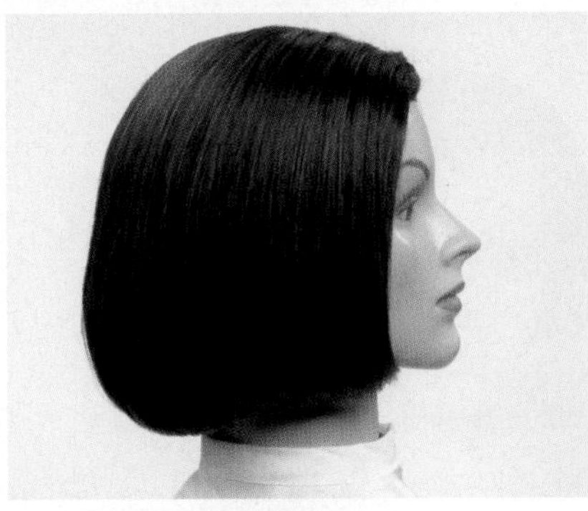

Figure 14-88 Side view

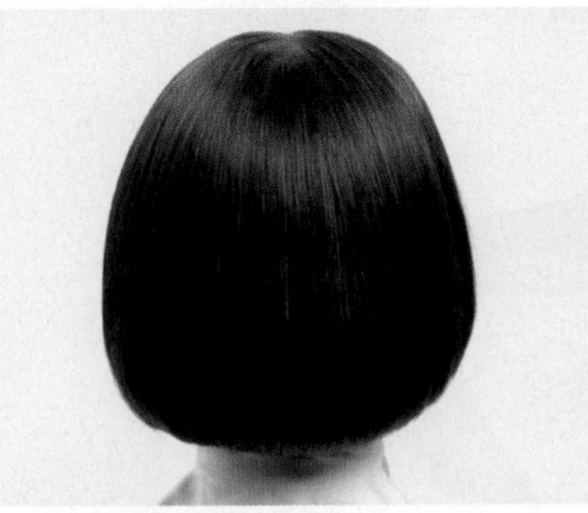

Figure 14-89 Back

OTHER BLUNT HAIRCUTS

The blunt haircut is the basis for many other classic cuts.

- In a classic A-line bob, a diagonal cutting line (finger angle) is used (Figure 14-88 through 14-90).
- In this longer blunt haircut (Figure 14-91), the bang has been left long and was cut with a horizontal finger angle. When blunt-cutting longer hair, hold the hair between the fingers with very little tension.
- Figure 14-92 illustrates a blunt haircut on curly hair. Note how the hair naturally "graduates" itself when it dries.
- In a classic pageboy, or "bowl" shape, the perimeter is curved, using a combination of horizontal and curved lines (Figure 14-93).

TIPS FOR BLUNT HAIRCUTS

- Always cut with minimal or no tension.
- Work with the natural growth patterns of the hair, keeping the client's head upright.
- Always comb the section twice before cutting, to ensure that you have combed the hair clean from the parting to the ends. If using the wide teeth of the comb while cutting, always comb the section first with the fine teeth, then turn the comb around, and re-comb with the wide teeth.

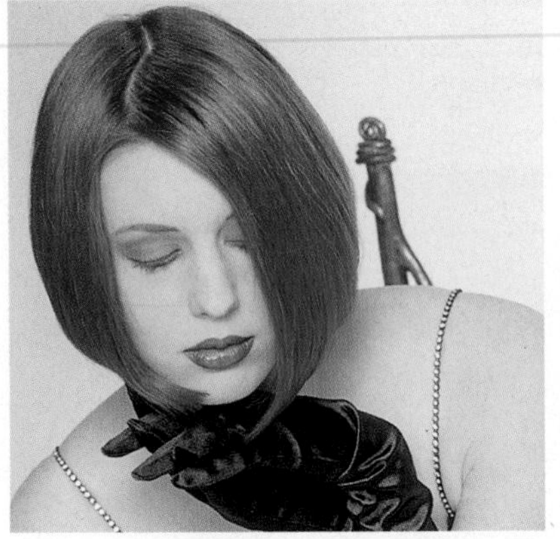

Figure 14-90 A-line bob.

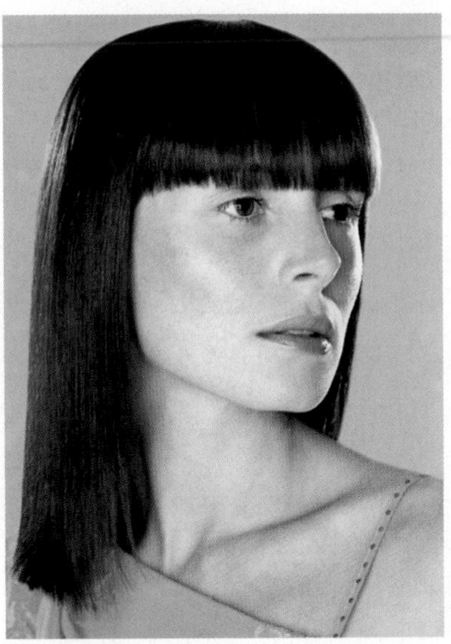

Figure 14-91 Longer blunt cut with one-length fringe.

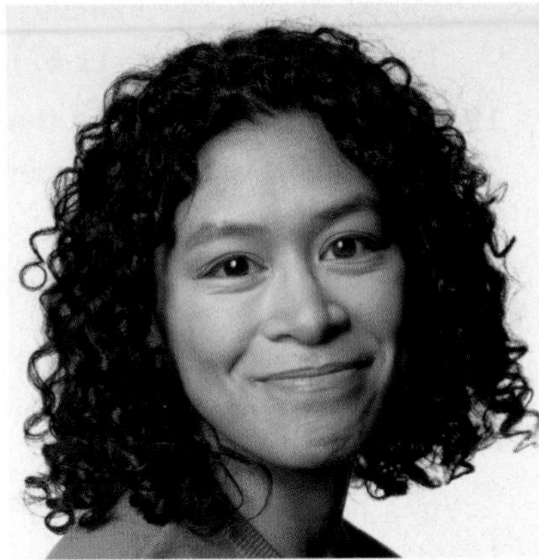

Figure 14-92 Blunt cut on curly hair.

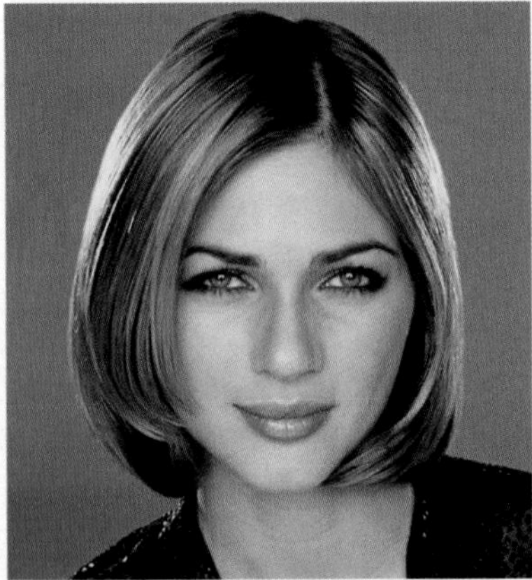

Figure 14-93 Classic blunt pageboy.

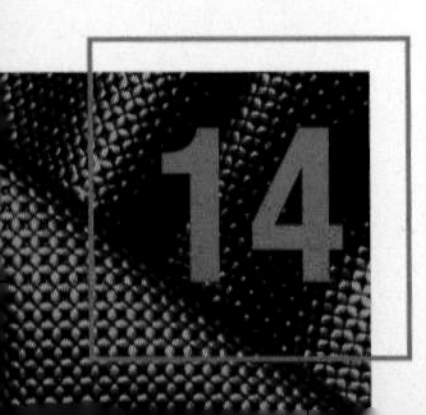

- Always maintain an even amount of moisture in the hair.
- Pay close attention to growth patterns in the crown and hairline.
- Take precautions to allow for the ears sticking out, to avoid getting a "hole."

GRADUATED (45-DEGREE) HAIRCUT

In this basic haircut, you will be working with a vertical cutting line and a 45-degree elevation as well as a 90-degree elevation. Although you will use a center part, keep in mind that this haircut can also work with a side part or a bang. You will be using a stationary guideline and a traveling guideline.

Remember, a stationary guideline is a guideline that does not move. All other sections are combed toward the guideline and are cut to match it. A traveling guideline moves with you as you work through the haircut.

Here's a great way to understand what a graduated haircut looks like. Hold a telephone book by the spine with the pages hanging down. The edges of the pages make a straight line, just like a blunt haircut (Figure 14-94). Now turn the book the other way, open it in the middle, and let the pages flop down on either side. The edges of the pages make a beveled line, just like a graduated haircut (Figure 14-95).

Here is another type of graduated haircut, created with different cutting angles. In the classic graduated bob made popular by Vidal Sassoon, diagonal sections and finger angles are used to create a rounded or beveled effect. This haircut begins in the back, using a 45-degree elevation throughout, and gradually incorporates the sides and top. If you find that the hairline grows up or toward the center, you can use the scissor-over-comb technique to blend it (Figures 14-96 and 14-97).

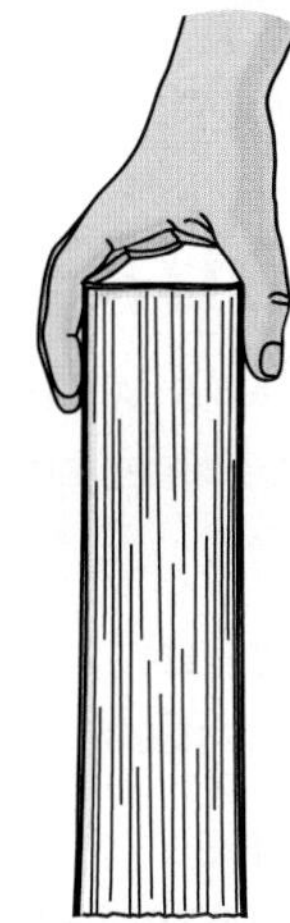

Figure 14-94 Straight or "blunt" hanging line.

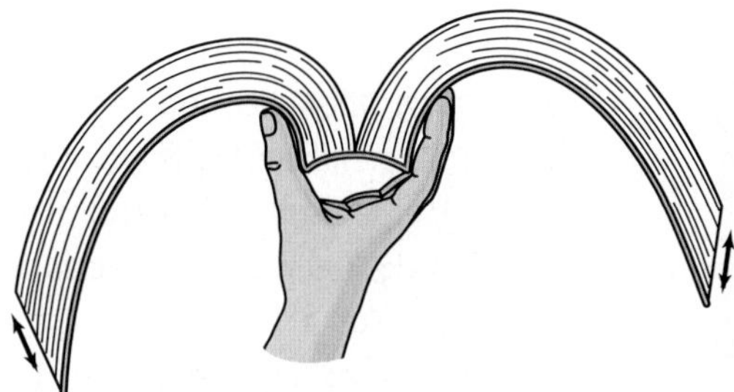

Figure 14-95 Beveled or "graduated" hanging line.

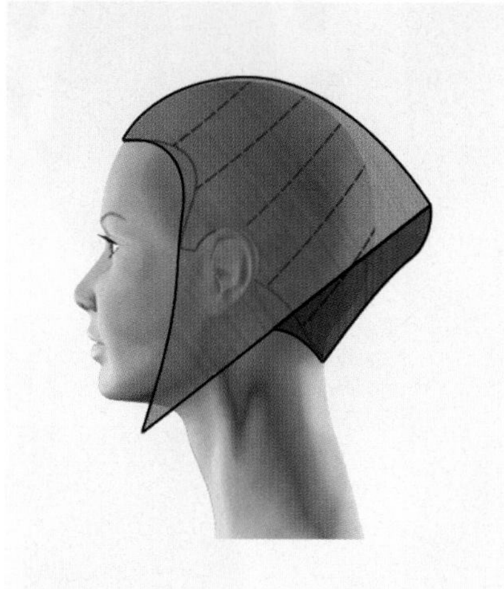

Figure 14-96 Graduated bob design.

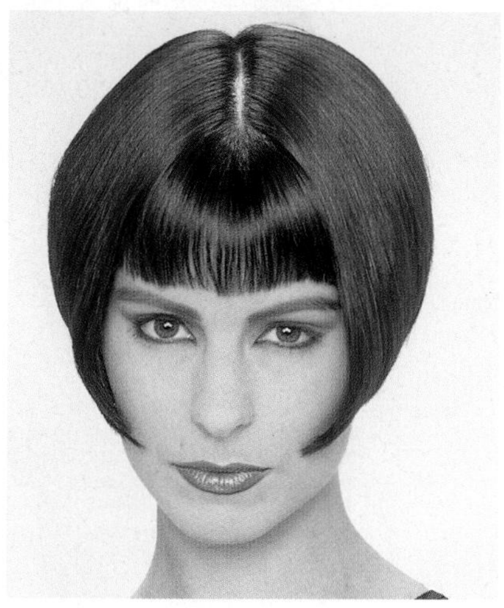

Figure 14-97 Finished graduated bob.

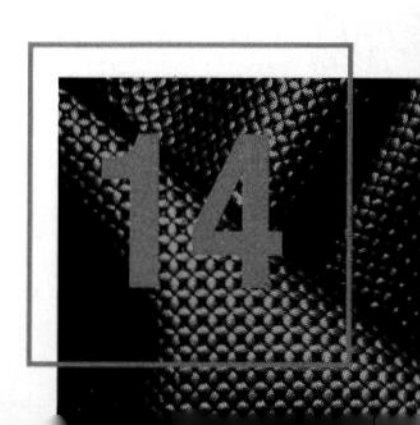

PROCEDURE 14-2

GRADUATED HAIRCUT

IMPLEMENTS AND MATERIALS

See list of implements and materials in "Blunt Haircut" procedure.

PREPARATION

Follow preparation steps in "Blunt Haircut" procedure.

PROCEDURE

1. **Part the hair.** Part the hair into six sections. Begin with a part from the front hairline just above the middle of each eyebrow back to the crown area, and clip the hair in place (Figure 14-98). Establish another part from the crown area where section one ends to the back of each ear, forming side sections two and three (Figure 14-99). Clip these sections in place. Part the hair down the center of the back to form sections four and five (Figure 14-100). Take a horizontal part from one ear to the other across the nape area about 1 inch (2.5 centimeters) above the hairline. This section (six) is your horizontal guide section (Figure 14-101).
2. **Create guideline.** Establish your guideline by first cutting the center of the nape section to the desired

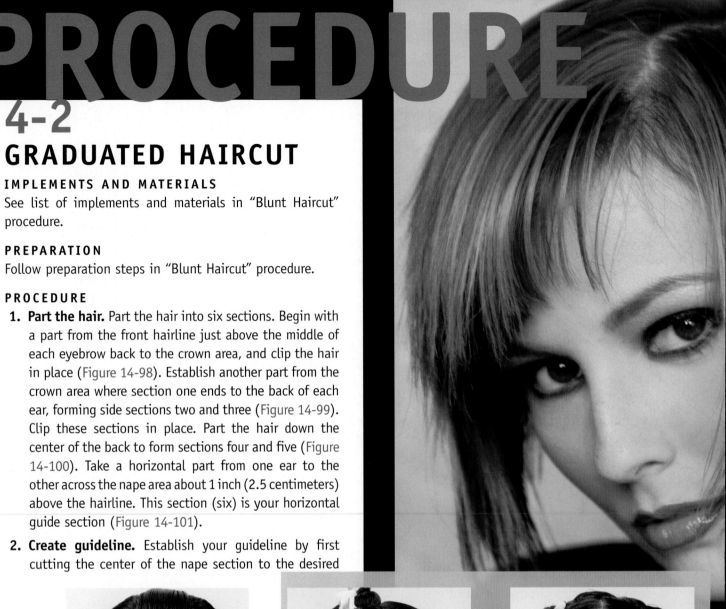

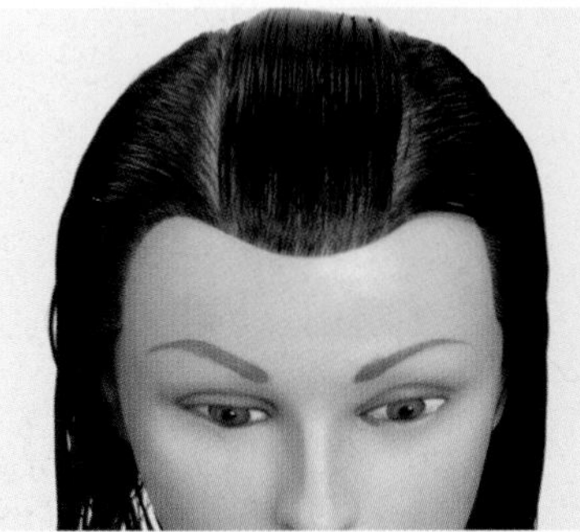

Figure 14-98 Part off section 1.

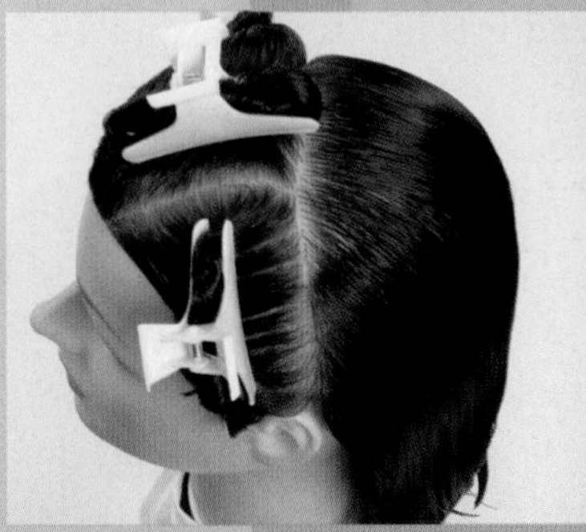

Figure 14-99 Form sections 2 and 3.

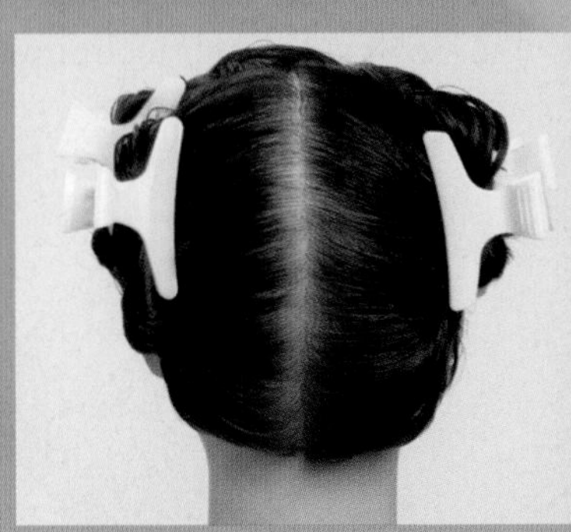

Figure 14-100 Form sections 4 and 5.

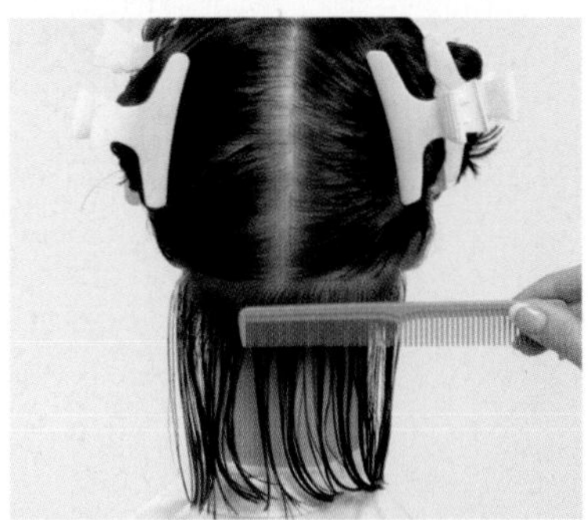

Figure 14-101 Horizontal guide.

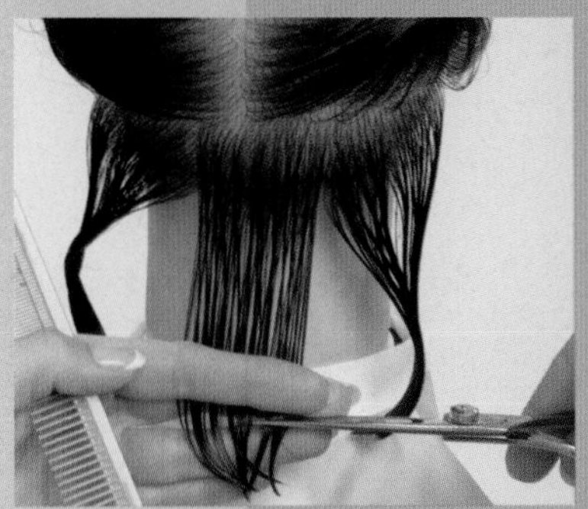

Figure 14-102 Cut the center nape section (guideline).

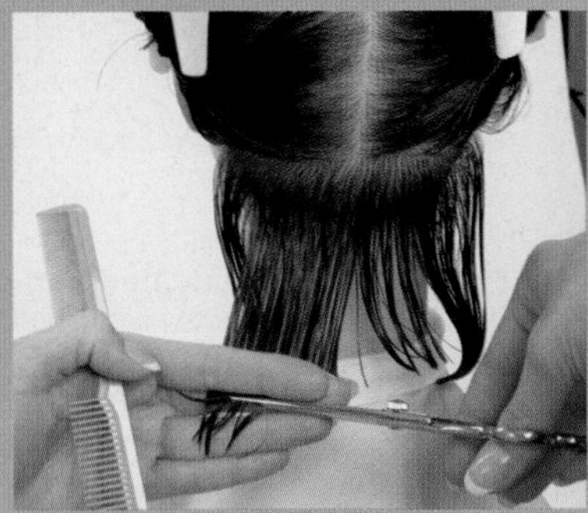

Figure 14-103 Finish cutting nape section.

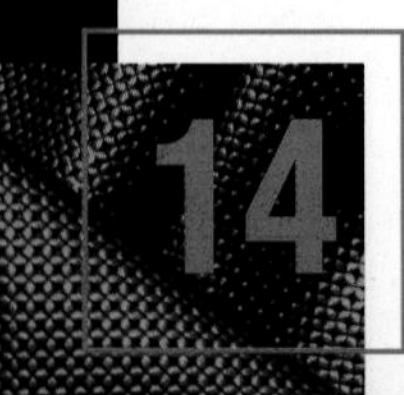

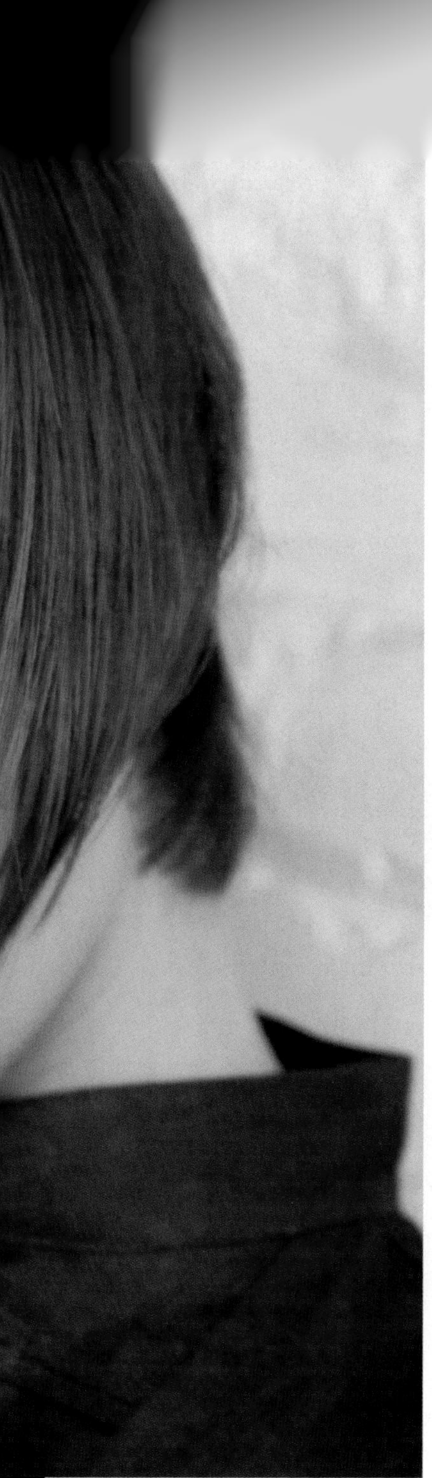

length. Use a horizontal cutting line parallel to the fingers (Figure 14-102). Cut the right and left sides of the nape section the same length as the center guideline (Figure 14-103).

3. **Measure and part off first section.** Working upward in the left back section, measure and part off the first horizontal section approximately 1 inch wide (Figure 14-104).
4. **Create vertical subsection.** Beginning at the center part, establish a vertical subsection approximately ½ inch (1.25 centimeters) wide. Extend the subsection down to include the nape guideline. Comb the subsection smooth at a 45-degree angle to the scalp (Figure 14-105). Hold your fingers at a 90-degree angle to the strand and cut (Figure 14-106).
5. **Cut horizontal section.** Proceed to cut the entire horizontal section by parting off vertical subsections and cutting in the same manner as Step 4. Check each section vertically and horizontally throughout the haircut. Each completed section will serve as a guideline for the next section.
6. **Part off.** Part off another horizontal section approximately 1 inch wide. Beginning at the center, create another vertical subsection that extends down and includes the previously cut strands (Figure 14-107). Comb the hair smoothly at a 45-degree elevation to the head. Hold the fingers and shears at a 90-degree angle to the subsection and cut (Figure 14-108). Cut the entire horizontal section this way. Make sure the second section blends evenly with the previously cut section.

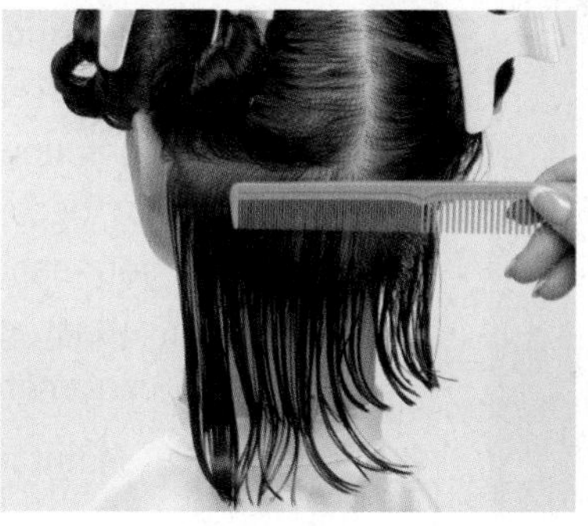

Figure 14-104 Measure off first horizontal section with comb.

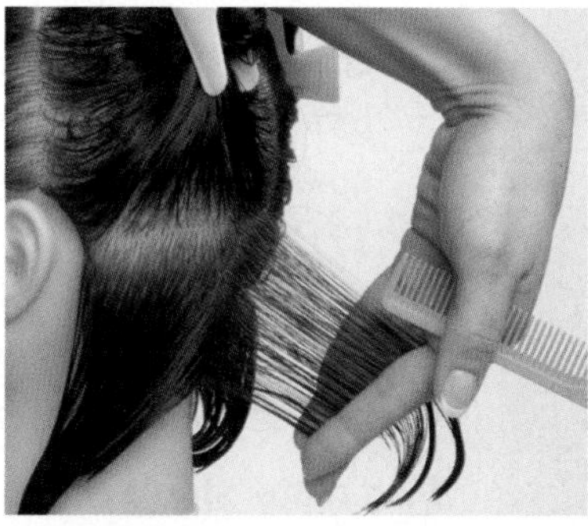

Figure 14-105 Comb first vertical subsection.

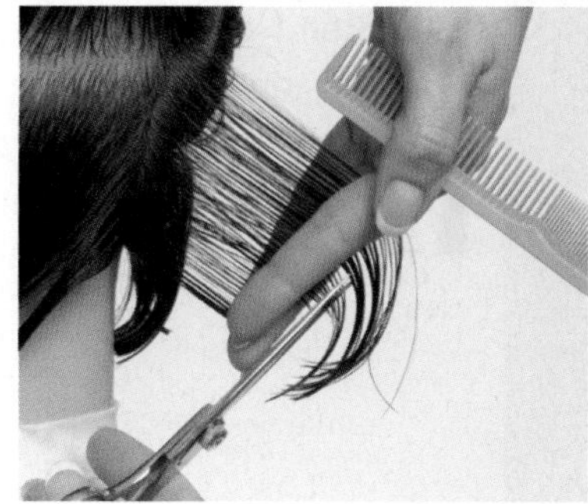

Figure 14-106 Cut first vertical subsection.

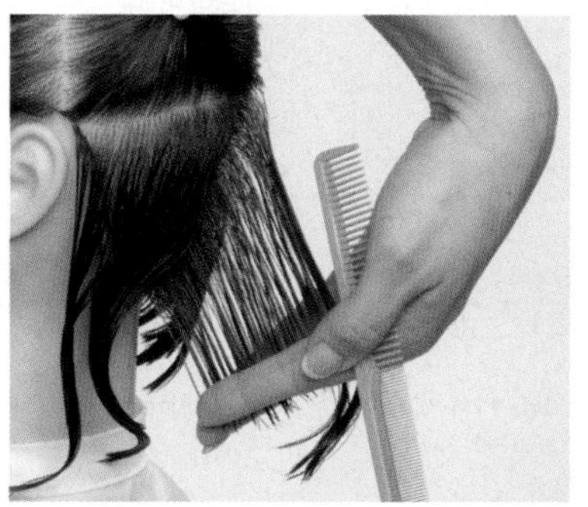

Figure 14-107 Create first vertical subsection in new section.

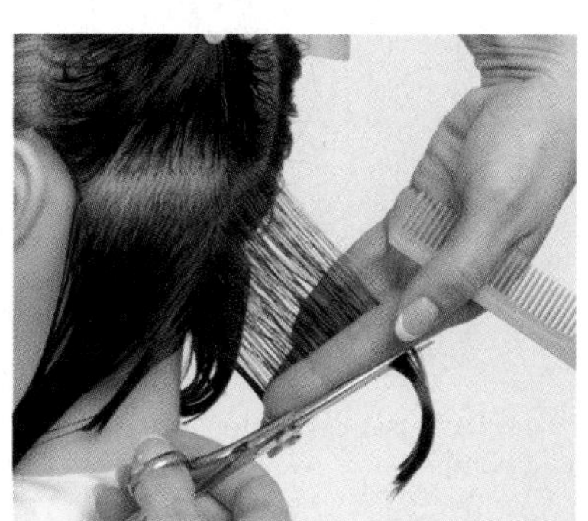

Figure 14-108 Cut subsection.

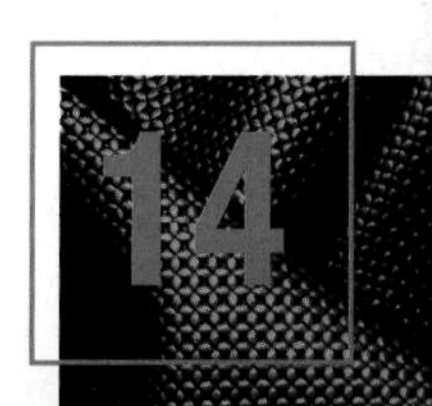

7. **Continue throughout left and rights sections.** Continue taking horizontal sections throughout the left and right back sections, and follow the same cutting procedure. The hair will gradually become longer as it reaches the apex. For example, if your nape guide was 2.5 inches (6.25 centimeters) long, your upper crown section will be approximately 6 inches (15 centimeters) long (Figure 14-109).
8. **Cut crown.** Maintain the length in the upper crown by holding each vertical subsection throughout the crown area at a 90-degree angle while cutting (Figure 14-110). After checking the back and crown for even blending, proceed to the left-side section.
9. **Create side guide.** Establish a narrow guide section on the left side at the hairline approximately ½ inch wide. The side guideline should be the same length as the nape (Figure 14-111). Move to the right side of the head and establish a matching guideline there. This will help you to be sure that both side sections will be the same length when the right side section is cut later (Figure 14-112).
10. **Create side section.** Establish a ½-inch side section that curves and follows the hairline above the ear back to the nape section. Smoothly comb the section, including the side guideline and part of the nape section (Figure 14-113).
11. **Blend nape and side.** Holding the hair with little or no tension, cut the hair from the nape guide to the side guide. Note that the fingers are held at a slight angle to connect the two guides (Figures 14-114 and 14-115).

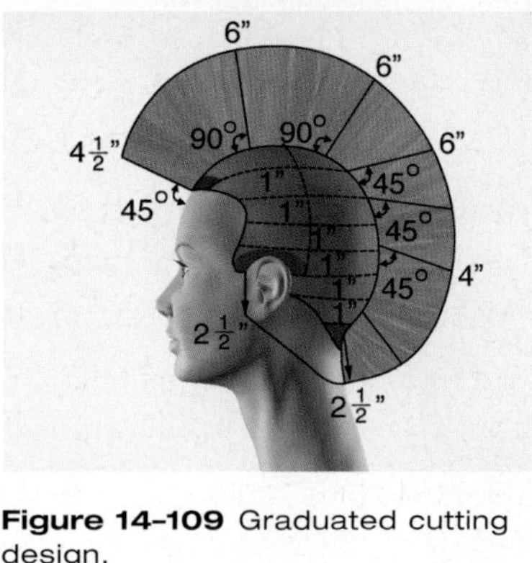

Figure 14-109 Graduated cutting design.

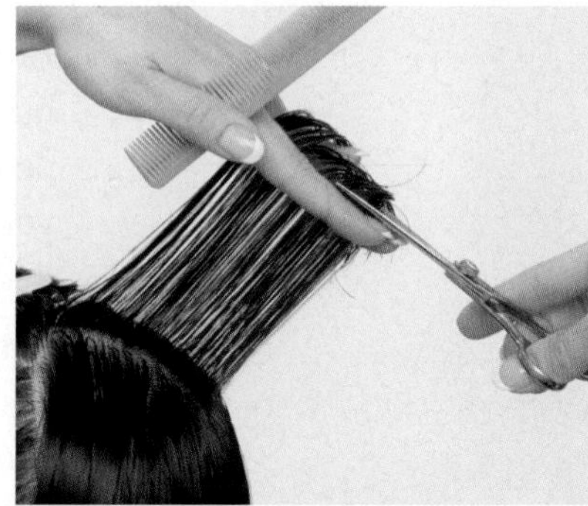

Figure 14-110 Cut hair in crown at 90 degrees.

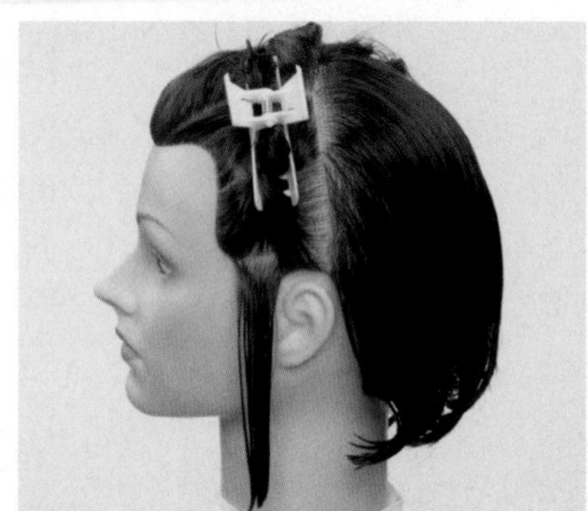

Figure 14-111 Establish guide section on the left.

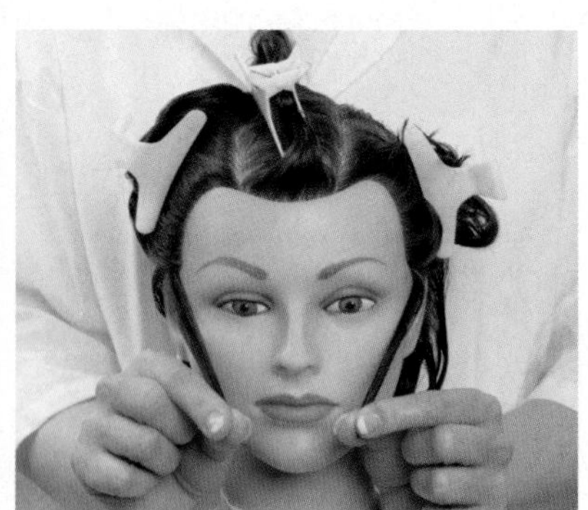

Figure 14-112 Check that both sections are the same length.

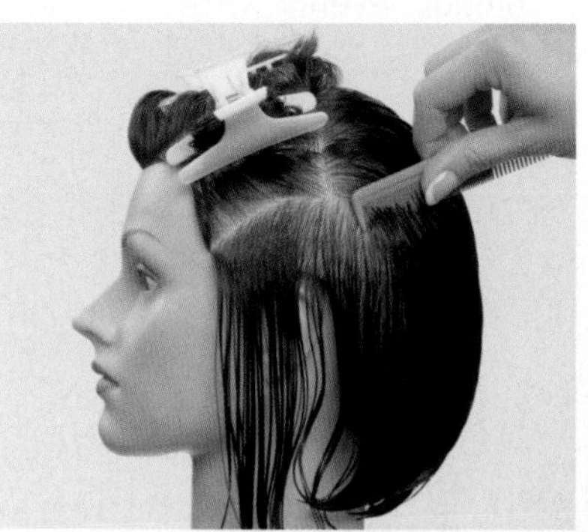

Figure 14-113 Establish side section.

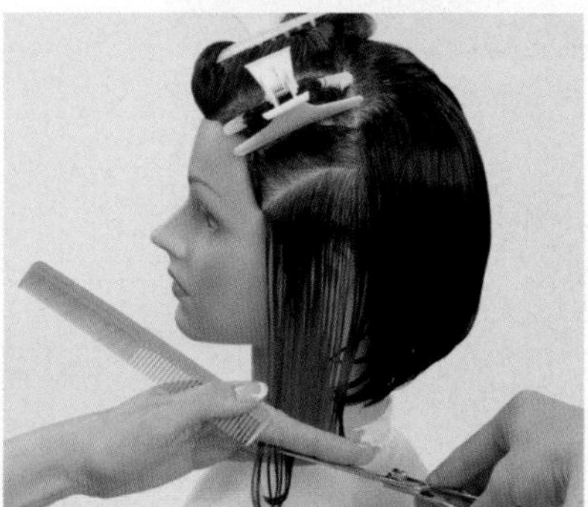

Figure 14-114 Cut hair from nape guide to side guide.

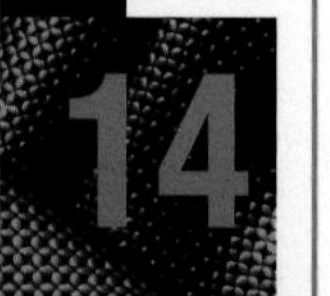

12. **Cut left side guide.** Establish a horizontal section on the left side. The width of this section will vary because of the irregular hairline around the ear (Figure 14-116).

13. **Cut ear guide.** Starting at the ear, part a ½-inch vertical subsection. Include the underlying guideline and a small portion of the nape section (Figure 14-117).

14. **Cut side section.** Continue following the same cutting procedure. Take vertical subsections, comb smooth, elevate at a 45-degree angle from the head, holding the fingers at a 90-degree angle to the hair. Cut the section even with the side guideline and nape section. Be sure to hold the vertical subsections straight out from the head at 45 degrees, not pulled to the right or left (Figure 14-118).

15. **Cut left side.** Continue establishing horizontal sections on the left side of the head and follow the same cutting procedure. Check each section horizontally to be sure the ends are evenly blended. Add hair from the back section when checking to ensure that the two sections are uniform in length.

16. **Blend side section.** When the left side section is complete, the hair in the uppermost part of the section should be the same length as those in the upper crown area. In the final 1-inch section, comb the vertical subsections and hold them at a 90-degree angle to the head. Position your fingers at 90 degrees to the hair and cut parallel to your fingers (Figure 14-119). Check the completed section horizontally to make sure the ends are even (Figure 14-120).

17. **Cut right side.** Move to the right side of the head and cut the hair in the same manner as you did on the left side, using the previously established guide. Once the back and both sides are complete, move to the bang and top areas.

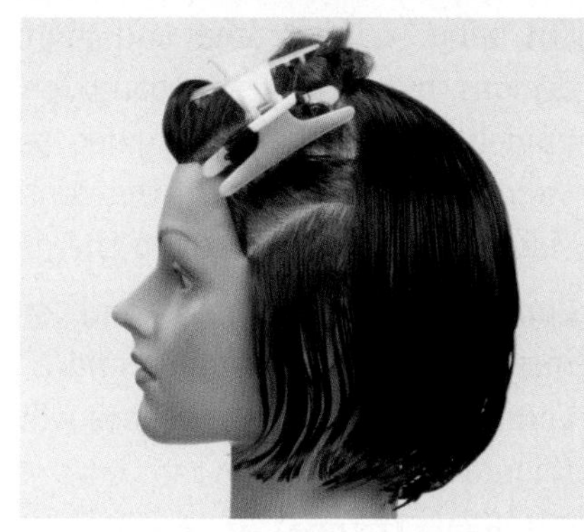

Figure 14–115 Finished side section.

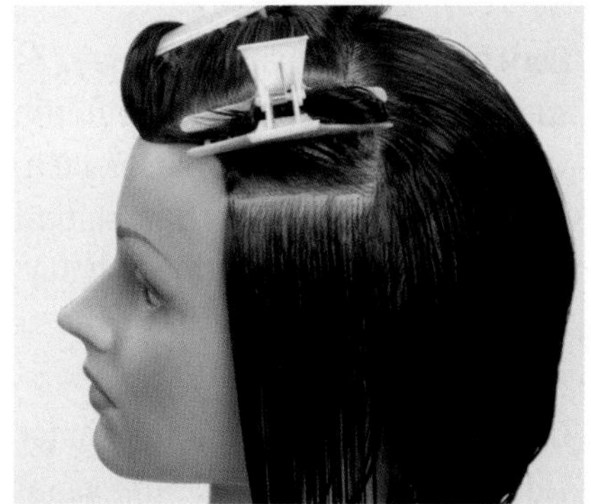

Figure 14–116 Establish horizontal section on left side.

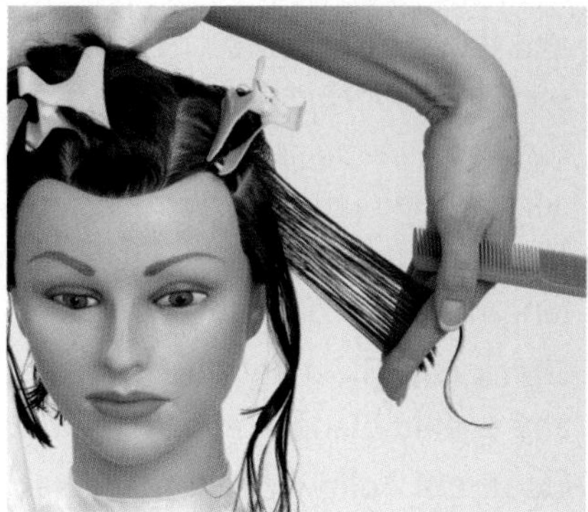

Figure 14–117 Part first vertical subsection.

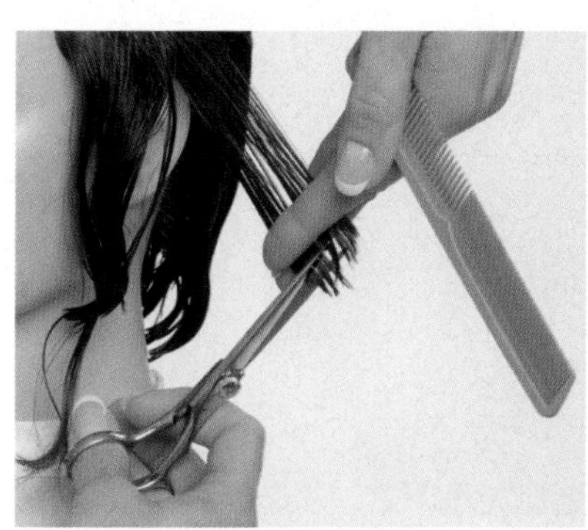

Figure 14–118 Hold vertical subsection straight out from the head at 45 degrees.

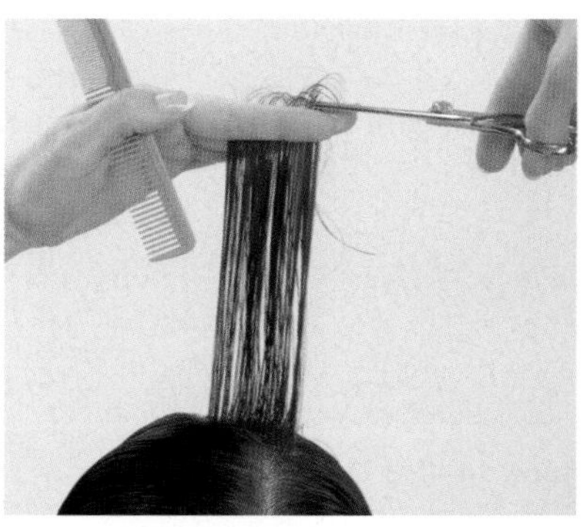

Figure 14–119 Blend subsections.

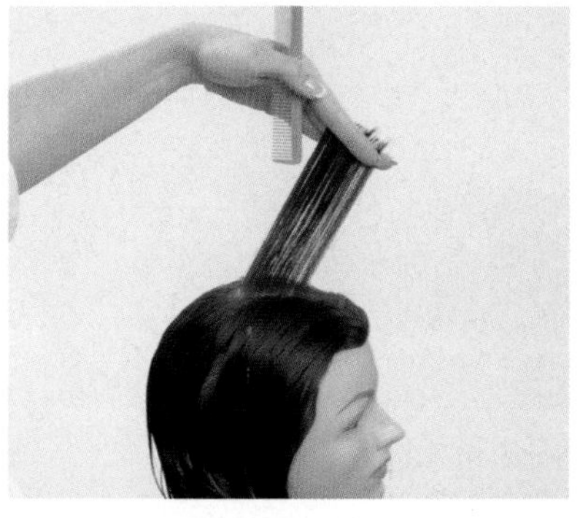

Figure 14–120 Cross-check section horizontally.

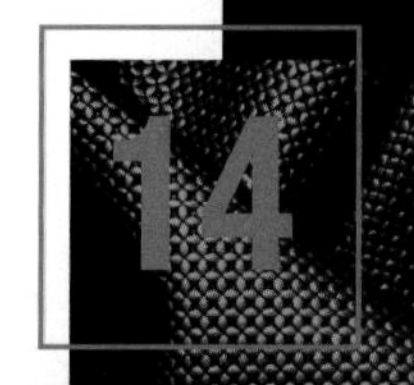

18. **Cut bang (fringe) area.** You can create a variety of bang (fringe) designs by cutting the bang length close to that of the side guideline. Create a bang guide section along the hairline about ½ inch wide. Starting at the center part and working on the left side of the forehead, cut to the desired length (Figure 14-121).
19. **Connect bang (fringe) and side.** Comb the bang section, including the center guide and a small portion of the side area. Connecting the two guidelines will determine the angle of the cut (Figure 14-122).
20. **Cut bang (fringe) at low elevation.** Cut this bang section at a low elevation. Check the cut for evenness and accuracy (Figure 14-123).
21. **Continue to cut bang (fringe).** Establish a 1-inch section parallel to the bang guideline. Beginning in the center, take narrow vertical subsections about ½ inch wide that include the guideline underneath. Comb the hair smooth and elevate from the head at 45 degrees. Continue this cutting procedure throughout the bang area (Figure 14-124). The fringe section should blend evenly with the side section.
22. **Cut right side.** Cut the remainder of the bang area on the right side of the head in the same manner as you did on the left side.
23. **Complete top section.** Finish the top section by taking ½-inch vertical subsections parallel to the center part. Hold the hair up from the head at a 90-degree angle. Include hair from the crown and bang area, and cut to blend the section with the two pre-cut sections. Continue cutting in this manner until the remainder of the top section is cut. Hold the hair up from the head at a 90-degree angle and check the completed cut. Trim any uneven ends. The bang guide gradually increases in length to the pre-established length in the top and crown areas (Figure 14-125).
24. **Check cut.** Blow-dry the haircut and view the de-sign, movement, and evenly blended ends (Figure 14-126).
25. **Clean up.** Follow cleanup and sanitation steps in "Blunt Haircut" procedure.

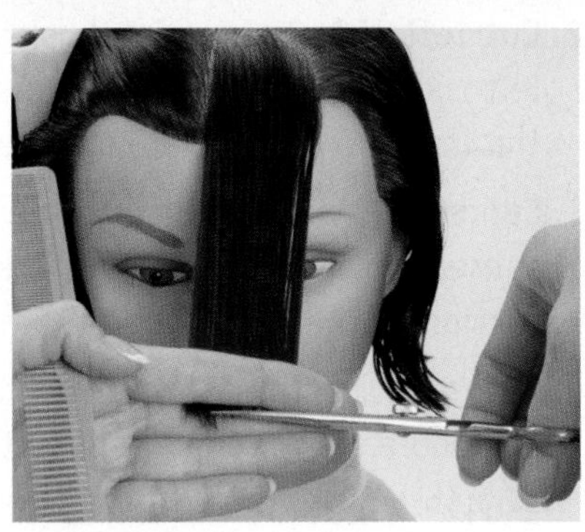

Figure 14-121 Cut bang guide section.

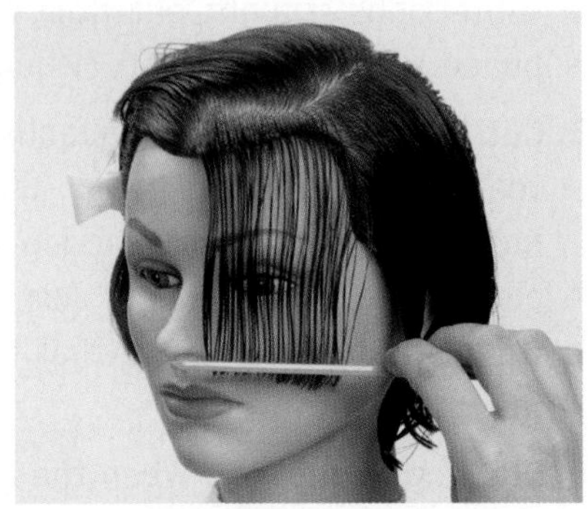

Figure 14-122 Comb bang section.

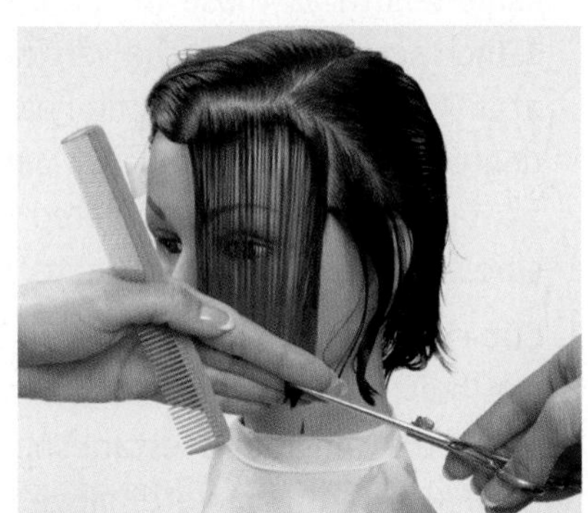

Figure 14-123 Cut bang section at low elevation.

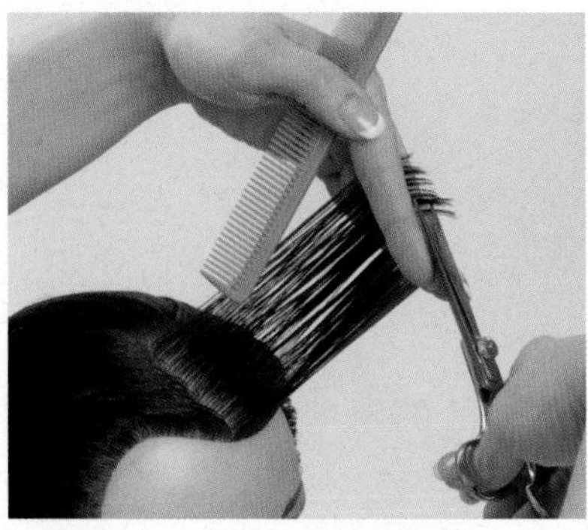

Figure 14-124 Cut vertical subsections in bang area.

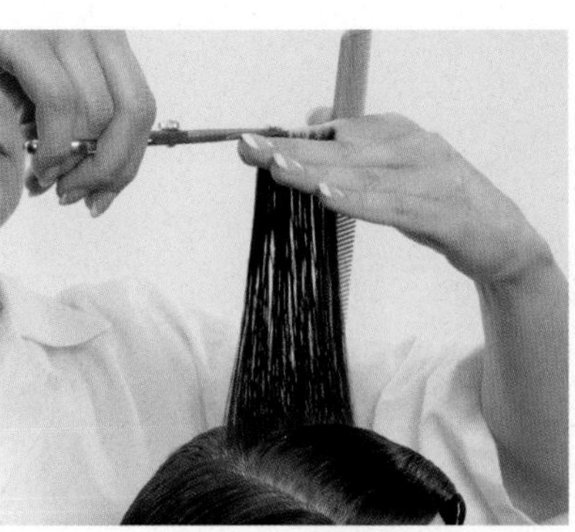

Figure 14-125 Cut top section.

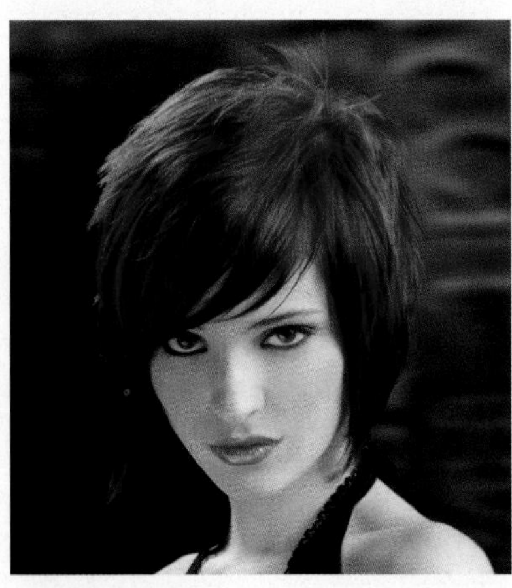

Figure 14-126 Finished graduated cut.

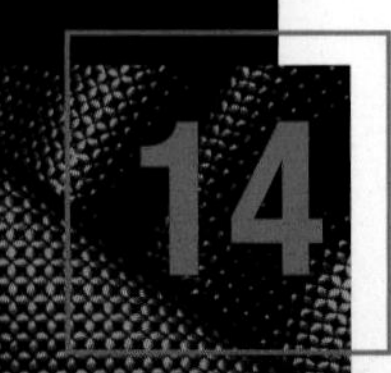

In the example in Figures 14-127, 14-128, and 14-129, you can see a shorter shape that has "rounded" weight. This haircut is created using diagonal partings that connect at the back of the ear. In front of the ear, the diagonal partings point down toward the face. Behind the ear, the diagonal partings point down toward the back. The sides are elevated and over-directed to the back of the ear, producing more length toward the face. The back is cut using a traveling guideline, with each section over-directed to the previous section.

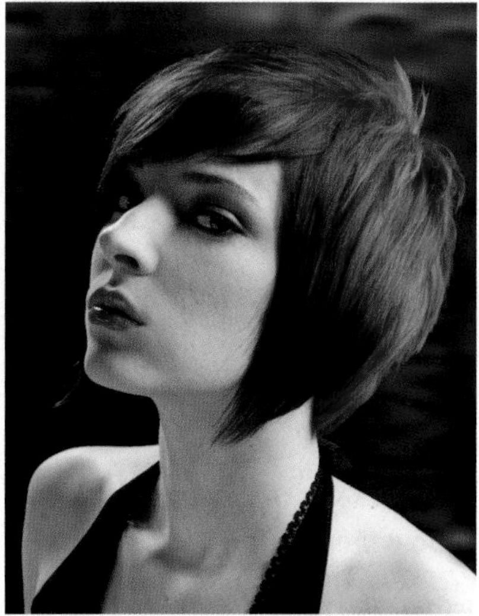

Figure 14-127 Finished graduated cut: side view.

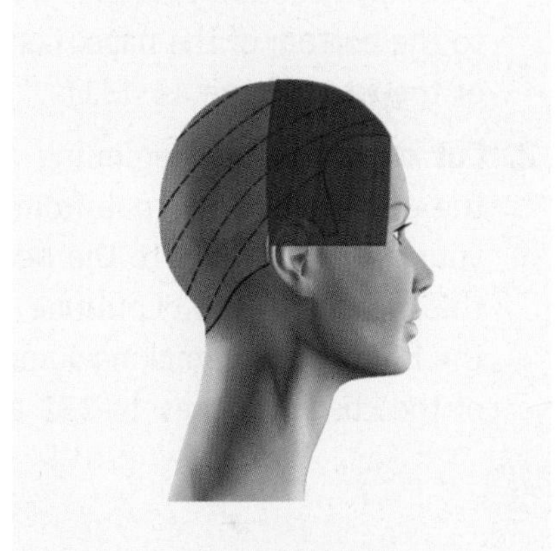

Figure 14-128 Classic (round) graduated cut: design.

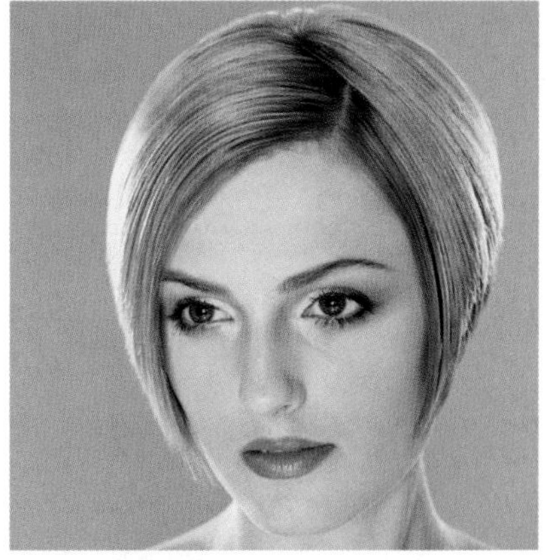

Figure 14-129 Finished classic (round) graduated cut.

TIPS FOR GRADUATED HAIRCUTS

- Heavier graduated haircuts (those cut with lower elevations) work well on hair that tends to "expand" when dry. Coarse textures and curly hair will appear to graduate more than straight hair. Keep your elevation below 45 degrees when working on these hair types.
- Fine hair is great for graduation. Because graduation builds weight, you can make thin or fine hair appear thicker and fuller. However, if hair is both fine and thin, avoid creating heavy weight lines. Softer graduation, using diagonal partings, will create a softer weight line. If hair has medium density but is fine in texture, it is safe to elevate more because there is enough density to support it.
- Check the neckline carefully before cutting the nape short. If the hairline grows straight up, you may want to leave the length longer and the graduation lower, so that it falls below the hairline. You can also blend in a tricky hairline by using the scissor-over-comb technique, which is explained later in this chapter.
- Always use the fine teeth of the comb and maintain even tension to ensure a precise line.

THE UNIFORM-LAYERED (90-DEGREE) HAIRCUT

The third basic haircut is the layered haircut created with **uniform layers.** All the hair is elevated to 90 degrees from the scalp and cut at the same length. Your guide for this haircut is an interior traveling guideline. An **interior guideline** is inside the haircut rather than on the perimeter. The resulting shape will appear soft and rounded, with no built-up weight or corners. The perimeter of the hair will fall softly, because the vertical sections in the interior reduce weight (Figure 14-130).

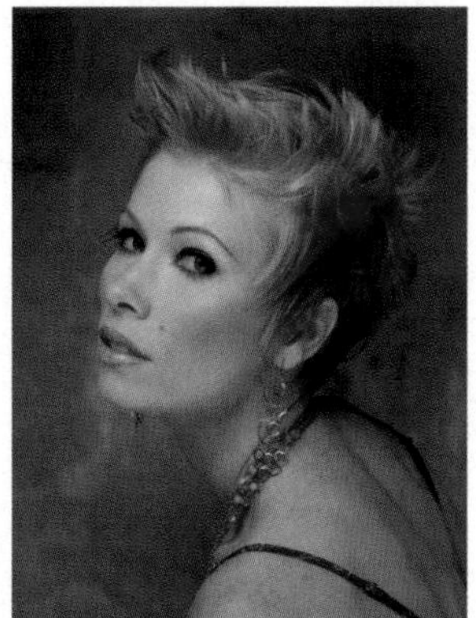

Figure 14-130 A uniform layered haircut

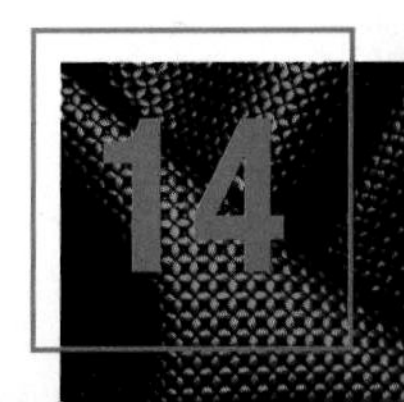

14-3

UNIFORM-LAYERED HAIRCUT (Figure 14-130)

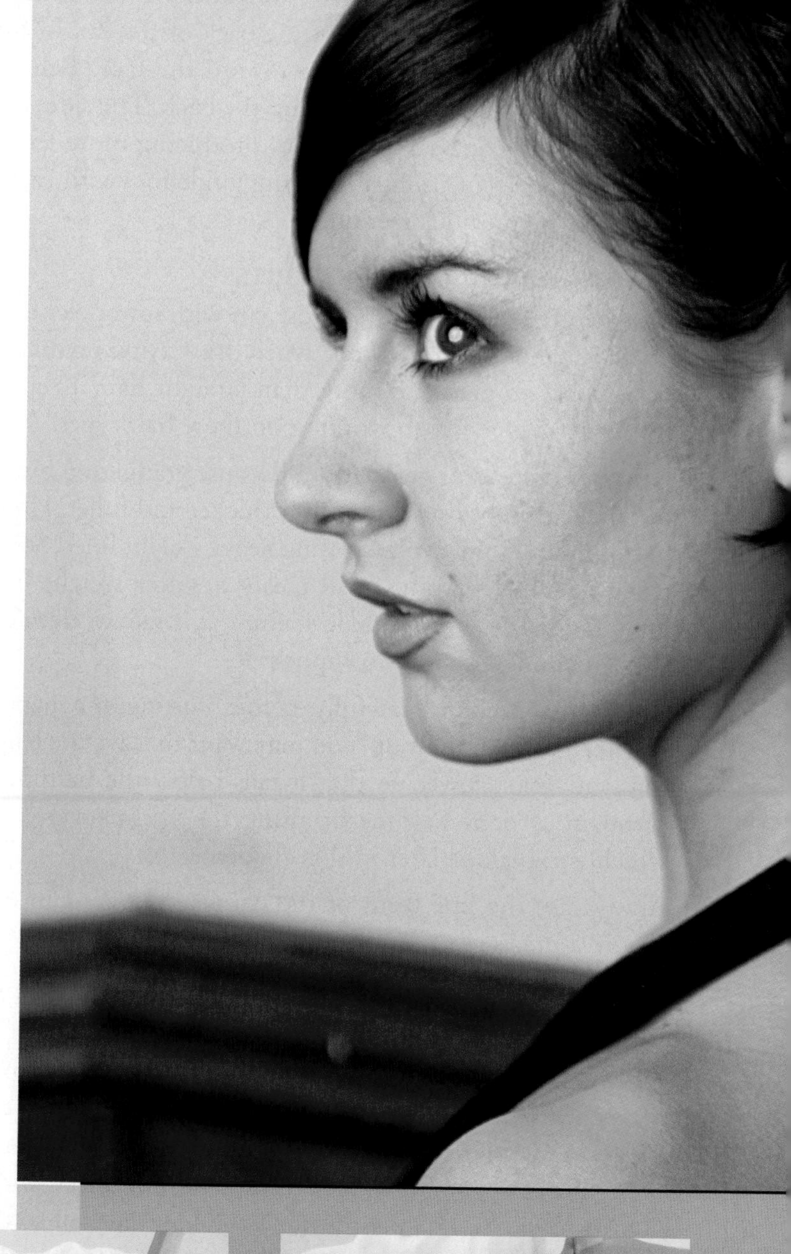

IMPLEMENTS AND MATERIALS

See list of implements and materials for "Blunt Haircut" procedure.

PREPARATION

Follow preparation steps in "Blunt Haircut" procedure.

PROCEDURE

1. **Create guideline.** To create the guideline, take two partings ½ inch (1.25 centimeters) apart, creating a section that runs from the front hairline to the bottom of the nape. Comb all other hair out of the way (Figure 14-131).
2. **Cut crown guide.** Beginning at the crown, comb the section straight out from the head, keeping your fingers parallel to the head form, and cut to the desired length. Continue working forward to the front hairline, making sure to stand to the side of the client (Figures 14-132 and 14-133).

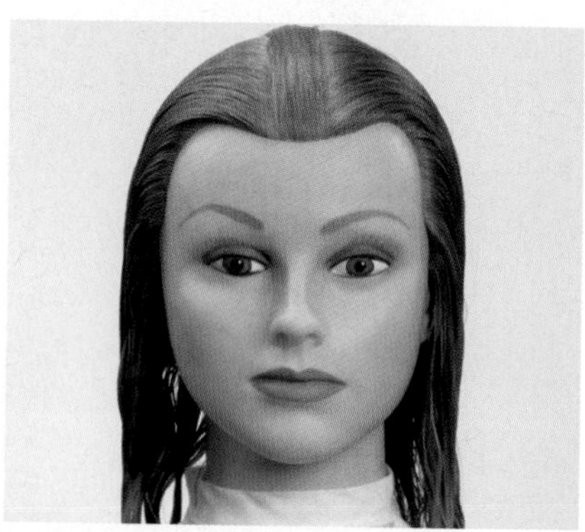

Figure 14-131 Part off guideline section.

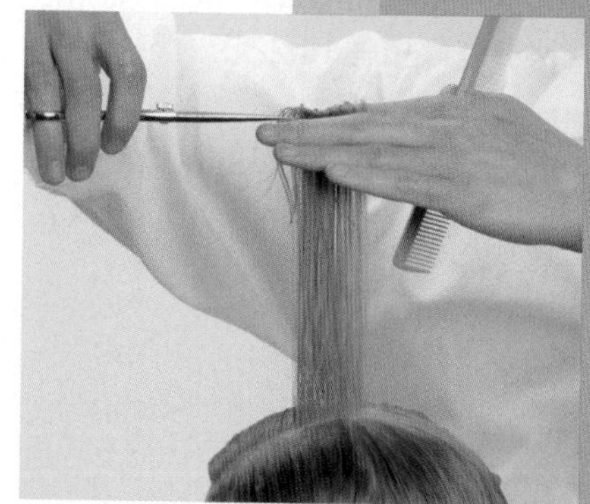

Figure 14-132 Part out first section in the crown and cut.

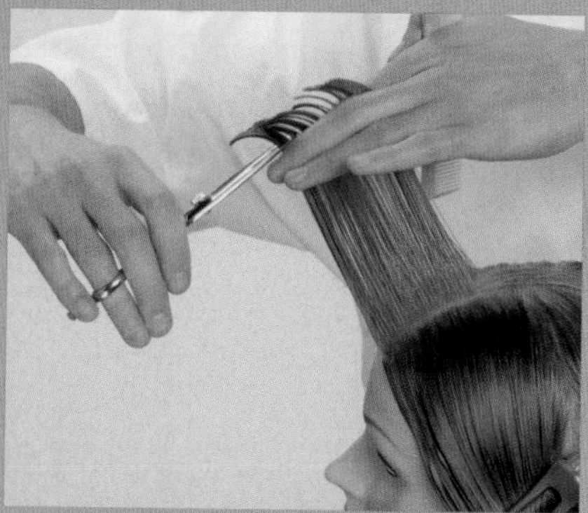

Figure 14-133 Cut front section.

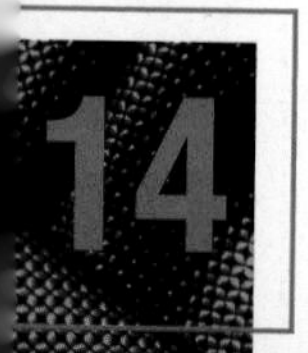

3. **Cut to nape.** Continue cutting the guideline from the crown to the nape, rounding off any corners as you go along and making sure that your fingers are parallel to the head form (Figures 14-134 and 14-135).
4. **Cut back section.** To maintain control and consistency while working through the haircut, separate the sides from the back by parting the hair from the apex to the back of the ear. Work through the back areas first. The parting pattern will be wedge-shaped, where each section begins at the same point in the crown and is slightly wider at the bottom of the nape (Figures 14-136 and 14-137).
5. **Cut right side first.** Work through the right side first. Take a vertical parting that begins at the crown and connects with the guideline, creating a vertical section that ends at the hairline. Keep the sections small to maintain control. Beginning at the crown and using the previously cut guideline, comb the new section to the guide, and elevate the hair straight out from the head, with no overdirection. Cut the line by keeping your fingers parallel to the head and matching the guideline (Figure 14-138).

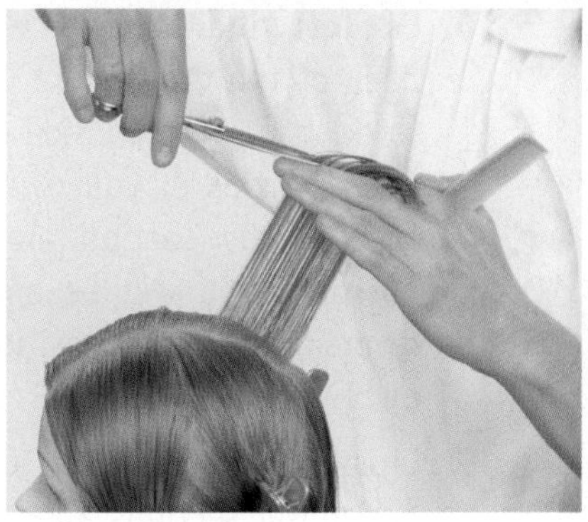

Figure 14–134 Connect crown to back.

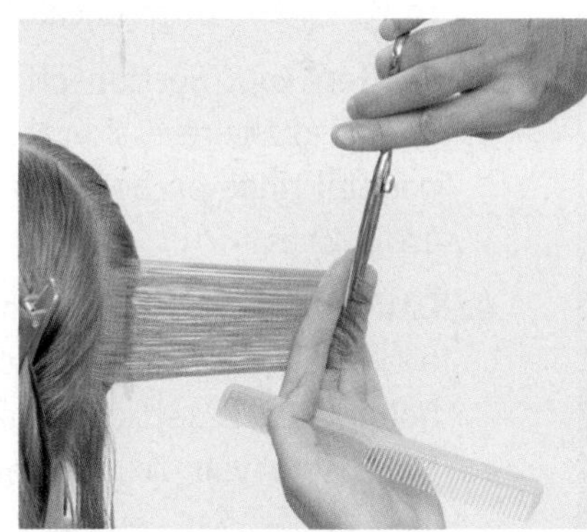

Figure 14–135 Connect back to nape.

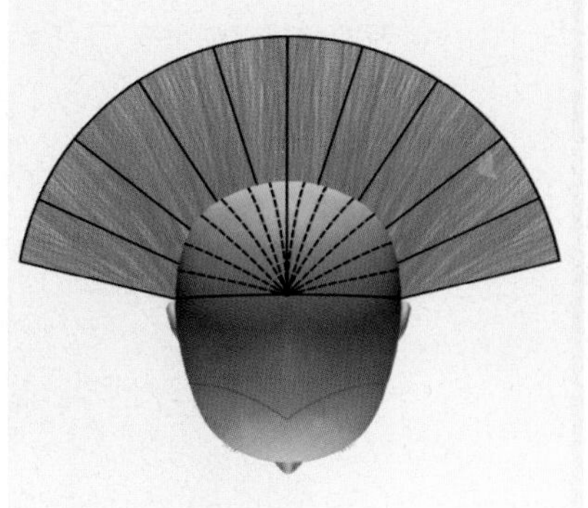

Figure 14–136 Wedge-shaped partings.

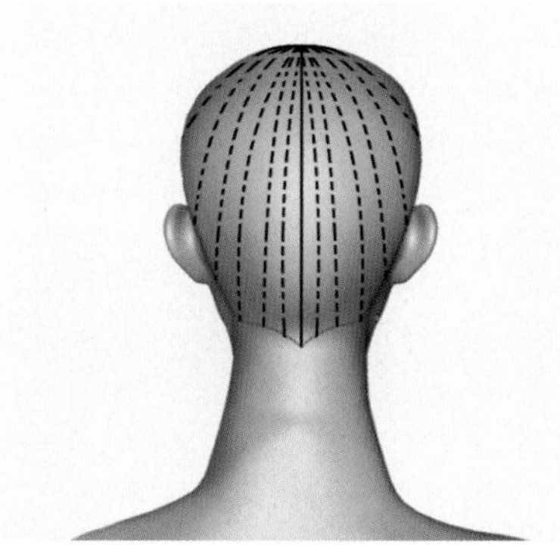

Figure 14–137 Wedge-shaped partings.

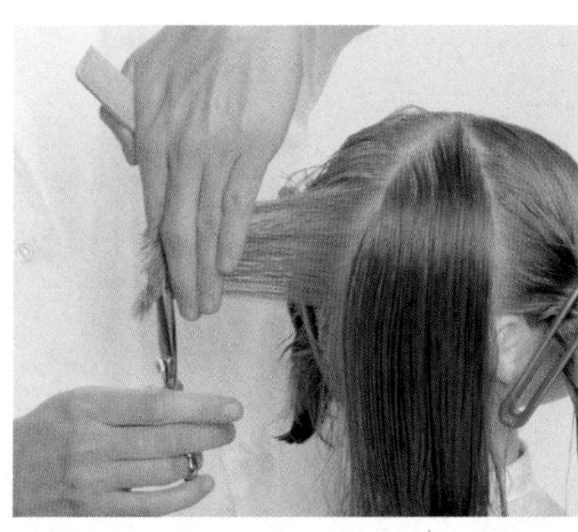

Figure 14–138 Cut second section on right back side.

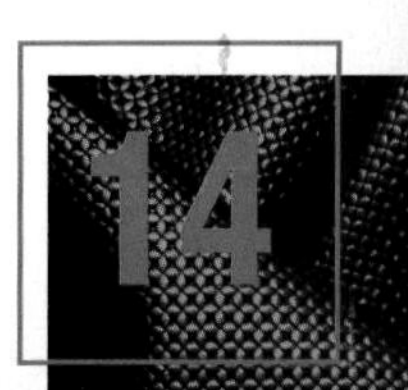

6. **Cut left side.** Continue working with a traveling guideline to the back of the ear (Figure 14-139). Repeat on the left side. When working on the left side of the back, shift your body position so that the tips of your shears are pointing down, and the fingers holding the section are pointing up. By shifting your hand position, you will be able to control the section. You will be reversing the hand position you used when you cut the right side of the back (Figure 14-140).
7. **Cross-check cut area.** Cross-check the entire back area. Take horizontal sections and elevate the hair at 90 degrees from the head. As you are checking, you should see a line that runs parallel to the shape of the head (Figure 14-141).
8. **Section top.** Section off the top area by taking a parting that begins at the recession area and ends at the crown, just above the parietal ridge on both sides. Clip the sides out of the way (Figure 14-142).
9. **Cut top.** Cut the top area using vertical partings. Using the previously cut center section as a guideline, connect to the crown, holding each section straight up at 90 degrees from the head. Make sure you do not overdirect the hair (Figures 14-143 and 14-144).

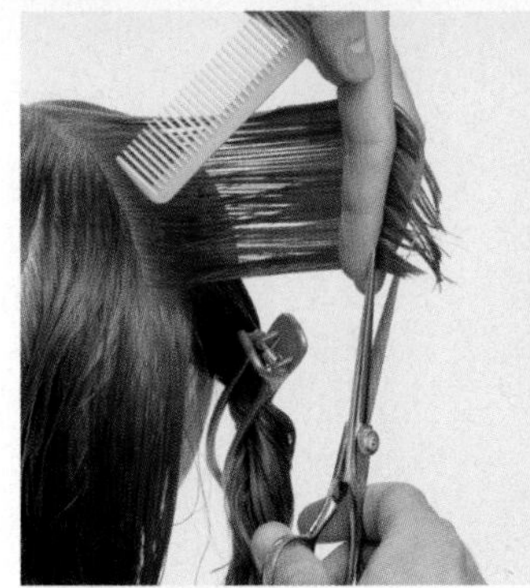

Figure 14-139 Cut section at back of the ear.

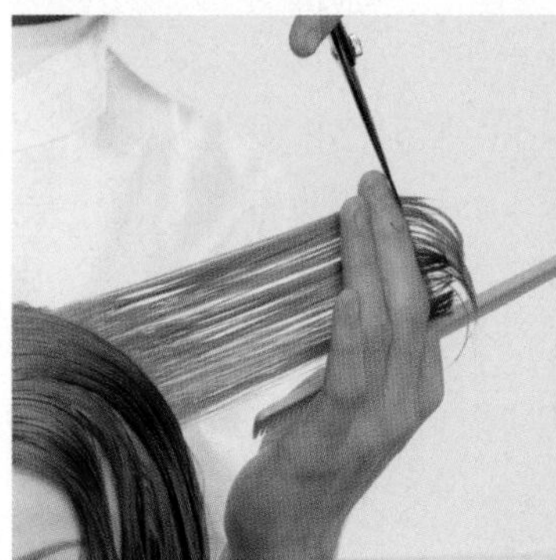

Figure 14-140 Shift hand position.

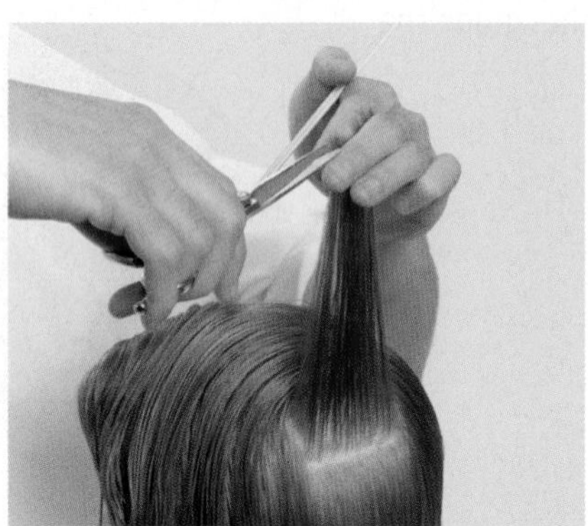

Figure 14-141 Cross-check back area.

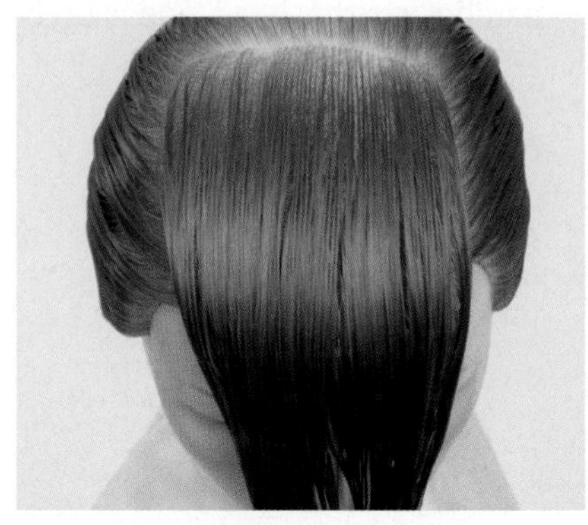

Figure 14-142 Section off the top area.

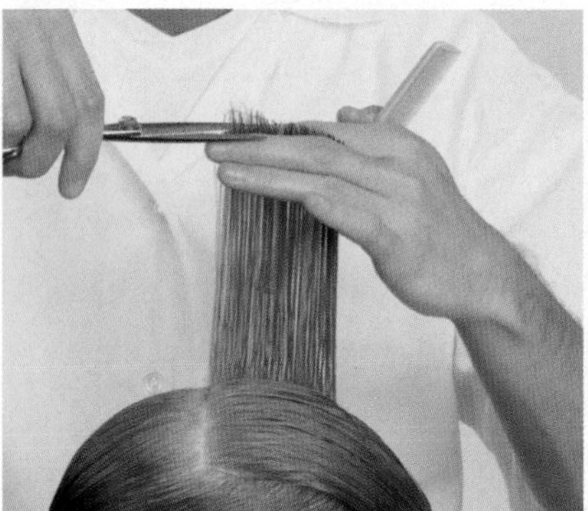

Figure 14-143 Match the first section to the guideline.

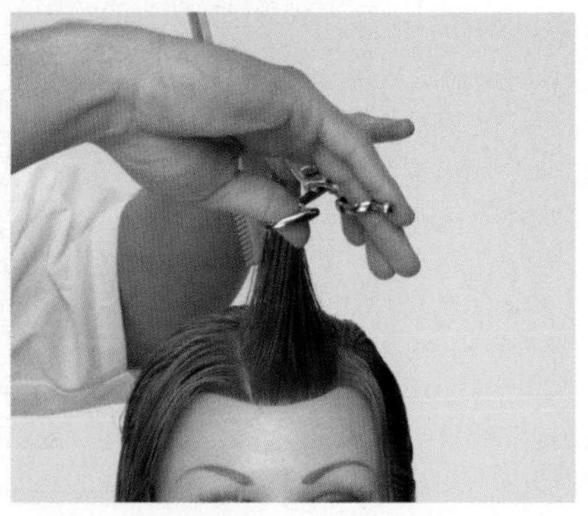

Figure 14-144 Complete last section of top area.

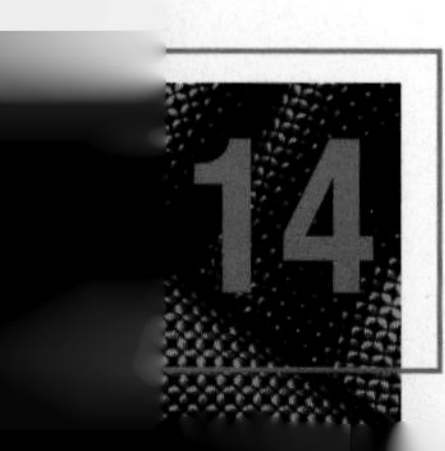

10. **Cross-check top.** Cross-check the top, using horizontal partings and elevating the hair 90 degrees from the head (Figure 14-145).
11. **Cut right side.** Now move to the right side. Work from the back of the ear toward the face, using vertical sections, and connect to the previous section at the back of the ear and the top. Comb the hair straight out from the head at 90 degrees, removing any corners as you go (Figures 14-146 and 14-147). Repeat on the left side, shifting body position so that the tips of your shears are pointing down, and the fingers holding the section are pointing up.
12. **Cross-check side.** Cross-check the side sections, using horizontal partings and combing the hair straight out at 90 degrees.
13. **Comb hair.** Comb the hair down. Note the soft perimeter and rounded head shape (Figure 14-148).
14. **Style hair.** Blow-dry the haircut using a vent brush to encourage movement, and complete (Figure 14-149 and 14-150).
15. **Clean up.** Follow cleanup and sanitation steps in "Blunt Haircut" procedure.

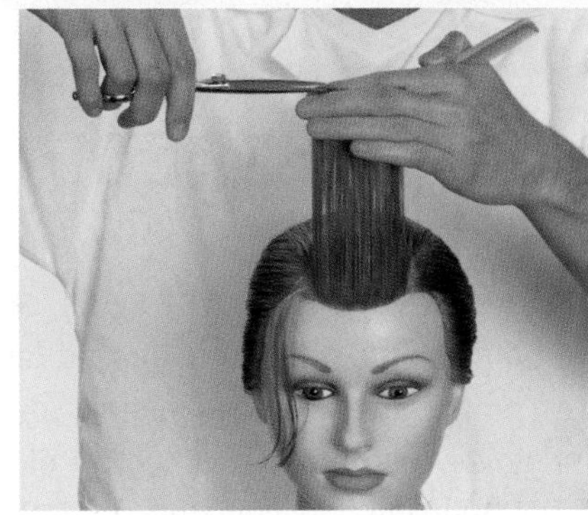

Figure 14-145 Cross-check the top.

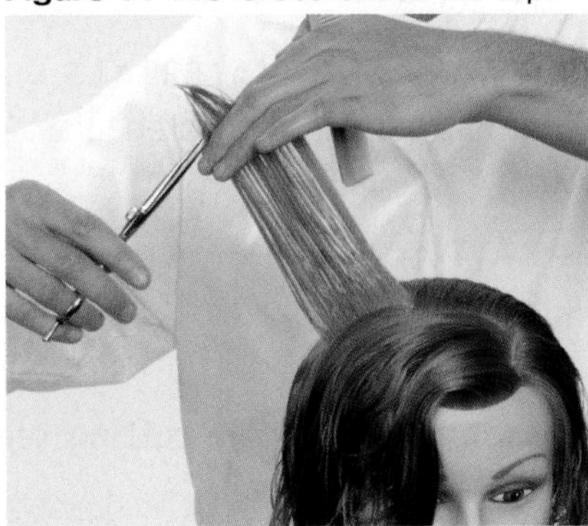

Figure 14-146 Connect at back of ear and top.

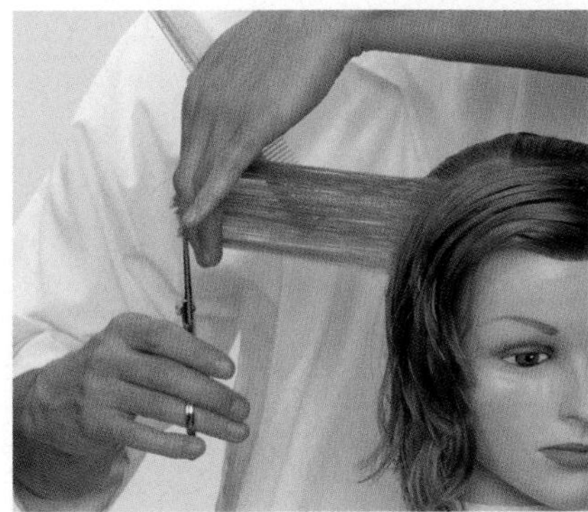

Figure 14-147 Connect lower portion of vertical section.

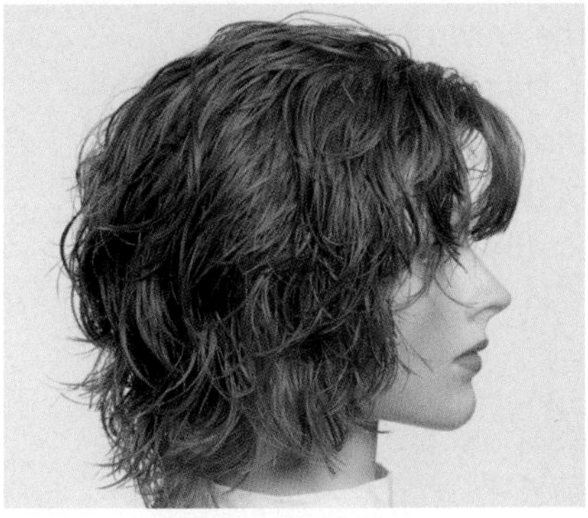

Figure 14-148 Finished haircut, wet profile.

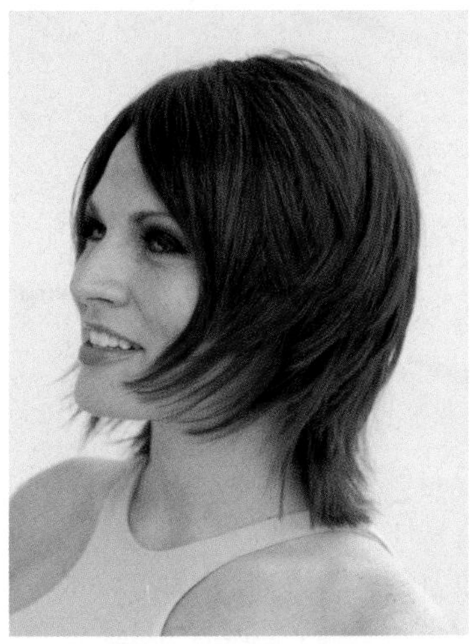

Figure 14-149 Finished uniform layered haircut: side view.

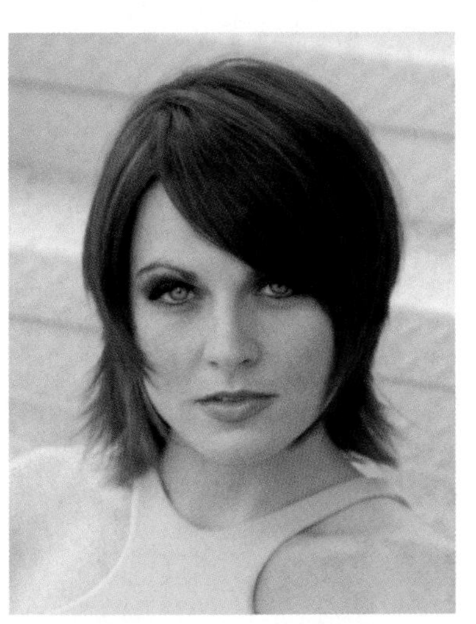

Figure 14-150 Finished uniform layered haircut.

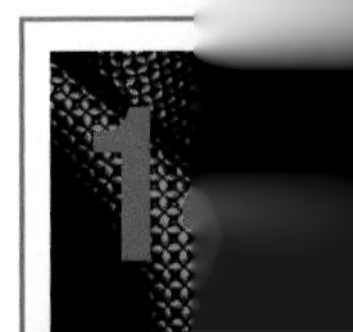

PROCEDURE 14-4

LONG-LAYERED HAIRCUT

LONG-LAYERED (180-DEGREE) HAIRCUT

In this haircut you will use increased layering, which features progressively longer layers. Your guide is an interior guide, beginning at the top of the head. All remaining hair will be elevated up (180 degrees) to match the guide.

IMPLEMENTS AND MATERIALS

See list of implements and materials in "Blunt Haircut" procedure.

PREPARATION

Follow preparation steps in "Blunt Haircut" procedure.

PROCEDURE

1. **Part the hair into five cutting sections** (Figure 14-151).
2. **Begin at crown.** Begin at the top of the crown by taking a ½ inch (1.25 centimeters) subsection across the head. Comb straight up from the head form and cut straight across (Figure 14-152).
3. **Cut top section.** Work to the front of the top section by taking a second ½-inch subsection. Direct the first subsection (guideline) to the second one and cut to the same length (Figure 14-153).
4. **Complete top.** Continue, using the previously cut subsection as your guideline to cut a new ½-inch subsection throughout the top section (Figure 14-154).
5. **Cut left side.** On the left front section, using ½-inch horizontal subsections, comb the hair straight up and match to the previously cut hair (guideline) in the top section (Figure 14-155). Continue working down the side, using ½-inch subsections until the hair no longer reaches the guide.

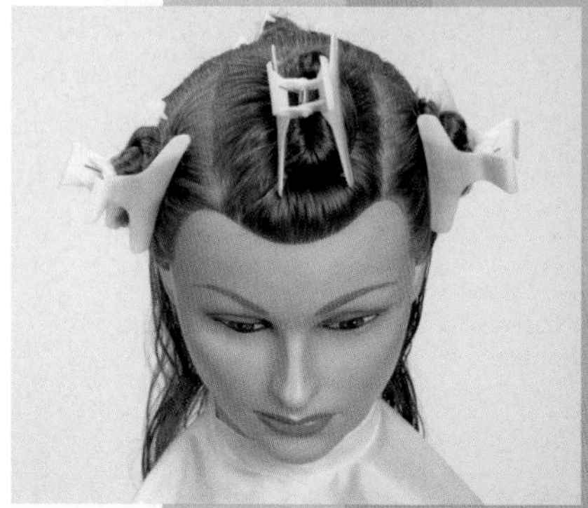

Figure 14-151 Five sections.

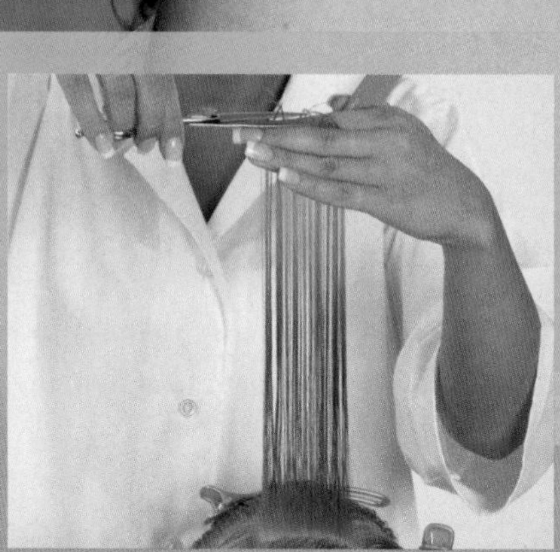

Figure 14-152 Cut the first subsection.

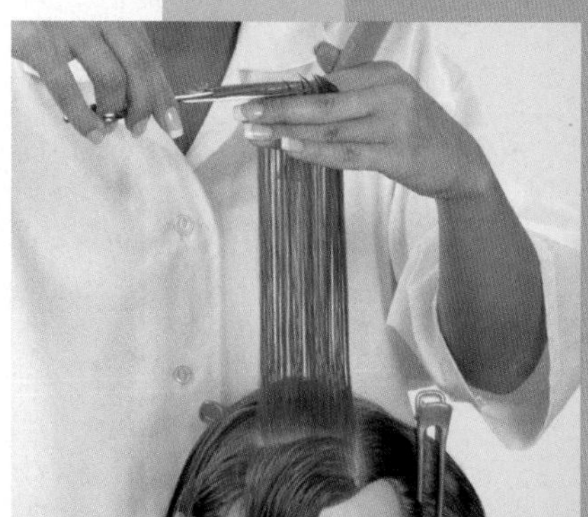

Figure 14-153 Cut the second subsection.

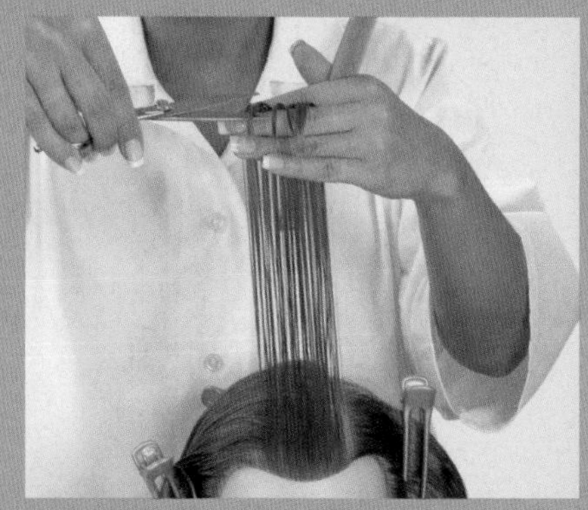

Figure 14-154 Continue cutting through top section.

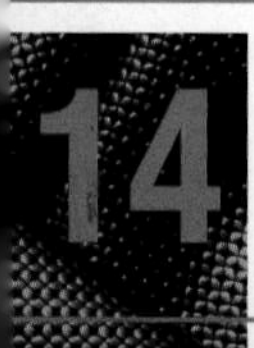

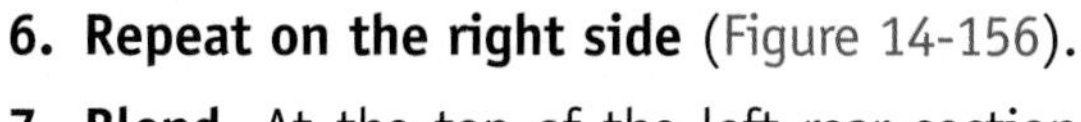

6. **Repeat on the right side** (Figure 14-156).
7. **Blend.** At the top of the left rear section, using ½-inch horizontal subsections, comb the hair straight up from the head form, matching the length to the top section (guideline) and cut straight across (Figure 14-157).
8. **Continue cutting.** Continue, using ½-inch horizontal subsections and working from top to bottom until the hair no longer reaches the guideline.
9. **Repeat on the right side until the hair no longer reaches the guideline** (Figure 14-158).
10. **Style hair.** Blow-dry the hair (Figure 14-159 through 14-161).

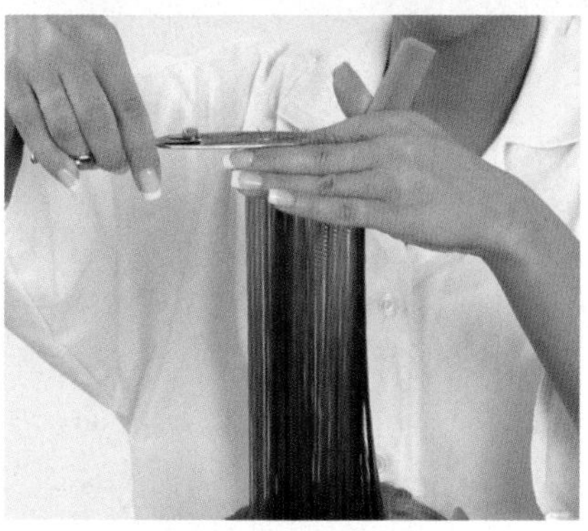

Figure 14-155 Match hair to guideline and cut.

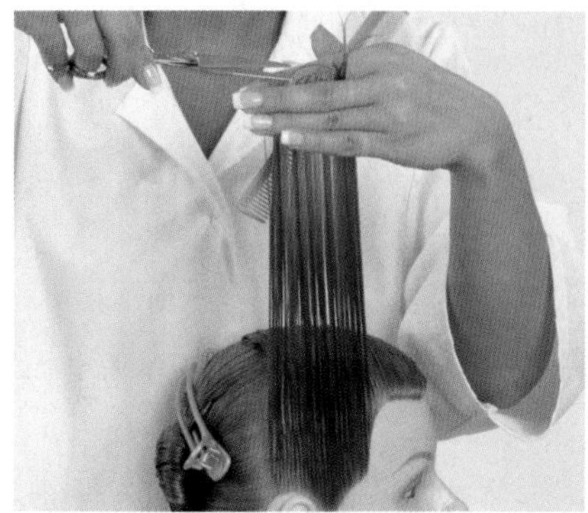

Figure 14-156 Repeat on the right side.

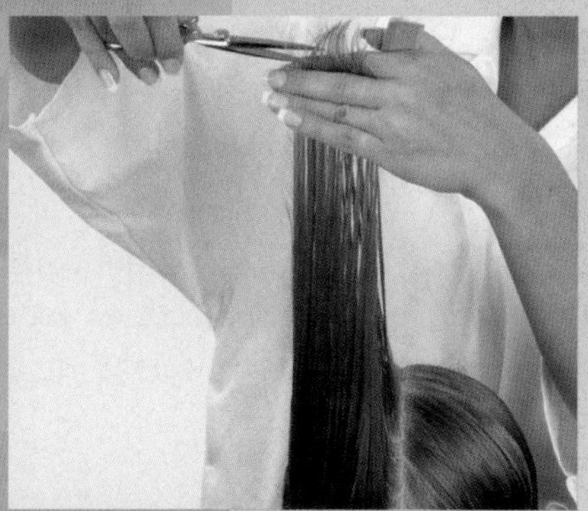

Figure 14-157 Cut left rear section.

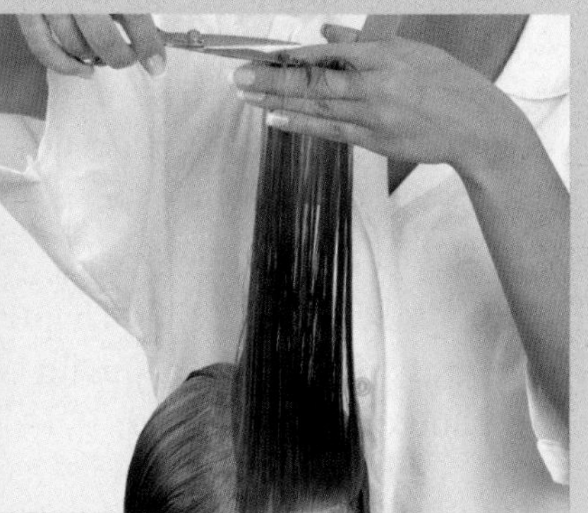

Figure 14-158 Work down the rear section.

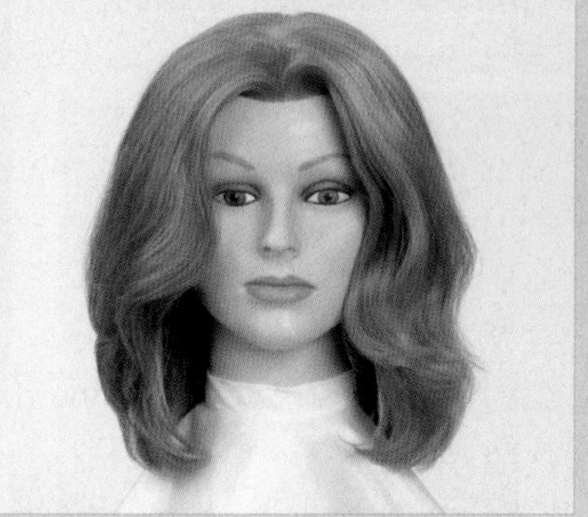

Figure 14-159 Finished long-layered haircut.

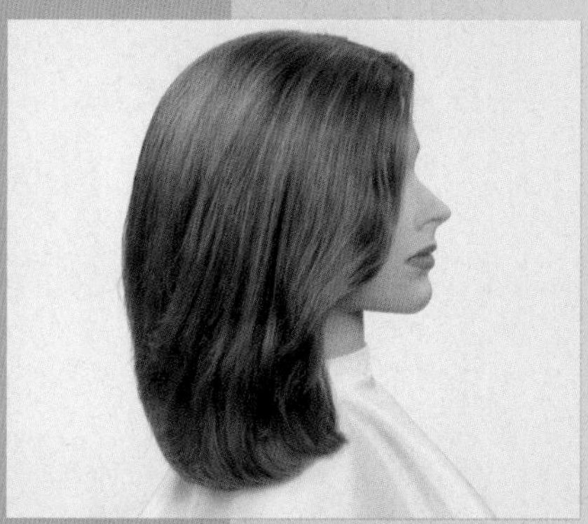

Figure 14-160 Finished long-layered haircut: Side view.

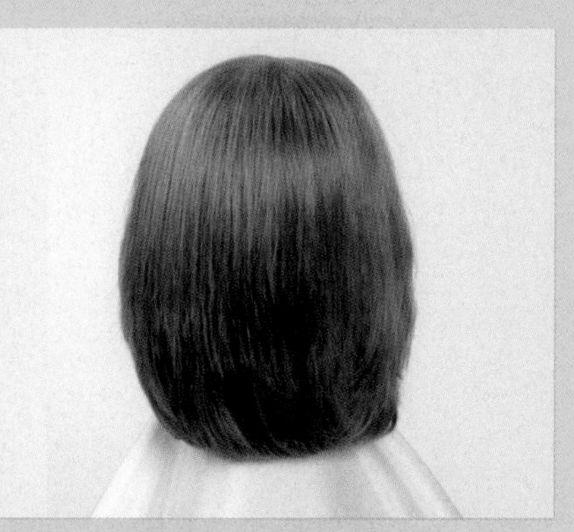

Figure 14-161 Finished long-layered haircut: Back.

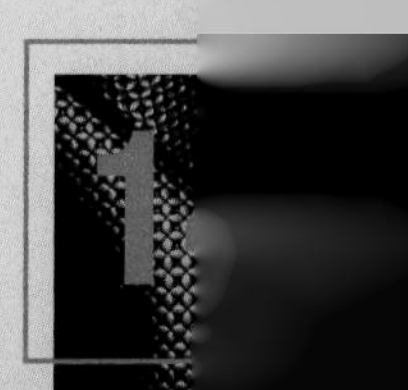

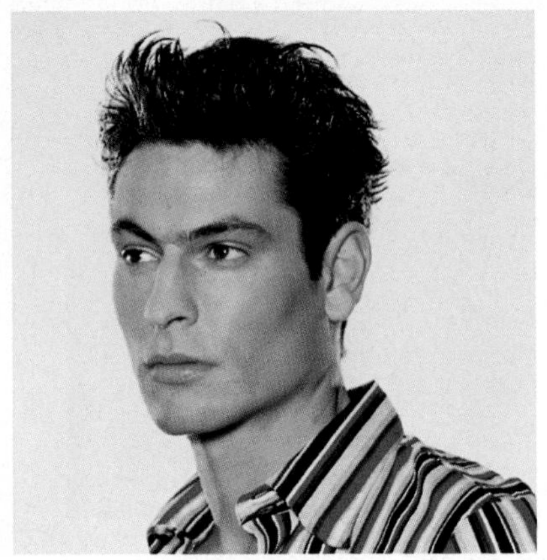

Figure 14-162 Short crop, men's cut.

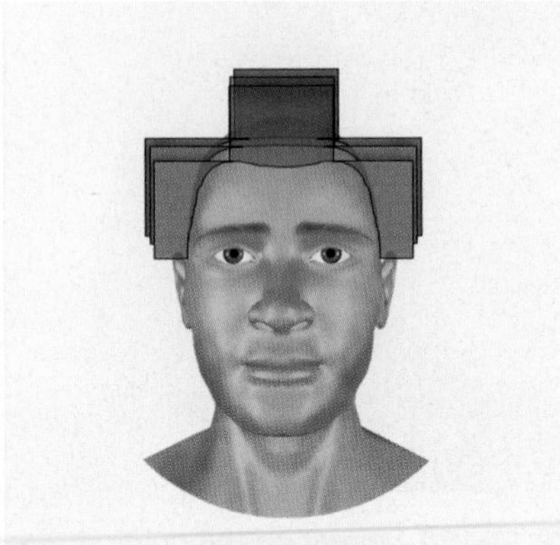

Figure 14-163 Basic men's haircut design.

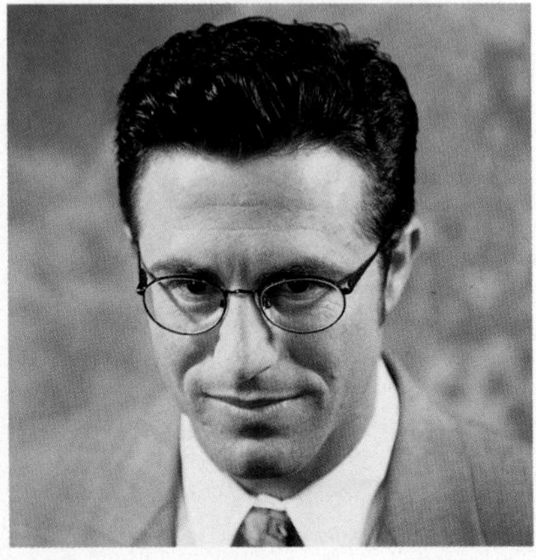

Figure 14-164 Basic men's haircut.

OTHER EXAMPLES OF LAYERED HAIRCUTS

There are many variations on the basic layered haircut.

- If you follow the uniform-layering technique but cut the hair much shorter, to 1 inch (2.5 centimeters) or so, you will create a "pixie," "crop," or "Caesar" haircut. This hairstyle is flattering on both men and women (Figure 14-162).
- If you follow the same method but keep the "corners" by keeping your fingers vertical and not following the head form, you can create a square shape, which is common in a man's basic haircut (Figures 14-163 and 14-164).
- You can create a layered haircut with longer perimeter lengths, otherwise known as a "shag," by cutting the top area the same as for uniform layers and then elevating the side and back sections straight up (180 degrees), blending them into the top lengths (Figures 14-165 and 14-166).

TIPS FOR LAYERED HAIRCUTS

- Cut the interior first. Then go back to the perimeter edges and cut stronger lines, cut out around the ears, and texturize where needed.
- When layering short hair, you will achieve the best results on medium to thicker densities. Cutting thin hair too short can expose the scalp.
- Coarse hair tends to stick out if cut shorter than 3 inches. This hair texture needs the extra length to hold it down.
- When working on longer layered shapes in which you want to maintain thickness at the bottom, remember to keep the top sections longer. Cutting the top layers too short will take too much hair away from the rest of the haircut, and may leave you with a collapsed shape that is stringy at the bottom.
- If the client has hair past the shoulder blades, use slide cutting (explained later in this chapter) to connect the top sections to the lengths. This will maintain maximum length and weight at the perimeter of the haircut.

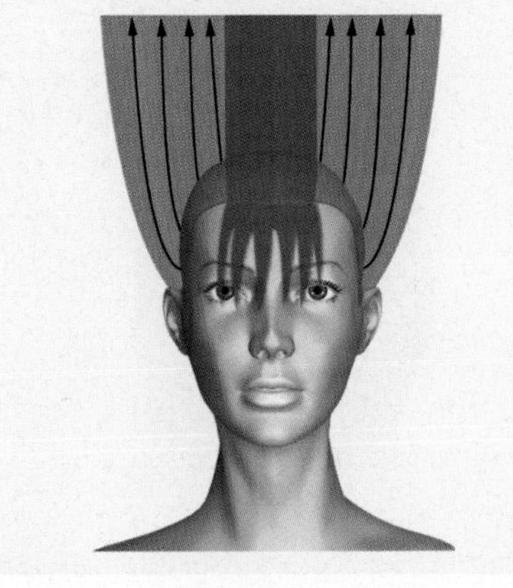

Figure 14-165 Long shag design.

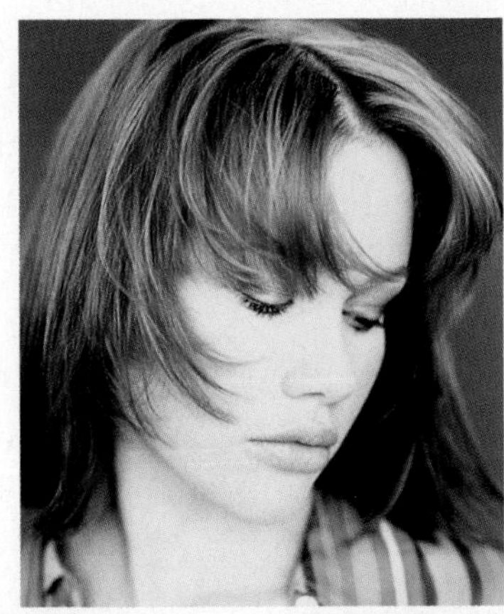

Figure 14-166 Long shag haircut.

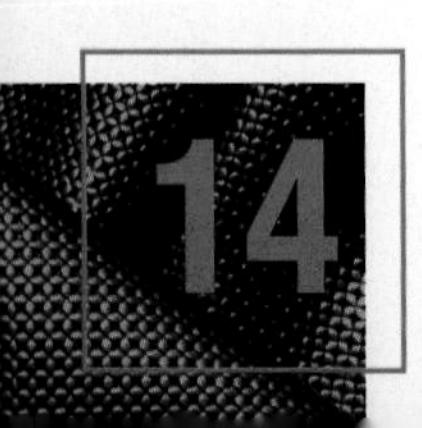

OTHER CUTTING TECHNIQUES

To go beyond the basic haircut, there are many techniques you can use to create different effects in hair. You can make wild hairlines calm down. You can make thick hair behave like thinner hair, fine hair appear fuller, create more movement, and add or reduce volume. You can also compensate for various growth patterns that exist in the same head of hair.

CUTTING CURLY HAIR

Curly hair can be a challenge to cut. Once you gain confidence, it can be a lot of fun to work with. However, it is important to understand how curly hair behaves after it has been cut and dried. Although you can apply any cutting technique to curly hair, you will get very different results than you would when cutting straight hair. Curl patterns can range from slightly wavy to extremely curly, and curly-haired clients may have fine, medium, or coarse textures, with density ranging from thin to thick.

TIPS FOR CUTTING CURLY HAIR

- Curly hair shrinks much more after it dries than straight hair. The curlier the hair, the more it will shrink. For every ¼ inch (0.6 centimeters) you cut when the hair is wet, it will shrink up to 1 inch (2.5 centimeters) when dry. Always keep this in mind when consulting with your client.
- Use minimal tension and/or the wide teeth of your comb. If you use a lot of tension when cutting curly hair, you will be stretching the wet hair even more, and making the hair shrink that much more when it dries.
- Curly hair naturally "graduates" itself. If the shape you want to create has strong angles, you need to elevate less than when working with straight hair.
- Curly hair expands more than straight hair. This means that you will generally need to leave lengths longer, which ultimately helps weigh the hair down and keeps the shape from ending up too short.
- In general, a razor should not be used on curly hair. Doing so weakens the cuticle and causes the hair to frizz.
- Choose your texturizing techniques carefully. Avoid using the razor, and work mostly with point cutting and free-hand notching to remove bulk and weight. (These techniques are discussed later in this chapter.)

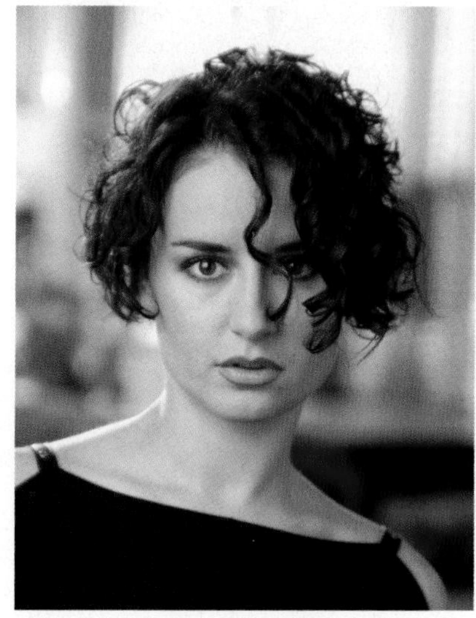

Figure 14-167 Blunt cut on curly hair.

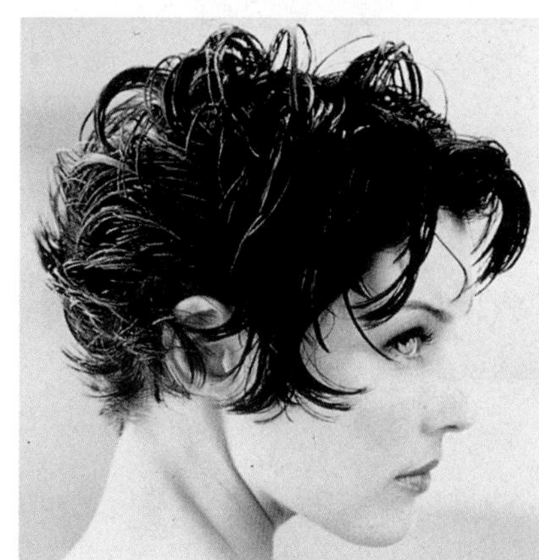

Figure 14-168 Graduated cut on curly hair.

EXAMPLES OF BASIC HAIRCUTS ON CURLY HAIR

Let us take a look at some basic haircuts, and how they work on curly hair. In Figure 14-167, note how the hair appears stacked, even though it was cut with a blunt technique. Although the hair was not elevated, it appears graduated. Note how the volume in the graduated haircut (Figure 14-168) is above the ears. The hair shrinks as it dries, resulting in a

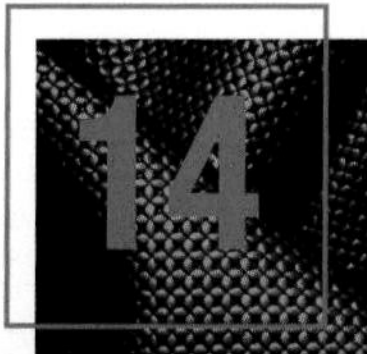

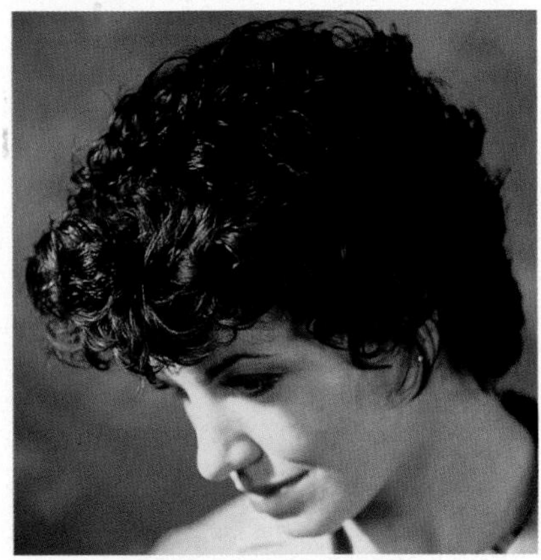

Figure 14-169 Uniform layered cut on curly hair.

weight line that has graduated itself even higher. In the next example (Figure 14-169), note the round shape. This is a uniform-layered cut on curly hair and was cut the same way as it was in Figure 14-149.

CUTTING THE BANGS (FRINGE)

Because much of our haircutting history comes from England, you will sometimes hear the word "fringe" used instead of "bangs." The two words mean basically the same thing. The bang or fringe area is the hair that lies between the two front corners, or approximately between the outer corners of the eyes (Figure 14-170).

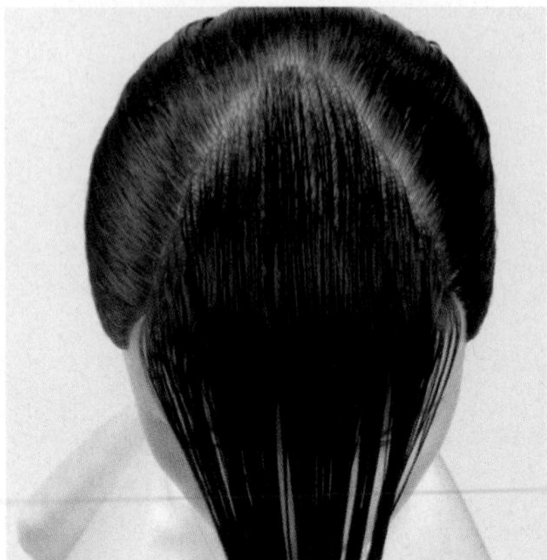

Figure 14-170 Bang area.

It is important to work with the natural **distribution** (where and how hair is moved over the head) when locating the bang area. Every head is different, and you need to make sure that you cut only the hair that falls in that area. Otherwise, you can end up with short pieces falling where they don't belong, which will ruin the lines of the haircut. When creating bangs (fringe), you do not always cut all the hair in this area, but you only cut more if you are blending into the sides or the top.

Let us have a look at a few types of bangs (fringe).

- In Figures 14-171 and 14-172, the bang is cut using a stationary guide, elevating at 90 degrees straight up from the head form.

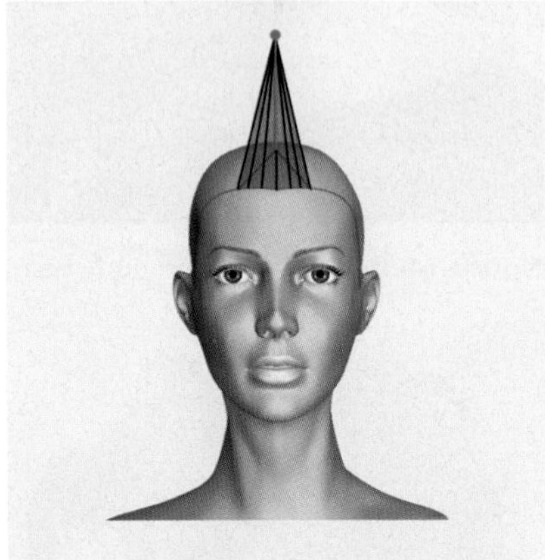

Figure 14-171 Layered bang design.

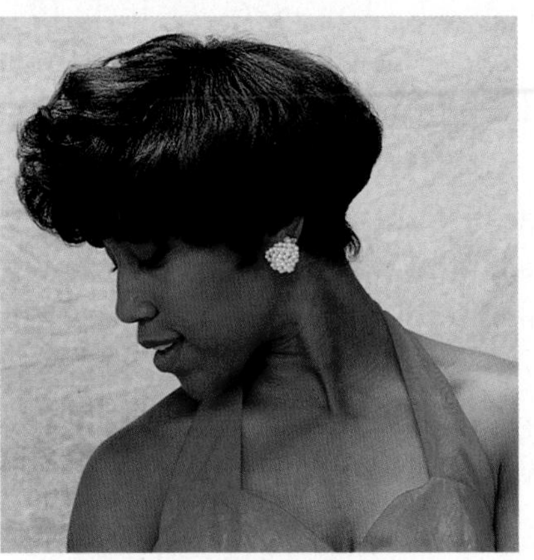

Figure 14-172 Layered bang cut.

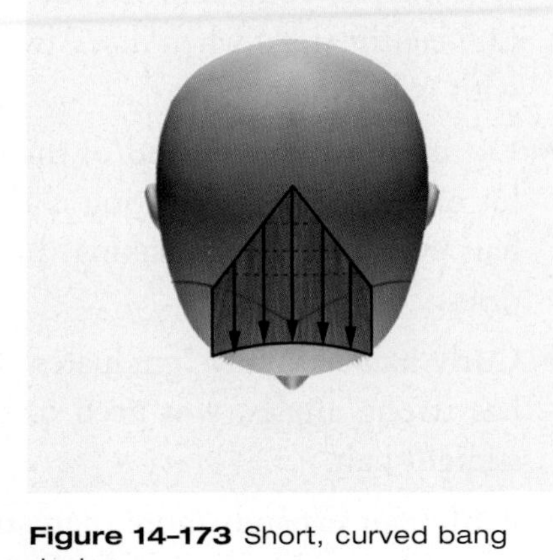

Figure 14-173 Short, curved bang design.

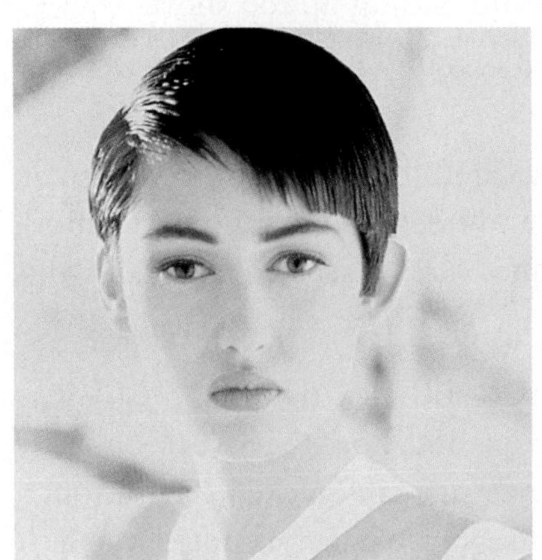

Figure 14-174 Short, curved bang cut.

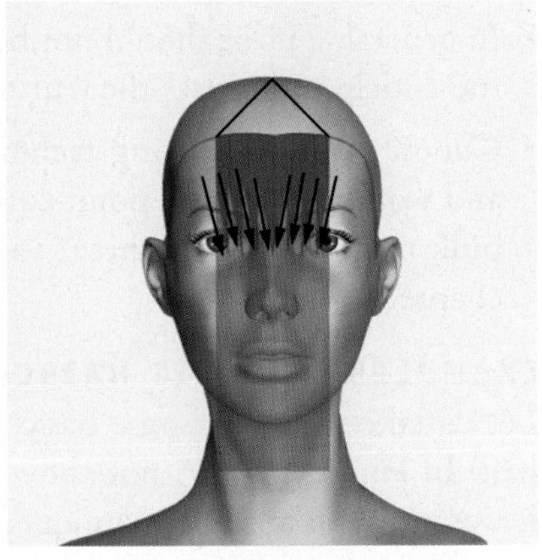

Figure 14-175 Long bang design.

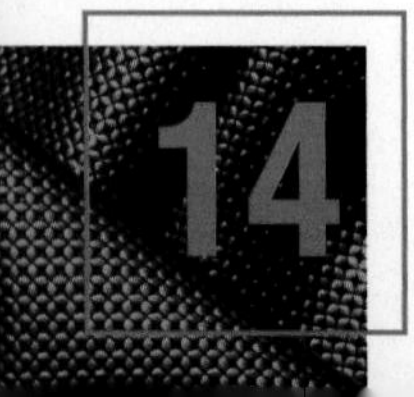

- A short bang makes a strong statement. In Figures 14-173 and 14-174, they are combined with a shorter layered haircut. Note that the line is curved. It has been cut with low elevation, so that it remains more solid and not too heavy.
- In Figures 14-175 and 14-176, the bang is very long and was cut with the slide-cutting technique to create a wispy effect.
- Sometimes only a few pieces are cut in the bang area, which keeps the hair out of the face. In this case, you will not be cutting all the hair in the bang area. You will cut only a small portion of this area and might even use a razor for that purpose (Figures 14-177 and 14-178).

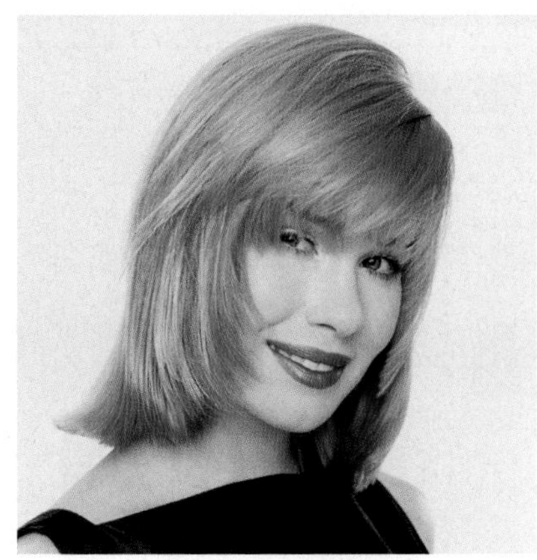

Figure 14-176 Long bang cut.

Depending on the haircut, a bang can be blended or not. If you are working with a blunt haircut and the bang is one length, you usually will not need to blend it in. If you are working with layered or graduated shapes, you may want to blend the length of the bang into the sides and/or the top (Figures 14-179 and 14-180).

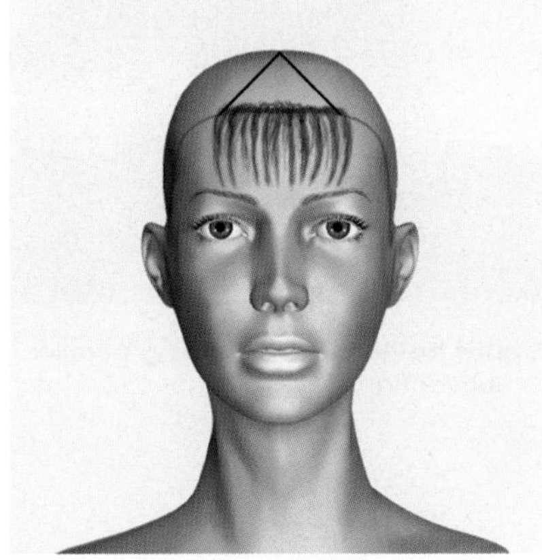

Figure 14-177 Wispy bang design.

RAZOR CUTTING

A razor cut gives a totally different result than other haircutting techniques. For instance, a razor cut gives a softer appearance than a shear cut. The razor is a great option when working with medium to fine hair textures. When you work with shears, the ends of the hair are cut blunt. When working with a razor, the ends are cut at an angle and the line is not blunt, which produces softer shapes with more visible separation, or a "feathered" effect, on the ends. With the razor, there is only one blade cutting the hair, and it is a much finer blade than the shears. With shears, there are two blades that close on the hair, creating blunt ends (Figure 14-181).

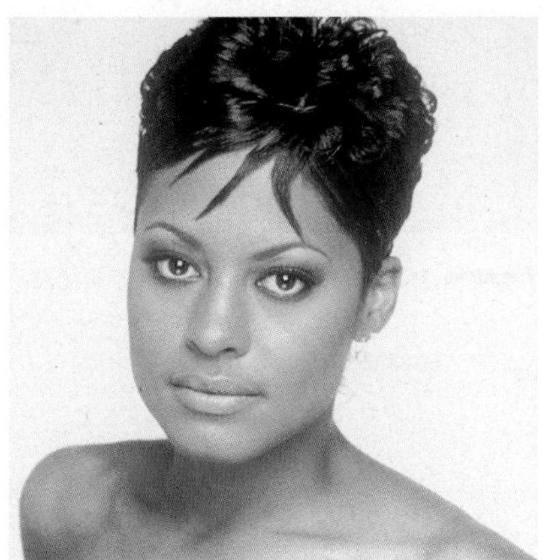

Figure 14-178 Wispy bang cut.

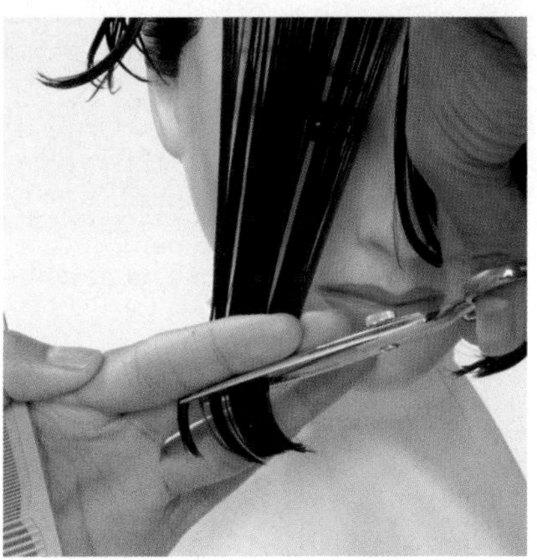

Figure 14-179 Blend bang to sides.

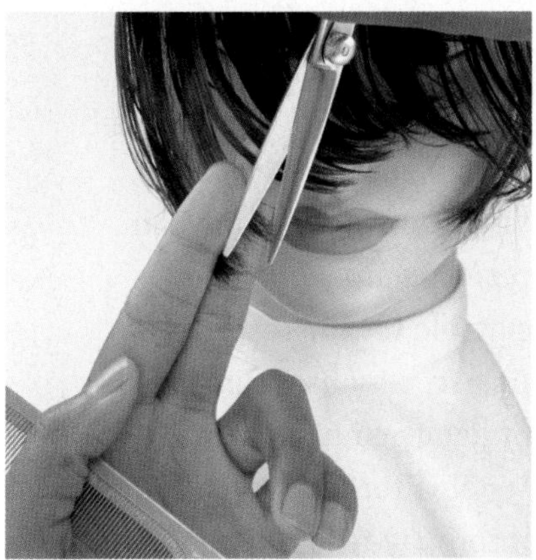

Figure 14-180 Blend bang to layered top.

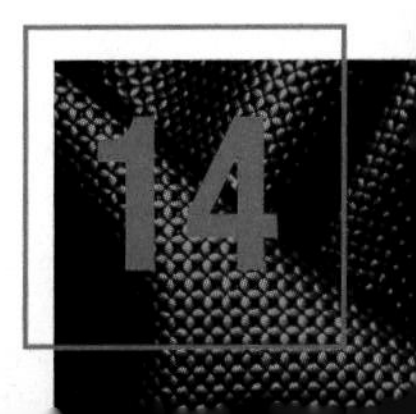

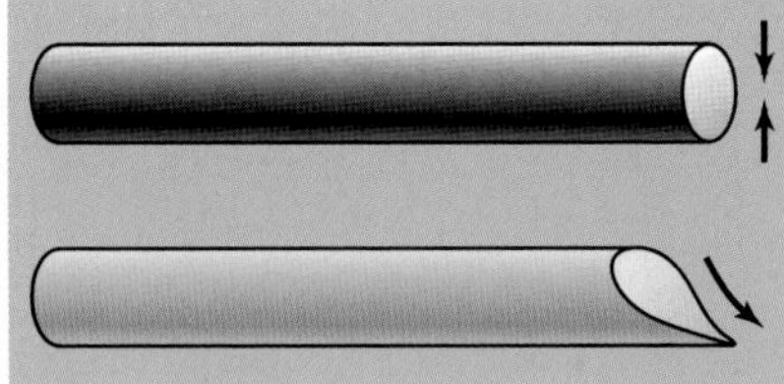

Figure 14-181 Razor-cut and shear-cut strands.

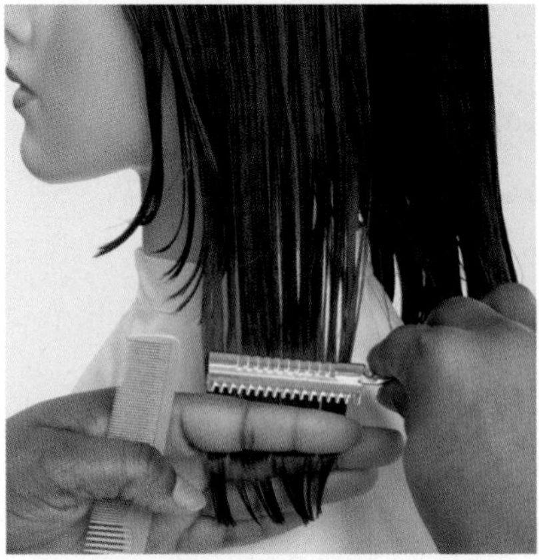

Figure 14-182 Razor cutting parallel to subsection.

Any haircut you can create with shears can also be done with the razor. You will be able to cut horizontal, vertical, and diagonal lines. The main difference is that the guide is above your fingers, whereas with shears the guide is usually below your fingers. Razor cutting is an entirely different experience from cutting with shears. The best way to get comfortable with the razor is to practice. Before cutting with a razor, review how to properly hold the razor in the "Tools, Safety, and Body Position" section of this chapter.

There are two commonly used methods for cutting with a razor. In the first method, the razor is kept parallel to the subsection (Figure 14-182). This technique is used to thin the ends of the hair, and the entire length of the blade is used. The other approach is to come into the subsection with the blade at an angle (about 45 degrees). Here you are using about one-third of the blade to make small strokes as you work through the subsection (Figure 14-183). If the blade is not entering the hair at an angle and you attempt to "push" the razor through the hair, you will be placing added stress on the hair, and risk losing control of the hair (Figure 14-184). Always remember that the blade needs to be at an angle when entering the hair.

When cutting a section, you usually move from top to bottom, or side to side, depending on the section and finger angle. Examples of razor techniques and hand positions on a vertical and horizontal subsection, respectively, are found in Figure 14-185 and Figure 14-186.

CAUTION

Always check with your instructor to see if the hair type you are working on is suitable for the razor. Coarse, wiry hair, curly hair, or damaged hair is not suitable for razor cuts. The razor may tend to make these hair types frizzier. Fine and medium hair textures in good condition are suitable for razor cuts.

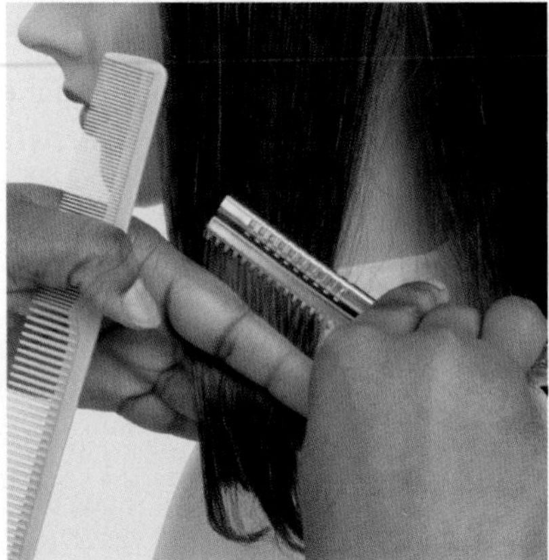

Figure 14-183 Razor cutting at a 45-degree angle.

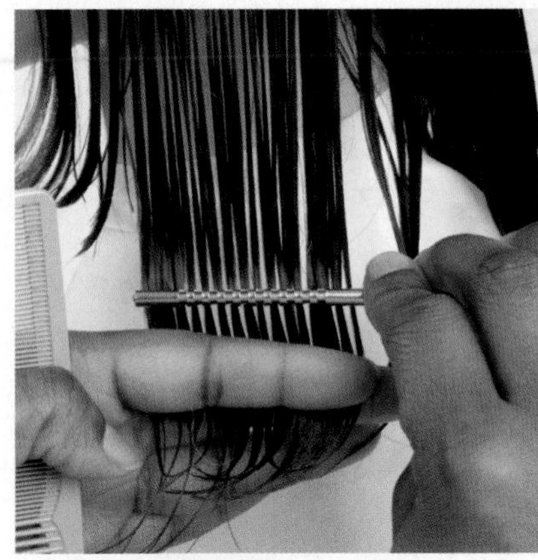

Figure 14-184 Incorrect razor angle.

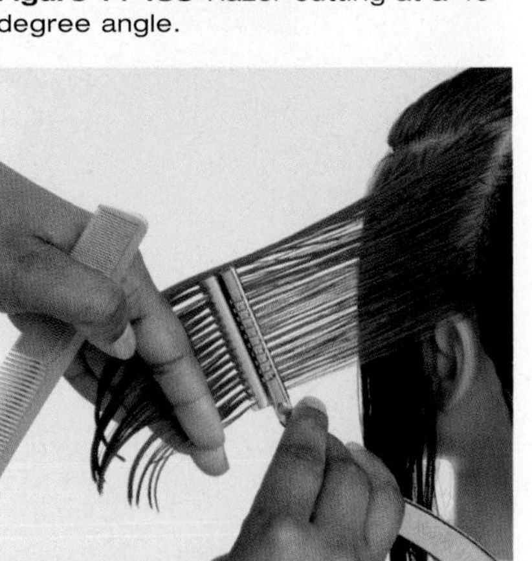

Figure 14-185 Hand position on vertical section.

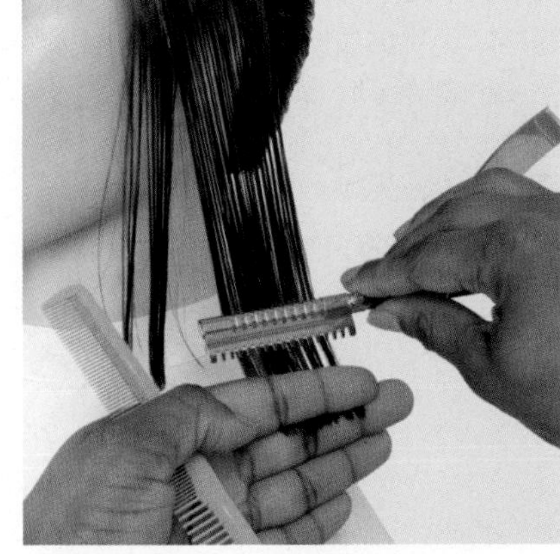

Figure 14-186 Hand position on horizontal section.

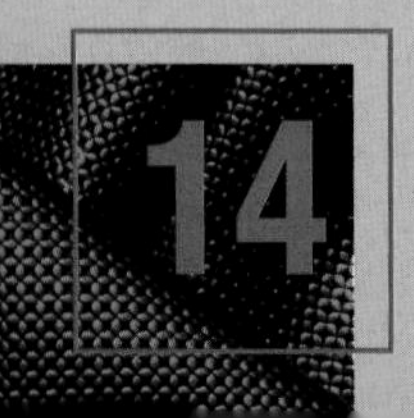

RAZOR CUTTING TIPS

- Always check with your instructor before performing a razor cut. Make sure that the hair is in good condition. For best results do not use a razor on curly hair, coarse wiry hair, or over-processed, damaged hair.
- Always use a guard.
- Always use a new blade. Working with a dull blade is painful for the client and puts added stress on the hair. Discard used blades in a puncture-proof container.
- Keep the hair wet. Cutting dry hair with a razor can make the hair frizz and may be painful to the client.
- Always work with the razor at an angle. Never force the razor through the hair.

SLIDE CUTTING

Slide cutting is a method of cutting or thinning the hair in which the fingers and shears glide along the edge of the hair to remove length. It is useful for removing length, blending shorter lengths to longer lengths, and texturizing. Slide cutting is a perfect way to layer very long hair and keep weight at the perimeter. Rather than opening and closing the shears, you keep them partially open as you "slide" along the edge of the section. This technique should only be performed on wet hair with very sharp shears.

There are two methods of holding the subsection when slide cutting. It is important to visualize the line you wish to cut before you begin (Figure 14-187). In one method, you hold the subsection with tension beyond the cutting line (Figure 14-188). In the other method, you place your shears on top of your knuckles, then use both hands to move simultaneously out the length to the ends.

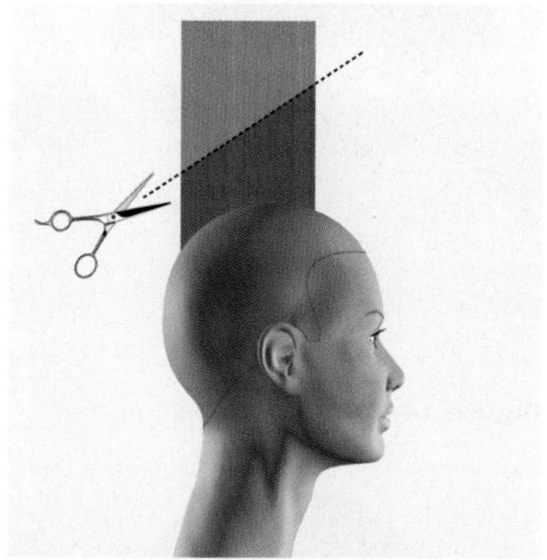

Figure 14-187 Visualize your cutting line first.

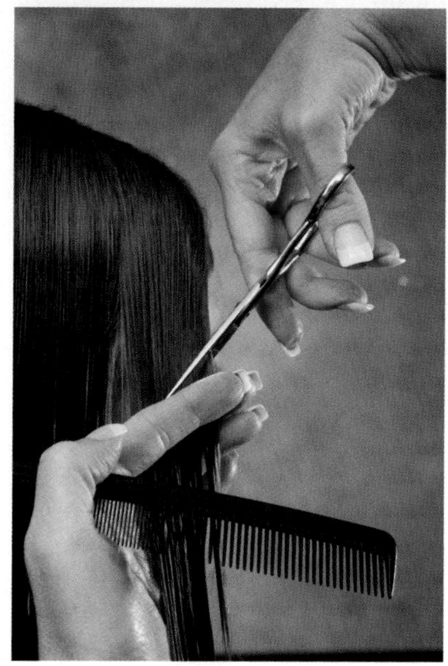

Figure 14-188 Slide cutting.

SCISSOR-OVER-COMB

Scissor-over-comb (also called shear-over-comb) is a barbering technique that has crossed over into cosmetology. In this technique, you hold the hair in place with the comb while you use the tips of the shears to remove length. Scissor-over-comb is used to create very short tapers and allows you to cut from an extremely short length to longer lengths. In most cases, you start at the hairline and work your way up to the longer lengths.

It is best to use this technique on dry hair, because then you can see exactly how much hair you are cutting and that helps you maintain control.

Lift (elevate) the hair away from the head using the comb, and allow the comb to act as your guide. Do not hold the hair between your fingers. Let the shear and comb move simultaneously up the head. It is important that one blade stays still and remains parallel to the spine of the comb as you move the thumb blade to close the shears. Try to cut with an even rhythm. Stopping the motion may cause "steps" or visible weight lines in the hair. Practice moving the comb and scissors simultaneously,

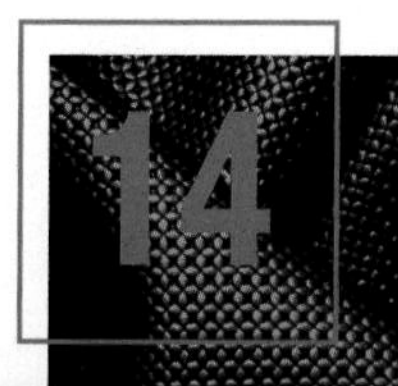

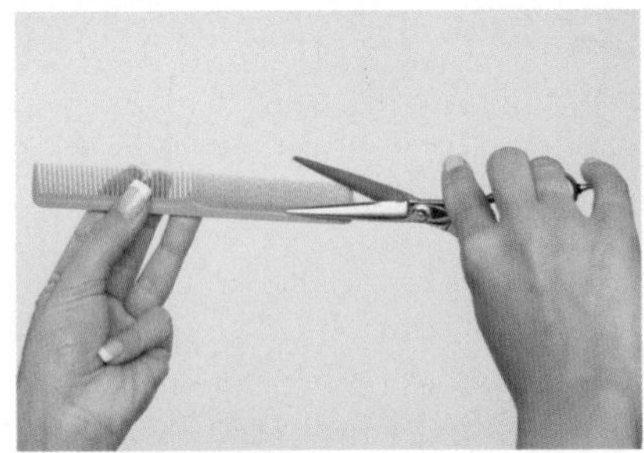

Figure 14-189 Scissor-over-comb technique.

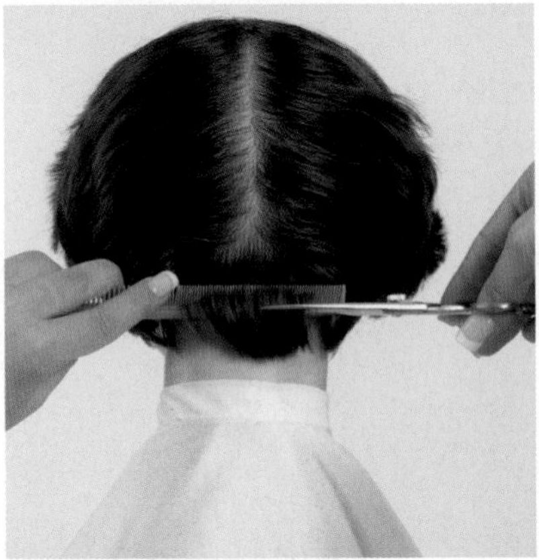

Figure 14-190 Comb position.

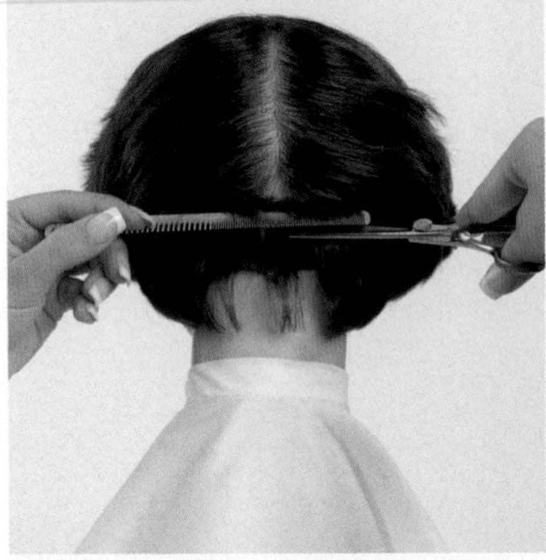

Figure 14-191 Reaching the weight line.

keeping the bottom blade still and opening and closing the shears with your thumb (Figure 14-189).

The basic steps when working with the scissor-over-comb technique are summarized below.

1. Stand or sit directly in front of the section you are working on. The area that you are cutting should be at eye level.
2. Place the comb, teeth first, into the hairline, and turn the comb so that the teeth are angled away from the head (Figure 14-190).
3. With the still blade parallel to the spine of the comb, begin moving the comb up the head, continually opening and closing the thumb blade smoothly and quickly.
4. Angle the comb farther away from the head as you reach the area you are blending to avoid cutting into the length (weight) (Figure 14-191).

SCISSOR-OVER-COMB TIPS

- Work with small areas at a time (no wider than the blade).
- Always start at the hairline and work up toward the length. You can run the comb through a previously cut section, on your way up to a new area.
- Cross-check by working across the area diagonally.
- Use a barber comb to cut areas very close (usually on sideburns and hairlines where the hair is cut close to the scalp). Switch to a regular cutting comb as you work up into the longer lengths.

TEXTURIZING

Texturizing is a technique often used in today's haircuts. **Texturizing** is the process of removing excess bulk without shortening the length. It can also be used to cut for effect within the hair length, causing wispy or spiky effects. The term "texturize" should not be confused with hair texture, which is the diameter of the hair strand itself.

Texturizing techniques can be used to add volume, remove volume, make hair "move," and blend one area into another. It can also be used to compensate for different densities that exist on the same head of hair.

Texturizing can be done with cutting shears, thinning shears, or a razor.

There are many texturizing techniques, and a number of them will be explained in this section. You will need to practice all the techniques, so that you can take the different effects they create and use them as needed on your clients.

TEXTURIZING WITH SHEARS

- **Point cutting** is a technique performed on the ends of the hair using the tips, or points, of the shears. This can be done on wet or dry hair. It is very easy to do on dry hair because the hair stands up and away from your fingers. Hold the hair 1 to 2 inches (2.5 to 5 centimeters) from the ends. Turn your wrist so that the tips of the scissors are

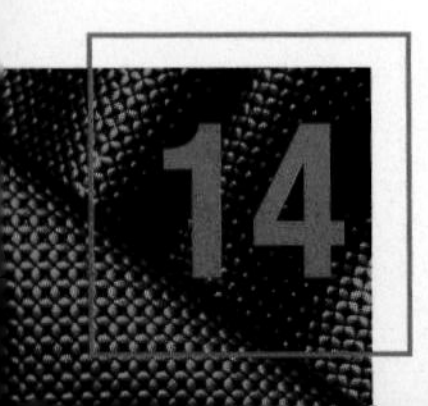

pointing into the ends. Open and close the scissors by moving your thumb as you work across the section. As you close the scissors, move them away from your fingers to avoid cutting yourself. Move them back in toward your fingers as you open them (Figure 14-192). Basically, you are cutting "points" in the hair. A more vertical angle of the shears removes less hair (Figure 14-193). The more diagonal the angle of the shears, the more hair is taken away and the chunkier the effect (Figure 14-194).

- **Notching** is another version of point cutting. Notching is more aggressive and creates a chunkier effect. Notching is done toward the ends. Hold the section about 3 inches (7.5 centimeters) from the ends. Place the tips of your shears about 2 inches (5 centimeters) from the ends. Close your shears as you quickly move them out toward the ends. If you are working on very thick hair, you can repeat the motion every 1/8 inch (0.3 centimeters). On medium to fine hair, place your "notches" farther apart. This technique can be done on wet or dry hair (Figure 14-195).
- **Free-hand notching** also uses the tips of the shears. Do not slide the shears, but simply snip out pieces of hair at random intervals. This technique is generally used on the interior of the section, rather than at the ends. It works well on curly hair, where you do not want to add too many layers, but rather where you want to release the curl and remove some density (Figure 14-196).

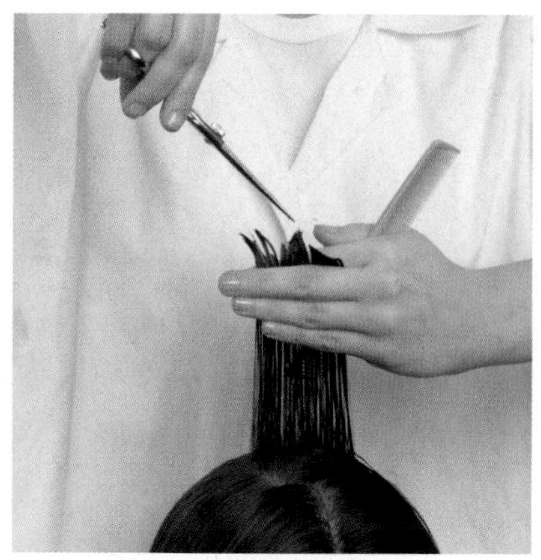

Figure 14-192 Point cutting.

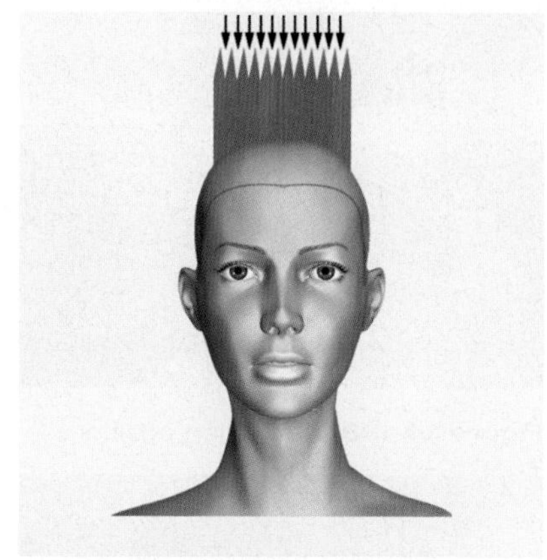

Figure 14-193 Point cutting with vertical angle of shears.

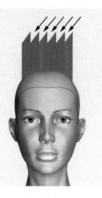

Figure 14-194 Point cutting with diagonal angle of shears.

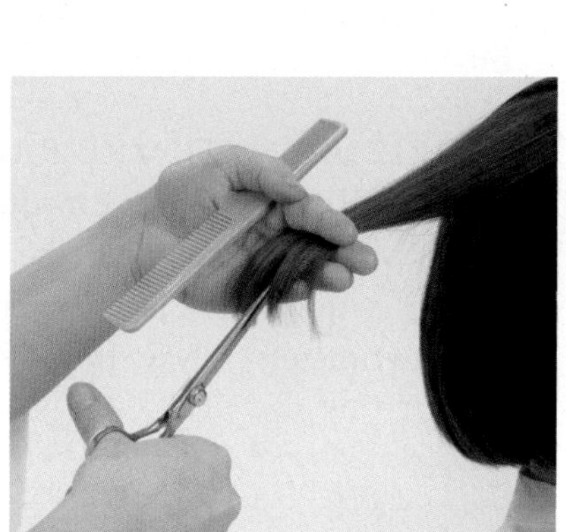

Figure 14-195 Notching.

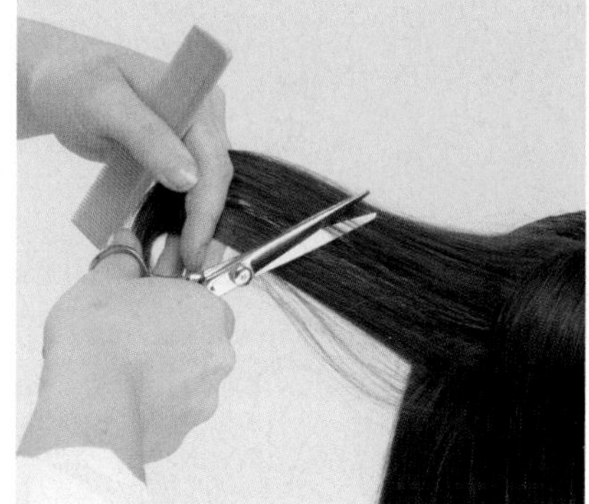

Figure 14-196 Free-hand notching.

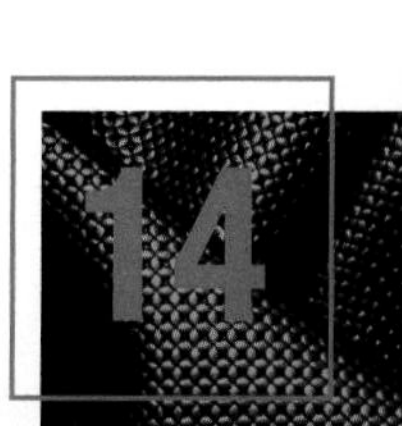

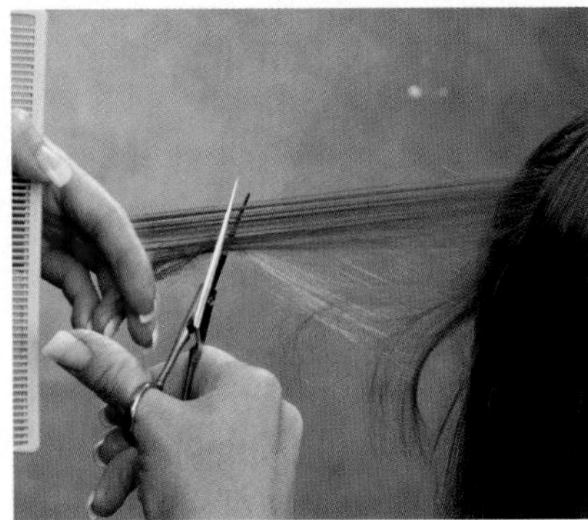

Figure 14-197 Slithering.

- **Slithering** or effilating is the process of thinning the hair to graduated lengths with shears. In this technique, the hair strand is cut by a sliding movement of the shears, with the blades kept partially opened (Figure 14-197). Slithering reduces volume and creates movement.
- **Slicing** is a technique that removes bulk and adds movement through the lengths of the hair. When slicing, never completely close the scissors. Use only the portion of the blades near the pivot. This prevents removing large pieces of hair (Figures 14-198 and 14-199). This technique can be performed within a subsection or on the surface of the hair with haircutting or texturizing shears (Figures 14-200 and 14-201). To slice an elevated subsection, work with either wet or dry hair. When slicing on the surface of the haircut, it is best to work on dry hair, because you can see exactly how much hair you are taking away.

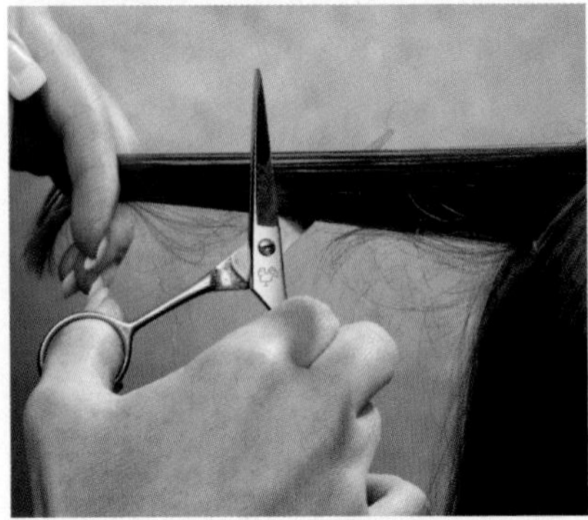

Figure 14-198 Ideal open position.

- **Carving** is a version of slicing that creates a visual separation in the hair. It works best on short hair (1½ to 3 inches [3.75 to 7.5 centimeters] in length). This technique is done by placing the still blade into the hair and resting it on the scalp. Move the shears through the hair, gently opening and partially closing the scissors as you move, thus "carving" out areas (Figure 14-202). The more horizontal your scissors, the more hair you remove; the more vertical, the less hair you remove.
- By carving the ends, you can add texture and separation to the perimeter of a haircut by holding the ends of a small strand of hair between your thumb and index fingers, and carving on the surface of that strand. Begin carving about 3 inches from the ends toward your fingers.

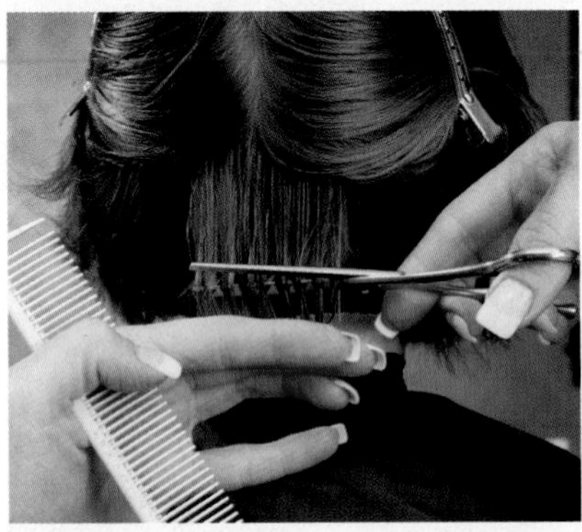

Figure 14-199 Slicing with shears.

TEXTURIZING WITH THE RAZOR

- **Removing weight.** You can use the razor to thin out the ends of the hair. On damp hair, hold the section out from the head, with your fingers at the ends. Place the razor flat to the hair, 2 to 3 inches (5 to 7.5 centimeters) away from your fingers. Gently stroke the razor,

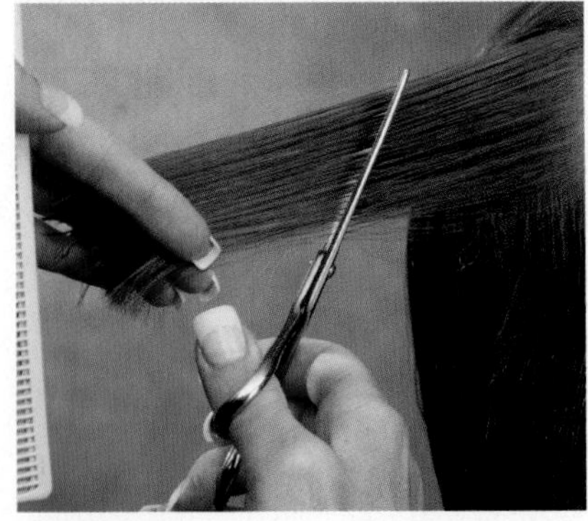

Figure 14-200 Slicing through a subsection with texturizing shears.

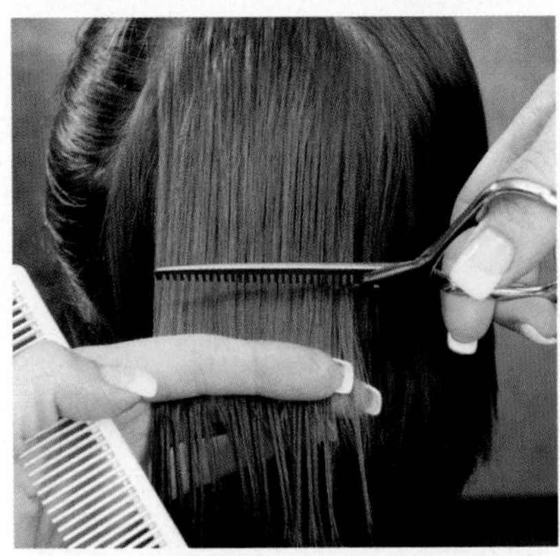

Figure 14-201 Slicing through the surface with texturizing shears.

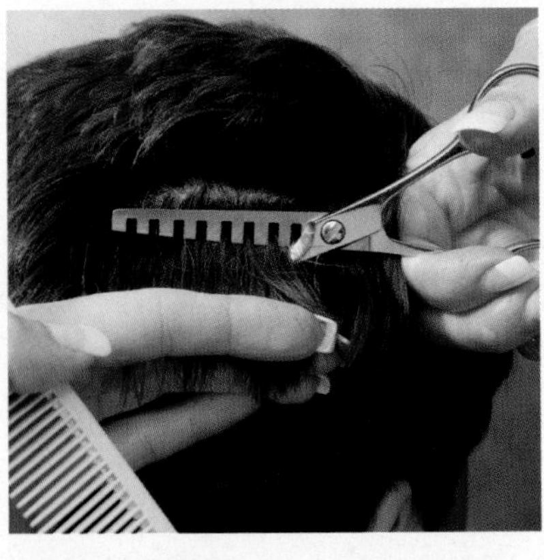

Figure 14-202 Carving through a short haircut

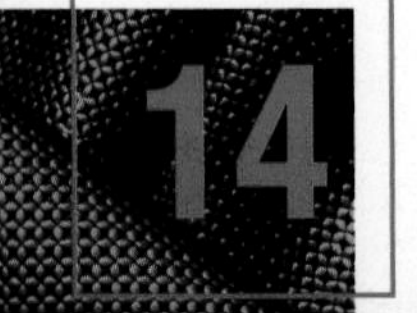

removing a thin "sheet" of hair from the area (Figure 14-203). This tapers the ends of the section, and can be used on any area of the haircut where this effect is desired.

- **Free-hand slicing.** This technique can be used throughout the section or at the ends, and should be done on wet hair. When working on the midshaft of the subsection, comb the hair out from the head, and hold it with your fingers close to the ends. With the tip of the razor, slice out pieces of hair. The more vertical the movement, the less hair you remove; the more horizontal the movement, the more hair you remove. This technique releases weight from the subsection, allowing it to move more freely.

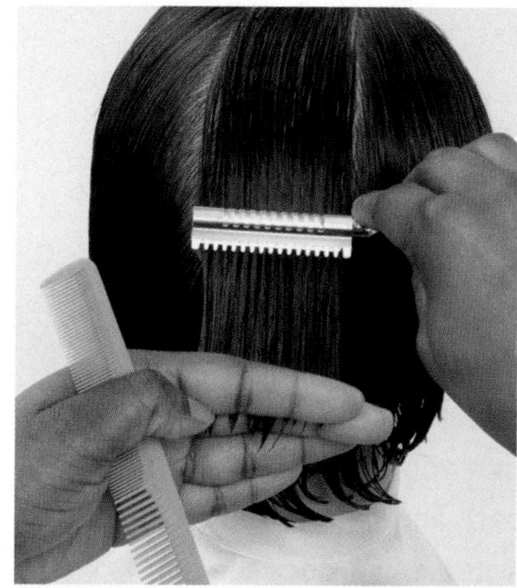
Figure 14-203 Thinning out the midsection.

TEXTURIZING WITH THINNING SHEARS AND RAZOR

- **Removing bulk (thinning).** Thinning shears were originally created for the purpose of thinning hair and blending. Many clients are afraid of the word "thinning." A better choice of words would be "removing bulk" or "removing weight." When using the thinning shears for this purpose, it is best to follow the same sectioning as in the haircut.

  Comb the subsection out from the head and cut it with the thinning scissors, at least 4 to 5 inches (10 to 12.5 centimeters) from the scalp (Figure 14-204). On longer lengths, you may need to repeat the process again as you move out toward the ends. On coarse hair textures, stay farther away from the scalp, as sometimes the shorter hairs will poke through the haircut. On blunt haircuts, avoid thinning the top surfaces, because you may see lines where the hair is cut with the thinning shears. When working on curly hair, it is best to use the free-hand notching technique rather than thinning shears.

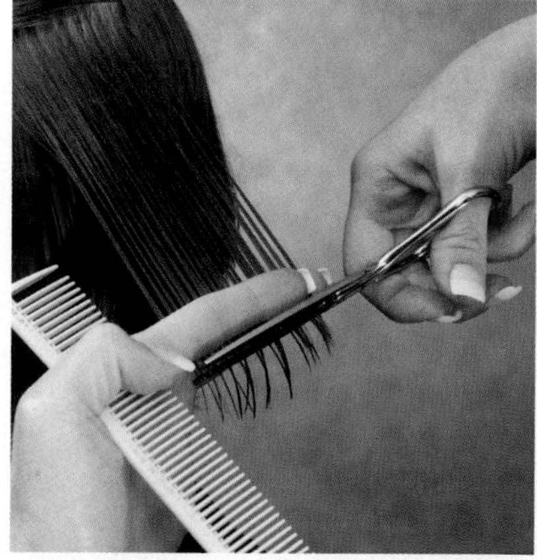
Figure 14-204 Thinning out the ends.

- **Removing weight from the ends.** You can also use thinning shears to remove bulk from the ends. This process works well on many hair textures. It can be used on both thin and thick hair, and it helps taper the perimeter of both graduated and blunt haircuts. Elevating each subsection out from the head, place the thinning shears into the hair at an angle and close the shears a few times as you work out toward the ends (Figure 14-205).

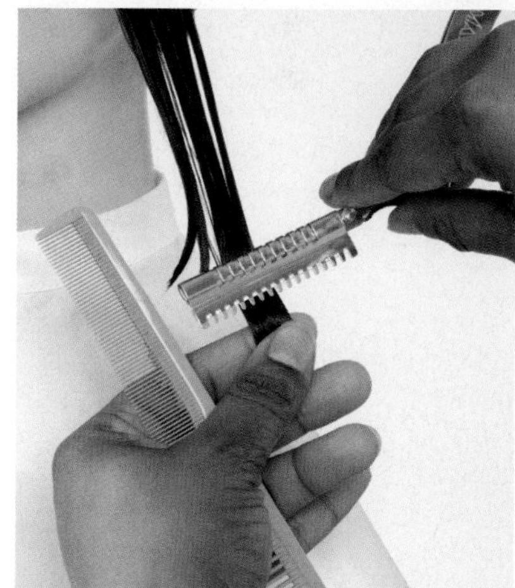
Figure 14-205 Tapering the ends with the razor.

- **Scissor-over-comb with thinning shears.** Practicing the scissor-over-comb technique with the thinning shears is a good way to master this technique. This technique is useful for blending weight lines on fine-textured hair, and can be used as well on thick and coarse texture haircuts that are cut very short, especially at the sides and the nape. It will help the hair lie closer to the head.
- **Other thinning shear techniques.** Any texturizing technique that can be performed with regular haircutting shears may also be performed with the thinning shears. When working on very fine or thin hair, try using the thinning shears for carving, point cutting, and slicing. This will help avoid over-texturizing and removing too much weight.
- **Free-hand slicing with razor.** You can also use free-hand slicing on the ends of the hair to produce a softer perimeter or to create separation

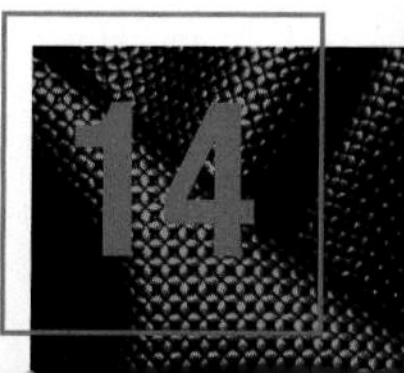

CAUTION

When thinning or texturizing hair, remember that you can always go back and remove more hair if necessary. Once the hair has been cut, it is impossible to replace, and you may have difficulty achieving the desired hairstyle.

throughout the shape (Figure 14-206). In this case, hold the ends of a small piece of hair in your fingertips. Beginning about 3 inches from your fingers, slice down one side of the piece toward your fingers (Figure 14-207).

- **Razor-over-comb.** In this technique, the comb and the razor are used on the surface of the hair. Using the razor on the surface softens weight lines and causes the area to lie closer to the head. This technique is used mainly on shorter haircuts. Here are two approaches: The first way is to place the comb into the hair, with the teeth pointing down, a few inches above the area on which you will be working. Make small, gentle strokes on the surface of the hair with the razor. Move the comb down as you move the razor down (Figure 14-208). This is a great technique for tapering in the nape area or softening weight lines.
- The second approach is referred to as **razor rotation,** it is very similar to razor-over-comb. The difference is that you make small circular motions. Begin by combing the hair in the direction you will be moving in. Place the razor on the surface of the hair. Then allow the comb to follow the razor, combing through the area just cut, and then comb back into the section or onto a new section. This helps soften the texture of the area and gives direction to the haircut (Figure 14-209).

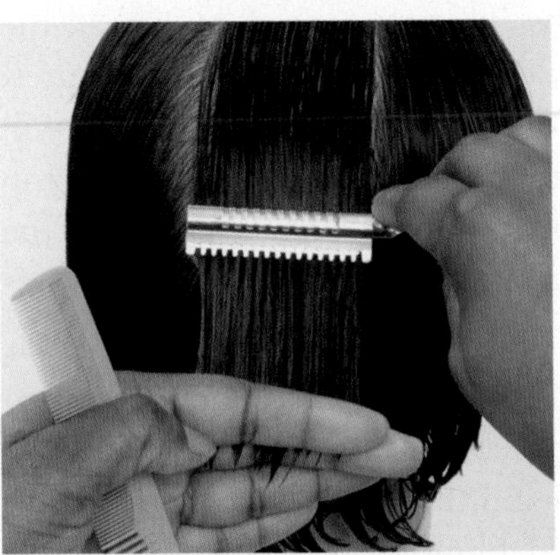

Figure 14-206 Slicing the midshaft.

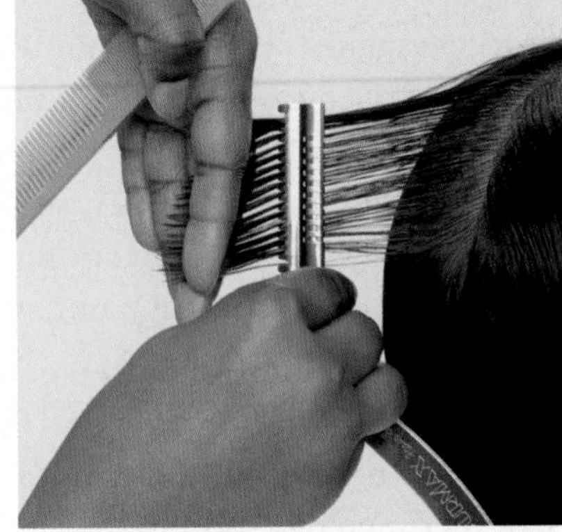

Figure 14-207 Slicing the perimeter.

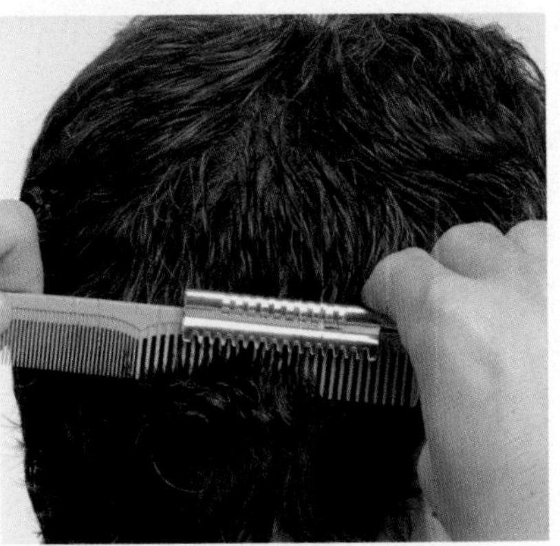

Figure 14-208 Razor-over-comb technique.

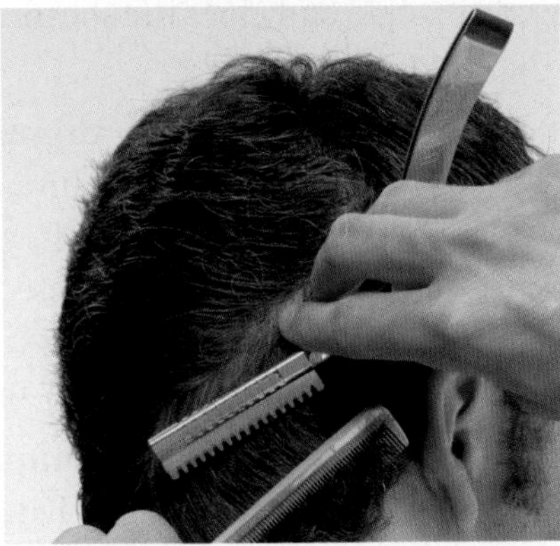

Figure 14-209 Razor rotation.

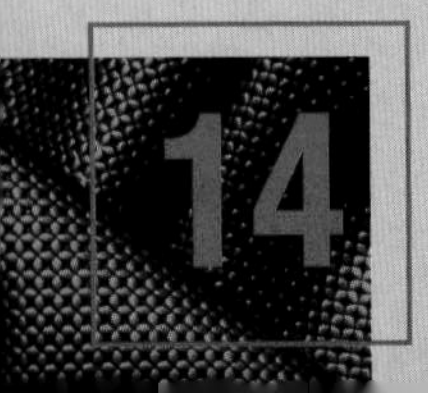

BASIC HAIRCUTS ENHANCED WITH TEXTURIZING TECHNIQUES

Examine these three basic haircuts and see how texturizing techniques have changed the appearance of each haircut.

1. Figure 14-210 shows a blunt haircut before freehand razor slicing, and Figure 14-211 shows the same haircut after free-hand razor slicing has been used.
2. Figure 14-212 shows a graduated haircut before free-hand scissors slicing, and Figure 14-213 shows the same haircut after free-hand shear slicing.
3. Figure 14-214 shows a uniform-layered haircut before, and Figure 14-215 shows the same haircut after notching on the ends and free-hand notching on the interior.

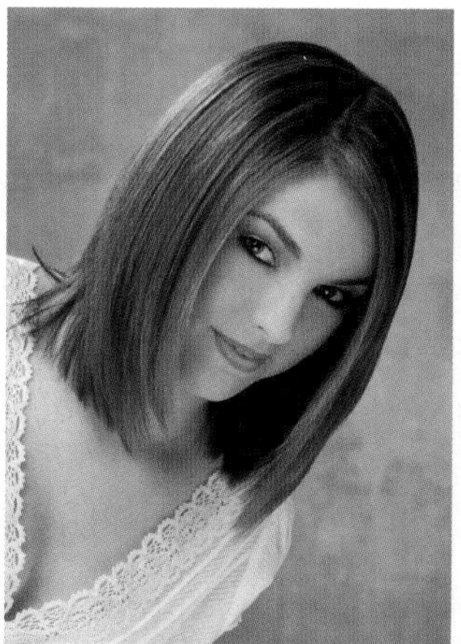

Figure 14-210 Blunt hair cut before texturizing.

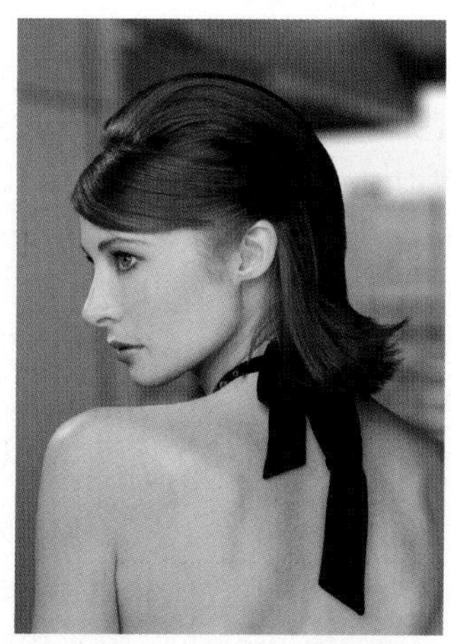

Figure 14-211 Texturized blunt haircut.

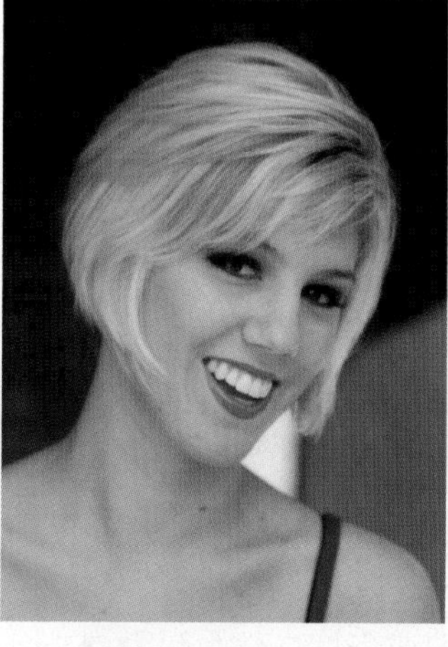

Figure 14-212 Graduated haircut before texturizing.

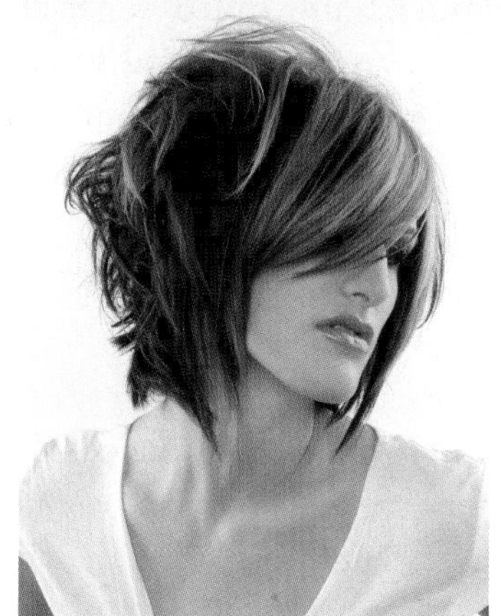

Figure 14-213 Texturized graduated haircut.

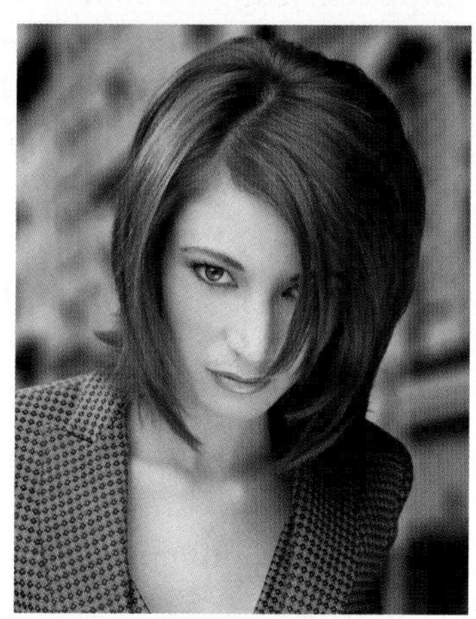

Figure 14-214 Uniform layered haircut before texturizing.

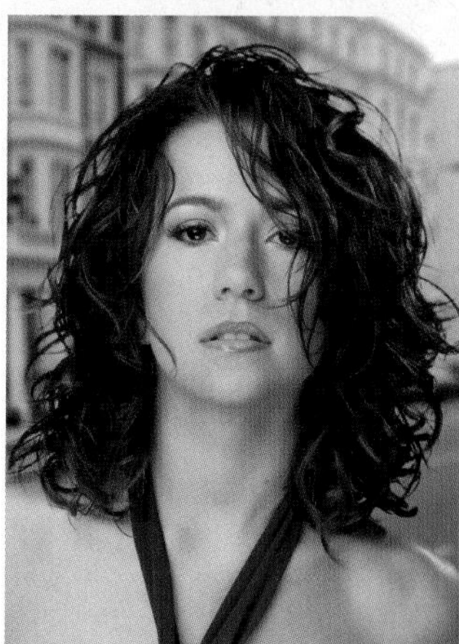

Figure 14-215 Texturized uniform layered haircut.

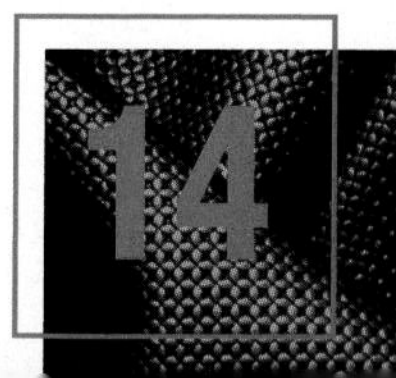

CLIPPERS AND TRIMMERS

Another type of tool that all stylists should be familiar with are clippers and trimmers, which offer solutions for many haircutting challenges.

Clippers are electric or battery-operated tools that cut the hair by using two moving blades held in place by a metal plate with teeth. The blade action is faster than the eye can see. Clippers are mainly used for cutting shorter haircuts, and can be used to create **tapers,** which sit very close to the hairline and gradually get longer as you move up the head. While men have been getting clipper cuts for many years, today clippers are being used in women's haircutting more and more. Clippers can be used as follows:

- Without length guards, to remove hair completely (great for cleaning up necklines and around the ears).
- Without length guards, to taper hairlines from extremely short lengths into longer lengths, using the **clipper-over-comb** technique (this technique is very similar to scissor-over-comb, except that the clippers move side to side across the comb rather than bottom to top).
- With length guards, which are attachments that fit over the blade plate and vary in size from ⅛ inch to 1 inch.

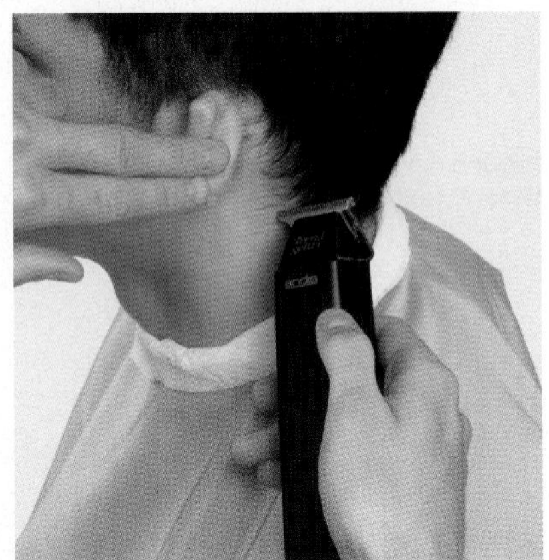

Figure 14-216 Trimmer cutting around the ear.

TOOLS FOR CLIPPER CUTTING

There are several tools to have on hand. When clipper cutting you will not need to use each tool for every haircut, but it is still important to understand when these tools are needed (see Figure 14-46.)

- **Clippers.** Clippers come in different shapes and sizes. They can be used with or without attachments. Trimmers, also called edgers, are usually cordless, smaller-sized clippers. They are mainly used to clean the necklines and around the ears (Figure 14-216). Clean clippers and trimmers after each use with a clipper brush. Apply one drop of clipper oil to the top of the blades while the clipper is running. Disinfect the detachable blade and heel after each use as well. Always follow the manufacturer's instructions for care and cleaning.
- **Length guard attachments.** When attached to the clippers, length guards allow you to cut all the hair evenly to that exact length. They range from ⅛ to 1 inch (.3 to 2.5 centimeters) wide, and can be used in different combinations to create different lengths.
- **Haircutting shears.** Used mainly for removing length and detailing the haircut.
- **Thinning shears.** Also called blending or tapering scissors, these are great for removing excess bulk and for blending one area with another.
- **Combs.** With a regular cutting comb, the wider-spaced teeth are intended for combing and cutting, while the finer-spaced teeth are used for detailing, scissor-over-comb, and clipper-over-comb techniques.

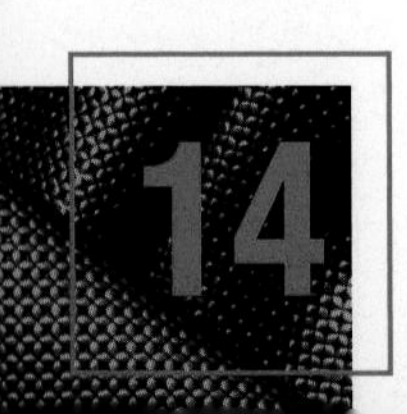

The classic barbering comb is often used in the nape, at the sides, and around the ears, and allows you to cut the hair very short and close to the head. The wide-toothed comb is used when cutting thicker and longer lengths, where detailing is not required.

BASIC CLIPPER TECHNIQUES

Basic techniques with clippers include clipper-over-comb and clipper cutting with length guard attachments.

CLIPPER-OVER-COMB

The clipper-over-comb technique allows you to cut the hair very close to the scalp and create a flat-top or square shape. The way you use the comb is the same as when you are working with scissor-over-comb. The main difference is that the clippers move across the comb, which requires that you keep the comb in position as you cut. The angle at which you hold the comb determines the amount of hair that is cut.

Clippers are more accurate when used on dry hair. Use the lever switch on the clipper or a numbered attachment to vary the distance that the clipper is held from the head.

Tips for working with the clipper-over-comb technique follow. This technique will be illustrated in the procedure for the men's basic clipper cut later in this chapter.

1. Stand directly in front of the section on which you are working. The area you are cutting should be at eye level.
2. Place the comb, teeth first, into the hairline, and turn the comb so that the teeth are angled slightly away from the head. Always work against the growth patterns of the hair to ensure that you are lifting the hair away from the head and cutting evenly.
3. Hold the comb stationary and cut the length against the comb, moving the clippers from right to left. (If you are left-handed, you will move the clippers left to right.)
4. Although your movements should be fluid, remember to stop momentarily to cut the section. Remove the comb from the hair and begin the motion again, using the previously cut section underneath as your guideline. Continue working up the head toward the weight or length.

CLIPPER CUTTING WITH ATTACHMENTS

Using the length guard attachments is a quick and easy way to create short haircuts. With practice, clipper-cutting with attachments allows you to create many different shapes. For example, you can use the ¼-inch guide on the nape and sides. Switch to the ½-inch guide as you reach the parietal area, which would maintain more length at the parietal area and produce a square shape.

TIPS FOR CLIPPER CUTTING

- Always work against the natural growth patterns, especially in the nape. This ensures that you are lifting the hair away from the head and cutting the hair evenly.

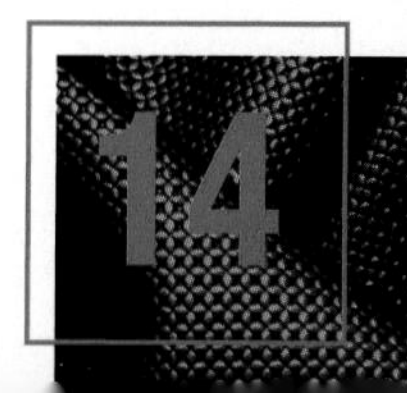

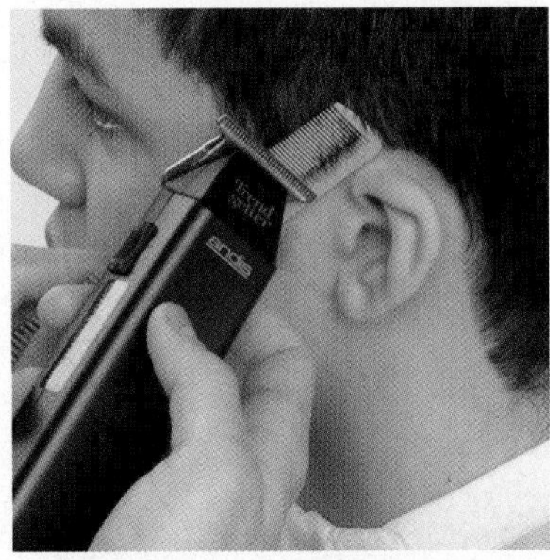

Figure 14-217 Arcing trimmer at front of the ear.

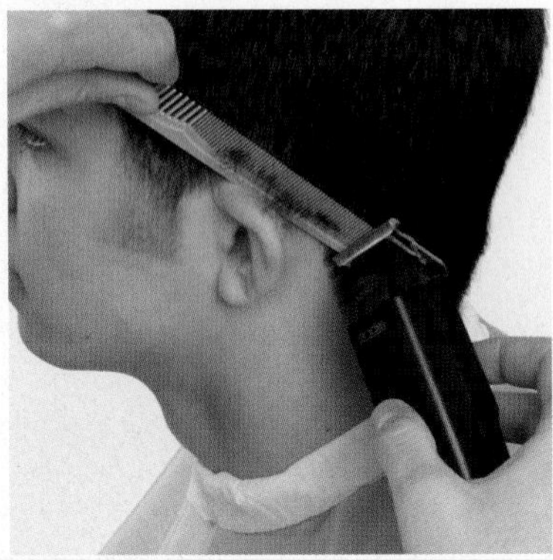

Figure 14-218 Arcing trimmer at back of ear with comb.

- Always work with small sections. When using the clipper-over-comb technique, do not try to cut all the way across the entire length of the comb. The area you are cutting should be no wider than 3 inches.
- When using the clipper-over-comb technique, the angle of the comb determines the length. If the comb is parallel to the head, you will cut the hair the same length as you move up the head. If the comb is angled away from the head as you move, you begin to increase length.

USING TRIMMERS

- Using trimmers around the ears. When cutting a clean line around the ears, use both hands to hold the edger sideways. Using just the outer edge on the skin, arc the edger up and around the ear (Figure 14-217). As you reach the area behind the ear, use the comb to hold the hair in place, and continue with the arcing motion (Figure 14-218).
- Using trimmers at the neckline. Clean up the hair on the neck that grows below the design line (Figure 14-219). Trimmers also help create more defined lines at the perimeter (Figure 14-220).

MEN'S BASIC CLIPPER CUT

In this cut, the hair is cropped close along the bottom and sides and longer as you travel up the head. The distance between the becomes longer as you travel up the head. The distance between the comb and the scalp determines the amount of hair to be cut. The clipper can be positioned horizontally, vertically, or diagonally.

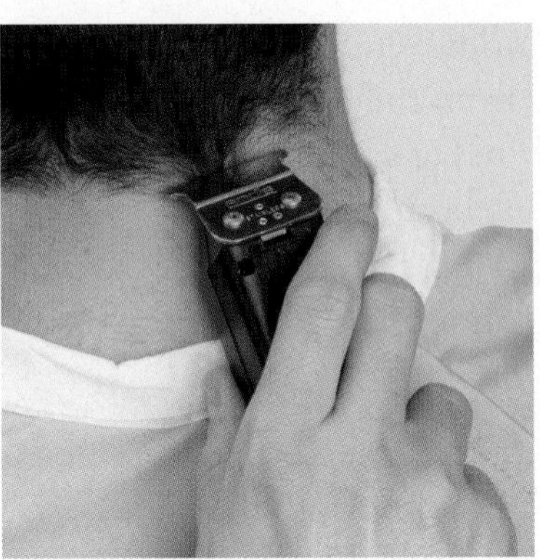

Figure 14-219 Cleaning up neck hair.

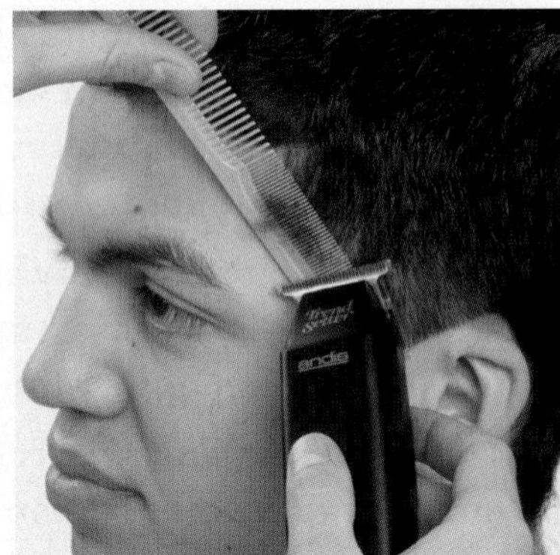

Figure 14-220 Edging line at side perimeter.

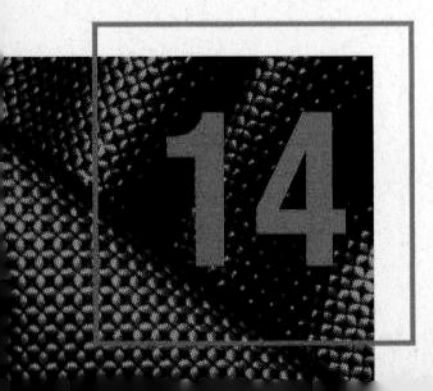

PROCEDURE 14-5

CLIPPER CUT

IMPLEMENTS AND MATERIALS

- Cutting cape
- Neck strip
- Haircutting comb
- Barber comb
- Haircutting scissors
- Clipper
- Trimmer
- Low-number guard attachment (optional)

PREPARATION

The hair should be clean and dry for this haircut (Figure 14-221).

PROCEDURE

1. **Part hair.** Make a horseshoe parting about 2 inches (5 centimeters) below the apex of the head, beginning and ending at the front hairline (Figure 14-222). Comb the hair above the part forward.
2. **Cut nape area.** Starting in the nape area, place the haircutting comb against the scalp, teeth up. Angle the comb against the scalp from 0 to 45 degrees, allowing for the natural contour of the head. Cut the hair that extends through the teeth of the comb (Figure 14-223).
3. **Cut back of head.** Repeat Step 3 as you move up the back of the head. Blend the lengths over the curve of the head by cross-cutting horizontally, from side to side (Figure 14-224). Shape the back center area first, from the nape to the parietal ridge. Then, still using the clipper-over-comb technique, cut both sides of the back from ear to ear.
4. **Blend.** Carefully blend the lengths over the curve of the head by cross-cutting.

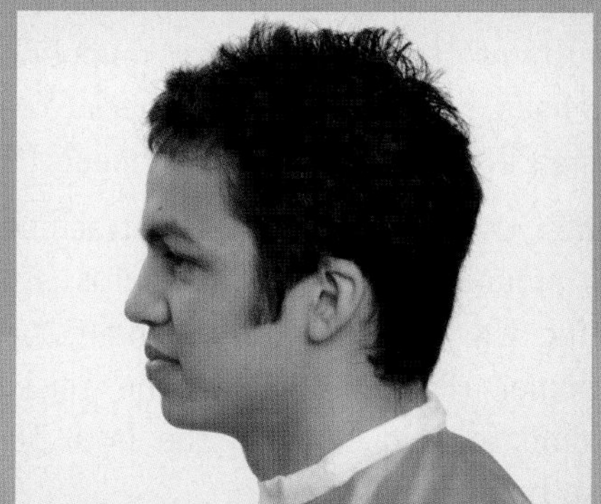

Figure 14-221 Client before clipper cut.

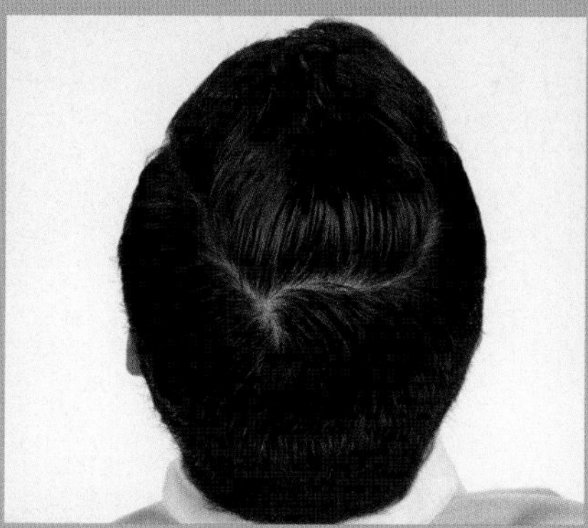

Figure 14-222 Make a horseshoe part.

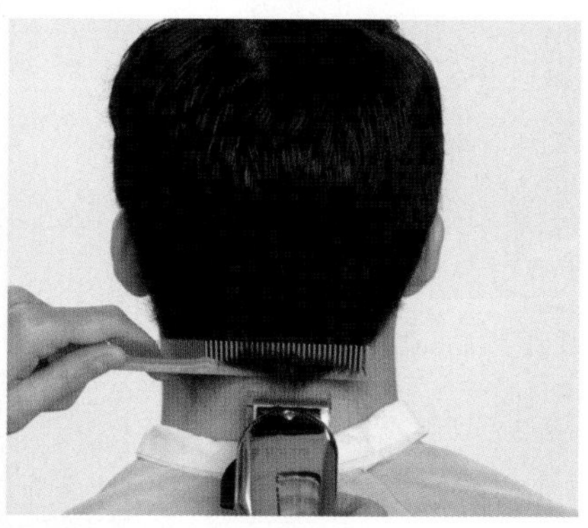

Figure 14-223 Cut at the nape.

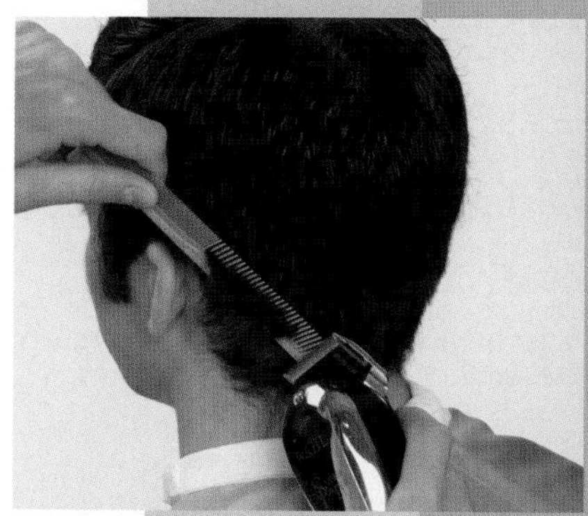

Figure 14-224 Cross-cut the back of the head.

5. Using a low-number length attachment on the clipper, cut up each side from the sideburn to the parietal ridge (Figure 14-225). The hair length will be very close to the scalp. If the client wants longer sides, the weight on the top will need to be blended.

6. **Create guide in crown.** Measure the distance between the eyebrows and the natural hairline to establish a guideline for the length in the crown area if the client wishes to keep hair out of the eyes (Figure 14-226).

7. **Cut guideline in crown.** Cut a narrow guideline at the crown end of the horseshoe parting. Determine the length by the forehead measurement (Figure 14-227).

   Beginning at the crown end, cut the top area with the clipper to the exact length of the initial crown guideline. As you move toward the forehead, over-direct the hair back toward the guideline in order to increase the length at the forehead (Figure 14-228).

8. **Cut around ears.** Using the clipper and attachment, shorten and shape the hair around the ears and sideburns (Figure 14-229). To blend or outline the perimeter of the haircut, you may use a clipper or trimmer (Figure 14-230). The scissor-over-comb or clipper-over-comb technique, using the front teeth of a barber comb, may also be used here.

9. **Clean up.** Follow cleanup and sanitation steps in "Blunt Haircut" procedure.

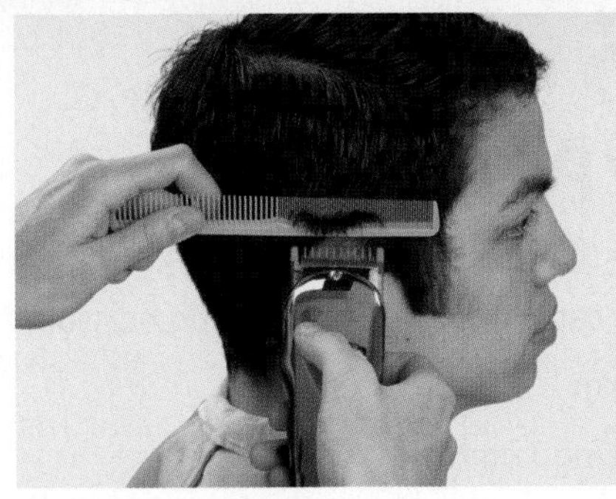

Figure 14-225 Cut from sideburn to parietal ridge.

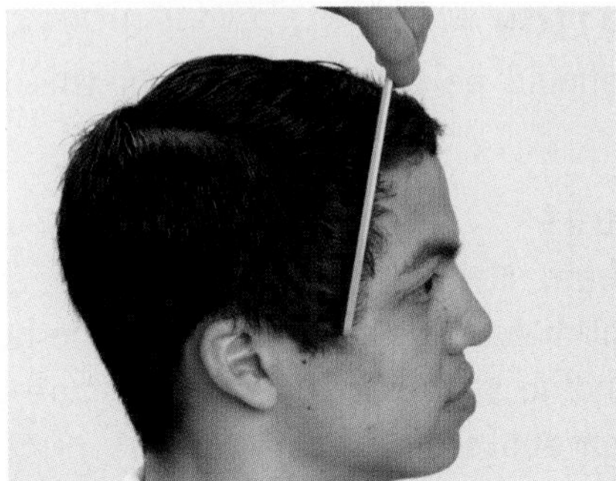

Figure 14-226 Measure from eyebrow to natural hairline.

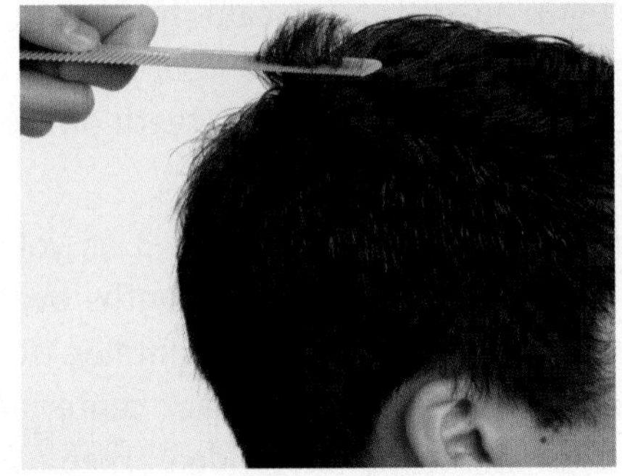

Figure 14-227 Cut guideline at crown.

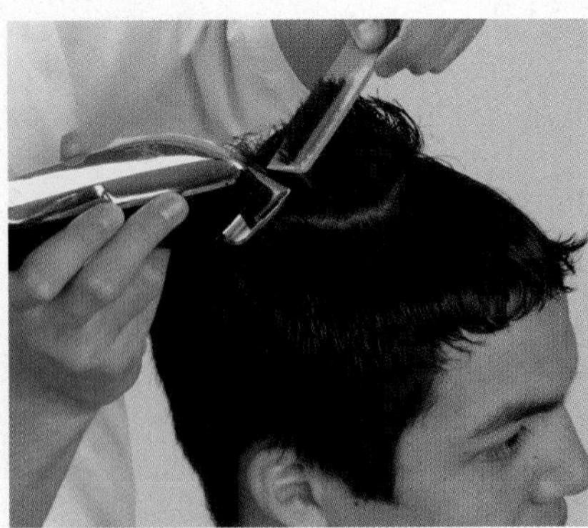

Figure 14-228 Bring hair toward guideline.

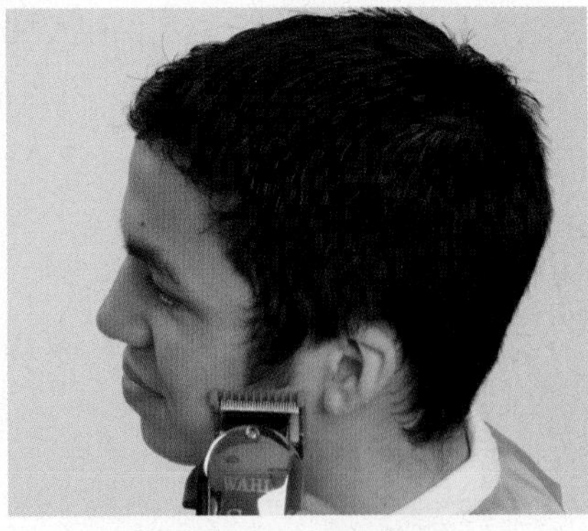

Figure 14-229 Shape hair around ears and sideburns.

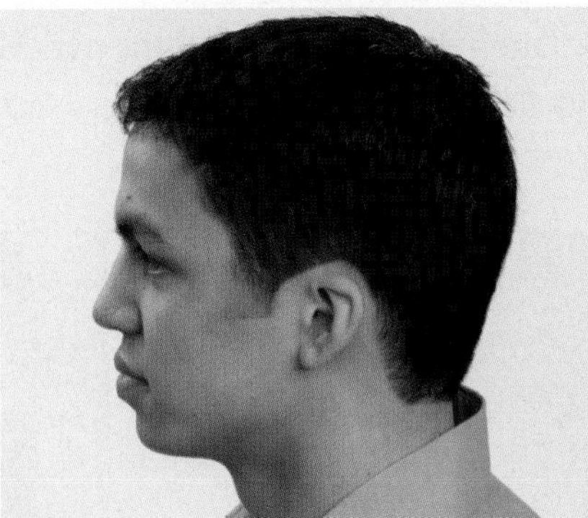

Figure 14-230 Finished clipper cut.

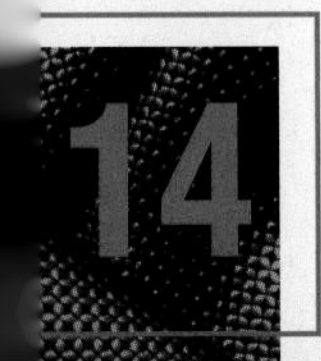

TRIMMING FACIAL HAIR

Clippers and trimmers can be used to trim beards and mustaches as well. The technique is very similar to scissor-over-comb and clipper-over-comb. When removing length, use the comb to control the hair, and always cut against the comb (Figure 14-231). You can also use the length guard attachments to trim a beard to the desired length (Figure 14-232). If you choose to use haircutting shears to trim facial hair, you may want to keep a less-expensive pair for this purpose because facial hair is very coarse and may dull your haircutting shears.

Some male clients have excess hair in or on their ears. When performing a haircut or trimming facial hair, always check the ears and ask the client if he would like you to remove any excess hair you may find. Carefully snip away the hair with your shears or trimmers, using extreme caution.

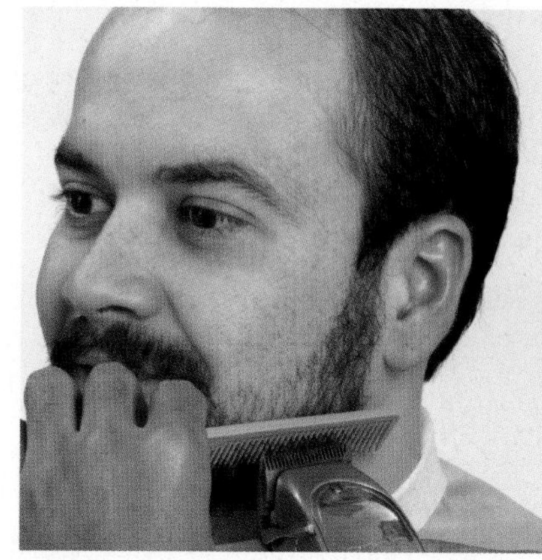

Figure 14-231 Trimming beard with clipper-over-comb.

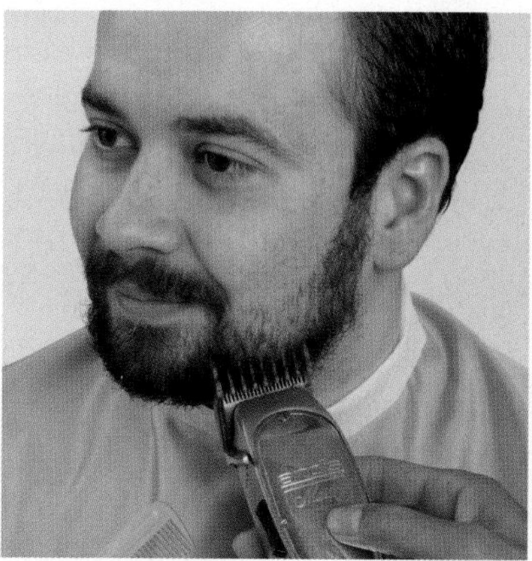

Figure 14-232 Trimming beard with clipper and guard.

REVIEW QUESTIONS

1. What are reference points and what is their function?
2. What are the main areas of the head and how do you find them?
3. Define elevation and describe the various effects it creates.
4. What is the difference between traveling and stationary guidelines, and when do you use each?
5. Define over-direction.
6. What are important considerations to discuss with a client during a haircutting consultation?
7. Explain the difference between hair density and hair texture.
8. Where are the danger zones in a haircut, and why do you need to be aware of them?
9. What is palm-to-palm cutting?
10. Explain the importance of proper posture and body position.
11. List disinfection and sanitation procedures that must be followed after performing every haircut.
12. Name and describe the four basic types of haircuts.
13. Define cross-checking.
14. Describe the scissor-over-comb technique.
15. Name and describe three different texturizing techniques performed with shears.

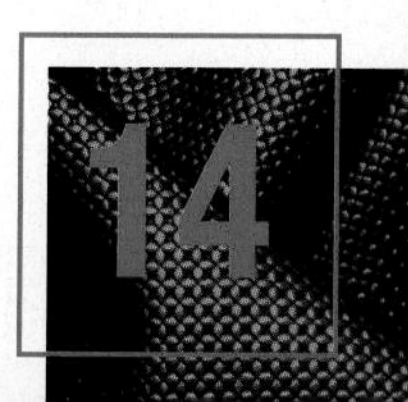

CHAPTER GLOSSARY

angle	Space between two lines or surfaces that intersect at a given point.
apex	Highest point on the top of the head.
bang (fringe)	Triangular section that begins at the apex and ends at the front corners.
beveling	Technique using diagonal lines by cutting hair ends with a slight increase or decrease in length.
blunt haircut	Haircut in which all the hair comes to one hanging level, forming a weight line or area; hair is cut with no elevation or over-direction; also referred to as a one-length, zero-elevation, or no-elevation cut.
carving	Haircutting technique done by placing the still blade into the hair and resting it on the scalp, and then moving the shears through the hair while opening and partially closing the shears.
clipper-over-comb	Haircutting technique similar to scissor-over-comb, except that the clippers move side to side across the comb rather than bottom to top.
cross-checking	Parting the haircut in the opposite way from which you cut it, to check for precision of line and shape.
crown	Area of the head between the apex and back of the parietal ridge.
cutting line	Angle at which the fingers are held when cutting, and ultimately the line that is cut; also known as finger angle, finger position, cutting position, cutting angle.
distribution	Where and how hair is moved over the head.
elevation	Angle or degree at which a subsection of hair is held, or lifted, from the head when cutting; also referred to as projection or lifting.
four corners	Points on the head that signal a change in the shape of the head, from flat to round or vice versa.
free-hand notching	Notching technique in which pieces of hair are snipped out at random intervals.
free-hand slicing	Technique used to release weight from the subsection, allowing the hair to move more freely.
graduated haircut	Graduated shape or wedge; an effect or haircut that results from cutting the hair with tension, low to medium elevation or over direction.
graduation	Elevation occurs when a section is lifted above 0 degrees.
growth pattern	Direction in which the hair grows from the scalp; also referred to as natural fall or natural falling position.
guideline	Section of hair, located either at the perimeter or the interior of the cut, that determines the length the hair will be cut; also referred to as a guide; usually the first section that is cut to create a shape.
hairline	Hair that grows at the outermost perimeter along the face, around the ears, and on the neck.

CHAPTER GLOSSARY

head form	Shape of the head, which greatly affects the way the hair falls and behaves; also called *head shape.*
interior	Inner or internal part.
interior guideline	Guideline that is inside the haircut rather than on the perimeter.
layered haircut	Graduated effect achieved by cutting the hair with elevation or over-direction; the hair is cut at higher elevations, usually 90 degrees or above, which removes weight.
layers	Create movement and volume in the hair by releasing weight.
line	Thin continuous mark used as a guide; can be straight or curved, horizontal, vertical, or diagonal.
long-layered haircut	Haircut in which the hair is cut at a 180-degree angle; the resulting shape has shorter layers at the top and increasingly longer layers toward the perimeter.
nape	Back part of the neck; the hair below the occipital bone.
notching	Version of point cutting in which the tips of the scissors are moved toward the hair ends rather than into them; creates a chunkier effect.
over-direction	Combing a section away from its natural falling position, rather than straight out from the head, toward a guideline; used to create increasing lengths in the interior or perimeter.
palm-to-palm	Cutting position in which the palms of both hands are facing each other.
parietal ridge	Widest area of the head, usually starting at the temples and ending at the bottom of the crown.
part/parting	Line dividing the hair to the scalp that separates one section of hair from another or creates subsections.
perimeter	Outer line of a hairstyle.
point cutting	Haircutting technique in which the tips of the shears are used to cut "points" into the ends of the hair.
razor-over-comb	Texturizing technique in which the comb and the razor are used on the surface of the hair.
razor rotation	Texturizing technique similar to razor-over-comb, done with small circular motions.
reference points	Points on the head that mark where the surface of the head changes or the behavior of the hair changes, such as ears, jawline, occipital bone, apex, and so on; used to establish design lines that are proportionate.
sections	To divide the hair by parting into uniform working areas for control.
scissor-over-comb	Haircutting technique in which the hair is held in place with the comb while the tips of the scissors are used to remove the lengths.

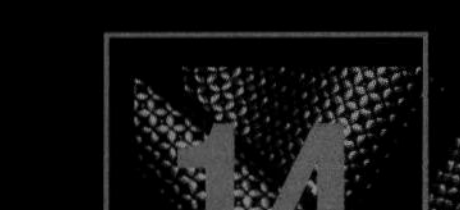

CHAPTER GLOSSARY

slicing	Technique that removes bulk and adds movement through the lengths of the hair; the shears are not completely closed, and only the portion of the blades near the pivot is used.
slide cutting	Method of cutting or thinning the hair in which the fingers and shears glide along the edge of the hair to remove length.
slithering (effilating)	Process of thinning the hair to graduated lengths with shears; cutting the hair with a sliding movement of the shears while keeping the blades partially opened; also called *effilating.*
stationary guideline	Guideline that does not move.
subsections	Smaller sections within a larger section of hair, used to maintain control of the hair while cutting.
tapers	Haircutting effect in which there is an even blend from very short at the hairline to longer lengths as you move up the head; "to taper" is to narrow progressively at one end.
tension	Amount of pressure applied when combing and holding a section, created by stretching or pulling the section.
texturizing	Removing excess bulk without shortening the length; changing the appearance or behavior of the hair through specific haircutting techniques, using shears, thinning shears, or a razor.
traveling guideline	Guideline that moves as the haircutting progresses, used often when creating layers or graduation.
uniform layers	Hair is elevated to 90 degrees from the scalp and cut at the same length.
weight line	Visual "line" in the haircut, where the ends of the hair hang together.

HAIRSTYLING

CHAPTER 15

chapter outline

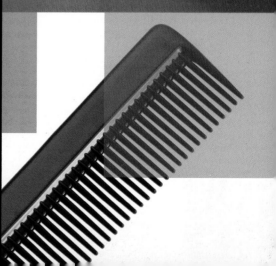

Learning Objectives

After completing this chapter, you will be able to:

- Demonstrate finger waving, pin curls, roller setting, and hair wrapping.
- Demonstrate various blow-dry styling techniques.
- Demonstrate three basic techniques of styling long hair.
- Demonstrate the proper use of thermal irons.
- Demonstrate various thermal iron manipulations and explain how they are used.
- Describe the three types of hair pressing.
- Demonstrate the procedures involved in soft pressing and hard pressing.

Key Terms

Page number indicates where in the chapter the term is used.

back-brushing pg. 321
back-combing pg. 321
barrel curls pg. 316
base pg. 310
blow-dry styling pg. 325
carved curls pg. 313
cascade or stand-up curls pg. 316
circle pg. 310
closed-center curls pg. 311
curl pg. 317
concentrator pg. 325
diffuser pg. 325
double press pg. 348
end curls pg. 345
finger waving pg. 304
finishing spray pg. 328
foam or mousse pg. 327
full-base curls pg. 346
full-stem curl pg. 311
gel pg. 327
hair pressing pg. 347
hair spray pg. 328
hair wrapping pg. 323
half base pg. 318
half-base curls pg. 346
half-stem curl pg. 310
hard press pg. 348
indentation pg. 318
liquid gels or texturizers pg. 327
medium press pg. 348
no-stem curl pg. 310
off base pg. 318
off-base curls pg. 346
on base pg. 318
open-center curls pg. 311
pomade or wax pg. 328
ribboning pg. 313
ridge curls pg. 313
rod pg. 336
shaping pg. 311
shell pg. 336
silicone pg. 328
skip waves pg. 313
soft press pg. 348
spiral curl pg. 345
stem pg. 310
straightening gel pg. 328
thermal waving and curling pg. 336
updo pg. 355
volume-base curls pg. 345
volumizer pg. 328
waving lotion pg. 305

The art of hairstyling or dressing the hair has always had a direct relation to the fashion, art, and life of the times. When you compare the ornate hair fantasies of Marie Antoinette and her court prior to the French revolution to the sleek bobs with finger waves and pin curls of a flapper during the 1920s and 1930s when "streamline modern" or "art deco" was the rage, you can see how a person's hairstyle reflects the period in which they live (Figure 15-1).

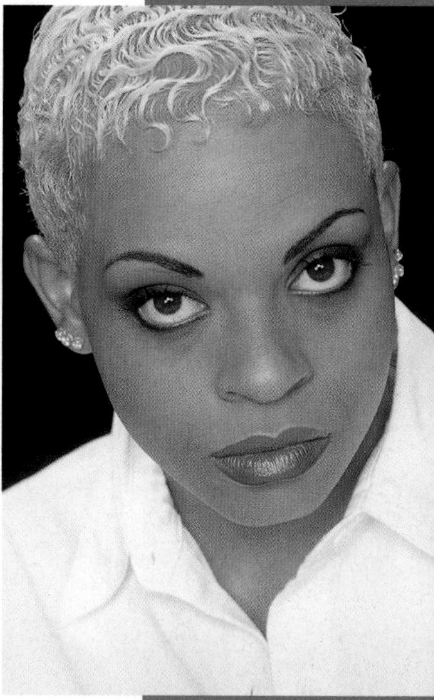

Figure 15-1 A modern look using finger waves.

With ready-to-wear clothing came wash-and-wear hair, misleading many hairstylists to believe that finishing hair was no longer necessary. With the exception of styling for formal occasions, many stylists have passed this important part of the hair experience into the hands of the client. It is our professional responsibility to educate clients in home care maintenance and styling options for their hair. No matter how great the haircut or haircolor, a client will often judge your work by the finished style.

Historical and technical knowledge of hairstyling will prepare you for the constant cyclical changes of fashion. Inspiration is often found in the past. Think retro—because what is out of style today may be back tomorrow. By learning the basic styling techniques, you will be ready and able to create what dreams are made of and to hear a satisfied client happily say, "This is what I always wanted."

CLIENT CONSULTATION

The client consultation is always the first step in the hairstyling process. Have your client look through magazines to find styles that she likes or, better yet, show her your portfolio of hairstyles. A picture is worth a thousand words. When deciding the best hairstyle, take into consideration all that you have learned in Chapter 12 regarding face shape, hair type, and lifestyle.

Often, you will be a creative problem solver. What if, on the client's last visit to another salon, she asked for a hairstyle that was not right for her

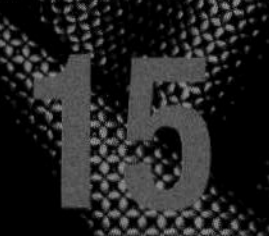

hair. Because the stylist did not suggest something more appropriate, the outcome was disastrous. Now you are being asked to "fix" the problem. If you can come up with a different style, one that is both flattering and easy to manage, she may become one of your most loyal clients.

WET HAIRSTYLING BASICS

Wet hairstyling tools include the following:

- Combs
- Brushes
- Rollers (plastic)
- Clips (duckbill, sectioning, finger waving, double prong, and single prong)
- Pins (bobby pins and hairpins)
- Clamps (sectioning clamps) (Figure 15-2)

FINGER WAVING

Finger waving is the process of shaping and directing the hair into an "S" pattern through the use of the fingers, combs, and waving lotion. Finger waving was all the rage back in the 1920s and1930s, which may have you wondering why you are being asked to learn this technique

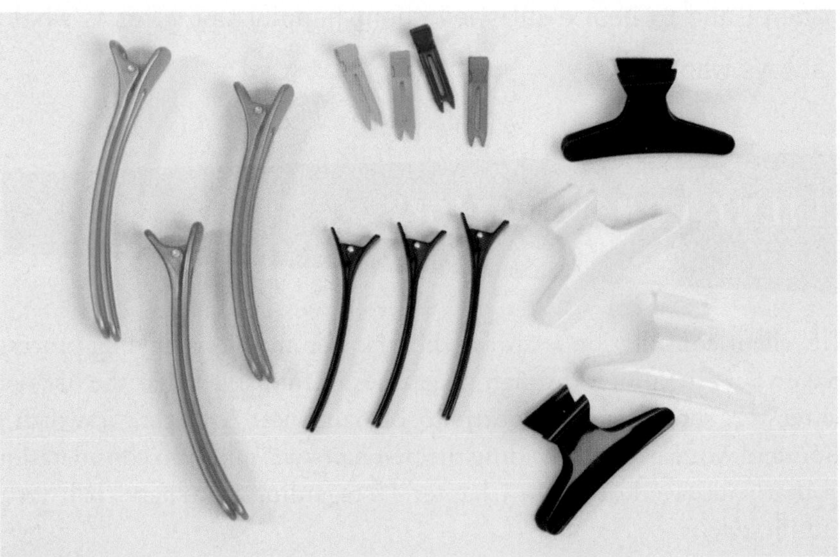

Figure 15-2 Clips (duckbill, sectioning, and double prong) and sectioning clamps.

today. In addition to its use in today's fashions, finger waving teaches you the technique of moving and directing hair. It also provides valuable training in molding hair to the curved surface of the head and is an excellent introduction to hairstyling.

FINGER WAVING LOTION

Waving lotion is a type of hair gel that makes the hair pliable enough to keep it in place during the finger waving procedure. It is traditionally made from karaya gum, taken from trees found in Africa and India. Karaya gum is diluted for use on fine hair, or it can be used in a more concentrated consistency on medium or coarse hair. A good waving lotion is harmless to the hair and does not flake when it dries. Be sure not use too much of it at any one time. You will know if you have used too much, as the hair will be too wet and the waving lotion will drip. Liquid styling gels are also commonly used in conjunction with finger waving, and in many cases, have phased out traditional karaya gum products.

OTHER METHODS OF FINGER WAVING

Instead of completing one side before beginning the other, you may want to complete the first ridge on one side of the head, and then move to the other side to form the first ridge on that side. After joining the two, you can then repeat in this manner until you are finished with the entire head.

In vertical finger waving, the ridges and waves run up and down the head. Horizontal finger waves are sideways and parallel around the head. The procedure is the same for both.

PROCEDURE 15-1

PREPARING THE HAIR FOR WET STYLING

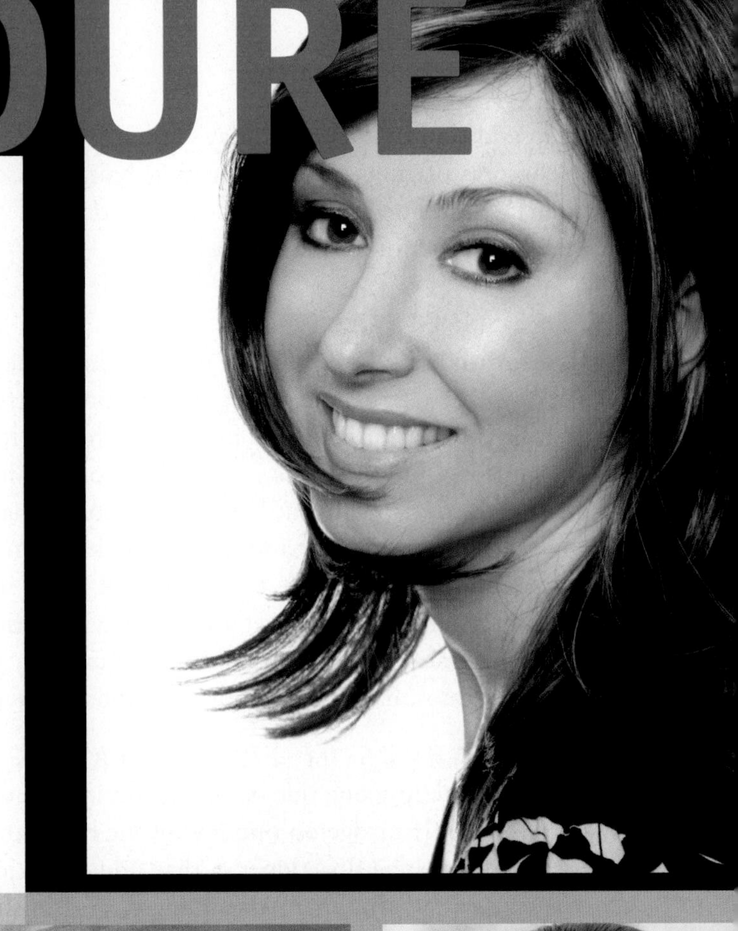

IMPLEMENTS AND MATERIALS

- Towels
- Plastic cape
- Shampoo
- Conditioner
- Neck strip

PREPARATION

1. Wash your hands with soap and warm water.
2. Perform the client consultation and hair analysis.
3. Drape the client for a shampoo service.
4. Shampoo the client's hair and condition if necessary.
5. Towel dry the hair.
6. Remove any tangles with a wide-tooth comb, starting at the ends and working up to the scalp.

If the client's natural part works with your hair design, use it. You can create a part anywhere on the head. If the client is more comfortable wearing it someplace else, or if your design works better with the part placed elsewhere, do it.

FINDING A NATURAL PART

1. Comb wet hair straight back from the hairline.
2. Push the hair gently forward with the palm of the hand (Figure 15-3).
3. Use your comb and other hand to separate the hair where it parts (Figure 15-4).

CREATING A PART

1. Lay the wide-tooth end of a styling comb flat at the hairline.
2. Draw the comb back to the end of the desired part (Figure 15-5).
3. Hold the hair with the index finger on one side of the part. Pull the rest of the hair down with the comb (Figure 15-6).

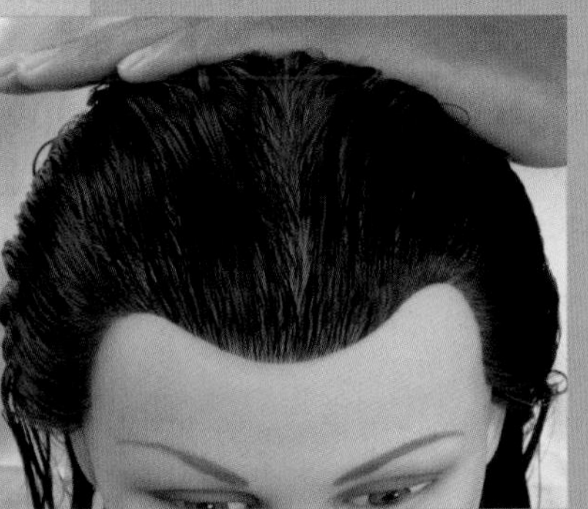

Figure 15-3 Push the hair forward.

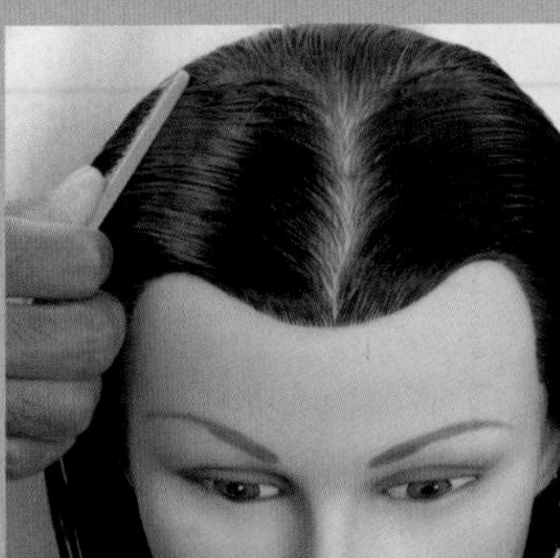

Figure 15-4 Find the natural part

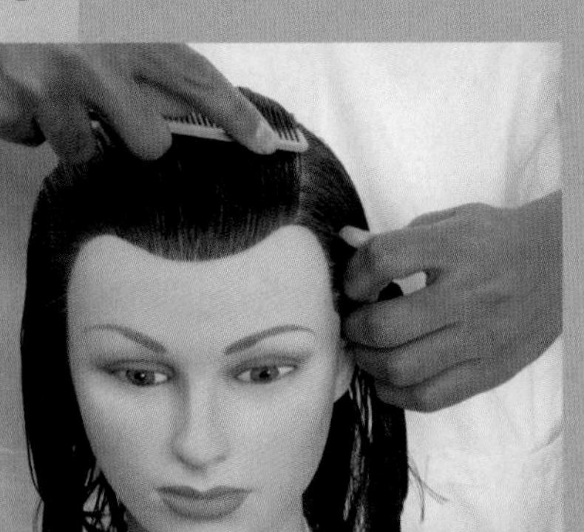

Figure 15-5 Part the wet hair.

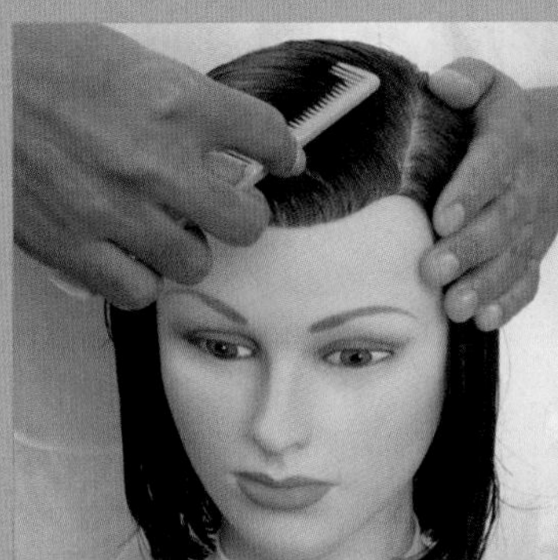

Figure 15-6 Comb the hair from part.

PROCEDURE 15-2

HORIZONTAL FINGER WAVING

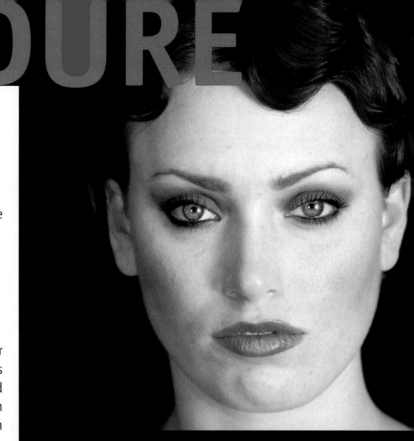

IMPLEMENTS AND MATERIALS

Use the list of implements and materials under preparing the hair for wet styling, and add the following:

- Styling comb
- Hairpins
- Waving lotion or styling gel
- Cotton or gauze
- Hairnet

PREPARATION

Follow the steps for preparing the hair for wet styling. Finger waves may be started on either side of the head. In this procedure, the hair is parted on the left side of the head and the wave is started on the right (heavy) side. Apply lotion to one side of the head at a time; this prevents it from drying and requiring additional applications.

PROCEDURE

1. **Part hair.** Part the hair, comb it smooth, and arrange it according to the planned style. Using the wide teeth of the comb will allow the hair to move more easily. Always follow the natural growth pattern when combing and parting the hair.
2. **Apply waving lotion.** Using an applicator bottle, apply waving lotion to the side of the hair you are working on while the hair is damp. Comb the lotion through the section (Figure 15-7).
3. **Start first wave.** Begin the first wave on the right side of the head. Using the index finger of your left hand as a guide, shape the top hair with a comb into the beginning of the S-shaping, using a circular movement. Starting at the hairline, work toward the crown in 1-$\frac{1}{2}$ to 2-inch (3.7 to 5 centimeters) sections at a time (Figure 15-8).
4. **Form first ridge.** To form the first ridge, place the index finger of your left hand directly above the position for the first ridge. With the teeth of the comb pointing slightly upward, insert the comb directly under the index finger. Draw the comb forward about 1 inch (2.5 centimeters) along the fingertip (Figure 15-9).
5. **Hold ridge in place.** With the teeth still inserted in the ridge, flatten the comb against the head in order to hold the ridge in place (Figure 15-10).

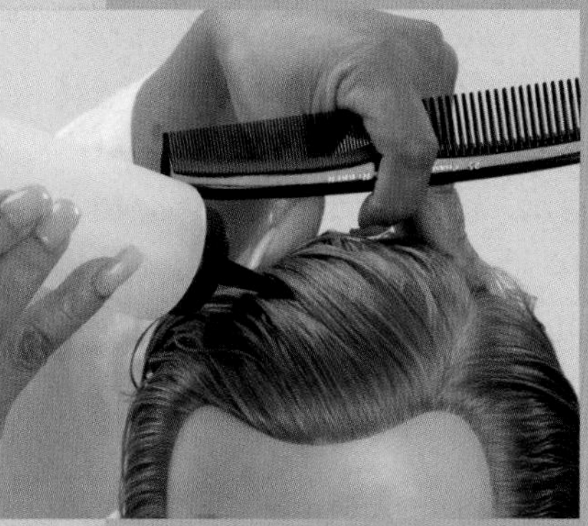

Figure 15-7 Comb waving lotion through the section.

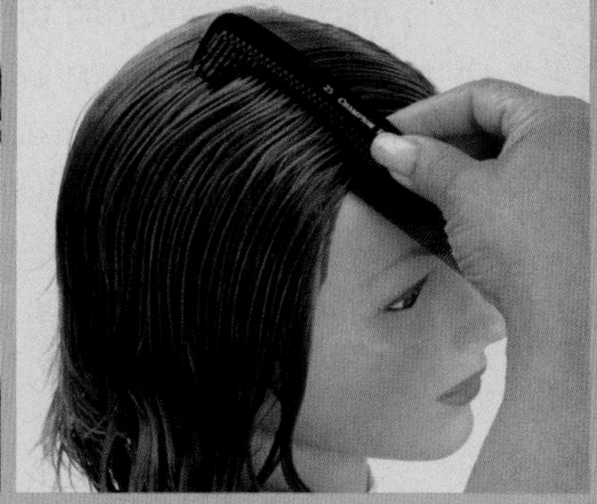

Figure 15-8 Shape the top area.

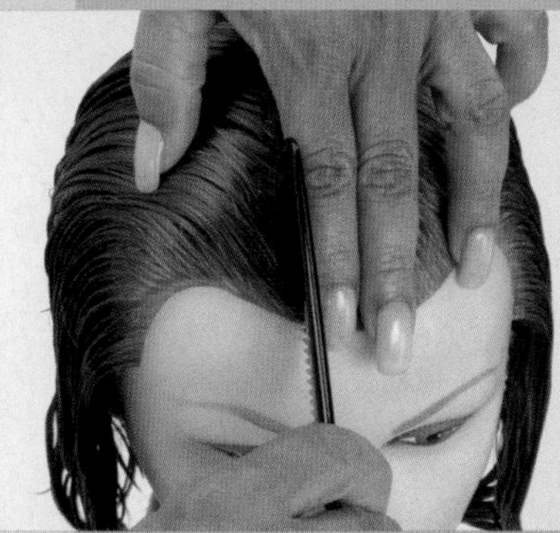

Figure 15-9 Draw hair toward the fingertip.

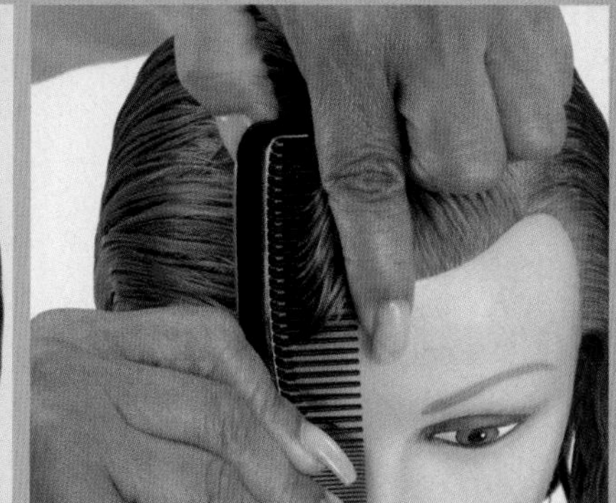

Figure 15-10 Flatten the comb against the head.

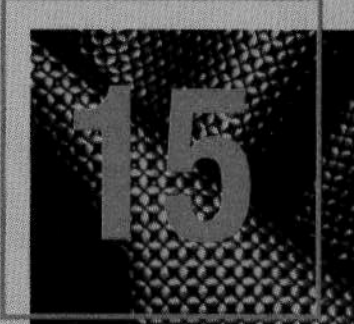

6. **Place finger above ridge.** Remove your left hand from the client's head and place your middle finger above the ridge with your index finger on the teeth of the comb. Draw out the ridge by closing the two fingers and applying pressure to the head (Figure 15-11). Do not try to increase the height or depth of a ridge by pinching or pushing with your fingers; such movements will create over-direction of the ridge and uneven hair placement.
7. **Form dip.** Without removing the comb, turn the teeth downward, and comb the hair in a semicircular direction to form a dip in the hollow part of the wave (Figure 15-12).
8. **Work to crown.** Follow this procedure, section by section, until the crown has been reached, where the ridge phases out (Figure 15-13). The ridge and wave of each section should match evenly, without showing separations in the ridge and the hollow part of the wave.
9. **Complete second ridge.** To form the second ridge, begin at the crown area (Figure 15-14). The movements are the reverse of those followed in forming the first ridge. Draw the comb from the tip of the index finger toward the base. All movements are followed in a reverse pattern until the hairline is reached, completing the second ridge (Figure 15-15).
10. **Begin third ridge.** Movements for the third ridge closely follow those used to create the first ridge. However, the third ridge is started at the hairline, and is extended back toward the back of the head (Figure 15-16).
11. **Complete side.** Continue alternating directions until the side of the head has been completed.

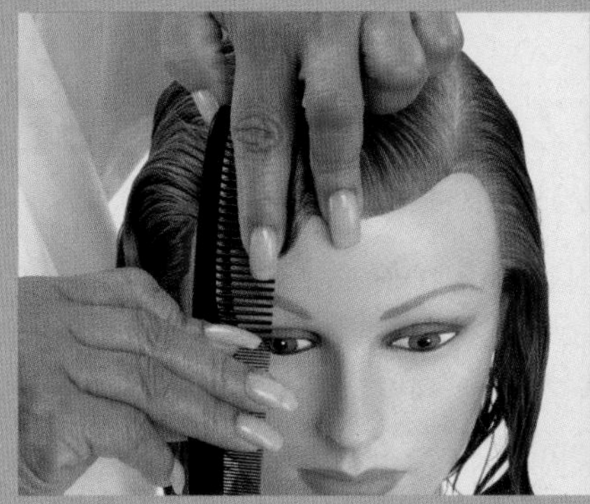

Figure 15-11 Emphasize the ridge.

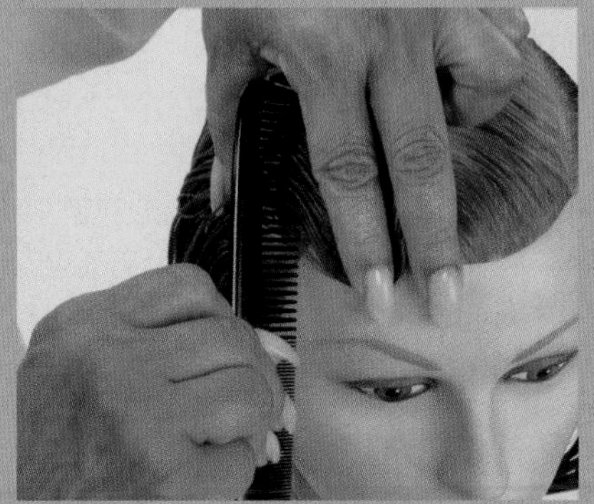

Figure 15-12 Comb hair in a semicircular direction.

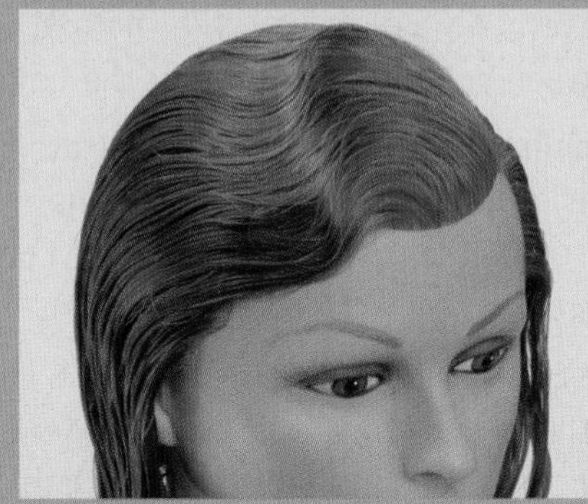

Figure 15-13 Completed first ridge.

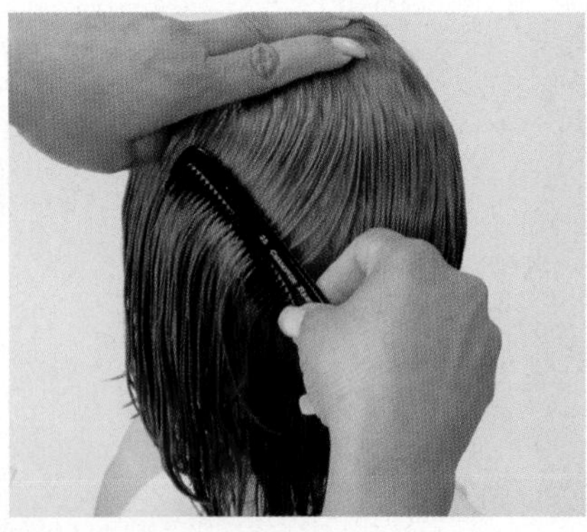

Figure 15-14 Start the second ridge.

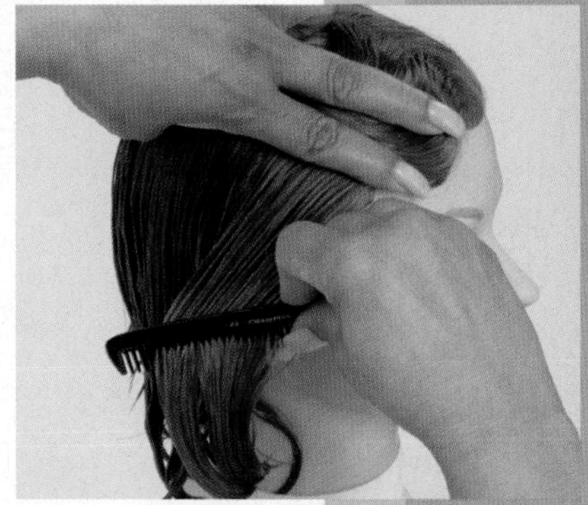

Figure 15-15 Completed second ridge.

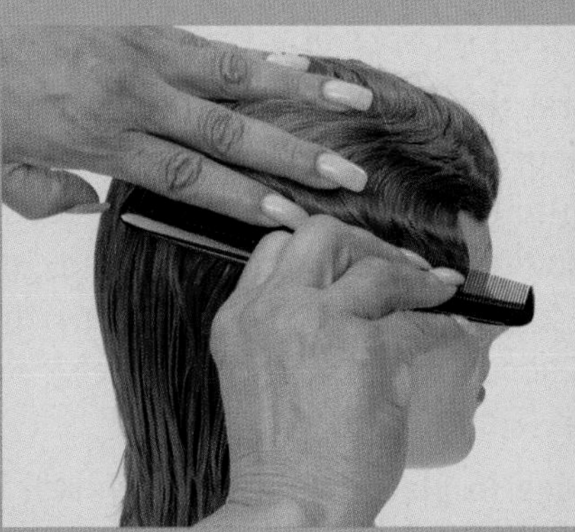

Figure 15-16 Start the third ridge.

12. **Complete light side.** Use the same procedure for the left (light) side of the head as you used for finger waving the right (heavy) side of the head. First, shape the hair by combing it in the direction of the first wave (Figure 15-17).
13. **Form first ridge.** Starting at the hairline, form the first ridge, section by section, until the second ridge of the opposite side is reached (Figure 15-18).
14. **Blend ridge and wave.** Both the ridge and the wave must blend without splits or breaks, with the ridge and wave on the right side of the head (Figure 15-19).
15. **Move to the left side.** Start with the ridge and wave in the back of the head and proceed, section by section, toward the left side of the face.
16. **Complete side.** Continue working back and forth until the entire side is completed (Figure 15-20).
17. **Dry hair.** Place a net over the hair, secure it with hairpins or clips if necessary, and protect the client's forehead and ears with cotton, gauze, or paper protectors while under the hood dryer. Adjust the dryer to medium heat and allow the hair to dry thoroughly.
18. **Cool hair.** Remove the client from under the dryer and let the hair cool down. Remove all clips or pins and the hairnet from the hair.
19. **Complete style. Comb-out** or brush the hair into a soft, waved hairstyle. Add a finishing spray for hold and shine (Figures 15-21 and 15-22). For a "retro" look, do not comb or brush the hair, but do consider adding a hair ornament such as a rhinestone clip in the hollow portion of a wave.

CLEANUP AND SANITATION

1. Disinfect brushes, combs, hairpins, clips, cape, and hairnet after each use.
2. Sanitize your workstation.
3. Wash your hands with soap and warm water.

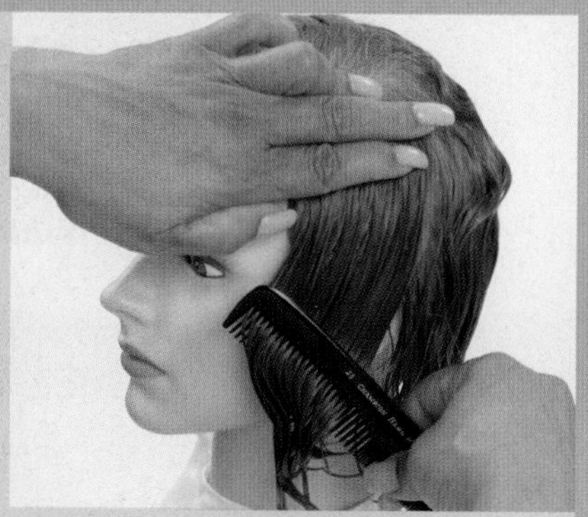

Figure 15-17 Shape the left side.

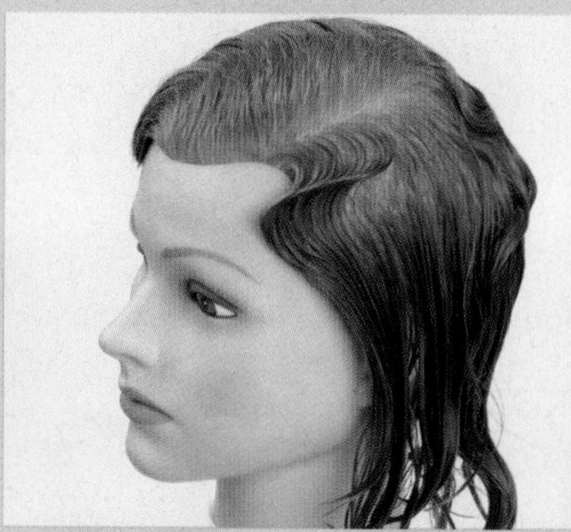

Figure 15-18 Start first ridge at hairline.

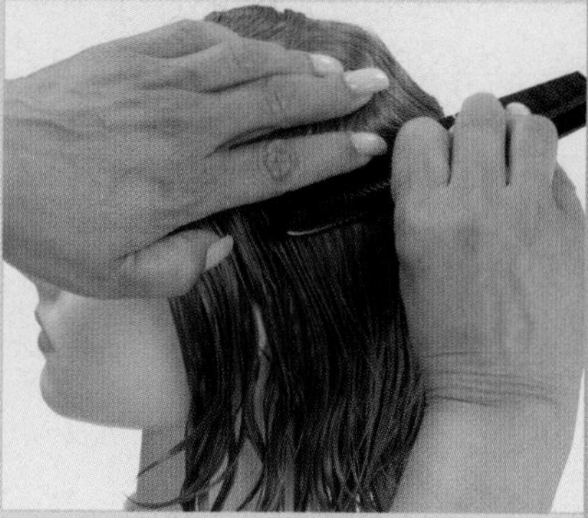

Figure 15-19 Ridge and wave matched in crown area.

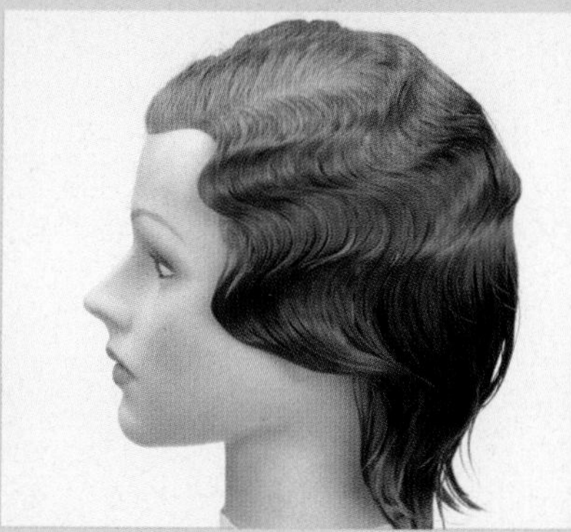

Figure 15-20 Left side completed.

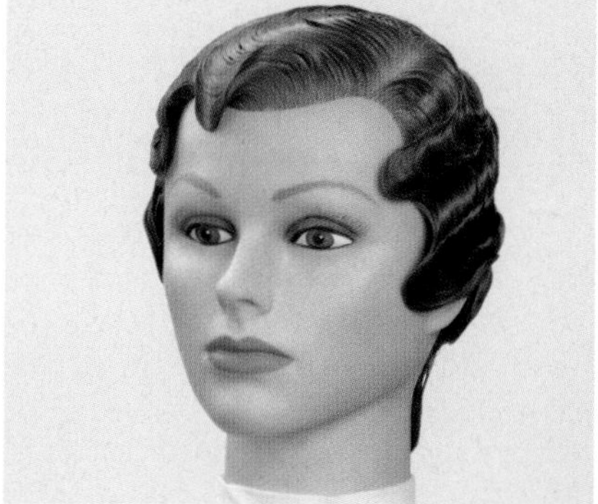

Figure 15-21 Finished hairstyle.

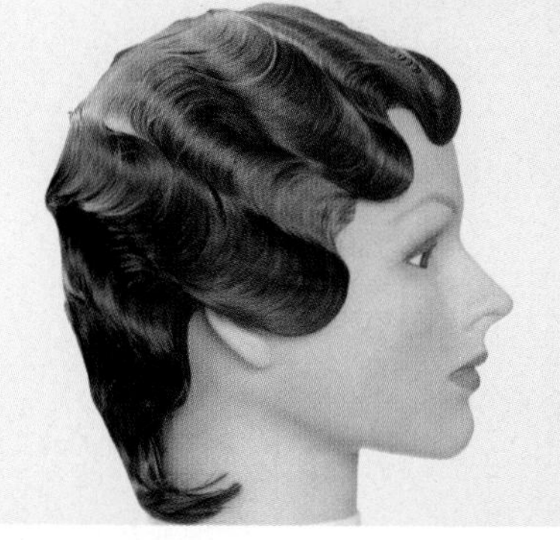

Figure 15-22 Side view.

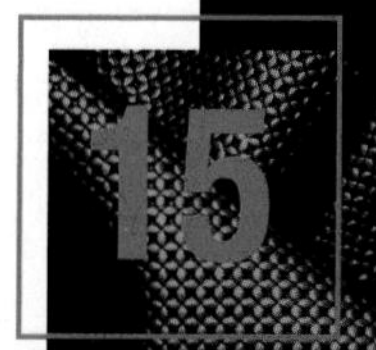

PIN CURLS

Pin curls serve as the basis for patterns, lines, waves, curls, and rolls that are used in a wide range of hairstyles. You can use them on all types of hair, including straight, permanent waved, or naturally curly hair. Pin curls work best when the hair is layered and is smoothly wound. This makes springy and long-lasting curls with good direction and definition.

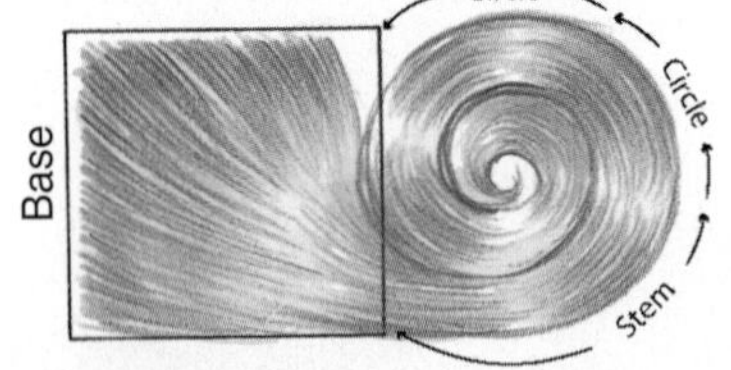

Figure 15-23 Parts of a curl.

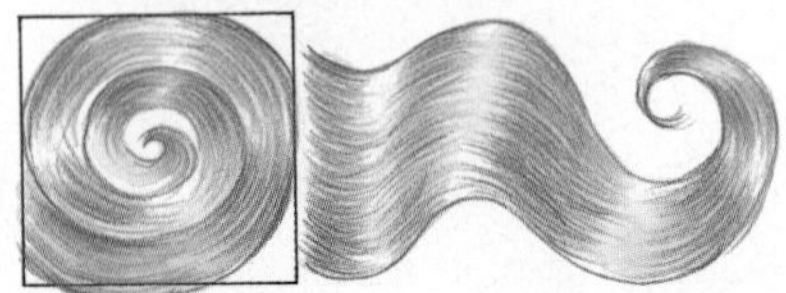
Figure 15-24 No-stem curl unwound.

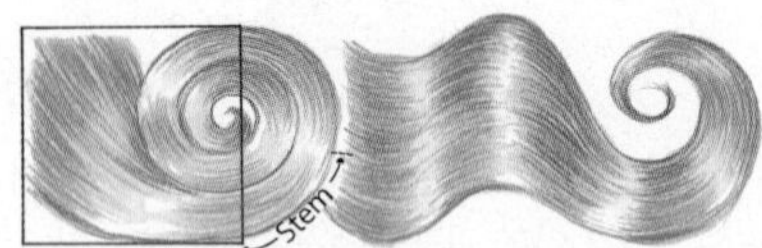

Figure 15-25 Half-stem curl opened out.

PARTS OF A CURL

Pin curls are made up of three principal parts: base, stem, and circle (Figure 15-23).

1. The **base** is the stationary (non-moving) foundation of the curl, which is the area closest to the scalp.
2. The **stem** is the section of the pin curl between the base and first arc (turn) of the circle that gives the curl its direction and movement.
3. The **circle** is the part of the pin curl that forms a complete circle. The size of the circle determines the width of the wave and its strength.

MOBILITY OF A CURL

The stem determines the amount of mobility, or movement, of a section of hair. Curl mobility is classified as no-stem, half-stem, and full-stem.

- The **no-stem curl** is placed directly on the base of the curl. It produces a tight, firm, long-lasting curl and allows minimum mobility (Figure 15-24).
- The **half-stem curl** permits medium movement; the curl (circle) is placed half off the base. It gives good control to the hair (Figure 15-25).

- The **full-stem curl** allows for the greatest mobility. The curl is placed completely off the base. The base may be a square, triangular, half-moon, or rectangular section, depending on the area of the head in which the full-stem curls are used. It gives as much freedom as the length of the stem will permit. If it is exaggerated, the hair near the scalp will be flat and almost straight. It is used to give the hair a strong, definite direction (Figure 15-26).

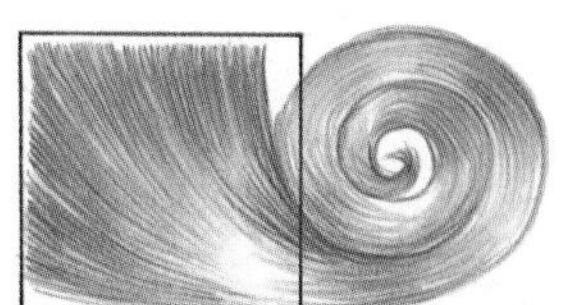

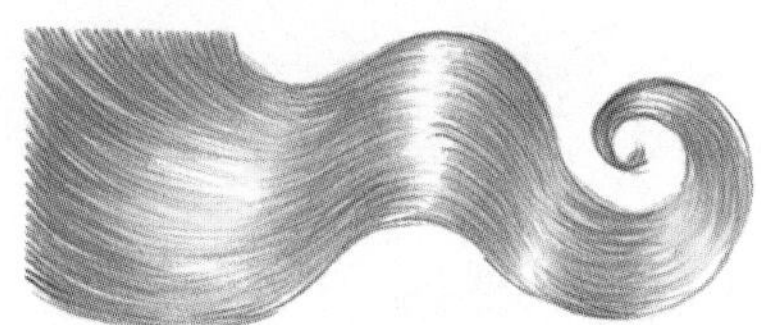

Figure 15-26 Full-stem curl opened out.

SHAPING FOR PIN CURL PLACEMENTS

A **shaping** is a section of hair that is molded in a circular movement in preparation for the formation of curls. Shapings are either open-end or closed-end. Always begin a pin curl at the open end, or convex side, of a shaping (Figures 15-27 and 15-28).

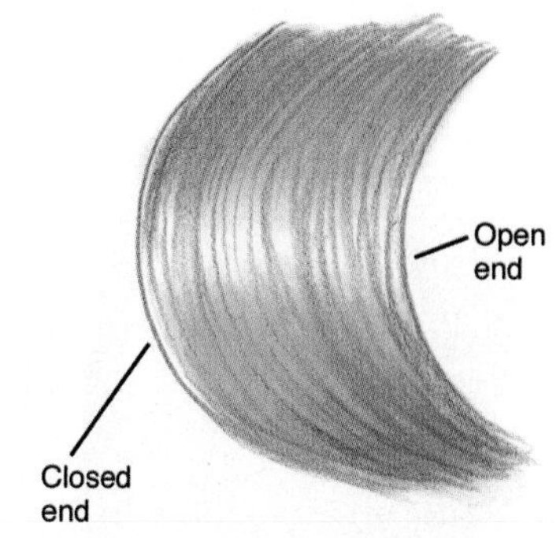

Figure 15-27 Closed and open ends of a curl.

OPEN- AND CLOSED-CENTER CURLS

Open-center curls produce even, smooth waves and uniform curls. **Closed-center curls** produce waves that get smaller in size toward the end. They are good for fine hair, or if a fluffy curl is desired. Note the difference in the waves produced by pin curls with open centers and those with closed centers. The width of the curl determines the size of the wave. If you make pin curls with the ends outside the curl, the resulting wave will be narrower near the scalp, and wider toward the ends (Figures 15-29 and 15-30).

CURL AND STEM DIRECTION

Curls may be turned toward the face, away from the face, upward, downward, or diagonally. The finished result will be determined by the direction the stem of the curl is placed.

The terms "clockwise curls" and "counterclockwise curls" are used to describe the direction of pin curls. Curls formed in the same direction as the movement of the hands of a clock are known as clockwise curls. Curls formed in the opposite direction are known as counterclockwise curls.

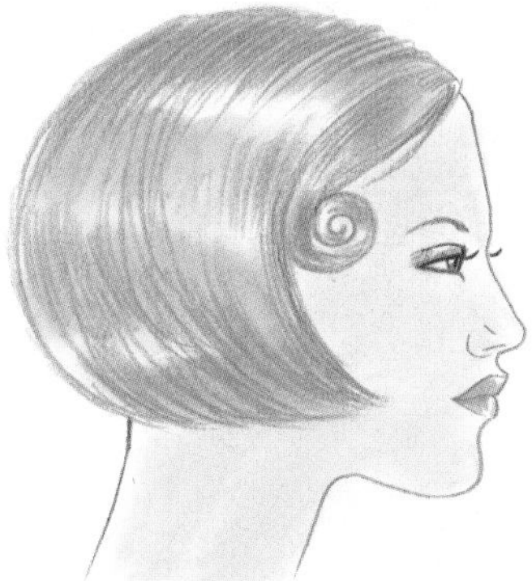

Figure 15-28 Curl in the shaping.

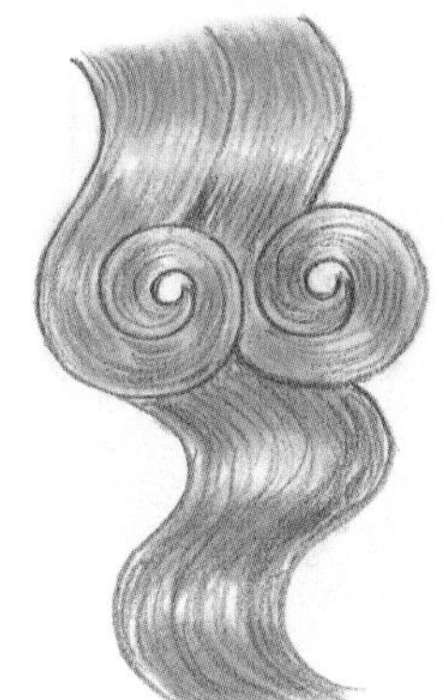

Figure 15-29 Curl with open center.

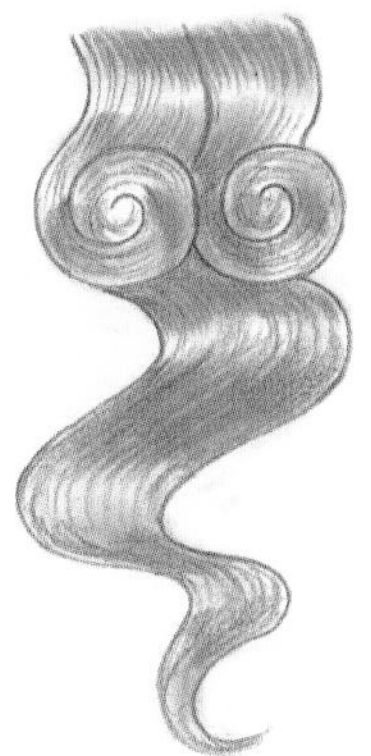

Figure 15-30 Curl with closed center.

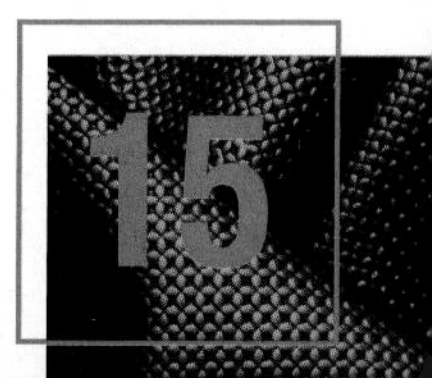

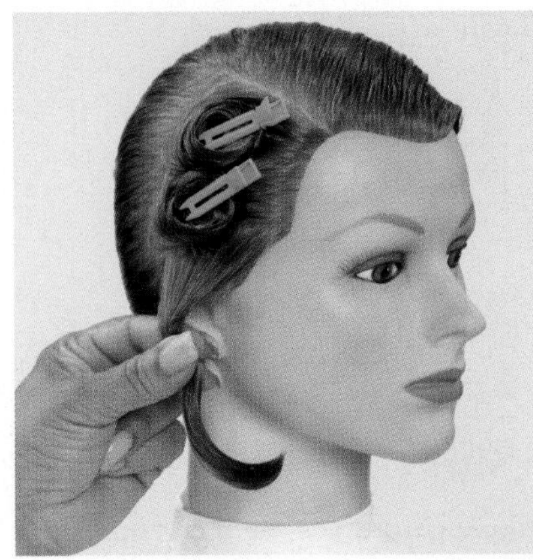

Figure 15-31 Rectangular base pin curls.

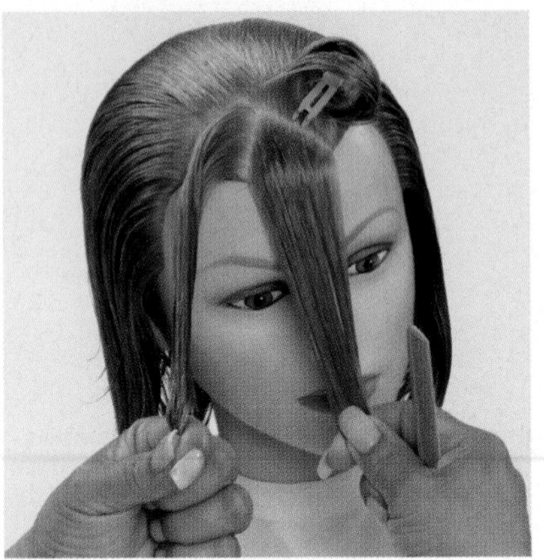

Figure 15-32 Triangular base pin curls.

BASE PIN CURL BASES OR FOUNDATIONS

Before you begin to make pin curls, divide the wet hair into sections or panels. Then subdivide each section into the type of base required for the various curls. The most commonly shaped base you will use is the arc base (half-moon or C-shape). Others are rectangular, triangular, or square.

To avoid splits in the finished hairstyle, you must use care when selecting and forming the curl base. When the sections of hair are as equal as possible, you will get curls that are similar to one another. Each curl must lie flat and smooth on its base. If it is too far off the base, the curl will lie loose away from the scalp. The shape of the base, however, does not affect the finished curl.

- *Rectangular base pin curls* are usually recommended at the side front hairline for a smooth, upsweep effect (Figure 15-31). To avoid splits in the comb-out, the pin curls must overlap.
- *Triangular base pin curls* are recommended along the front or facial hairline to prevent breaks or splits in the finished hairstyle. The triangular base allows a portion of the hair from each curl to overlap the next, and can be combed into a wave without splits (Figure 15-32).
- *Arc base pin curls,* also known as half-moon or C-shape base curls, are carved out of a shaping. Arc base pin curls give good direction and may be used at the hairline or in the nape (Figure 15-33).
- *Square base pin curls* are suitable for curly hairstyles without much volume or lift. They can be used on any part of the head and will comb out with lasting results. To avoid splits in the comb-out, stagger the sectioning as shown in the illustration (square base, brick-lay fashion) (Figure 15-34).

PIN CURL TECHNIQUES

There are various methods used to make pin curls. We will illustrate several methods below, but your instructor might demonstrate other methods that are equally correct.

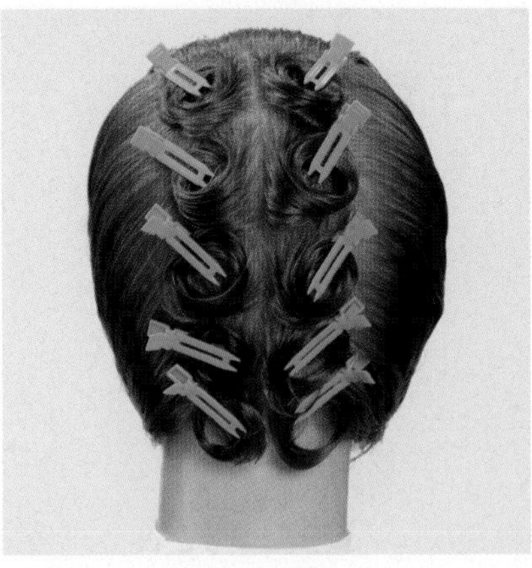

Figure 15-33 Arc base pin curls.

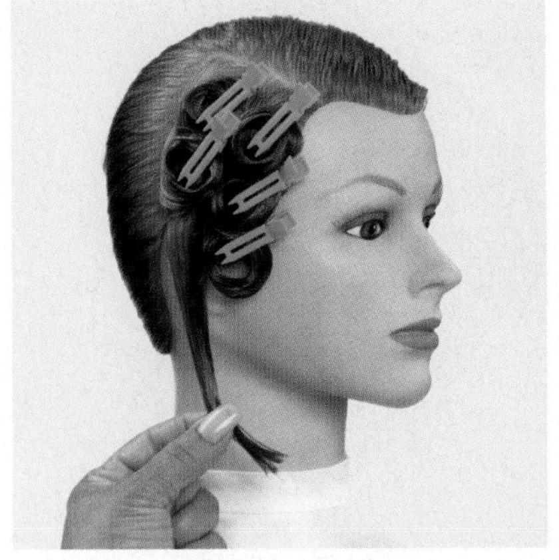

Figure 15-34 Square base pin curls.

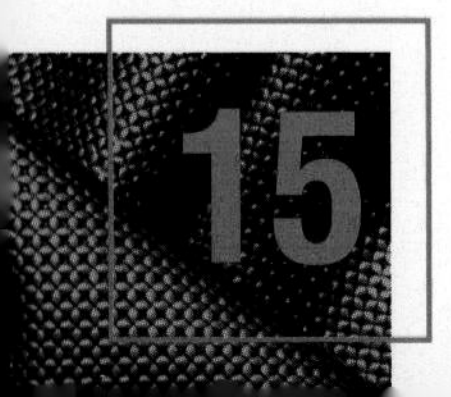

One important technique to learn is called **ribboning,** which involves forcing the hair between the thumb and the back of the comb to create tension. You can also ribbon hair by pulling the strands while applying pressure between your thumb and index finger out toward the ends of the strands.

CARVED OR SCULPTURED CURLS

Pin curls sliced from a shaping and formed without lifting the hair from the head are referred to as **carved curls** (or sculptured curls).

DESIGNING WITH PIN CURLS

- To create a wave, use two rows of pin curls. Set one row clockwise, and the second row counterclockwise (Figures 15-35 and 15-36).
- **Ridge curls** are pin curls placed immediately behind or below a ridge to form a wave (Figures 15-37 and 15-38).
- **Skip waves** are two rows of ridge curls, usually on the side of the head.

They create a strong wave pattern with well-defined lines between the waves. This technique represents a combination of finger waving and pin curls (Figures 15-39 and 15-40).

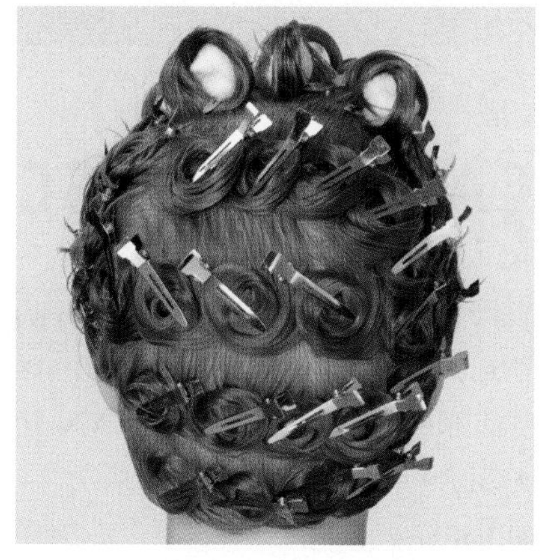

Figure 15-35 Setting pattern for wave.

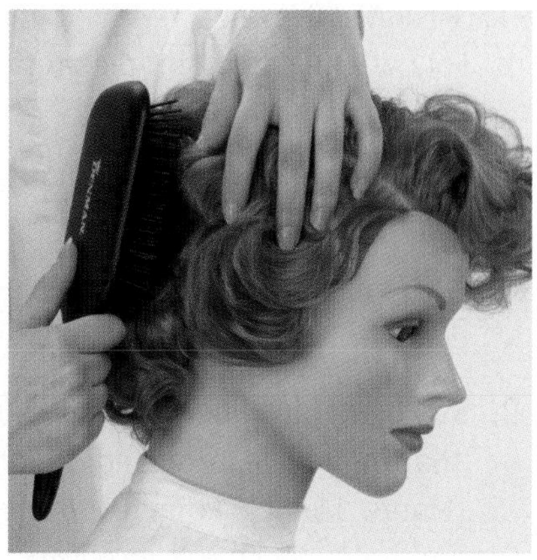

Figure 15-36 Comb-out of wave setting.

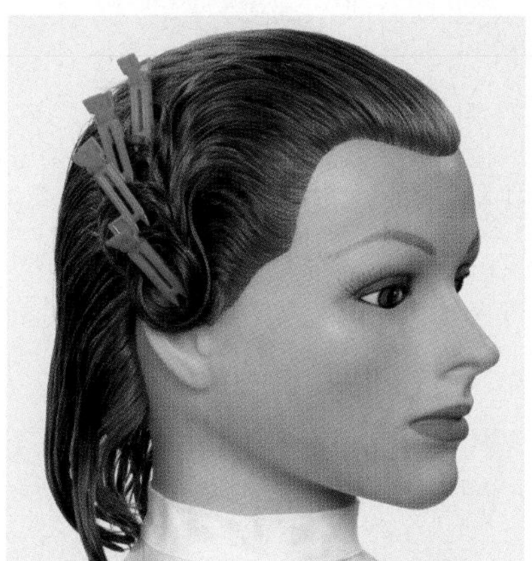

Figure 15-37 Setting pattern for ridge curl.

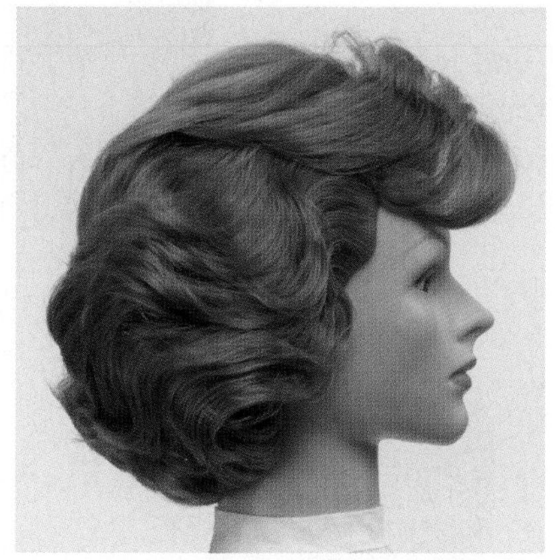

Figure 15-38 Comb-out for ridge curl.

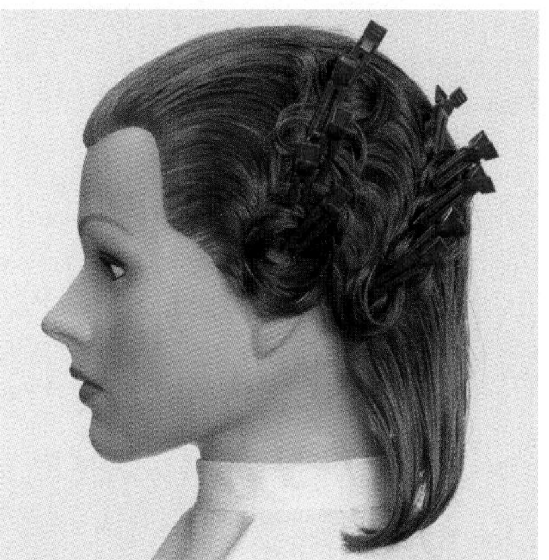

Figure 15-39 Setting pattern for skip wave.

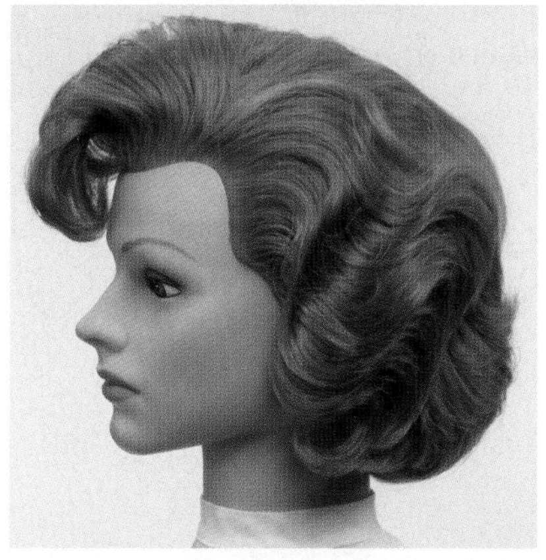

Figure 15-40 Comb-out of skip wave setting.

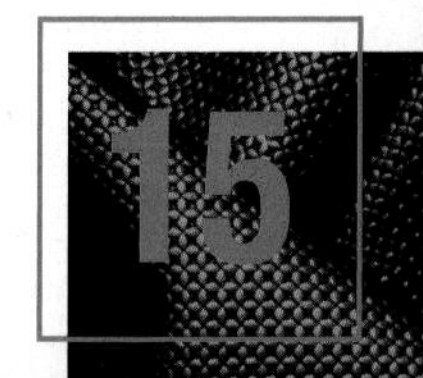

PROCEDURE 15-3

CARVED OR SCULPTED CURLS

IMPLEMENTS AND MATERIALS

Use the list of implements and materials for preparing the hair for wet styling and add the following:

- Styling comb
- Setting lotion
- Double or single prong clips

PREPARATION

1. Follow the steps in preparing the hair for wet styling.
2. Apply a gel or setting lotion and comb the hair smoothly.

PROCEDURE

1. Form the first shaping (Figure 15-41).
2. **Start making curls at the open end of the shaping.** Slice a strand to create the first curl (Figure 15-42). Point your left index finger down and hold the strand in place.
3. Ribbon the strand (Figure 15-43).
4. Wind the curl forward, keeping the hair ends inside the center of the curl (Figure 15-44).
5. Hold the curl in the shaping and anchor it with a clip (Figure 15-45).

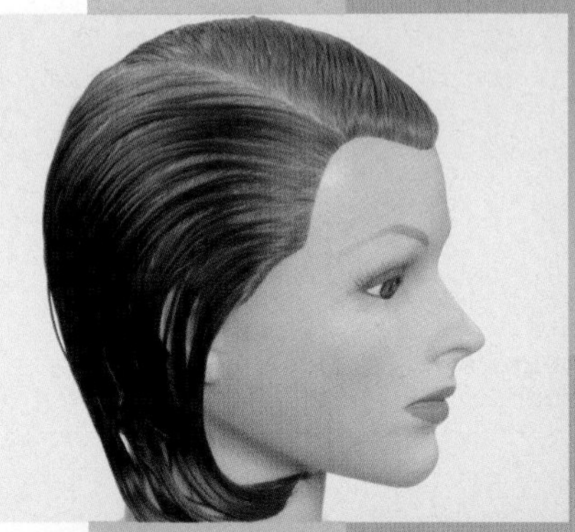

Figure 15-41 Form the first shaping.

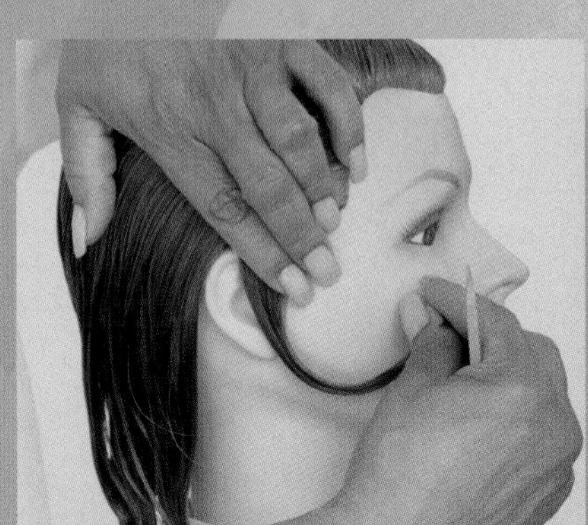

Figure 15-42 Slicing.

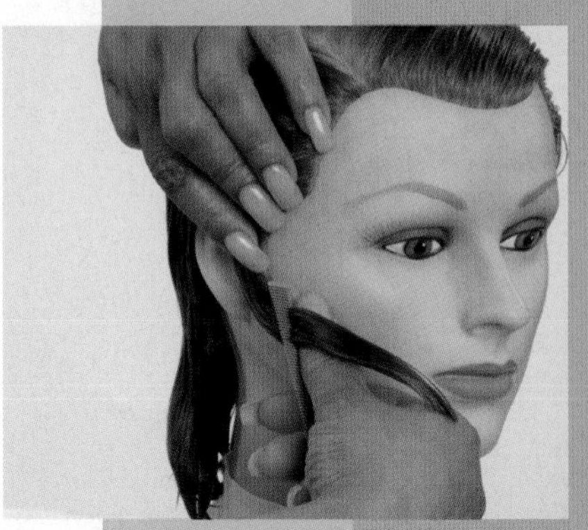

Figure 15-43 Ribbon the strand.

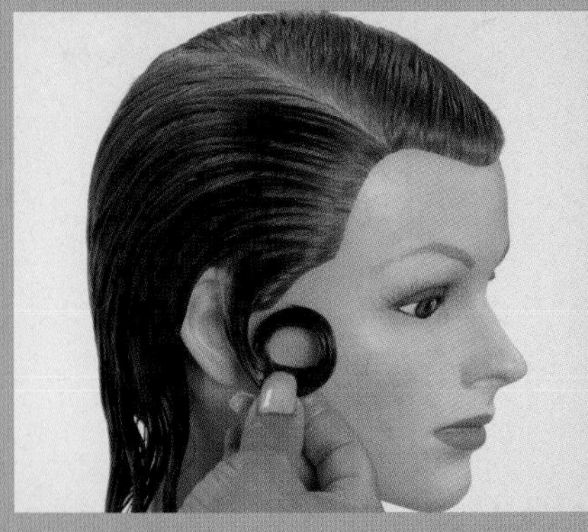

Figure 15-44 Wind the curl.

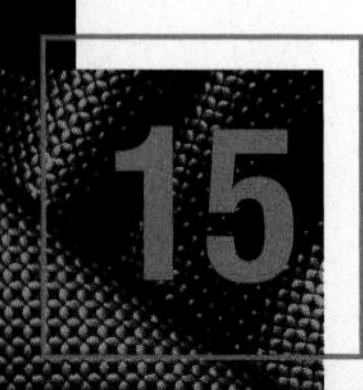

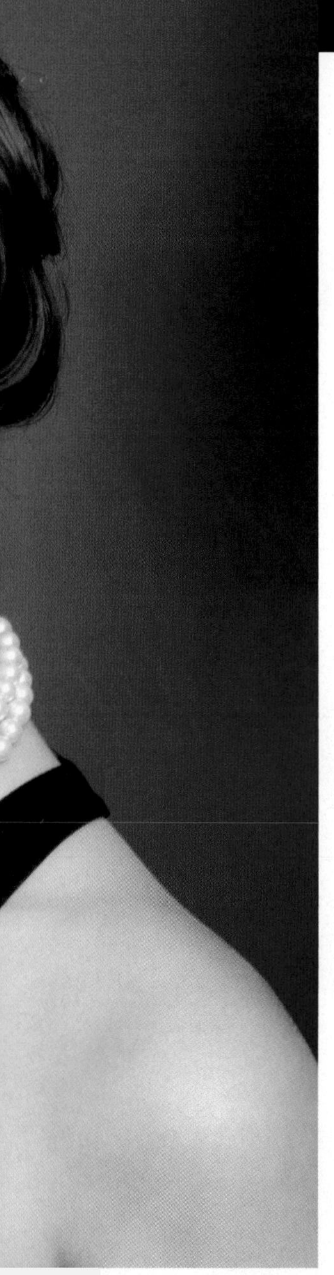

ANCHORING PINS

Follow the steps below to anchor pin curls correctly so that the curls hold firmly where you have placed them. This will allow you to comb the hair into the style you have planned.

1. **Anchor the clip.** To anchor pin curls, start at the open end of the curl. This is the side opposite the stem (Figure 15-46).
2. **The clip should enter the circle parallel to the stem.** Open the clip and place one prong above, and one prong below one side of the circle. The upper prong should enter the hair in the center of the circle. The curl should be in the gap between the prongs. To avoid an indentation ("dent") in the curl, do not pin across the circle (Figures 15-47 and 15-48).
3. **Place cotton.** If any clips touch the skin, place cotton between the skin and the clip to keep the skin from burning when the client is placed under the hood dryer.

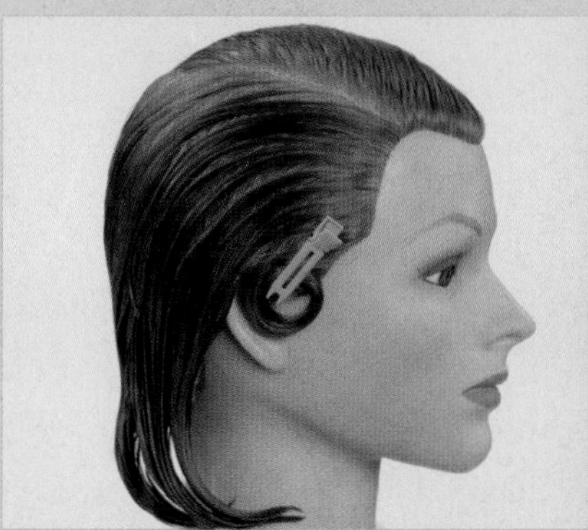

Figure 15-45 Anchor the curl.

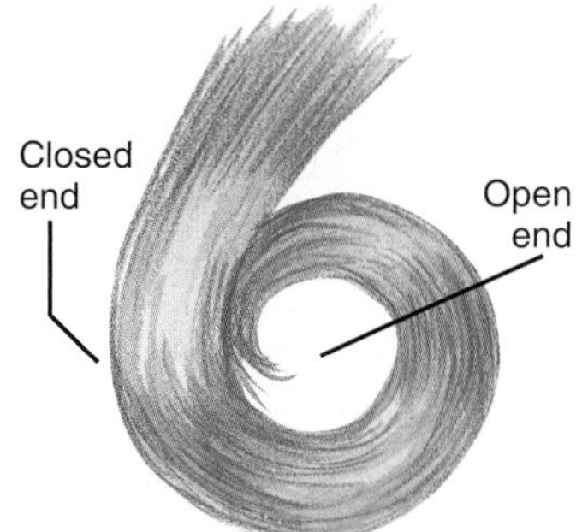

Figure 15-46 Closed and open ends of curl.

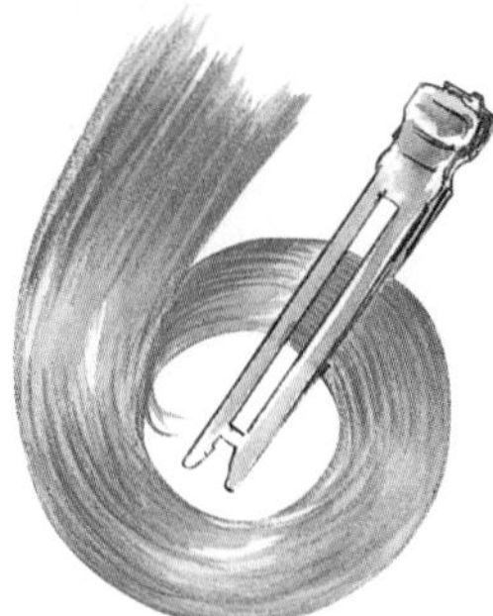

Figure 15-47 Correct placement of clip.

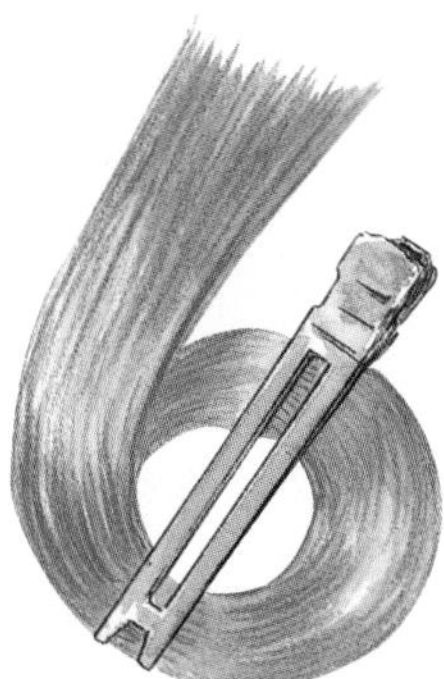

Figure 15-48 Incorrect placement of clip.

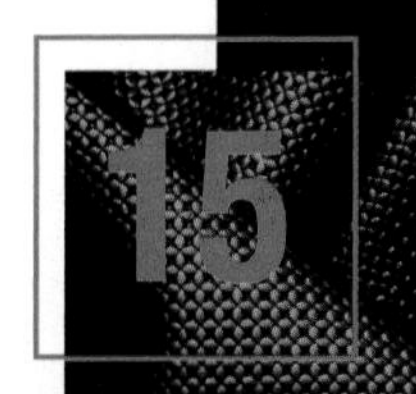

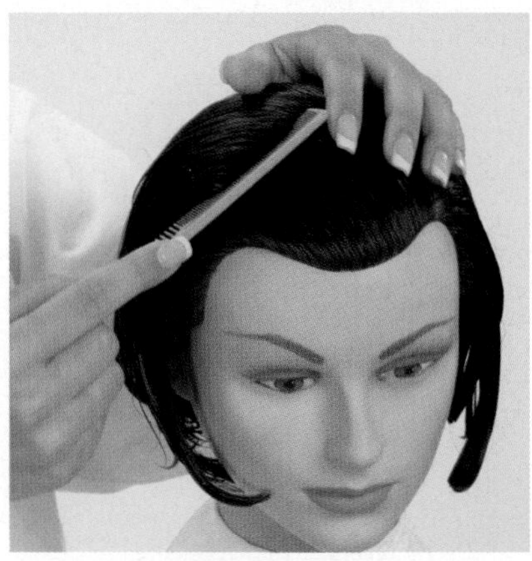

Figure 15-49 Comb, divide, and smooth section.

CREATING VOLUME WITH PIN CURLS

One of the best things about pin curls is they can add volume to the hair. Two types of pin curls that are particularly effective in this respect follow:

- **Cascade** or **stand-up curls,** which are used to create height in the hair design. They are fastened to the head in a standing position to allow the hair to flow upward and then downward. The size of the curl determines the amount of height in the comb-out (Figures 15-49 through 15-55).
- **Barrel curls,** which have large center openings and are fastened to the head in a standing position on a rectangular base. They have the same effect as stand-up pin curls. A barrel curl is similar to a roller, but does not have the same tension as a roller when it is set.

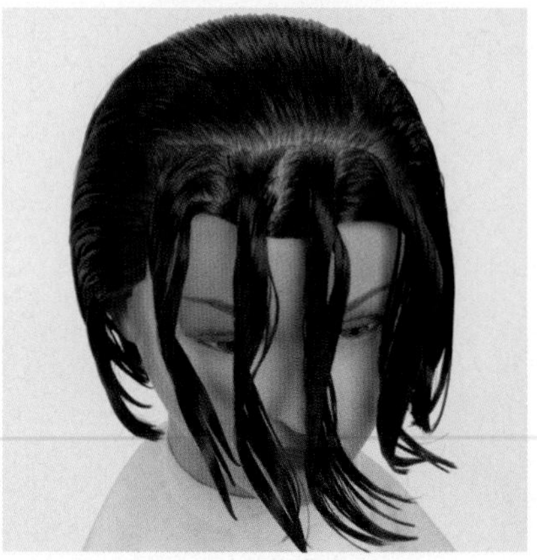

Figure 15-50 Divide section into strands.

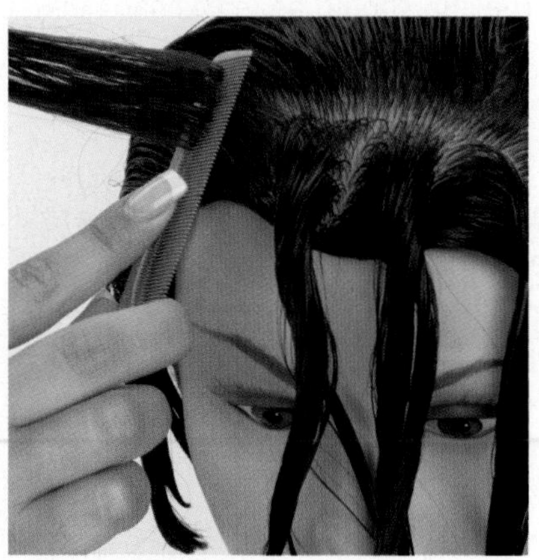

Figure 15-51 Ribbon the strand.

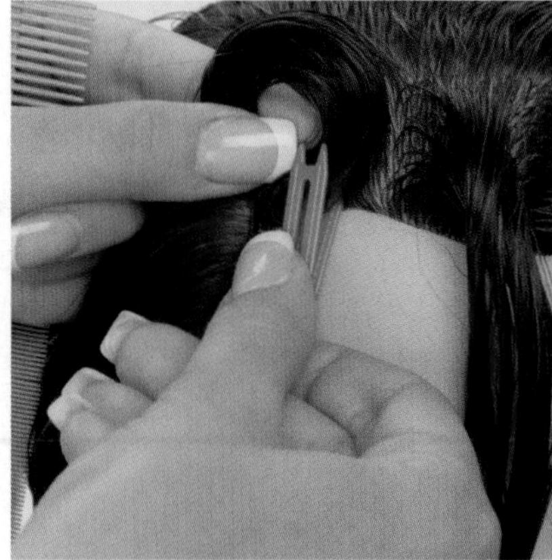

Figure 15-52 Direct the strand.

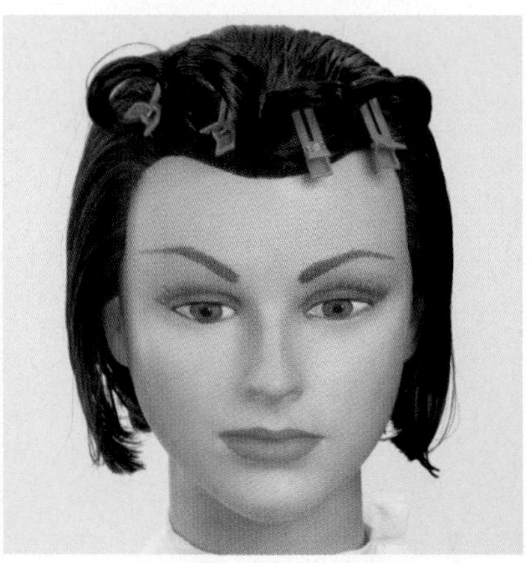

Figure 15-53 Anchor curl at base.

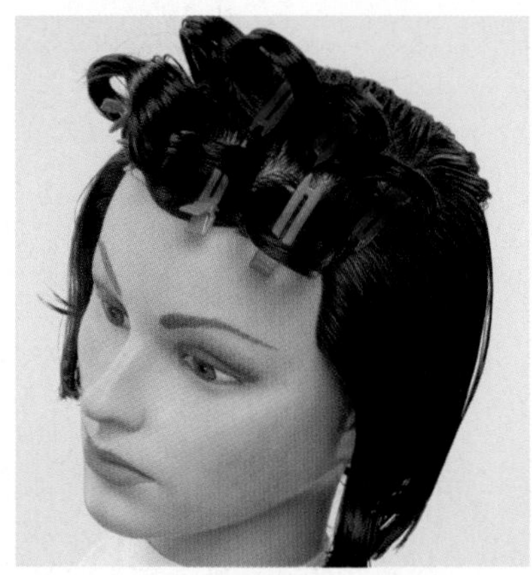

Figure 15-54 Top setting.

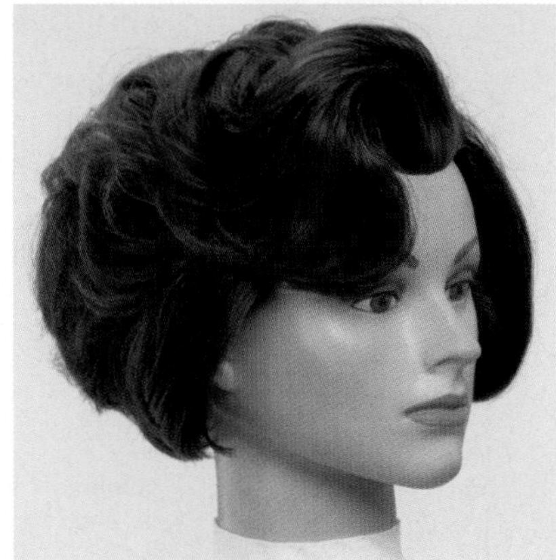

Figure 15-55 Comb-out as you would a roller set.

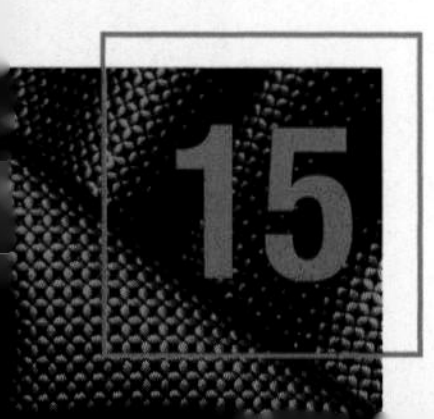

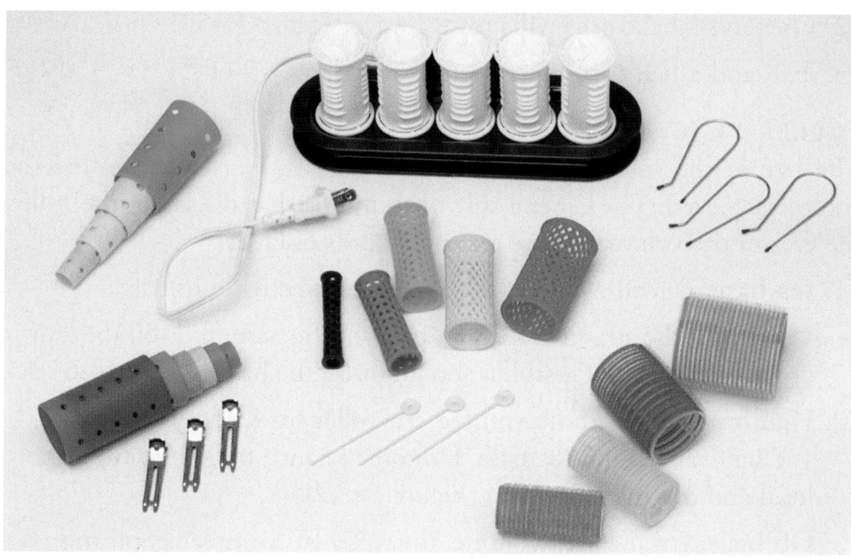

Figure 15-56 Rollers: plastic, mesh, hot, and Velcro.

ROLLER CURLS

Rollers are used to create many of the same effects as stand-up pin curls.

Rollers have the following advantages over pin curls.

- Because a roller holds the equivalent of two to four stand-up curls, the roller is a much faster way to set the hair.
- The hair is wrapped around the roller with tension, which gives a stronger and longer-lasting set.
- Rollers come in a variety of shapes, widths, and sizes, which broadens the creative possibilities for any style (Figure 15-56).

PARTS OF A ROLLER CURL

It is important for you to be able to identify the three parts of a roller curl (Figure 15-57).

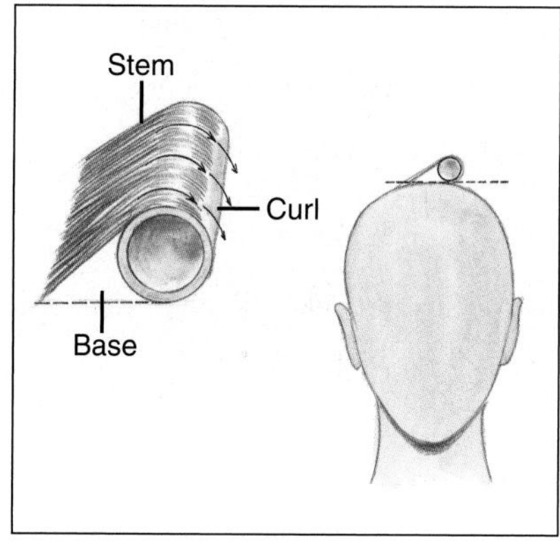

Figure 15-57 Parts of a roller curl.

- **Base.** The panel of hair on which the roller is placed. The base should be the same length and width as the roller. The type of base affects the volume.
- **Stem.** The hair between the scalp and the first turn of the roller. The stem gives the hair direction and mobility.
- **Curl** or circle. The hair that is wrapped around the roller. It determines the size of the wave or curl.

CHOOSING YOUR ROLLER SIZE

The relationship between the length of the hair and the size of the roller will determine whether the result will be a C-shape, wave, or curl. These three shapes are created as follows.

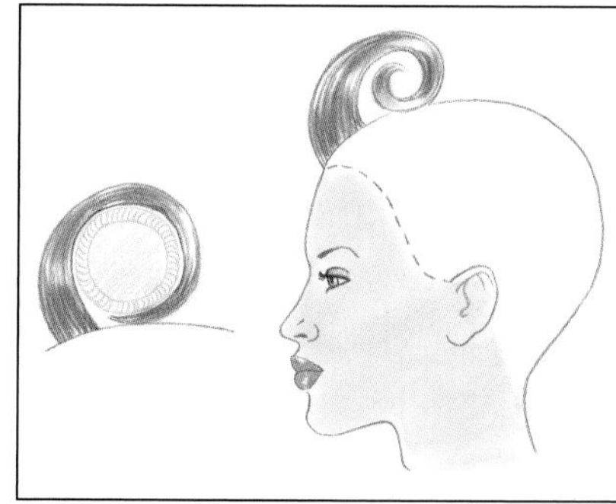

Figure 15-58 C-shaped curl.

1. One complete turn around the roller will create a C-shape curl (Figure 15-58).

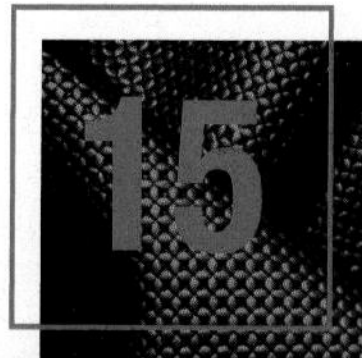

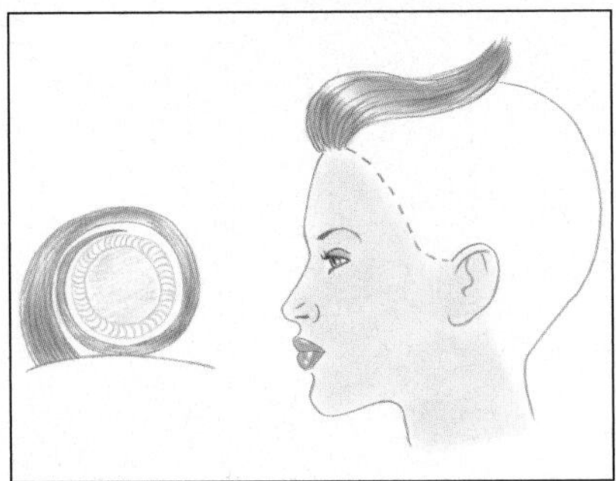
Figure 15-59 Wave.

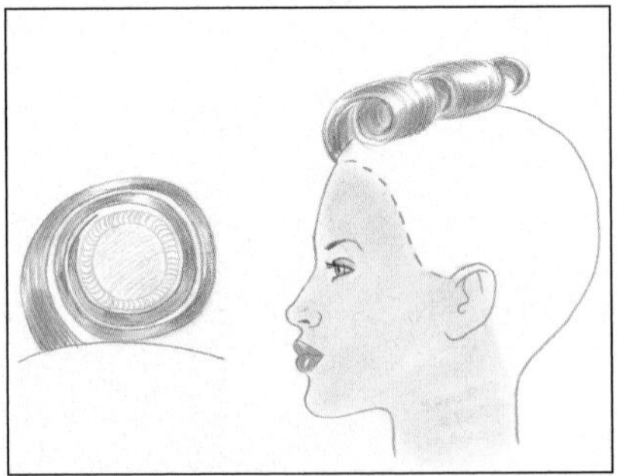
Figure 15-60 Curl.

2. One-and-a-half turns will create a wave (Figure 15-59).
3. Two-and-a-half turns will create curls (Figure 15-60).

ROLLER PLACEMENT

The size of the roller, and how it sits on its base, will determine the volume achieved. The general rule of thumb is that the larger the roller, the greater the volume. There are three kinds of bases.

1. **On base.** For full volume, the roller sits directly on its base.

   Overdirect the strand slightly in front of the base, and roll the hair down to the base. The roller should fit on the base (Figure 15-61).
2. **Half base.** For medium volume, the roller sits halfway on its base, and halfway behind the base. Hold the strand straight up from the head and roll the hair down (Figure 15-62).
3. **Off base.** For the least volume, the roller sits completely off the base. Hold the strand 45 degrees down from the base and roll the hair down (Figure 15-63).

ROLLER DIRECTION

The placement of rollers on the head usually follows the movement of the finished style. For versatility in styling, a downward directional wrap gives options to style in all directions—under, out, forward, or back, while still maintaining volume. To reduce volume bringing movement back in to the head, use indentation curl placement.

Indentation is the point where curls of opposite directions meet forming a recessed area. This is often found in flip styles or in bangs (fringes) with a dip or wave movement. This can be achieved using rollers, curling irons, or a round brush.

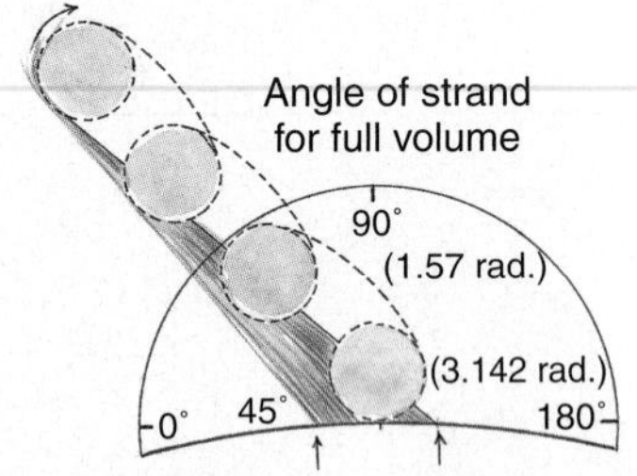

Figure 15-61 On base roller: full volume.

HOT ROLLERS

Hot rollers are to be used only on dry hair. They are heated either electrically or by steam, and are a great time-saver in the salon. Follow the same setting patterns as with wet setting, but allow the hot roller to stay on the hair for about 10 minutes. A thermal protector can be sprayed on the hair before setting. The result is a curl that is less strong than a wet set curl but stronger and longer lasting than can be achieved using a curling iron.

Also available are spray-on products to apply to each section of hair to create a stronger set.

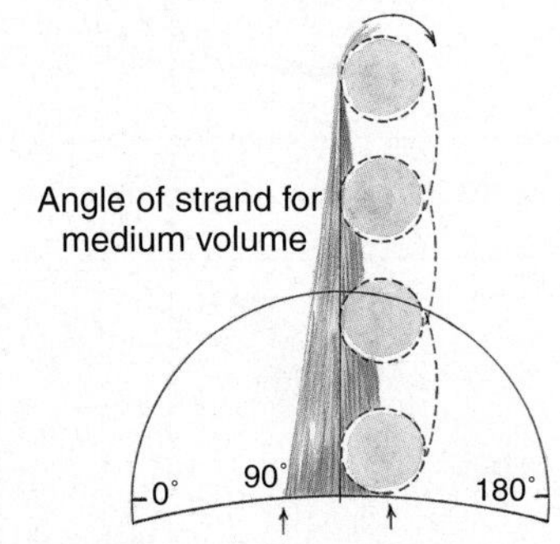

Figure 15-62 One-half base roller: medium volume.

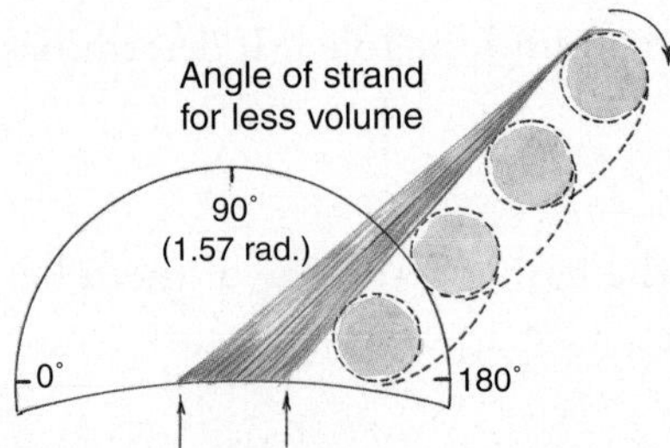

Figure 15-63 Off-base roller: less volume.

PROCEDURE 15-4

WET SET WITH ROLLERS

IMPLEMENTS AND MATERIALS

Use the list of implements and materials under preparing the hair for wet styling and add the following:

- Plastic rollers of various sizes
- Setting or styling lotion
- Clips (double or single prong)
- Tail comb

PREPARATION

1. Follow the steps under preparing the hair for wet styling.
2. Apply a setting or styling lotion.

PROCEDURE

1. **Comb the hair in the direction of the setting pattern.** Shapings may be used to accent the design.
2. **Comb and smooth hair.** Starting at the front hairline, part off a section the same length and width as the roller. Choose the type of base according to the desired volume. Comb the hair out from the scalp to the ends, using the fine teeth of the comb. Repeat several times to make sure that the hair is smooth (Figure 15-64).

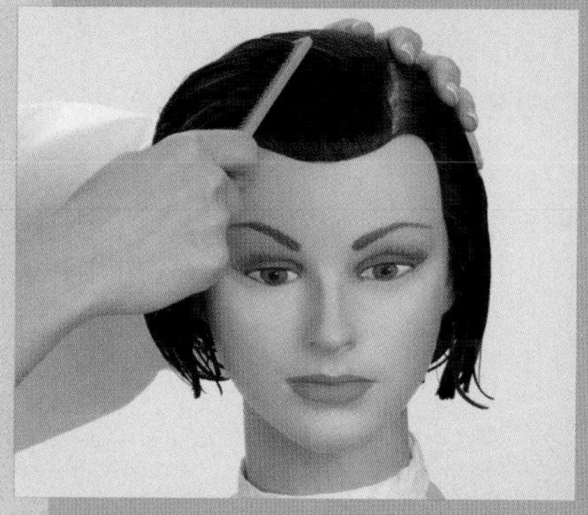

Figure 15-64 Comb section from scalp to ends.

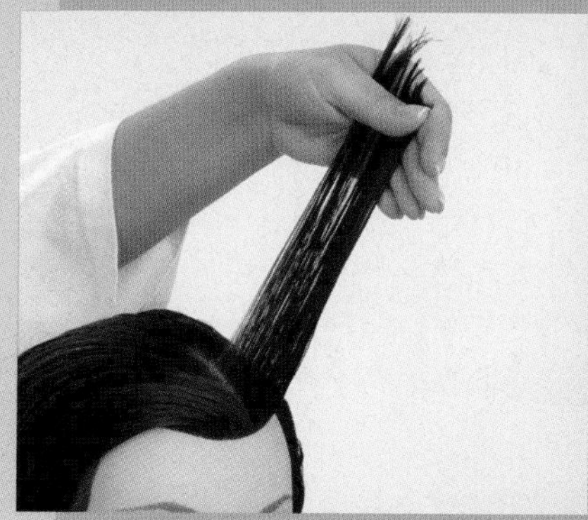

Figure 15-65 Right way to hold hair.

Here's a TIP

Some stylists find using a tail comb is easier for creating sections and subsections.

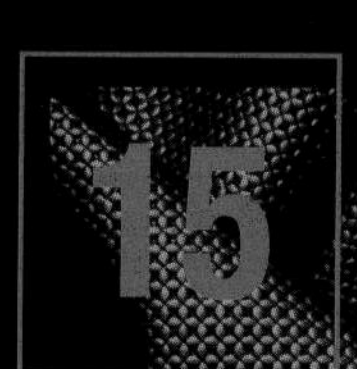

3. **Hold the hair.** Hold the hair with tension between the thumb and middle finger of the left hand. Place the roller below the thumb of the left hand. Do not bring the ends of the hair together (Figure 15-65). Wrap the ends of the hair smoothly around the roller until the hair catches and does not release.
4. **Roll hair.** Place the thumbs over the ends of the roller and roll the hair firmly to the scalp (Figure 15-66).
5. **Clip the roller securely to the scalp hair** (Figure 15-67). Roll the remainder of the hair according to the desired style.
6. **Place the client under a hood dryer.** Set the dryer at a temperature that is comfortable for the client.
7. **Dry the hair.** When the hair is dry, allow it to cool, then remove the rollers (Figure 15-68 and Figure 15-69).
8. **Style hair.** Comb out and style the hair as desired.

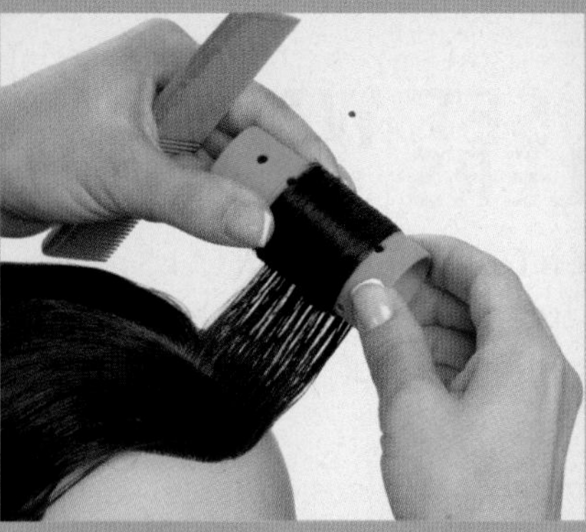

Figure 15-66 Wind the roller.

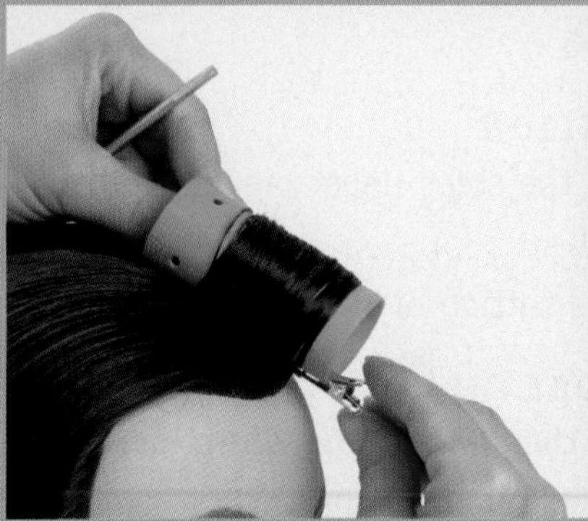

Figure 15-67 Clip the roller.

Here's a TIP

When clipping the roller, it is important to secure the roller properly to the head. A loose roller will lose its tension, resulting in a weak set. If the clip is placed at an angle against the hair, the sharp metal edge can cause the hair to break. Hold the roller against the scalp, maintaining the tension. Open the clip and slide it into the center of the roller. Place one end under the roller and one end inside the roller.

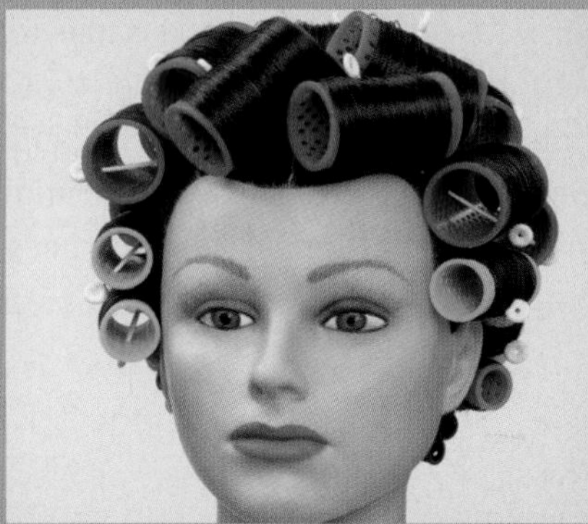

Figure 15-68 Finished roller set.

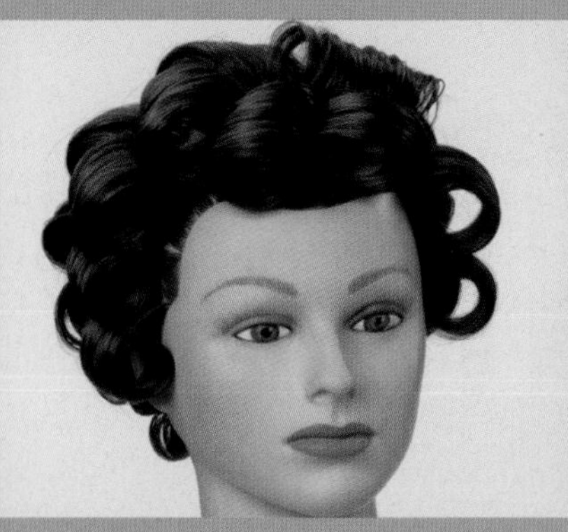

Figure 15-69 Remove the rollers.

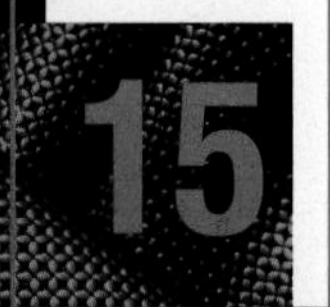

VELCRO ROLLERS

Velcro rollers are not allowed by the state board of some states and provinces due to the difficulty of sanitizing them properly. Check with your regulatory agency to determine if you can use them.

As with hot rollers, Velcro rollers are used only on dry hair. Using them on wet hair will snag and pull the hair. If you have a client who needs more body than can be achieved with a round brush, and less volume than a hot roller or wet set will produce, try Velcro rollers. When they are used after the hair is blow-dried, they may provide just the amount of volume you are looking for.

Velcro rollers need to stay in the hair for only 5 to 10 minutes, depending on how much set you want in the hair. Follow the same setting patterns as with wet setting, but keep in mind that no clipping is necessary to secure the roller. The Velcro fabric grips the hair well and stays in place on its own.

Mist the entire head with hairspray, and then either place the client under a hooded dryer for 5 to 10 minutes, or use the diffuser attachment on your blow-dryer for the recommended time to give a soft set to the hair. For an even softer look, do not apply heat after the rollers are put in, just have your client sit for a few minutes. This would be a good time to instruct the client on how she can repeat the process at home in order to maintain the style.

Always remove any hair from Velcro and electric rollers after use. See Chapter 5 for instructions on disinfecting rollers.

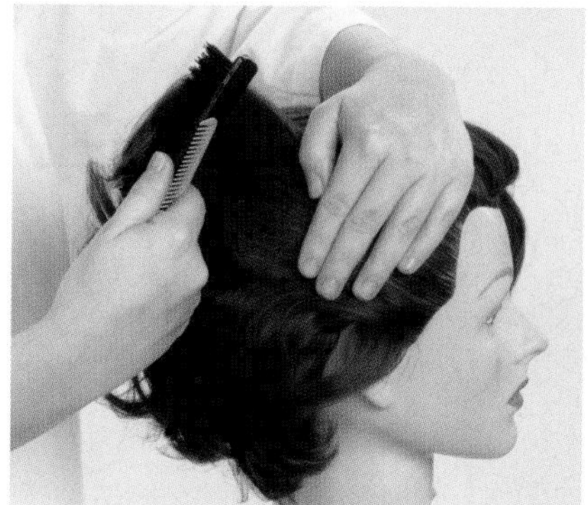

Figure 15-70 Brush out the hair.

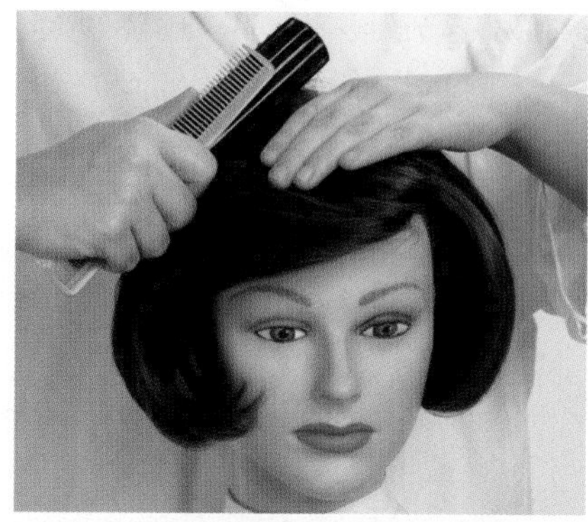

Figure 15-71 Direct hair into desired pattern.

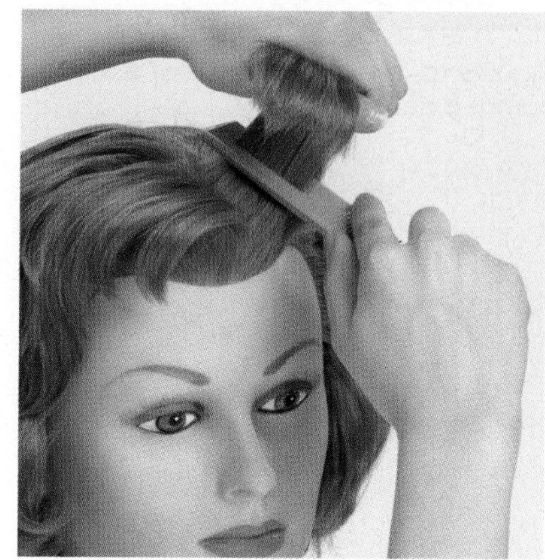

Figure 15-72 Insert comb.

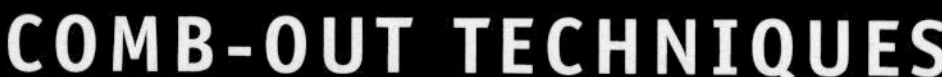

COMB-OUT TECHNIQUES

A good set leads to a good comb-out (Figure 15-70). For successful finishes, learn how to shape and mold the hair, and then practice fast, simple, and effective methods for comb-outs (Figure 15-71). If you follow a well-structured system of combing out hairstyles, you will save time and get more consistent results.

BACK-COMBING AND BACK-BRUSHING TECHNIQUES

Back-combing and back-brushing are the best ways to lift and increase volume, as well as to remove indentations caused by roller setting. **Back-combing,** also called teasing, ratting, matting, or French lacing, involves combing small sections of hair from the ends toward the scalp, causing shorter hair to mat at the scalp and form a cushion or base. **Back-brushing,** also called ruffing, is used to build a soft cushion or mesh two or more curl patterns together for a uniform and smooth comb-out.

During the 1950s and 1960s, women typically had their hair wet-set and combed out, and the set would last an entire week with back-

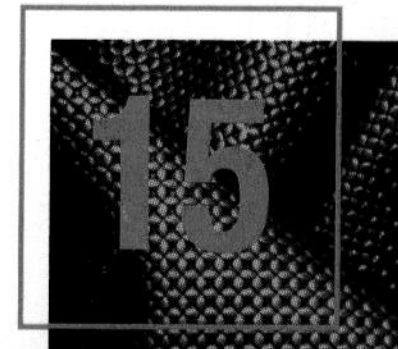

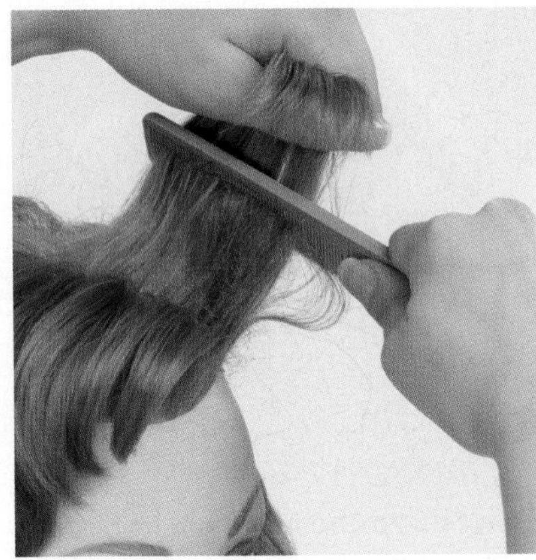

Figure 15-73 Press comb down.

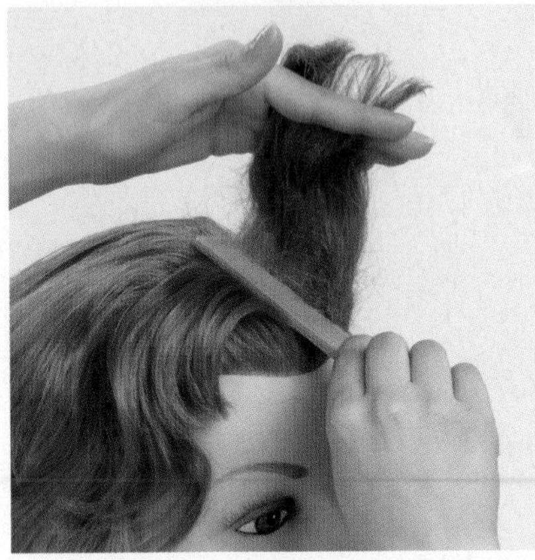

Figure 15-74 Create base of back-combed hair.

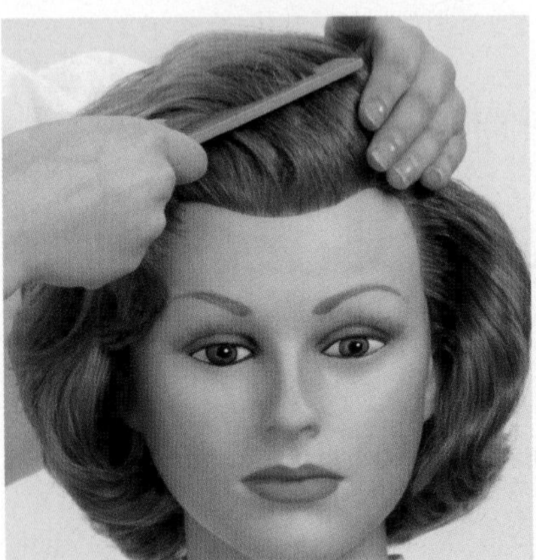

Figure 15-75 Smoothing hair with comb.

combing and back-brushing. Now these techniques are used for styling updos, or to add a little height to a hairstyle, after hot roller setting or blow-drying.

BACK-COMBING TECHNIQUE

1. **Section hair.** Starting in the front, pick up a section of hair no more than 1 inch thick and no more than 2 to 3 inches (5 to 7.5 centimeters) wide.
2. **Insert comb.** Insert the fine teeth of your comb into the hair at a depth of about 1½ inches (3.75 centimeters) from the scalp (see Figure 15-72 on page 321).
3. **Press comb down.** Press the comb gently down to the scalp, rotating it down and out of the hair. Repeat this process, working up the section until the desired volume is achieved (Figure 15-73).
4. **Create a cushion.** If you wish to create a cushion (base), the third time you insert the comb, use the same rotating motion but firmly push the hair down to the scalp. Slide the comb-out of the hair (Figure 15-74).
5. **Repeat for volume.** Repeat this process, working up the strand until the desired volume is achieved.
6. **Smooth hair.** To smooth the hair that is back-combed, hold the teeth of a comb, or the bristles of a brush, at a 45-degree angle pointing away from you, and lightly move it over the surface of the hair (Figure 15-75).

BACK-BRUSHING TECHNIQUE

1. **Hold strand.** Pick up and hold a strand straight out from the scalp.
2. **Place brush.** Maintaining a slight amount of slack in the strand, place a teasing brush or a grooming brush near the base of the strand. Push and roll the inner edge of the brush with the wrist until it touches the scalp.
3. **Roll brush.** For interlocking to occur, the brush must be rolled (Figure 15-76).

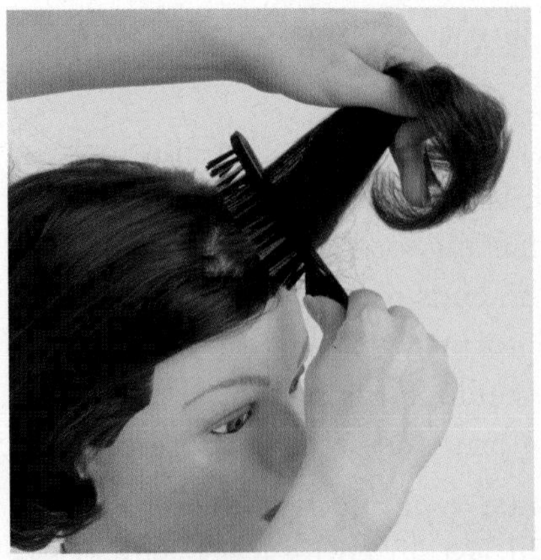

Figure 15-76 Roll brush.

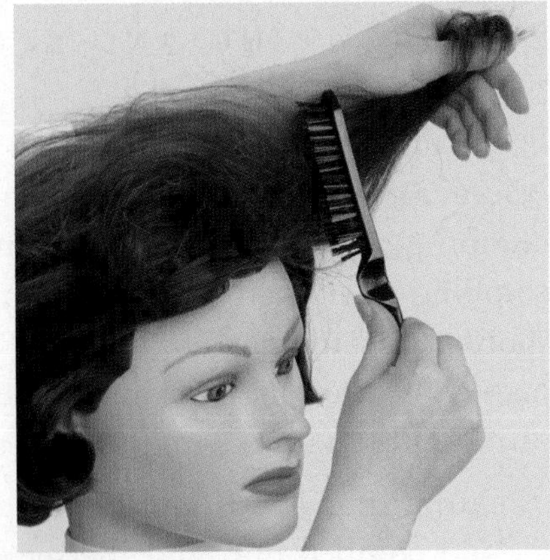

Figure 15-77 Remove brush.

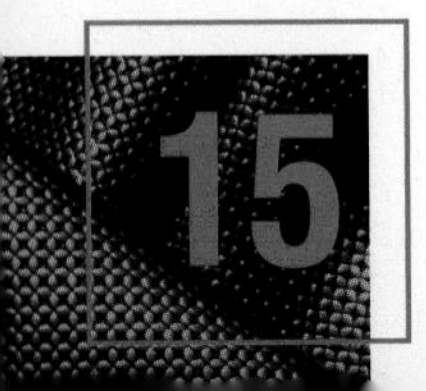

4. **Roll brush.** Then remove the brush from the hair with a turn of the wrist, peeling back a layer of hair (Figure 15-77). The hair will be interlocked to form a soft cushion at the scalp.
5. **Blend hair.** You can create softness and evenness of flow by blending, smoothing, and combing (Figure 15-78). Avoid exaggerations and overemphasis. Finished patterns should reflect rhythm, balance, and smoothness of line.
6. **Complete styling.** Final touches make hairstyles look professional, so take your time. After completing the comb-out, you can use the tail of a comb to lift areas where the shape and form are not as full as you want them to be (Figure 15-79). Every touch during the final stage must be very lightly done. When you have completed your finishing touches, check the entire set for structural balance and then lightly spray the hair with a finishing spray (Figure 15-80).

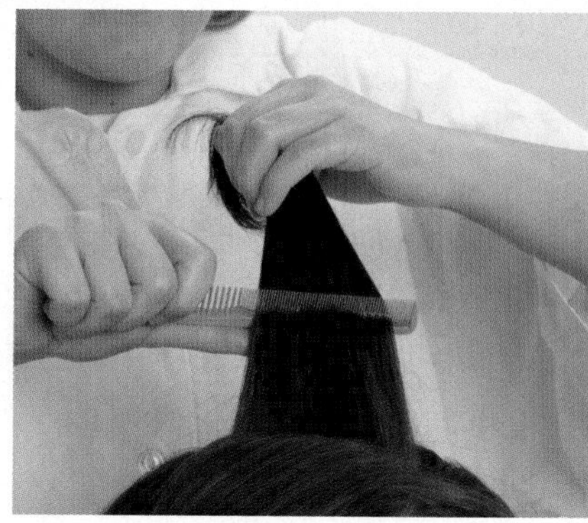

Figure 15-78 Blend sections with back-combing.

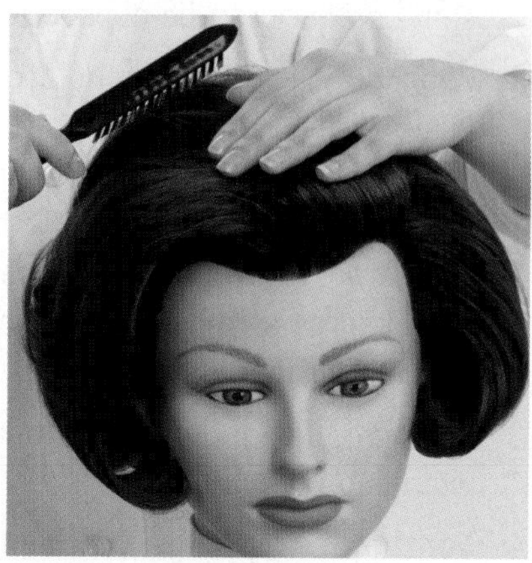

Figure 15-79 Finished style.

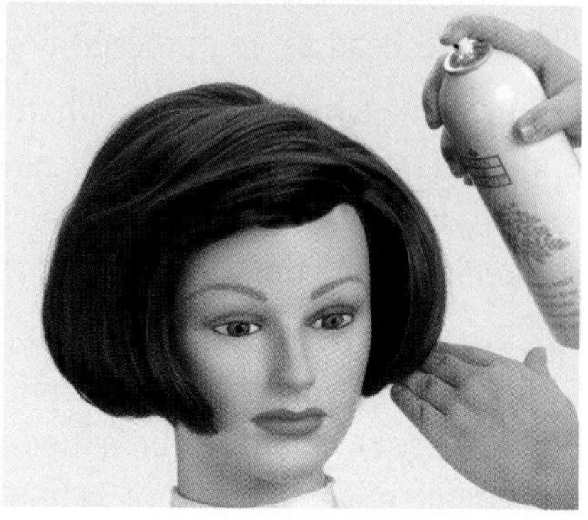

Figure 15-80 Apply finishing spray to complete style.

CLEANUP AND SANITATION

1. Discard the neck strip and place the cape in the laundry.
2. Thoroughly remove all hair from brushes and combs and disinfect.
3. Disinfect rollers, clips, and picks.
4. Sanitize your workstation.
5. Wash your hands with soap and warm water.

HAIR WRAPPING

Hair wrapping is used to keep curly hair smooth and straight, while still retaining a beautiful shape. Just as hair is wrapped around a roller to give it a smooth, rounded contour, you can wrap curly hair around the head to create this same effect. When wrapping hair, very little volume is attained because the hair at the scalp is not lifted. If height is desired, you can place large rollers directly at the crown, with the remainder of the hair wrapped around the head.

Wrapping can be done on wet or dry hair. On curly hair, wet wrapping creates a smooth, sleek look. For very curly hair, press it first, then do a dry hair wrapping.

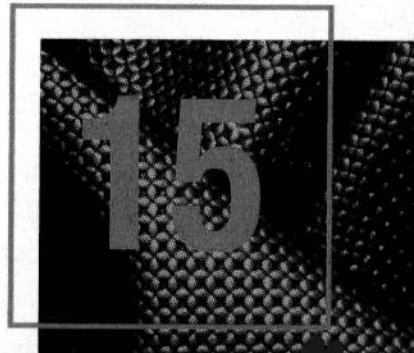

PROCEDURE 15-5

HAIR WRAPPING

IMPLEMENTS AND MATERIALS

- Gel or silicone shine
- Boar-bristle brush
- Duckbill clips
- Neck strip
- Bobby pins

1. **Apply styling product.** If the hair is wet, a light gel can be applied before wrapping. If the hair is dry, a silicone shine product can be applied for a glossy comb-out.
2. **Wrap outer perimeter.** Hold one hand at the top of the head. Using the brush in a pivot motion, wrap the hair on the outer perimeter of the head (Figure 15-81). Do not brush or push the hair to the back; the correct way is to always brush the hair clockwise around the head. Think of the head as a roller. Your job is to smooth the hair in a circular motion around it.
3. **Clip hair.** Use duckbill clips to keep the hair in place while wrapping (Figure 15-82).
4. **Continue wrapping.** Continue wrapping the hair in a clockwise direction around the head. Follow the brush with your hand, smoothing down the hair and keeping it tight to the head as you proceed (Figure 15-83).
5. **Protect wrapped hair.** When all the hair is wrapped, stretch a neck strip around the head so that it overlaps at the ends. Secure the wrapped strip with a bobby pin and remove the clips (Figure 15-84).
6. **Dry hair.** If you have been working on dry hair, leave the hair wrapped for about 15 minutes. If the hair was wet, place the client under a hooded dryer until the hair is completely dry, usually 45 minutes to 1 hour, depending on the hair length. The longer the hair is wrapped, the smoother it will be (Figure 15-85).

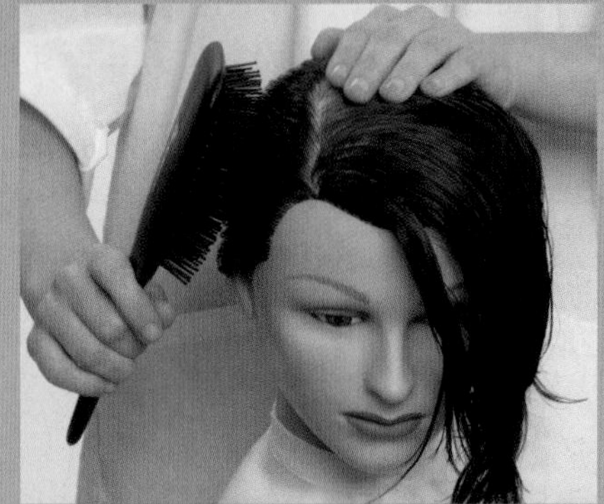

Figure 15-81 Wrap first section.

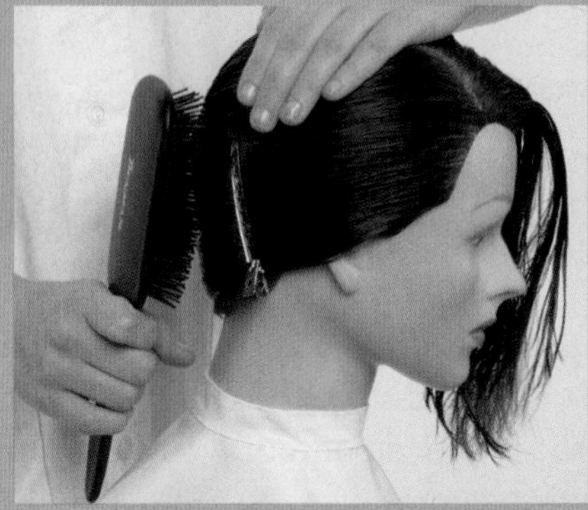

Figure 15-82 Hold wrapped hair with duckbill clips.

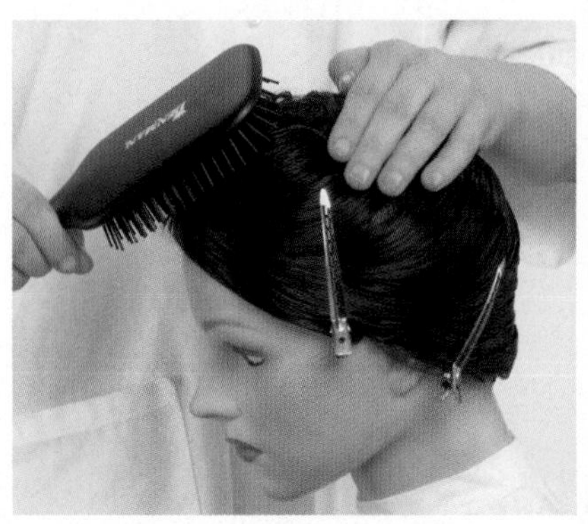

Figure 15-83 Continue wrapping hair.

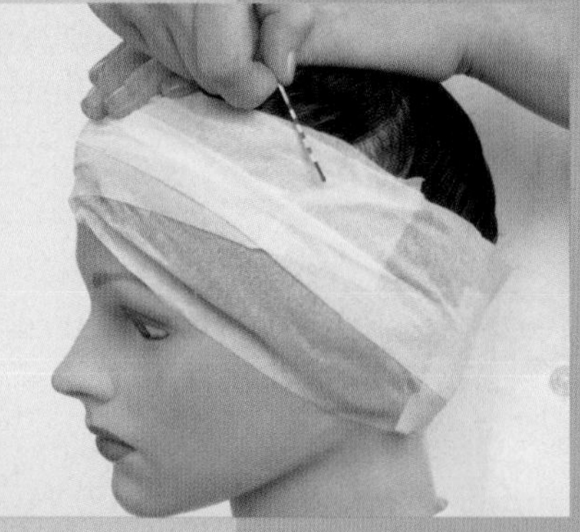

Figure 15-84 Wrap neck strip around hair.

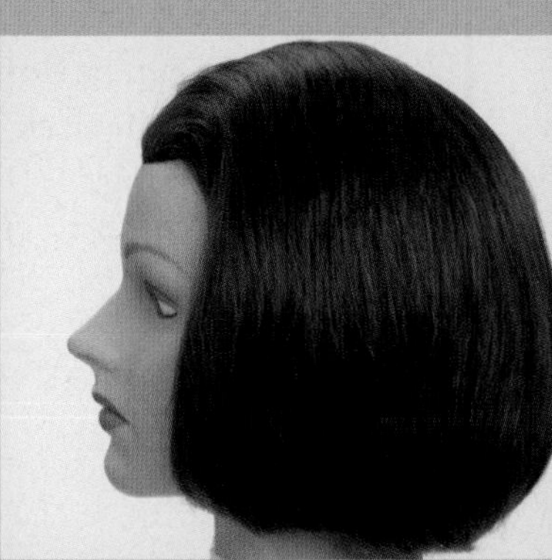

Figure 15-85 Finished style.

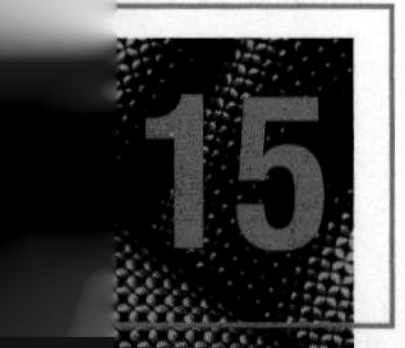

BLOW-DRY STYLING

Blow-dry styling—the technique of drying and styling damp hair in one operation—has revolutionized the hairstyling world. Today, women desire hairstyles that require the least time and effort to maintain. The selection of styling tools, techniques, and products must relate to the client's lifestyle. Is she capable of styling her own hair, and how much time will she have to do it? As the stylist, it is your responsibility to guide and educate the client through this process. To do so, you must first learn all about the tools and products available to you. Remember, the client's first impression of the haircut you have done will be determined by the quality of the blow-dry.

TOOLS FOR BLOW-DRY STYLING

The following are the basic tools used for blow-drying techniques.

THE BLOW-DRYER

A blow-dryer is an electrical appliance designed for drying and styling hair. Its main parts are a handle, slotted nozzle, small fan, heating element, and speed/heat controls. Some also come with cooling buttons. The temperature control switch helps to produce a steady stream of air at the desired temperature. The blow-dryer's nozzle attachment, or **concentrator,** is a directional feature that creates a concentrated stream of air.

The **diffuser** attachment causes the air to flow more softly, and helps to accentuate or keep textural definition (Figure 15-86).

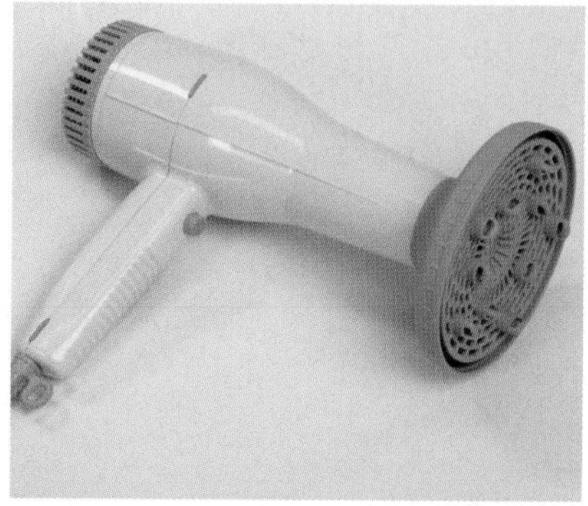

Figure 15-86 Blow-dryer and diffuser.

To keep your blow-dryer as safe and effective as possible, make sure that it is always perfectly clean and free of dirt, oil, and hair before using. Dirt or hair in the blow-dryer could cause extreme heat and burn the hair. The air intake at the back of the dryer must also be kept clear at all times. If the intake is covered and air cannot pass through freely, the dryer element will burn out prematurely.

COMBS AND PICKS

Combs and picks are designed to distribute and part the hair. They come in a wide variety of sizes and shapes to adapt to many styling options (Figure 15-87). The length and spacing of the teeth may vary from one comb to another. Teeth that are closely spaced remove definition from the curl and create a smooth surface; widely spaced teeth shape larger sections of hair for a more textured surface. Combs with a pick at one end lift the hair away from the head.

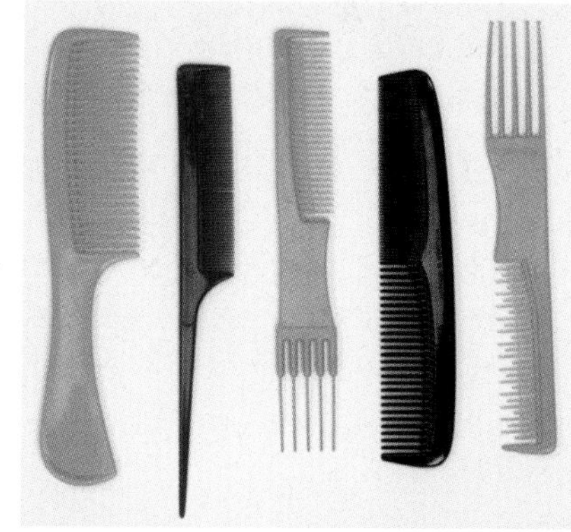

Figure 15-87 From left to right: wide-tooth comb, fine-tooth tail comb, styling comb with metal pins, finger wave comb, teasing comb.

BRUSHES

When choosing a styling brush, take into account the texture, length, and styling needs of the hair that you are working with. Brushes come in many sizes, shapes, and materials (Figure 15-88).

- A *classic styling brush* is a half-round, rubber-based brush. These brushes typically have either seven or nine rows of round-tipped nylon

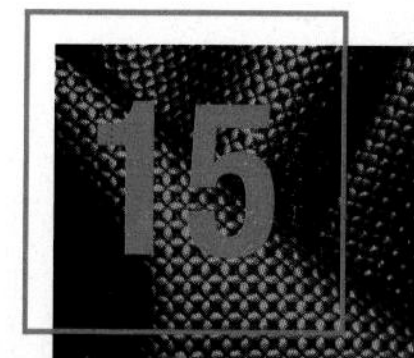

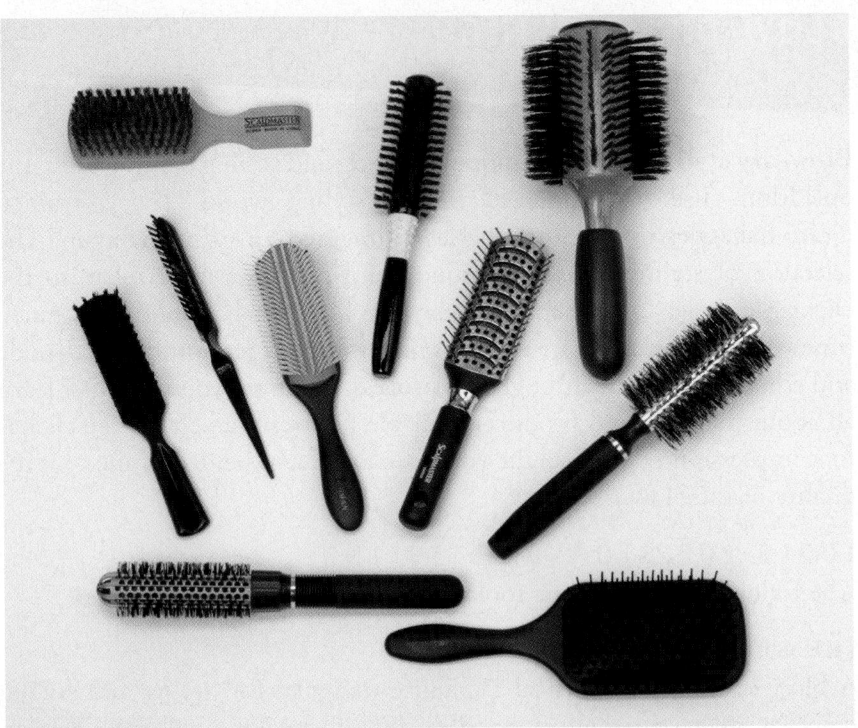

Figure 15–88 Brushes: paddle brush, grooming brush, teasing brush, classic plastic styling brush, vent brush, round brushes.

bristles. They are heat-resistant and antistatic, and ideal for smoothing and untangling all types of hair. While they are perfect for blow-drying precision haircuts where little volume is desired, they are less suitable for smooth classic looks.

- *Paddle brushes,* with their large, flat bases, are well suited for mid- to longer-length hair. Some have ball-tipped nylon pins and staggered pin patterns that help to keep the hair from snagging.
- *Grooming brushes* are generally oval with a mixture of boar and nylon bristles. The boar bristles help distribute the scalp oils throughout the hair shaft, giving it shine. The nylon bristles stimulate the circulation of blood to the scalp. They are particularly useful for adding polish and shine to fine to medium hair, and are great for combing out updos.
- *Vent brushes,* with their ventilated design, are used to speed up the blow-drying process, and are ideal for blow-drying fine hair and adding lift at the scalp.
- *Round brushes* come in various diameters. The client's hair should be able to wrap twice around the brush. Round brushes often have natural bristles, sometimes with nylon mixed in for better grip. Smaller brushes add more curl; larger brushes straighten the hair and bevel the ends of the hair. Medium round brushes can be used to lift the hair at the scalp. Some round brushes have metal cylinder bases so that the heat from the blow-dryer is transferred to the metal base, creating a stronger curl that is similar to those produced with an electric roller. Always use the cooling button on the blow-dryer before releasing the section to "set" the hair into the new shape.

- A *teasing brush* is a thin nylon styling brush that has a tail for sectioning, along with a narrow row of bristles. Teasing brushes are perfect for back-combing hair, and then using the sides of the bristles to smooth it into the desired style.

SECTIONING CLIPS

Sectioning clips are usually metal or plastic, and have long prongs to hold wet or dry sections of hair in place. It is important to keep whatever wet hair you are not working on sectioned off in clips so that the wet hair does not sit over the dry hair, especially when drying long hair.

STYLING PRODUCTS

Styling products can be thought of as "liquid tools." They give a style more hold and can add shine and curl, or take curl away. When used correctly, they can greatly enhance a style.

With so many styling products on the market, stylists need to carefully consider their options before applying one of these products to the hair. First, how long does the style need to hold? Under what environmental conditions—dryness, humidity, wind, sun—will the client be wearing the style? You also must consider the type of hair—fine, coarse, straight, curly—when deciding on a product. Heavier products work by causing strands of hair to cling together, adding more pronounced definition, but they can also weigh the hair down, especially fine hair. Styling products range from a light to very firm hold. Determine the amount of support desired and choose accordingly.

TYPES OF STYLING PRODUCTS

Foam or **mousse** is a light, airy, whipped styling product that resembles shaving foam. It builds moderate body and volume into the hair. Massage it into damp hair to highlight textural movement, or blow-dry it straight for styles when body without texture is desired. Foam is good for fine hair because it does not weigh the hair down. It will hold for 6 to 8 hours in dry conditions. Conditioning foams are excellent for drier, more porous hair.

Gel is a thickened styling preparation that comes in a tube or bottle. Gels create the strongest control for slicked or molded styles, and distinct texture definition when spread with the fingers. When brushed out, it creates long-lasting body. Firm-hold gel formulations may overwhelm fine hair because of the high resin content. This is not a concern if fine hair is molded into the lines of the style, and does not get brushed through when dry.

Similar to firm-hold gels, **liquid gels** or **texturizers** are lighter and more viscous (liquid) in form. They allow for easy styling, defining, and molding. With brushing, they add volume and body to the style. Good for all hair types, they offer firmer, longer hold for fine hair with the least amount of heaviness, and give a lighter, more moderate hold for normal or coarse hair types. Home-care recommendation of styling products represents a natural retailing opportunity in the salon. As you style the client's hair, talk about the products you are using to achieve the desired look, and why. Have the client hold the product while you demonstrate the uses and benefits of each product. Most clients are eager to learn

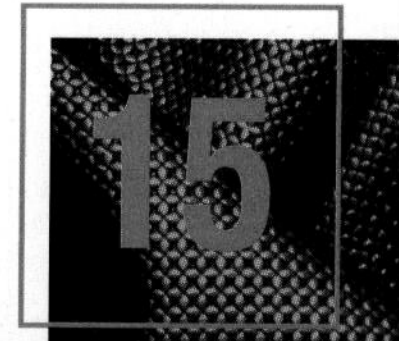

any and all styling "secrets" by discussing and recommending professional products as you use them.

When **straightening gel** is applied to damp hair ranging from wavy to extremely curly, and blown dry, it creates a smooth, straight look that provides the most hold in dry outdoor conditions. It counters frizzy hair by coating the hair shaft and weighing it down. Of course, this is a temporary solution that will last only from shampoo to shampoo, and may become undone in extremely humid conditions.

When sprayed into the base of fine, wet hair, **volumizers** add volume to the shape, especially at the base, when the hair is blown dry. When a vent brush or round brush is used, and the hair is not stretched too tightly around the brush, even more volume can be achieved. You may want to add a light gel or mousse to the rest of the hair for more hold, but be careful to avoid the base of the hair when applying the product.

Pomade or **wax** adds considerable weight to the hair by causing strands to join together, showing separation in the hair. Used on dry hair, this makes the hair very easy to mold. It allows greater manageability. It should be used sparingly on fine hair because of the weight. As a man's grooming product, pomade is excellent on short hair.

Silicone adds gloss and sheen to the hair, while creating textural definition. Nonoily silicone products are excellent for all hair types, either to provide lubrication and protection to the hair while blow-drying, or finishing at the very end to add extra shine. When applied like hair spray, spray shines add shine without weight, so they are useful for all hair types.

Hair spray or **finishing spray** is applied in the form of a mist to hold a style in position. It is the most widely used hairstyling product. Available in both aerosol and pump containers, and in a variety of holding strengths, it is useful for all hair types. Finishing spray is used when the style is complete and will not be disturbed.

PROCEDURE 15-6

BLOW-DRYING SHORT, LAYERED, CURLY HAIR TO PRODUCE SMOOTH AND FULL FINISH

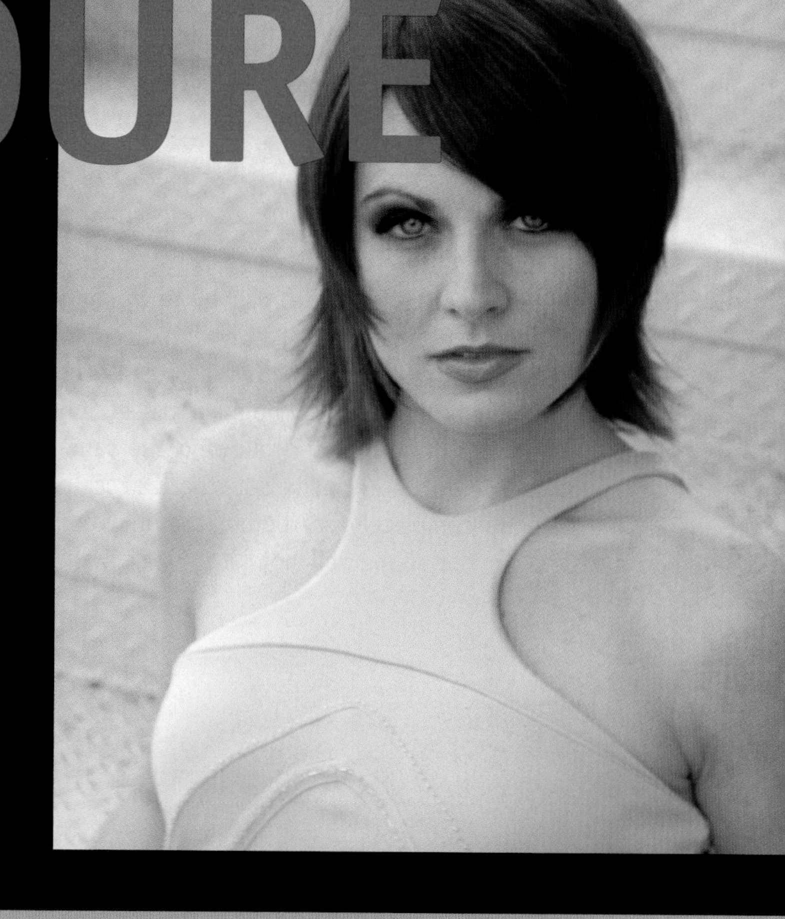

IMPLEMENTS AND MATERIALS

- Blow-dryer with attachments
- Styling product
- Wide-tooth comb
- Round brush
- Styling cape
- Neck strip
- Sectioning clips

PREPARATION FOR ALL HAIR TYPES

1. **Shampoo hair.** After shampooing, return the client to the seated position and comb out any tangles in the hair. Remove excess moisture from the hair by blotting with a towel.
2. **Drape.** Place a clean neck strip on the client and drape with a cutting or styling cape.
3. **Escort the client to the styling chair.**

PROCEDURE

1. **Apply styling product.** Distribute styling product through the hair with your fingers, and comb through with a wide-tooth comb.
2. **Mold hair.** Using the comb, mold the hair into the desired shape while still wet (Figure 15-89).
3. **Achieve volume.** For volume and lift similar to that which you would get from a roller set, use a small round brush. Apply a mousse or spray volumizer at the base. Section and part the hair according to the amount of volume desired (Figure 15-90).
4. **Insert the round brush at the base of the curl.** The degree of lift determines the type of volume you will achieve. Using the techniques that you have learned in roller setting, dry each section either full base or half base. For maximum lift, insert the brush on base and direct the hair section up at a 125-degree angle (Figure 15-91). Roll the hair down to the base with medium tension (Figure 15-92). Direct the stream of air from the blow-dryer over the curl in a back-and-forth motion.

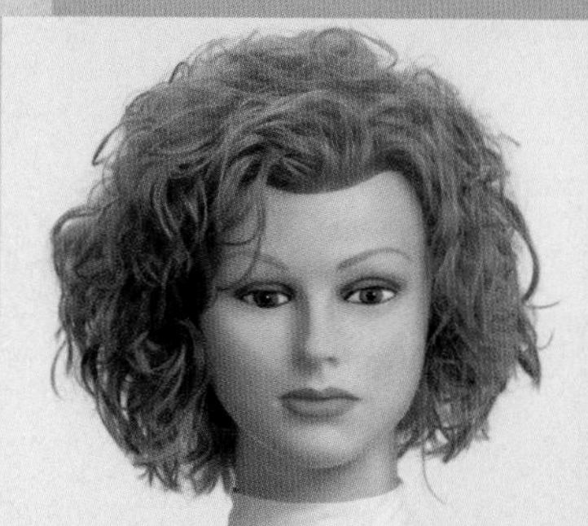

Figure 15-89 Mold the hair into the shape it will take when dry.

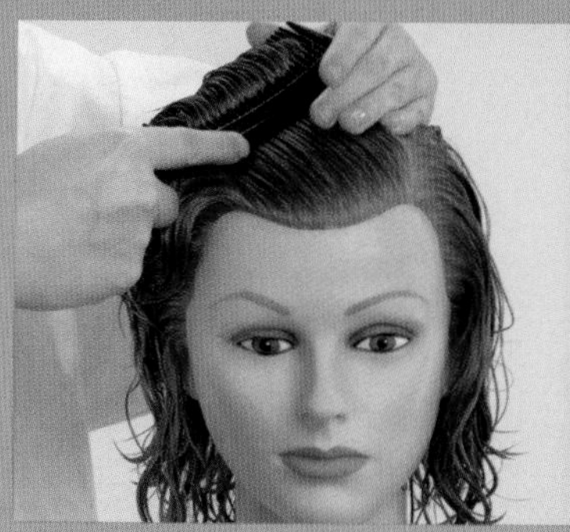

Figure 15-90 Section the hair for blow-drying.

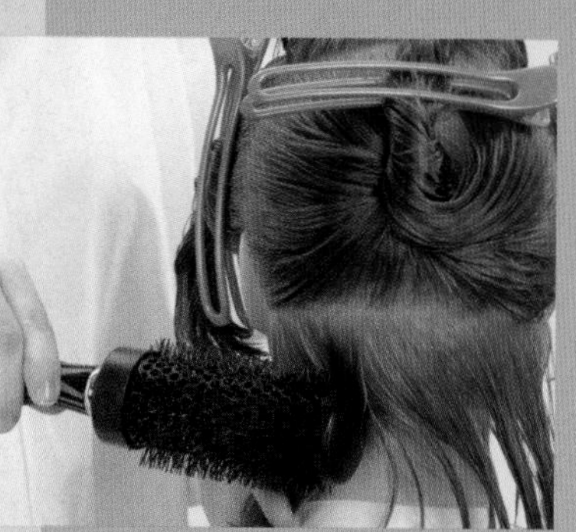

Figure 15-91 Direct the hair upward.

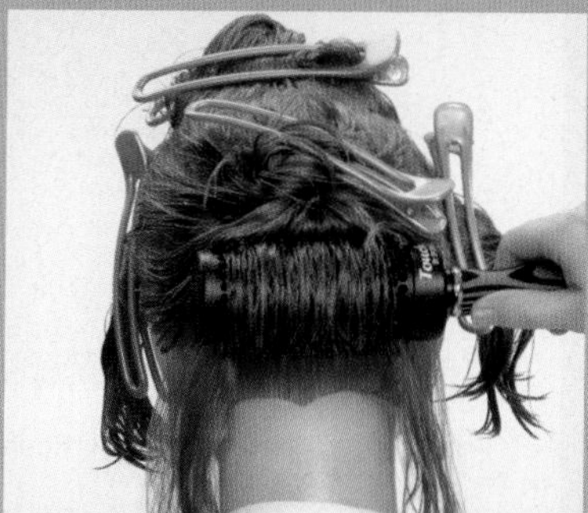

Figure 15-92 Roll the hair to the base.

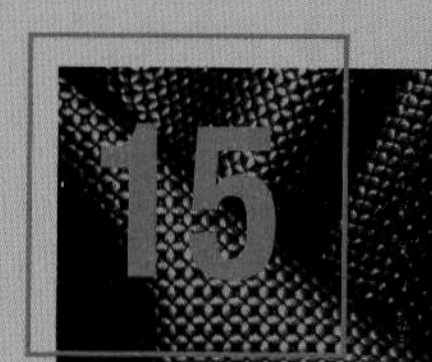

5. **Dry section.** When the section is completely dry, press the cooling button and cool down the section to strengthen the curl formation.
6. **Release brush.** Release the brush by unwinding the section from the brush. (Pulling it out could cause the hair to get tangled in the brush.) For less lift at the scalp, begin by holding the section at a 70- to 90-degree angle, following the same procedure (Figure 15-93). Make sure that the scalp and hair are completely dry before combing out the style, or the shape will not last. Finish with hair spray (Figure 15-94).

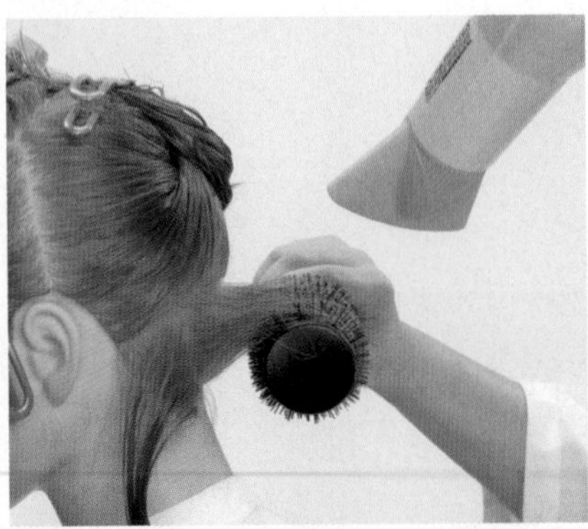

Figure 15-93 Full base section for blow-drying.

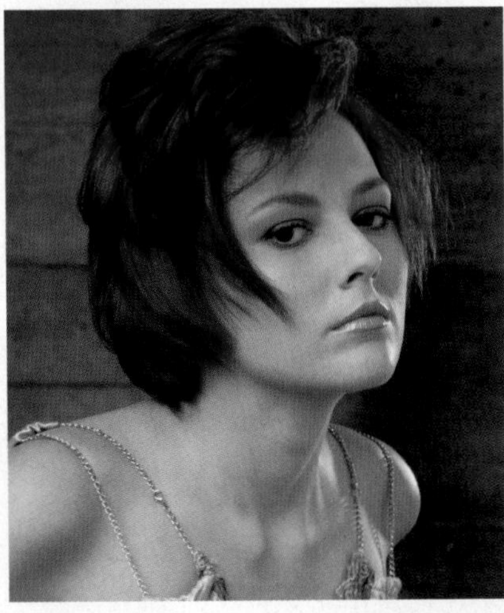

Figure 15-94 Finished style.

CAUTION

Never hold the blow-dryer too long in one place. Always direct the hot air away from the client's scalp to avoid scalp burns. Direct it from the scalp toward the ends of the hair. The hot air should flow in the direction in which the hair is wound; improper technique will rough up the hair cuticle and give the hair a frizzy appearance.

Move the blow-dryer in a constant back-and-forth motion unless you are using the cooling button cool a section.

Because hair stretches easily when it is wet, partially towel-dry the ha before blow-drying, especially damaged or chemically treated hair. T is not necessary if you ar cutting the hair before y blow-dry it, as the hair w already be partially dry d to the amount of time it takes to cut it.

PROCEDURE 15-7

BLOW-DRY SHORT, CURLY HAIR IN IT'S NATURAL WAVE PATTERN

1. **Use diffuser.** Attach the diffuser to the blow-dryer.
2. **Apply gel.** Apply a liquid gel on the client's hair.
3. **Direct hair.** With a wide-tooth comb or your fingers, encourage the hair into the desired shape (Figure 15-95).
4. **Diffuse hair.** Diffuse the hair gently, pressing the diffuser on and off the hair without over manipulating the hair, until each area of the head is dry (Figure 15-96).
5. **Relax curl.** To relax or soften the curl, slowly and gently run your fingers through the curl when the hair is almost dry.
6. **Tighten curl.** For a tighter curl, scrunch the hair by placing your hand over a section of hair while it is being diffused, forming a fist with the hair in your hand (Figure 15-97). Using a pulsing motion, release and repeat until the section is dry.
7. **Add shine.** For more shine, finish with a silicone spray or product to add the desired shine (Figure 15-98).

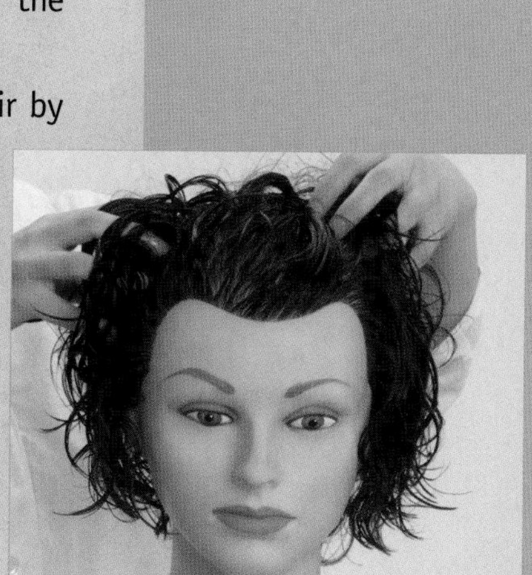

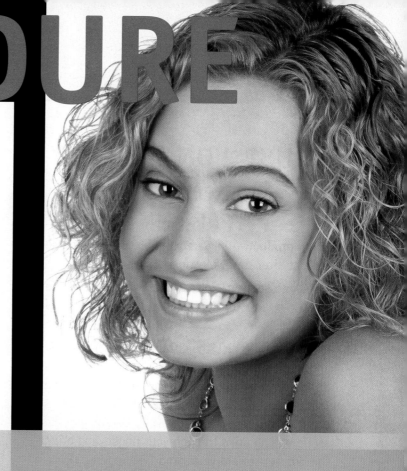

Figure 15-95 Comb hair into desired shape.

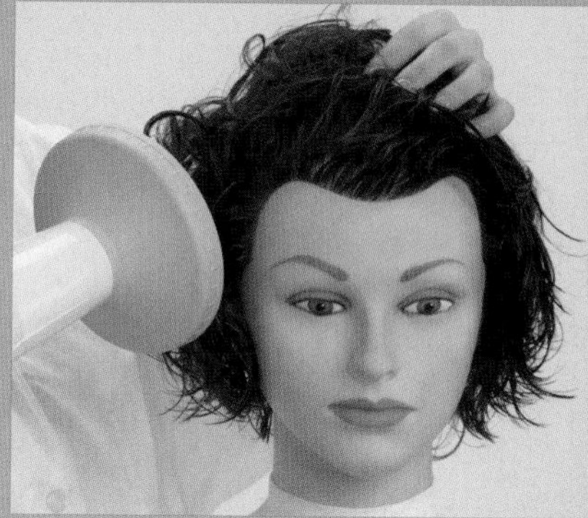

Figure 15-96 Hair being diffused.

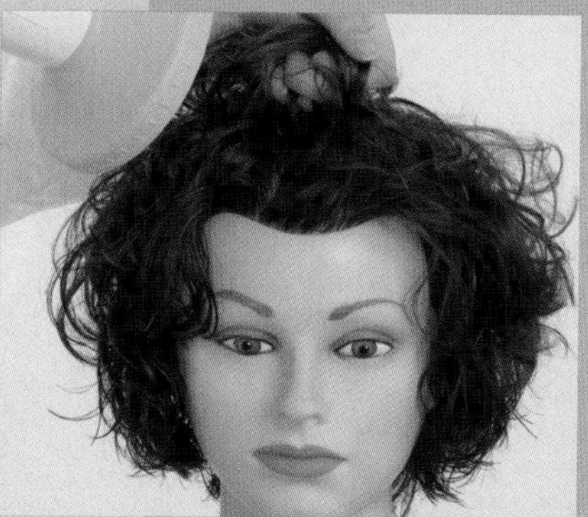

Figure 15-97 Scrunch the hair.

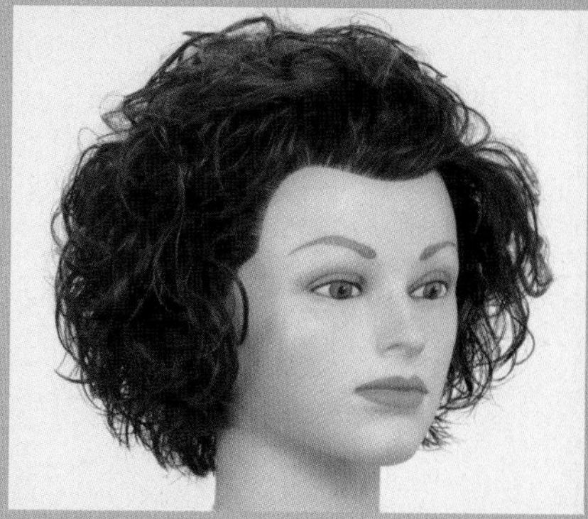

Figure 15-98 Finished hairstyle.

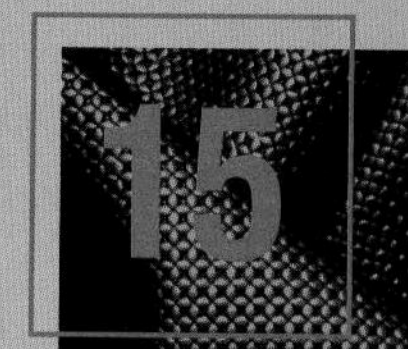

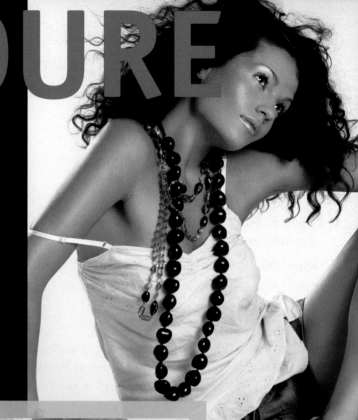

PROCEDURE 15-8

DIFFUSE LONG, CURLY OR EXTREMELY-CURLY HAIR IN ITS NATURAL WAVE PATTERN

1. **Apply product.** Apply a styling product or silicone product after towel-blotting hair.
2. **Work one section.** For easier control, section the hair and work on one particular section at a time.
3. **Use diffuser.** Attach the diffuser to the blow-dryer and diffuse the hair by letting the hair sit on top of the diffuser and pulsing the dryer toward the scalp and then away, repeating until the section is dry (Figure 15-99). Alternatively, gently run the section being dried through your fingers and bring the diffuser toward your hand (Figure 15-100).

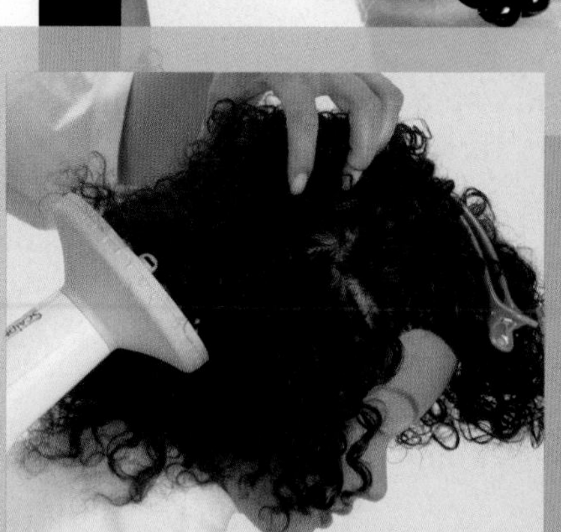

Figure 15-99 Using a diffuser.

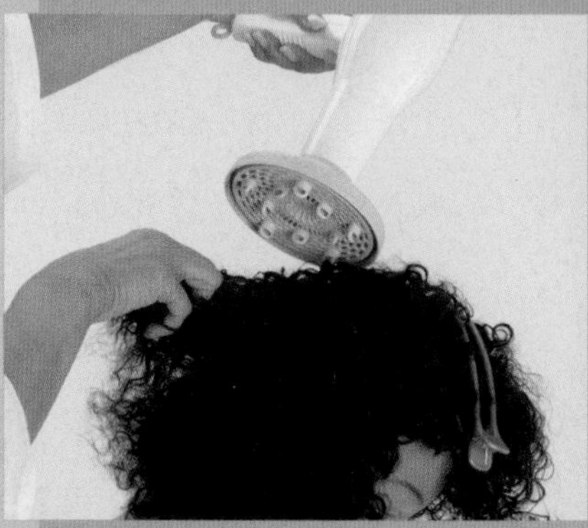

Figure 15-100 Another way to use a diffuser.

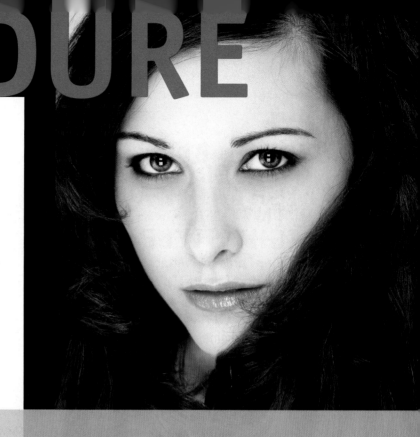

PROCEDURE 15-9

BLOW-DRY STRAIGHT OR WAVY HAIR WITH MAXIMUM VOLUME

1. **Apply styling product.** Apply a mousse, volumizing spray, or lightweight gel to dampen the hair.
2. **Use brush.** Using a vent brush or classic styling brush, distribute the hair into the desired shape.
3. **Begin at the nape.** Build your shape from the bottom up, working from the nape up toward the crown. When you begin at the nape, hold the wet hair above the nape in a sectioning clip (Figure 15-101).
4. **Insert the brush in the hair at the scalp.** While turning the brush downward and away from the scalp, allow the brush to pick up a section of hair and begin drying. Direct the airflow towards the top of the brush, moving in the desired direction (Figure 15-102).
5. **Work a section at a time.** Work in sections, lifting and drying the sections and then brushing them in the desired direction when they are completely dry. Repeat all over the head, directing the hair at the sides either away or forward (Figure 15-103). The bang (fringe) area could be dried either onto the forehead or away from the face.
6. **Finish styling.** Use an appropriate styling product to achieve the desired finish (Figures 15-104 and 15-105).

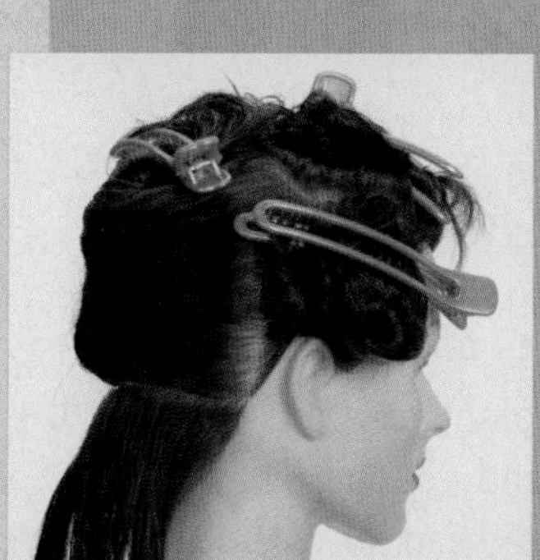

Figure 15–101 Clip hair above nape to begin drying.

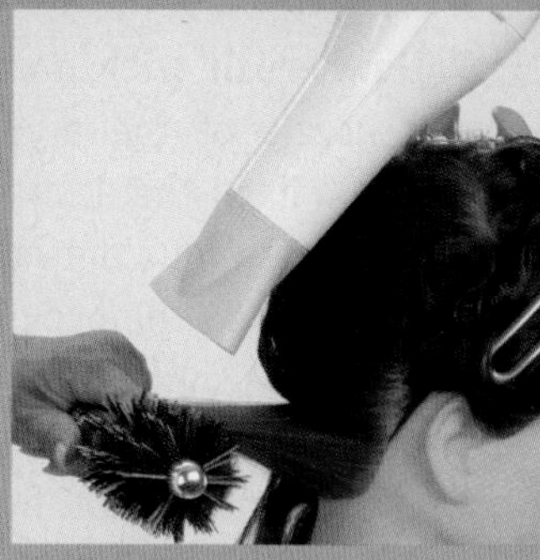

Figure 15–102 Lift the hair from the nape.

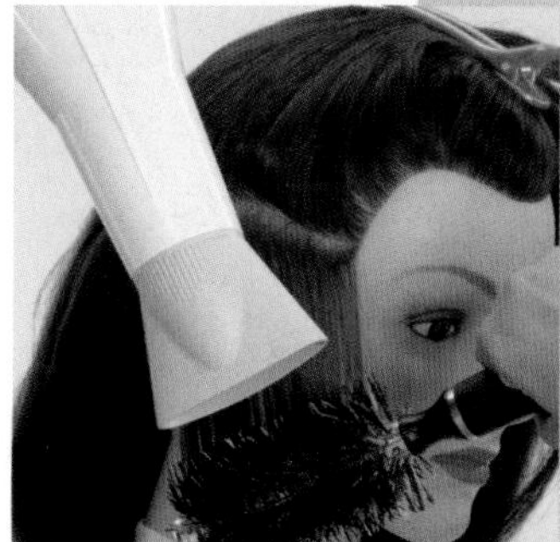

Figure 15–103 Brush hair in the desired direction.

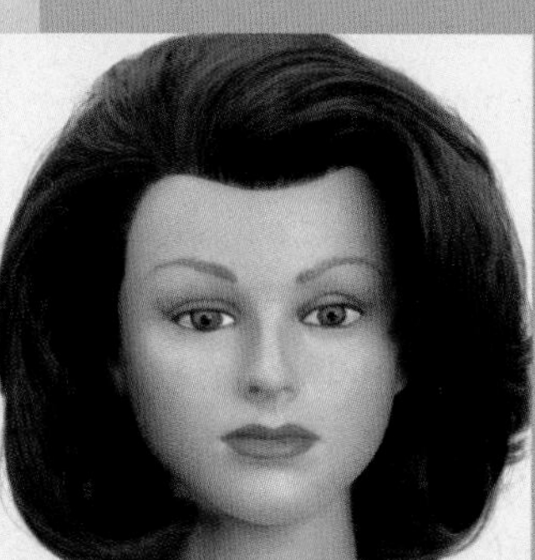

Figure 15–104 Finished style.

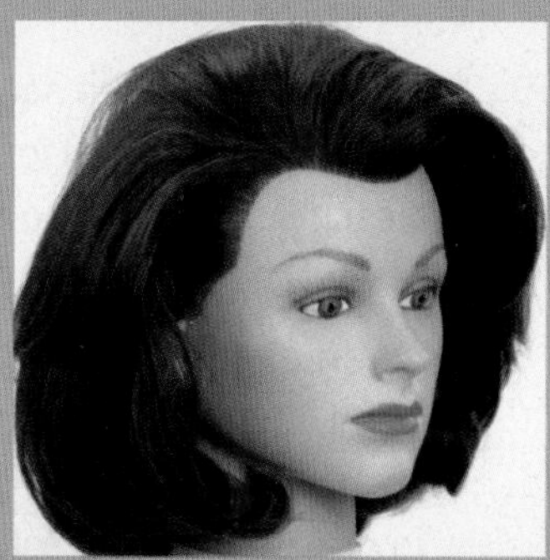

Figure 15–105 Side view of finished style.

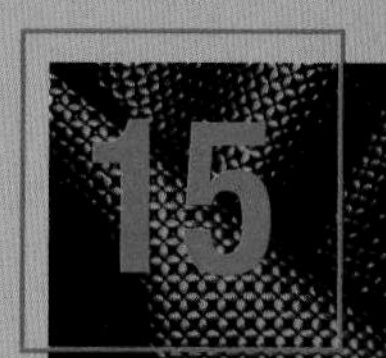

PROCEDURE 15-10

BLOW-DRY BLUNT OR LONG LAYERED, STRAIGHT TO WAVY HAIR INTO A STRAIGHT STYLE

1. **Apply styling product.** Attach the nozzle or concentrator attachment to the blow-dryer for more controlled styling. Part and section the hair so that only the section you are drying is not in clips. Apply a light gel or a straightening gel (Figure 15-106).
2. **Start at nape.** Using 1-inch subsections, start your first section at the nape of the neck and use a classic styling brush to dry the hair straight and smooth. Place the brush under the first section and hold the hair low (Figure 15-107).
3. **Follow brush with nozzle.** Follow the brush with the nozzle of the dryer while bending the ends of the hair in the desired direction, either under or flipped outward. Continue using the same technique working up to the occipital area in 1-inch sections. To keep the shape flat and straight, continue using low elevation. For more lift and volume, hold the section straight out from the head or overdirect upward (Figure 15-108).
4. **Work up to the crown,** continuing to take 1-inch sections. On the longer sections toward the top of the crown, you could switch to a paddle brush, using the curve of the brush to add bend to the ends of the hair.
5. **Cool hair.** After each section is blown dry, follow by using the cooling button on the blow-dryer to help set each section and to keep it smooth. For a fuller look, switch to a round brush.
6. **Dry hair above the ear.** Continue by subdividing the hair on the side, and start with the section above the ear. Continue working in 1-inch sections. Hold at a low elevation and follow with the nozzle of the dryer facing toward the ends. Bend the ends under by turning the brush for a rounded edge, or outward for a flipped edge (Figures 15-109 and 110).

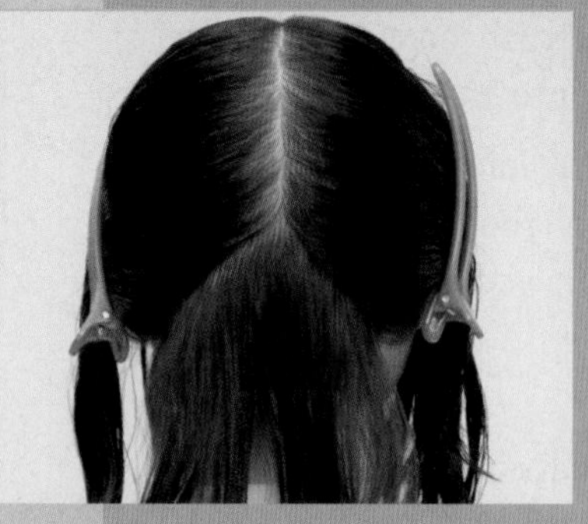

Figure 15-106 Hair sectioned for drying.

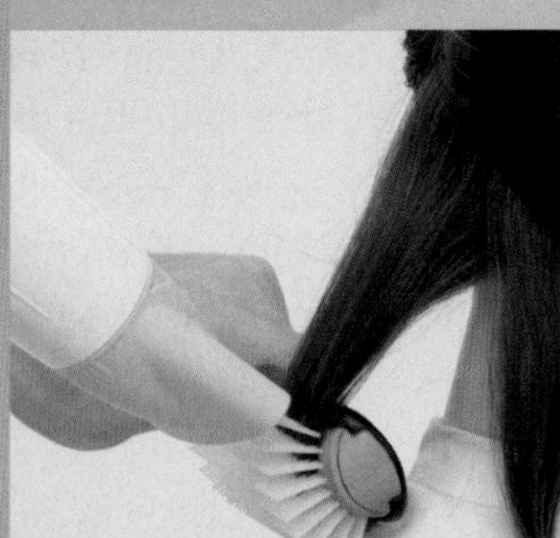

Figure 15-107 Hold the hair at lo elevation.

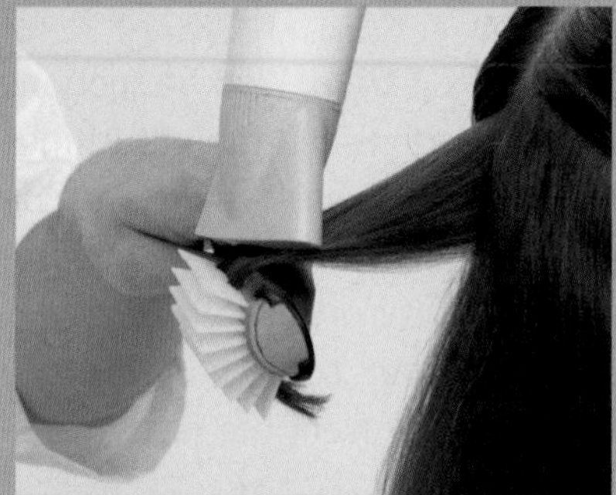

Figure 15-108 Hold the section straight out from the head.

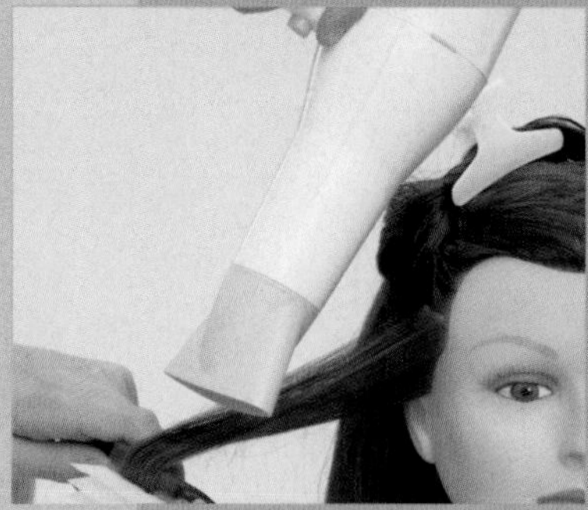

Figure 15-109 Side section turned under.

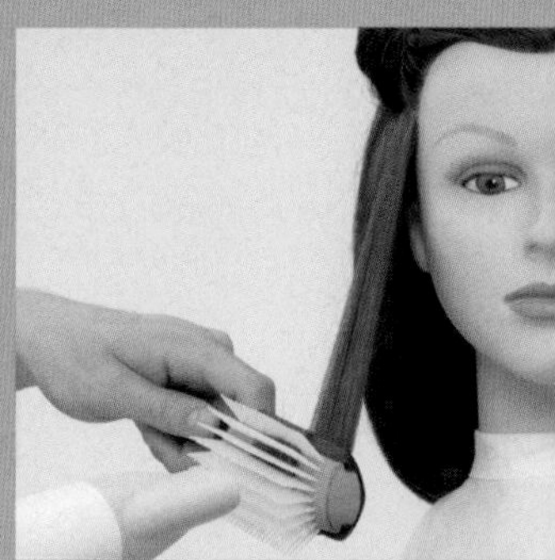

Figure 15-110 Side section flip out.

7. **Dry hair at top of head.** Work in the same manner across the top. If there is a bang (fringe), dry it in the desired direction. To dry the bang (fringe) straight and onto the forehead, point the nozzle of the dryer down over the bang (fringe) and dry it straight using your fingers or a classic styling brush to direct the hair (Figure 15-111).
8. **Direct bang (fringe).** To direct the bang (fringe) away from the face, brush the bang (fringe) back and push the hair slightly forward with the brush, creating a curved shaping (Figures 15-112 and 15-113). Place the dryer on a slow setting and point the nozzle toward the brush. When dry, the bang (fringe) will fall away from the face and slightly to the side, for a soft look (Figures 15-114 and 15-115).

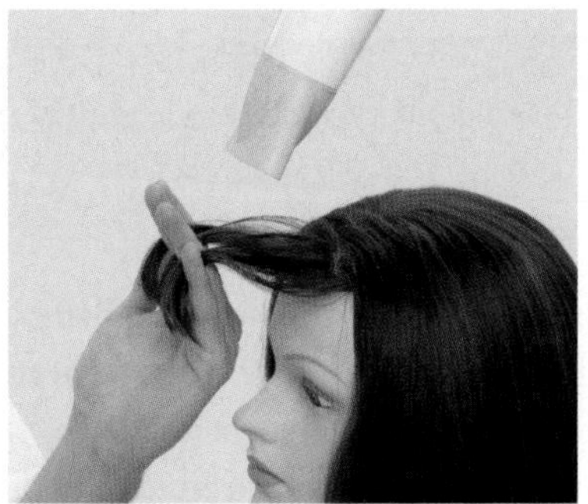

Figure 15-111 Dry bang (fringe) straight.

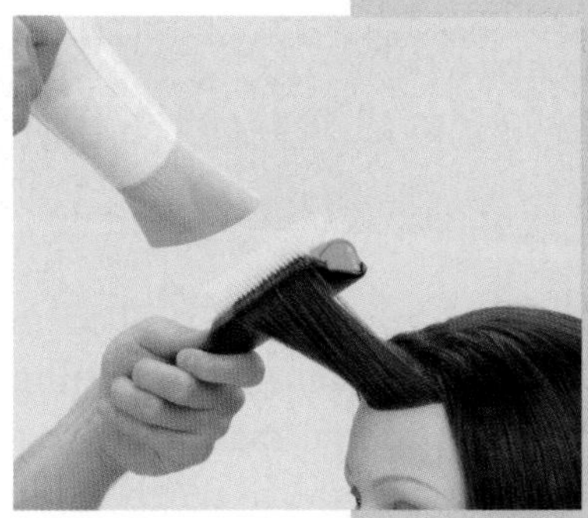

Figure 15-112 Brush bang (fringe) away.

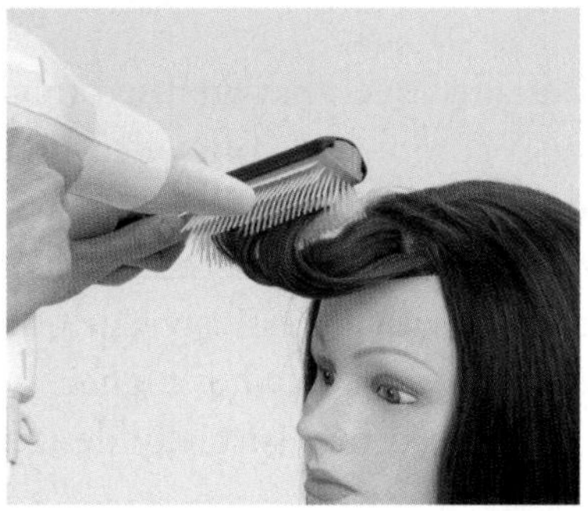

Figure 15-113 Curve section forward with nozzle facing section.

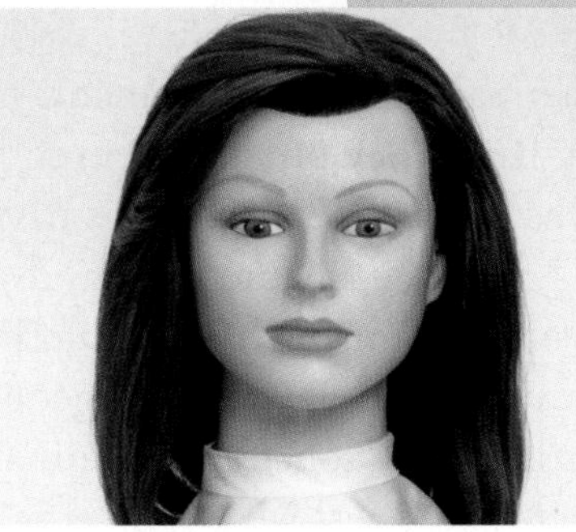

Figure 15-114 Finished style.

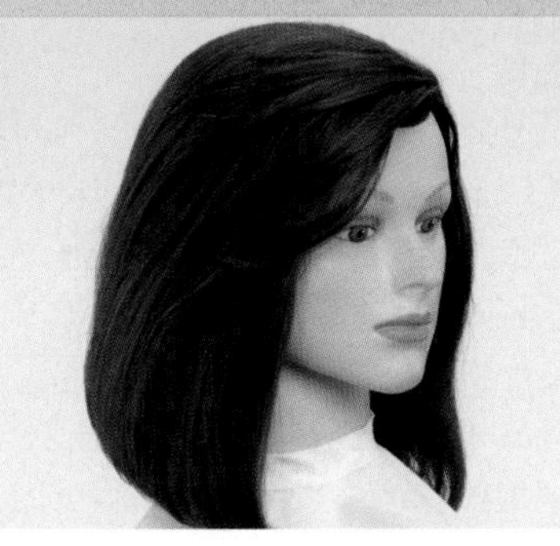

Figure 15-115 Side view of finished style.

CLEANUP AND SANITATION

1. Discard the neck strip.
2. Thoroughly clean brushes of any loose hair and disinfect them.
3. Clean the blow-dryer and remove any dust from the air intake area or filter.
4. Sanitize your workstation.
5. Wash your hands with soap and warm water.

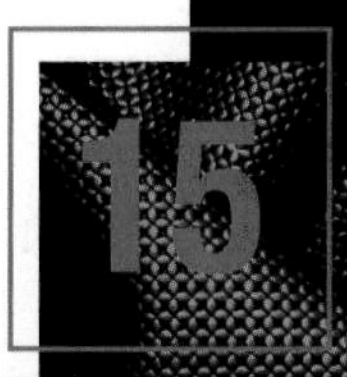

To blow-dry curly hair into a straight style, follow the preceding method. You may want to apply a straightening gel, and then use the largest round brush the hair length will allow. More tension will have to be applied to pull each 1-inch section straight. Be careful to keep the dryer moving in a back-and-forth motion at all times.

If the hair is fragile or damaged, this method is not recommended. Consider an alternate method such as wrapping the hair.

GRADUATED HAIRCUTS

Graduated haircuts have either long- or short-layered interiors. To blow-dry graduated haircuts, use the same basic blow-drying techniques presented in the previous sections, choosing the technique that best suits the length of the hair you are working on.

THERMAL HAIRSTYLING

Thermal waving (also called marcel waving) and **thermal curling** ar methods of waving and curling straight or pressed hair using therma irons and special manipulative techniques on dry hair (Figure 15-116) These irons, which can be either electrical or stove-heated, have beer modernized so successfully that they are more popular today than eve before. Manipulative techniques are basically the same for electric iron or stove-heated irons.

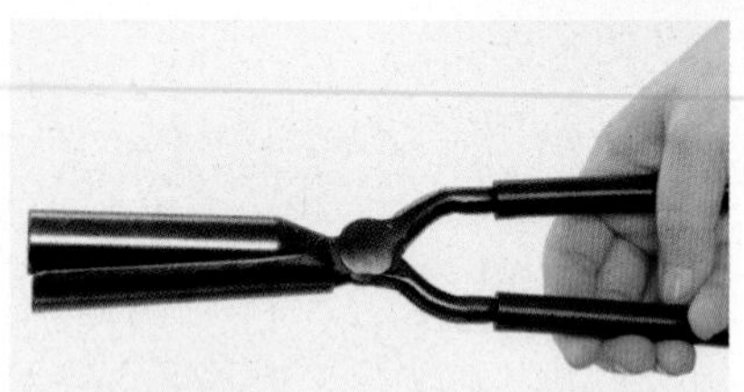

Figure 15-116 Conventional thermal (marcel) iron.

THERMAL IRONS

Thermal irons are implements made of quality steel that are used to cur dry hair. They provide an even heat that is completely controlled by th stylist. Electric curling irons have cylindrical barrels ranging from ½ incl to 3 inches in diameter (Figure 15-117). Nonelectrical thermal irons ar favored by many stylists catering to clients with excessively curly hai because of the larger range of barrel or rod sizes and higher hea capabilities. Nonelectric thermal irons are heated in a specially designe electric or gas stove (Figure 15-118).

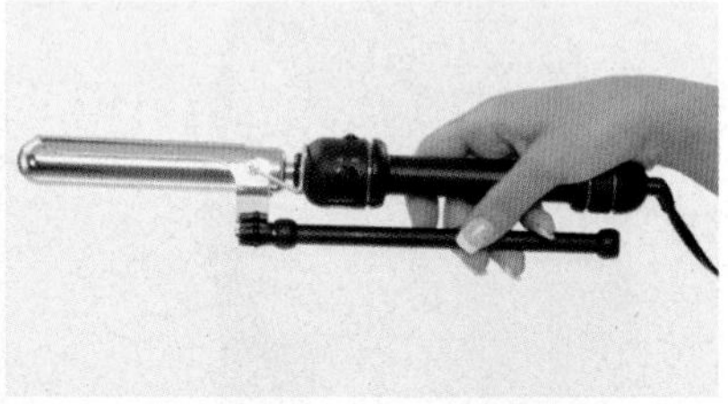

Figure 15-117 Electric thermal iron.

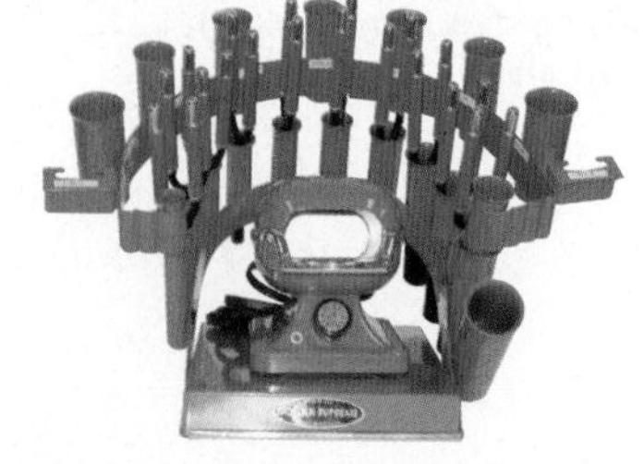

Figure 15-118 A modern stove-heated thermal iron and stove.

All thermal irons have four basic parts: (1) rod handle, (2) shell handle (3) barrel or **rod** (cylinder), and (4) **shell** (the clamp that presses the hai against the barrel) (Figure 15-119).

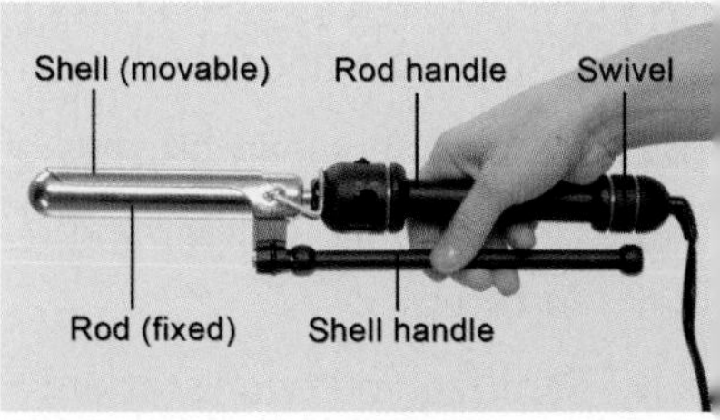

Figure 15-119 The parts of a thermal iron.

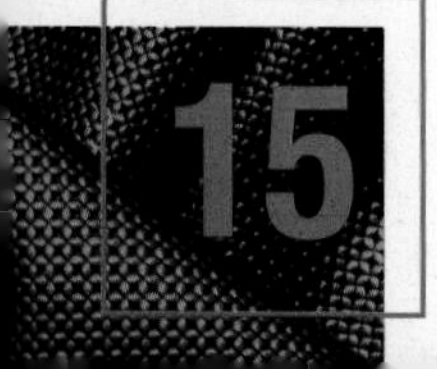

FLAT IRONS

Flat irons have two hot plates ranging in size from ½ inch to 3 inches across. Flat irons with straight edges are used to create smooth, straight styles, even on very curly hair. Flat irons with beveled edges can be manipulated to bend or cup the ends. The edge nearest the stylist is called the inner edge; the one farthest from the stylist is called the outer edge. Modern technology is constantly improving electric curling and flat irons, including adding infinite heat settings for better control, constant heat even on high settings, ergonomic grips, and lightweight designs for ease of handling.

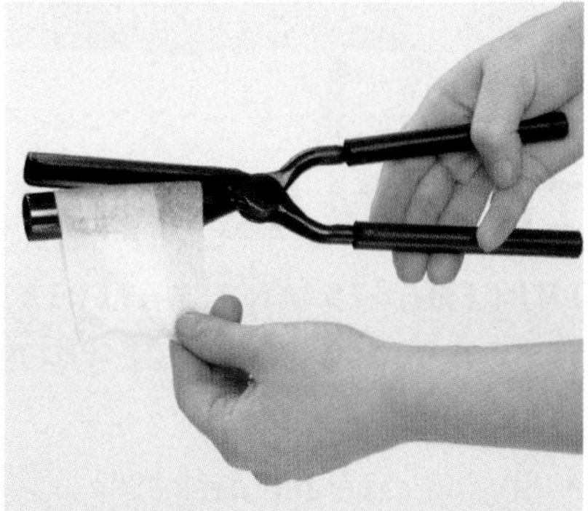

Figure 15-120 Testing the heat of a thermal iron.

PREPARATION

1. Drape the client; shampoo and towel-dry the hair.
2. Re-drape the client with a neck strip and styling cape.
3. Apply the appropriate styling product that will give the hair a lot of hold. Blow-dry the hair.

TESTING THERMAL IRONS

After heating the iron to the desired temperature, test it on a piece of tissue paper or a damp towel. Clamp the heated iron over this material and hold for 5 seconds. If it scorches or turns brown, the iron is too hot (Figure 15-120). Let it cool a bit before using. An overly hot iron can scorch the hair, and discolor white hair. Remember that fine, lightened, or badly damaged hair withstands less heat than normal hair.

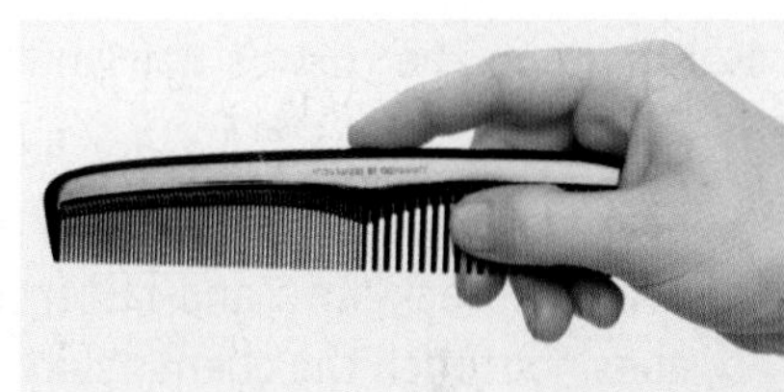

Figure 15-121 Holding the comb.

CARE OF THERMAL IRONS

To remove dirt, oils, and product residue, dampen a towel or rag and wipe down the barrel of the iron with a soapy solution containing a few drops of ammonia. If you are using a nonelectrical thermal iron, immerse the barrel in this solution. Do not do this when your iron is turned on, or is still cooling down from a previous styling service.

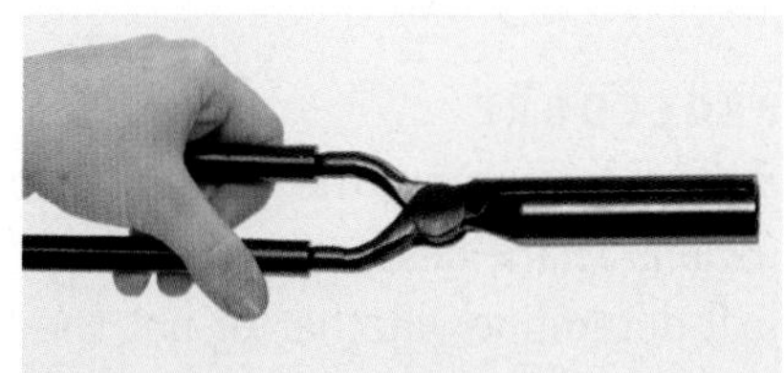

Figure 15-122 Rolling the iron.

COMB USED WITH THERMAL IRONS

The comb should be about 7 inches (17.5 centimeters) long, made of hard rubber or another nonflammable substance, and should have fine teeth to firmly hold the hair.

Hold the comb between the thumb and all four fingers of the left hand, with the index finger resting on the backbone of the comb for better control and one end of the comb resting against the outer edge of the palm. This position ensures a strong hold and a firm movement (Figure 15-121).

CAUTION

When using thermal irons on chemically straightened hair, be cautious and test the heat of the iron to avoid causing breakage.

MANIPULATING THERMAL IRONS

Hold the iron in a comfortable position that gives you complete control. Grasp the handles of the iron in your right hand—in the left hand if you are left-handed—far enough away from the joint to avoid the heat. Place your three middle fingers on the back of the lower handle, your little finger in front of the lower handle, and your thumb in front of the upper handle.

The best way to begin to practice manipulative techniques with thermal irons is by rolling the cold iron in your hand, first forward and then backward. This rolling movement should be done without any sway or motion in the arm; only the fingers are used as you roll the handles in either direction (Figure 15-122).

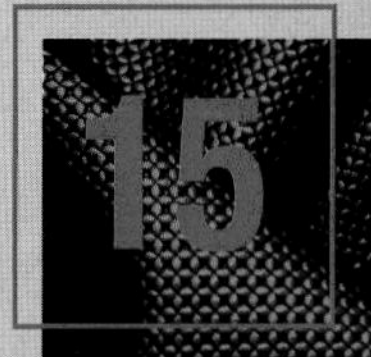

15-11 THERMAL WAVING

IMPLEMENTS AND MATERIALS

Thermal waving requires no setting creams or lotions.

- Shampoo
- Styling cape and neck strip
- Hard rubber comb (fine-toothed)
- Conventional (marcel) or electric irons

PREPARATION

1. **Shampoo** the client's hair and dry it completely.
2. **Drape the client** for a dry hair service; secure a neck strip around the client's neck. Place a cape over the neck strip and fasten it so that the cape does not touch the client's skin. Fold the uncovered portion of the neck strip down over the cape.
3. **Heat the iron.**
4. **Blow dry hair.**

PROCEDURE

Before beginning the waves, comb the hair in the general shape desired by the client. The natural growth will determine whether or not the first wave will be a left-moving wave or a right-moving wave. The procedure described here is for a left-moving wave.

1. **Comb the hair** thoroughly, following its directional growth.
2. **Part hair.** With the comb, pick up a strand of hair about 2 inches (5 centimeters) in width. Insert the iron in the hair with the groove facing upward (Figure 15-123).
3. **Turn iron.** Close the iron and give it a ¼ turn forward (away from you). At the same time, draw the hair with the iron about ¼ inch (.625 centimeters) to the left, and direct the hair ¼ inch (.625 centimeters) to the right with the comb (Figure 15-124).

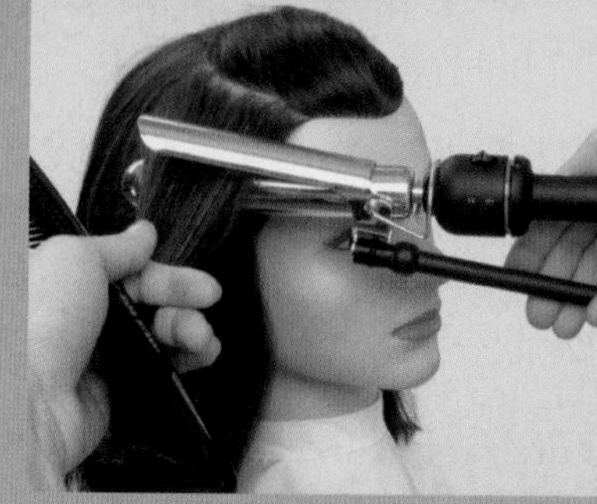

Figure 15-123 Insert iron in the hair.

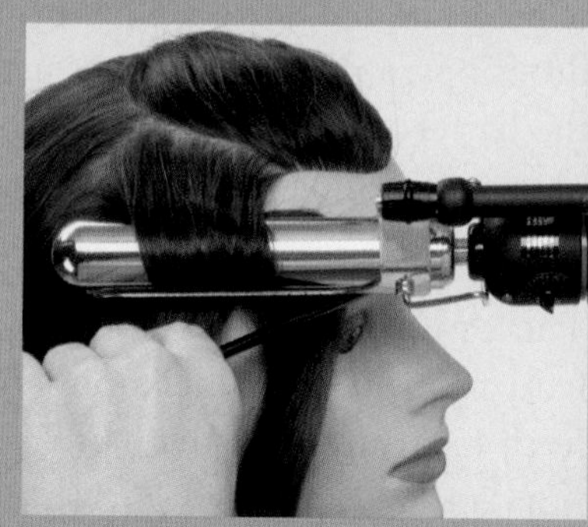

Figure 15-124 Direct the hair to the right with the comb.

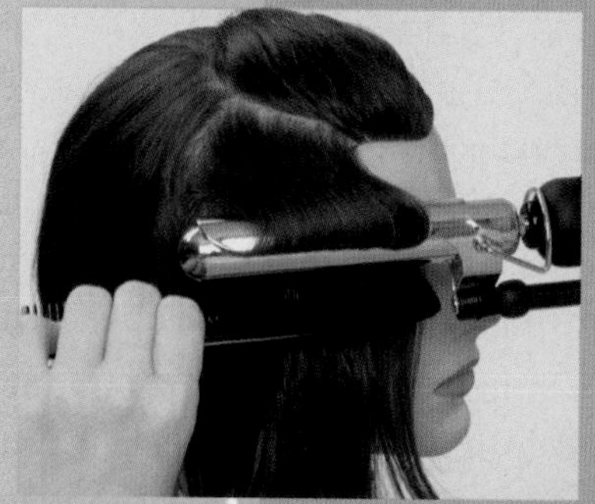

Figure 15-125 Roll the iron one full turn forward.

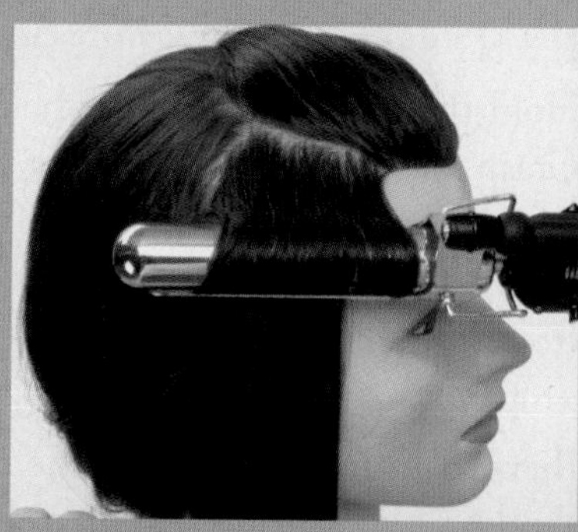

Figure 15-126 Reverse movement.

4. **Roll iron.** Roll the iron one full turn forward and away from you (Figure 15-125). When doing this, keep the hair uniform with the comb. You will find that the hair has rolled on a slight slant on the prong of the iron. Keep this position for a few seconds in order to allow the hair to become sufficiently heated throughout.
5. **Reverse movement.** Reverse the movement by simply unrolling the hair from the iron and bringing it back into its first resting position (Figure 15-126). When this movement is completed, you will find the comb resting somewhat away from the iron.
6. **Open iron.** Open the iron with your little finger and place it just below the ridge or crest by swinging the rod of the iron toward you, and then closing it (Figure 15-127). The outer edge of the groove should be directly underneath the ridge just produced by the inner ridge.
7. **Draw the hair.** Keeping the iron perfectly still, direct the hair with the comb upward about 1 inch (2.5 centimeters), thus forming the hair into a half circle (Figure 15-128). Remember that in order to perform Step 7 properly, you do not move the comb from the position explained in Step 6.
8. **Roll iron.** Without opening the iron, roll it a half turn forward and away from you (Figure 15-129). In this movement, keep the comb perfectly still and unchanged.
9. **Slide iron.** Slide the iron down about 1 inch (2.5 centimeters) (Figure 15-130). This movement is accomplished by opening the iron slightly, gripping it loosely, and then sliding it down the strand.
10. **Begin second ridge.** After completing step 9, you will find the iron and comb in the correct position to make the second ridge. This is the beginning of a right-moving wave, in which the hair is directed opposite to that of a left-moving wave.
11. **Wave next strand.** After completely waving one strand of hair, wave the next strand to match. Pick up the strand in the comb and include a small section of the waved strand to guide you as you form a new wave (Figure 15-131). When waving the second strand

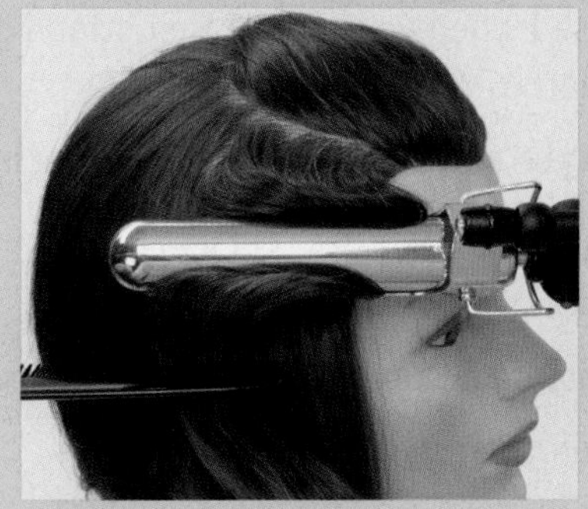

Figure 15-127 Start to form the curl.

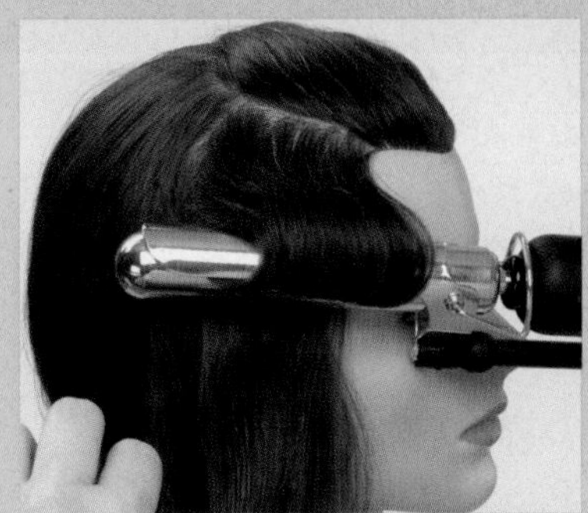

Figure 15-128 Form the hair into a half circle.

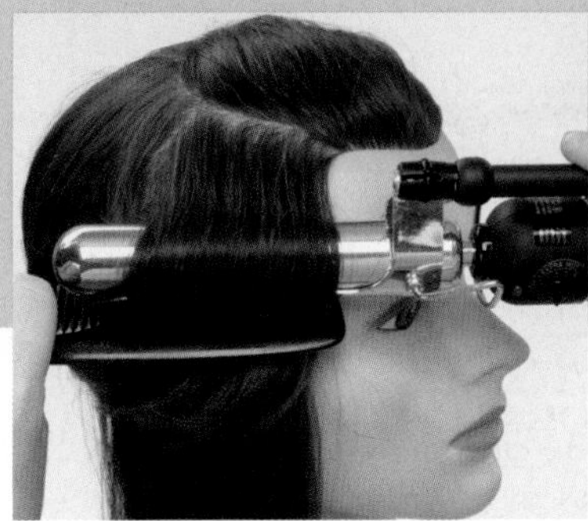

Figure 15-129 Roll iron one-half turn forward.

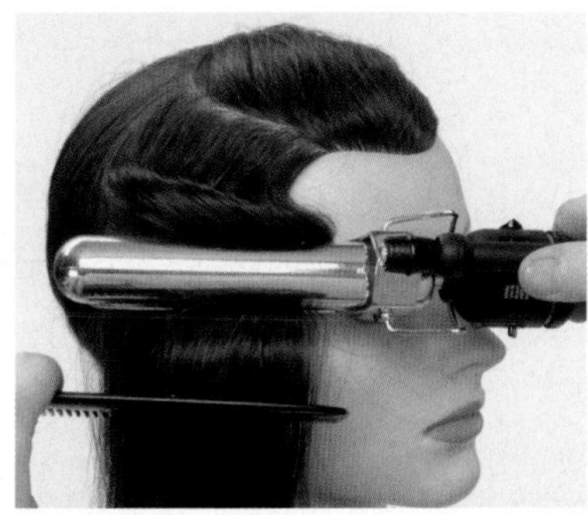

Figure 15-130 Slide iron down.

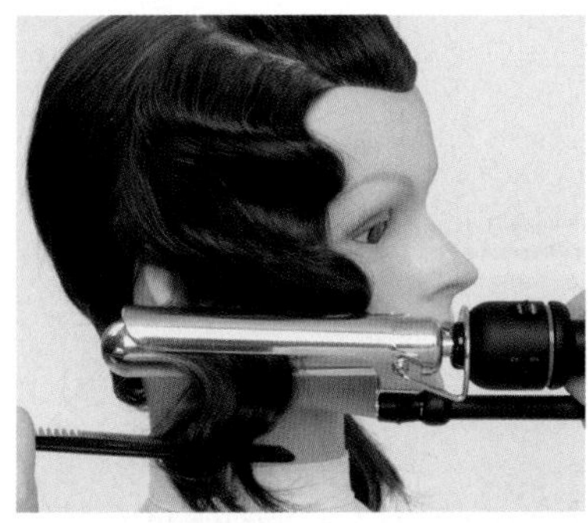

Figure 15-131 Matching the wave.

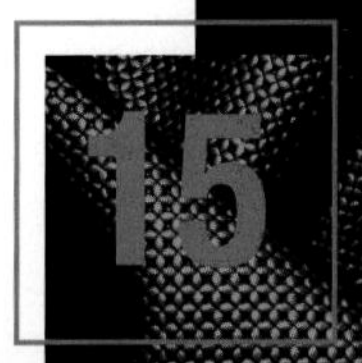

of hair, be sure to use the same comb-and-iron movements you used when waving the first strand of hair. This will make the waves match.

12. **Style and finish the hair as desired** (Figure 15-132).

CLEANUP AND SANITATION

1. Discard the neck strip.
2. Disinfect combs and other implements.
3. Sanitize your workstation.
4. Wash your hands with soap and warm water.

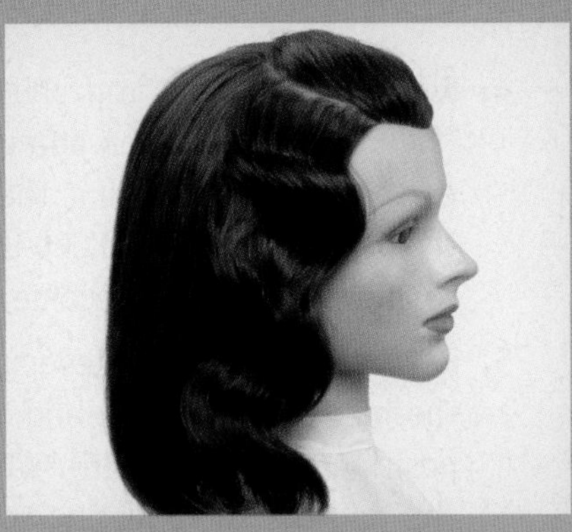

Figure 15-132 Finished thermal waved style.

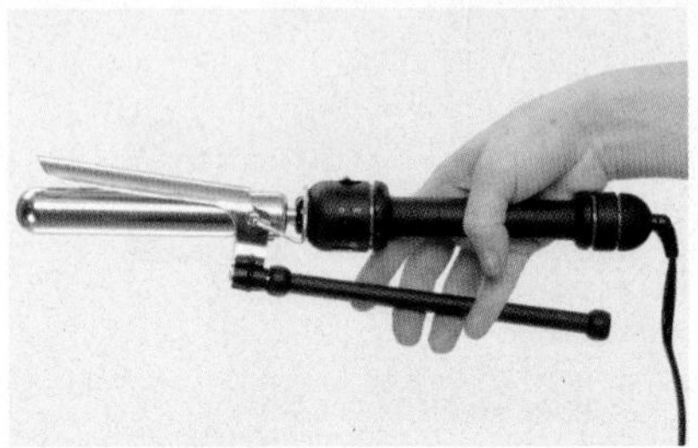

Figure 15-133 Use the little finger to open the clamp.

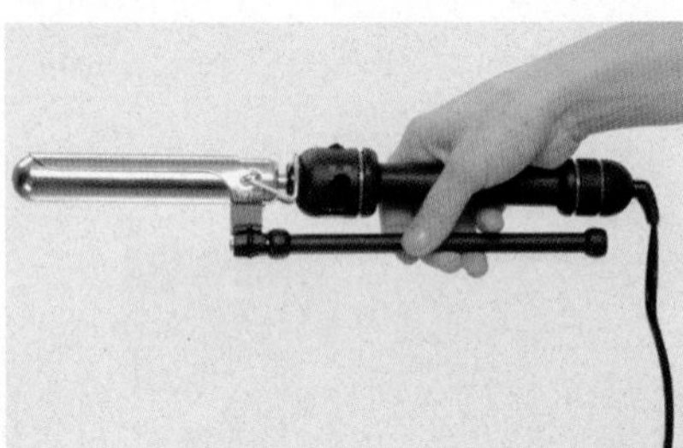

Figure 15-134 Use three middle fingers to close and manipulate the iron.

TEMPERATURE

There is no single correct temperature used for the iron when thermal curling or thermal waving the hair. The temperature setting for an iron depends on the texture of the hair, whether it is fine or coarse, or whether it has been lightened or tinted. Hair that has been lightened or tinted, as well as white hair, should be curled and waved with a gentle heat. As a rule, coarse and gray hair can withstand more heat than fine hair.

THERMAL CURLING WITH ELECTRIC THERMAL IRONS

A modern thermal iron and a comb are all you need to give your client curls. Thermal curling, which requires no setting gels or lotions, may be used to great advantage on the following:

- *Straight hair.* Permits quick styling. Thermal curling eliminates working with wet hair and does away with the need for rollers and a long hairdrying process.
- *Pressed hair.* Permits styling the hair without the danger of its returning to its former extremely curly condition. Thermal curling prepares the hair for any desired style.
- *Wigs and hairpieces* (human hair). Presents a quick and effective method for styling.

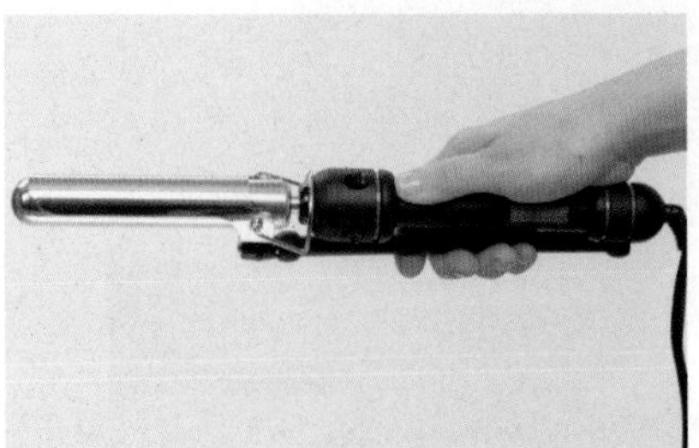

Figure 15-135 Shift thumb when manipulating the iron.

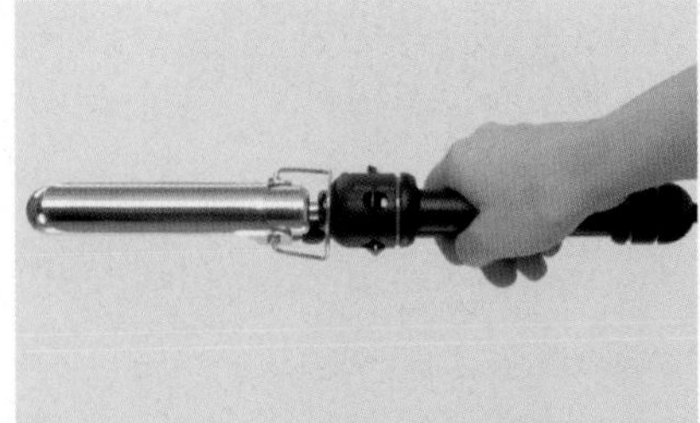

Figure 15-136 Close shell and make a one-quarter turn downward.

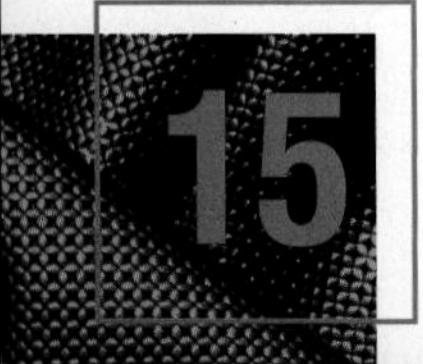

CURLING IRON MANIPULATIONS

The following is a series of basic manipulative movements for using curling irons. Most other curling iron movements are variations of these basic movements (Figures 15-133 through 15-139). Some stylists prefer to use just the little finger, or the little finger plus the ring finger, for this purpose. Either method is correct. The method of holding the iron is a matter of personal preference. Choose the one that gives you the greatest ease, comfort, and control of movement.

If you want to get really good at using curling irons, the key is to practice manipulating them. Always practice with cold irons. The following four exercises are designed to help you learn the most effective ways to use an iron.

1. Since it is important to develop a smooth rotating movement, practice turning the iron while opening and closing it at regular intervals. Practice rotating the iron in both directions—downward (toward you) and upward (away from you) (Figure 15-140).
2. Practice releasing the hair by opening and closing the iron in a quick, clicking movement.
3. Practice guiding the hair strand into the center of the curl as you rotate the iron. This exercise will ensure that the end of the strand is firmly in the center of the curl (Figure 15-141).
4. Practice removing the curl from the iron by drawing the comb to the left, and the rod to the right (Figure 15-142). Use the comb to protect the client's scalp from burns.

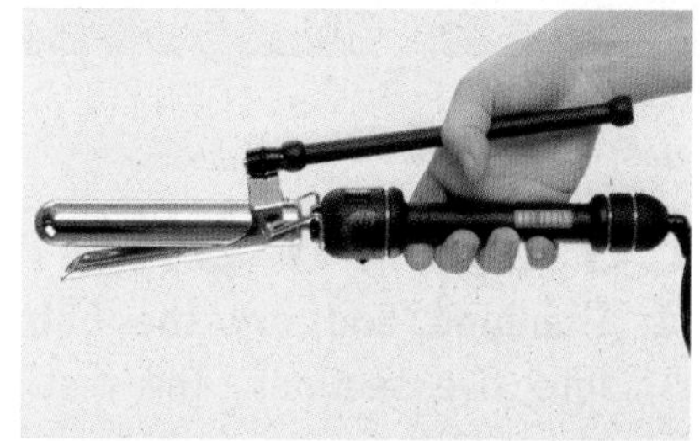

Figure 15-137 Iron has made a half turn. Use thumb to open clamp and relax hair tension.

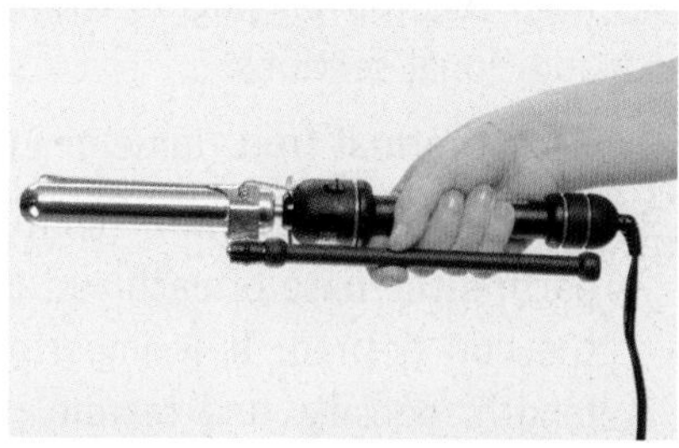

Figure 15-138 Rotate iron to three quarters of a complete turn.

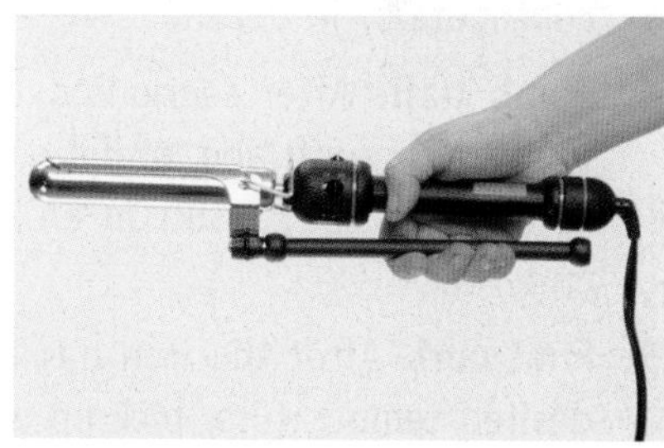

Figure 15-139 Full turn.

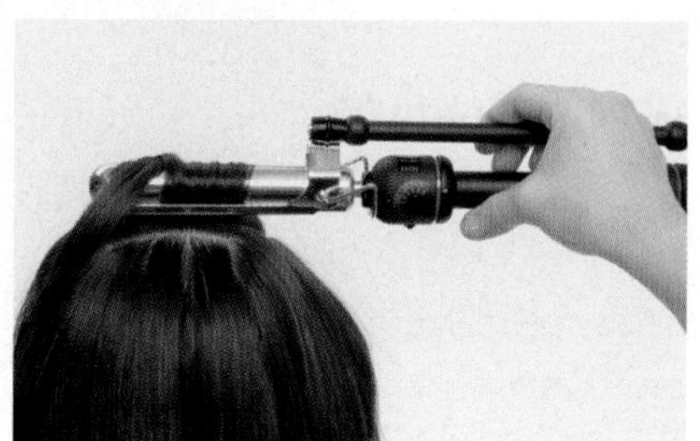

Figure 15-140 Rotate while opening and closing the iron.

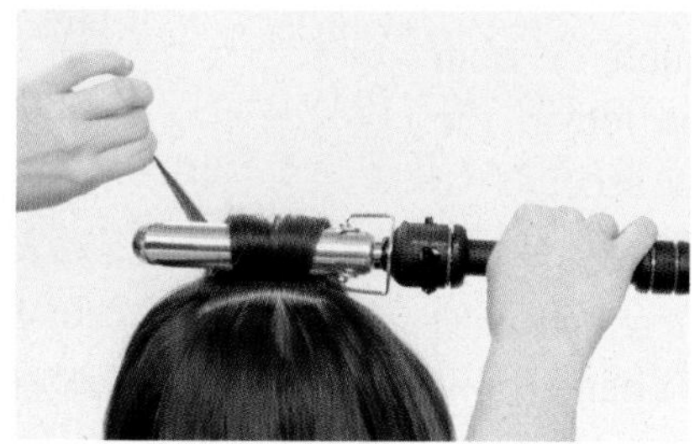

Figure 15-141 Guide the hair strand into the center of curl while rotating the iron.

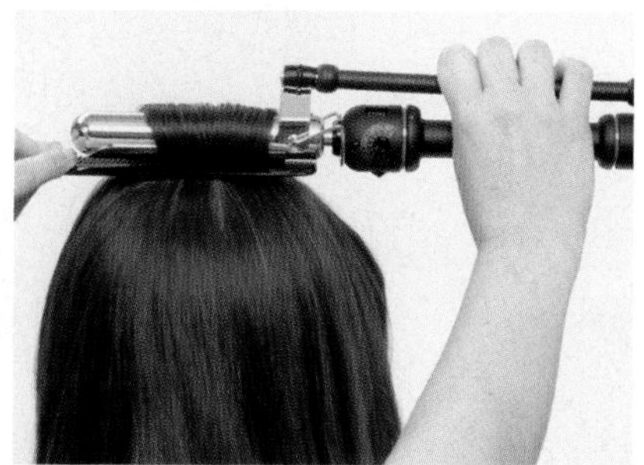

Figure 15-142 Remove curl using the comb as you guide.

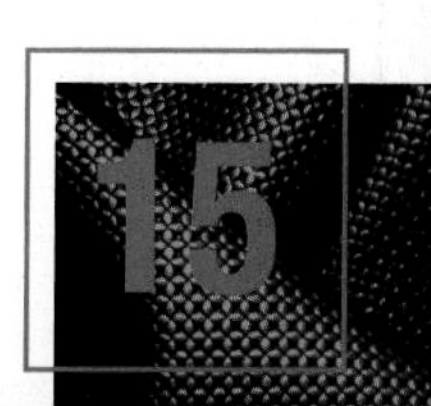

PROCEDURE 15-12

CURLING SHORT HAIR

1. **Shampoo and dry the hair.** Divide the head into five sections. The first section should be about 2½ inches (6.25 centimeters) wide, and extend from the center of the forehead to the nape of the neck. Divide the two side panels in half, from the top parting to the neck, to create four additional sections.
2. **Heat thermal iron** (large or jumbo size).
3. **Section and part hair.** Begin by sectioning and parting the base of each curl to match the size of the curl desired. It is important to consider hair length, density, and texture. The base is usually about 1½ inches to 2 inches (3.75 centimeters to 5 centimeters) in width, and ½ inch (1.25 centimeters) in depth.
4. **Comb hair.** After sectioning off the base, comb the hair smooth and straight out from the scalp. Loose hairs may result in an uneven and ragged curl.
5. **First curl.** After the iron has been heated to the desired temperature, pick up a strand of hair and comb it smoothly. With the groove on top, insert the iron about 1 inch (2.5 centimeters) from the scalp, and pull the hair over the rod in the direction of the curl. Hold for a few seconds to form a base (Figure 15-143).
6. **Turn iron.** Hold the ends of the hair strand with your thumb and two fingers of your left hand (right hand if you are left-handed), using a medium degree of tension. Turn the iron downward (toward you) with your right hand (Figure 15-144).
7. **Open and close the iron rapidly as you turn, to prevent binding.** Guide the ends of the strand into the center of the curl as you rotate the iron (Figure 15-145).
8. **Remove curl.** The result of this procedure will be a smooth, finished curl, with the ends firmly fixed in the center. Remove the iron from the curl (Figure 15-146).

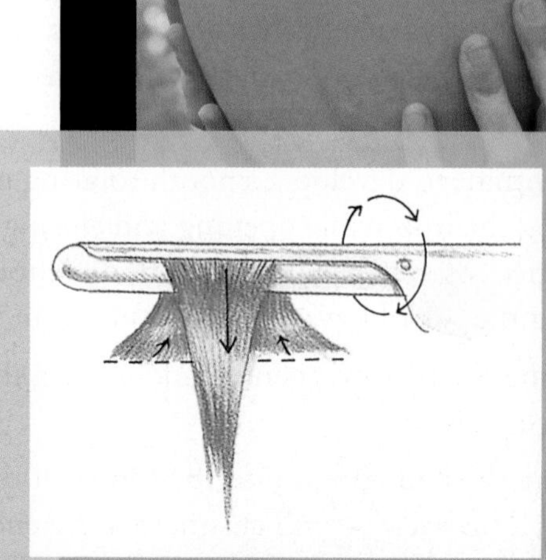

Figure 15-143 Form a base.

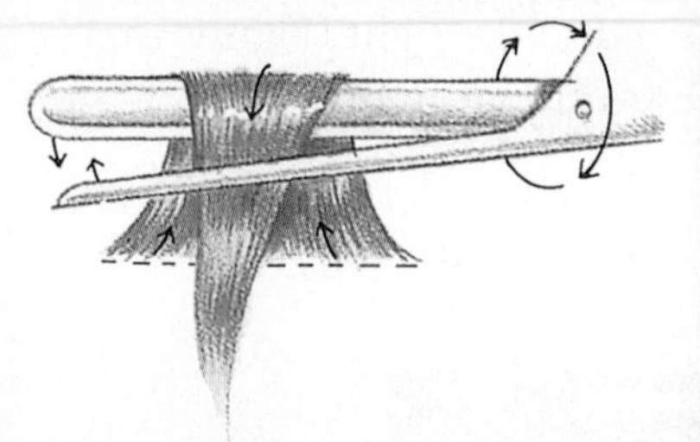

Figure 15-144 Turn iron.

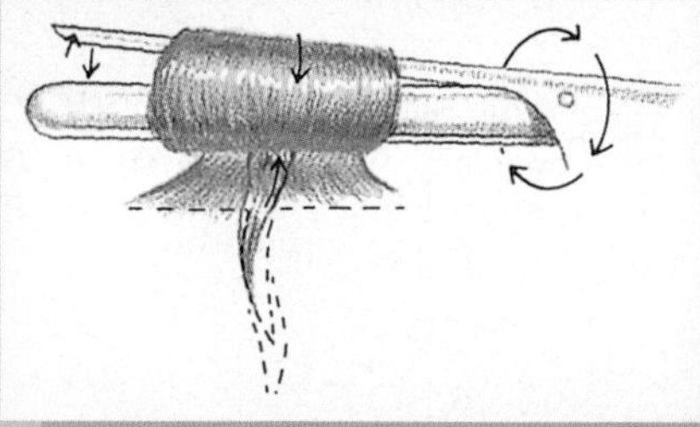

Figure 15-145 Rotate the iron and guide the ends of strand into the center.

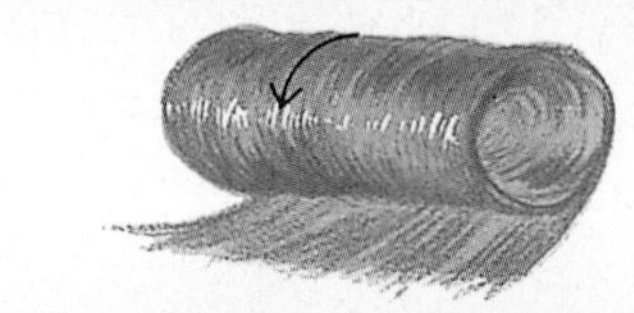

Figure 15-146 Finished curl.

PROCEDURE 15-13

CURLING MEDIUM-LENGTH HAIR

1. **Section hair.** Section and form the base of the curl as described for short hair.
2. **Insert hair into iron.** Insert the hair into the open iron at the scalp. Pull the hair over the rod in the direction of the curl and close the shell. Hold the iron in this position for about 5 seconds to heat the hair, and then slide the it up to 1 inch (2.5 centimeters) from the scalp. The shell must be on top (Figure 15-147).
3. **Turn iron.** Turn the iron downward a half revolution. Then pull the end of the strand over the rod to the left, directing the strand toward the center of the curl (Figure 15-148).
4. **Direct ends.** Complete the revolution of the iron, and continue directing the ends toward the center (Figure 15-149).
5. **Make another complete revolution of the iron.** The entire strand has now been curled with the exception of the ends. Enlarge the curl by opening the shell. Insert the ends of the curl into the opening created between the shell and the rod (Figure 15-150).
6. **Close the shell and slide the iron toward the handles.** This technique will move the ends of the strand into the center of the curl. Rotate the iron several times to even out the distribution of the hair in the curl (Figure 15-151).
7. **Smooth the ends.** When the curl is formed and the ends are freed from between the rod and the shell, make one complete revolution of the iron inside the curl. This smoothes the ends and loosens the hair away from the iron. Use the comb to help remove the curl from the iron. Slowly draw the iron in one direction, while drawing the hair in the opposite direction with the comb. To protect the client during the curling process, use the comb between the scalp and the iron.

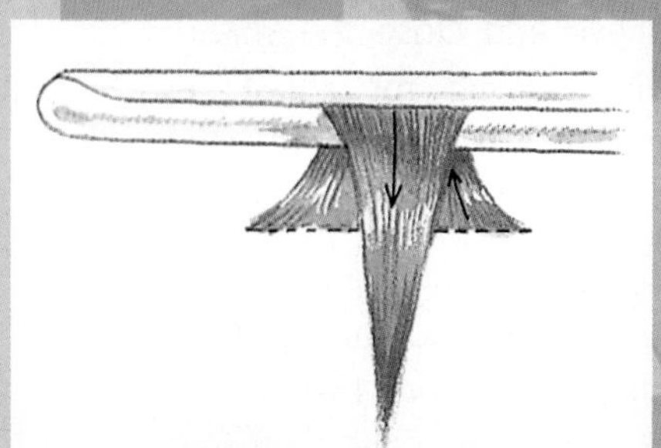

Figure 15-147 Insert hair into the open iron at scalp.

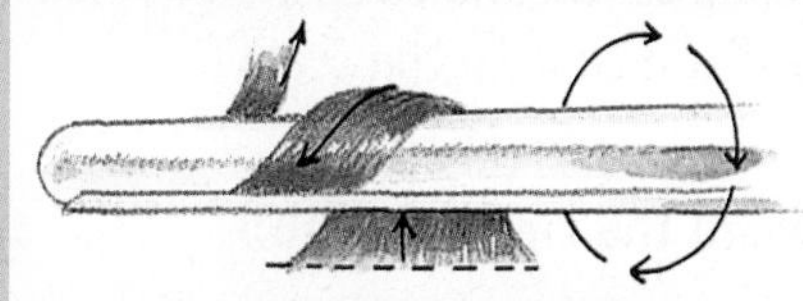

Figure 15-148 Turn iron downward a half revolution.

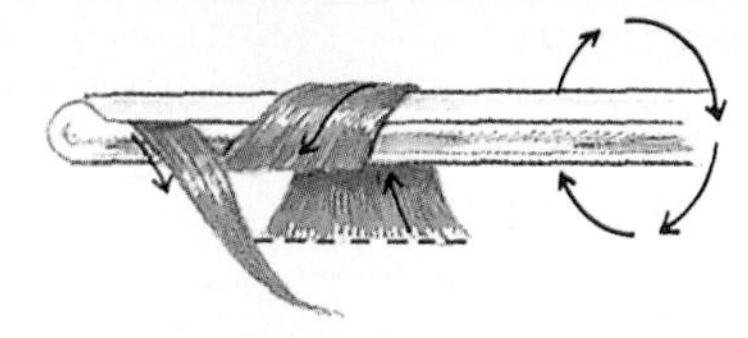

Figure 15-149 Complete revolution of iron.

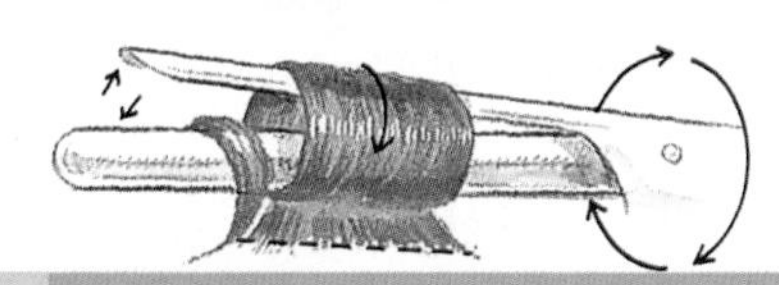

Figure 15-150 Make another complete revolution.

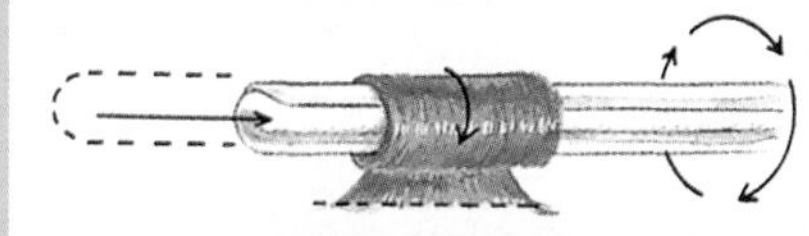

Figure 15-151 Close the shell and slide the iron toward the handles.

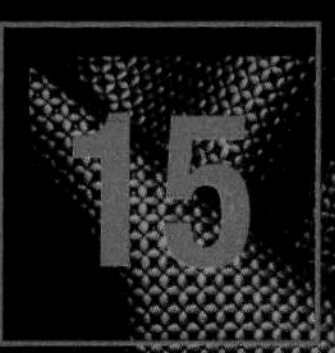

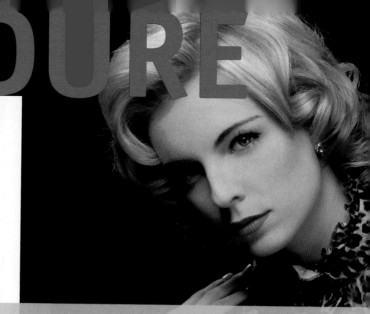

PROCEDURE 15-14

CURLING HAIR (USING TWO LOOPS OR "FIGURE 8")

1. **Section hair.** Section and form the base of the curl as described for short hair.
2. **Insert hair.** Insert the hair into the open iron about 1 inch (2.5 centimeters) from the scalp. Pull the hair over the rod in the direction in which the curl is to move and close the shell. Hold the iron in this position for about 5 seconds, in order to heat the hair. Hold the strand of hair with a medium degree of tension (Figure 15-152).
3. **Roll iron.** Roll the iron under; click and roll it until the groove is facing you (Figure 15-153).
4. **Pick up ends.** With the left hand, pick up the ends of the hair (Figure 15-154).
5. **Roll and click iron.** Continue to roll and click the iron, keeping it the same distance from the scalp (Figure 15-155).
6. **Draw the hair strand toward the tip of the iron** (Figure 15-156).
7. **Draw strand, push iron.** Draw the strand a little to the right and, at the same time, push the iron slightly to the left (Figure 15-157).
8. **Form two loops.** By pushing the iron forward, and pushing the hair with the left hand, you will form two loops around the closed iron, with the ends of the strand extending out between the loops (Figure 15-158).
9. **Roll and click iron.** Roll under and click the iron until the ends of the hair disappear (Figure 15-159).
10. **Rotate iron.** Rotate the iron several times to even out the distribution of the hair in the curl and to facilitate the movement of the curl off the iron.

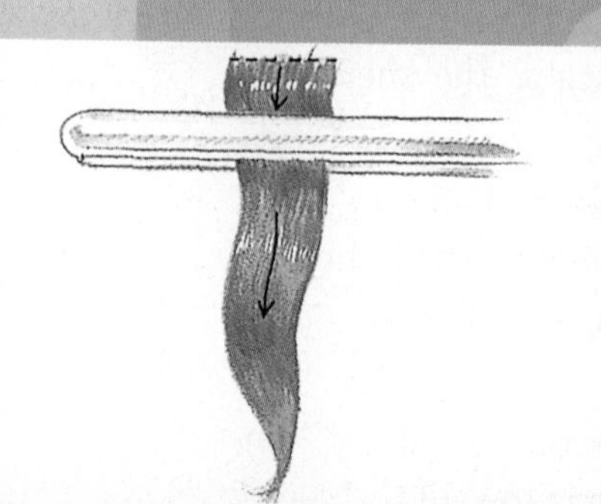

Figure 15–152 Insert hair 1 inch (2.5 centimeters) from scalp.

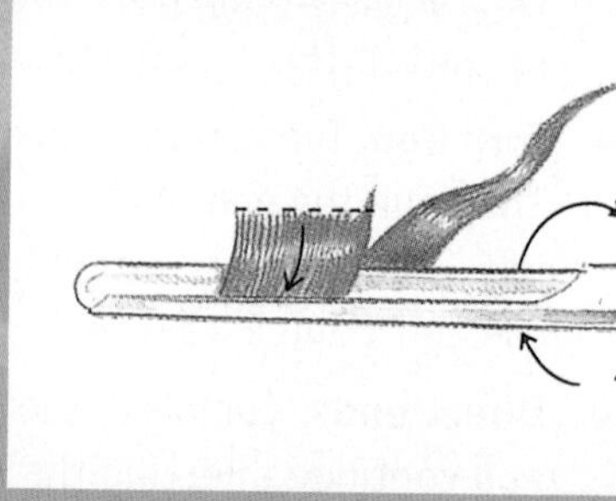

Figure 15–153 Roll iron under.

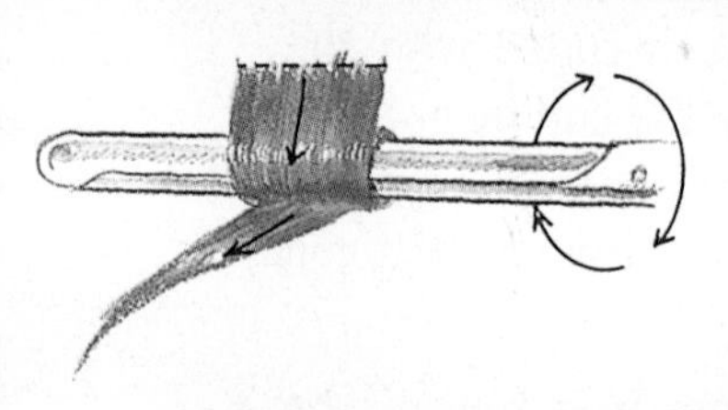

Figure 15–154 Pick up ends of hair.

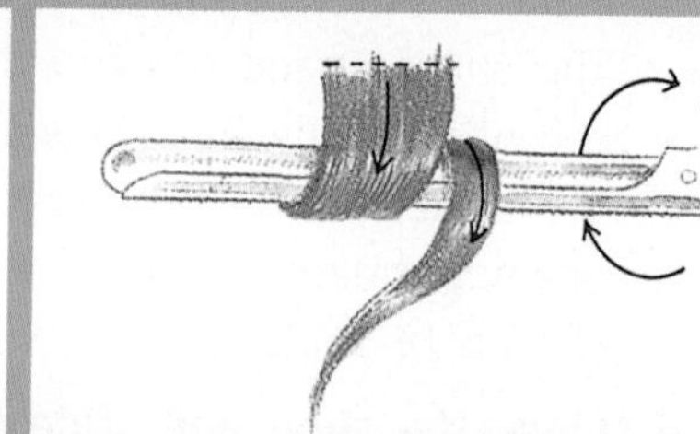

Figure 15–155 Continue to roll iron.

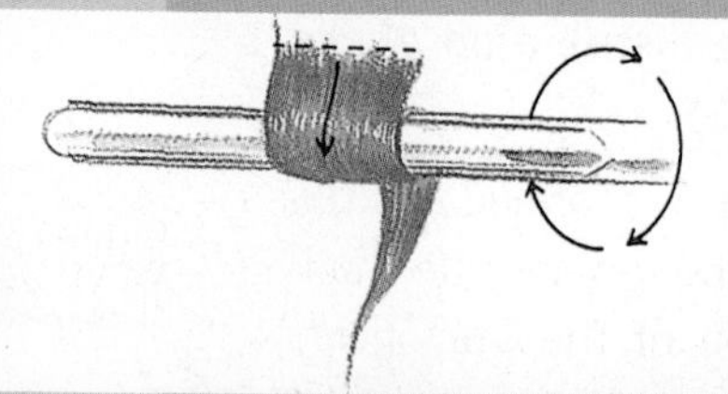

Figure 15–156 Draw hair strand toward the point of the iron.

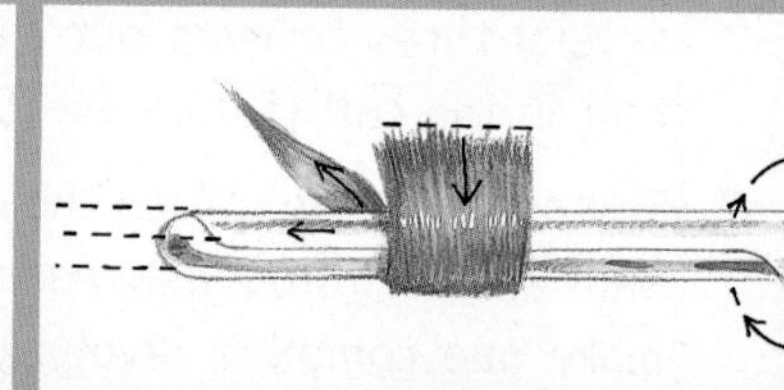

Figure 15–157 Draw strand right, pu[sh] iron left.

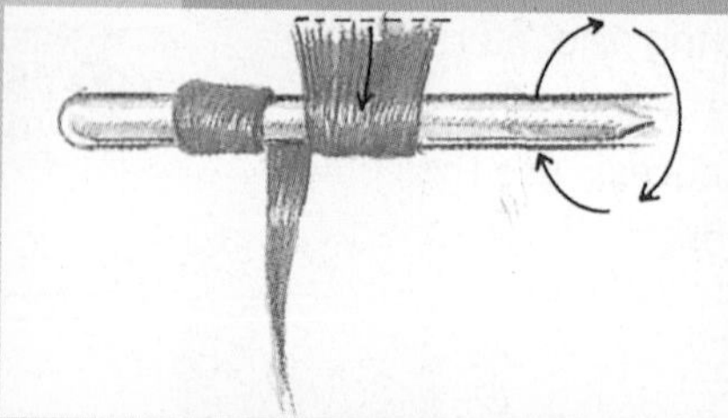

Figure 15–158 Form two loops around the closed iron.

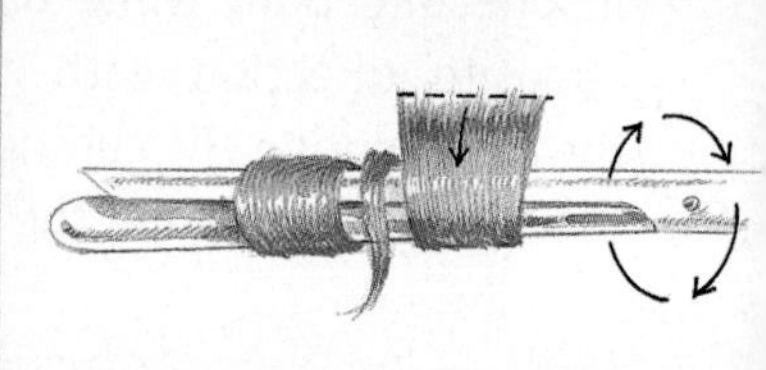

Figure 15–159 Roll the iron until all t[he] hair ends disappear.

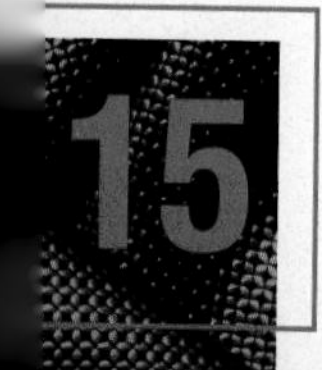

OTHER TYPES OF CURLS

There are a number of other curls you can use for your styling purposes. The **spiral curl** is a method of curling the hair by winding a strand around the rod. It creates hanging curls suitable for medium to long hairstyles. To create a spiral curl, part the hair into as many sections as there will be curls and comb smooth. Insert the iron at an angle, with the bowl (groove) on top near the base of the strand, and rotate the iron until all the hair is wound (Figures 15-160 and 15-161). Hold the curl in this position for 4 to 5 seconds, and remove the iron in the usual manner (Figure 15-162 and 15-163).

End curls can be used to give a finished appearance to hair ends. Long, medium-length, or short hair may be styled with end curls. The hair ends can be turned under or over, as desired. The position of the curling iron, and the direction of its movements, will determine whether the end curls will turn under or over (Figure 15-164 and 15-165).

VOLUME THERMAL IRON CURLS

Volume thermal iron curls are used to create volume or lift in a finished hairstyle. The degree of lift desired determines the type of volume curls to be used.

VOLUME-BASE THERMAL CURLS

Volume-base curls provide maximum lift or volume, since the curl is placed very high on its base. Section off the base as described. Hold the curl strand at a 135-degree angle. Slide the iron over the strand about ½ inch (1.25 centimeters) from the scalp. Wrap the strand over the rod with medium tension.

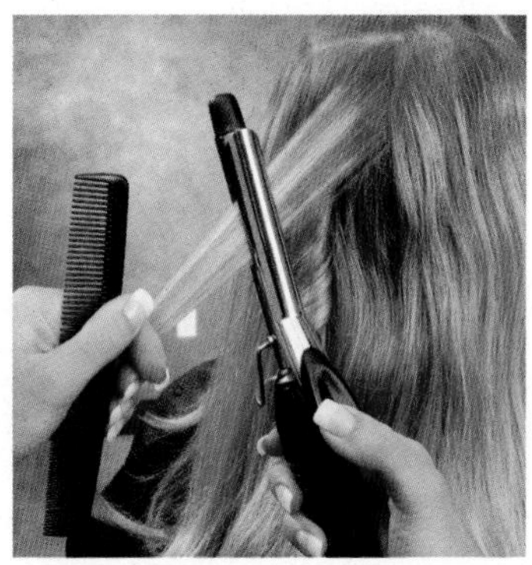

Figure 15-160 Insert iron at an angle.

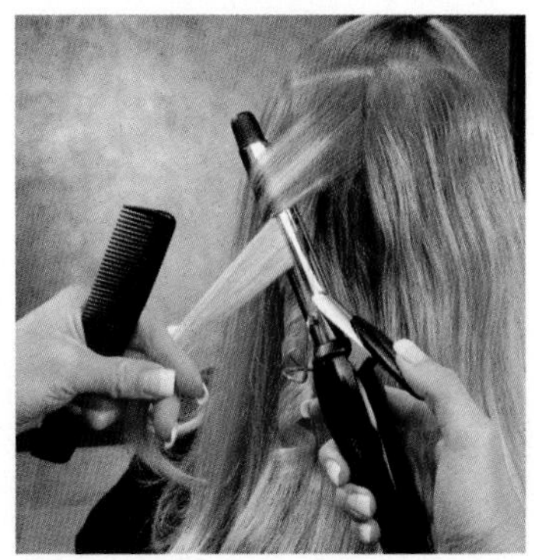

Figure 15-161 Rotate iron until hair is wound.

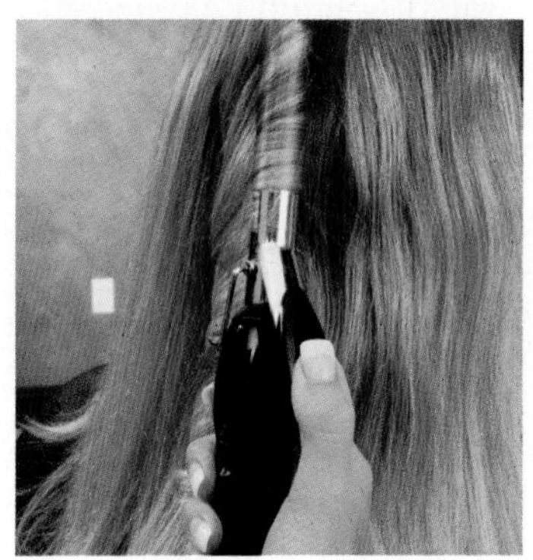

Figure 15-162 Hold curl in position.

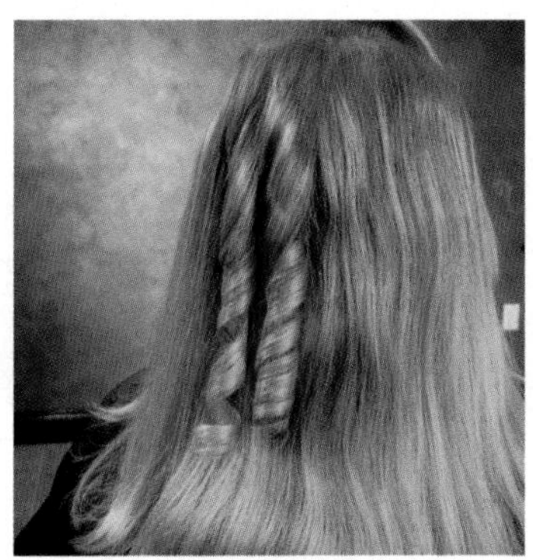

Figure 15-163 Finished curl.

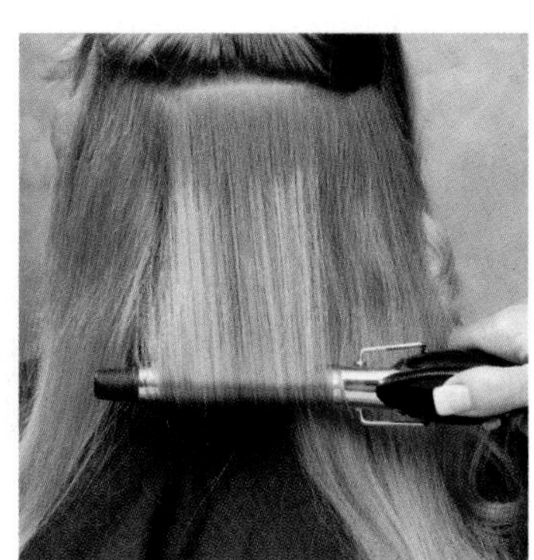

Figure 15-164 Turn iron under.

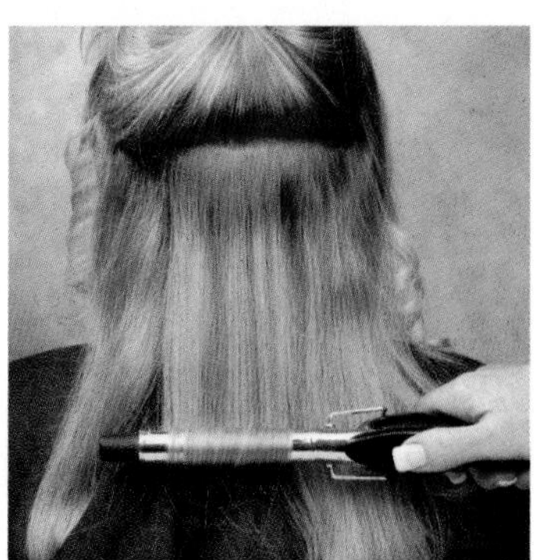

Figure 15-165 Turn iron over.

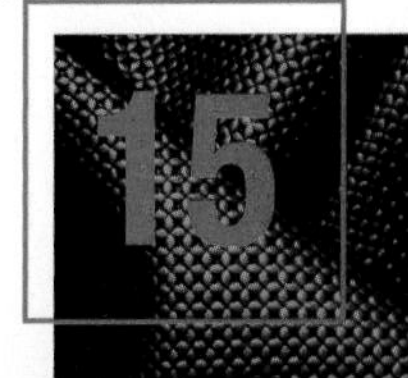

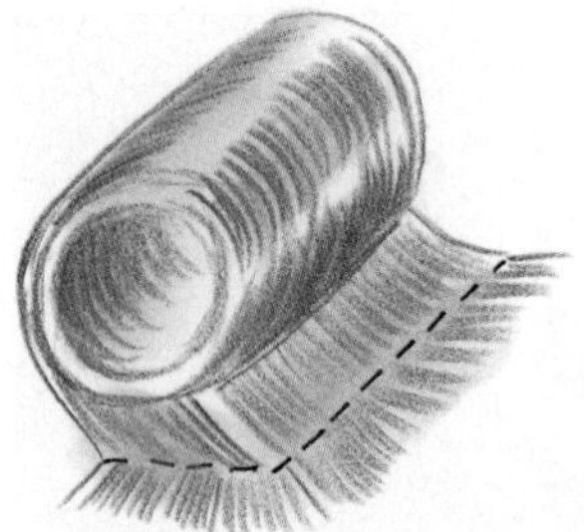

Figure 15-166 Volume-base curl.

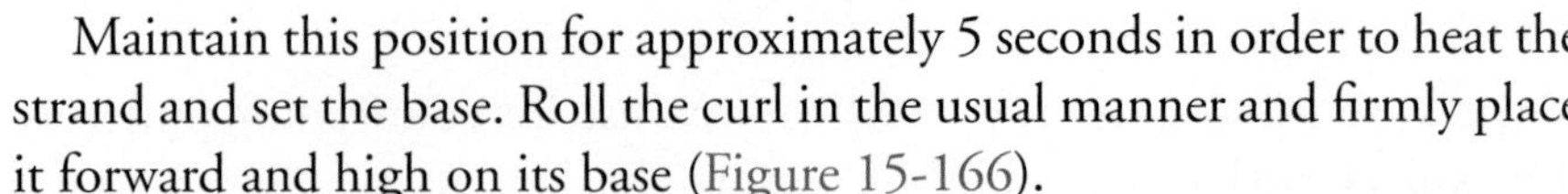

Maintain this position for approximately 5 seconds in order to heat the strand and set the base. Roll the curl in the usual manner and firmly place it forward and high on its base (Figure 15-166).

FULL-BASE THERMAL CURLS

Full-base curls provide a strong curl with full volume. Section off the base as described. Hold the hair strand at a 125-degree angle. Slide the iron over the hair strand about ½ inch (1.25 centimeters) from the scalp. Wrap the strand over the rod with medium tension. Maintain this position for about 5 seconds to heat the strand and set the base. Roll the curl in the usual manner, and place it firmly in the center of its base (Figure 15-167).

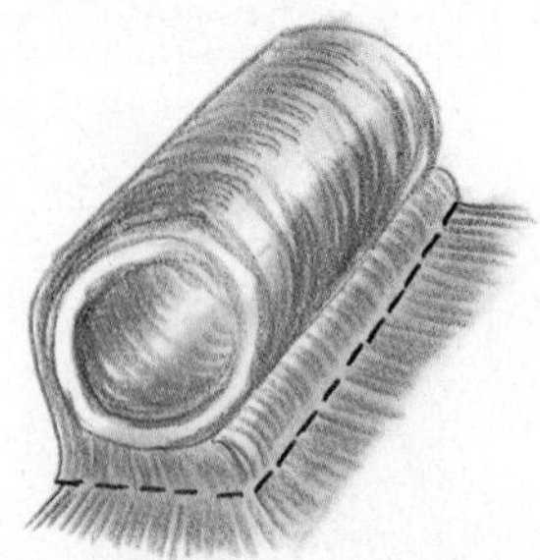

Figure 15-167 Full-base curl.

HALF-BASE THERMAL CURLS

Half-base curls provide a strong curl with moderate lift or volume. Section off the base as described. Hold the hair at a 90-degree angle. Slide iron over the hair strand about ½ inch (1.25 centimeters) from the scalp. Wrap the strand over the rod with medium tension. Maintain this position for about five seconds to heat the strand and set the base. Roll the curl in the usual manner, and place it half off its base (Figure 15-168).

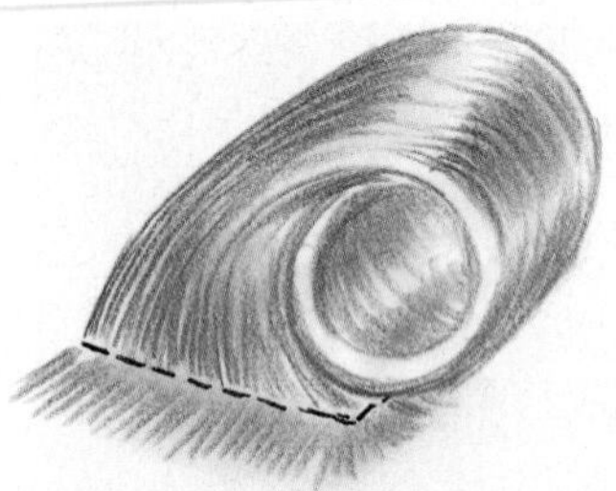

Figure 15-168 Half-base curl.

OFF-BASE THERMAL CURLS

Off-base curls offer a curl option with only slight lift or volume. Section off the base as described previously, holding the hair at a 70-degree angle. Slide the iron over the hair strand about ½ inch (1.25 centimeters) from the scalp. Wrap the strand over the rod with medium tension. Maintain this position for about five seconds to heat the strand and set the base. Roll the curl in the usual manner, and place it completely off its base (Figure 15-169).

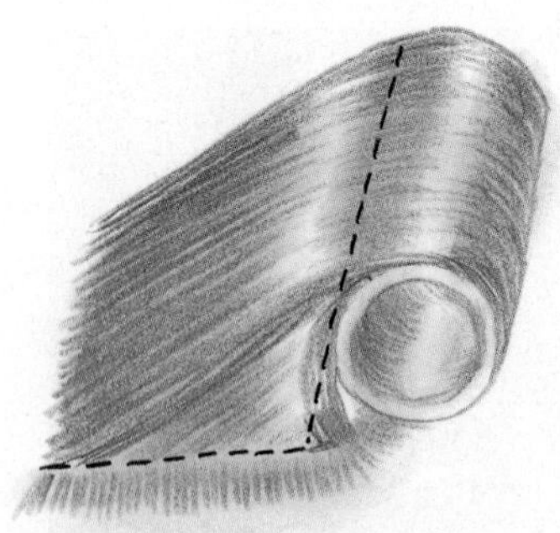

Figure 15-169 Off-base curl.

FINISHED THERMAL CURL SETTINGS

For best results when giving a thermal setting, clip each curl in place until the whole head is complete and ready for styling (Figure 15-170). Brush the hair, working up from the neckline and pushing the waves into place as you progress over the entire head. If the hairstyle is to be finished with curls, do the bottom curls last (Figures 15-171 through 15-173).

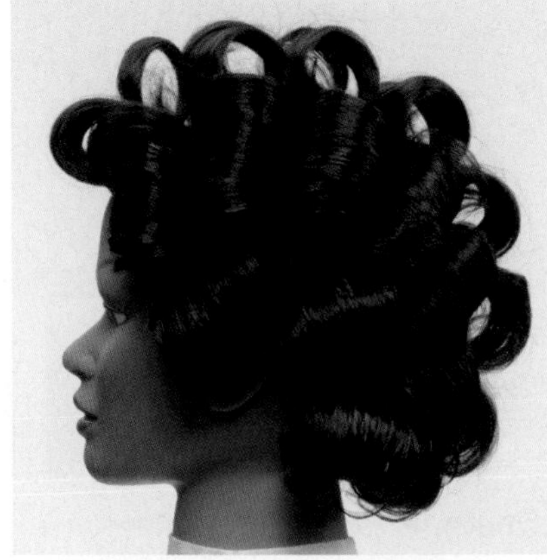

Figure 15-170 Completely curled head, side view.

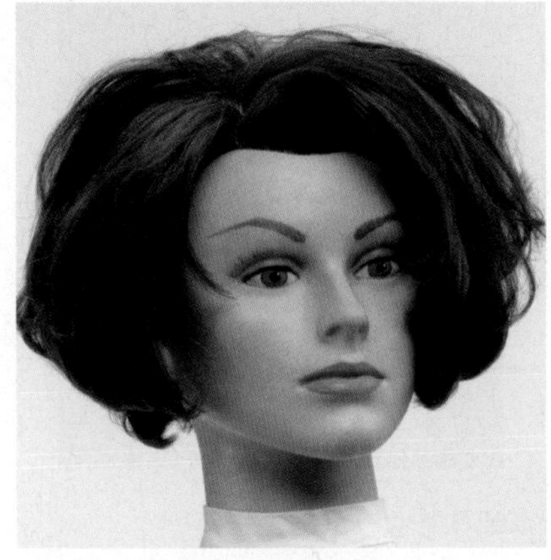

Figure 15-171 Finished thermal-curled short hairstyle.

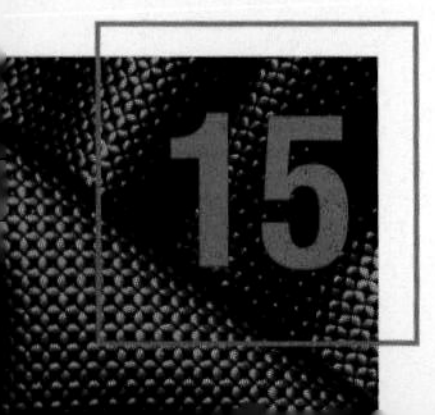

SAFETY MEASURES

1. Use thermal irons only after receiving instruction in their use.
2. Keep thermal irons clean.
3. Do not overheat the iron, because this can damage the ability of the iron to hold heat uniformly.
4. Test the temperature of the iron on tissue paper or a damp towel before placing it on the hair. This will safeguard against burning the hair.
5. Handle thermal iron carefully to avoid burning yourself or the client.
6. Place hot irons in a safe place to cool. Do not leave them where someone might accidentally come into contact with them and be burned.
7. When heating a conventional iron, do not place the handles too close to the heater. Your hand might be burned when removing the iron.
8. Make sure the iron is properly balanced in the heater, or it might fall and be damaged or injure someone.
9. Use only hard rubber or nonflammable combs. Celluloid combs must not be used in thermal curling, as they are flammable.
10. Do not use metal combs; they can become hot and burn the scalp.
11. Place a comb between the scalp and the thermal iron when curling or waving hair to prevent burning the scalp.
12. The client's hair must be clean and completely dry to ensure a good thermal curl or wave.
13. Do not allow the hair ends to protrude over the iron; this causes fishhooks (hair that is bent or folded).
14. When ironing lightened, tinted or relaxed hair, always use a gentle heat setting.

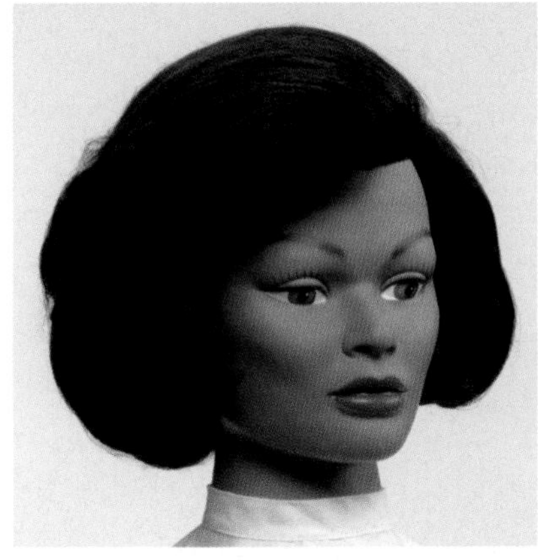

Figure 15-172 Finished thermal-curled medium-length hairstyle.

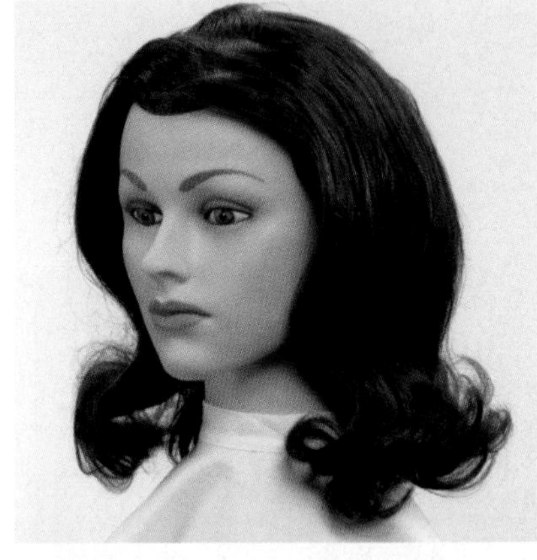

Figure 15-173 Finished thermal-curled long hairstyle.

THERMAL HAIR STRAIGHTENING (HAIR PRESSING)

Hair straightening, or pressing, is a popular service that is very profitable in the salon. When properly done, **hair pressing** temporarily straightens extremely curly or unruly hair by means of a heated comb. A pressing generally lasts until the hair is shampooed. (Permanent hair straightening is covered in Chapter 18.) Hair pressing also prepares the hair for additional services, such as thermal curling and croquignole thermal curling (the two-loop or "Figure 8" technique). A good hair pressing leaves the hair in a natural and lustrous condition, and is not harmful to the hair (Figure 15-174).

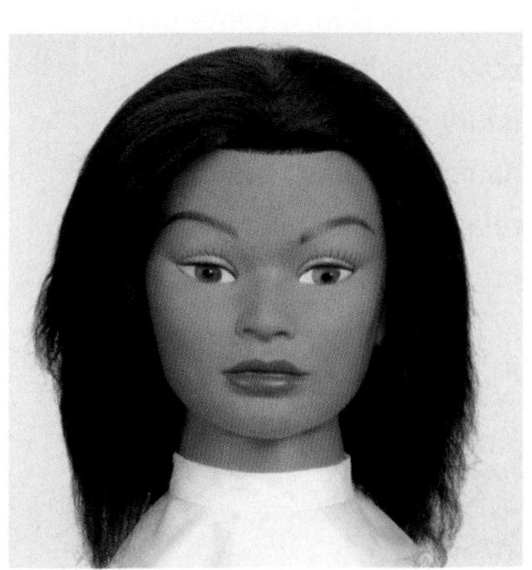

Figure 15-174 Pressed hairstyle.

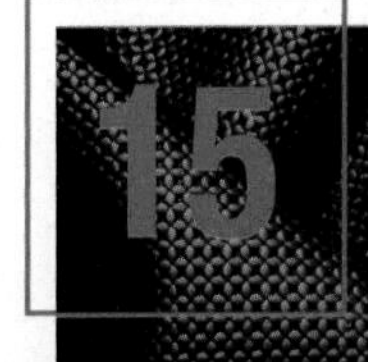

There are three types of hair pressing:

1. **Soft press,** which removes about 50 to 60 percent of the curl, is accomplished by applying the thermal pressing comb once on each side of the hair.
2. **Medium press,** which removes about 60 to 75 percent of the curl, is accomplished by applying the thermal pressing comb once on each side of the hair, using slightly more pressure.
3. **Hard press,** which removes 100 percent of the curl, is accomplished by applying the thermal pressing comb twice on each side of the hair. A hard press can also be done by first passing a hot thermal iron through the hair. This is called a **double press.**

ANALYSIS OF HAIR AND SCALP

Before you press a client's hair, you will need to analyze the condition of the hair and scalp. If the client's hair and scalp are not healthy, you should give appropriate advice concerning corrective treatments. In the case of scalp skin disease, it is not the cosmetologist's job to diagnose the condition, but rather to advise the client to see a dermatologist. If the hair shows signs of neglect or abuse caused by faulty pressing, lightening, or tinting, recommend a series of conditioning treatments. Failure to correct dry and brittle hair can result in hair breakage during hair pressing. Burned hair strands cannot be conditioned.

Remember to check your client's hair for elasticity and porosity. Under normal conditions, if a client's hair has good elasticity, it can be stretched to about 50 percent of its original length before breaking. If the porosity is normal, the hair will return to its natural wave pattern when it is wet or moistened.

A careful analysis of the client's hair should cover the following points:

- Wave pattern
- Length
- Texture (coarse, medium, fine)
- Feel (wiry, soft, or silky)
- Elasticity
- Color (natural, faded, streaked, gray, tinted, lightened)
- Condition (normal, brittle, dry, oily, damaged, or chemically treated)
- Condition of scalp (normal, flexible, or tight)

It is important that the cosmetologist be able to recognize individual differences in hair texture, porosity, elasticity, and scalp flexibility. Guided by this information, the cosmetologist can determine how much pressure the hair and scalp can handle without breakage, hair loss, or burning from a pressing comb that may not be adjusted to the correct temperature.

HAIR TEXTURE

Variations in hair texture have to do with the diameter of the hair (coarse, medium, or fine) and the feel of the hair (wiry, soft, or silky). Touching the client's hair, and asking about specific hair characteristics, will help you determine the best way to treat the hair.

CAUTION

Under no circumstances should hair pressing be given to a client who has a scalp abrasion, a contagious scalp condition, a scalp injury, or chemically damaged hair. Chemically relaxed hair should not be pressed.

Coarse, extremely curly hair has qualities that make it difficult to press. Coarse hair has the greatest diameter, and during the pressing process it requires more heat and pressure than medium or fine hair.

Medium curly hair is the normal type of hair that cosmetologists deal with in the beauty salon. No special problem is presented by this type of hair, and it is the least resistant to hair pressing.

Fine hair requires special care. To avoid hair breakage, less heat and pressure should be applied than for other hair textures.

Wiry, curly hair may be coarse, medium, or fine and feels stiff, hard, and glassy. Because of the compact construction of the cuticle cells, it is very resistant to hair pressing and requires more heat and pressure than other types of hair.

SCALP CONDITION

The condition of the client's scalp can be classified as normal, tight, or flexible. If the scalp is normal, proceed with an analysis of hair texture and elasticity. If the scalp is tight and the hair coarse, press the hair in the direction in which it grows to avoid injury to the scalp. The main difficulty with a flexible scalp is that the cosmetologist might not apply enough pressure to press the hair satisfactorily.

RECORD CARD

Be sure to keep a record of the results of your hair and scalp analysis, as well as all pressing treatments performed on a client. It is also a good idea to question the client about any lightener, tint, gradual colors (metallic), or other chemical treatment that have been used on her hair. A release statement should be used for hair pressing, as with all services that help protect the stylist from responsibility from accidents or damages. (See Figure 4-4 on page 39 for an example of a release statement on the client consultation card.)

CONDITIONING TREATMENTS

Effective conditioning treatments involve special cosmetic preparations for the hair and scalp, thorough brushing, and scalp massage. Applying a conditioning treatment usually results in better hair pressing.

A tight scalp can be made more flexible by the systematic use of scalp massage or hair brushing. The client benefits because there is better circulation of blood to the scalp.

Once you become adept at the basic styles presented in this chapter, you will want to experiment and create your own styles. Each client's hair represents more possibilities for creativity. That is why having a mannequin at home to duplicate the looks you see in magazines is such an important part of keeping current. Trends change quickly, and you need to always be able to offer the latest to your clients.

PRESSING COMBS

There are two types of pressing combs: regular and electric. Both should be constructed of good-quality stainless steel or brass. The handle is usually made of wood since wood does not readily absorb heat.

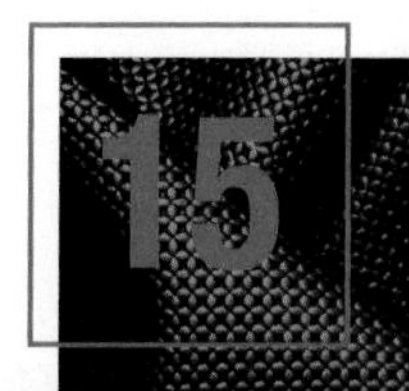

The space between the teeth of the comb varies with the size and style of the comb. A comb with more space between the teeth produces a coarse or open-looking press, while a comb with less space produces a smoother press.

Pressing combs also vary in size. Shorter combs are used to press short hair; longer combs are used to press long hair.

It may be a good idea to temper a new brass pressing comb. Tempering allows the brass to hold heat evenly along the entire length of the comb, which gives better results when used on your clients' hair.

Another good reason to temper is to burn off any polish the manufacturer may have used to coat the comb. If the polish is not burned off, the comb may stick to the hair, causing scorching and breakage.

To temper a new pressing comb, heat the comb until it is extremely hot. Coat the comb in petroleum or pressing oil. Let it cool down naturally, and then rinse under hot running water to remove the oil.

HEATING THE COMB

Depending on what they are made of, combs vary in their ability to accept and retain heat. Regular pressing combs may be designed as electrical appliances or heated in electric or gas stoves. (Figure 15-175). While being heated in a gas stove, the teeth should face upward and the handle should be kept away from the fire.

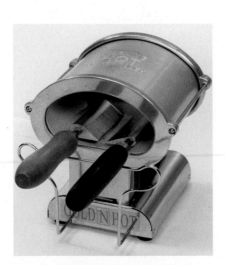

Figure 15-175 Electric heater for pressing combs.

After heating the comb to the proper temperature, test it on a piece of light paper. If the paper becomes scorched, allow the comb to cool slightly before applying it to the hair.

Electric pressing combs are available in two forms. One comes with an "on" and "off" switch; the other is equipped with a thermostat that has a control switch indicating high or low degrees of heat.

There is available a straightening comb attachment that fits the nozzle of a standard hand-held dryer. While it is less damaging than either an electric comb or an oven-heated comb, it may also be less effective.

CLEANING THE COMB

The pressing comb will perform more efficiently if it is kept clean. Wipe the comb clean of loose hair, grease, and dust before and after every use. The intense heat keeps the comb sterile, once all loose hair or clinging dirt is removed.

With a stove-heated pressing comb (nonelectrical), remove the carbon by rubbing the outside surface and between the teeth with a fine steel wool pad or fine sandpaper. Then place the metal portion of the comb in a hot baking soda solution for about 1 hour; rinse and dry. The metal will acquire a smooth and shiny appearance.

PRESSING OIL OR CREAM

Prepare the hair for a hair pressing treatment by first applying pressing oil or cream. Both of these products have the following effects:

- Make hair softer
- Prepare and condition the hair for pressing

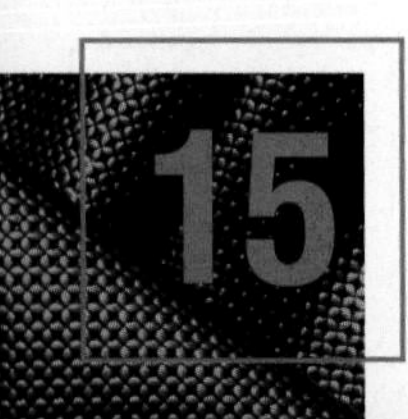

PROCEDURE 15-15

SOFT PRESSING FOR NORMAL CURLY HAIR

IMPLEMENTS AND MATERIALS

- Shampoo
- Towels
- Shampoo and styling capes
- Neck strip
- Pressing comb
- Clips
- Pressing oil or cream
- Hairbrush and comb
- Spatula
- Pomade
- Thermal iron

PREPARATION

1. Drape the client for shampooing.
2. Shampoo, rinse, and towel-dry the client's hair.
3. Drape the client for thermal styling, using a neck strip and styling cape.
4. Apply pressing oil or cream (some stylists prefer to apply pressing oil or cream to the hair after it has been completely dried) (Figure 15-176).
5. Dry hair thoroughly (blow-drying will leave the hair more manageable than hood drying).
6. Comb and divide the hair into four main sections and pin them up (Figure 15-177).

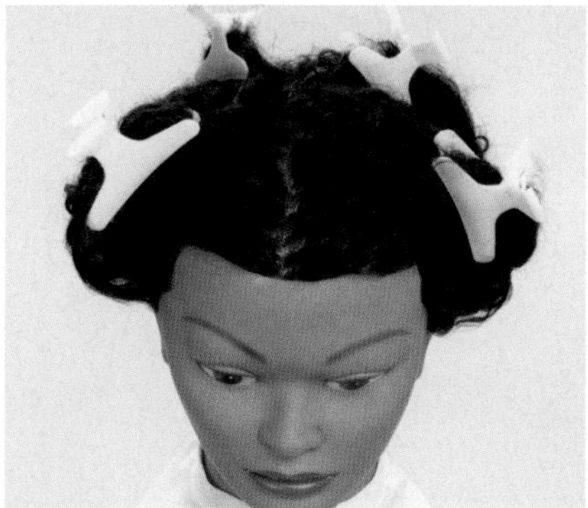

Figure 15-177 Divide hair into four sections.

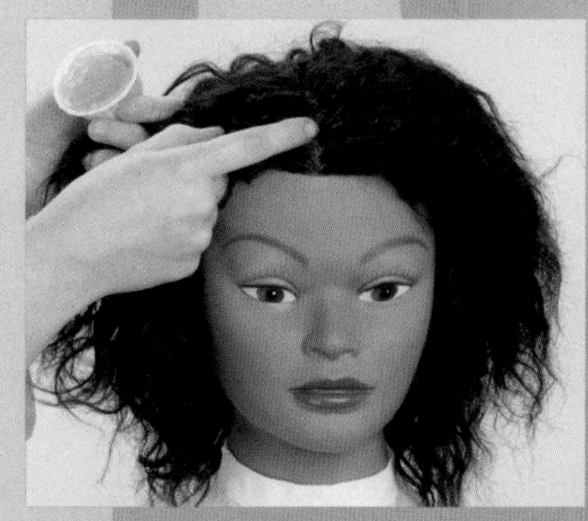

Figure 15-177 Apply pressing oil or cream to the client's hair.

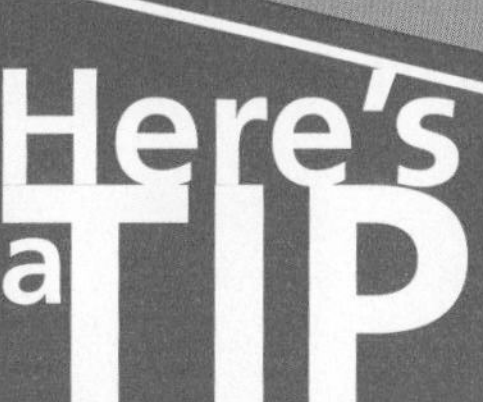

Subdivide the sections into 1-inch to 1½ inch (2.5 to 3.75 centimeters) partings, depending on the texture and density of the hair. For medium-textured hair of average density, use subsections of average size. For coarse hair with greater density, use smaller sections to ensure complete heat penetration and effectiveness.

For thin or fine hair with sparse density, use larger sections.

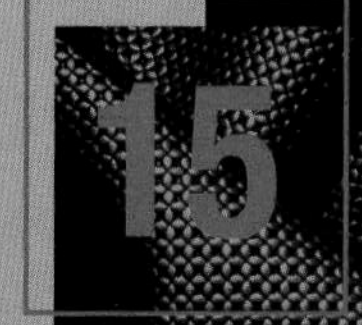

The following procedure is one of several ways to give a hair pressing treatment. Keep in mind that you can adjust the procedure according to the methods your instructor demonstrates.

1. Heat the pressing comb.
2. **Unpin section.** Unpin one section of the hair at a time and subdivide into smaller partings. Beginning at the right side of the head, work from front to back (some stylists prefer to start at the back of the head and work forward) (Figure 15-178).
3. If necessary, apply pressing oil evenly and sparingly over the small hair sections.
4. **Test temperature of iron.** Test the temperature of the heated pressing comb on a white cloth or white paper to determine heat intensity before you place it on the hair (Figure 15-179).
5. **Lift end of hair.** Lift the end of a small hair section with the index finger and thumb of the left hand and hold it upward, away from the scalp.
6. **Insert teeth of comb.** Holding the pressing comb in the right hand, insert the teeth of the comb into the top side of the hair section (Figure 15-180).
7. **Draw out comb.** Draw out the pressing comb slightly, and make a quick turn so that the hair strand wraps itself partly around the comb. The back rod of the comb actually does the pressing (Figure 15-181).

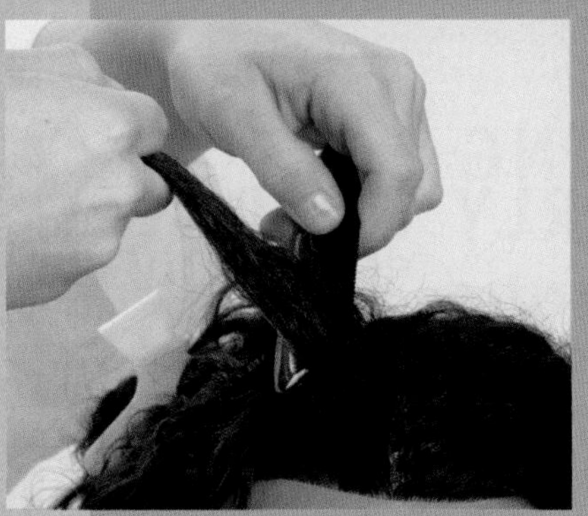

Figure 15-178 Unpin one section.

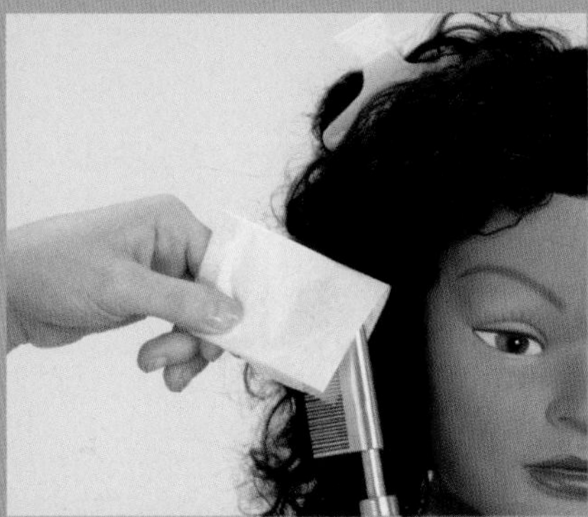

Figure 15-179 Test heated pressing comb.

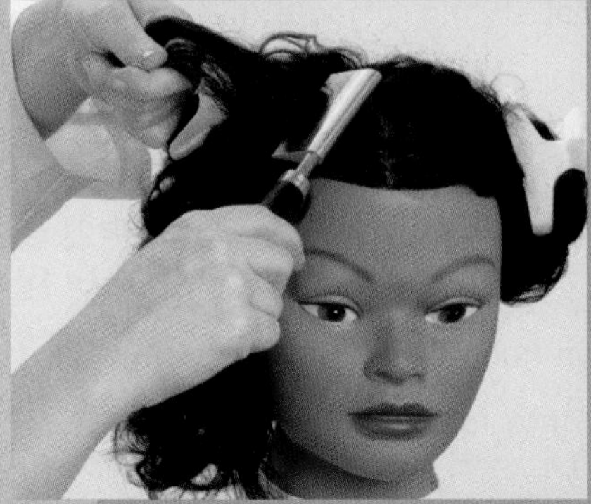

Figure 15-180 Insert comb into top side of hair section.

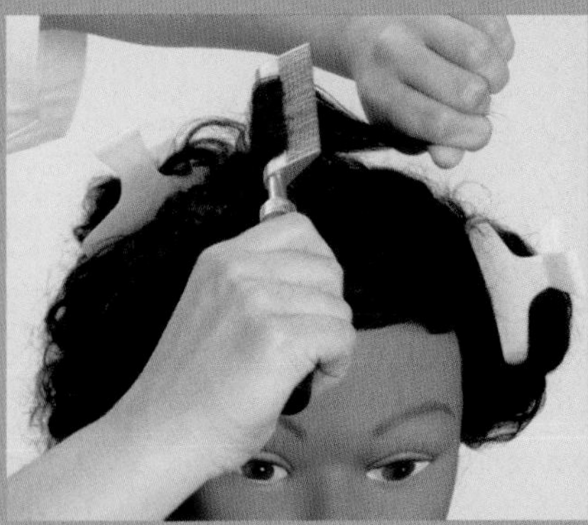

Figure 15-181 Press hair strand with back rod of comb.

8. **Press through hair strand.** Press the comb slowly through the hair strand until the ends of the hair pass through the teeth of the comb (Figure 15-182).
9. Bring each completed hair section over to the opposite side of the head (Figure 15-183).
10. **Continue.** Continue Steps 4 to 8 on both sections on the right side of the head, and then do the same on both sections on the left side.
11. **Apply pomade.** Apply a little pomade to the hair near the scalp and brush it through the hair. If desired, the hair can be curled with a curling iron at this time.
12. Style and comb the hair according to the client's wishes (Figure 15-184).

CLEANUP AND SANITATION

1. Discard disposable items. Disinfect brush and comb.
2. Clean the pressing comb (see Procedure 5-1 Disinfecting Nonelectrical Tools and Equipment in chapter 5)
3. Sanitize your workstation.
4. Wash hands with soap and warm water.

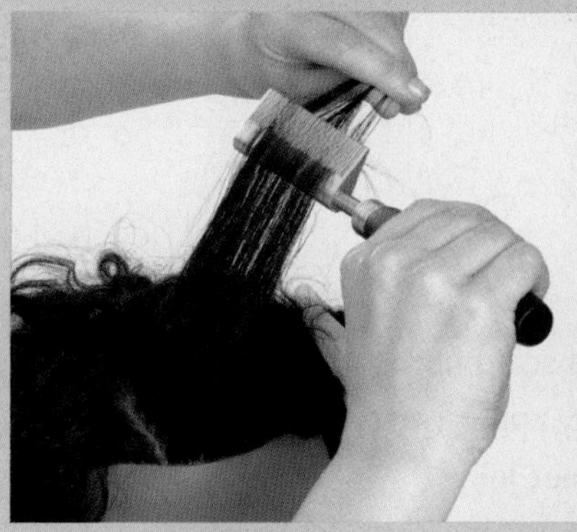

Figure 15-182 Bring pressing comb through ends of hair.

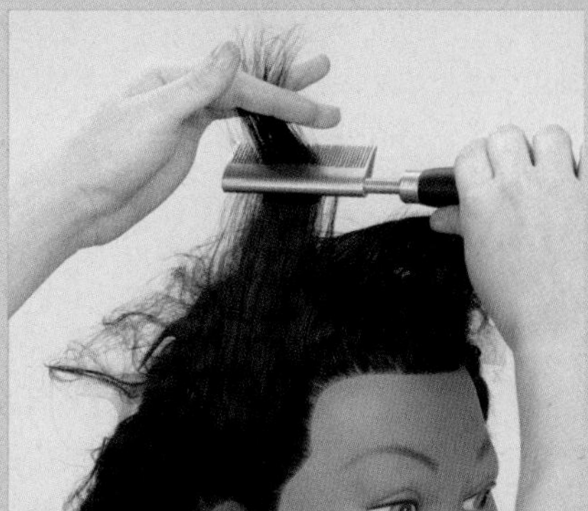

Figure 15-183 Bring finished section to one side.

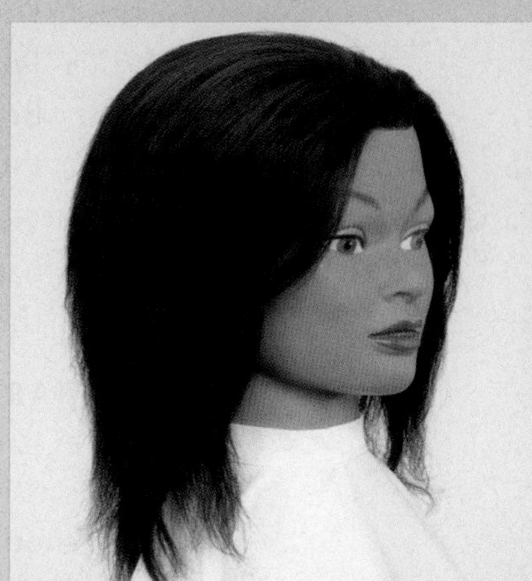

Figure 15-184 Finished pressed hairstyle.

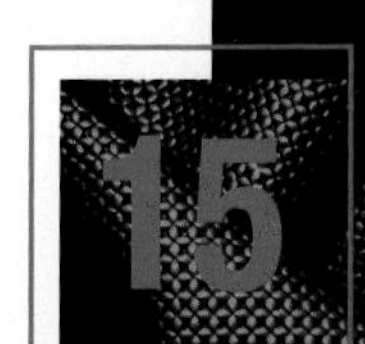

CAUTION

In case of a scalp burn, immediately apply 1-percent gentian violet jelly.

- Help prevent the hair from burning or scorching
- Help prevent hair breakage
- Condition the hair after pressing
- Add sheen to pressed hair
- Help hair stay pressed longer

REMINDERS AND HINTS ON ALL PRESSING

Good judgment should be used to avoid damage, with consideration always given to the texture of the hair and condition of the scalp. The client's safety is ensured only when the stylist observes every precaution and is especially careful during the actual hair pressing. Listed below are do's and don'ts:

- Avoid excessive heat or pressure on the hair and scalp.
- Avoid too much pressing oil on the hair (it attracts dirt and makes the hair look greasy and artificial).
- Avoid perfumed pressing oil near the scalp if the client is allergic.
- Avoid overly frequent hair pressing.
- Keep the comb clean at all times.
- Avoid overheating the pressing comb if using a stove.
- Test the temperature of the heated comb on a white cloth or paper before applying it to the hair.
- Adjust the temperature of the pressing comb to the texture and condition of the client's hair.
- Use the heated comb carefully to avoid burning the skin, scalp, or hair.
- Prevent the smoking or burning of hair during the pressing treatment by drying the hair completely after it is shampooed, and avoiding excessive application of pressing oil over the hair.
- Use a moderately warm comb to press short hair on the temples and back of the neck. You may also use a temple comb, which is about half the size of a regular pressing comb.

HARD PRESS

A hard press is only recommended when the results of a soft press are not satisfactory. The entire comb press procedure is repeated. Pressing oil should be added to hair strands only if necessary. A hard press is also known as a double-comb press.

TOUCH-UPS

Touch-ups are sometimes necessary when the hair becomes curly again due to perspiration, dampness, or other conditions. The process is the same as for the original pressing treatment, with the shampoo omitted.

SAFETY PRECAUTIONS

Two types of injuries that can occur in hair pressing:

1. Injuries that are the immediate result of hair pressing and that cause physical damage, such as burned hair that breaks off, burned scalp that causes either temporary or permanent loss of hair, and burns on the ears and neck that form scars.

2. Injuries that are not immediately evident but can later cause physical damage, such as a skin rash if the client is allergic to pressing oil, or the breaking and shortening of the hair due to many frequent hair pressings.

SPECIAL CONSIDERATIONS

You should take certain precautions and safeguards when dealing with the following special situations.

- Pressing fine hair. Follow the same procedure as for normal hair, while avoiding the use of a hot pressing comb or too much pressure. To avoid hair breakage, apply less pressure to the hair near the ends. After completely pressing the hair, style it.
- Pressing short, fine hair. Extra care must be taken at the hairline. When the hair is extra short, the pressing comb should not be too hot because the hair is fine and will burn easily; a hot comb can also cause accidental burns, which are very painful and can cause scars. In the event of an accidental burn, immediately apply 1-percent gentian violet jelly to the burn.
- Pressing coarse hair. Apply enough pressure so that the hair remains straightened.
- Pressing tinted, lightened, or gray (unpigmented) hair. This hair requires special care. Lightened or tinted hair might require conditioning treatments, depending on the extent to which it has been damaged. Gray hair may be particularly resistant. To obtain good results, use a moderately heated pressing comb applied with light pressure. Avoid excessive heat as discoloration or breakage can occur.

STYLING LONG HAIR

An **updo** is a hairstyle with the hair arranged up and off the shoulders, and secured with implements such as hairpins, bobby pins, and elastics. Clients usually request updos for special occasions such as weddings, proms, and evening events. A few popular updo styles are described below.

- **Chignon.** A true classic that has been popular for centuries. It is created out of a simple ponytail and can be dressed up with flowers or ornaments, or kept simple. If the client's hair is very straight and silky, you will have to first set the hair for 10 minutes in electric rollers, or the style will not last. If the hair is wavy or curly, blow-dry the hair straight. If it is extremely curly, you could press the hair first, or leave it natural for a textured-looking chignon.
- **Basic French twist.** This elegant, sleek look can go anywhere. If you are working on straight, fine hair, you may want to first set the hair in electric or Velcro rollers to give it more body.

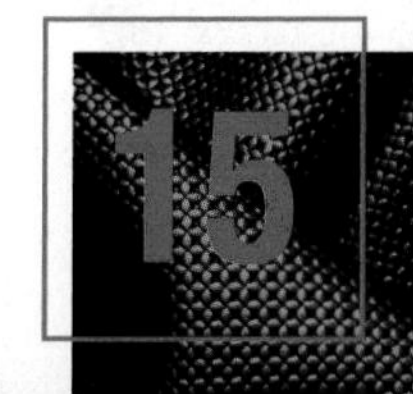

- **Classic French twist.** The traditional way to style a French twist, mostly for weddings and black-tie events. The shape is much larger than the basic twist, and you can be more creative with the front area. When executing an updo, always inspect the shape you are building from every angle to make sure that it is well balanced and well proportioned.

CLIENT CONSULTATION

As always, consult with the client first to make sure you understand what she has in mind. Have on hand magazines that show a lot of updos, such as bridal magazines, or keep a folder of pictures clipped from magazines at your station that show current styles. If you are doing a pre-bridal consultation with a bride, always suggest that she come in with her headpiece, so that she can try several styles, to see how they look. Take photographs to help decide which style she likes best. Classic styles are timeless and are better for brides; leave the latest trend for the bridesmaids. This suggestion will be appreciated years later. Keep the photo of the chosen style so that you can duplicate it for her big day.

CHIGNON

IMPLEMENTS AND MATERIALS

- Neck strip
- Styling cape
- Electric or Velcro rollers
- Grooming or teasing brush
- Bobby pins, hairpins
- Elastics
- Working hair spray
- Finishing spray
- Curling iron
- Tail comb

PREPARATION

1. Drape the client; shampoo and towel-dry the hair.
2. Redrape the client with a neck strip and styling cape.
3. Apply the appropriate styling product that will give the hair a lot of hold. Blow-dry the hair, smoothing it with a brush for a sleek finish.
4. Set hair in electric rollers or Velcro rollers, depending on the amount of curl or volume you may need.

PROCEDURE

1. **Part hair.** Using a grooming bristle brush, part the hair on whichever side you choose, and brush it into a low ponytail at the nape (Figure 15-185).
2. **Secure ponytail.** Secure the ponytail with an elastic band, keeping the hair as smooth as possible. Use the side of the bristles on the brush to smooth the hair. Place two bobby pins onto the band and spread them apart, one on each side (Figure 15-186). Place one bobby pin in the base of the ponytail. Stretch the band around the ponytail base. Place the second bobby pin in the base. Lock the two pins together (Figure 15-187).
3. **Part the hair.** Part a small section of hair from the underside of the ponytail, wrap it around the ponytail to cover the elastic, and secure with a bobby pin underneath (Figure 15-188).

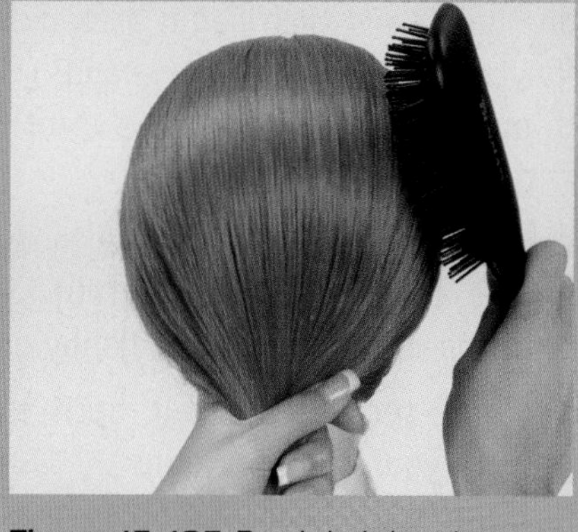

Figure 15-185 Brush hair into low ponytail.

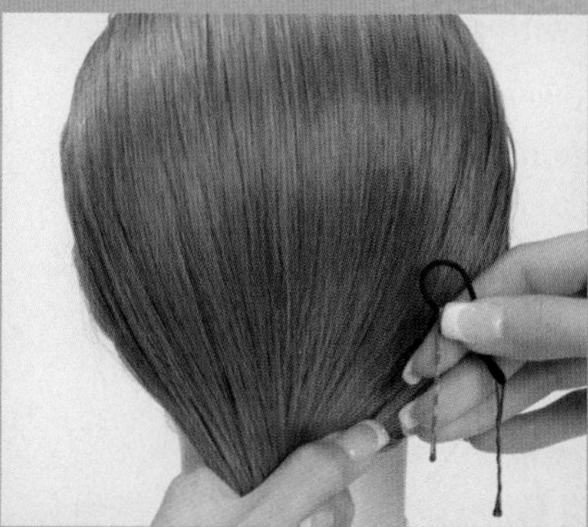

Figure 15-186 Elastic band and bobby pins.

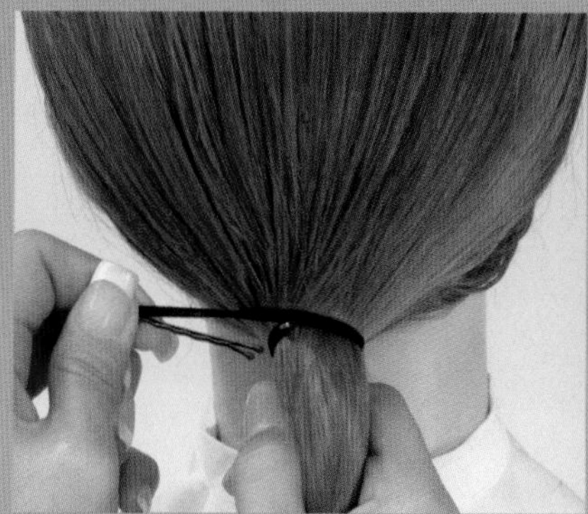

Figure 15-187 Lock bobby pins together around ponytail base.

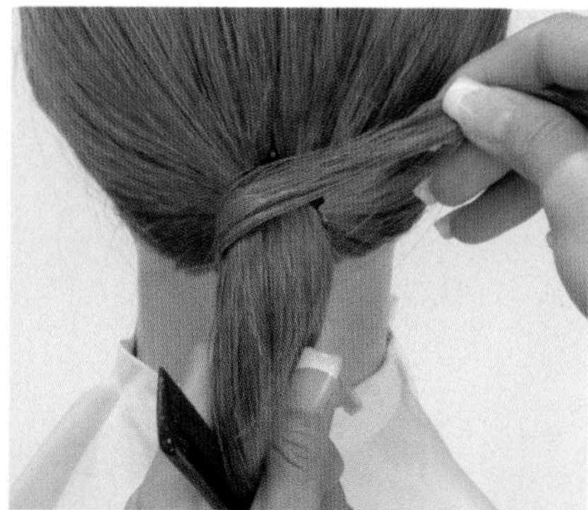

Figure 15-188 Pin-wrapped section under.

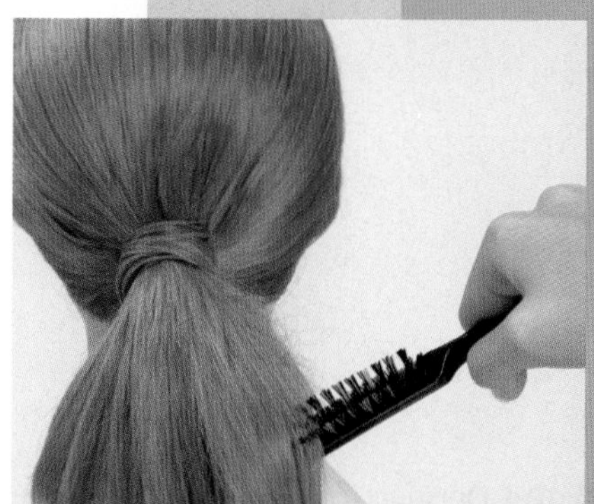

Figure 15-189 Back-brush the ponytail.

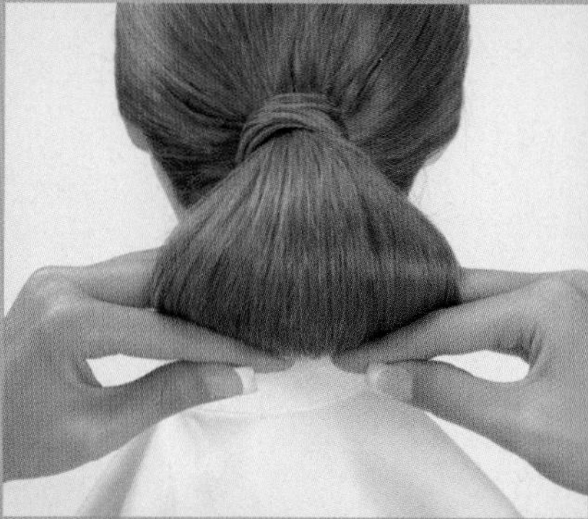

Figure 15-190 Roll the hair toward the head.

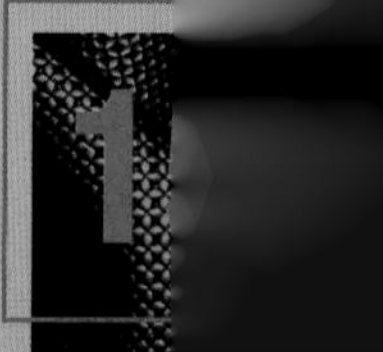

4. **Smooth and back-brush.** Smooth out the ponytail and hold it with one hand, and then begin back-brushing from underneath the ponytail with your other hand (Figure 15-189). Gently smooth out the ponytail after back-brushing, using the sides of the bristles.
5. **Roll under and secure.** Roll the hair under and toward the head to form the chignon (Figure 15-190). Secure on the left and right undersides of the roll with bobby pins (Figure 15-191).
6. **Fan out and secure.** Fan out both sides by spreading the chignon with your fingers (Figure 15-192). Secure with hairpins, pinning close to the head. Use bobby pins if more hold is needed (Figure 15-193).
7. Finish with a strong finishing spray.
8. Add flowers or a hair ornament to dress up the chignon (Figures 15-194 and 195).

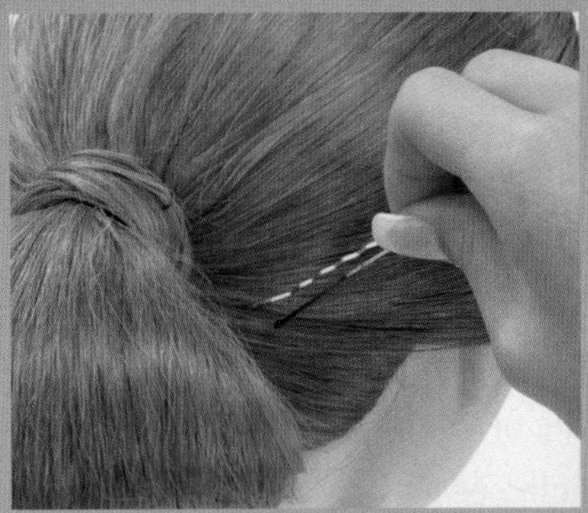

Figure 15-191 Pin the right side.

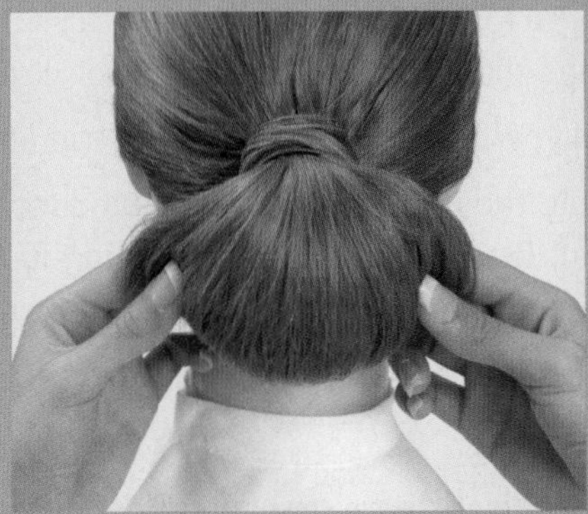

Figure 15-192 Spread out the sides.

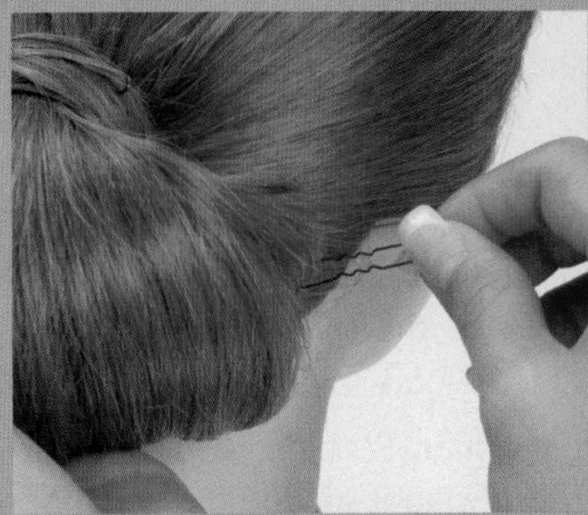

Figure 15-193 Pin the sides.

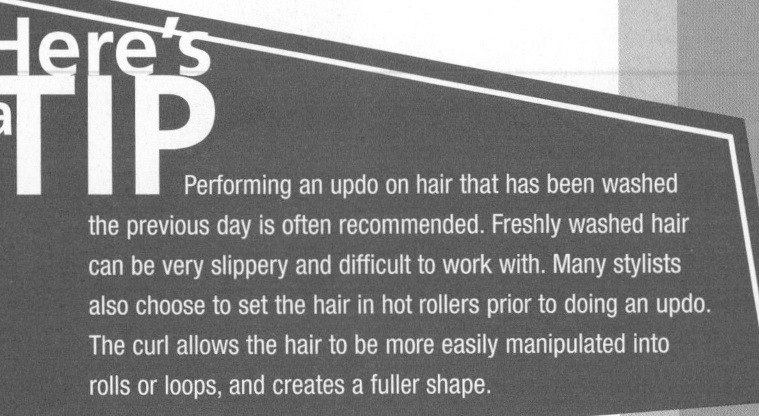

Here's a TIP Performing an updo on hair that has been washed the previous day is often recommended. Freshly washed hair can be very slippery and difficult to work with. Many stylists also choose to set the hair in hot rollers prior to doing an updo. The curl allows the hair to be more easily manipulated into rolls or loops, and creates a fuller shape.

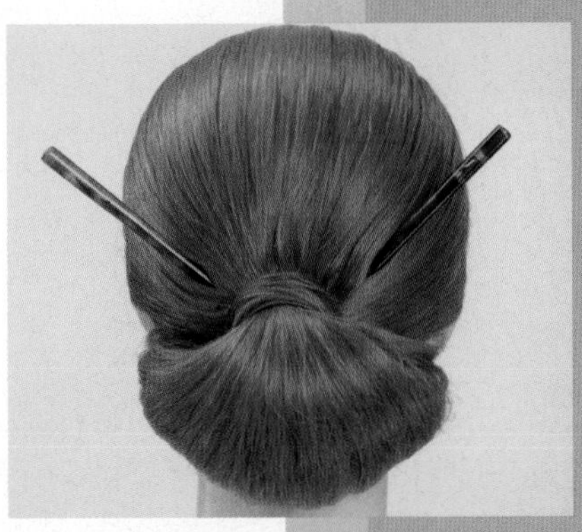

Figure 15-194 Finished chignon.

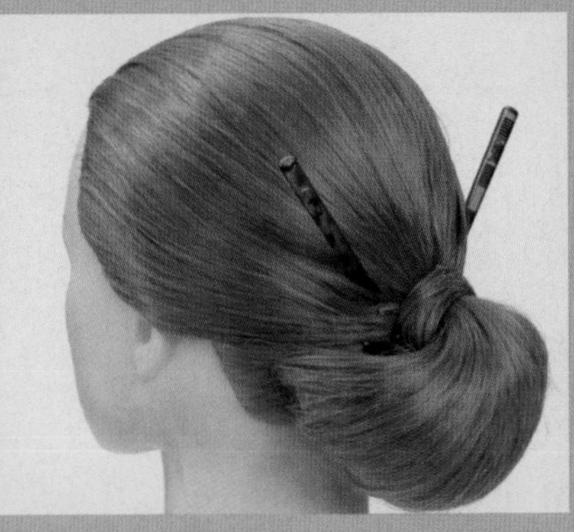

Figure 15-195 Side view of finished chignon.

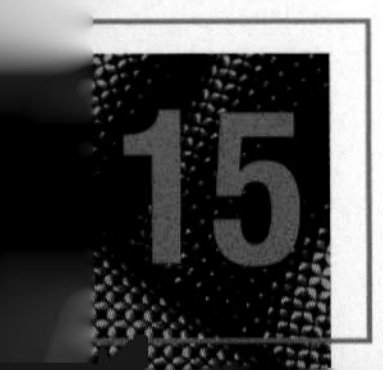

PROCEDURE 15-17

BASIC FRENCH TWIST

IMPLEMENTS AND PREPARATION

Same as for chignon.

PROCEDURE

1. Brush all the hair smoothly into a ponytail at the occipital bone (Figure 15-196).
2. **Reach in front.** With your free hand, reach in front of the hand that is holding the ponytail, with the thumb pointing down toward the client's nape (Figure 15-197).
3. **Move hair inward and upward.** Grab the ponytail with your thumb still pointing down and twist the hair in the direction in which your palm is facing, moving the hair inward and upward (Figure 15-198).
4. **Twist the hair.** As you move toward the crown, twist the hair into a funnel shape and secure the twist with hairpins by pinning into the seam, making sure not to expose the pins (Figures 15-199 and 200).
5. Tuck the ends into the top of the funnel of the twist near the crown (Figures 15-201 and 15-202).
6. **Fan out hair ends.** For a less formal or younger look, let the hair ends fan out and fall loosely over the sides of the twist, instead of tucking them into the top of the twist. Another option is to form curls, loops, or knots with the hair at the top of the twist (Figure 15-203).

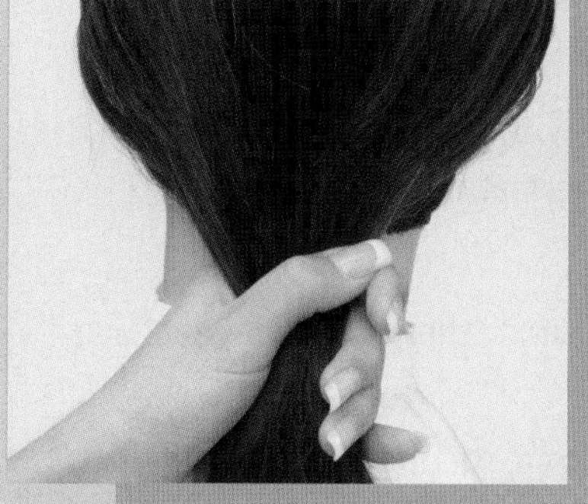

Figure 15-196 Brush hair out from the occipital.

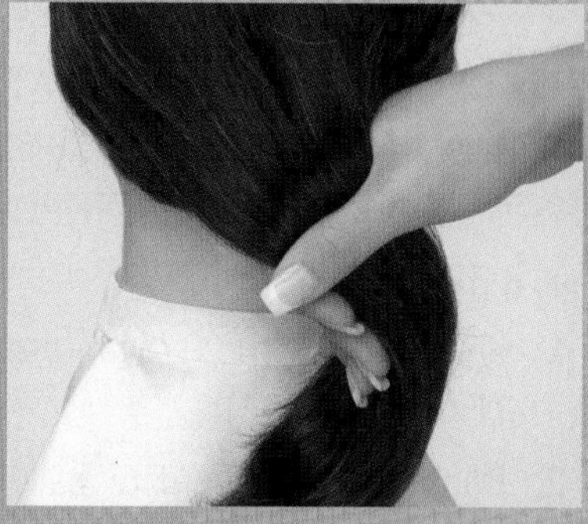

Figure 15-197 Reach over and grab the ponytail.

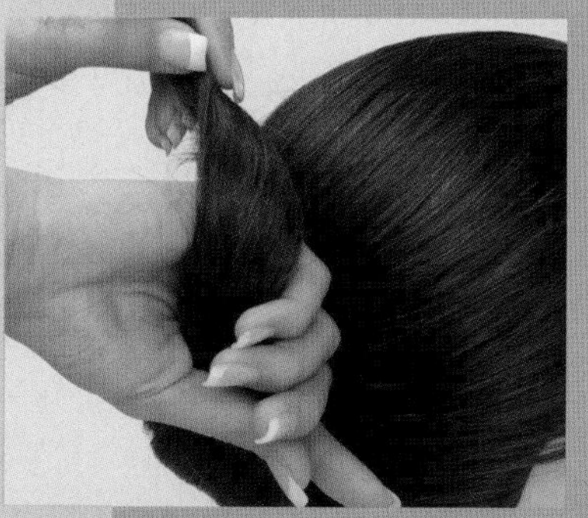

Figure 15-198 Twist the hair.

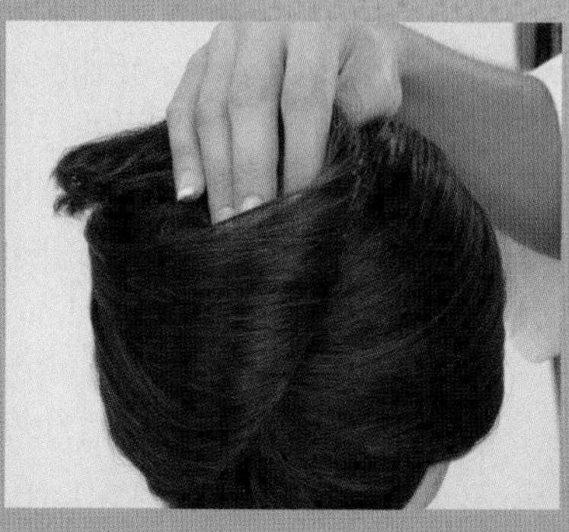

Figure 15-199 Create a funnel.

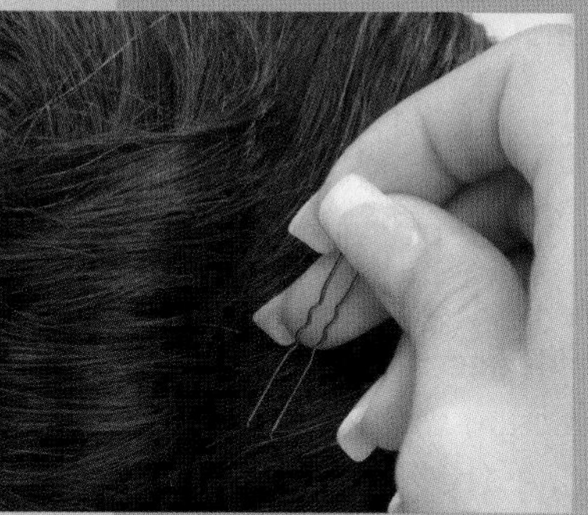

Figure 15-200 Pin into the seam.

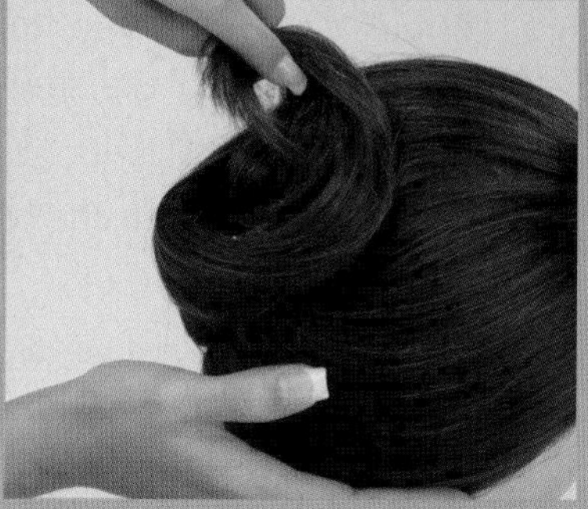

Figure 15-201 Tuck the ends into the top of the twist.

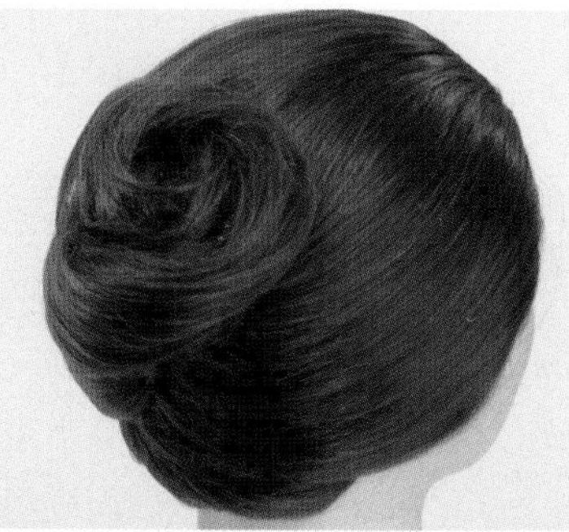

Figure 15-202 Completed basic French twist.

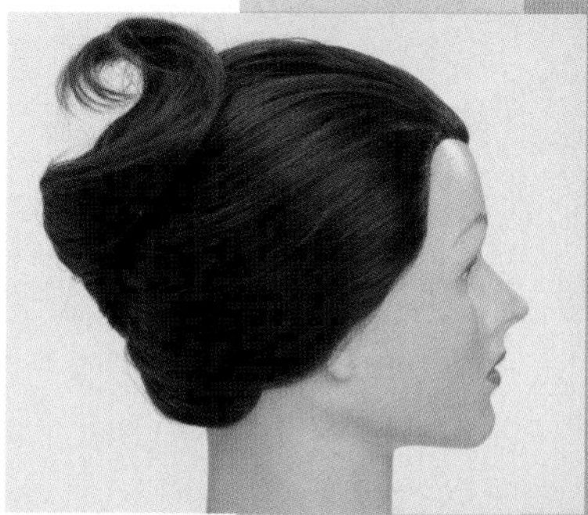

Figure 15-203 Option: form loops at the top of the twist.

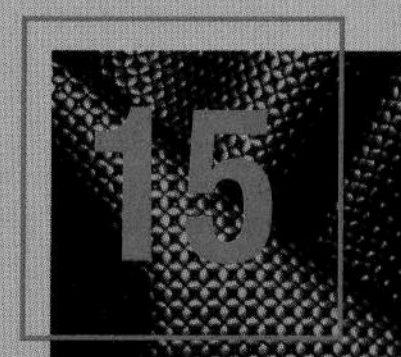

PROCEDURE 15-18

CLASSIC FRENCH TWIST

IMPLEMENTS AND PREPARATION

Same as for chignon. Set the hair with a wet set or, if you wish to save time, electric rollers or thermal irons.

PROCEDURE

1. Section off the crown area and the two side sections (Figure 15-204).
2. Back-comb the entire back area, taking vertical sections (Figure 15-205).
3. **Smooth hair.** Using the side bristles of a grooming brush or a teasing brush, gently smooth all the hair of the back section to one side of the head (in this example all the hair will move to the left). Hold the hair to that side by reaching over the client's head with your free hand.
4. **Pin hair.** Begin pinning the hair at the center of the nape, moving upward with bobby pins. Overlap the pins by criss-crossing them to lock into place. Repeat until you reach the back of the crown (Figure 15-206).
5. **Twist hair at nape.** With the brush, bring the hair from the left side over the center-line and twist from the center of the nape. Move upward and inward, tucking the ends into the fold as you move up, to create a funnel shape. Secure with hairpins into the seam as you move up, hiding the pins in the seam (Figure 15-207).
6. Tuck all the ends into the top of the twist and pin (Figure 15-208).
7. **Twist hair at side.** Move to a side section and lightly back-brush the section. Twist the section with the seam facing the back of the head, covering the part as you twist. Secure with a bobby pin at the top of the side section, leaving the ends out (Figures 15-209 and 15-210).

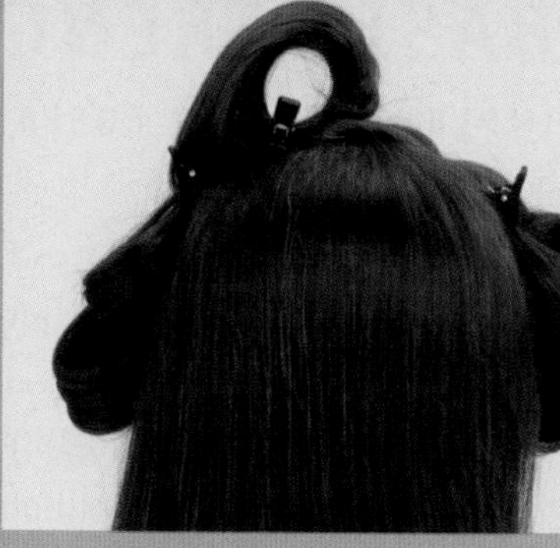

Figure 15-204 Sections.

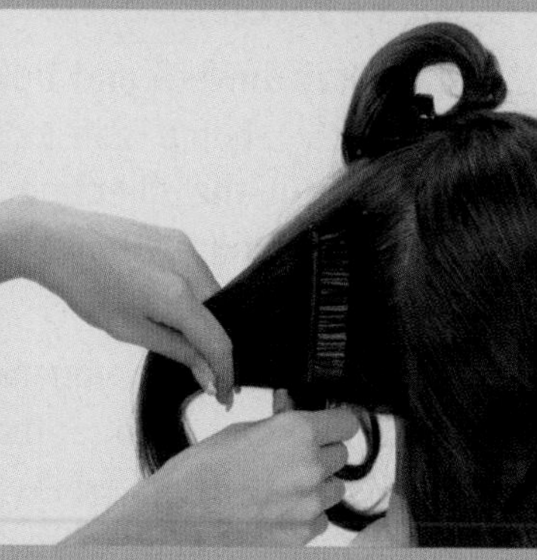

Figure 15-205 Back-comb vertical section.

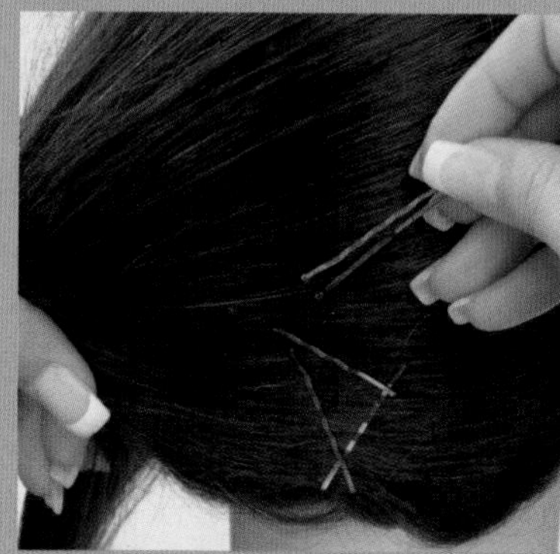

Figure 15-206 Criss-cross the bob pins.

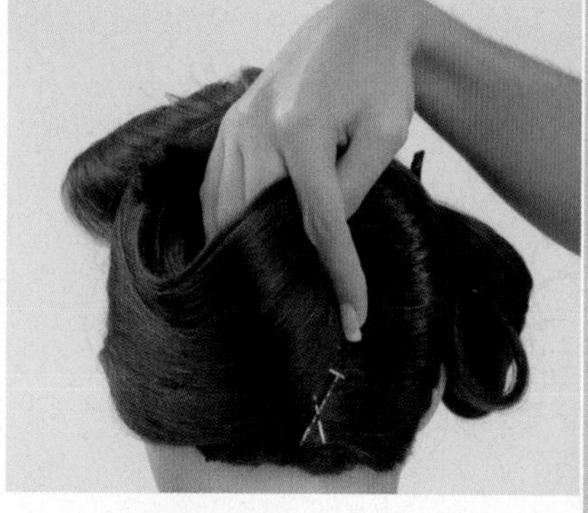

Figure 15-207 Twist and pin the hair.

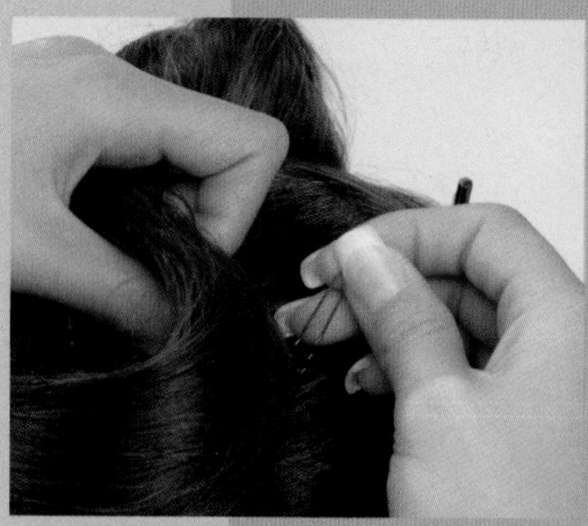

Figure 15-208 Completed center section.

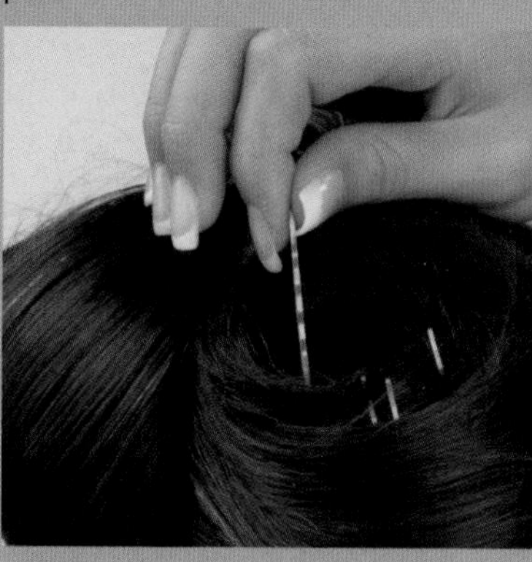

Figure 15-209 Twist the section.

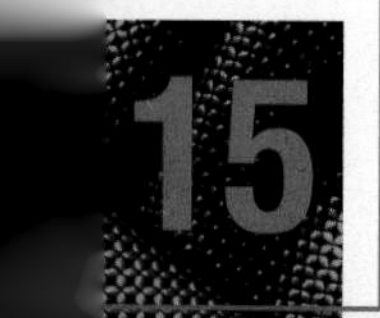

8. Repeat on the other side.
9. **Make three subsections.** Remove the sectioning clip from the top section. Make three subsections horizontally across the top of the head (Figure 15-211).
10. **Slice out a subsection.** Beginning with the section closest to the back of the crown, slice out a subsection about a third of the width of the horizontal section (Figure 15-212).
11. **Secure section.** Back-brush and smooth the subsection, using the sides of the brush bristles. Loop the section over your fingers and secure at the base of the loop on the scalp with a bobby pin. Take care not to expose the pin (Figure 15-213).
12. **Pin the loops.** Take the other two sections and form looped curls in the same manner. Pin the loops as close to the top of the twist as you can get, checking for balance and proportion.
13. Repeat with the center horizontal section, making two or three looped curls, depending on what the density of the hair will allow (Figure 15-214).
14. **Twist, loop, and pin side.** Go back to the side area, and with the hair remaining out from the side, twist, loop, and pin. Again, check in your mirror for balance and proportion.
15. **Style fringe.** Style the section in the front near the bangs (fringe) as you wish. This section could also be brought back and added to the other looped curls if your client is comfortable with all her hair off her face, or sweep the hair loosely to the side and leave the ends hanging softly down. Here is where your creativity comes into play as you make the best design decision for your client (Figures 15-215, 15-216, 15-217).
16. Spray with a firm-hold finishing spray, and check to make sure there are no exposed pins.

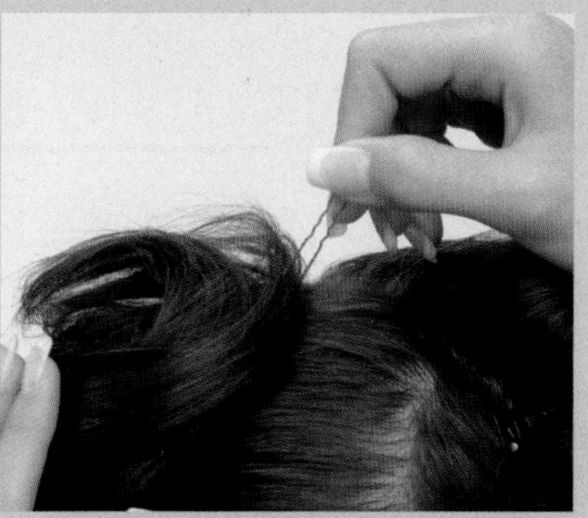

Figure 15-210 Pin the top.

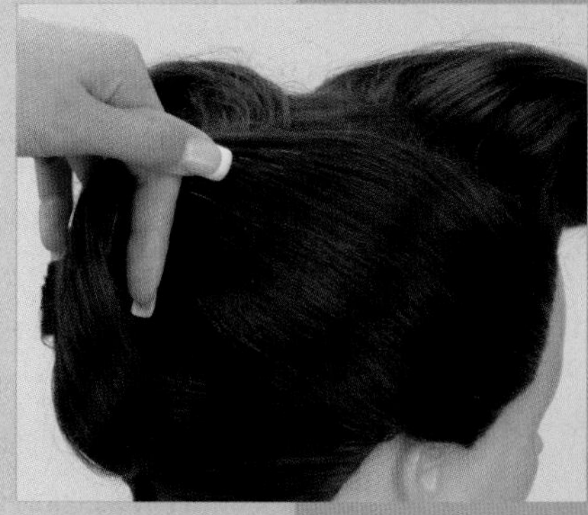

Figure 15-211 Subsections on top of the head.

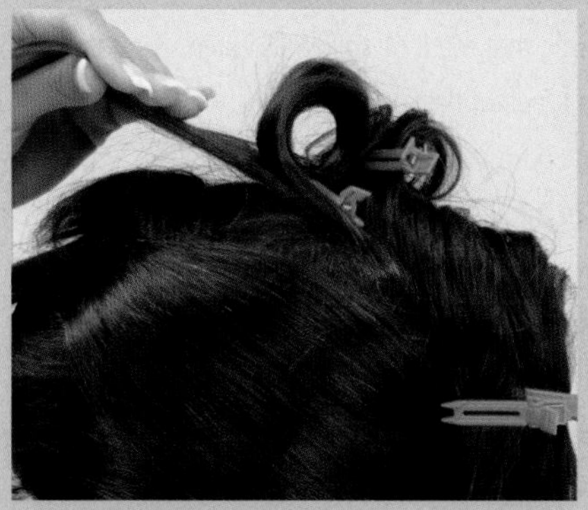

Figure 15-212 Hold out a third of the back section.

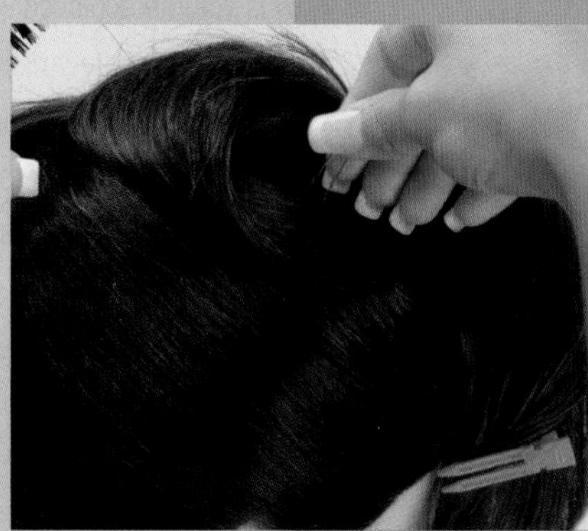

Figure 15-213 Loop hair over fingers.

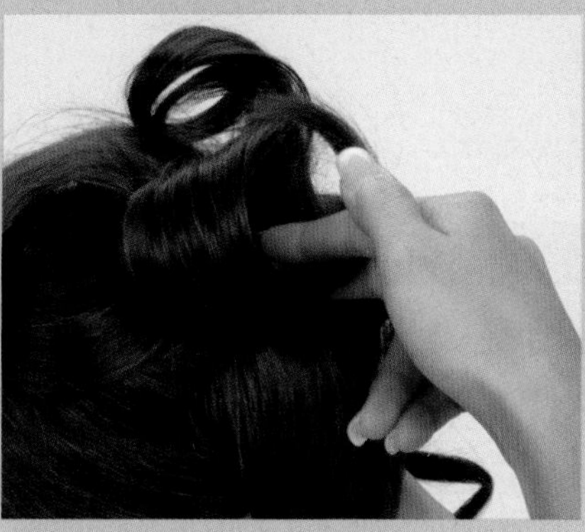

Figure 15-214 Loop the center section.

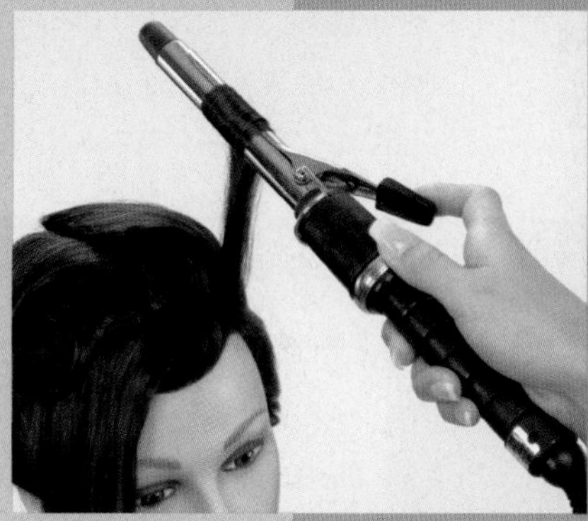

Figure 15-215 Front section curled back.

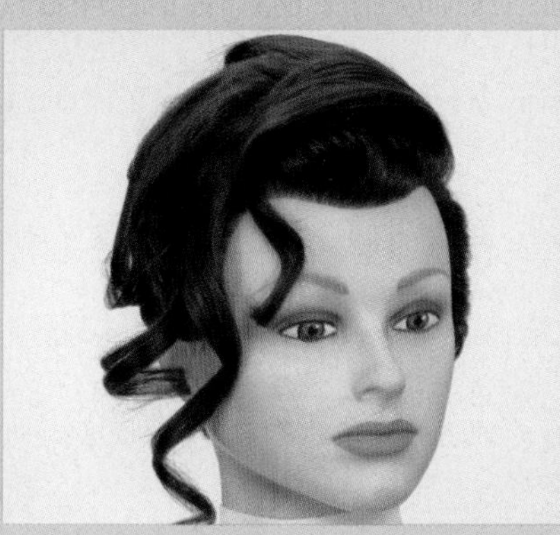

Figure 15-216 Finished classic French twist.

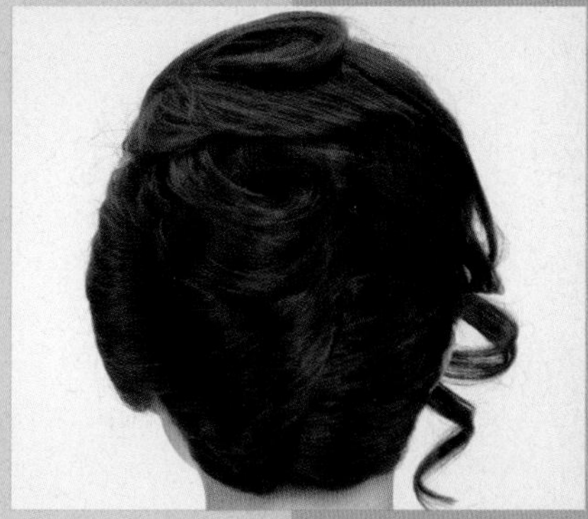

Figure 15-217 Side view of finished classic French twist.

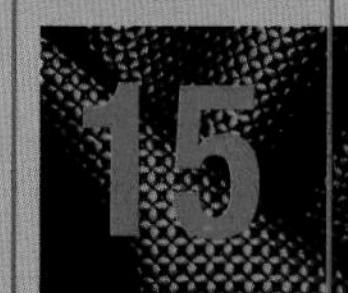

REVIEW QUESTIONS

1. What is the purpose of finger waving?
2. What are the three parts of a pin curl?
3. Name the four pin curl bases and their uses.
4. Describe the three kinds of roller curl bases and the uses of each.
5. What is the purpose of back-combing and back-brushing?
6. How can you avoid burning the client's scalp during blow-drying?
7. List and describe the various styling products used in blow-dry styling.
8. How is volume achieved with thermal curls?
9. List at least 10 safety measures that must be followed when using thermal irons.
10. Name and describe the three types of hair presses.
11. How do you test the pressing comb before beginning a service?
12. What are the considerations in a hair and scalp analysis prior to hair pressing?
13. Under what circumstances should hair not be pressed?
14. List at least four safety measures that must be followed when pressing the hair.

CHAPTER GLOSSARY

back-brushing	Technique used to build a soft cushion or mesh two or more curl patterns together for a uniform and smooth comb-out; also called ruffing.
back-combing	Combing small sections of hair from the ends toward the scalp, causing shorter hair to mat at the scalp and form a cushion or base; also called teasing, ratting, matting, or French lacing.
barrel curls	Pin curls with large center openings, fastened to the head in a standing position on a rectangular base.
base	Stationary, or nonmoving, foundation of a pin curl, which is the area closest to the scalp; the panel of hair on which a roller is placed.
blow-dry styling	Technique of drying and styling damp hair in a single operation.
carved curls	Pin curls sliced from a shaping and formed without lifting the hair from the head.
cascade or stand-up curls	Pin curls fastened to the head in a standing position to allow the hair to flow upward and then downward.
circle	The part of the pin curl that forms a complete circle; also, the hair that is wrapped around the roller.
closed-center curls	Pin curls that produce waves that get smaller toward the end.

CHAPTER GLOSSARY

curl	Hair that is wrapped around the roller; also called circle.
concentrator	Nozzle attachment of a blow-dryer; directs the air stream to any section of the hair more intensely.
diffuser	Blow-dryer attachment that causes the air to flow more softly and helps to accentuate or keep textural definition.
double press	Technique of passing a hot curling iron through the hair before performing a hard press.
end curls	Used to give a finished appearance to hair ends either turned under or over.
finger waving	Process of shaping and directing the hair into in a pattern of "S"-shaped waves through the use of the fingers, combs, and waving lotion.
finishing spray	Hairspray used to lock in a style after completion.
foam or mousse	A light, airy, whipped styling product that resembles shaving foam and builds moderate body and volume into the hair.
full-base curls	Thermal curls that sit in the center of their base; strong curls with full volume.
full-stem curl	Curl placed completely off the base; allows for the greatest mobility.
gel	Thickened styling preparation that comes in a tube or bottle and has a strong hold.
hair pressing	Method of temporarily straightening extremely curly or unruly hair by means of a heated iron or comb.
hair spray	A styling product applied in the form of a mist to hold a style in position; available in a variety of holding strengths.
hair wrapping	A technique used to keep curly hair smooth and straight.
half base	Position of a curl or a roller one-half off its base, giving medium volume and movement.
half-base curls	Thermal curls placed half off their base; strong curls with moderate lift or volume.
half-stem curl	Curl (circle) placed half off the base; permits medium movement and gives good control to the hair.
hard press	Technique that removes 100 percent of the curl by applying the pressing comb twice on each side of the hair.
indentation	The point where curls of opposite directions meet forming a recessed area.
liquid gels or texturizers	Styling products that are lighter and more viscous or sticky than firm-hold gels, used for easy styling, defining, and molding.
medium press	Technique removing 60 percent to 75 percent of the curl by applying a thermal pressing comb once on each side of the hair using slightly more pressure than in the soft press.
no-stem curl	Curl placed directly on its base; produces a tight, firm, long-lasting curl and allows minimum mobility.
off base	The position of a curl or a roller completely off its base for maximum mobility and minimum volume.

CHAPTER GLOSSARY

off-base curls	Thermal curls placed completely off their base; have only slight lift or volume.
on base	Position of a curl or roller directly on its base for maximum volume; also called full base.
open-center curls	Pin curls that produce even, smooth waves and uniform curls.
pomade or wax	Styling products that add considerable weight to the hair by causing strands to join together, showing separation in the hair.
ribboning	Technique of forcing the hair between the thumb and the back of the comb to create tension.
ridge curls	Pin curls placed immediately behind or below a ridge to form a wave.
rod	Round, solid prong of a thermal iron.
shaping	Section of hair that is molded in a circular movement in preparation for the formation of curls.
shell	The clamp that presses the hair against the barrel or rod of a thermal iron.
silicone	Styling product ingredient that adds gloss and sheen to the hair while creating textural definition.
skip waves	Two rows of ridge curls, usually on the side of the head.
soft press	Technique of pressing the hair to remove 50 to 60 percent of the curl by applying the thermal pressing comb once on each side of the hair.
spiral curl	Method of curling the hair by winding a strand around the rod.
stem	Section of the pin curl between the base and first arc (turn) of the circle that gives the circle its direction and movement; the hair between the scalp and the first turn of the roller.
straightening gel	Styling product applied to damp hair that is wavy, curly, or extremely curly, and then blown-dry; relaxes the hair for a smooth, straight look.
thermal irons	An implement comprised of a rod handle, shell handle, barrel or rod, and shell that is made of quality steel used to dry hair using heat.
thermal waving and curling	Methods of waving and curling straight or pressed hair using thermal irons and special manipulative curling techniques on dry hair.
updo	Hairstyle in which the hair is arranged up and off the shoulders.
volume-base curls	Thermal curls placed very high on their base; provide maximum lift or volume.
volumizer	Styling product that adds volume to the shape, especially at the base, when the hair is blow-dried.
waving lotion	Type of hair gel that makes the hair pliable enough to keep it in place during the finger waving procedure.

BRAIDING & BRAID EXTENSIONS CHAPTER 16

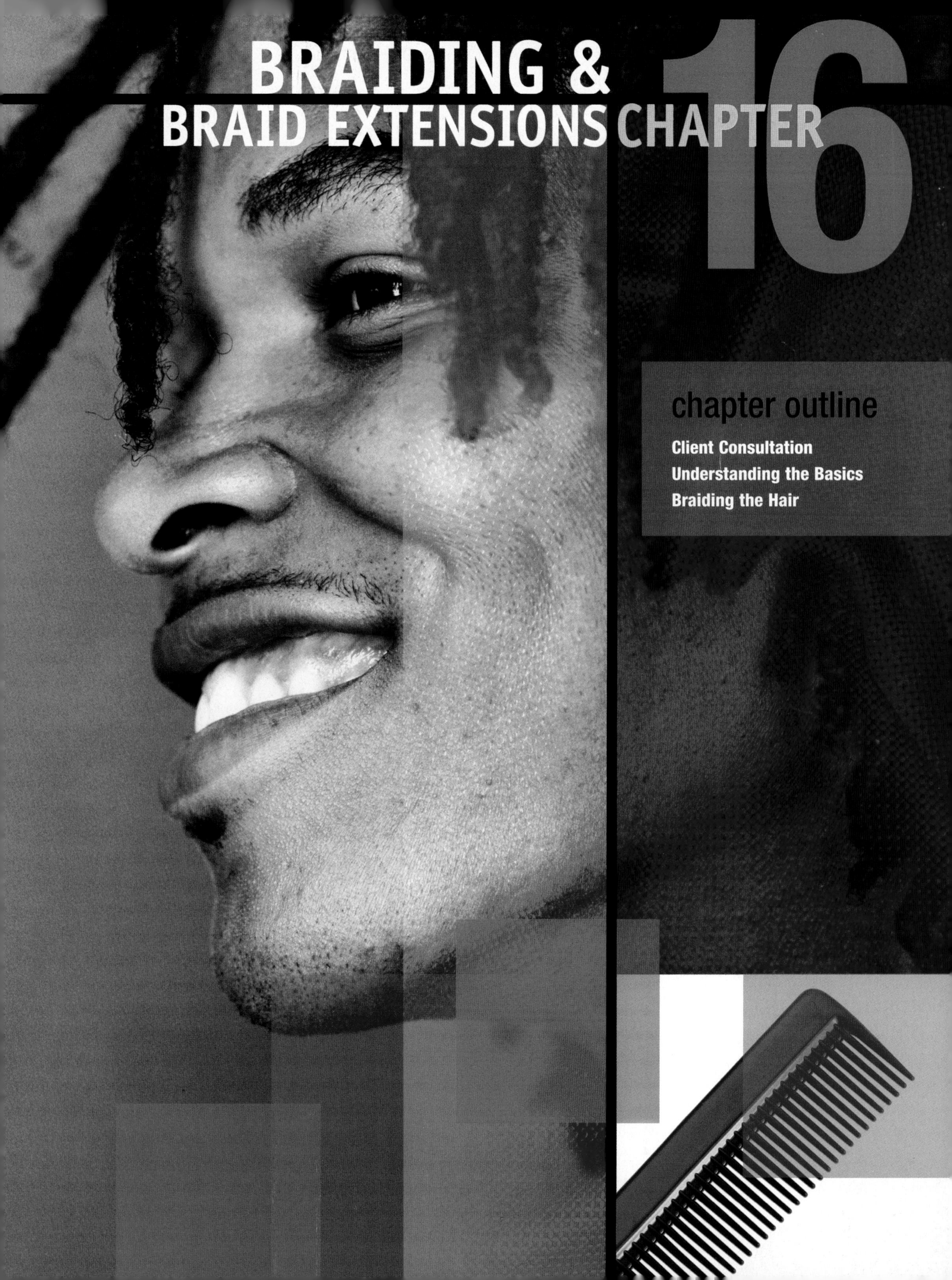

chapter outline

Learning Objectives

After completing this chapter, you will be able to:

- **Perform a client consultation and hair analysis with respect to hair braiding.**
- **Explain how to prepare the hair for braiding.**
- **Demonstrate the procedures for the invisible braid, rope braid, and fishtail braid.**
- **Demonstrate the procedures for single braids, with and without extensions.**
- **Demonstrate the procedures for cornrowing, with and without extensions.**

Key Terms

Page number indicates where in the chapter the term is used.

cornrows or canerows
pg. 383

fishtail braid
pg. 375

invisible or inverted braid
pg. 374

locks or dreadlocks
pg. 392

natural hairstyling
pg. 367

rope braid
pg. 375

single braids
pg. 375

visible braid
pg. 374

From its origins in Africa to its widespread use today, hair braiding has always played a significant role in grooming and beauty practices. In some African tribes, the statement made by a person's braiding went beyond mere appearance or fashion. Different styles of braiding signified a person's social status within the community. The more important a person was, the more elaborate his or her braiding would be. Today, braiding styles continue to communicate important signals about a person's self-esteem and self-image (Figure 16-1).

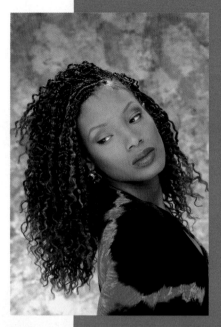

Figure 16-1 A contemporary braiding style.

Hair braiding reached its peak of social and aesthetic significance in Africa, where it has always been regarded as an art form to be handed down from generation to generation. This art form can require an enormous investment of time, with some elaborate styles taking up to an entire day to complete. Because braiding is so time consuming, it is regarded in many African cultures as an opportunity for women to socialize and form relationships.

In recent years, braiding salons have sprung up in many urban areas in the United States. These salons practice what is commonly known as **natural hairstyling,** which uses no chemicals or dyes, and does not alter the natural curl or coil pattern of the hair. While the origins of natural hairstyling are rooted in African-American heritage, people of all ethnicities can appreciate its beauty and versatility. In the 21st century, natural hairstyling has brought a new and diverse approach to hair care. It can be elaborate, or elegant yet simple. In all cases, offering your clients many different styles of braiding can inspire your creativity as a hair artist, and create a greater sense of client loyalty.

Some braiding styles can take many hours to complete. These more complex styles are not "disposable" hairdos to be casually washed away or brushed out. In fact, with proper care, a braiding pattern can last up to 3 months, with 6 to 8 weeks being preferable to preserve the health of the hair. The investment in time and money is high for both the client and stylist. As a stylist, the last thing you want is to spend hours on a braiding style, and have the client reject it and demand that all the braids be removed. Giving your clients a quality consultation is the best way to avoid misunderstandings and ensure a happy ending to every natural styling service. Always fill out a client card during the initial consultation, and update it every time the client returns.

CLIENT CONSULTATION

HAIR ANALYSIS

During the consultation, you will also be analyzing the condition of your client's hair and scalp. In terms of natural styling, you must be particularly aware of the texture (Figure 16-2). When we talk about braiding and other natural hairstyling, texture refers to the following three qualities.

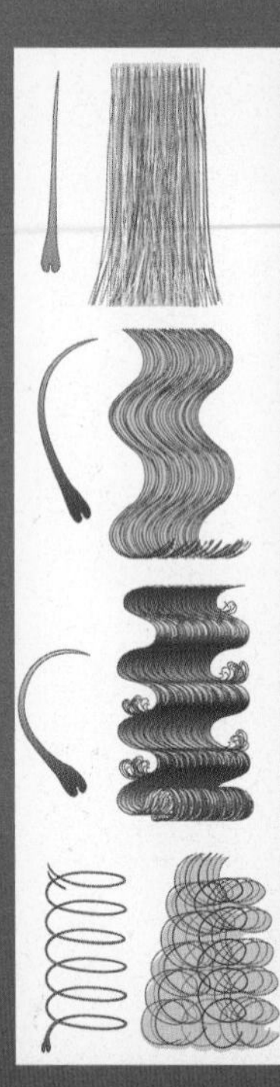

Figure 16-2 Wave pattern or coil onfiguration.

1. *Diameter of the hair.* Is the hair coarse, medium, or fine?
2. *Feel.* Does the hair feel oily, dry, hard, soft, smooth, coarse, or wiry?
3. *Wave pattern* or *coil configuration.* Is the hair straight, wavy, curly, or coiled?

Regarding the wave pattern, a coil is a very tight curl. It is spiral in formation and, when lengthened or stretched, resembles a series of loops. For the purposes of this chapter, "textured hair" has a tight coil pattern.

In addition to texture, consider the following:

- Density. Look for areas where the hair is thin.
- Condition. Check for damage and breakage from previous braids or chemical services.
- Length. Make sure that the hair is physically long enough to execute the braiding style.
- Check the condition of the scalp to ensure that it is healthy and properly cared for.

Carefully checking the hair and scalp is essential for a good outcome. If the hair has extremely thin areas, for instance, the braid thickness will be noticeably different in these areas. In addition, damaged hair should not be braided since it will further stress the hair. Because everyone has thinner, finer hair around the hairline, you should never choose styles that place direct tension in this area.

FACIAL SHAPES

When you assist the client in choosing a braid style, an important consideration is to determine what best complements the client's most attractive features. During the consultation, you should first observe the facial structure and any distinct facial features of the client. You will need to understand and appreciate the distinct characteristics of various ethnic groups, all of whom have their own particular brand of beauty.

As you have already learned, part of your role as a hairstylist is to recognize various facial shapes and features, accentuate attractive features, and try to camouflage less attractive features. The following list offers a general description of flattering braid styles for certain facial types and features:

- *Oval.* Most braided styles are appropriate for this facial shape (Figure 16-3).
- *Round.* When styling, add height to create the illusion of thinness (Figure 16-4). Updo braiding styles can also add length to the face. Braided styles with waves or full curls frame the face and help to create balance.
- *Square.* To create the illusion of length and to soften facial lines, choose full styles that frame the face around the forehead, temples, and jawline (Figure 16-5). Wisps of hair or a tapered fringe also help to soften angular lines.
- *Diamond.* Create styles that are full around the forehead or jawline to help create a more oval appearance (Figures 16-6 and 16-7). Full bangs (fringe) or partial bangs (fringe) will help counter a narrow forehead. Keep braids close to the head along the cheekbones to visually narrow this area. Avoid updo styles and styles that move away from the cheeks or hairline.
- *Triangular (pear-shaped).* Soft fringes around the forehead will camouflage a small forehead without closing up the face (Figures 16-8 and 16-9). Styles that frame the cheekbones and are close to the ears, or go behind the ears, can reduce a wide chin line.

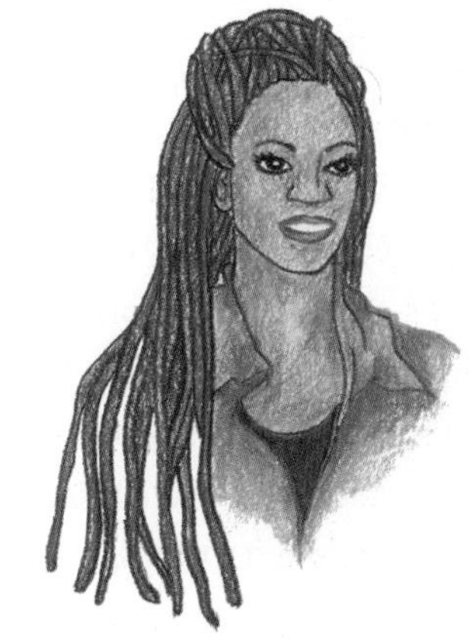

Figure 16-3 Oval face shape

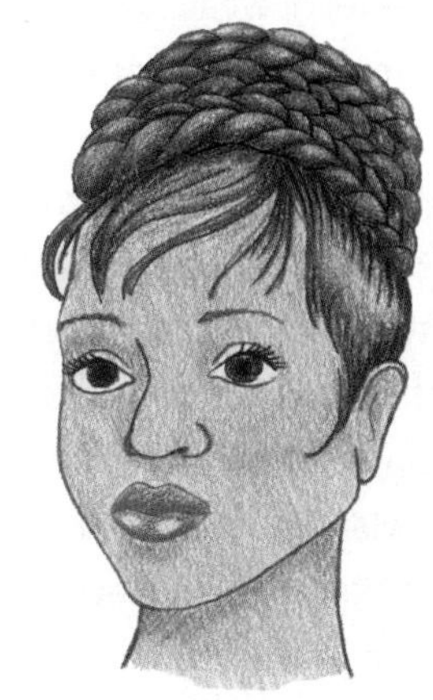

Figure 16-4 Round face shape.

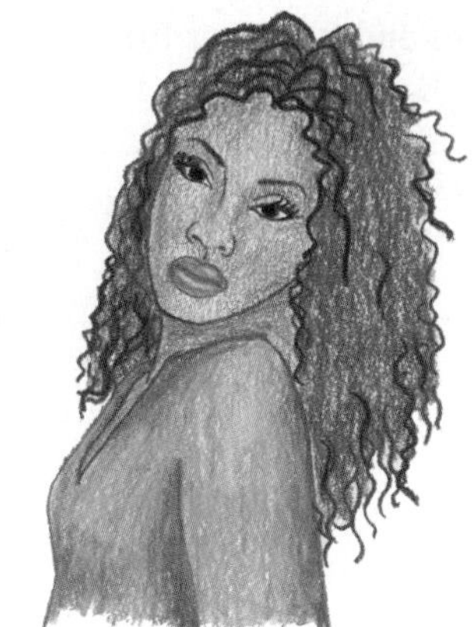

Figure 16-5 Square face shape.

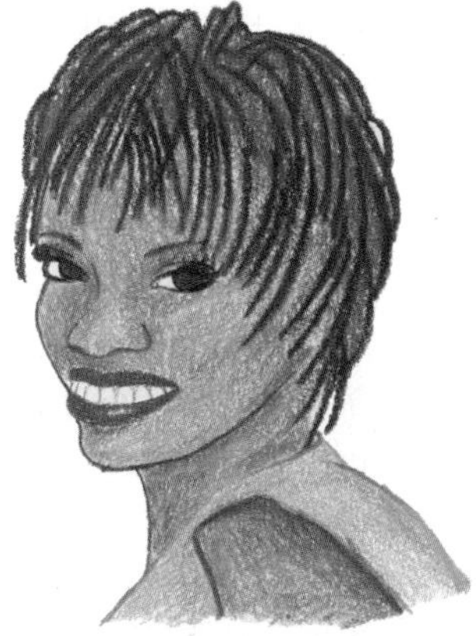

Figure 16-6 Diamond face shape.

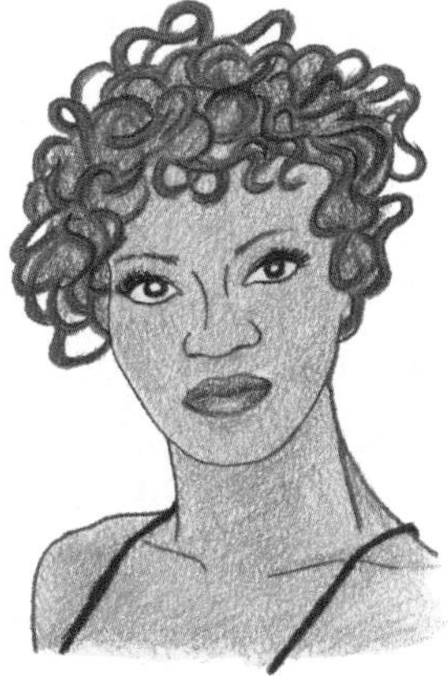

Figure 16-7 Fullness around the forehead helps balance a diamond-shaped face.

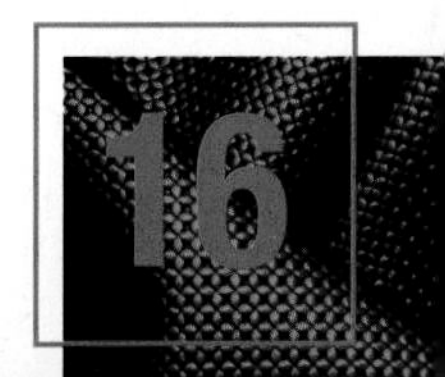

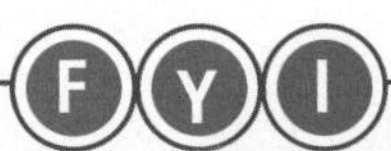

Hair is referred to as "natural" or "virgin" if it has had no physical abuse, as well as no previous coloring or lightening or other chemical treatments. Styles used in natural hairstyling include braid extensions, twists (two strands overlapped to form a "candy cane" effect), weaving, wrapping, and locks, also called African locks or dreadlocks. (State regulatory agencies may define natural hairstyling in different ways.) For African Americans, these styles are a proud acknowledgment of their cultural heritage. However, their use is not limited to African Americans. People today borrow and enjoy styles and traditions from many different cultures.

- *Inverted Triangle (heart-shaped).* Minimize the width of the forehead by styling with partial bangs (fringe) and/or braids that frame the face. This will add fullness around the chin.
- *Oblong.* Creating full styles can make the face appear shorter or wider. Soft, partial bangs (fringe) or wisps of curls along the face can also soften facial lines. Braids should be kept to a medium length. Avoid middle parts because they add length to a long, narrow face.

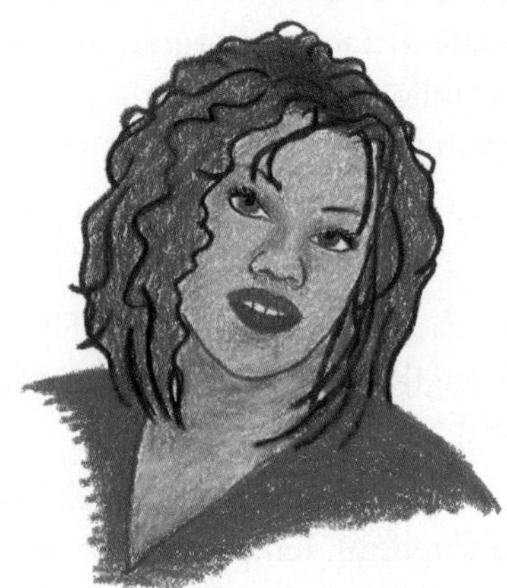

Figure 16-8 Triangular face shape.

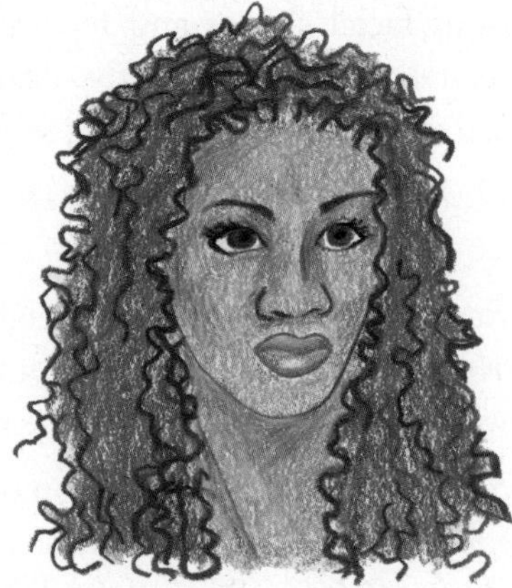

Figure 16-9 Braiding styles that hug the cheekbones help balance a triangular-shaped face.

UNDERSTANDING THE BASICS

Before exploring the various braiding techniques, it is important to have a good grasp of braiding basics. These include the tools you will be using, the materials you will be working with, and the factors involved in styling wet and dry hair.

TOOLS FOR BRAIDING

Artists are only as good as their tools, and this adage applies equally to cutting, coloring, or creating natural hairstyles. No matter what length and texture the hair might be, certain tools are essential in order to master various braiding techniques (Figures 16-10 and 16-11).

- *Boar-bristle brush (natural hairbrush).* Best for stimulating the scalp as well as removing dirt and lint from locks. Nylon-bristle brushes are not as durable, and many snag the hair. Soft nylon brushes may be an option for fine, soft hair around the hairline.

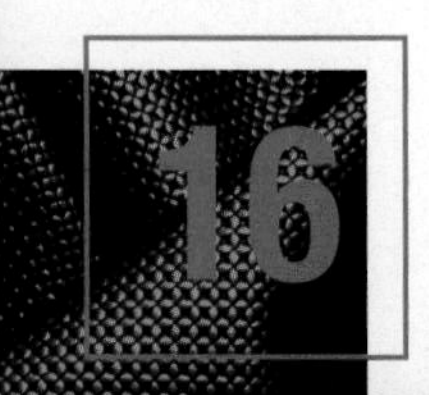

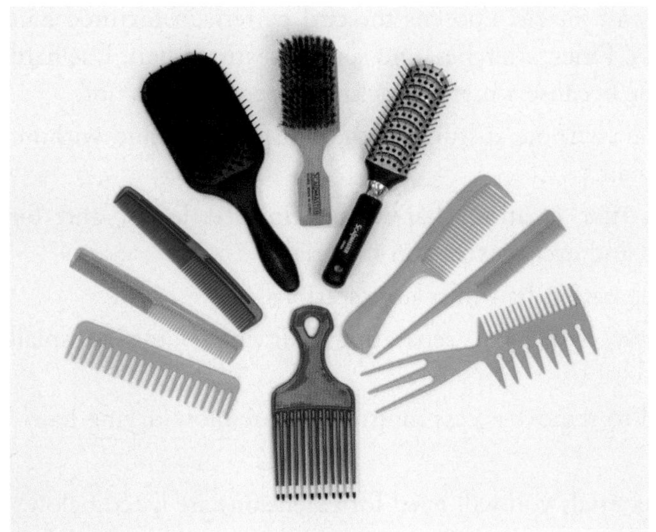
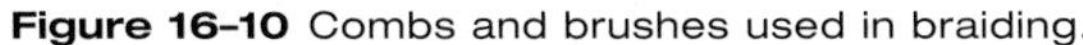

Figure 16–10 Combs and brushes used in braiding.

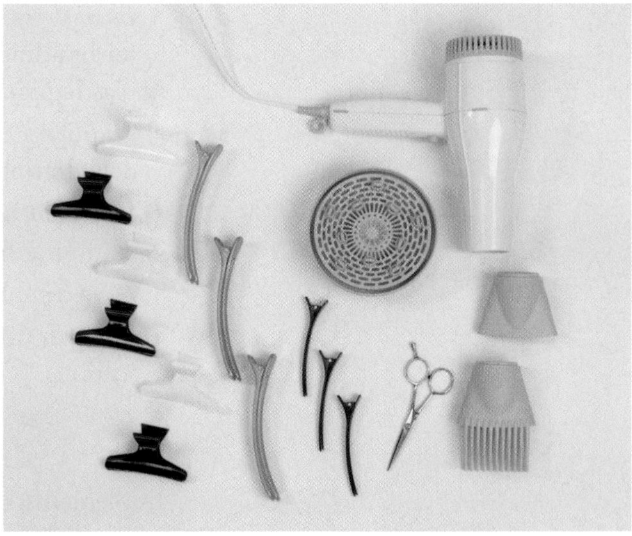

Figure 16–11 Clips, blow-dryer, diffuser concentrator, nozzle and scissors.

- *Square paddle brush.* Good for short textured hair and long straight hair to release tangles, knots, and snarls. Square paddle brushes are "pneumatic" because they have a cushion of air in the head that makes the bristles collapse when they encounter too much resistance. This is key to preventing breakage in fragile African-American hair.
- *Vent brush.* Has a single or double row of widely spaced pins with protective tips to prevent tearing and breaking the hair. Vent brushes are used to gently remove tangles on wet wavy or dry curly hair, as well as on human hair extensions. Always check the protective tips before using a vent brush on the hair. If even one is missing, discard the brush.
- *Wide-tooth comb.* Available in a variety of shapes and designs, these combs ply through hair with little snarling. The teeth, which range in width from medium to large, have long rounded tips to avoid scratching the scalp. The distance between the teeth is the most important feature of this comb; larger spacing allows textured hair to move between the rows of teeth with ease.
- *Double-tooth comb (detangling comb).* Separates the hair as it combs, making it an excellent detangling tool for wet curly hair.
- *Tail comb.* Excellent for design parting, sectioning large segments of hair, and opening and removing braids.
- *Finishing comb.* Usually 8 to 10 inches in length, this tool is used while cutting and works well on fine or straight hair.
- *Cutting comb.* For cutting small sections. Should be used only after the hair is softened and elongated with a blow-dryer.
- *Pick with rounded teeth.* Useful for lifting and separating textured hair. This tool has long, widely spaced teeth and is commonly made of metal, plastic, or wood.

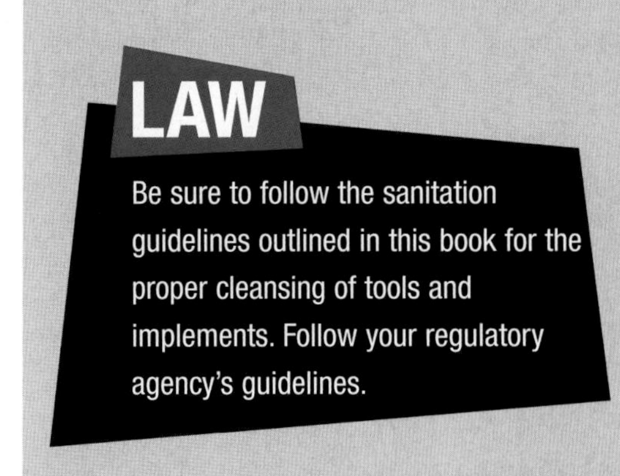

LAW

Be sure to follow the sanitation guidelines outlined in this book for the proper cleansing of tools and implements. Follow your regulatory agency's guidelines.

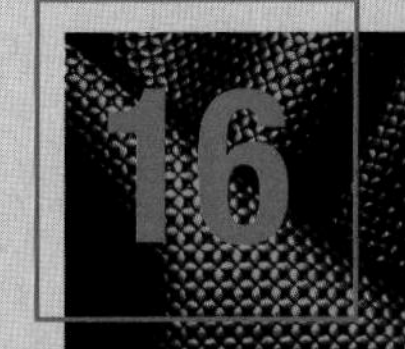

- *Blow-dryer with pick nozzle.* Loosens the curl pattern in textured hair for braiding styles. Dries, stretches, and softens textured hair. Use hard plastic pick nozzle because a metal attachment becomes too hot.
- *Diffuser.* Dries hair without disturbing the finished look and without dehydrating the hair.
- *Five-inch scissors.* For creating shapes and finished looks, and for trimming fringes and excess extension material.
- *Long clips.* For separating hair into large sections.
- *Butterfly and small clips.* For separating hair into large or small sections.
- *Hood dryer.* Used to remove excess moisture before blow-drying hair.

Implements and materials you will need for extensions are listed below.

- *Extension fibers.* Kanekalon, nylon, rayon, human hair, yarn, lin, and yak.
- *Hackle.* A board of fine, upright nails through which human hair extensions are combed; used for detangling or blending colors and highlights.
- *Drawing board.* Flat leather pads with very close, fine teeth that sandwich the human hair extensions. The pads are weighed down with books, and the required amount of hair is extracted without loosening and disturbing the rest of the hair during the process of braiding.

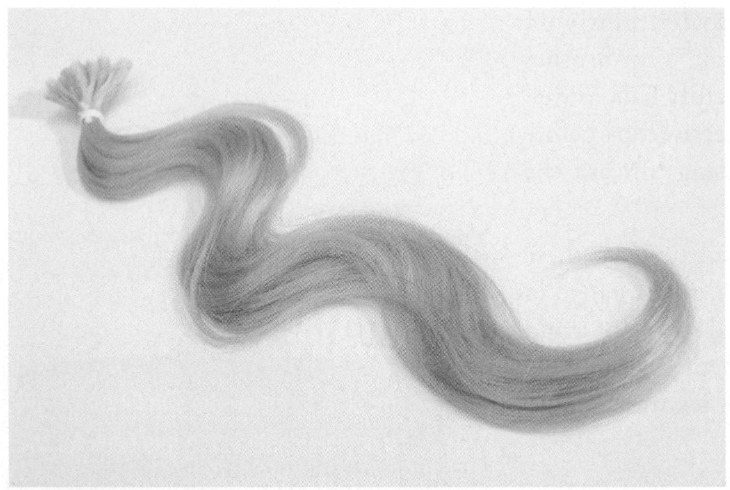

Figure 16-12 Human hair is the gold standard for hair extensions.

MATERIALS FOR EXTENSIONS

A wide variety of fibers are available for the purpose of extending hair. It is important to keep in mind that the fibers you use will largely determine how successful and durable the extension will be. Although it may seem like a good idea to buy the least expensive product, in the long run this may not prove to be the most economical solution, especially if you are buying hair fabric in large quantities. You may get stuck with a lot of material, for instance, that does not give you the results you desire. When buying a new product, buy in small quantities and test the fiber on a mannequin before using it on a client.

The following materials are most commonly used for hair extensions:

- *Human hair.* Human hair is the gold standard for hair extensions. Unfortunately, the human hair market can be a confusing and sometimes deceptive business. Most human hair is imported from Asia, with little information about how it was processed, or even if it is 100% human hair. This makes it very important to only deal with suppliers who you know and trust (Figure 16-12).
- *Kanekalon.* A manufactured synthetic fiber of excellent quality, Kanekalon has a texture similar to extremely curly or coiled hair types. It does not reflect light, which means it has less shine, but it comes in

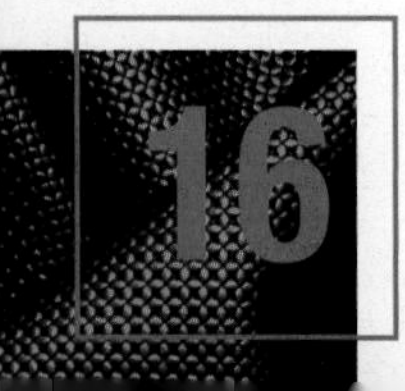

a variety of colors and is versatile and easy to match with natural hair colors. Durable, soft, and less inclined to tangle than other synthetics, Kanekalon holds up to shampooing and styling. It costs more than most synthetics, but is a better-quality product. It feels smooth to both the client's scalp and your fingers (Figure 16-13).

- *Nylon or rayon synthetic.* This product is less expensive than Kanekalon and is available in varying qualities. It reflects light and leaves the hair very shiny. A drawback of nylon and rayon is that both of these fibers have been known to cut or break the hair. Repeated shampooing will make these extensions less durable. In addition, they will melt if high heat is applied, such as a hot blow-dryer.
- *Yarn.* Traditional yarn used to make sweaters and hats is now being used to adorn hair. It can be made of cotton or a nylon blend, and is very inexpensive and easy to find. Yarn is light, soft, and detangles easily. It is available in many colors, does not reflect light, and gives the braid a matte finish. While yarn may expand when shampooing, it will not slip from the base, making it durable for braids. The one caution when purchasing yarn is that some products may appear jet black in the store, and show a blue or green tint in natural light.
- *Lin.* This beautiful wool fiber imported from Africa has a matte finish and comes only in black and brown. Lin comes on a roll and is used in any length and size. Keep in mind that this cotton-like fabric is very flammable.
- *Yak.* This strong fiber comes from the domestic ox found in the mountains of Tibet and Central Asia. Yak hair is shaved and processed to use alone or blended with human hair. Mixing human hair with yak hair helps to remove the manufactured shine (Figure 16-14).

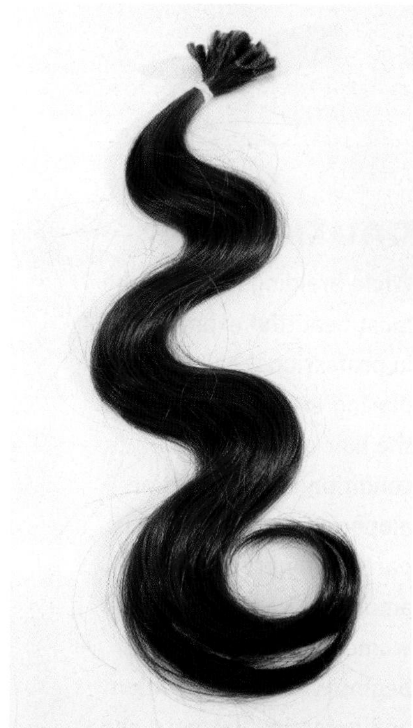

Figure 16-13 Kanekalon is a top-of-the-line synthetic fiber used for hair extensions.

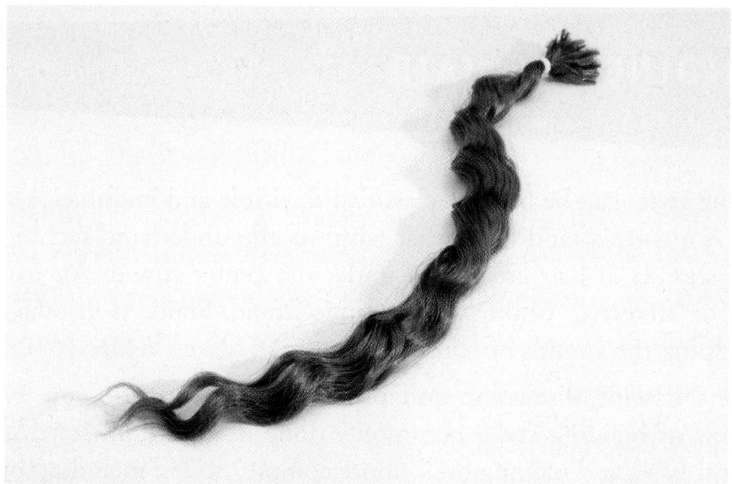

Figure 16-14 Yak blends beautifully with human hair.

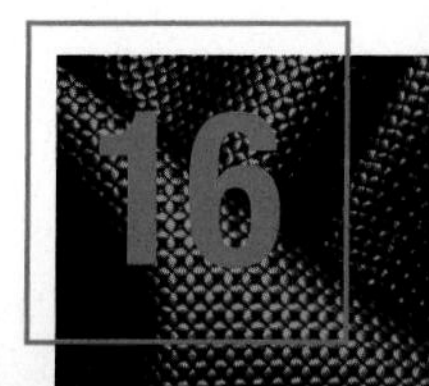

CAUTION

While braiding is one of the most beautiful expressions in professional hairstyling, placing excessive tension on the hair can lead to a condition called "traction alopecia." This condition is particularly prevalent among African-American women and children. It begins with scalp irritation and excessive flakiness, and eventually leads to hair loss, particularly around the hairline. Wearing excessively tight braids (tight enough to pull the hair or impede circulation to the scalp) over a prolonged period of time can lead to permanent hair loss.

WORKING WITH WET OR DRY HAIR

In general, it is best to braid curly hair when it is dry. When curly hair is braided wet, it shrinks and recoils as it dries. This shrinkage may create excess pulling and scalp tension. When the hair dries tightly around the braid, the tension can lead to breakage or hair loss from pulling or twisting. If you are using a style that requires your client's hair to be wet while being manipulated, you must allow for shrinkage, thereby avoiding damage to the hair.

Straight, resistant hair is best braided slightly damp or very lightly coated with a wax or pomade to make it more pliable. After you shampoo the client's hair, towel blot without rubbing or tension, using several towels if necessary. Apply a leave-in conditioner to make combing the hair easier. Begin combing at the ends of the fibers and gently work out the tangles while moving upward toward the scalp. Use a wide-tooth or detangling comb for this purpose, and then blow-dry the hair. Wax, pomades, pastes, or lotions can be used to hold the hair in place for a finished look. Brush the hair with a large paddle brush, beginning at the ends as you do with a comb.

Textured hair presents certain challenges when styling. It is very fragile both wet and dry. Because most braiding styles require the hair to be dry, blow-drying is the most effective way to prepare the hair for the braiding service. Not only does blow-drying quickly dry the hair, it softens it in the process, making it more manageable for combing and sectioning. Blow-drying also loosens and elongates the wave pattern, while stretching the hair shaft length. This is great for short hair, allowing for easier "pick up" and manipulation of the hair. Make sure to control the hair while blow-drying to prevent frizzing!

BRAIDING THE HAIR

Braiding styles can be broadly classified as visible and invisible. A **visible braid** is a three-strand braid that employs the underhand technique in which strands of hair are woven under the center strand. An **invisible braid** or **inverted braid,** also a three-strand braid, is produced by overlapping the strands of hair on top of each other (Figure 16-15).

The following discussion and procedures will provide you with an overview of braiding styles commonly done in the salon, starting with the most basic and moving on to more complex styles, including braided extensions (Figure 16-16).

INVISIBLE BRAID

The invisible braid uses an overhand pick-up technique. It can be done on the scalp, or off the scalp, with or without extensions. This style is ideal for long hair, but it can also be executed successfully on hair with long layers. If you are dealing with straight, layered hair, apply a light coating

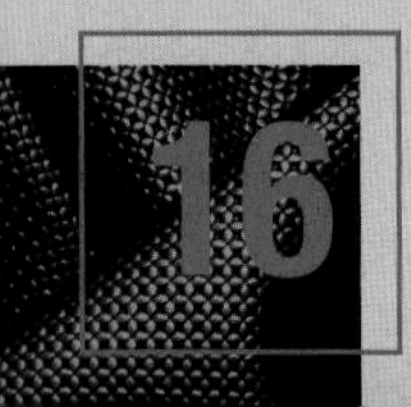

of wax or pomade to the hair to help hold shorter strands in place. Procedure 16-2 demonstrates one braid down the back of the head.

ROPE BRAID

The **rope braid** (Procedure 16-3) is made with two strands that are twisted around each other. It can be done on hair that is all one length, as well as on long, layered hair. Remember to add to both sides before you twist the right side over the left.

FISHTAIL BRAID

The **fishtail braid** (Procedure 16-4) is a simple two-strand braid in which hair is picked up from the sides and added to the strands as they are crossed over each other. It is best done on non-layered hair that is at least shoulder length.

SINGLE BRAIDS

The terms **single braids,** box braids, and individual braids all refer to free-hanging braids, with or without extensions that can be executed with either an underhand or overhand stitch. Single braids can be used with all hair textures and in a variety of ways. For instance, two or three single braids added to a ponytail or chignon can be a lovely evening look.

The partings or subsections for single braids can be square, triangular, or rectangular. The parting determines where the braid is placed, and how it moves. Single braids can move in any direction, so make sure to braid in the direction you want them to go. As you are braiding, you are styling and shaping the finished look. The procedure for medium-to-large single braids is done with an underhand stitch.

Extensions for single braids come in a wide range of sizes and lengths, and are integrated into the natural hair using the three-strand underhand technique. Fiber for extensions can be selected from synthetic hair, yarn, or human hair; the selection is vital in determining the finished style. Braiding must be consistent and close together.

As part of the consultation step, open the package of extension fibers and show them to the client to verify that the color is correct. Remove the fibers from the package and, if necessary, cut them to the desired length. Place half the extension fibers in the bottom portion of the drawing board and "sandwich" them with the upper portion of board. To secure the hair extensions, place a heavy object on top of the board, such as a large book. This allows you to easily extract the appropriate amount of fibers for the braids. Hair extensions can also be separated and dispensed by a free-hand method.

CAUTION

If you notice a scalp disorder while performing a hair and scalp analysis prior to braiding, be sure to advise your client to seek medical attention.

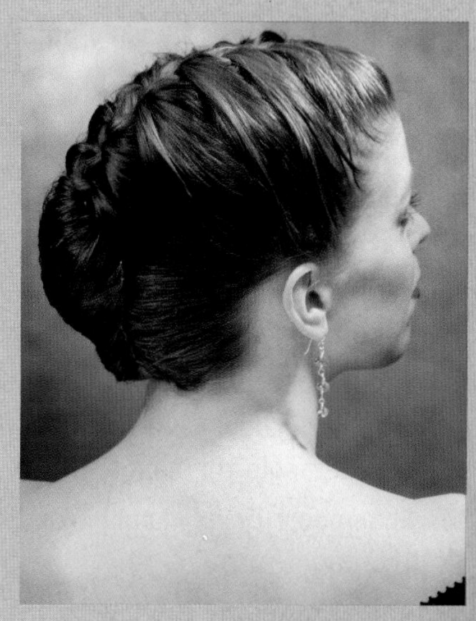

Figure 16–15 Braided French twist

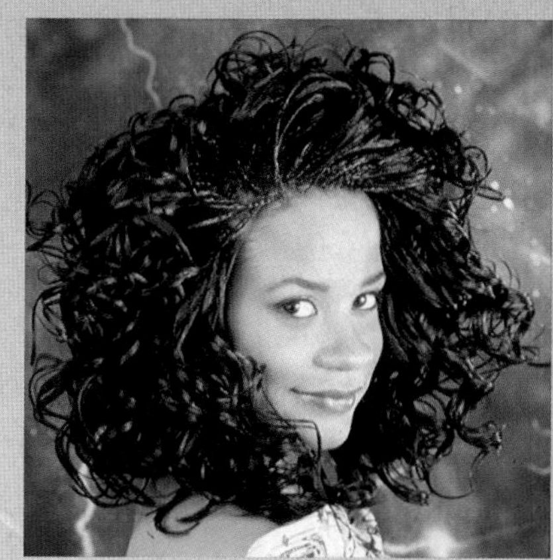

Figure 16–16 Micro-braiding is a popular, time-consuming service offered by expert natural hairstylists.

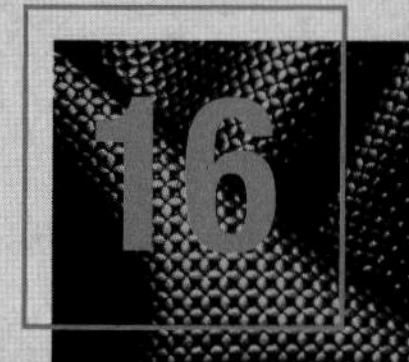

PROCEDURE 16-1

PREPARING TEXTURED HAIR FOR BRAIDING

IMPLEMENTS AND MATERIALS

- Shampoo cape
- Neck strip
- Towels
- Shampoo
- Conditioner (protein or moisturizing)
- Tail comb with large rounded teeth
- Detangling solution (four parts water to one part cream rinse or oil) in spray bottle
- Butterfly clips
- Blow-drying cream or lotion with oil or glycerine base

PREPARATION

1. Wash your hands.
2. Perform a client consultation and hair and scalp analysis (Figure 16-17).
3. Drape the client for a shampoo. If necessary, comb and detangle the hair.
4. Shampoo, rinse, apply conditioner, and rinse thoroughly.
5. Gently towel-dry the hair.

PROCEDURE

1. **Part ear to ear.** Part damp hair from ear to ear across crown. Use butterfly clips to separate front section from back section (Figure 16-18).
2. **Sectioning.** Part back of head into four to six sections. For thick textured hair, make more sections to allow for increased ease and control. For thinner hair, use fewer sections. The front half of the head where hair is less dense can be sectioned in three or more sections. Separate the sections with clips.
3. **Comb and detangle.** Beginning on left section in the back, start combing the ends of the hair first, working your way up to the base of the scalp. Lightly spray each section as you go along with

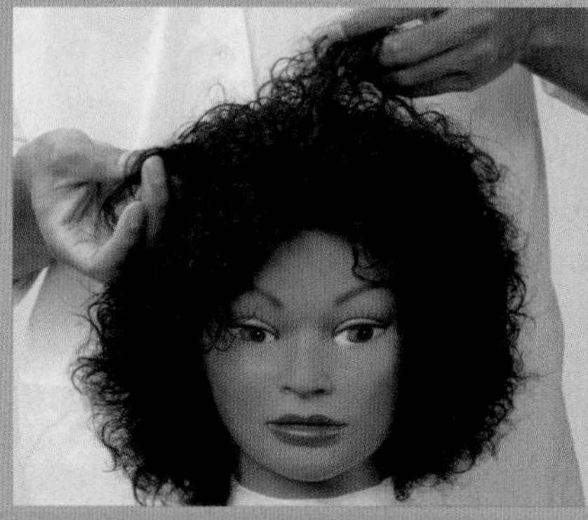

Figure 16-17 Scalp analysis.

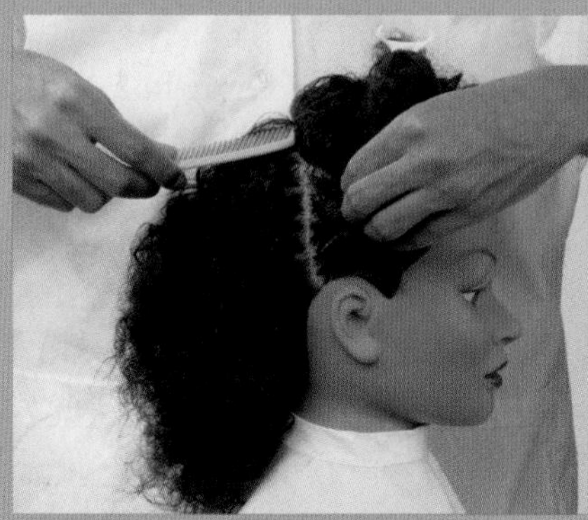

Figure 16-18 Part the hair across the crown.

detangling solution if needed. The combing movement should be fast and rhythmic, but not create tension on the scalp. Use a picking motion to comb through the hair (Figure 16-19).

4. **Divide and twist.** After combing thoroughly, divide section into two equal parts and twist them together to the end and hold section in place (Figure 16-20).
5. **Repeat Steps 4 and 5.** Continue with the other sections of the hair until the entire head is sectioned.
6. **Remove moisture.** Place client under a medium heat hood dryer for 5 to 10 minutes to remove excess moisture.
7. **Open combed section.** Open one of the combed sections. Using fingers, apply blow-drying cream to hair from scalp to ends (Figure 16-21).
8. **Blow-dry.** Using a pick nozzle attachment on blow-dryer, hold hair down and away from client's head as you begin drying. Use comb-out motion with the pick, always pointing the nozzle away from client (Figure 16-22). As ends relax and stretch, work the blow-dryer, with heat blowing downward, toward scalp. Blowing directly on scalp can cause a burn or discomfort. The hair is now ready to braid (Figure 16-23).

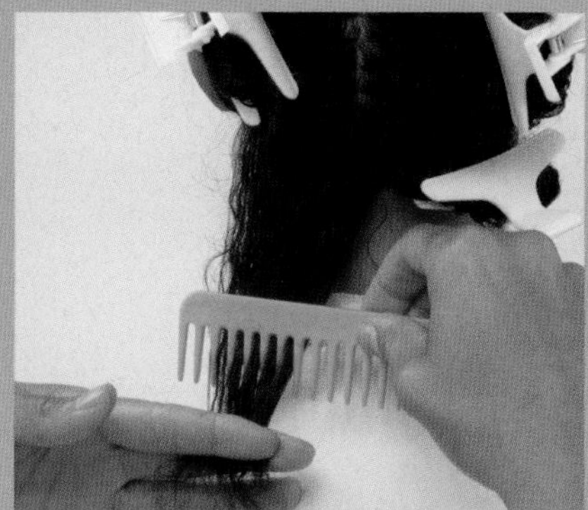

Figure 16-19 Comb the section.

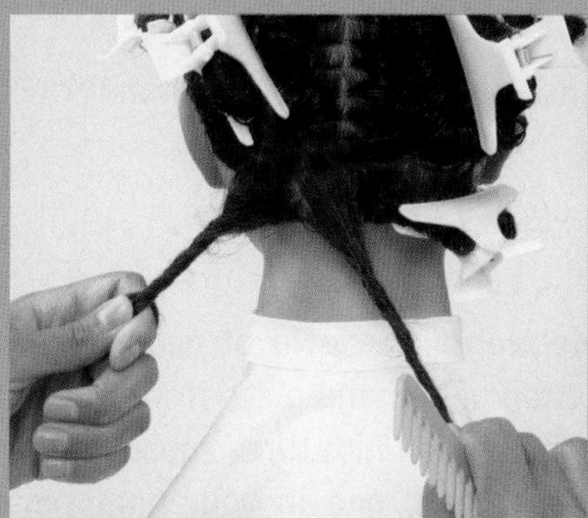

Figure 16-20 Twist the two parts of the section.

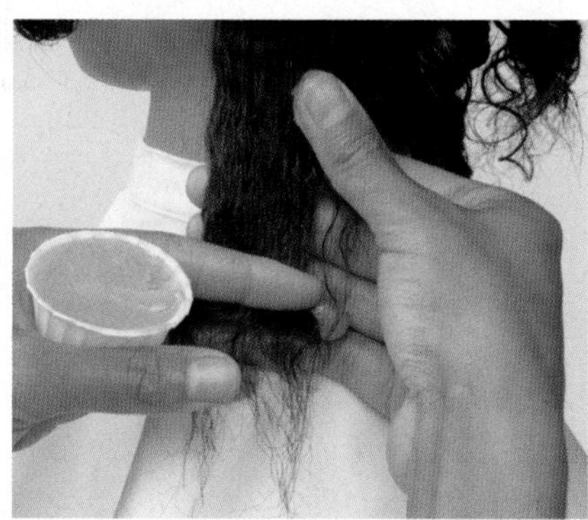

Figure 16-21 Apply blow-drying cream to hair.

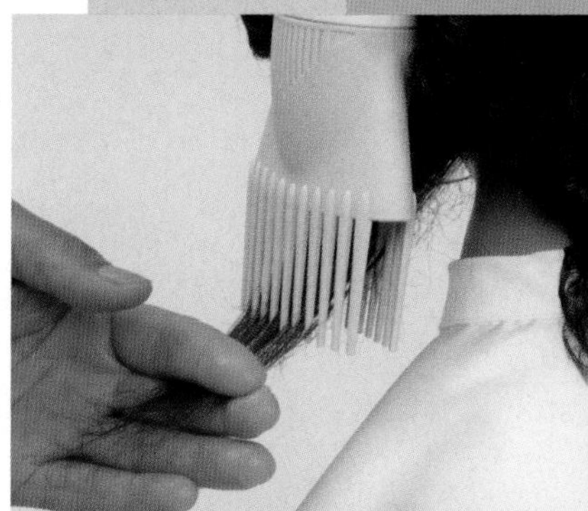

Figure 16-22 Blow-dry the section.

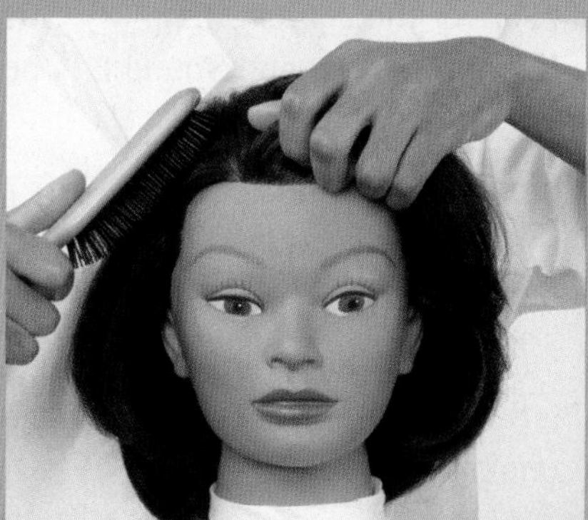

Figure 16-23 Hair prepared for braiding.

PROCEDURE 16-2

INVISIBLE BRAID

IMPLEMENTS AND MATERIALS

- Styling cape
- Neck strip
- Rubber band or fabric-covered elastic
- Tail comb

PREPARATION

1. Wash your hands.
2. Perform a client consultation and hair and scalp analysis (Figure 16-17 on page 376).
3. Drape the client for a shampoo. If necessary, comb and detangle the hair.
4. Shampoo, rinse, apply conditioner, and rinse thoroughly.
5. Gently towel-dry the hair.

PROCEDURE

1. **Take three sections.** At crown of head, take a triangular section of hair and place it in your left hand. Divide the section into three equal strands, two in your left hand, one in your right hand (Figure 16-24).
2. **Cross right strand.** Place your fingers close to the scalp for a tight stitch. For a looser stitch, move away from the scalp. Cross the right strand (1) over the center strand (2). Strand 1 is now in the new center, and Strand 2 is now on the right (Figure 16-25).
3. **Cross left strand.** Cross the left strand (3) over the center section and place it in your right hand.
4. **Separate strands.** Place all three strands in your left hand with your fingers separating the strands (Figure 16-26).

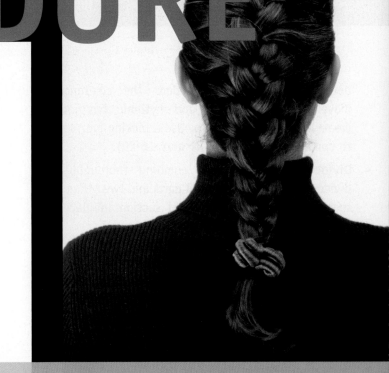

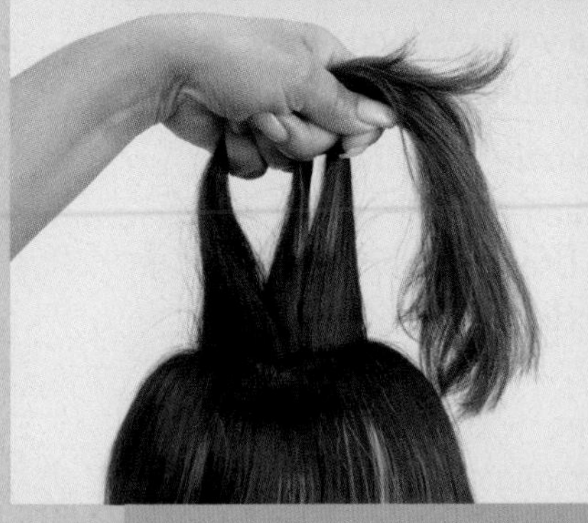

Figure 16-24 Divide section into three equal strands.

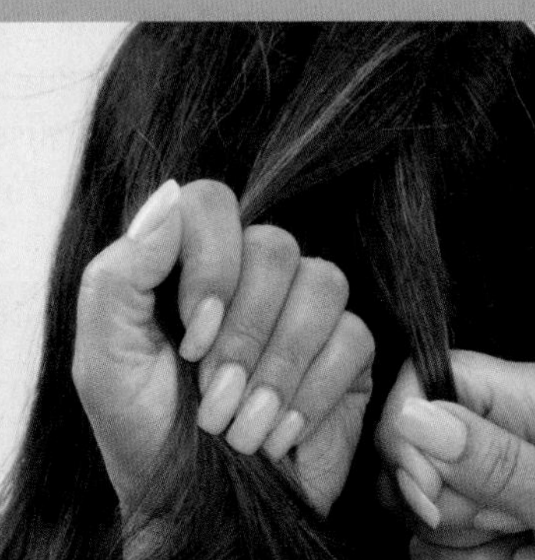

Figure 16-25 Cross right strand ov center strand.

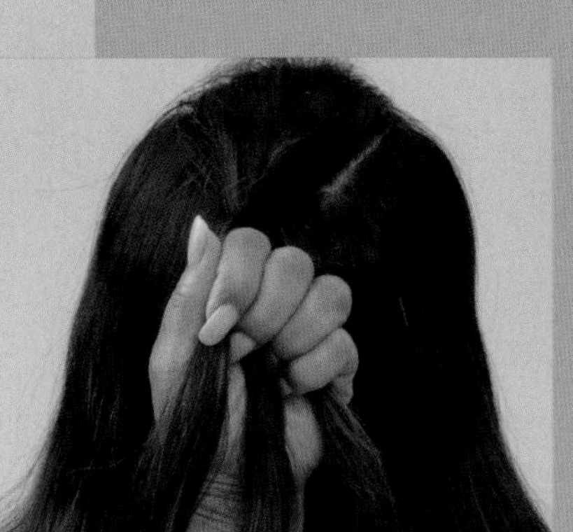

Figure 16-26 Place strands in left hand.

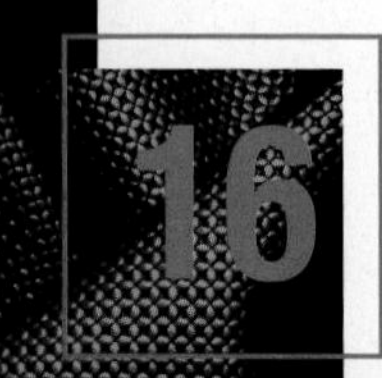

5. **Pick up strand.** With your right hand, pick up a 1-inch x 1-inch section of hair on the right side. Add to strand 2 in your left hand (Figure 16-27).
6. **Cross combined strands.** Take the combined strands in your right hand and cross them over the center strand. Place all the strands in your right hand (Figure 16-28).
7. **Add section.** With your left hand, pick up a 1-inch section on the left side. Add this section to the left outer strand (1) in your right hand (Figure 16-29).
8. **Cross combined strands.** Take the combined strands and cross them over the center strand (Figure 16-30).
9. **Pick up right side.** Place all three sections in your left hand, pick up the right side, and add to the outer strand (3) (Figure 16-31).
10. **Move down head alternating pick-up movements.** Remember that the outer strands are added to and then crossed over the center. Continue these movements until the braid is complete. Secure the braid with a rubber band, then with a ribbon or other accessory for a finished style (Figure 16-32).

CLEANUP AND SANITATION

1. Disinfect all implements.
2. Place capes and towels in hamper for laundering.
3. Sanitize your workstation.
4. Wash your hands with soap and warm water.

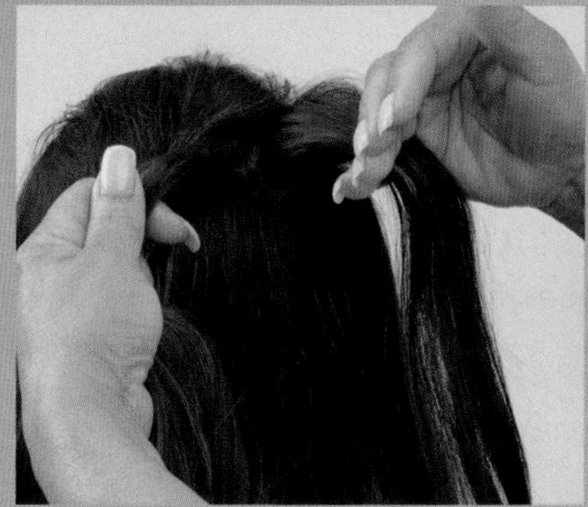
Figure 16-27 Add hair to the right strand

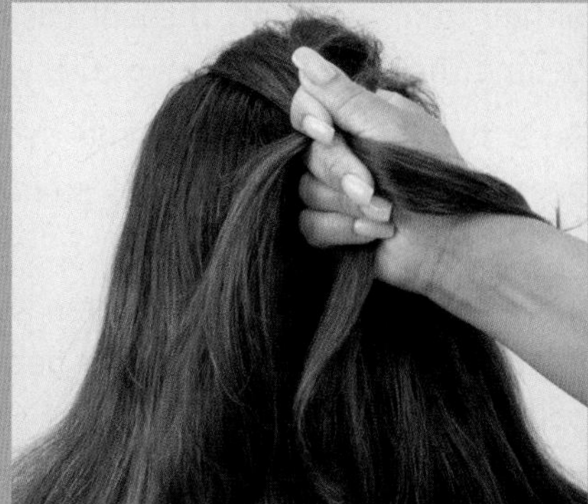
Figure 16-28 Place strands in right hand.

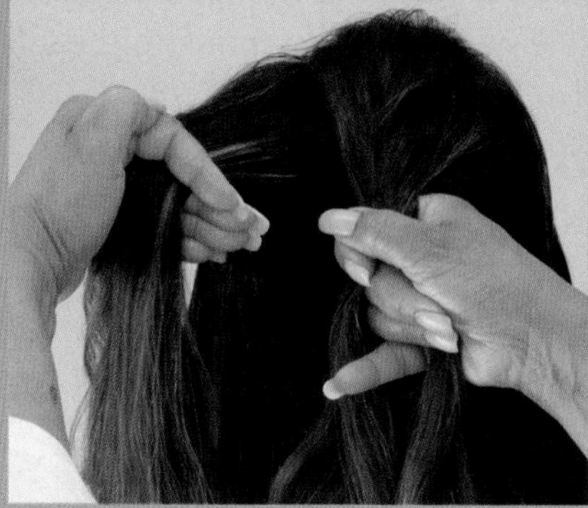
Figure 16-29 Add hair to outer right strand.

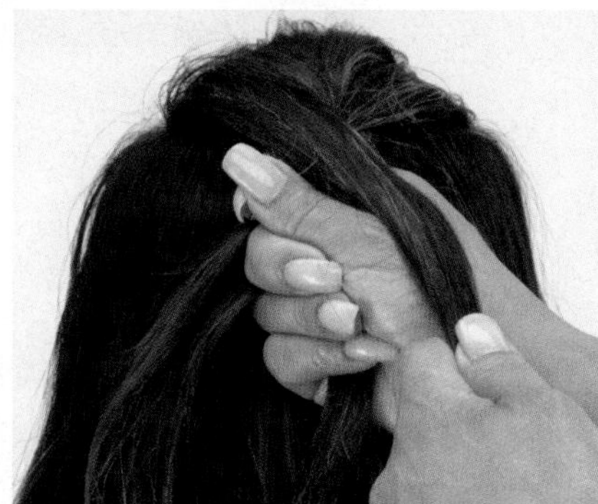
Figure 16-30 Cross combined strand over center strand.

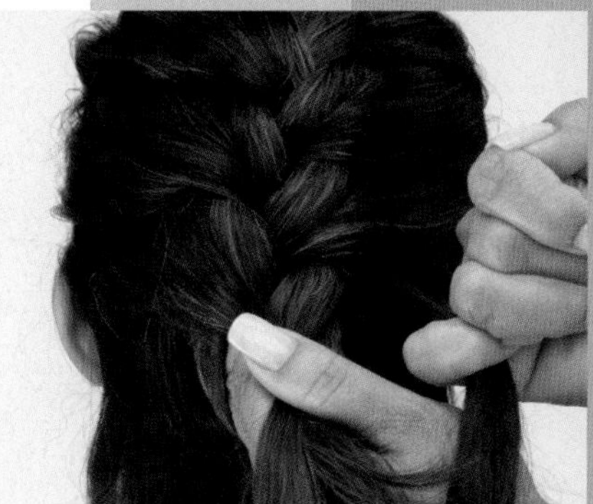
Figure 16-31 Add hair to outer right strand.

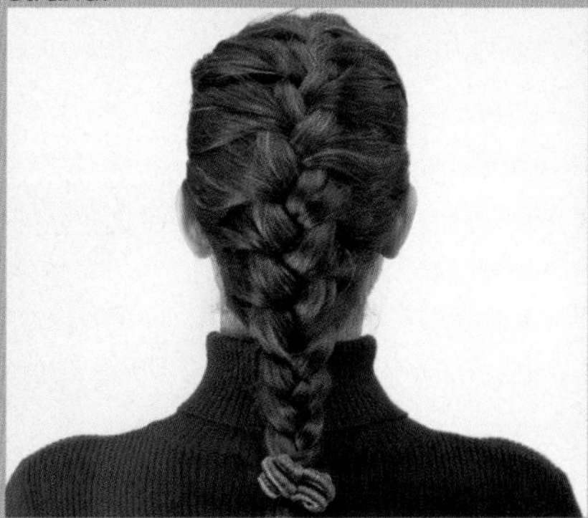
Figure 16-32 Finished invisible braid.

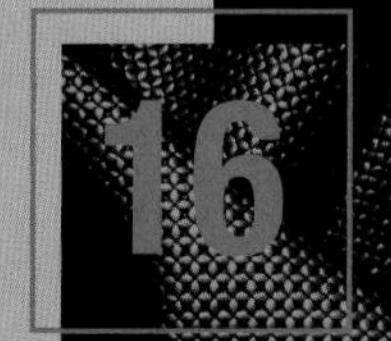

PROCEDURE 16-3

ROPE BRAID

IMPLEMENTS AND MATERIALS

Same as for the invisible braid.

PREPARATION

Same as for the invisible braid.

PROCEDURE

1. **Take triangular section.** Take a triangular section of hair from the front. If client has a fringe, begin behind the fringe (Figure 16-33).
2. **Take two strands.** Divide the section into two equal strands. Cross the right strand over the left strand (Figure 16-34).
3. **Place strands.** Place both strands in your right hand with your index finger in between and your palm facing upward (Figure 16-35).
4. **Twist clockwise.** Twist the left strand two times clockwise (toward the center) (Figure 16-36).
5. **Pick up section.** Pick up a 1-inch section from the left side. Add this section to the left strand (Figure 16-37).
6. **Place strands.** Put both strands in your left hand with the index finger in between and your palm up (Figure 16-38).
7. **Add strand.** Pick up a 1-inch section from the right side and add it to the right strand (Figure 16-39).

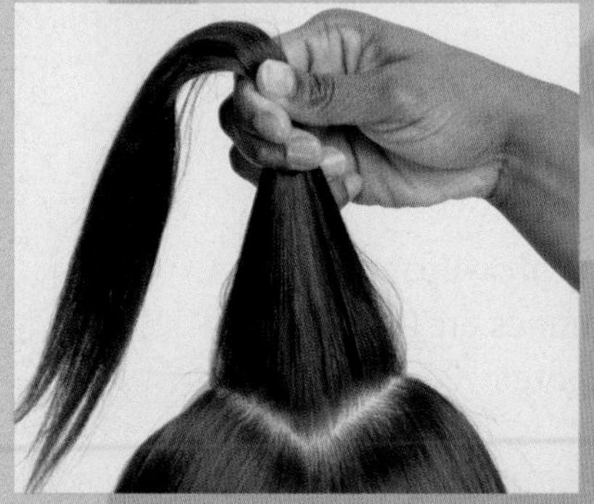

Figure 16-33 Take a triangular section of hair.

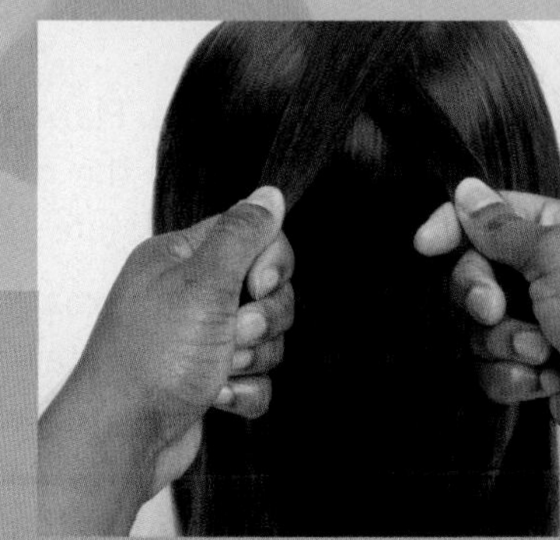

Figure 16-34 Cross the right stra over the left strand.

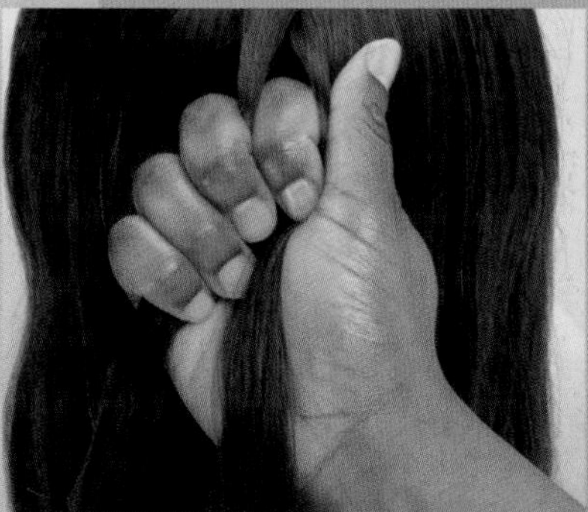

Figure 16-35 Place both strands in your right hand.

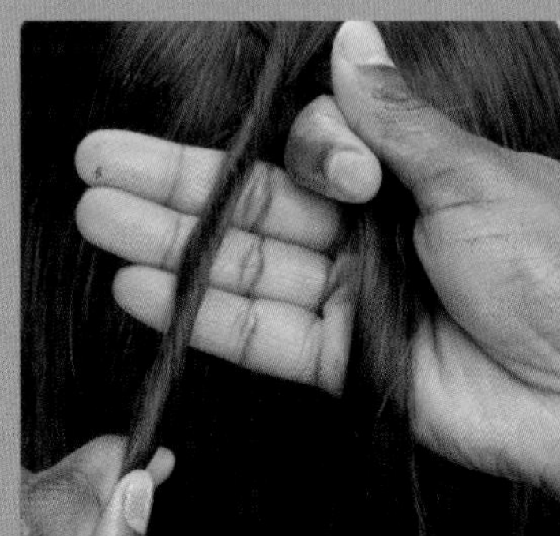

Figure 16-36 Twist left strand.

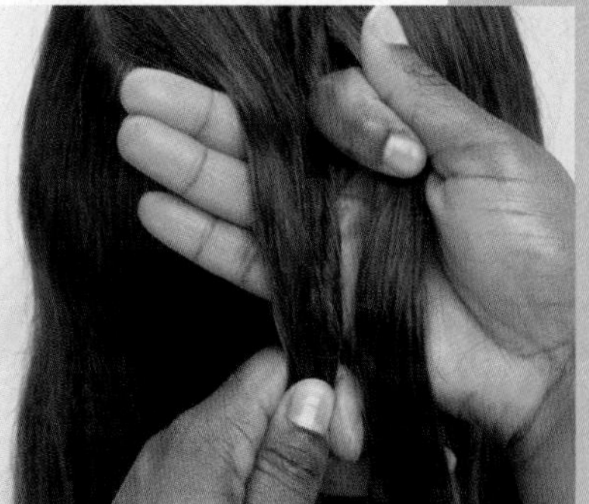

Figure 16-37 Add to left strand.

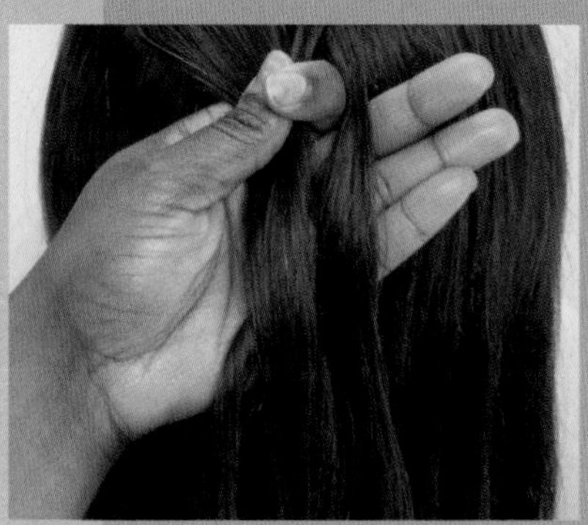

Figure 16-38 Put both strands in your left hand.

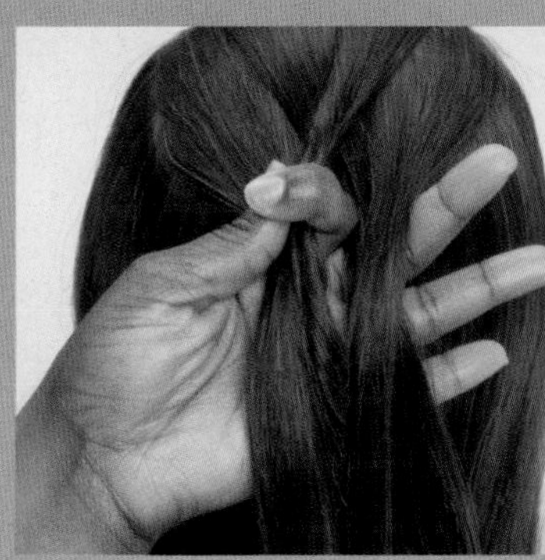

Figure 16-39 Twist hand toward left.

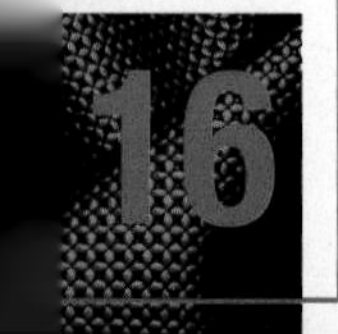

8. **Place strands.** Put both strands in your right hand with your index finger in between and your palm up (Figure 16-40).
9. **Twist counterclockwise.** With your hand in this position, twist toward the left (counterclockwise) until your palm is facing down (Figure 16-41).
10. **Repeat Steps 3 through 9.** Work toward the nape until the style is complete. Secure with a rubber band (Figure 16-42).
11. **Create rope ponytail.** When you run out of sections to pick up, another option is to create a rope ponytail with the remaining hair. Twist the left strand clockwise (to the right) two or three times. Place the strands in your right hand, index finger in between and palm up (Figure 16-43). Twist the palm down (counterclockwise), right hand over left (Figure 16-44). Repeat these steps until you reach the end of the hair. Secure ends with a rubber band (Figure 16-45).
12. **Sanitation.** Follow cleanup and sanitation procedures for invisible braid.

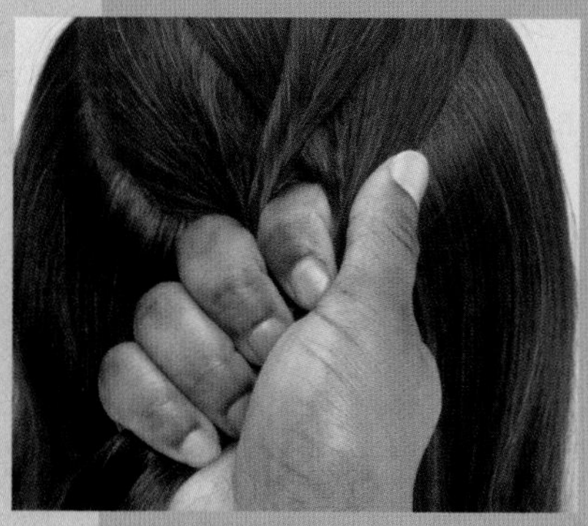

Figure 16–40 Add to the right strand.

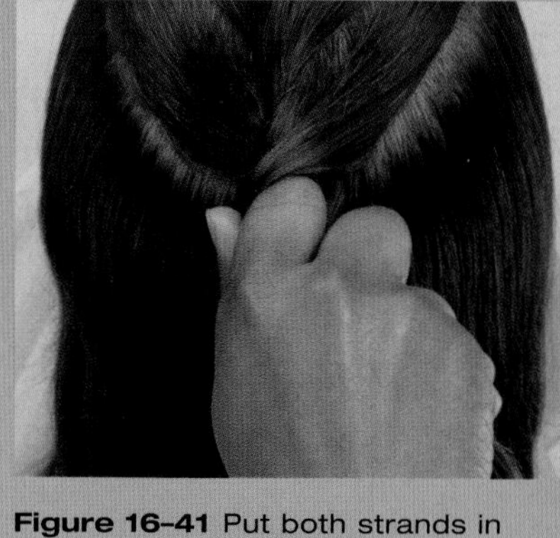

Figure 16–41 Put both strands in your right hand.

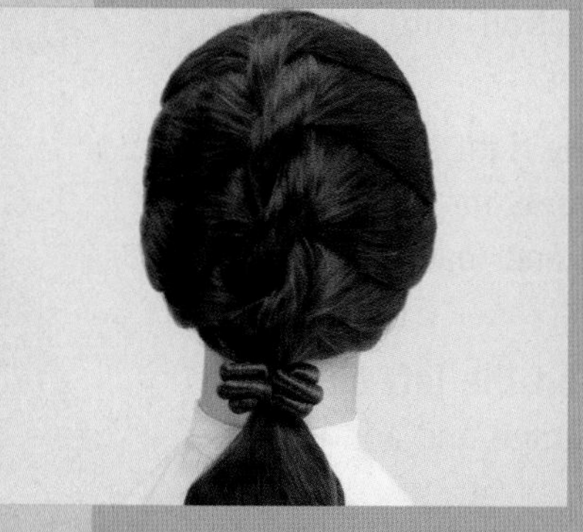

Figure 16–42 Finished rope braid.

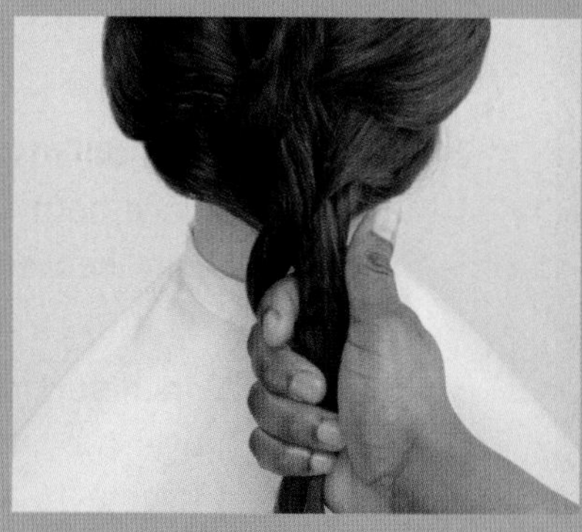

Figure 16–43 Place two strands in right hand.

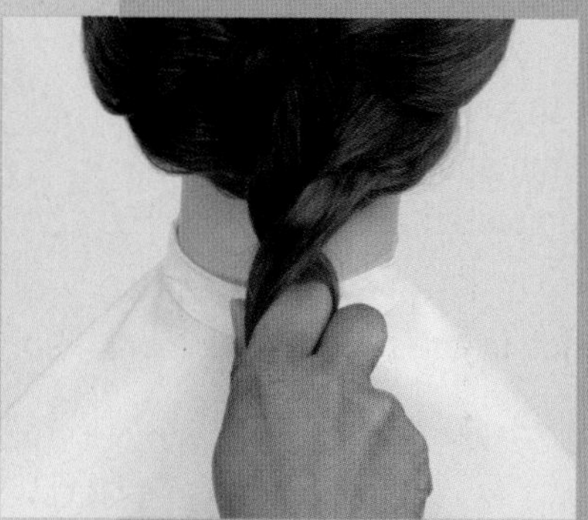

Figure 16–44 Twist hand counterclockwise.

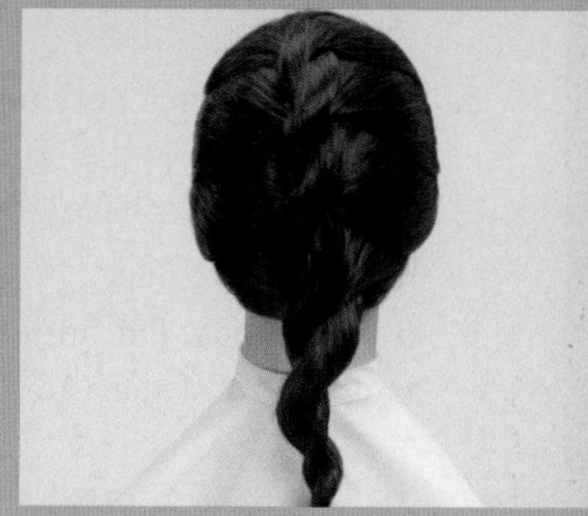

Figure 16–45 Finished rope ponytail.

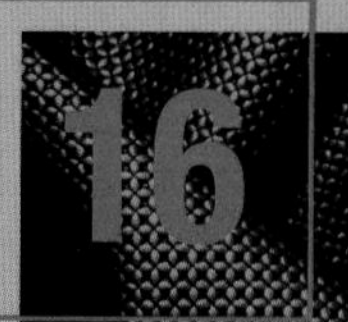

PROCEDURE 16-4

FISHTAIL BRAID

IMPLEMENTS AND MATERIALS

Same as for invisible braid.

PREPARATION

Same as for invisible braid.

PROCEDURE

1. **Take front section.** Take a triangular section from the front. If the client has a fringe, begin behind the fringe. Divide this section into two equal strands (Figure 16-46).
2. **Cross right strand.** Cross the right strand over the left strand. Place both strands in the right hand, index finger in between and palm up (Figure 16-47).
3. **Pick up a 1-inch section on the left side.** Cross this section over the left strand and add it to the right strand (Figure 16-48).
4. **Place strands.** Put both strands in the left hand, index finger in between and palm up (Figure 16-49).
5. **Pick up a 1-inch section on the right side.** Cross this section over the right strand and add it to the left strand. You have now completed an X shape (Figure 16-50).
6. **Place strands.** Put both strands in the right hand, as in Step 2 (Figure 16-51).

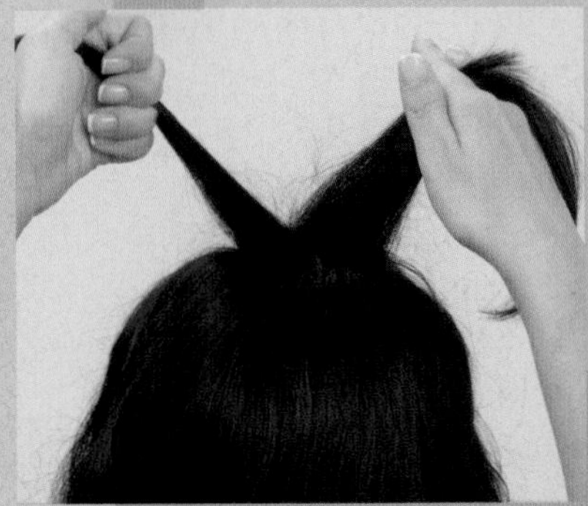

Figure 16–46 Divide section into two equal strands.

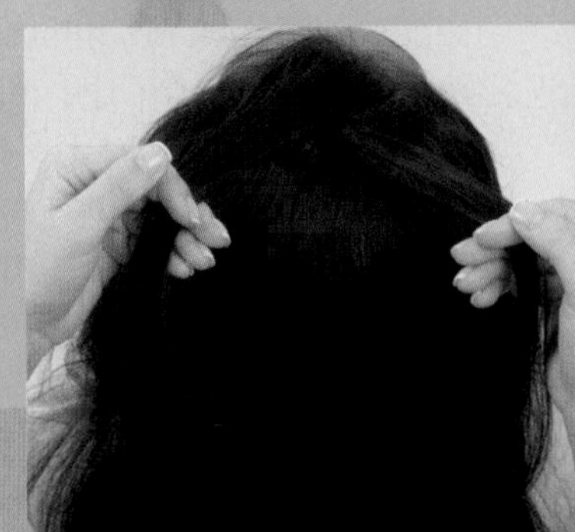

Figure 16–47 Cross right strand over left strand.

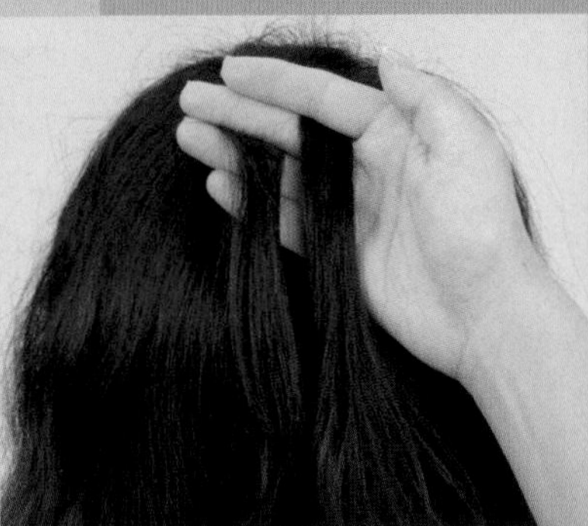

Figure 16–48 Place both strands in right hand.

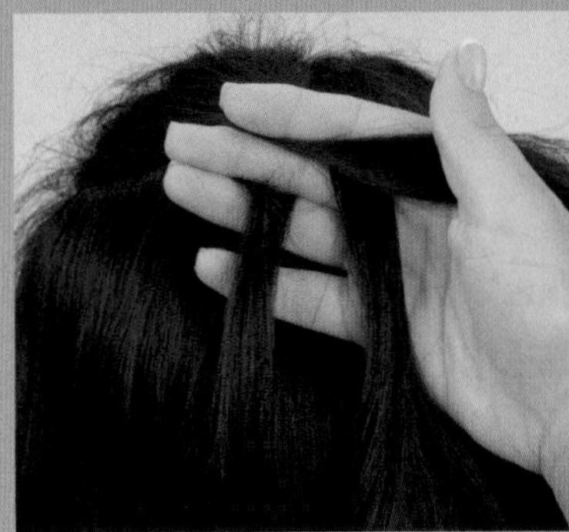

Figure 16–49 Add hair from the lef side, finger in between and palm u

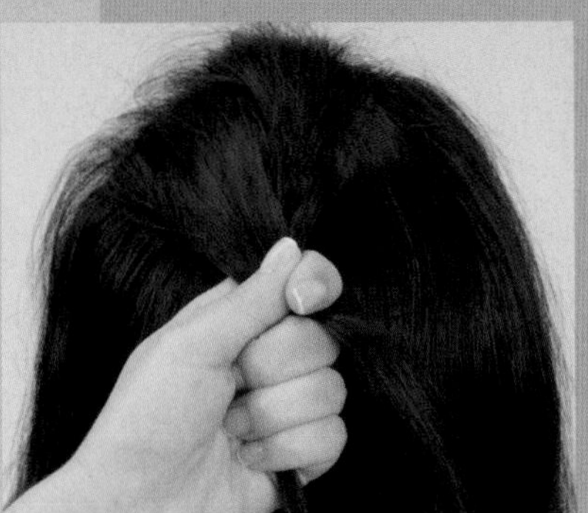

Figure 16–50 Put both strands in left hand.

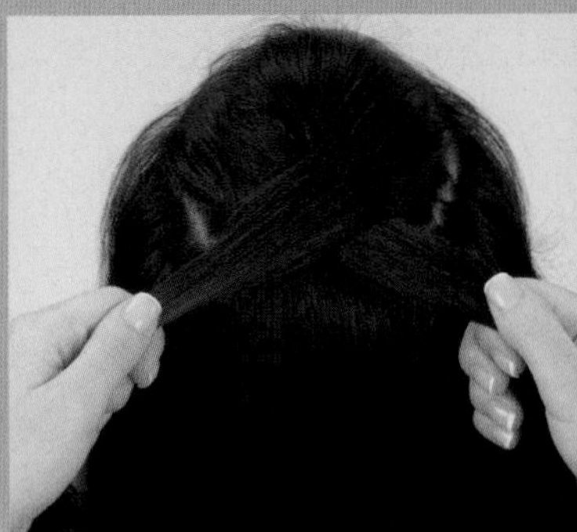

Figure 16–51 Add hair from the rig side.

7. **Repeat steps 3 through 6.** Move your hand down toward the nape with each new section picked up. When you run out of sections, secure the hair with a rubber band (Figures 16-52 and 16-53).
8. **Sanitation.** Follow cleanup and sanitation procedures for invisible braid.

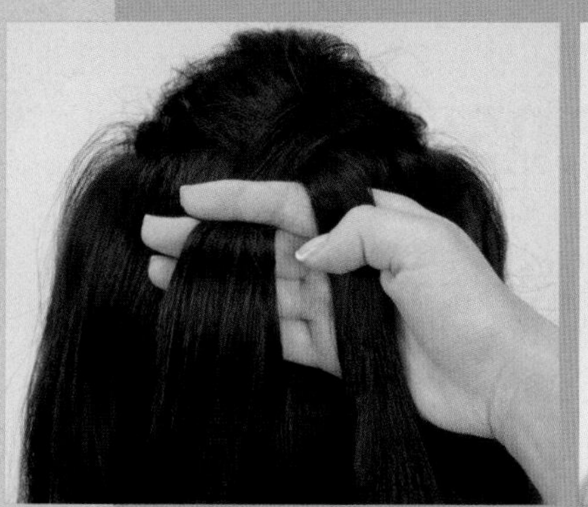

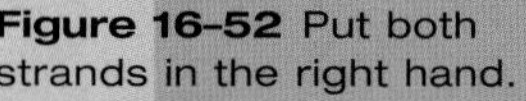

Figure 16-52 Put both strands in the right hand.

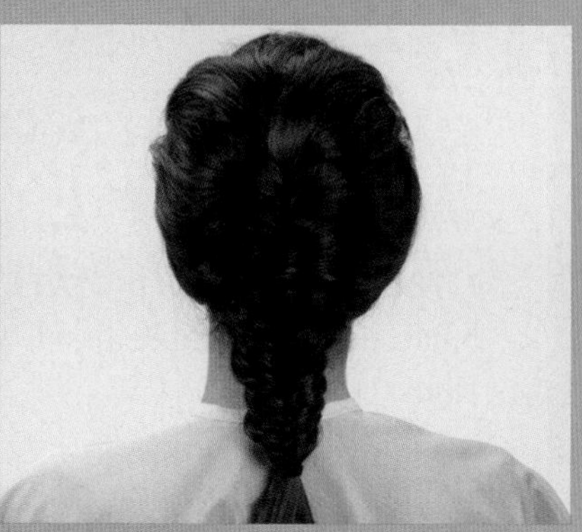

Figure 16-53 Finished fishtail braid.

CORNROWS

The fundamentals of braiding start with the classic cornrow technique. **Cornrows,** also called **canerows,** are narrow rows of visible braids that lie close to the scalp. They are created with a three-strand, on-the-scalp braid technique. Consistent and even partings are the foundation of beautiful cornrows. Learning to create these partings requires patience and practice. Using a mannequin to practice will help develop your speed, accuracy, and finger and wrist dexterity.

Cornrows are worn by men, women, and children, and can be braided on hair of various lengths and textures. For long straight hair, large cornrows are a fashionable and elegant hairstyle. Designer cornrows have become increasingly popular, with elaborate designs that demonstrate the stylist's skill and creative expression. The flat contoured styles can last several weeks when applied without extensions, and up to 2 months when applied with extensions.

CORNROWS WITH EXTENSIONS (FEED-IN METHOD)

Extensions can be applied to cornrows or individual braids with the feed-in method. In this method, the braid is built up strand by strand. Excess amounts of extension material can place too much weight on the fragile areas of the hairline and will tighten and pull the hair to leave an unrealistic finished look. By properly applying the correct tension when using the feed-in method, the braid stylist can eliminate the artificial look and prevent breakage.

The traditional cornrow is flat, natural, and contoured to the scalp. The parting is important because it defines the finished style. The feed-in method creates a tapered or narrow base at the hairline. Small pieces or strips of extension hair are added to fill in the base, bringing the adjoining braids closer together. This technique takes longer to perform than traditional cornrowing. However, a cornrow achieved by the feed-in method will last longer, look more natural, and will not place excessive tension on the hairline. There are several different ways to start a cornrow and feed in extension pieces.

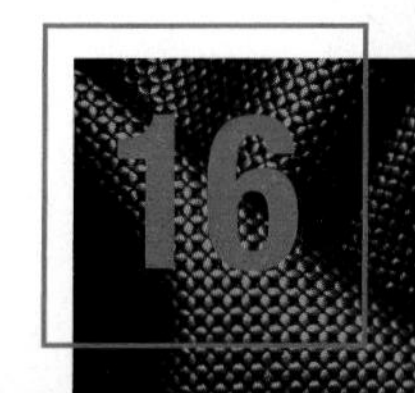

PROCEDURE 16-5

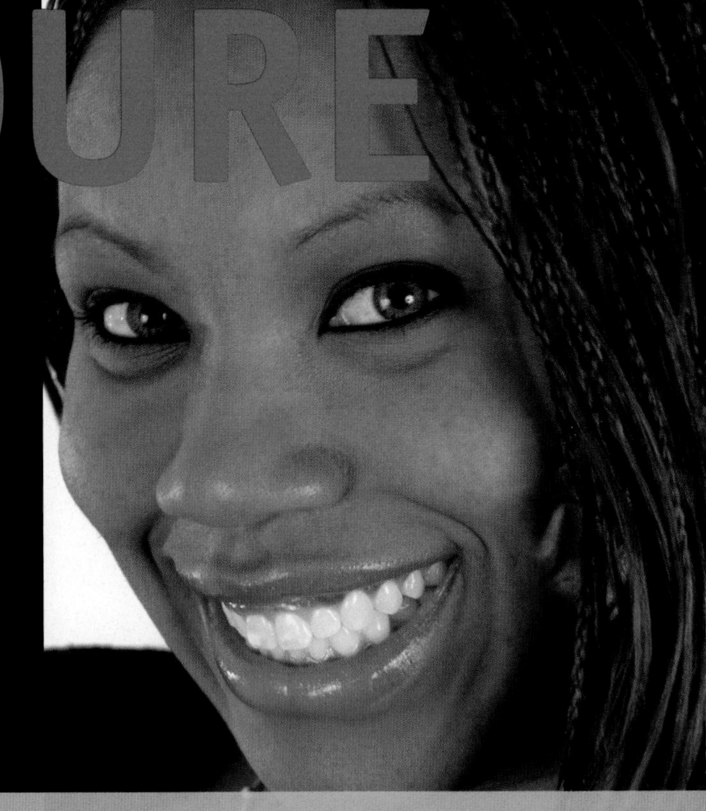

SINGLE BRAIDS WITHOUT EXTENSIONS

IMPLEMENTS AND MATERIALS

Same as for invisible braid, with the following additions:

- Light essential oil
- Butterfly clips
- Small rubber bands (optional)
- Oil sheen
- Bobby pins

PREPARATION

Same as for invisible braid.

PROCEDURE

1. **Apply essential oil.** Apply a light essential oil to the scalp and massage the oil into the scalp and throughout the hair.
2. **Ear to ear parting.** Divide the hair in half by parting from ear to ear across the crown. Clip away the front section (Figure 16-54).
3. **Determine direction.** Based on the style that you and the client have selected, determine the size and direction of the base of the braid.
4. **Take back section.** Part a diagonal section in the back of the head about 1 inch wide, taking into account the texture and length of the client's hair (Figure 16-55).
5. **Divide into strands.** Divide the section into three even strands. Place your fingers close to the base. Cross the left strand under the center strand and then cross the right strand under.

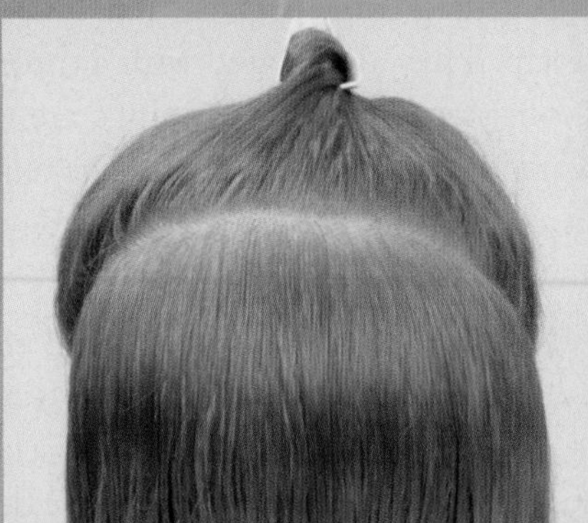

Figure 16-54 Divide hair into two main sections.

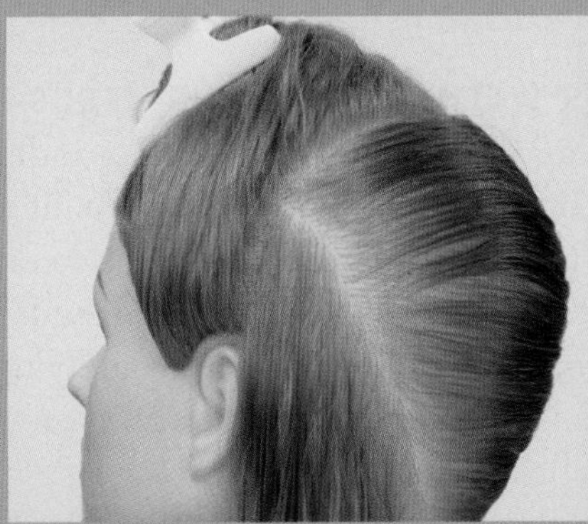

Figure 16-55 Part diagonal section.

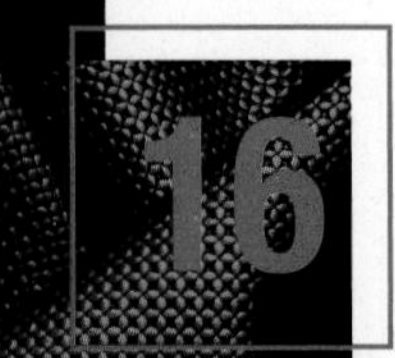

6. **Pass strands.** Pass the outer strands under the center strands, moving down the braid to the end (Figure 16-56).
7. **Continue braiding.** Move to the next section. Repeat the braiding movement by passing the alternating outside strands under the center strand. Maintain an even tension on all strands.
8. **Repeat braiding.** Continue procedure until the back is completed. Repeat in the front section (Figures 16-57 and 16-58).
9. **Work on speed and accuracy.** Try to build up speed and accuracy to create straight and even braids. Rubber bands are optional to finish each braid.
10. **Apply oil sheen.** Apply an oil sheen product as desired by your client for a shiny finished look (Figure 16-59).
11. **Sanitation.** Follow cleanup and sanitation procedures for invisible braid.

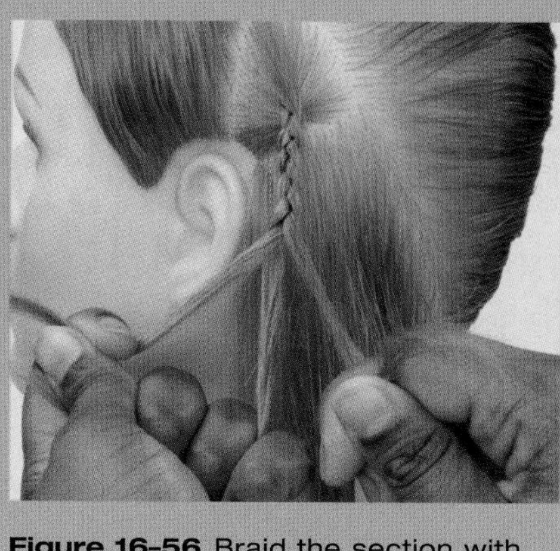

Figure 16-56 Braid the section with underhand stitch.

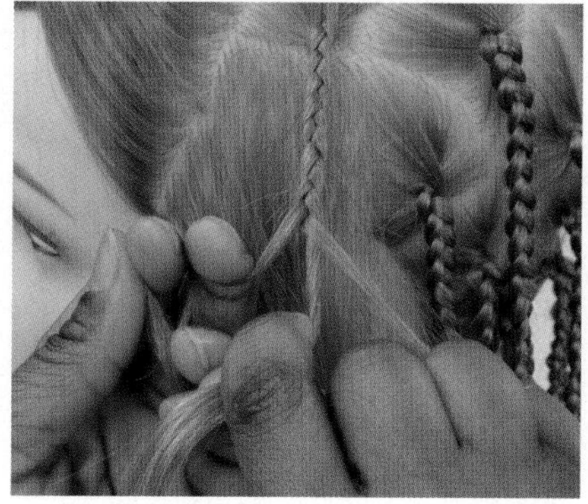

Figure 16-57 Braid the first section in the front.

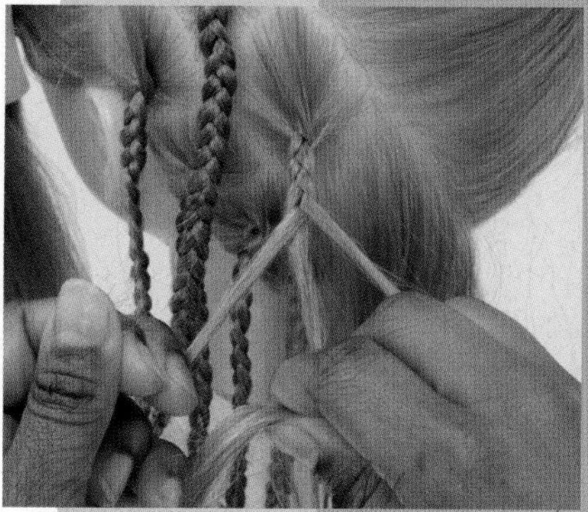

Figure 16-58 Braid the next section in the back.

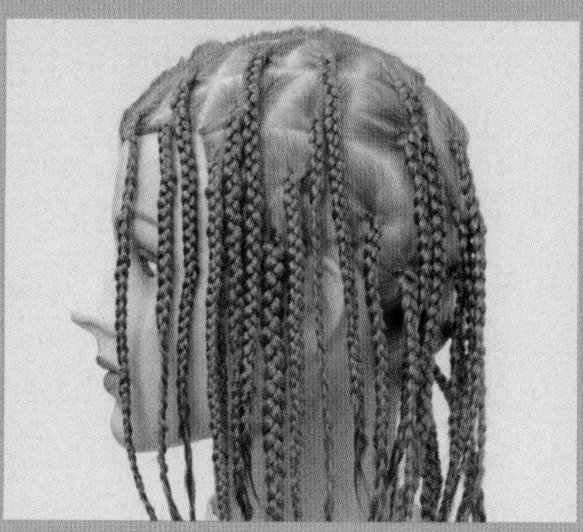

Figure 16-59 Finished single braids.

PROCEDURE 16-6

SINGLE BRAIDS WITH EXTENSIONS

IMPLEMENTS AND MATERIALS

Same as for single braids, with the following additions:

- Extension fibers
- Drawing board (optional)

PREPARATION

1. Shampoo, comb, and blow-dry the client's hair.
2. Prepare the extension fibers.

PROCEDURE

1. **Ear to ear parting.** Part the hair across the crown from ear to ear. Clip away the front section (Figure 16-60).
2. **Ear to nape parting.** Part a diagonal section in the back of the head, at about a 45-degree angle, from the ear to the nape of the neck. For a medium-size braid, this section can be from 1/4 inch (0.6 centimeters) to 1 inch (2.5 centimeters) wide depending on the texture and length of the client's hair (Figure 16-61).
3. **Create diamond-shaped base.** Using vertical parts to separate the base into subsections, create a diamond-shaped base (Figure 16-62).
4. **Select extensions.** Select the appropriate amount of extension fibers from the drawing board. The extension should always be proportional to the section that it is being applied to. For tapered ends, gently pull extension fibers at both sides so that the ends are uneven. Then fold the fibers in half (Figure 16-63).
5. **Divide into three sections.** Divide the natural hair into three equal sections. Place the folded extension on top of the natural hair, on the outside and center portions of the braid (Figure 16-64).

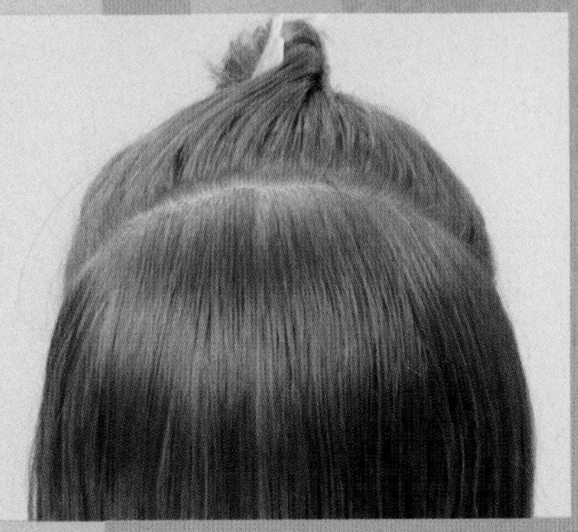

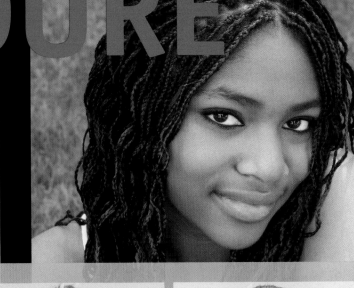

Figure 16-60 Part the hair across the crown.

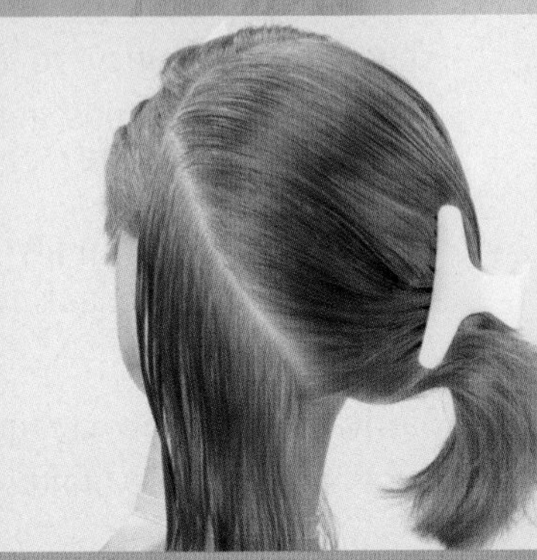

Figure 16-61 Part a diagonal sectio

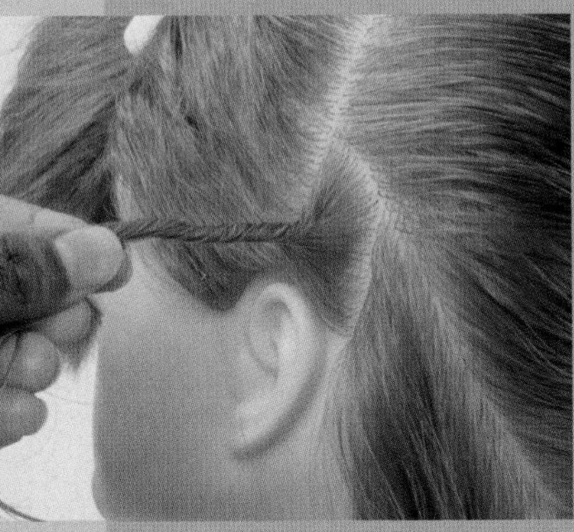

Figure 16-62 Create diamond-shaped base.

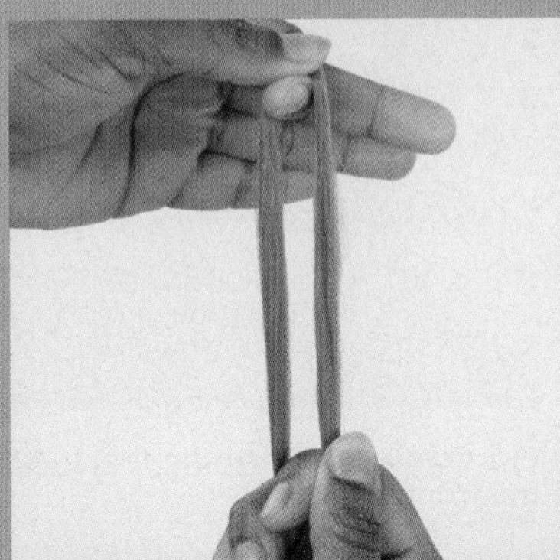

Figure 16-63 Fold extension fibers half.

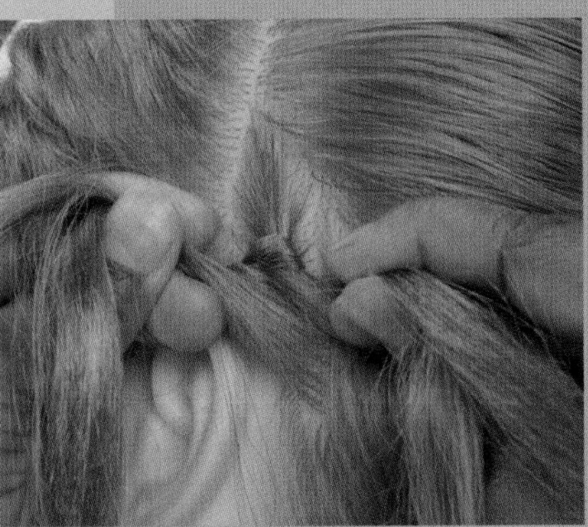

Figure 16-64 Place extension fibers on natural hair.

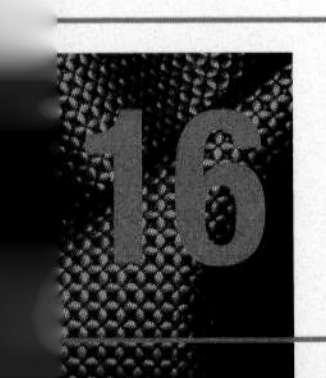

6. **Underhand movement.** Once the extension is in place, begin the underhand braiding movement. Remember that the outer strands should cross under the center strand. Each time you pass an outer strand under the center strand, bring the center strand over tightly so that the outside strand stays securely in the center. As you move down the braid, keep your fingers close to the stitch, so that the braid remains tight and straight (Figure 16-65).
7. **Braid.** Continue braid to the desired length.
8. **Continue with next section.** The next section should be above the previous section on a diagonal part, moving toward the ear. After several sections have been completed, alternate the diagonal partings so that a V-shaped pattern forms in the back of the head (Figure 16-66).
9. **Part above ear in front.** Once the back is finished, create a diagonal or horizontal parting above the ear in the front (Figure 16-67). As you get closer to the hairline, be aware of the amount of extension hair that is applied to the hairline. Do not add excessive amounts of fiber into a fragile hairline. The fiber should always be proportionate to the hair that it is being applied to (Figures 16-68 and 16-69).
10. **Remove loose ends.** After the entire head has been braided, remove all loose hair ends from the braid shaft with scissors.
11. **Finish ends.** Spray hair ends with water to activate the wave in human hair extensions (Figure 16-70).
12. **Sanitation.** Follow cleanup and sanitation procedures for invisible braid.

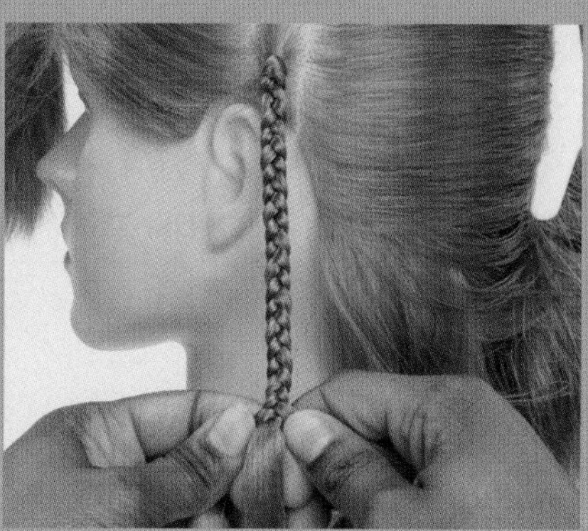
Figure 16-65 Braid the section.

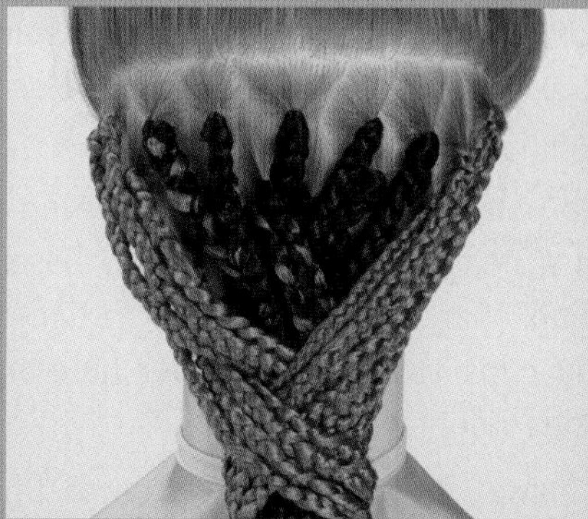
Figure 16-66 "V" pattern.

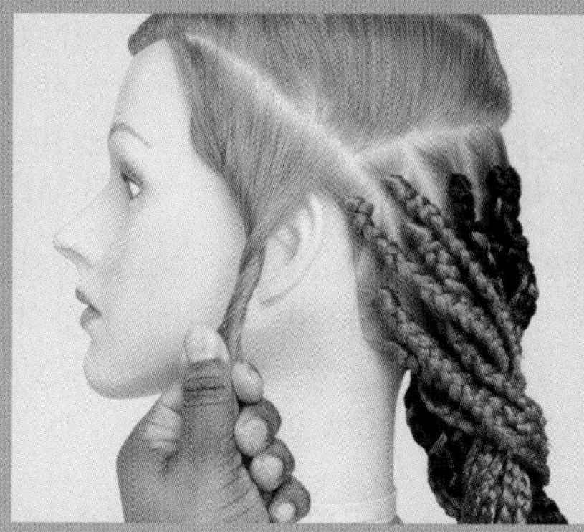
Figure 16-67 Create parting above the ear.

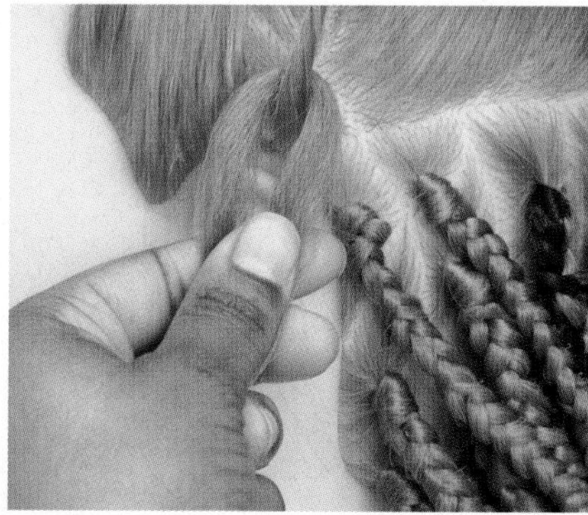
Figure 16-68 Work down the braid.

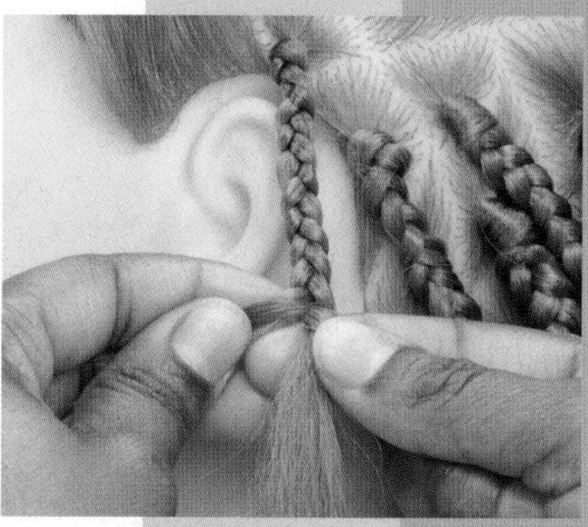
Figure 16-69 Add extension fibers.

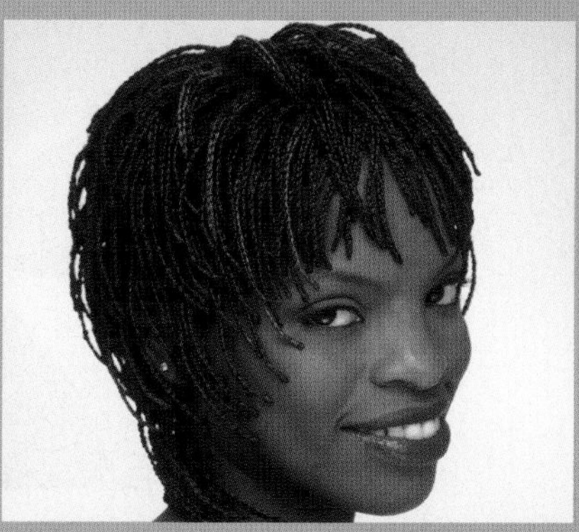
Figure 16-70 A finished style.

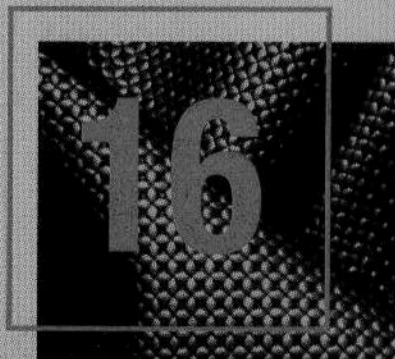

PROCEDURE 16-7

BASIC CORNROWS

IMPLEMENTS AND MATERIALS

Same as for single braids.

PREPARATION

Same as for single braids.

PROCEDURE

1. **Determine direction and size.** Depending on desired style, determine the correct size and direction of the cornrow base. With tail comb, part hair into 2-inch (5-centimeter) sections and apply a light essential oil to the scalp. Massage oil throughout scalp and hair (Figure 16-71).
2. **Create a panel.** Start by taking two even partings to form a neat row for the cornrow base. With a tail comb, part the hair into a panel, using butterfly clips to keep the other hair pinned to either side (Figure 16-72).
3. **Divide panel and cross left strand.** Divide the panel into three even strands. To ensure consistency, make sure that strands are the same size. Place fingers close to the base. Cross the left strand (1) under the center strand (2). The center strand is now on the left and strand (1) is the new center (Figure 16-73).
4. **Cross the right strand.** Cross the right strand (3) under the center strand (1). Passing the outer strands under the center strand this way creates the underhand cornrow braid (Figure 16-74).

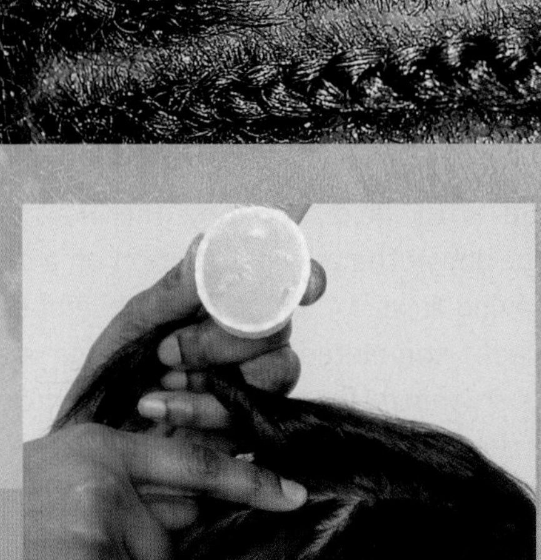

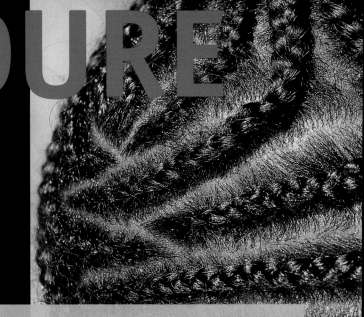

Figure 16-71 Massage essential oil through hair.

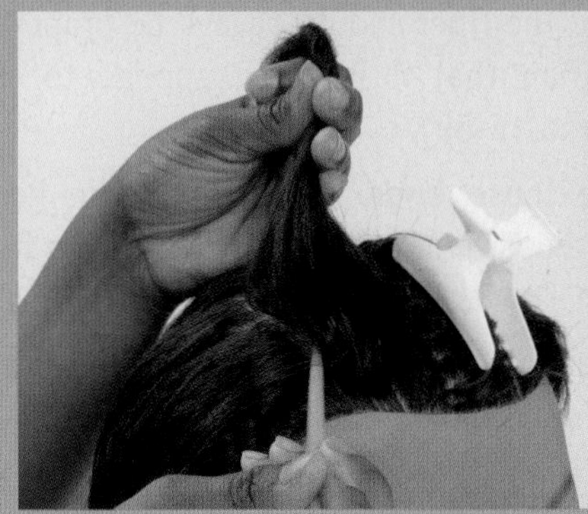

Figure 16-72 Part out a panel.

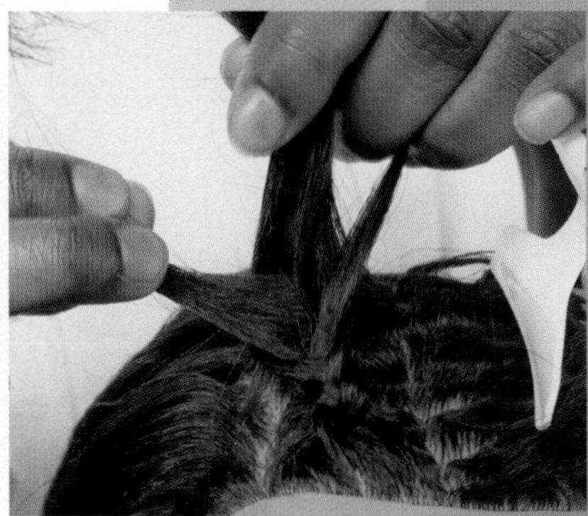

Figure 16-73 Pass left strand under center strand.

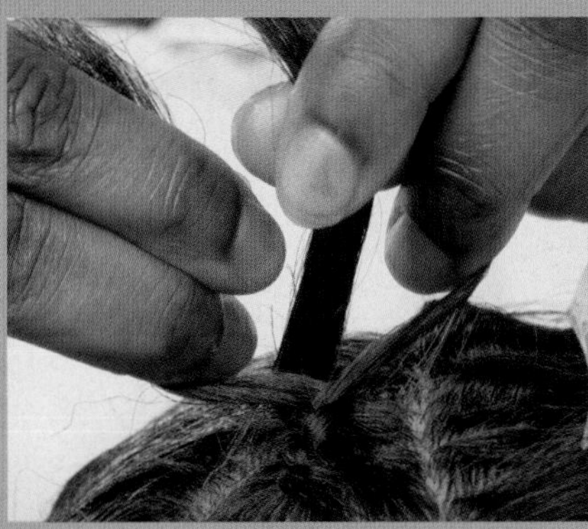

Figure 16-74 Pass right strand under center strand.

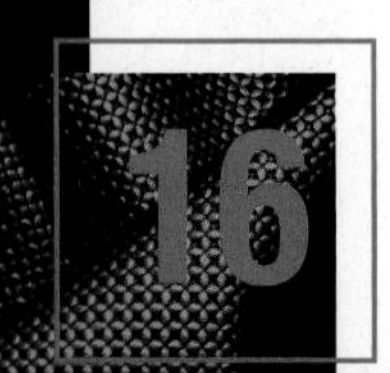

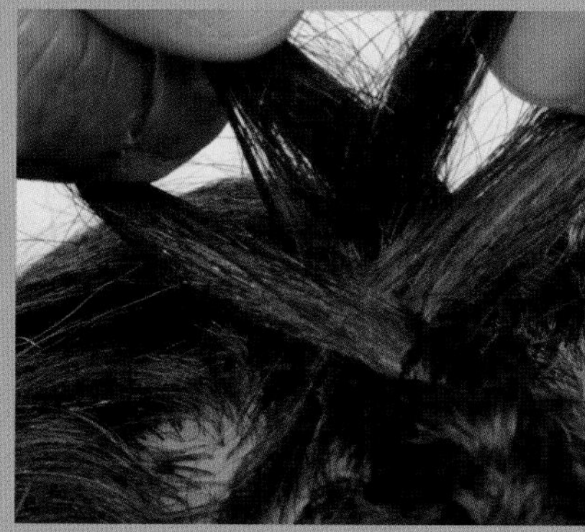
Figure 16-75 Add hair to left outer strand.

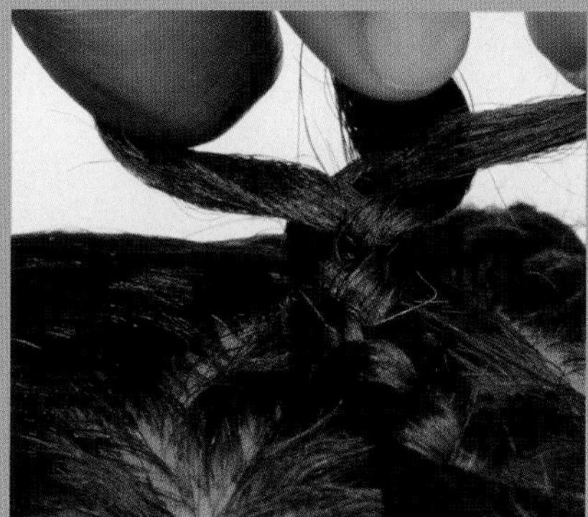
Figure 16-76 Add hair to right outer strand.

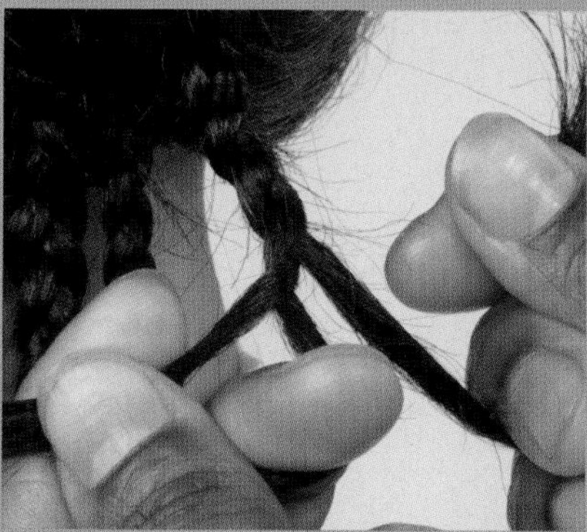
Figure 16-77 Braid cornrow to end.

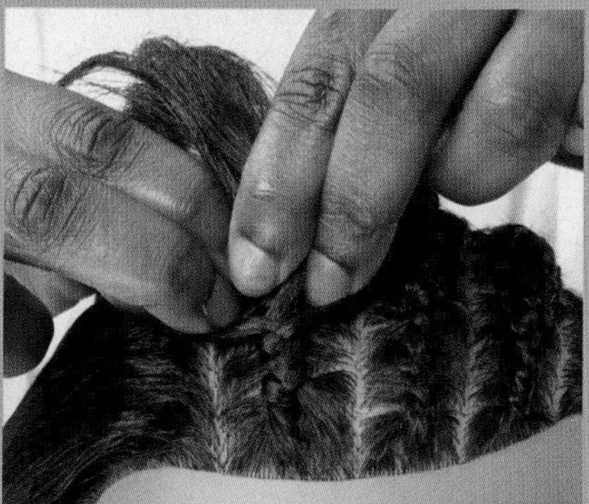
Figure 16-78 Braid next cornrow.

5. **Add to outer strand.** With each crossing under or revolution, pick up from the base of the panel a new strand of equal size and add it to the outer strand before crossing it under the center strand (Figure 16-75).
6. **Continue braiding and add to outer strand.** As you move along the braid panel, pick up a strand from the scalp with each revolution, and add it to the outer strand before crossing it under, alternating the side of the braid on which you pick up the hair (Figure 16-76).
7. **Add new strands.** As new strands are added, the braid will become fuller. Braid to the end.
8. **Braid to ends.** Simply braiding to the ends can finish the cornrow; small rubber bands can be used to hold the ends in place (Figure 16-77). Other optional finishes, such as singeing, are considered advanced methods and require special training.
9. **Braid next panel.** Braid the next panel in the same direction and in the same manner. Keep the partings clean and even (Figure 16-78).
10. **Repeat until all the hair is braided.** Apply oil sheen for a finished look (Figure 16-79).
11. **Sanitation.** Follow cleanup and sanitation procedures for invisible braid.

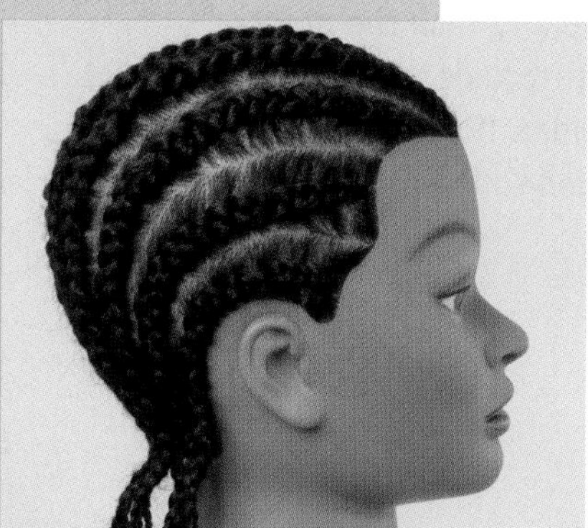
Figure 16-79 Finished cornrows.

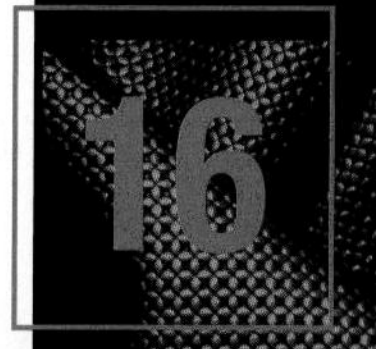

PROCEDURE 16-8

CORNROWS WITH EXTENSIONS

IMPLEMENTS AND MATERIALS

Same as for single braids with extensions.

PREPARATION

Same as for single braids with extensions.

PROCEDURE

1. **Part and oil.** With tail comb, part the hair into 2-inch (5-centimeter) sections and apply light essential oil to the scalp. Massage the oil throughout the scalp and hair.
2. **Part off base.** Starting at the hairline, part off a cornrow base in the desired direction (Figure 16-80). No extension is added at the starting point. If the hair extension is required because of a thinning hairline, apply minute amounts, as small as 5 to 10 strands. Divide the natural hair into three equal strands.
3. **First revolution.** With the first revolution, cross strand 1 under strand 2 (Figure 16-81).
4. **Second revolution.** On the second revolution, the right strand 3 crosses under strand 1. Pick up a small portion of natural hair and add it to the outer strand during the revolution (Figure 16-82).
5. **Introduce extension fiber.** After several revolutions and pick-ups of the natural hair, you can introduce small amounts of extension fiber, perhaps 10 to 20 fibers. To avoid bulk or knots, the amount of extension should be proportionately less than the size of the base. Fold the fibers in the middle and tuck the point in between two adjoining strands of natural hair (Figure 16-83). The folded fibers will form two portions, which are added to the center and

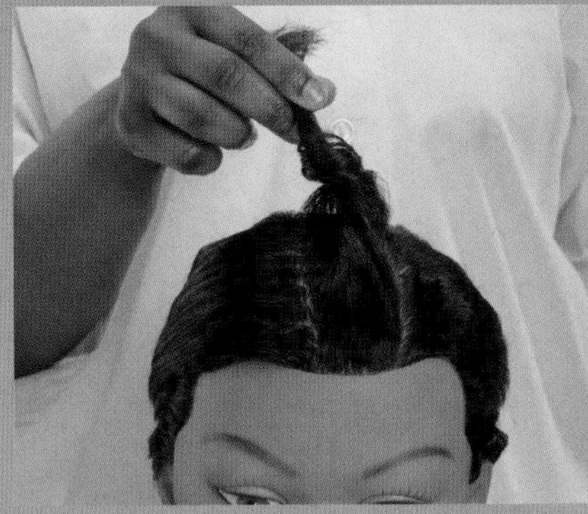

Figure 16-80 Part off cornrow base.

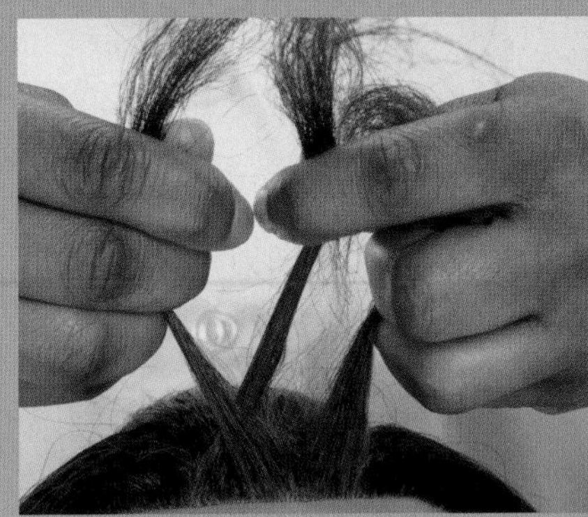

Figure 16-81 Cross outer strand under center strand.

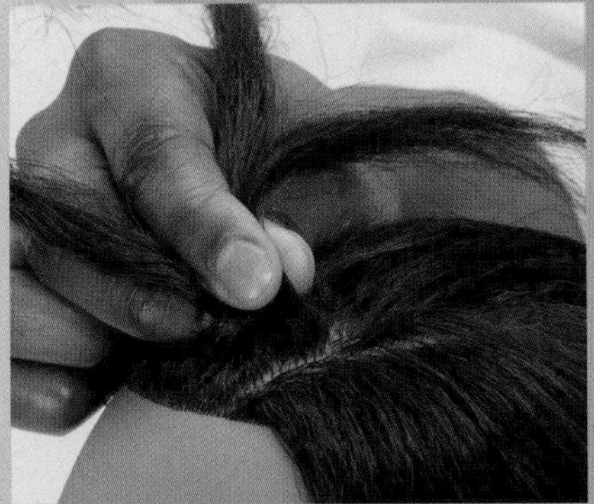

Figure 16-82 Add hair to outer strand.

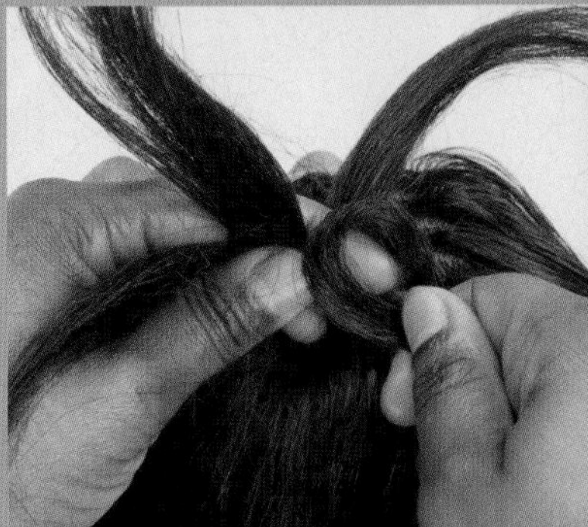

Figure 16-83 Tuck folded extension fibers into cornrow.

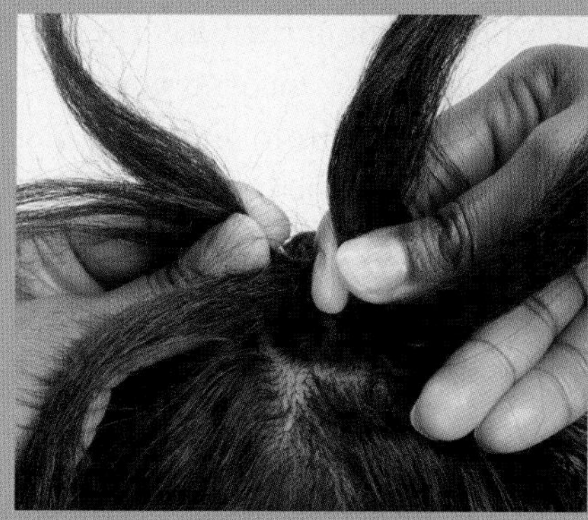

Figure 16-84 Add sides of extensions to center and outer strands.

outer strands before the next pick-up and revolution (Figure 16-84). Do not forget to continue picking up natural hair with each revolution in order to execute the cornrow (Figures 16-85 and 16-86).

6. **Repeat until all the hair is braided** (Figure 16-87).
7. **Sanitation.** Follow cleanup and sanitation procedures for invisible braid.

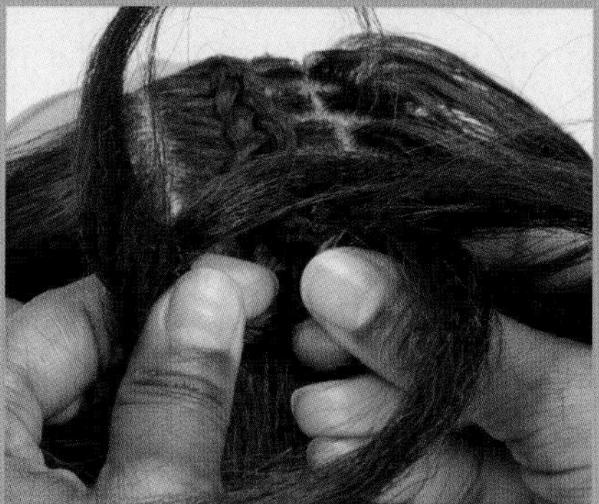

Figure 16-85 Pick up natural hair.

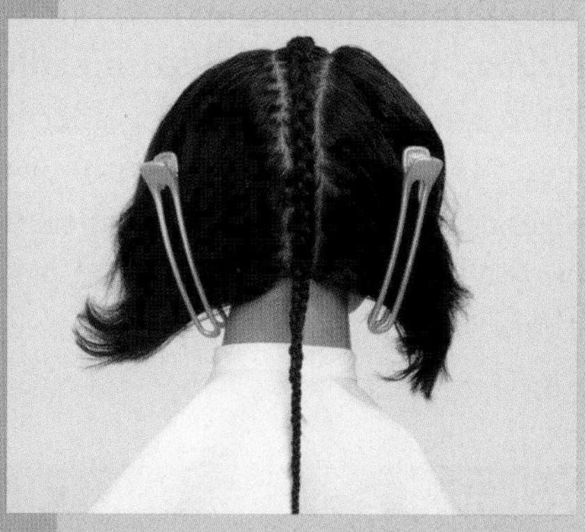

Figure 16-86 Braid to end of strand.

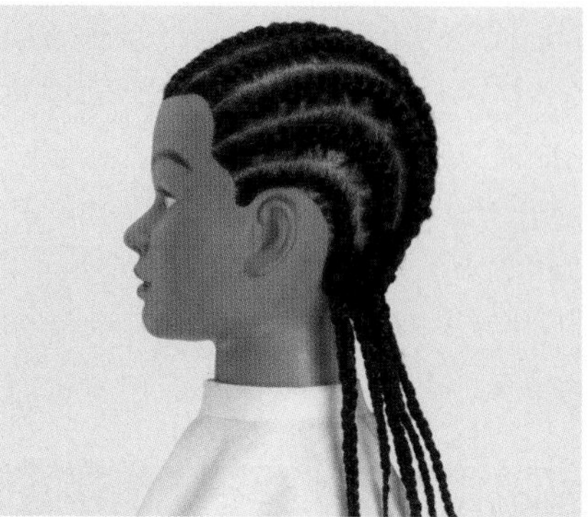

Figure 16-87 Finished style.

Here's a TIP

For a professional finish, always trim any ends that may stick up through the braid. Holding your scissors flat, move up the shaft as you trim, making sure that you avoid cutting into the braid.

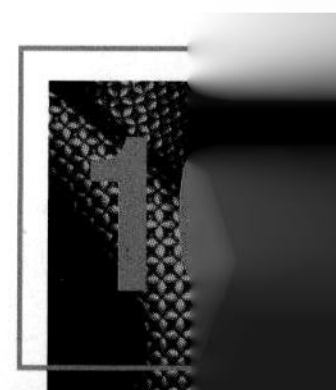

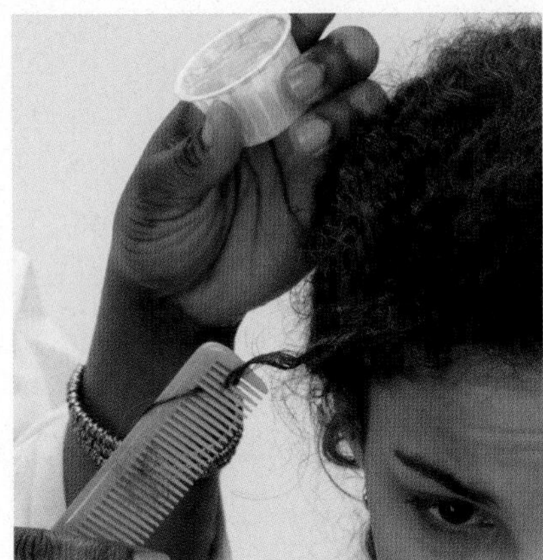
Figure 16-88 Spiral the hair with the comb.

During the cornrow process, when picking up hair at the base, the hair directly underneath the previous revolution must be incorporated into the braid. The hair that you pick up must never come from another panel or be extended up into the braid from a lower part of the braid. The same is true when executing any braid technique. Overextending or misplacing the beginning of the extension leaves the hair exposed and unsupported, which can lead to breakage and hair loss in that area. This is particularly true when adding extensions at the hairline. If the extension is not made secure by two or three revolutions before picking up, it may shift away from the point of entry.

LOCKS

The ultimate in natural hair care is the textured richness offered by hair locking. **Locks,** also called **dreadlocks,** are natural textured hair that is intertwined and meshed together to form a single or separate network of hair. Hair locking is done without the use of chemicals. The hair locks in several slow phases, which can take from six months to a year depending on the length, density, and coil pattern of the hair (see Figure 16-88 and Table 16-1).

	DEVELOPMENT PHASES OF LOCKS
PHASE	Characteristics
Phase 1	Hair is soft and is coiled into spiral configurations. The coil is smooth and the end is open. The coil has a shiny or a glossy texture.
Prelock Stage, Phase 2	Hair begins to interlace and mesh. The separate units begin to "puff up" and expand in size. The units are no longer glossy or smooth.
Sprouting Stage, Phase 3	A bulb can be felt at the end of each lock. Interlacing continues.
Growing Stage, Phase 4	Hair begins to regain length. Lock may still be frizzy, but also solid in some areas.
Maturation Stage, Phase 5	Locks are closed at the ends, dense and dull, and do not reflect light.
Atrophy Stage, Phase 6	Lock is totally closed at the end. Hair is tightly meshed, giving the hair a rope-like cylinder shape, except where there is new growth at the base. After several years of maturation, the lock may start to weaken or come apart at the ends.

Table 16-1 Developmental Phases of Locks

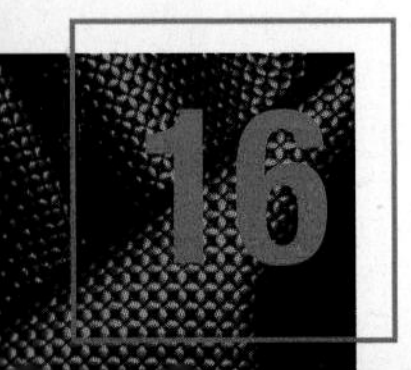

Locks are more than just a hairstyle; they are a cultural expression. There are several ways to cultivate locks, such as double twisting, wrapping with cord, coiling, braiding, or simply by not combing or brushing the lock. As demonstrated by the Rastafarians of Jamaica, leaving the hair to its own natural course will cause it to lock. Cultivated African locks have symmetry and balance.

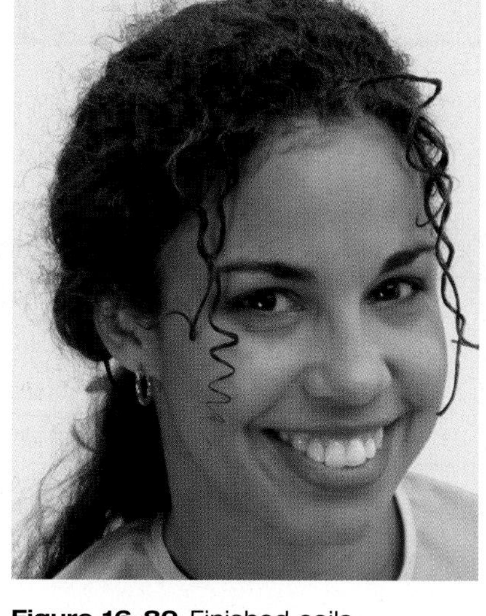

Figure 16-89 Finished coils.

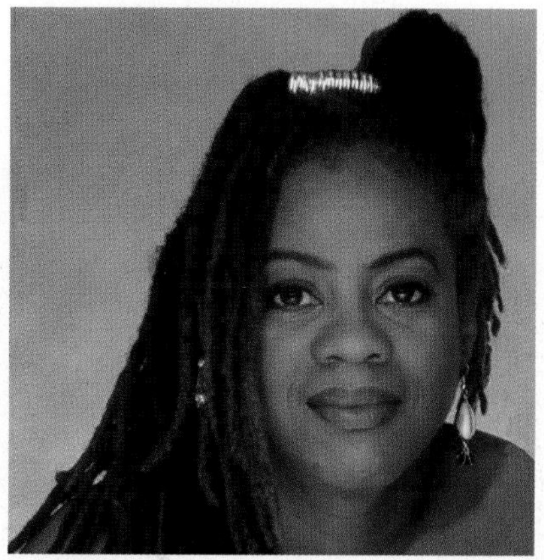

Figure 16-90 Locks.

The three basic methods of locking follow:

1. *The comb technique.* Particularly effective during the early stages of locking while the coil is still open, this method involves placing the comb at the base of the scalp and, with a rotating motion, spiraling the hair into a curl. With each revolution, the comb moves down until it reaches the end of the hair shaft. It offers a tight coil and is excellent on short (1-inch to 3-inch) hair (Figures 16-89 and 16-90).
2. *The palm roll.* This method is the gentlest on the hair and guides it through all the natural stages of locking. Palm rolling takes advantage of the hair's natural ability to coil. This method involves applying gel to dampened subsections, placing the portion of hair between the palms of both hands, and rolling in a clockwise or counterclockwise direction (Figure 16-91). With each revolution, as you move down the coil shaft, the entire coil is formed (Figure 16-92). Partings can be directional, horizontal, vertical, or brick-layered. Decorative designs and sculpting patterns are some of the creative options you can choose.
3. *Braids or extensions.* Another effective way to start locks involves sectioning the hair for the desired size of lock and single braiding the hair to the end. Synthetic hair fiber, human hair fiber, or yarn can be added to a single braid to form a lock. After several weeks, the braid will grow away from the scalp, at which time the palm roll method can be used to cultivate the new growth to form a lock.

Shaping dreadlocks takes patience and commitment on the part of clients. In the beginning, they must have frequent professional hair shapings to ensure a good outcome.

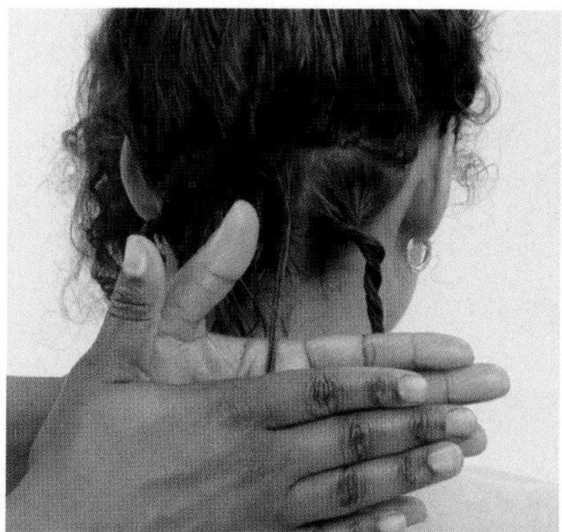

Figure 16-91 Roll the hair between the palms.

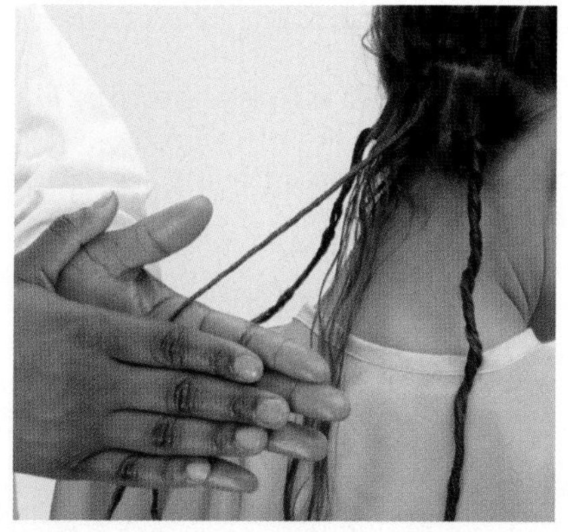

Figure 16-92 Roll down the coil shaft.

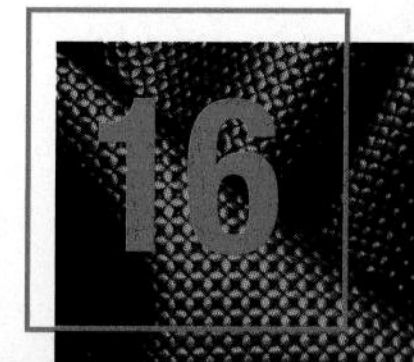

REVIEW QUESTIONS

1. What is meant by "natural hairstyling"?
2. In the context of braiding, what are the three qualities that determine hair texture?
3. What is a coil?
4. What six materials are most commonly used for hair extensions?
5. Why does textured (extremely curly or coiled) hair require special preparation before braiding?
6. What is the difference between a visible and invisible braiding style?
7. Describe rope and fishtail braids.
8. Explain the basic procedure for creating single braids.
9. Explain the methods of cornrowing with and without extensions.
10. Name the three basic methods of hair locking.

CHAPTER GLOSSARY

cornrows or canerows	Narrow rows of visible braids that lie close to the scalp; created with a three-strand, on-the-scalp braid technique.
fishtail braid	Simple two-strand braid in which hair is picked up from the sides and added to the strands as they are crossed over each other.
invisible or inverted braid	Three-strand braid produced by overlapping the strands of hair on top of each other.
locks or dreadlocks	Natural textured hair that is intertwined and meshed together to form a single or separate network of hair.
natural hairstyling	Hairstyling that uses no chemicals or tints and does not alter the natural curl or coil pattern of the hair.
rope braid	Braid made with two strands that are twisted around each other.
single braids	Free-hanging braids, with or without extensions, that can be executed either underhand or overhand; also called individual or box braids.
visible braid	Three-strand braid made by the underhand technique, in which the strands of hair are woven under the center strand.

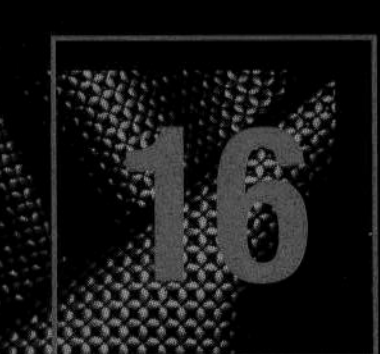

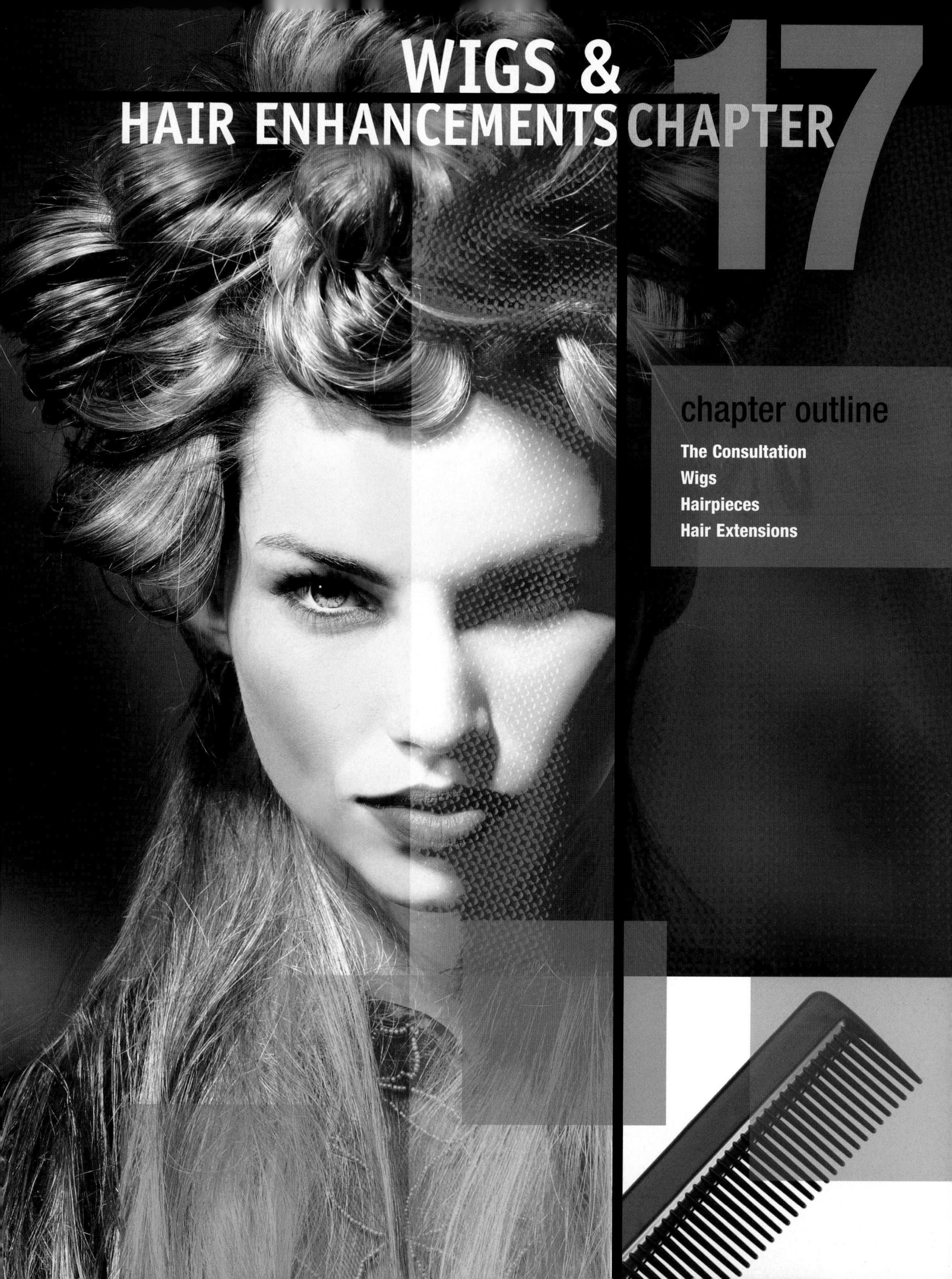
WIGS &
HAIR ENHANCEMENTS
CHAPTER
17
chapter outline
The Consultation
Wigs
Hairpieces
Hair Extensions

Learning Objectives

After completing this chapter, you will be able to:

- List the elements of a client consultation for wig services.
- Explain the differences between human hair and synthetic wigs.
- Describe the two basic categories of wigs.
- Demonstrate the procedure for taking wig measurements.
- Demonstrate the procedure for putting on a wig.
- Describe the various types of hairpieces and their uses.
- Explain the various methods of attaching extensions.

Key Terms

Page number indicates where in the chapter the term is used.

block
pg. 404

bonding
pg. 417

cap wigs
pg. 403

capless wigs
pg. 403

fallen hair
pg. 403

fusion
pg. 418

hair extensions
pg. 416

hairpiece
pg. 400

hand-tied wigs or *hand-knotted wigs*
pg. 403

integration hairpiece
pg. 413

machine-made wigs
pg. 404

semi-hand-tied wigs
pg. 404

toupee
pg. 413

track-and-sew method
pg. 416

turned hair
pg. 402

wefts
pg. 403

wig
pg. 400

From the very beginning of recorded history, wigs have played an important role in the world of fashion. The ancient Egyptians shaved their heads with bronze razors and wore heavy black wigs to protect themselves from the sun. In ancient Rome, women wore wigs made from the prized blond hair of barbarians captured from the north. In 18th-century England, men wore wigs, called "perukes," to indicate that they were in the army or navy, or engaged in the practice of law.

Wigs and hair additions play an equally important role in today's fashion-conscious world. Specialists in hair additions and enhancements are increasingly in demand, working on runway and hair shows, and print and video shoots (Figures 17-1 and 17-2). For the millions of people who suffer from extreme thinning or total hair loss, today's natural-looking wigs can make them feel much better about their appearance. Imagine how gratifying it would be to help a cancer patient who has suffered hair loss to feel better about her appearance. Or, you could offer help to a client who is going through premature hair loss and is feeling anxious about it. With the right knowledge and practice, you can use your skills in hair enhancement to bring a satisfying new dimension to many people's lives.

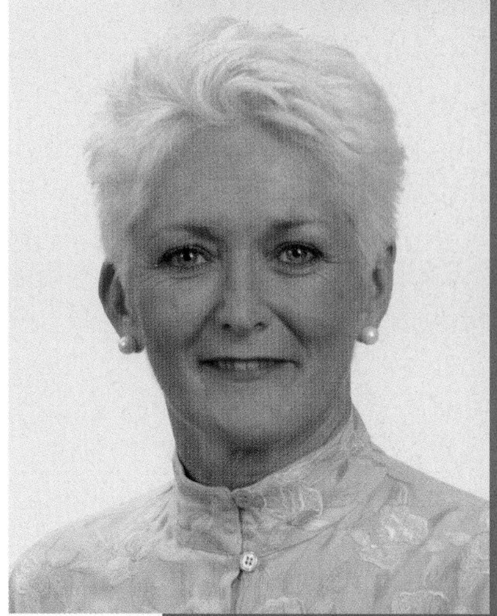

Figure 17-1 Client before fitting with a wig.

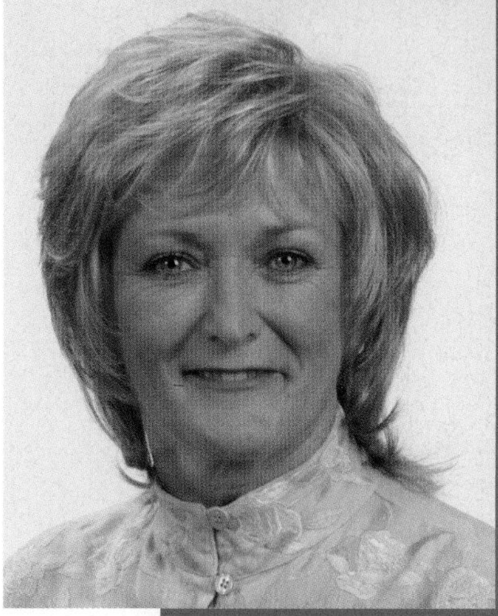

Figure 17-2 The same client, transformed.

THE CONSULTATION

As with other salon services, the client consultation for wig services is designed to offer some degree of protection for both you and the client (Figure 17-3). Your client may have big dreams that he or she feels can be made into reality by a wig or hairpiece. You can offer your client a makeover, but the results will always be limited by reality. This needs to be fully understood at the beginning. If not understood, both client and practitioner may suffer disappointment and frustration.

A wig service can also be a large financial and emotional investment for the client. Often, the decision to wear a wig results from the client's hair loss. You need to understand your client's motivation in seeking a wig service to make sure that the client will be satisfied in the end.

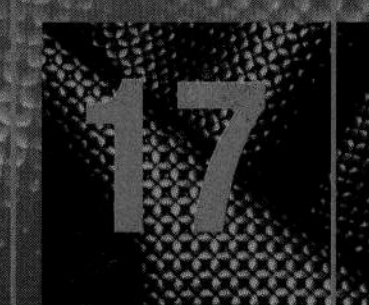

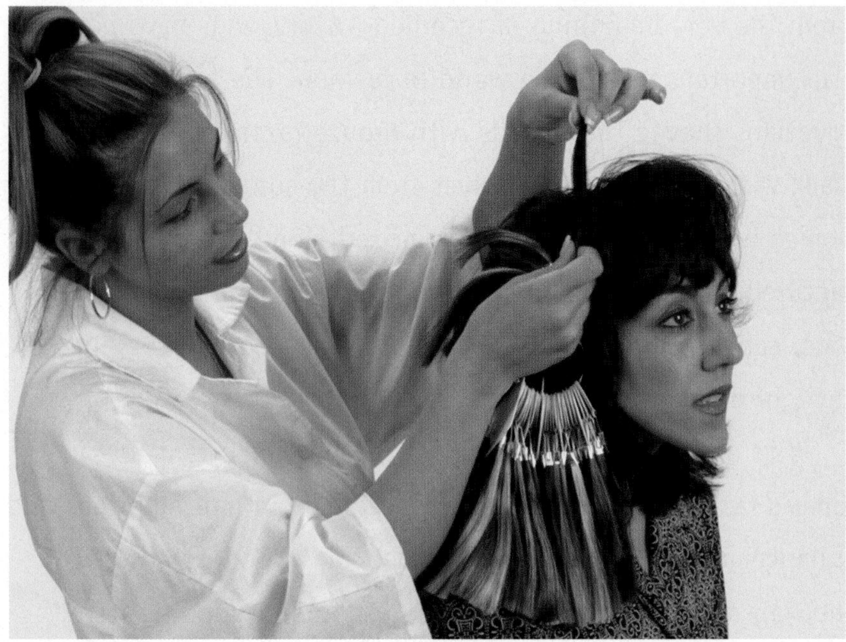

Figure 17-3 Client consultation.

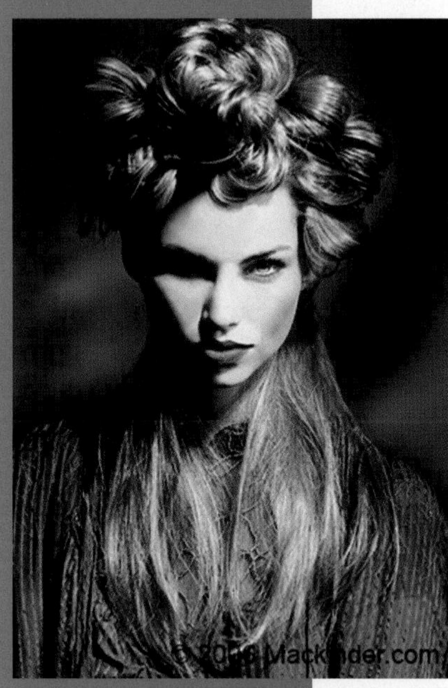

Figure 17-4 Wigs can add a dramatic touch.

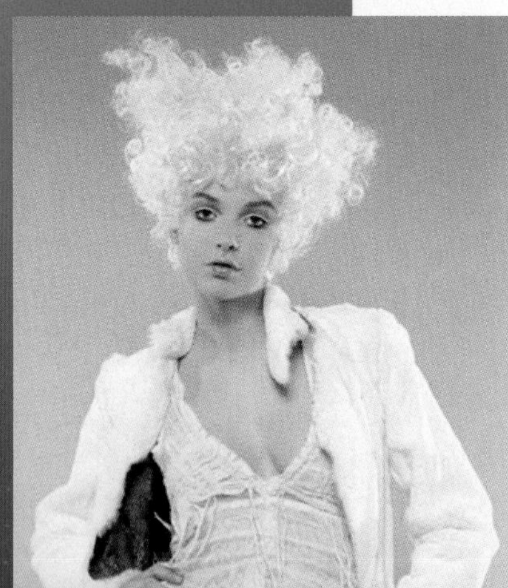

Figure 17-5 Wigs can be whimsical.

Conduct your consultation with understanding and sensitivity. Make a person-to-person connection that conveys a positive attitude. Keep in mind that regardless of the client's motivation for trying a hair enhancement—a social event, to cover up hair loss, or just for fun—the client is likely to feel a little nervous about it (Figures 17-4 and 17-5). Concerns may include how she looks, how her spouse will feel about it, whether people will know the hair is not the client's own, and how much money it will cost. The point of the consultation is to cut through the doubts and fears with genuine communication. Your best tool for achieving good communication is the following "key point checklist":

1. Determining need and desire.
   - Does your client plan to use the addition as a fashion accessory?
   - Will it be used for a wedding, prom, or some other special occasion?
   - Is the client looking to create instant glamour for herself?
   - Will the main reason of the addition be to disguise thinning hair or hair loss due to illness?
   - Will the hair addition be used in film work, TV, theater, fashion shows, or photo shoots?
2. Matching the style with the client.
   - Determine your client's personality type. The introverted client often likes to "play it safe" with a style that is natural and does not draw too much attention to the hair addition. Her goal is to enhance what she already has. The extroverted client is bold and adventurous and may be looking for a change. She is often drawn to the more stylized hair additions that are dramatic.

- Consider your client's age. If she is young, she may want a playful style. If she is mature, she may prefer a more natural style.
- Consider your client's personal image. Is it corporate? Trendy? Classic? Country? Glamorous? Cute? Athletic?
- Take note of the client's job or career. If she works in a health club, for instance, she can get away with a look that may be out of place in a bank.

3. Finding the right balance.
   - Study your client's bone structure and body type. Step back and take a look at the big picture. Keep in mind the rule of classic proportions: the ratio of head size to body should be about 1 to 7. The added hair must not overwhelm the client, unless it is part of a theatrical look.
   - When adding hair, it is best to conduct your consultation with the client in her street clothes, not caped and gowned. Capes offer excellent protection when performing a service, but they can also camouflage the client's body type and mask proportions. You want to make sure that the style you envision will work with the client's "look."
4. Working with the client's hair type.
   - You will need to determine hair texture in order to blend the artificial hair with the natural hair.
   - Be aware of natural hairlines and growth patterns, which will influence your choice of wig, hairpiece, or extensions.
   - The condition of the natural hair will determine how much of the real hair you decide to show and how much you decide to cover up.
   - Check the hair density. Does the client have a full head of hair and simply want an alternative look, or is the client's hair thinning and patchy?
5. Selecting the appropriate hair addition.
   - Among the hair addition options you will be bringing to your client's attention are wigs (human or synthetic, custom-made, or ready-to-wear), hair extensions (temporary, clip-in, or semi-permanent), or hairpieces (falls, ponytails, switches, wiglets, braids, ponytail wraps) and toupees.
   - Is the addition temporary or semi-permanent? Does the client want to maintain the look through salon services or home maintenance? How long will the client be wearing the wig? Are there serious health issues involved that might determine the length of time that the wig will be worn?
   - What environmental factors are involved? Consider humidity and exposure, for instance. You might want to suggest a synthetic hairpiece for a client in Florida, because it will not frizz in high humidity.

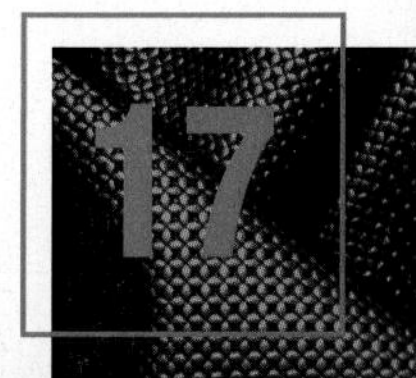

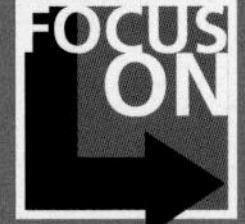

Focus on . . .
Client Care

In addition to wearing wigs for fun and versatility, many clients experience hair loss due to a serious illness or the treatment for a disease (e.g., cancer). Be attuned to your client's emotional state about his/her well-being and be sensitive to the client's need for a private consultation.

- Use a sample color ring to identify the correct color match for your client.
- Have on hand various product photos and brochures from which your client can make a selection. It is also good to keep samples of the products themselves for your client to see and feel.
- Will the wig or hairpiece need to be custom cut or colored?

6. Budgetary concerns.
   - What is the client's budget? This is often the biggest factor in choosing a product.
   - Using catalogs and price lists, be prepared to educate the client on the features and benefits of the various price points (high, medium, and low).
   - Establish salon service fees for custom cutting, coloring, and styling of hair additions.
7. Other available creative options. Do not neglect to call your client's attention to the following services that you can provide:
   - Custom cutting.
   - Color, perming, setting, and styling of wigs, hairpieces, and extensions.
   - Styling maintenance program that will educate the client in the use of styling products.

WIGS

A **wig** can be defined as an artificial covering for the head consisting of a network of interwoven hair. When wearing a wig, the client's hair is completely concealed (100-percent coverage). If a hair addition does not fully cover the head, it is classified as a **hairpiece,** which is a small wig used to cover the top or crown of the head (Figure 17-6).

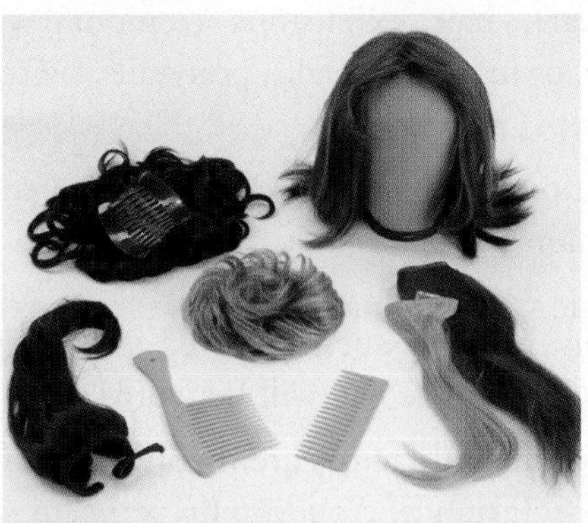

Figure 17-6 Wigs and hairpieces come in a wide range of styles and colors.

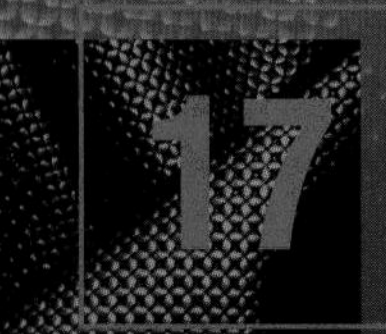

HUMAN HAIR VERSUS SYNTHETIC HAIR

What is the fastest way to tell if a strand of hair is a synthetic product or real human hair? Pull the strand out of the wig or hairpiece and burn it with a match. Human hair will burn slowly, giving off a distinctive odor. A strand of synthetic fiber, on the other hand, will either "ball up" and melt, extinguishing itself (a characteristic of a synthetic like Kanekalon), or will continue to flame and burn out very quickly (typical of polyester). In either case, it will not give off an odor.

How can you determine whether real hair or a synthetic is best for your client? Both have advantages and disadvantages.

ADVANTAGES OF HUMAN HAIR WIGS

- More realistic appearance than synthetic wigs.
- Greater durability.
- Same styling and maintenance requirements as natural hair. Human hair wigs can be custom colored and permed to suit the client, and they tolerate heat from a blow-dryer, curling iron, or hot rollers.

DISADVANTAGES OF HUMAN HAIR WIGS

- Human hair reacts to the climate the way that natural hair does. Depending on what type of hair it is, it may frizz or lose its curl in humid weather.
- After shampooing, the hair needs to be reset. This can be a challenge for the client who intends to maintain the wig at home.
- The color will oxidize, meaning that it will fade with exposure to light.
- The hair will break and split just like human hair if mistreated by harsh brushing, back-combing, or excessive use of heat.

ADVANTAGES OF SYNTHETIC WIGS

- Over the years, the technology of producing synthetic fibers has greatly improved. Wigs made of modacrylic are particularly strong and durable. Top-of-the-line synthetics like Kanekalon, a modacrylic fiber, simulate protein-rich hair, with a natural lustrous look and feel. These synthetics are so realistic they can even fool stylists.
- Synthetic wigs are a great value. Not only are they very realistic, but they are also less expensive than real hair. Both style and texture are set into the hair. Ready-to-wear wigs are very easy for the client to maintain at home. Shampooing in cold water will not change the style, nor will exposure to extreme humidity.
- Most synthetic ready-to-wear wigs are cut according to the latest styles, with the cut, color, and texture already set. The only work you may be required to do is some detailing or custom trimming.
- The colors are limitless, ranging from natural to wild fantasy shades. Again, price is a factor here. The cheaper wigs tend to be more solid in color (less tone-on-tone) and the fiber is coarser (polyester based). The high-end products are a mix of many shades, with highlights and lowlights for a natural effect.

Did You Know

In 1989 the Cosmetic, Toiletry, and Fragrance Association (CTFA) founded the CTFA Foundation, a charitable organization, and established the Look Good . . . Feel Better program to help cancer patients deal with hair loss. For more information about working with or helping clients with hair loss due to illness, visit the Look Good . . . Feel Better website at www.lookgoodfeelbetter.org or call 1-800-395-LOOK.

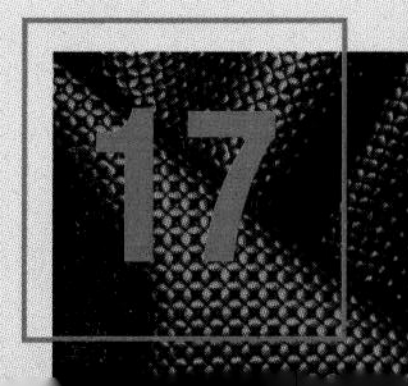

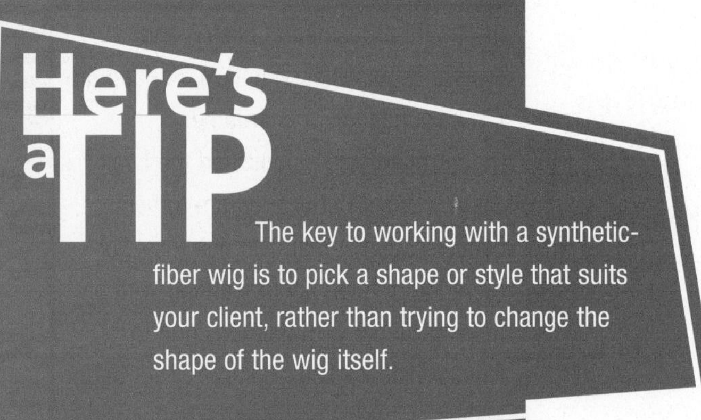

The key to working with a synthetic-fiber wig is to pick a shape or style that suits your client, rather than trying to change the shape of the wig itself.

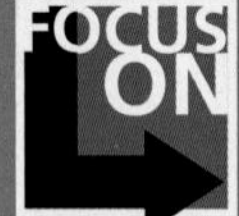

Focus on . . . Cost

To the average consumer, the "deals" at the local wig store may look good. But that apparent deal could be a mix of animal hair and human hair, and one washing could mat the wig into a big ball. The most realistic wigs, such as those used in film work, might be valued at thousands of dollars. Your client will not necessarily need something of this grade, but you must still pay attention to quality. As a professional, you must educate your client and recommend only well-made products. Remember, when you recommend anything, you are putting your reputation on the line.

- Synthetic colors will not fade or oxidize, even when exposed to long periods in the sun.

DRAWBACKS OF SYNTHETIC WIGS

- Synthetic hair cannot be exposed to extreme heat (curling irons, hot rollers, or the high heat of blow-dryers).
- Coloring synthetic fibers is not recommended, as traditional haircolor will not work on them.
- Sometimes synthetic wigs are so shiny that they may not look natural. Also, if they are thick, they will look unnatural on a fine-haired client. Price often has a lot to do with how natural a synthetic wig can look.

QUALITY AND COST

As seen here, there are pros and cons for human-hair and synthetic wigs. The bottom line in both cases is that you get what you pay for.

Ultimately, your success in working with any hair addition will be determined by the quality of the product itself. Do not be fooled by imitations. Cheap wigs may be great for "fun moments" or to practice cutting on, but in other situations they can look tacky and unattractive.

The most expensive wigs are those made of human hair. Pricing varies as follows:

- *European hair* is at the top of the line. Virgin hair is the most costly; color-treated hair is second in cost.
- *Hair from India and Asia,* the two regions that provide most of the human hair commercially available, are next in cost. Indian hair is usually available in lengths from 12 inches to 16 inches. Asian hair is available in lengths of 12 inches to 28 inches. Indian hair is naturally wavy; Asian hair is naturally straight.
- *Human hair mixed with animal hair* is next. The animal hair may be angora, horse, yak, or sheep hair. Yak hair is taken from the animal's belly and is the purest of whites. Its natural color lends itself to adding fantasy colors, which attract teenagers. Mixed-hair products are often used in theatrical or fashion settings.

There are several important questions to ask when selecting a wig for the client.

- Is the wig made of human hair, animal hair, a mix of both, or is it synthetic?
- Is the hair colored, or in its natural state (virgin hair)?
- If the hair is human hair, is it graded in terms of strength, elasticity, and porosity?
- Is the cuticle intact? Cuticle-intact hair is more expensive, as the hair has been "turned." In **turned hair,** the root ends are arranged to prevent the hair from tangling. The root end of every hair strand is sewn into the base so that the cuticles of all hair strands slope in the

same direction (Figure 17-7). The hair is in better condition and is much easier to work with. Turning is a tedious, time-consuming process that increases the cost of the wig.

- Is the hair **fallen hair,** meaning hair that has been shed from the head and perhaps gathered from a hairbrush, as opposed to hair that has been cut? Fallen hair is not turned, and the cuticle is removed so that it will not lock and mat. This hair tends to be less expensive.
- Is the hair tangle-free? If the cuticle has been removed, this often means you cannot condition the hair, for it will tend to mat.
- What is the condition of the hair? Has it been bleached? Can it be colored? Has it been colored with metallic dye?
- Will the hair match the client's hair? Should you be blending to match?
- Can the hair be permed?
- If the client is going to maintain her hair at home, will the wig last a reasonable amount of time (4 to 6 months if in continual use)?

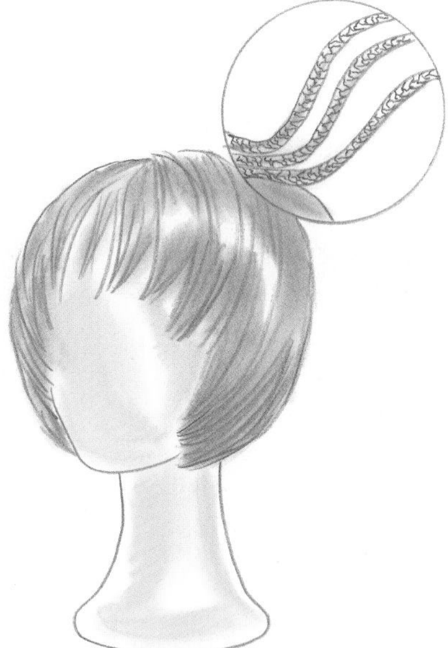

Figure 17-7 Turned hair.

TYPES OF WIGS

There are two basic categories of wigs: cap and capless.

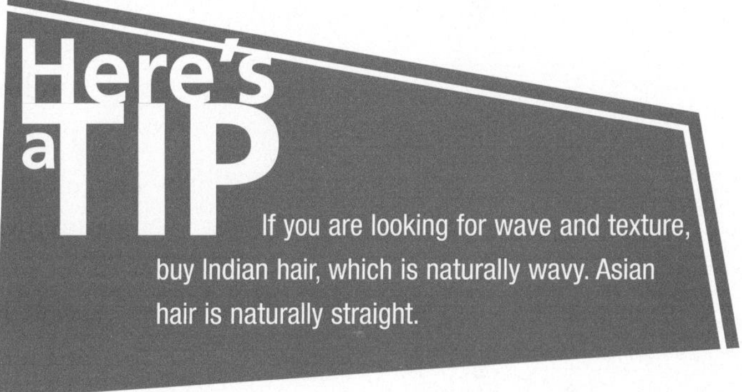

Here's a TIP
If you are looking for wave and texture, buy Indian hair, which is naturally wavy. Asian hair is naturally straight.

Cap wigs are constructed with an elasticized mesh-fiber base to which the hair is attached. They are made in several sizes and require special fittings. More often than not, cap wigs are hand-knotted. The front edge of a cap wig is made of a material that resembles the client's scalp, along with a lace extension and a wire support, used at the temples for a snug, secure fit. Hair is hand-tied under the net ("under-knotted") to conceal the cap edge. The side and back edges contain wire supports, elastic, and hooks for a secure fit. Also available are latex molded cap wigs, which are prostheses for special need clients.

Capless wigs are machine-made. The hair (human or artificial) is woven into long strips called **wefts.** Rows of wefts are sewn to elastic strips in a circular pattern to fit the head shape. Capless wigs are more popular than cap wigs as they are ready-to-wear and less expensive.

The capless wig is a frame of connected wefts with open areas. Compare a nylon stocking to a fishnet stocking: one has a closed framework (the cap wig), and the other is open (capless). Due to their construction and airiness, capless wigs are extremely light and comfortable to wear (Figure 17-8).

In general, capless wigs or caps that allow the scalp to breathe are healthier, as they prevent excess perspiration. A cap wig is best for a client with extremely thin hair, or no hair. If you put a capless wig on a bald client, her scalp will show through.

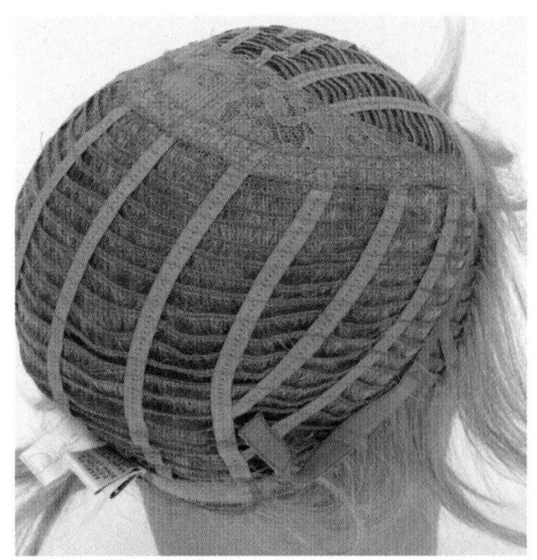

Figure 17-8 A capless wig.

METHODS OF CONSTRUCTION

- **Hand-tied** or **hand-knotted wigs.** These wigs are made by inserting individual strands of hair into a mesh foundation and knotting them

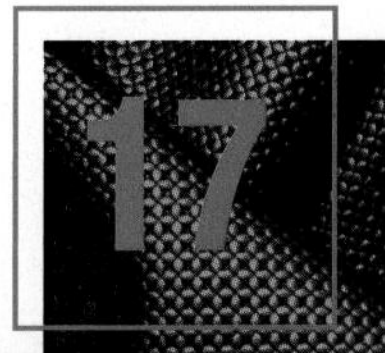

with a needle. Hand-tying is done particularly around the front hairline and the top of the head. These wigs have a natural, realistic look and are wonderful for styling. The hand-tied method most closely resembles actual human hair growth, with flexibility at the roots. There is no definite direction to the hair; it can be combed in almost any direction.

- **Semi-hand-tied wigs.** These wigs are constructed with a combination of synthetic hair and hand-tied human hair. Reasonably priced, they offer a natural appearance and good durability.
- **Machine-made wigs.** The least expensive option, these wigs are made by feeding wefts through a sewing machine, then sewing them together to form the base and shape of the wig. They have the disadvantage of the wefting direction, which restricts styling options. Some hairstylists can become overly creative with this type of wig and cut it to the point of no return. Another aspect of these wigs is their "bounce-back" quality. Even after shampooing, the style returns.

It is important to be aware of the artificial growth patterns of a wig. Wig construction will determine the direction in which you style the hair. The most flexible and versatile of all patterns is the hand-tied wig. Machine-made wigs are sewn in a specific direction, offering no versatility. If you like the style, this is a good thing; if you do not, you have a problem. Make sure you like the direction of the style, and work within that framework.

TAKING WIG MEASUREMENTS

The creation of a custom-made wig begins with taking the client's measurements. Use a soft tape measure, keeping it close to the head without pressure.

Always keep a written record of the client's head measurements and forward a copy to the wig dealer or manufacturer. You should include precise specifications of hair shade, quality of hair, length of hair, and type of hair part and pattern.

If the wig is ready-to-wear, no measuring will be needed, because it can be adjusted by tightening the straps, or the elastic in the nape. Ready-to-wear wigs are more common in the salon, mostly because of the price difference. But every wig needs to be adjusted to the head and custom styled or trimmed to suit the client.

BLOCKING THE WIG

A **block** is a head-shaped form, usually made of canvas-covered cork or Styrofoam, on which the wig is secured for fitting, cleaning, coloring, and styling. Canvas blocks are available in six sizes, from 20 inches (50 centimeters) to 22- inches (56.25 centimeters). The block is best attached to your work area with a swivel clamp, which allows for greater control.

PUTTING ON THE WIG

One of the most important steps in the wig service is instructing the client on how to put on the wig. Start by educating the client on the correct method for preparing her hair before placing the wig. The client's skill at securing her hair under the wig cap and making it flat and even will determine how well the wig sits on her head. Two methods for preparing the hair are the hair wrap and pin curls (Procedure 17-1).

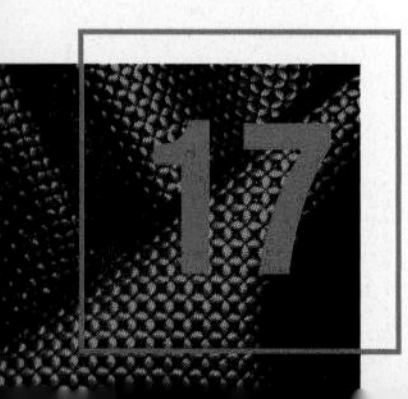

PROCEDURE 17-1

TAKING WIG MEASUREMENTS

IMPLEMENTS AND MATERIALS

- Styling cape
- Neck strip
- Boar-bristle brush
- Duckbill clips
- Cloth measuring tape

PREPARATION

1. Client consultation.
2. Drape the client with a styling cape and neck strip for a dry hair service.
3. Brush the hair down smoothly and pin it as flatly and tightly to the scalp as possible (Figure 17-9).

PROCEDURE

1. Measure the circumference of the head. Place the tape completely around the head, starting at the hairline in the middle of the forehead. Place the tape above the ears, around the back of the head, and return to the starting point (Figure 17-10).
2. Beginning from the hairline at the middle of the forehead, measure over the top to the nape of the neck. Bend the head back and measure to the point where the wig will ride on the base of the skull at the nape (Figure 17-11).
3. Measure from ear to ear, across the forehead (Figure 17-12).
4. Measure from ear to ear, over the top of the head (Figure 17-13).

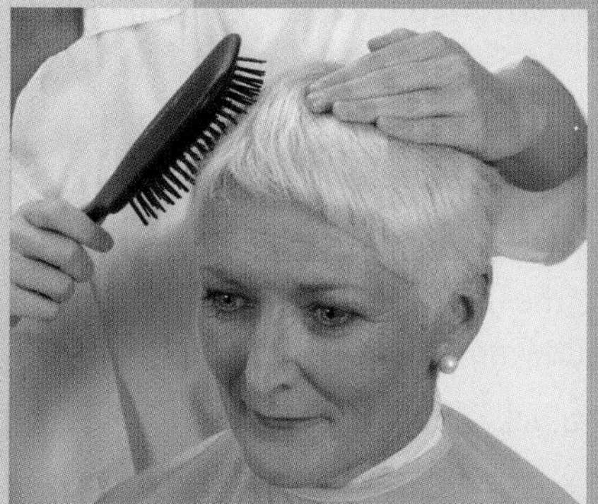

Figure 17-9 Brush hair down smoothly.

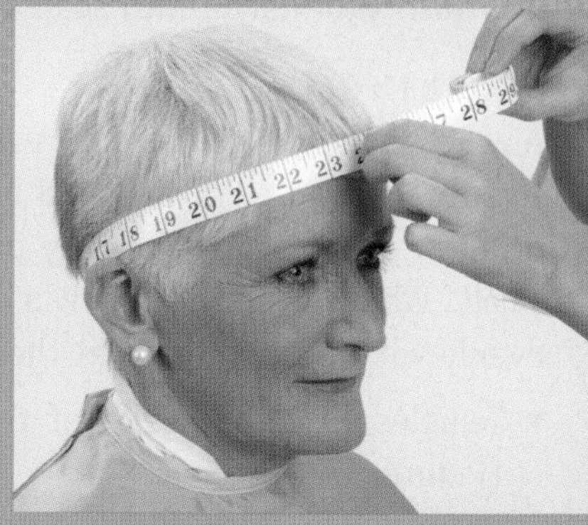

Figure 17-10 Measure circumference of head.

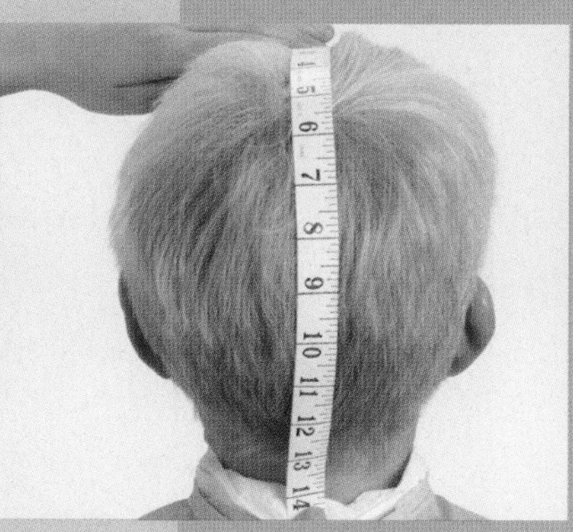

Figure 17-11 Measure from middle of front hairline to nape.

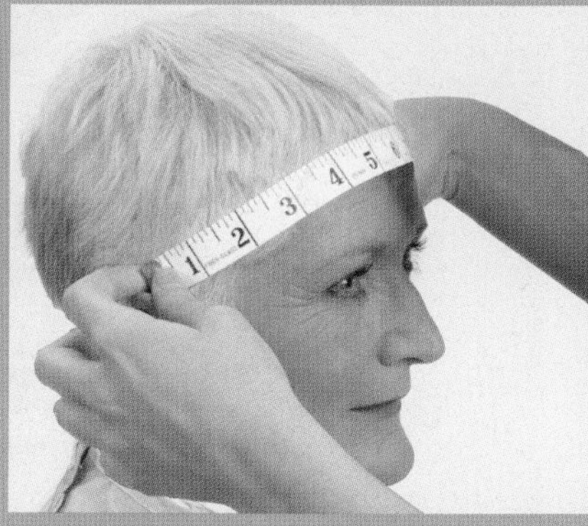

Figure 17-12 Measure across forehead.

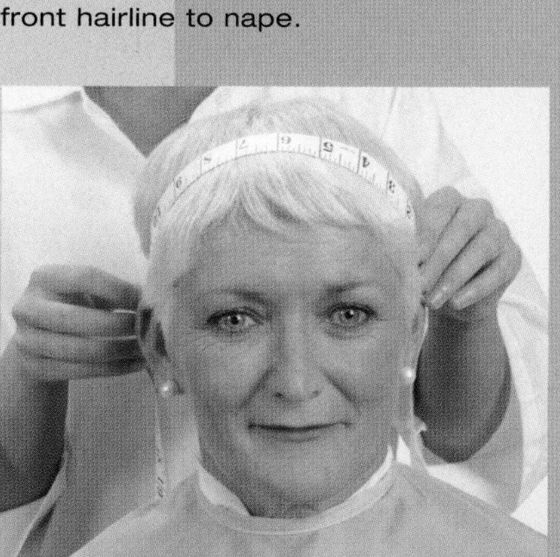

Figure 17-13 Measure top of head.

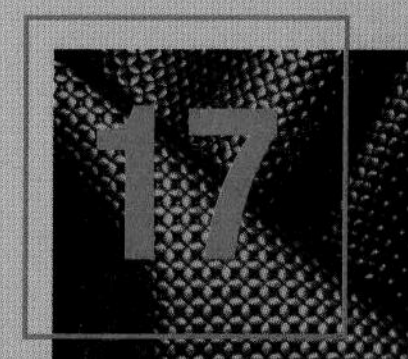

5. Place the tape across the crown and measure from temple to temple (Figure 17-14).
6. Measure the width of the nape line, across the nape of the neck (Figure 17-15).

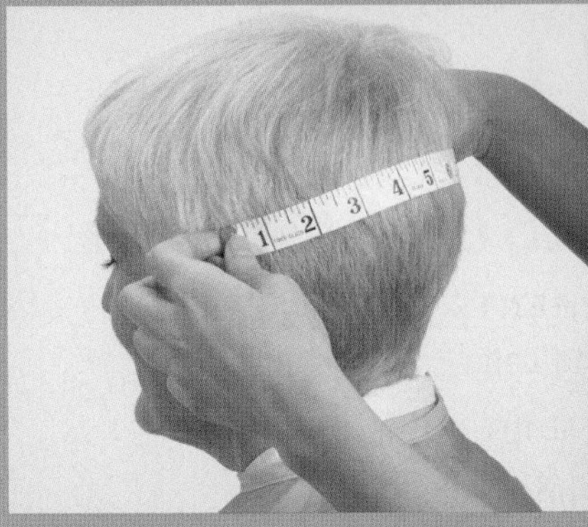

Figure 17-14 Measure from temple to temple.

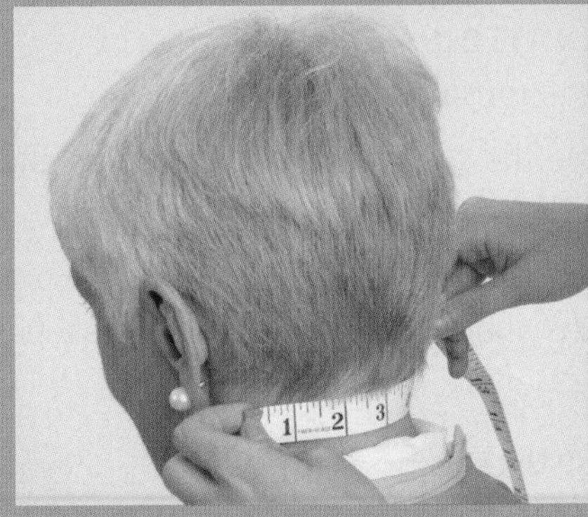

Figure 17-15 Measure width of nape line.

CLEANUP AND SANITATION

1. Disinfect all implements and store in appropriate containers.
2. Discard neck strip and place cape in hamper for laundering.
3. Sanitize your workstation.
4. Wash your hands with soap and warm water.

BLOCKING THE WIG

Always fit the wig to the right size of block. Do not try to stretch a wig to fit it onto a block that is too large or allow a wig to hang loosely on a block that is too small. When mounting the wig on the block, pin it evenly with T-shaped pins at the following points:

- Temples (use the seams of the block as a guide) (Figure 17-16)
- Above each ear (Figure 17-17)
- Each corner of the nape (Figure 17-18)

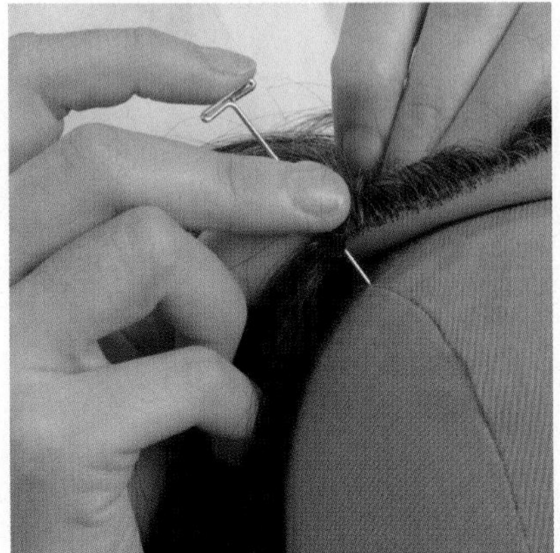

Figure 17-16 Pin at each temple.

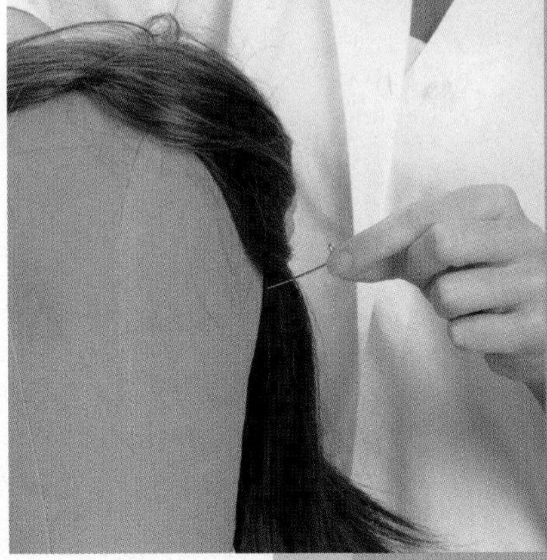

Figure 17-17 Pin above each ear.

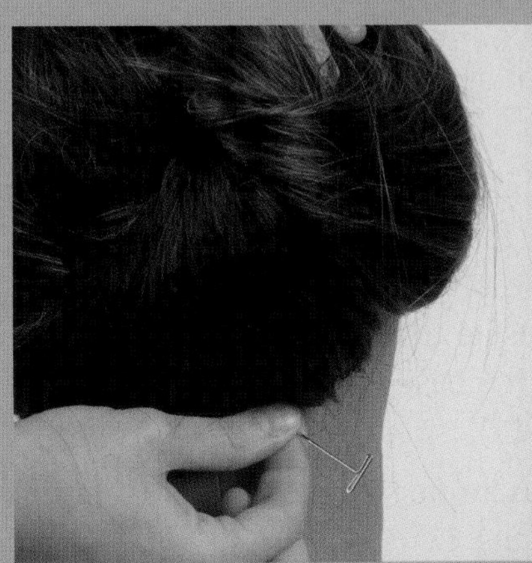

Figure 17-18 Pin each corner of the nape.

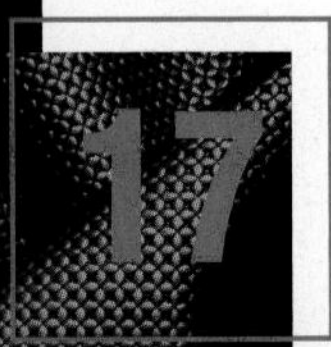

PROCEDURE 17-2

PUTTING ON THE WIG

IMPLEMENTS AND MATERIALS

- Styling cape and neck strip
- Comb
- Hairpins
- Bobby pins
- Wig cap
- Wig

PREPARATION

1. Client consultation (Figure 17-19).
2. Drape the client for a dry hair service with a styling cape and neck strip.

PROCEDURE FOR PIN CURLS

1. Brush the hair smooth.
2. Take large sections of the hair and wrap them into flat pin curls, keeping the base of each pin curl as flat and smooth as possible (Figures 17-20 and 17-21).

PROCEDURE FOR HAIR WRAP

1. Section off a large triangular section at the crown and pin this hair out of the way (Figure 17-22).
2. Taking small sections, brush the client's hair all around the head, as if you were setting the hair on a big roller, with the head as the roller (Figure 17-23).

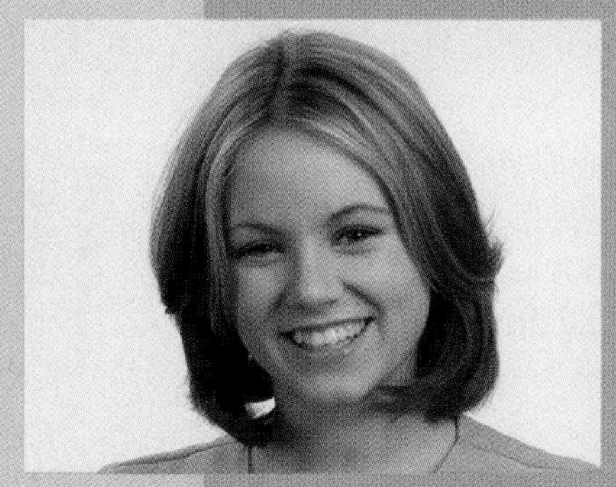

Figure 17-19 Client before draping.

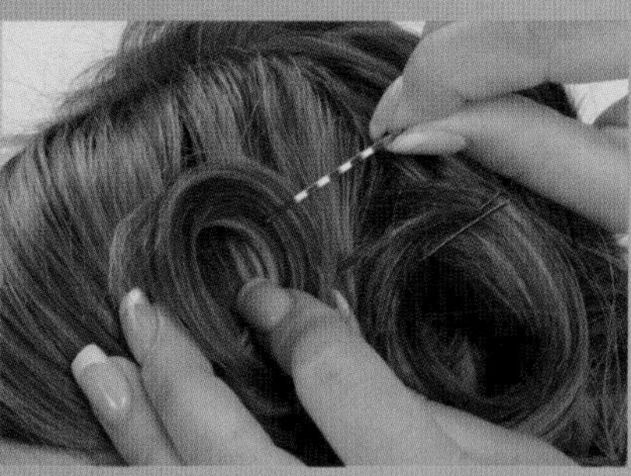

Figure 17-20 Arrange the hair in large pin curls.

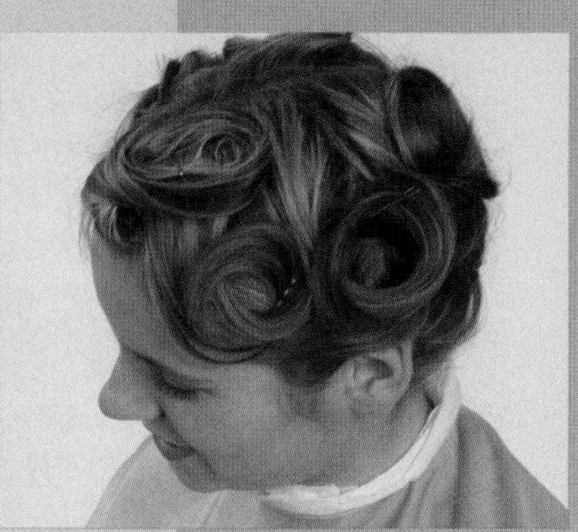

Figure 17-21 All the hair in pin curls.

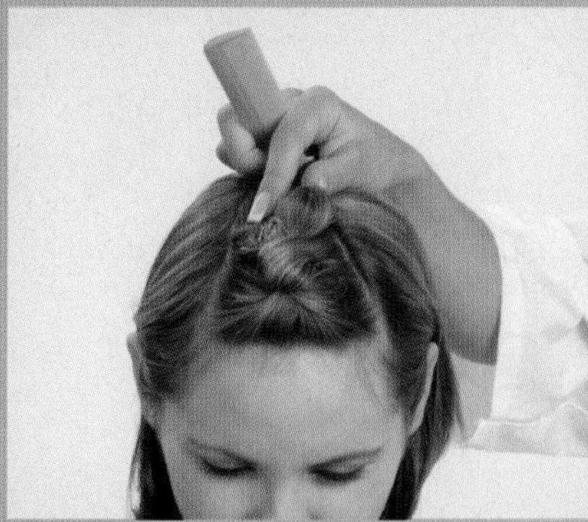

Figure 17-22 Section off triangle at crown.

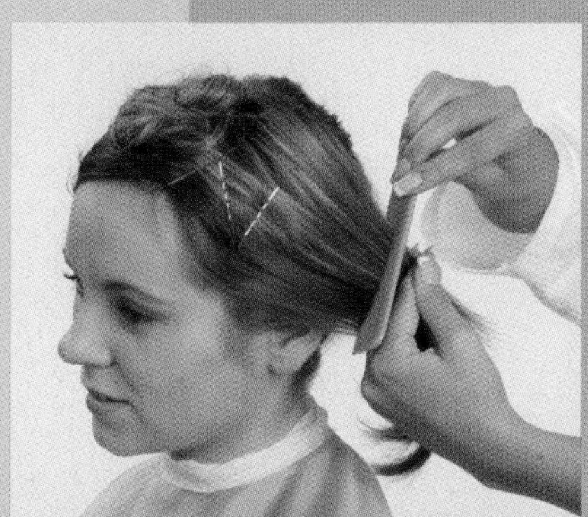

Figure 17-23 Wrap the hair around the head.

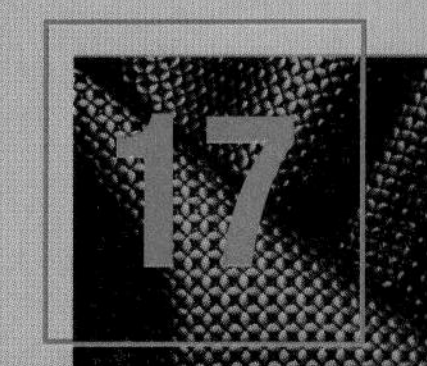

3. Pin the hair in place. You may pull a wig cap over the hair if desired (Figure 17-24).

PROCEDURE FOR PUTTING ON THE WIG

1. Holding the front of the wig against the forehead with one hand, use your other hand to gently slide the wig back onto the head (Figure 17-25).
2. Hold the edge in front of the ears and pull it down, making sure that the wig is sitting straight (Figure 17-26).
3. If the wig is loose, tighten it by adjusting the elastic and hooks at the nape. You may have to tighten it off the head and then refit it on the client (Figures 17-27 and 17-28).
4. If the client has long or thick hair, you may need some extra pins to lock the wig deeper into place, as the client's hair could push the wig up. For clients with thin or short hair, additional pinning is not usually necessary.

CLEANUP AND SANITATION

Follow cleanup and sanitation procedures for measuring the wig.

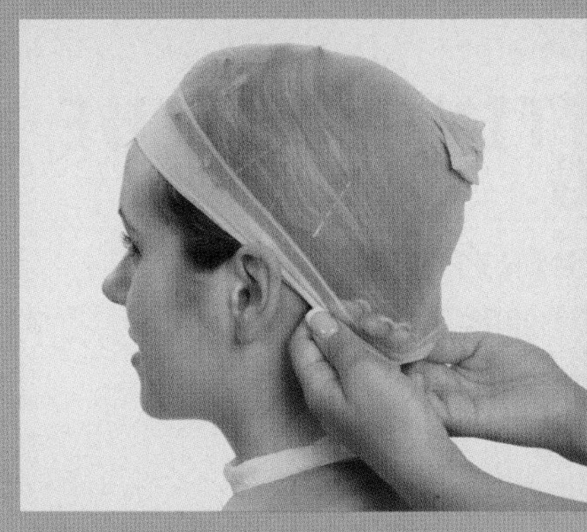

Figure 17-24 Wig cap over wrapped hair.

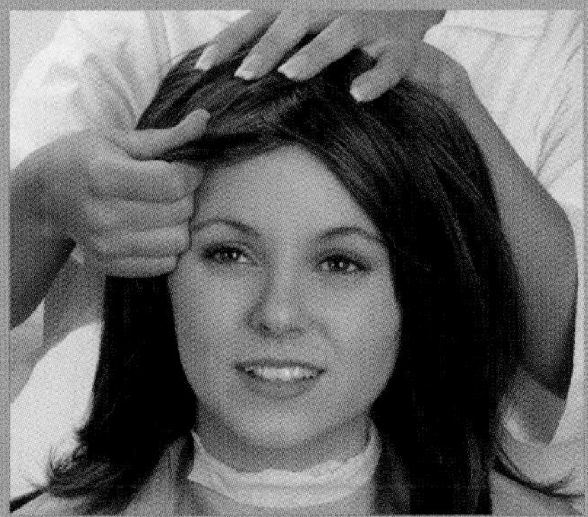

Figure 17-25 Pull the wig on front to back.

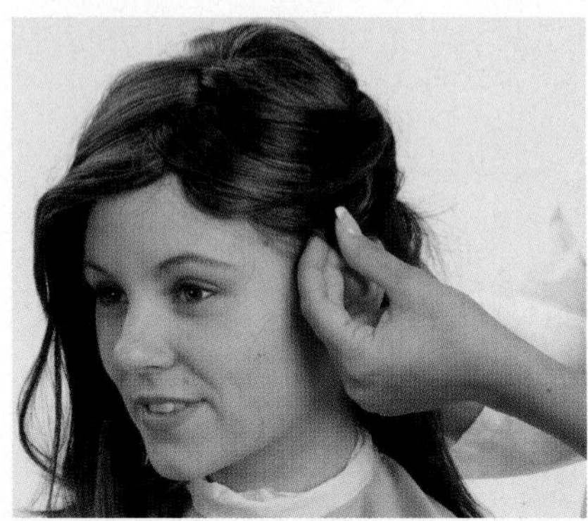

Figure 17-26 Pull the wig down at the sides.

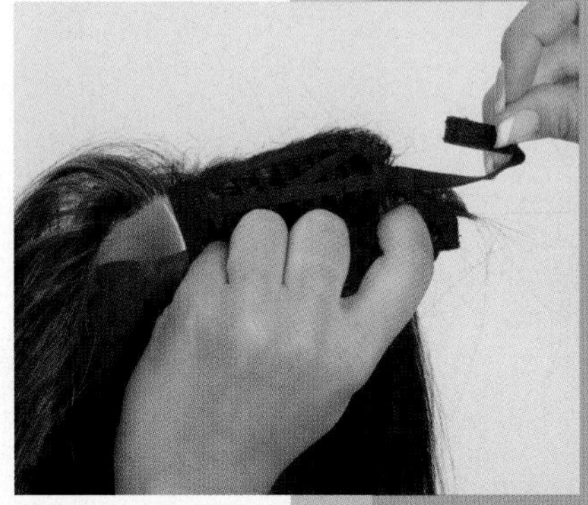

Figure 17-27 Tighten the wig off the client's head.

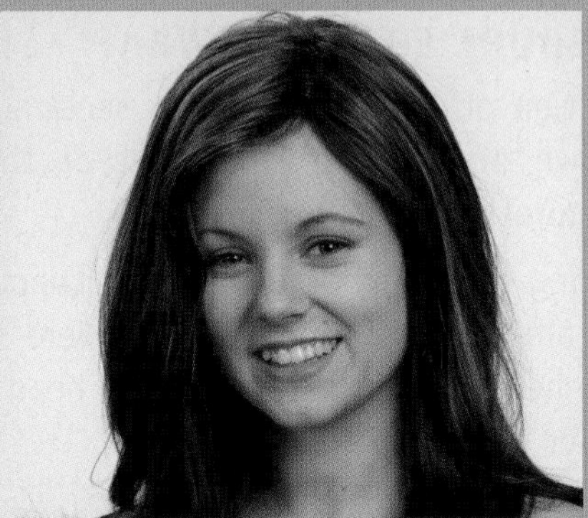

Figure 17-28 A well-fitted wig.

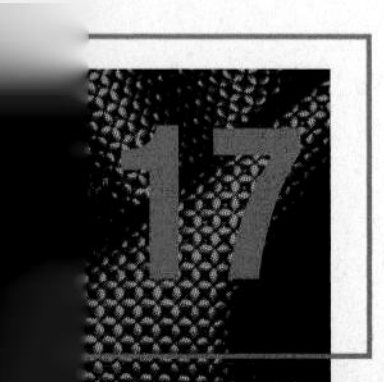

CUTTING THE WIG

When cutting a wig, generally your goal is to make the hair look more realistic. As you know, the hair on the human head has many lengths. Even when hair is cut to one length, internally there are various stages of hair growth. Hair that is 1 month old and hair that is years old exist on the same head. The stylist should try to achieve this natural look in the wig. The most effective way to do this is to taper the ends when cutting the wig. The more solid the shape, the more unnatural the hair will look.

When cutting and trimming wigs, you can follow the basic methods of haircutting—blunt, layered, and graduated—using the same sectioning and elevations as on a real head of hair. Or you may do what many top stylists prefer to do, which is to cut free-form on dry hair. The wig should be placed on the block for cutting, but the comb-out and finishing should be done on the client's head.

Free-form cutting moves from longer to shorter lengths, always working toward the weight. Vertical sections create lightness. Diagonal sections create a rounder beveled edge. Horizontal sections build heavier weight (Figures 17-29 to 17-31).

To use this visual approach, begin by cutting a small section and observe how the hair falls. Your next step will be based on how the hair responds.

Draw a diagram of the silhouette or have handy a photo image for reference. These will work as a kind of blueprint for you to follow.

Free-form cutting is usually done on dry hair, which allows you to see more easily how the hair will fall. When the hair is wet, it can be hard to judge how the hair will lie.

To practice wig cutting, buy two inexpensive, ready-to-wear wigs in the same style. Take a photo for reference purposes. Draw a diagram of the sections, indicating how you are going to cut the wigs. This way, you can rehearse your plan before even picking up the shears.

Begin your practice with the "shadow cut." Trim the wigs following the original design that has been precut into the wig, but cut the first wig wet. Then air-dry it and evaluate the style. Trim the second wig, following the same style, but this time cut it dry. Take photos of both results and evaluate the looks you have achieved with both dry and wet cutting.

You will discover that the wet cutting method was more controlled and technical, while the dry cutting method was freer and more abstract. Often, the more abstract method results in a cut that looks more realistic. What do you think?

Repeat the above exercise with a razor, thinning shears, and standard haircutting shears using the tapering method only. Compare the results.

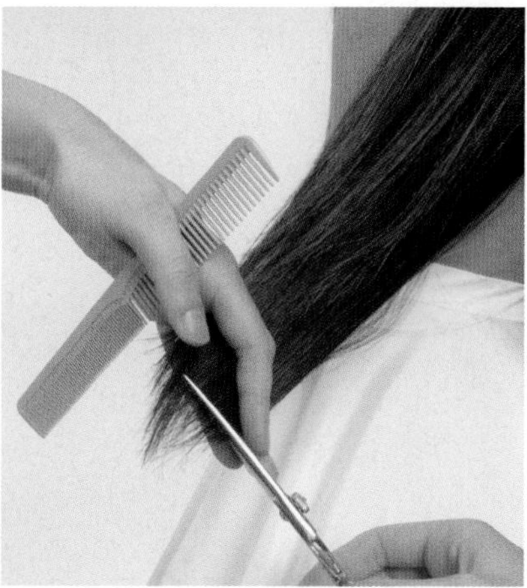

Figure 17-29 Free-form cutting with vertical sections.

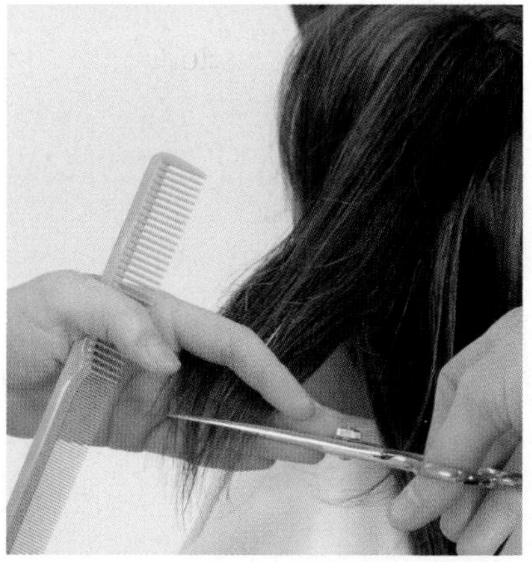

Figure 17-30 Free-form cutting with diagonal sections.

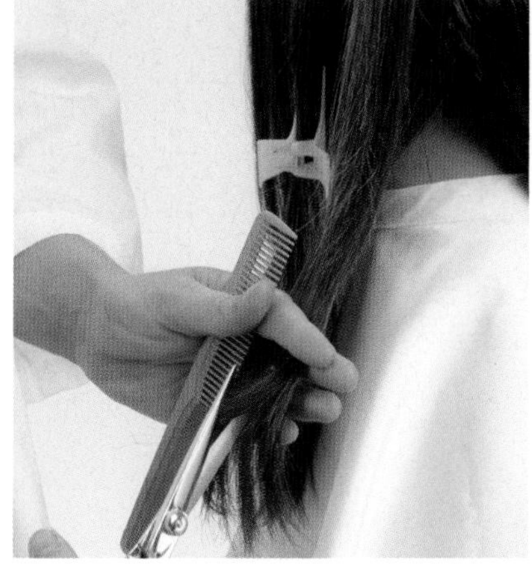

Figure 17-31 Free-form cutting with horizontal sections.

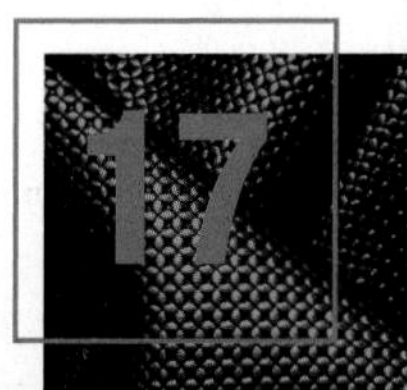

STYLING THE WIG

The important thing to remember when you are styling a wig is that you must never lose sight of the big picture. Some stylists get overly involved in the wig, as if it is a creation that exists apart from the client. This is the wrong approach. A great stylist works with the total person, not just the head. When you have finished styling the wig, step back and ask the client to stand up and walk around so that you can check for balance and proportion and make corrections accordingly.

Most of the hair you will be working with is chemically treated, so it needs to be handled gently. You will achieve the best styling results by following these guidelines:

- When using heat on human hair, always set the styling tool on low.
- Treat the hair gently and kindly; do not pull it, or otherwise treat it carelessly.
- Traditionally, brushes made with natural boar bristles have been regarded as the best for use on human hair. Their soft bristles are preferred to the sharp-edged synthetic bristles that can damage hair. Today, however, you will find many synthetic brushes that have smooth, rounded plastic teeth, more like a comb, and they are excellent and economical choices. Keep in mind that the key with any brush or comb is to be gentle, for hair can be easily damaged.

Use a block for all your coloring, perming, setting, and basic cut outlining. The combing-out and finishing touches for most modern cuts should be completed on the client's head in order to achieve proper balance and personalization.

Remember that most clients come into the salon looking for a natural look. Making a wig look believable is very challenging, and to do it well is truly an art form. The areas that must appear the most convincing are the crown, the part, and the hairline. Sometimes, crowns and parts look more natural when they are flat to the head; other times it looks more natural to fluff up these areas and direct the emphasis away. This will be determined by the style. A general rule is to follow the direction of the knotting and weave, as preset by the wig maker. If you fight the direction, the results may look odd.

STYLING TIPS FOR THE HAIRLINE

- Choose styling products that have been formulated for color-treated hair. These will work the best, and are the kindest to human hair. Just remember that whatever you put into the hair will eventually have to be shampooed out.
- Back-comb gently around the hairline. The fluffy effect softens the hairline.
- Release the client's hair around the hairline and cut and blend it into the wig hair.

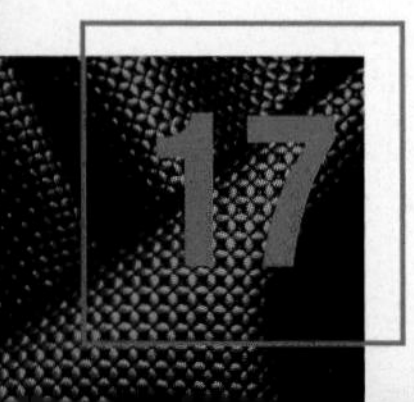

- The best test to gauge how realistic the wig looks is to use the "wind test." This test simulates the situation of a client walking outside with the wind blowing the hair off her face. Gently blow around the client's face with a blow-dryer set at cool and low and observe how the hairline looks. Does it seem realistic? If so, point out the results to the client, who may be feeling insecure about whether the wig looks natural enough (Figure 17-32).

When styling a wig, do not try to make it look perfect. Little imperfections help achieve a realistic look. Use your hands rather than a brush for a more natural look (Figure 17-33). Do not plaster the hair down, because it looks artificial.

CAUTION

Harsh handling will damage wig hair. Unlike hair on the human head, wig hair will not grow back. If you treat a wig carelessly, it will have a short life.

CLEANING THE WIG

To clean any wig, always follow the manufacturer's instructions. If shampooing is recommended, use a gentle shampoo, such as one you would use for color-treated hair. Avoid any harsh shampoos with a sulfur base, such as dandruff shampoos.

COLORING WIGS AND EXTENSIONS

All synthetic haircolors used for wigs and hairpieces are standardized according to the 70 colors on the haircolor ring used by wig and hairpiece manufacturers. The colors range from black to the palest blond. As most commercially available hair originates in either India or China, the natural color level is 0, or black. It is very difficult to lift level 0 to level 10 (see Chapter 19 for a discussion of hair color levels). White yak hair is an excellent base to add fantasy colors that appeal to younger clients.

If you are going to custom color the hair, use hair that has been decolorized (bleached) through the lifting process, not with metallic dyes. Check with the manufacturer.

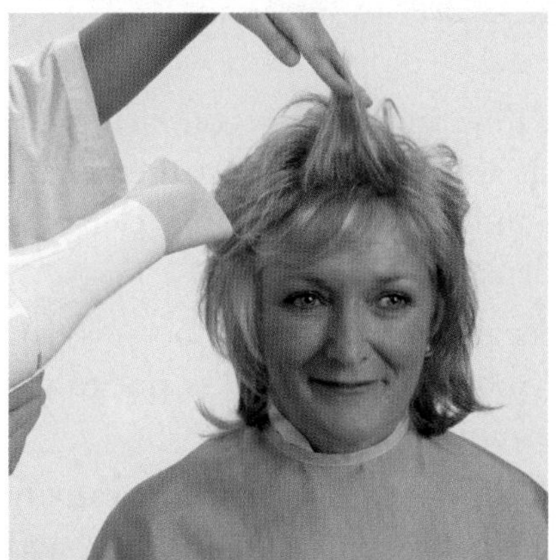

Figure 17-32 The wind test.

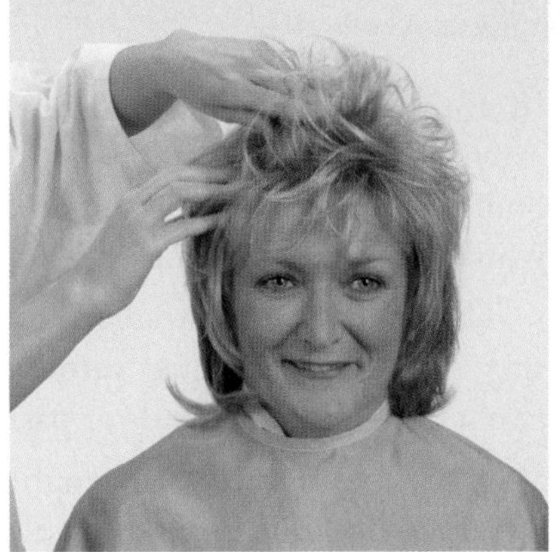

Figure 17-33 Style with the fingers for a natural look.

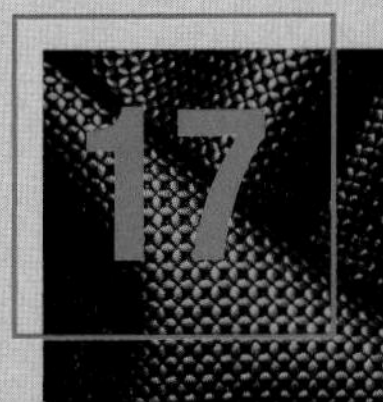

As in all disciplines, you must first learn the rules before you break them. Good colorists are not afraid to make mistakes, because they know how to correct them. The principles that guide the coloring of natural hair are also applied to the art of coloring wigs and hair extensions.

First, check to see if the cuticle is intact. Hair in which the cuticle is absent is very porous and will react to color in an extreme manner. Always strand test the hair prior to a full-color application. Use semi-permanent, demi-permanent, glaze, rinse, or color mousse products. Use permanent haircolor on human hair wigs; unless the hair is porous, in which case semi-permanent color is the better choice (see Chapter 19 for descriptions and procedures).

When coloring a human hair wig or hairpiece, conduct regular color checks every 5 to 10 minutes. Remember that the hair you are working on did not come from one head, but from many different heads, and can be unpredictable. It may be easier to color the client's hair to match a hairpiece than to color the piece itself.

PERMING THE WIG

If you want to perm a wig made of human hair to match the client's natural wave pattern, you need to know how the hair was colored. Was it decolorized (bleached) or dyed with metallic dye? Do not perm hair that has been colored with a metallic dye.

The permanent wave must be performed with the wig off the client's head. Cover the head form with plastic to protect it from the chemical solutions, pin the wig securely to the head form, and perm as you would a normal head of hair (see Chapter 18 for perming procedures).

HAIRPIECES

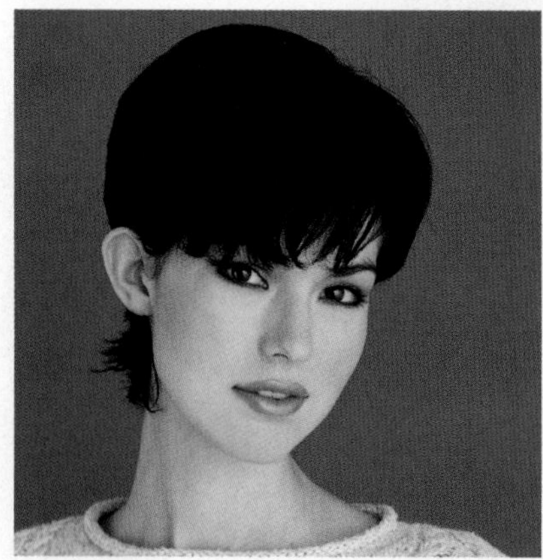

Figure 17-34 Hairpieces can look very natural.

In 18th-century France, women wore towering hairdos complete with extensions and various apparatuses such as springs to adjust the height. Some of these coiffures were 3 feet high and had elaborate visual elements worked into them such as ships or gardens.

They were often untouched for weeks at a time. The bad news is that they sometimes attracted vermin. The moral of this story is not to get swept up in current trends or passing fashions.

Always be aware of the strength of "classic design." Too much creativity can often backfire. Keep it simple, remembering that "less is more," and try not to let yourself get carried away.

Hairpieces are another important area of hair additions. A hairpiece gives 20- to 70-percent coverage (Figure 17-34). Hairpieces sit on top of the client's hair, and are usually attached by temporary methods (they are not worn to sleep at night).

Many wig companies offer ready-to-wear, low-maintenance hairpieces that serve as an introduction to the world of wigs, as well as a good retail

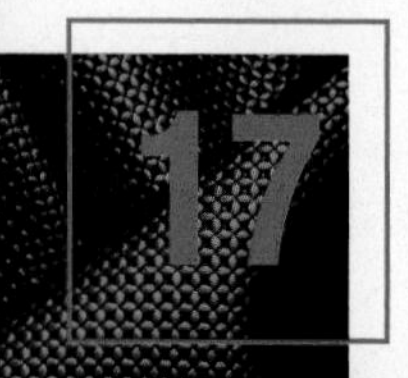

item in the salon. Some hairpieces are easily blended into long hair, others into shorter hair. Some add natural-looking height or volume, while others add length. They can be placed just about anywhere on the head.

The client's hair can be prepared in a number of ways before the hairpiece is attached. It can be tied into a ponytail or bun or twisted into a French twist. It can be blended with the hairpiece or serve as a base for it.

Temporary attachment methods include interlocking combs, flexible wire combs, elastic, claw clips, and even Velcro. In one versatile hairpiece, hair wefts are wrapped around elastic and resemble a cloth scrunchie. Some hairpieces are constructed on a weft base and are attached with flexible combs around the front and nape. Others that are attached by a semi-permanent method are called integration hairpieces.

When it comes to hairpieces, there are many ways to go wrong. Too much hair on a small body frame will make the client look out of balance. An ill-fitting hairpiece may draw negative attention.

It is easy to lose perspective when you are working with hairpieces. Too much focused concentration can get you into trouble and lead you to overwork the style. When you finally step back, you may discover that you have created an alarmingly large shape. Remember, "less is more."

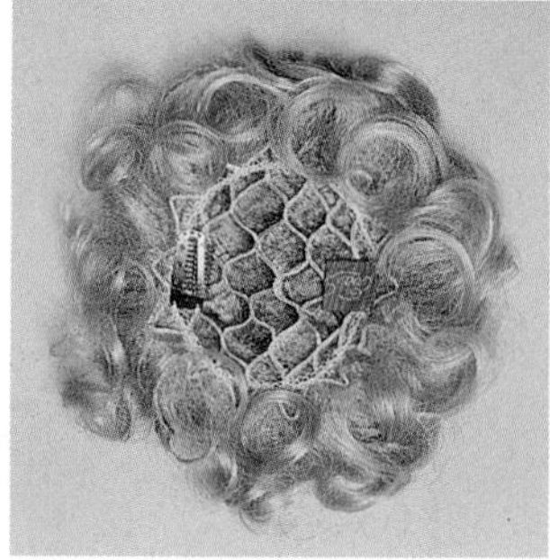

Figure 17-35 Integration hairpiece.

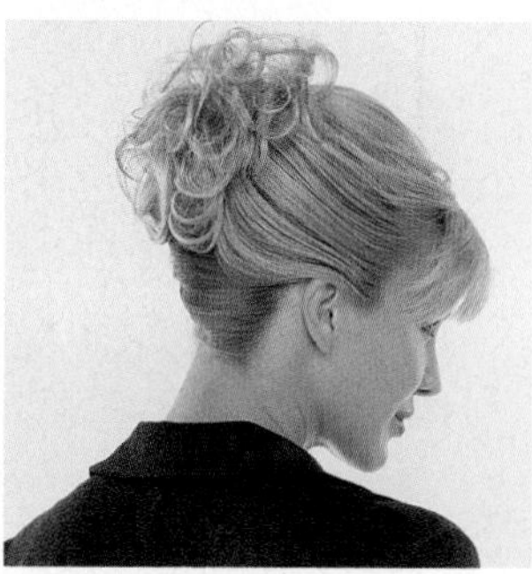

Figure 17-36 An integration hairpiece is easy to wear.

INTEGRATION HAIRPIECES

An **integration hairpiece** has openings in the base through which the client's own hair is pulled to blend with the hair (natural or synthetic) of the hairpiece. These hairpieces are very lightweight, natural-looking products that add length and volume to the client's hair. If your client is wearing hair extensions and would like a change, the integration hairpiece can be a good alternative. It is also recommended for clients with thinning hair, but not for those with total hair loss, as the scalp is likely to show through (Figures 17-35 and 17-36).

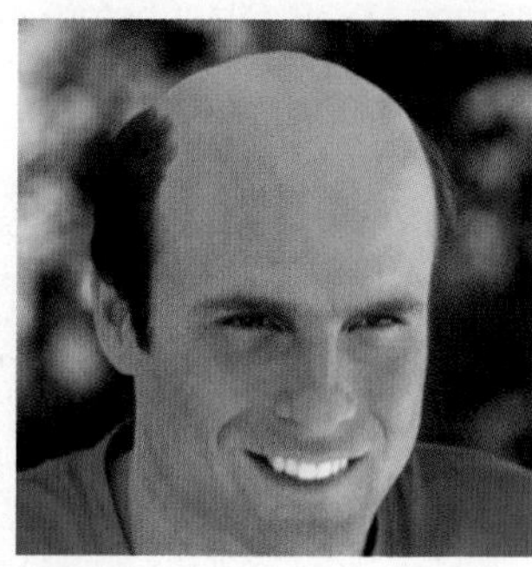

Figure 17-37 Male hair enhancement client.

TOUPEES

While men usually are the clients for toupees, women also wear these hairpieces. A **toupee** is a small wig used to cover the top and crown of the head. The fine net base is usually the most appropriate material for the client with severe hair loss. There are two ways to attach toupees: temporary (tape or clips) or semi-permanent (weaving, tracks, adhesive, or sewing).

Most wearers of toupees prize the confidence gained from wearing an authentic-looking hairpiece, and are prepared to pay a high price for it. The best toupees are custom designed. The top manufacturers offer in-depth instruction for those interested in learning this specialty service (Figures 17-37 and 17-38).

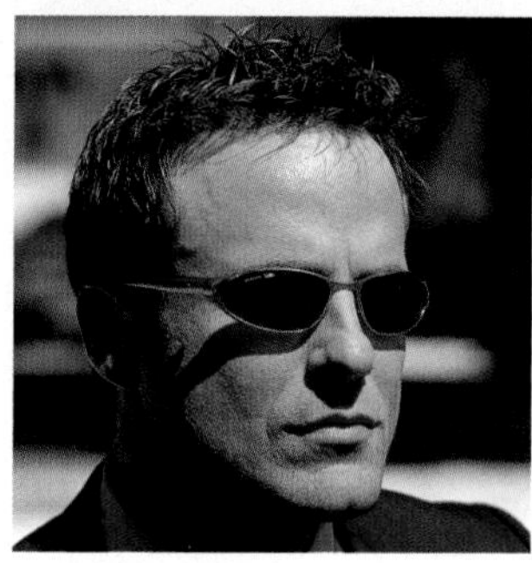

Figure 17-38 The same client fitted with a toupee.

FASHION HAIRPIECES

Fashion hairpieces are a great salon product for special occasions or for use as fashion accessories. They are especially popular in the bridal business.

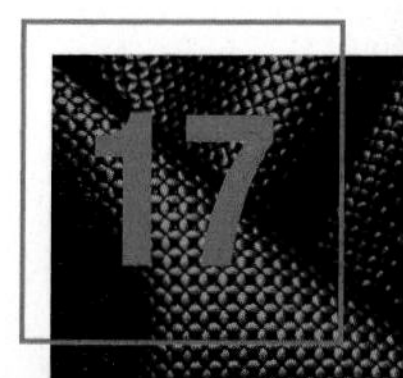

These hairpieces vary in size and are constructed on a stiff net base. They are attached, on a temporary basis, with hairpins, clips, combs, bobby pins, or elastic. Three of these attachment methods are illustrated here.

- The wraparound ponytail is a long length of wefted hair that covers 10 to 20 percent of the head. It is used as a simple ponytail or in chignons. It is particularly useful for the client who can just get her own hair into a ponytail (Figures 17-39 to 17-43).

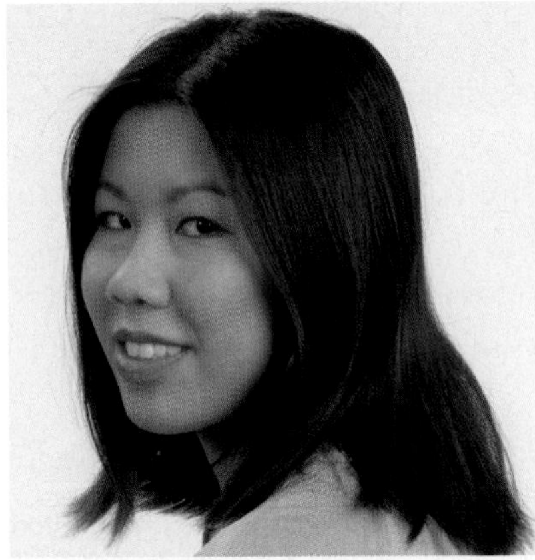

Figure 17-39 Client before fitting with a wraparound ponytail.

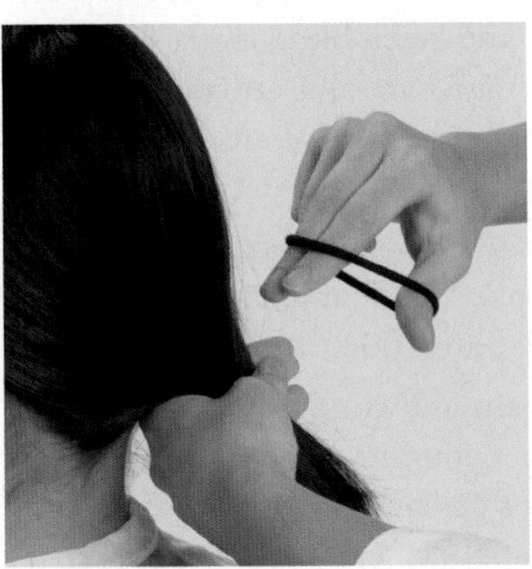

Figure 17-40 Client's own ponytail.

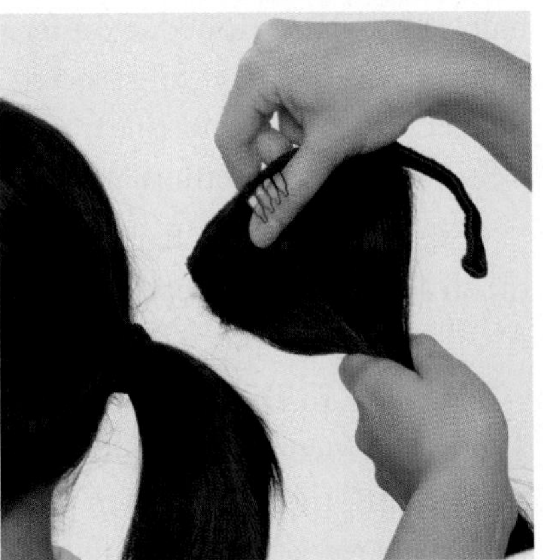

Figure 17-41 Attaching the hairpiece.

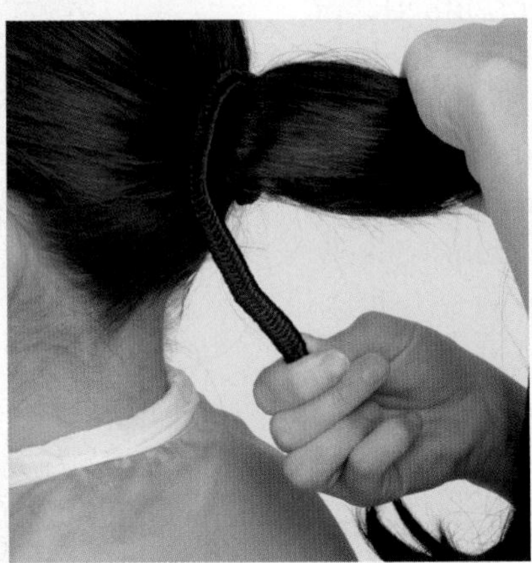

Figure 17-42 Wrapping the band around the ponytail base.

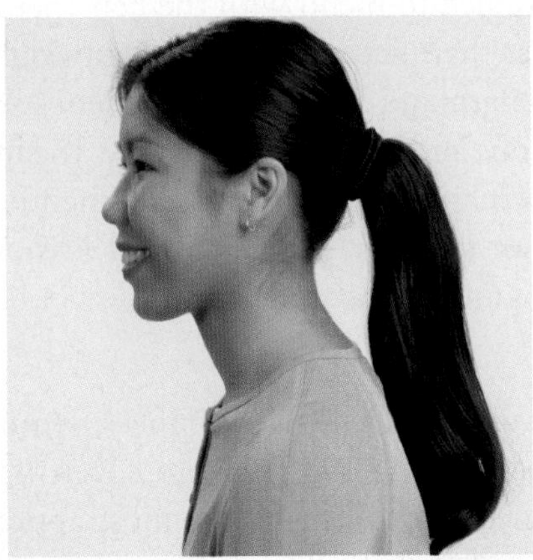

Figure 17-43 A "new," much longer ponytail.

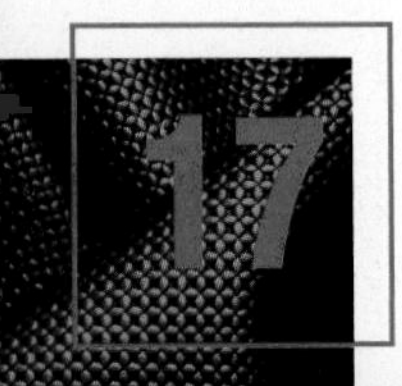

- A cascade of curls is attached with combs (Figures 17-44 to 17-48).
- A hair wrap is mounted on an elastic loop. It is further secured to the client's own hair with hairpins (Figures 17-49 to Figure 17-52).

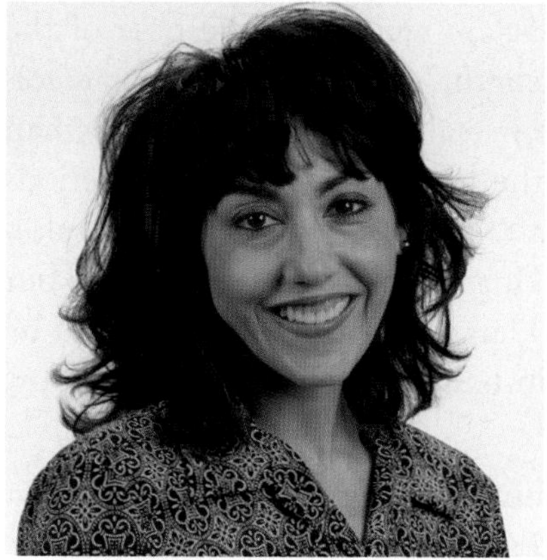

Figure 17-44 Client before fitting with comb-attached curls.

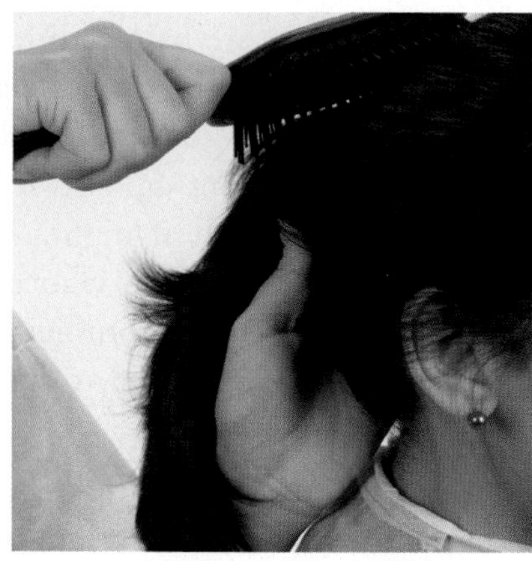

Figure 17-45 Brushing the client's hair into a ponytail.

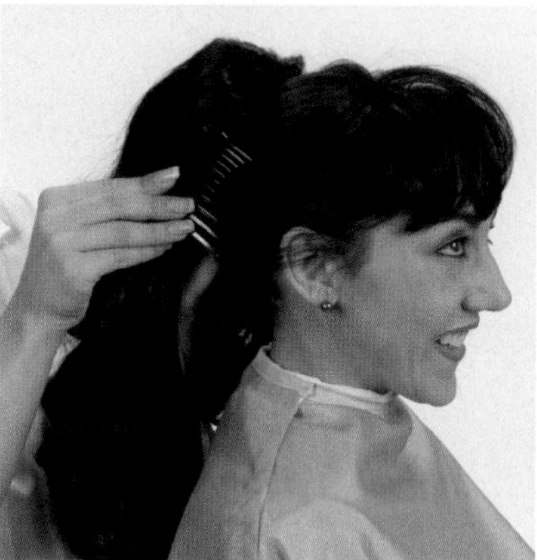

Figure 17-46 Attaching the combs.

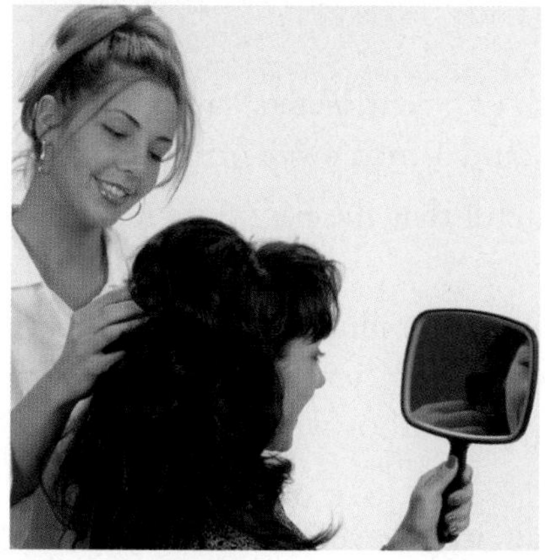

Figure 17-47 Adjusting the hairpiece.

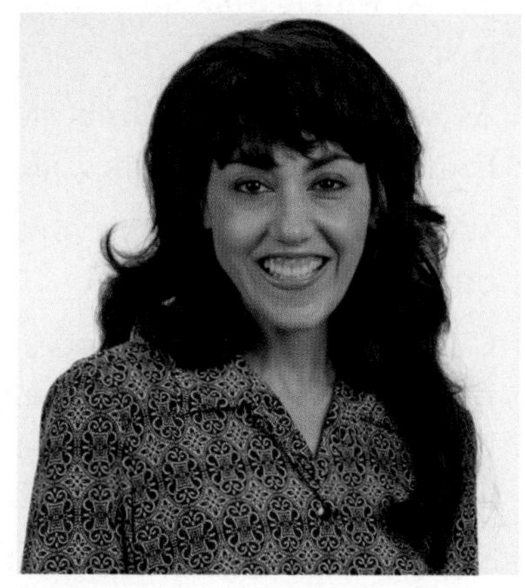

Figure 17-48 Cascade of curls.

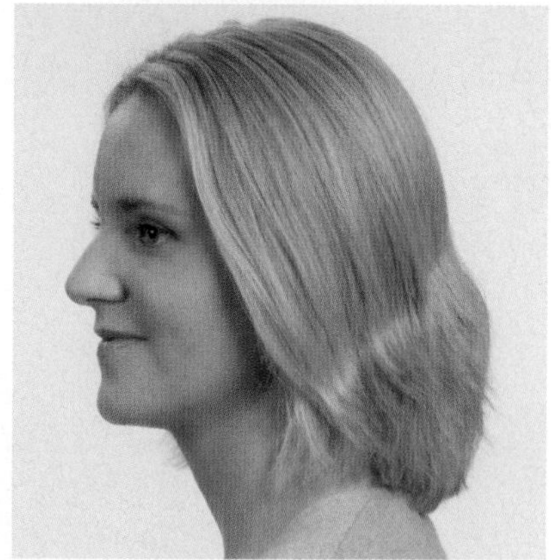

Figure 17-49 Client before fitting with a hair wrap.

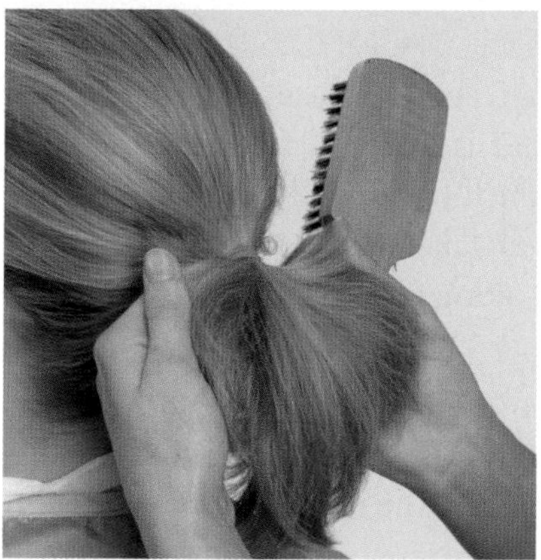

Figure 17-50 Brushing client's hair into a ponytail.

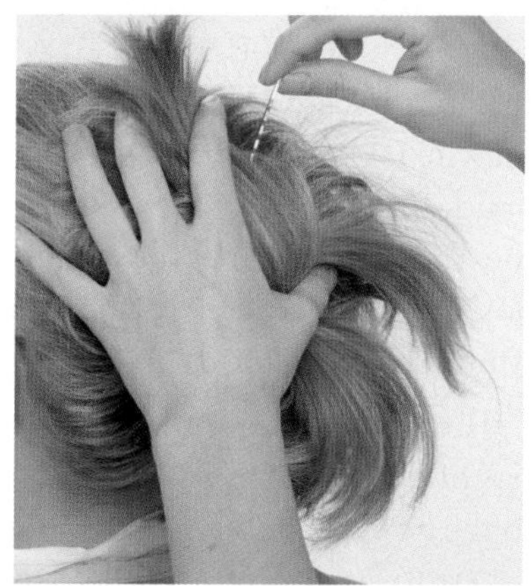

Figure 17-51 Securing the hairpiece with hairpins.

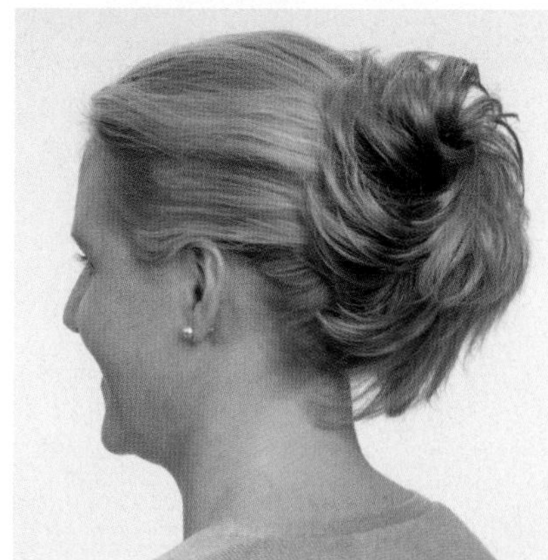

Figure 17-52 An easy, dressed-up look.

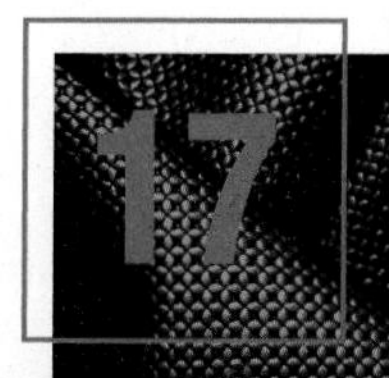

FOCUS ON Focus on . . . Sharpening Your Skills

In order to achieve a natural look, it is crucial that you blend the client's hair with the hairpiece. You must match up both the color and the wave pattern. If the client has naturally wavy hair, it may be wiser to find a wave pattern that matches her own. To match the color, use the color ring. The color selection of most lines of hairpieces is very broad and very easy to match to the client's hair. You cannot color the hairpiece, so any custom coloring to achieve a match must be performed on the client's hair.

HAIR EXTENSIONS

Hair extensions are hair additions that are secured to the base of the client's natural hair in order to add length, volume, texture, or color. Extensions offer a better blending of real and artificial hair than hairpieces. Extensions are also left in the hair for much longer periods and are not removed at night. They are an increasingly popular salon service, not only for clients who are looking for something "different" but also for those suffering from hair loss. Hair extensions are often used by celebrities who never seem to have thin hair, and can "magically" grow their hair long overnight.

Manufacturers generally offer training in the attachment of hair extensions, but there are certain general guidelines to keep in mind.

- Start by deciding whether you are adding length, thickness, or both.
- Know which final style you are striving for. Map out your desired style.
- As a general rule of thumb, stay 1 inch (2.5 centimeters) away from the hairline at the front, sides, and nape, and 1 inch away from the part.
- With very thin hair, you must be careful that the base does not show through.
- Curly hair tends to expand and can give the illusion of being thicker than it really is. When working with curly hair, you will need to determine whether you are matching the curl or whether you wish to add another curl pattern to the hair.
- Straight thin hair and curly thin hair may have similar density, but curly hair will appear thicker. This means you may not need to put as many extensions in curly hair as in straight hair.

TRACK-AND-SEW ATTACHMENT METHOD

In the **track-and-sew method,** hair extensions are secured at the base of the client's own hair by sewing. The hair is attached to an on-the-scalp braid, or cornrow, which serves as the track (Figure 17-53). The angle of the track determines how the hair will fall. You may position tracks horizontally, vertically, or diagonally, or along curved lines that follow the contours of the head.

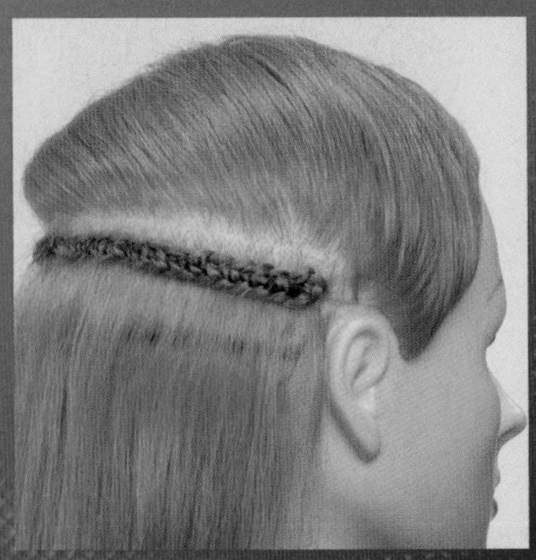

Figure 17-53 Cornrow track.

Partings are determined according to the style you have chosen. The size of the sections is determined by the amount of hair that will be added to the head. Plan the tracks so that the ends of the braids will be hidden. It is best to position the tracks 1 inch (2.5 centimeters) behind the hairline to ensure proper coverage.

When sewing the extension onto a track, use only a blunt, custom-designed needle, either straight or curved. These blunt ends will help avoid damage to the hair and will protect you and the client as well. Extensions can be sewn to the track using a variety of stitches.

- *Lock stitch.* Cut a length of thread double the length of the weft being sewn. Pass the needle through the weft to connect it to the track (Figure 17-54). Pull the thread through to create a loop. Pass the needle though the loop and wrap the thread around the needle (Figure 17-55). Pull the loop tight to form a lock stitch to secure the ends of the weft to the track (Figure 17-56). This stitch can also be used over the entire length of the track in evenly spaced stitches.
- *Double-lock stitch.* This stitch is much like the lock stitch, but the thread is wound around the needle twice to create the double lock. It is used in the same ways as the lock stitch.
- *Overcast stitch.* This simple, quick stitch can be used to secure the entire length of the weft to the track. Pass the needle under both the track and the weft, and then bring it back over to make a new stitch (Figure 17-57). Moving along the track, repeat the stitch until you reach the end of the track. Complete with a lock stitch for security (Figure 17-58).

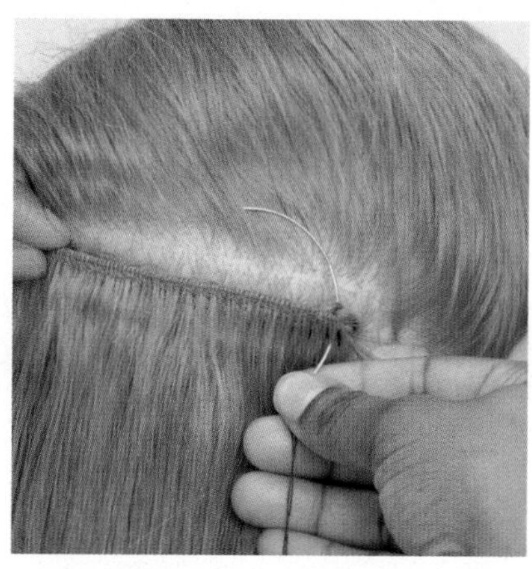

Figure 17-54 Sew weft to track.

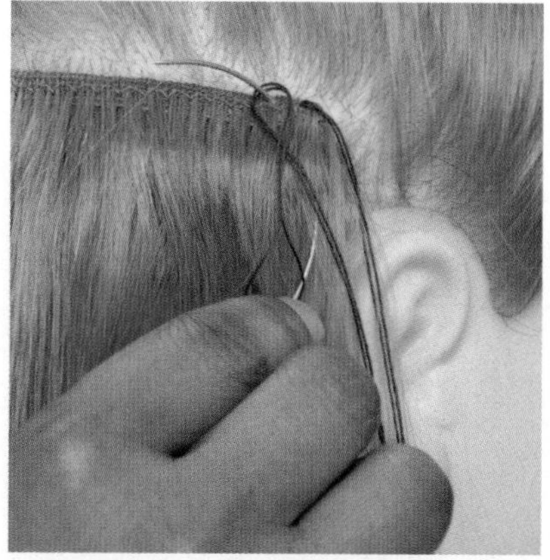

Figure 17-55 Wrap thread around needle.

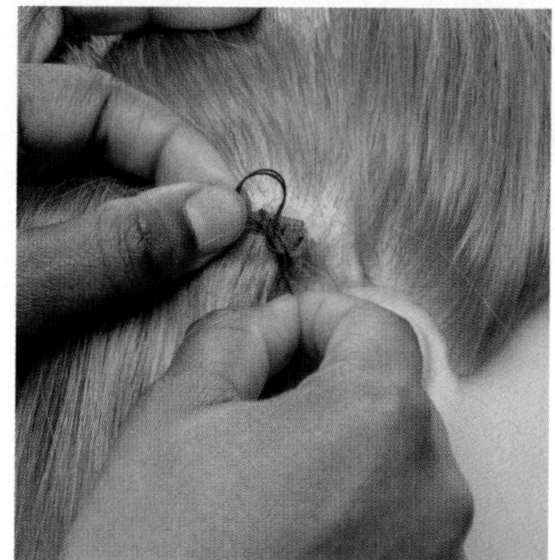

Figure 17-56 Form lock stitch.

BONDING METHOD

Bonding involves attaching hair wefts or single strands with an adhesive or a glue. This glue uses an applicator "gun" (not the kind available in crafts stores), but a special tool created specifically for bonding.

Bonded hair sits snugly on the head, and is fast to apply. There is, however, a certain degree of slippage. Generally, the bonding product lasts from 2 to 4 weeks, depending on factors such as the frequency of shampooing, the oiliness or dryness of the scalp, and the quality of the products used. This means that the client will need to be on a maintenance program that requires salon visits as often as every 2 weeks. One advantage of bonding is that the client can shampoo the hair with the wefts in, as long as it is done gently.

Bonding can be offered at a very affordable price, as the time it takes to complete the service is approximately 10 to 20 minutes, depending on your experience.

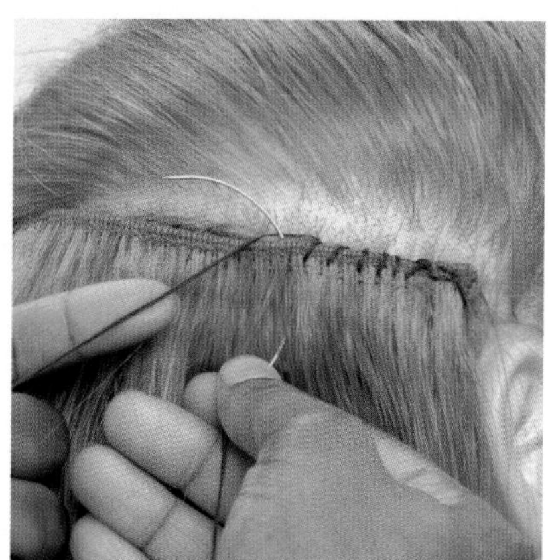

Figure 17-57 Finished overcast stitches.

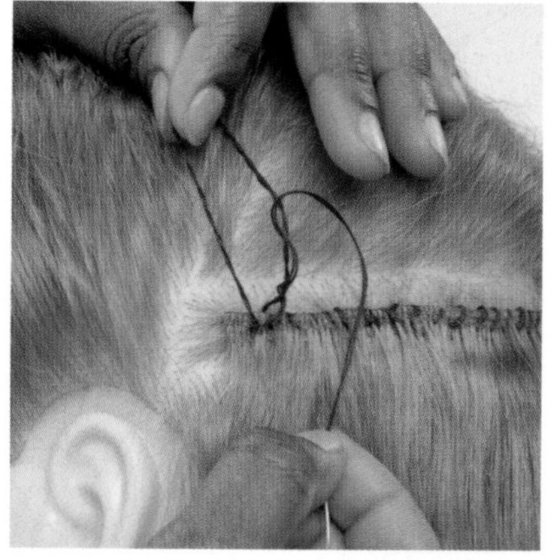

Figure 17-58 Completed line of overcast stitching.

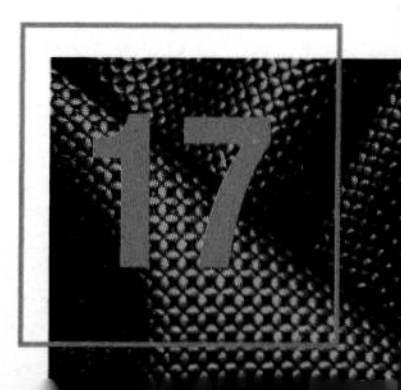

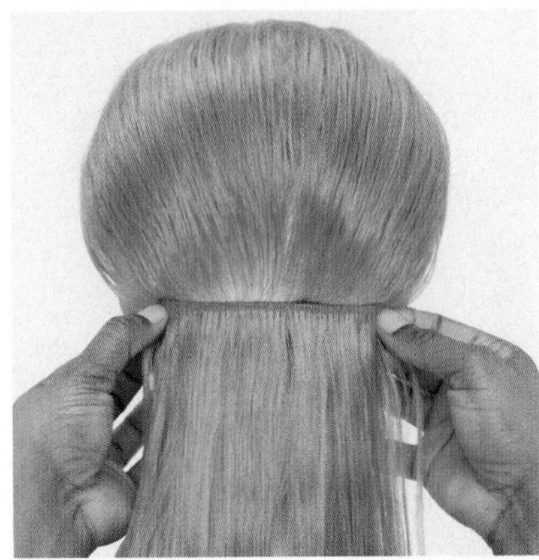

Figure 17-59 Measure weft against parting.

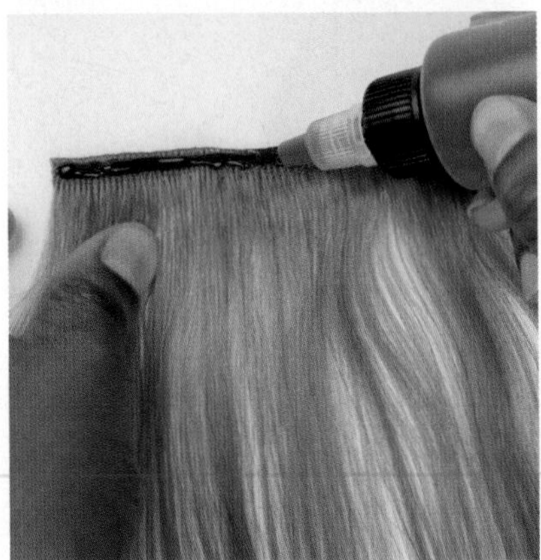

Figure 17-60 Apply adhesive to base of weft.

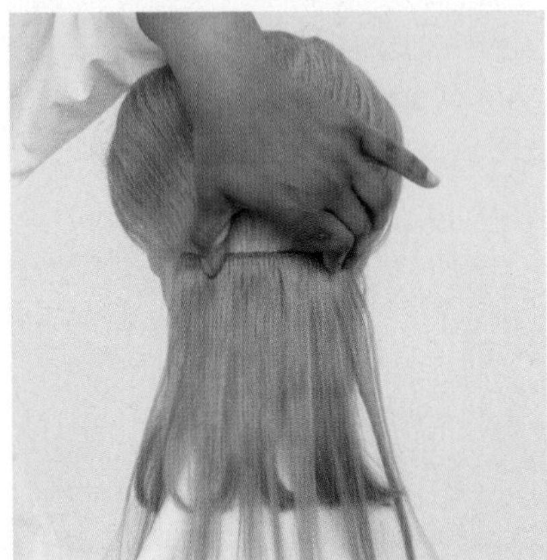

Figure 17-61 Press weft to parting.

The bonding procedure generally begins by sectioning off the hair at the nape. Measure the first weft against the parting, ¼ inch to ½ inch (0.6 to 1.25 centimeters) from the hairline (Figure 17-59). Lay the weft on a flat surface and carefully apply adhesive along the base (Figure 17-60). Use a consistent amount of adhesive—too much will ooze on the head, and too little will fail to adhere. Lightly press the weft against the clean parting (Figure 17-61). Hold for approximately 20 seconds, gently tugging to make sure that the weft has adhered. You may use a blow-dryer, set on low to medium heat, to help seal the bond (Figure 17-62). Proceed to the next section, working upward on the head, until the desired length and volume are achieved.

Care must be taken when bonding to avoid working too close to the crown or the parting, or the weft will show through. Working 1 inch (2.5 centimeters) away from the hairline will also keep the wefts from showing. Remember that hair is not a static material; it has a natural swing and it moves. When the wind blows, it should be the hairline that shows, not the wefts.

Bonded wefts are removed by dissolving the adhesive bond with oil or bond remover.

Some clients may have an allergic reaction to the ingredients in the bonding adhesive. Always perform a patch test prior to the application of bonded extensions.

FUSION METHOD

In the **fusion** method of attaching extensions, extension hair is bonded to the client's own hair with a bonding material that is activated by the heat from a special tool. This method, while expensive, harmonizes with the client's natural hair with no uncomfortable and unattractive attachment sites. The bonds are light and comfortable to wear, and the hair moves like real hair and is easy to maintain (Figure 17-63). The attachment lasts up to 4 months, almost twice as long as other methods. Removal is quick and painless. The fusion method requires certification training.

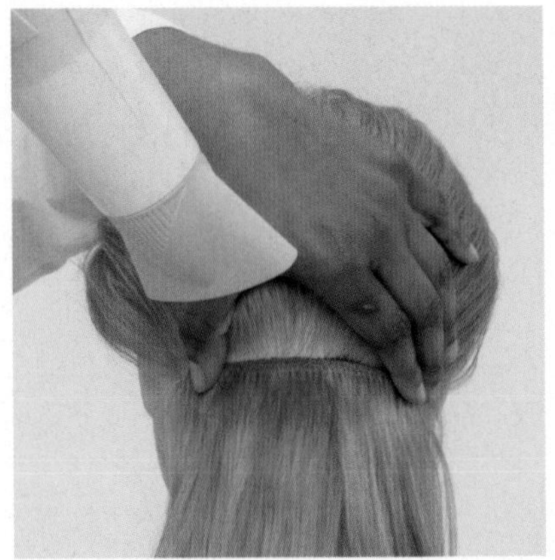

Figure 17-62 Using a blow-dryer can help seal the bond.

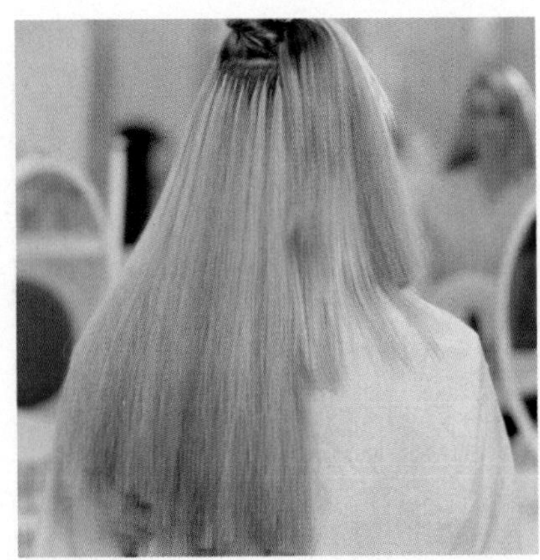

Figure 17-63 Fused extensions.

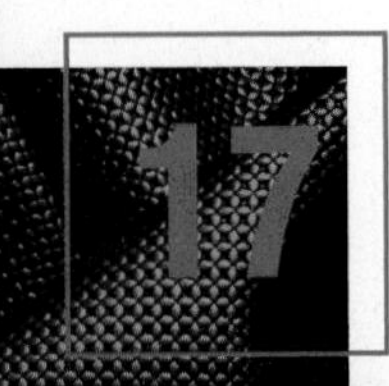

Fusion may be the best choice for clients with fine, limp hair. Bonding and tracking can create bulk at the base, which is not a problem on hair with texture and fullness, but may be too bulky and obvious with fine hair.

The fusion procedure involves wrapping a keratin-based strip around both the client's hair and the extension. The heating element is applied until the bonding agent has softened, and the bond is rolled between the fingers until both natural and added hair have adhered.

HAIR FOR SALE

Hairpieces are a great retail product for the salon. They can be displayed in fun, creative ways, and because they are fairly easy to attach and remove, they almost sell themselves, particularly to younger, more adventurous clients. Retailing hair additions and related home-care products can mean substantial additional income for you.

To be effective always keep the following guidelines in mind:

- Identify the client's needs.
- Explain why it would be worthwhile for the client to make the investment.
- Describe the features and benefits of the products you recommend.
- Discuss product performance and cost.
- Always believe in your recommendations and stand by your products.

To be the best, work only with the best. Work with one or two companies that offer a good range of human and synthetic hair, high-quality products, good customer service, and first-rate support and product education through training, seminars, and videos. Always stick with companies that stand by their products.

A FINAL THOUGHT-PRACTICE, PRACTICE, PRACTICE

Working with hair additions can be one of the most exciting, challenging, and lucrative areas of cosmetology. But to become skilled at this work, you need to practice. The more you do, the better you will become. The better you become, the more you will be able to help people look good and feel good about themselves. There is a great satisfaction in being able to do that, particularly when working with people who have suffered the trauma of hair loss, and may have given up hope that they could look good again (Figure 17-64).

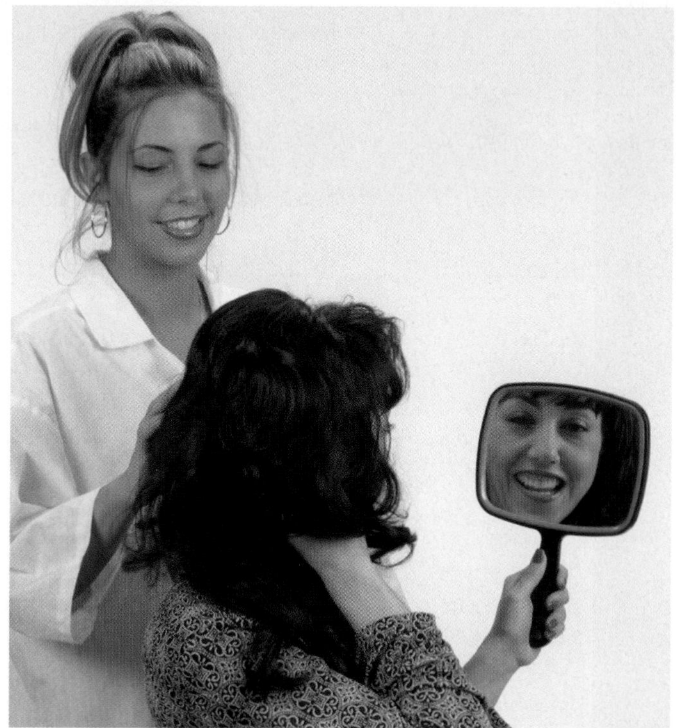

Figure 17-64 A wig specialist and her satisfied client.

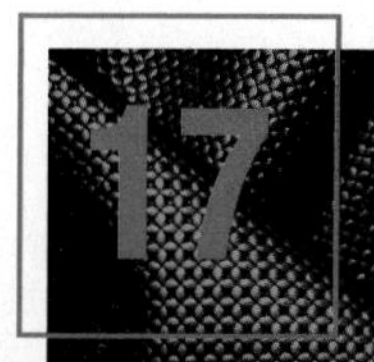

REVIEW QUESTIONS

1. List the seven key points you should cover in a client consultation for wig services.
2. Define wig, hairpiece, and hair extensions.
3. What are some advantages of human hair wigs? Of synthetic wigs?
4. Name and describe the two basic categories of wigs.
5. List the measurements that must be taken when measuring a client for a wig.
6. List at least three guidelines for styling a wig.
7. What is an integration hairpiece?
8. Name at least three methods for attaching hairpieces.
9. Name three methods for attaching hair extensions.

CHAPTER GLOSSARY

block	Head-shaped form, usually made of canvas-covered cork or Styrofoam, to which the wig is secured for fitting, cleaning, coloring, and styling.
bonding	Method of attaching hair extensions in which hair wefts or single strands are attached with an adhesive or a glue gun.
cap wigs	Wigs consisting of elasticized mesh-fiber bases to which the hair is attached.
capless wigs	Machine-made wigs in which rows of wefts are sewn to elastic strips in a circular pattern to fit the head shape.
fallen hair	Hair that has been shed from the head or gathered from a hairbrush, as opposed to hair that has been cut.
fusion	Method of attaching extensions in which extension hair is bonded to the client's own hair with a bonding material that is activated by heat from a special tool.
hair extensions	Hair additions that are secured to the base of the client's natural hair in order to add length, volume, texture, or color.
hairpiece	Small wig used to cover the top or crown of the head; does not fully cover the head; toupee.
hand-tied wigs or hand-knotted wigs	Wigs made by inserting individual strands of hair into mesh foundations and knotting them with a needle.
integration hairpiece	Hairpiece with an opening in the base through which the client's own hair is pulled to blend with the hair (natural or synthetic) of the hairpiece.

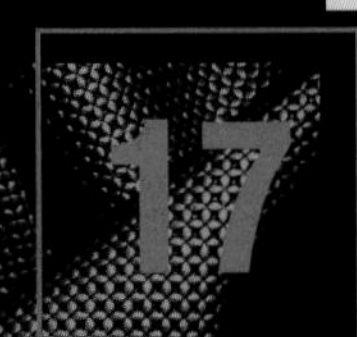

CHAPTER GLOSSARY

machine-made wigs	Wigs made by machine by feeding wefts through a sewing machine, and then sewing them together to form the base and shape of the wigs.
semi-hand-tied wigs	Wigs constructed with a combination of synthetic hair and hand-tied human hair.
toupee	Small wig used to cover the top or crown of the head.
track-and-sew method	Attachment method in which hair extensions are secured at the base of the client's own hair by sewing.
turned hair	Wig hair in which the root end of every hair strand is sewn into the base so that the cuticles of all hair strands slope in the same direction.
wefts	Strips of human or artificial hair woven by hand or machine onto a thread.
wig	Artificial covering for the head consisting of a network of interwoven hair.

18 CHAPTER CHEMICAL TEXTURE SERVICES

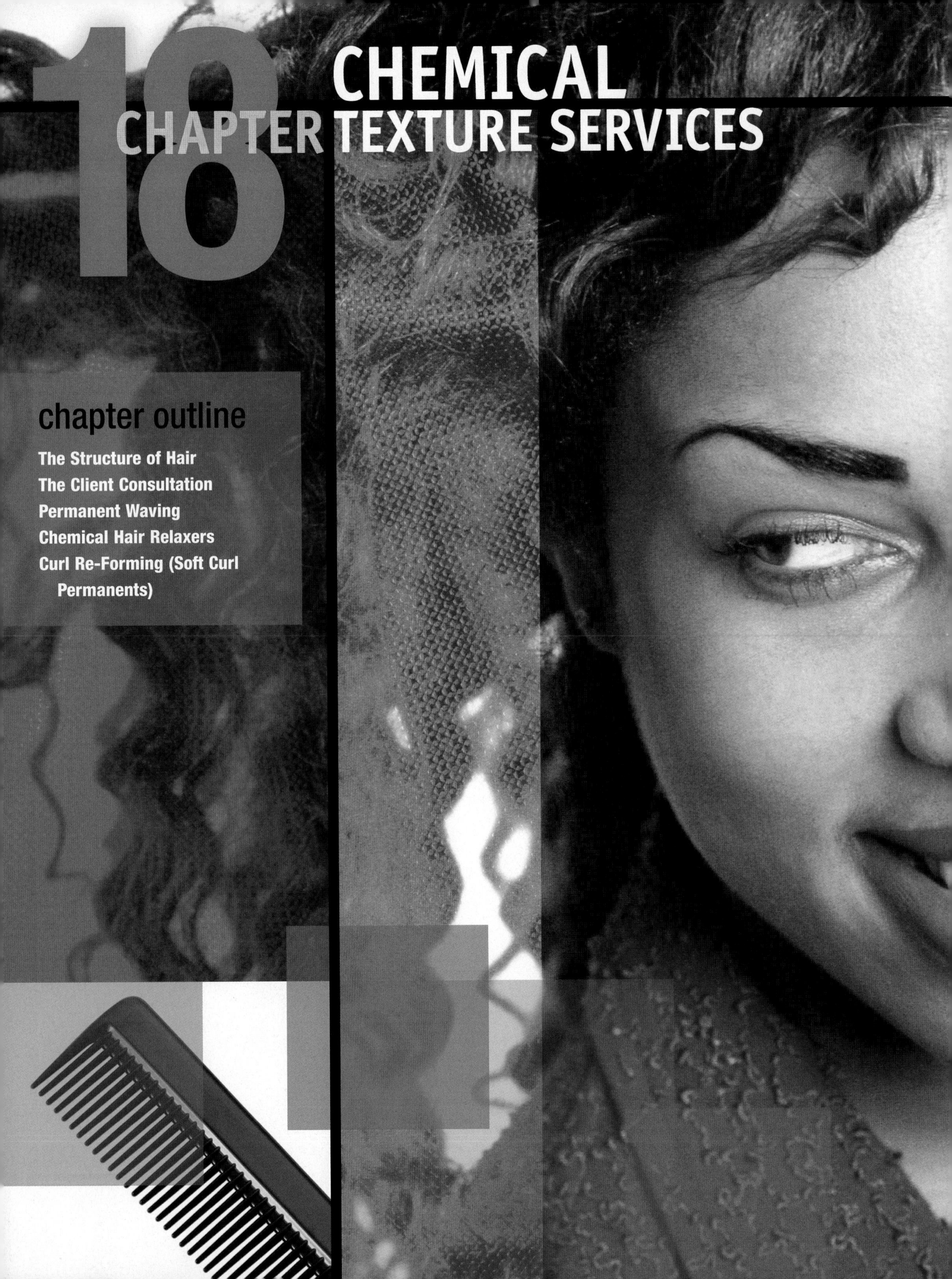

chapter outline

Learning Objectives

After completing this chapter, you will be able to:

- **List the factors of hair analysis for chemical texture services.**
- **Explain the physical and chemical actions that take place during permanent waving.**
- **List and describe the various types of permanent waving solutions.**
- **Demonstrate basic wrapping procedures: straight set, curvature wrap, bricklay wrap, weave wrap, double-rod wrap, and spiral wrap.**
- **Describe the procedure for chemical hair relaxing.**
- **Understand the difference between hydroxide relaxers and thio relaxers.**
- **Understand the difference between hydroxide neutralizers and thio neutralizers.**
- **Explain the basic procedure for a curl re-forming service.**

Key Terms

Page number indicates where in the chapter the term is used.

acid-balanced waves pg. 437

alkaline waves or cold waves pg. 436

amino acids pg. 426

ammonia-free waves pg. 438

ammonium thioglycolate (ATG) pg. 436

base cream or *protective base cream* pg. 461

base control pg. 443

base direction pg. 434

base placement pg. 433

base relaxers pg. 461

base sections pg. 433

basic perm wrap pg. 443

bookend wrap pg. 432

bricklay perm wrap pg. 443

chemical hair relaxing pg. 458

chemical texture services pg. 424

concave rods pg. 431

cortex pg. 424

croquignole perms pg. 434

curvature perm wrap pg. 443

disulfide bonds pg. 426

double flat wrap pg. 432

double-rod (piggyback) technique pg. 444

endothermic waves pg. 438

end papers or end wraps pg. 432

exothermic waves pg. 438

glyceryl monothioglycolate (GMTG) pg. 436

half off-base placement pg. 434

hydrogen bonds pg. 427

hydroxide neutralization pg. 460

hydroxide relaxers pg. 459

lanthionization pg. 460

loop or circle rod pg. 432

low-pH waves pg. 438

medulla pg. 424

metal hydroxide relaxers pg. 460

no-base relaxers pg. 461

normalizing lotions pg. 462

off-base placement pg. 434

on-base placement pg. 433

peptide bonds or end bonds pg. 426

polypeptide chains pg. 426

salt bonds pg. 427

side bonds pg. 426

single flat wrap pg. 432

soft bender rods pg. 432

soft curl permanent pg. 470

spiral perm wrap pg. 434

straight rods pg. 432

thioglycolic acid pg. 436

thio neutralization pg. 441

thio relaxers pg. 459

thio-free waves pg. 438

true acid waves pg. 437

weave technique pg. 443

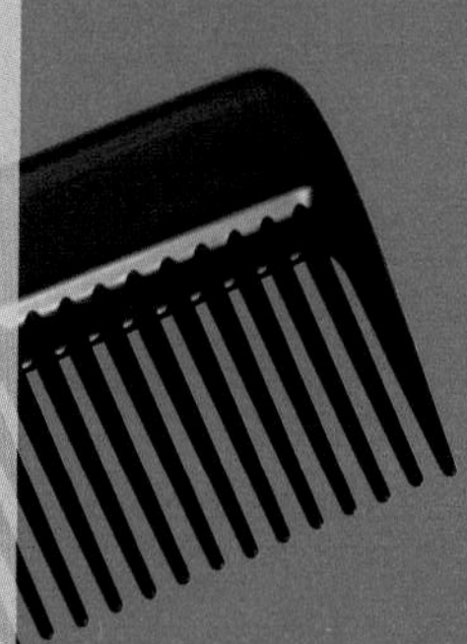

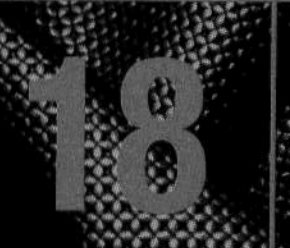

Chemical hair texture services give you the ability to permanently change the hair's natural wave pattern, and offer your client a variety of styling options that would not be possible otherwise. Texture services can be used to curl straight hair, straighten overly curly hair, or to soften coarse, straight hair and make it more pliable (Figure 18-1).

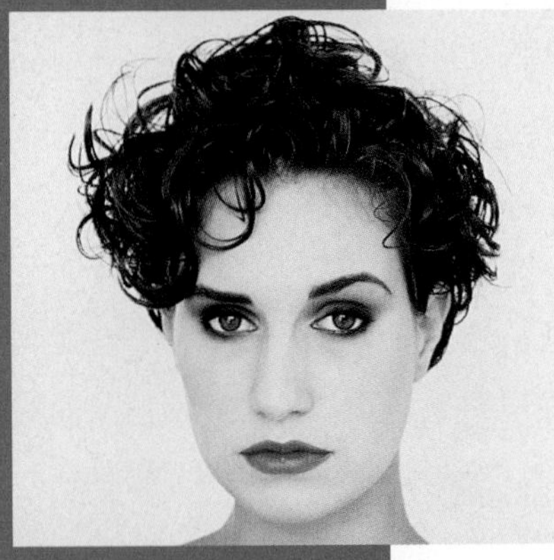
Figure 18-1 Permanent waving is one kind of chemical texture service.

Chemical texture services include the following:

1. Permanent waving—Adding wave or curl to the hair
2. Relaxing—Removing curl, leaving it smooth and wave-free
3. Curl Re-forming (soft curl permanents)—Loosening overly curly hair, such as turning tight curls into loose curls or waves

Because of the large number of people who wish to smooth their curls, or give their straight hair better body, mastering the techniques in this chapter will allow you to greatly expand your potential as a stylist.

THE STRUCTURE OF HAIR

Because all chemical texture procedures involve chemically and physically changing the structure of the hair, this chapter begins by reviewing the structure and purpose of each layer of the hair.

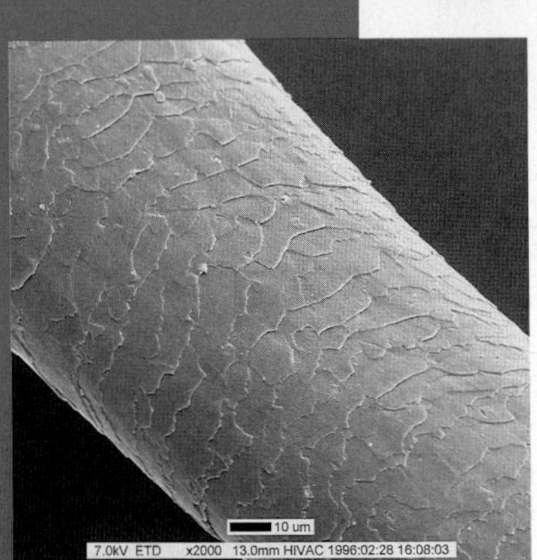

Figure 18-2 A healthy cuticle is compact and lays tight against the hair strand. It protects the hair from damage, and makes it appear smooth and shiny.

Cuticle. Tough exterior layer of the hair. It surrounds the inner layers, and protects the hair from damage. Although the cuticle is not directly involved in the texture or movement of the hair, texture chemicals must penetrate through the cuticle to their target in the cortex in order to be effective (Figures 18-2 and 18-3).

Cortex. Middle layer of the hair, located directly beneath the cuticle layer. The cortex is responsible for the incredible strength and elasticity of human hair. Breaking the side bonds of the cortex makes it possible to change the natural wave pattern of the hair.

Medulla. Innermost layer of the hair and is often called the pith or core of the hair. The medulla does not play a role in chemical texture services and may be missing in fine hair.

IMPORTANCE OF PH IN TEXTURE SERVICES

The term **pH** literally means *potential of hydrogen.* The symbol pH represents the quantity of hydrogen ions. The pH scale measures the acidity and alkalinity of a substance by measuring the quantity of hydrogen

18

ions it contains. The pH scale has a range from 0 to 14. A pH of 7 is neutral, a pH below 7 is acidic, and pH above 7 is alkaline. The natural pH of hair is between 4.5 and 5.5. Chemical texturizers raise the pH of the hair to an alkaline state in order to soften and swell the hair shaft. This action lifts the cuticle layer, and allows the solution to reach the cortex layer where restructuring takes place. Coarse, resistant hair with a strong, compact cuticle layer requires a highly alkaline chemical solution. Porous, damaged, or chemically treated hair requires a less alkaline solution.

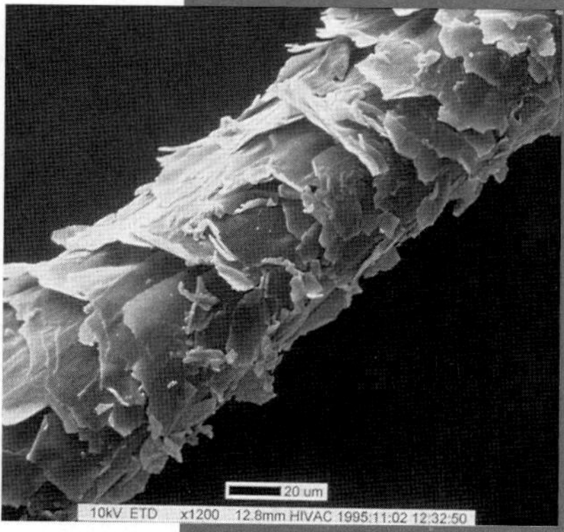

Figure 18–3 A damaged cuticle is chipped and does not lay tight against the hair shaft. Because it cannot adequately protect the hair against damage, the hair becomes rough, dull, and prone to split ends and breakage.

To understand how a chemical texturizer changes the structure of hair, it is important to understand the basic building blocks of hair (Figures 18-4 to 18-8).

Keratin proteins are made of long chains of amino acids linked together end to end like beads. The chemical bonds that link amino acids together are called peptide (PEP-tyd) bonds or end bonds. These chains of amino acids linked by peptide bonds are called polypeptides. Keratin proteins are made of long, coiled, polypeptide chains, which in turn are comprised of amino acids.

The Amino Acid Content of Hair

All the protein structures of hair are made from these eighteen amino acids:

Cysteic acid	Aspartic acid	Threonine
Arginine	Serine	Glutamic acid
Proline	Glycine	Alanine
Valine	Cystine	Methionine
Isoleucine	Leucine	Tyrosine
Phenylalanine	Lysine	Histidine

Figure 18–4 Amino acids are the building blocks of proteins.

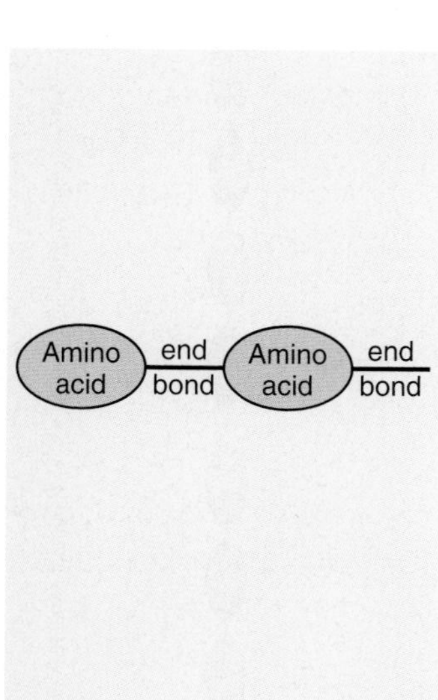

Figure 18–5 Peptide bonds (end bonds) link amino acids together in long chains.

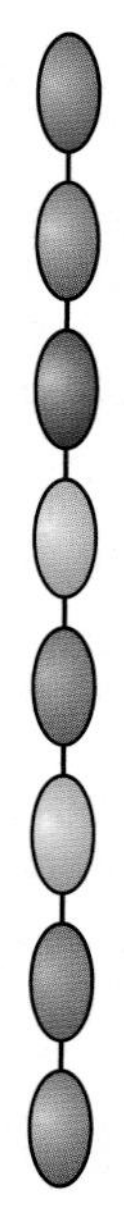

Figure 18–6 Polypeptide chains are formed when amino acids link together.

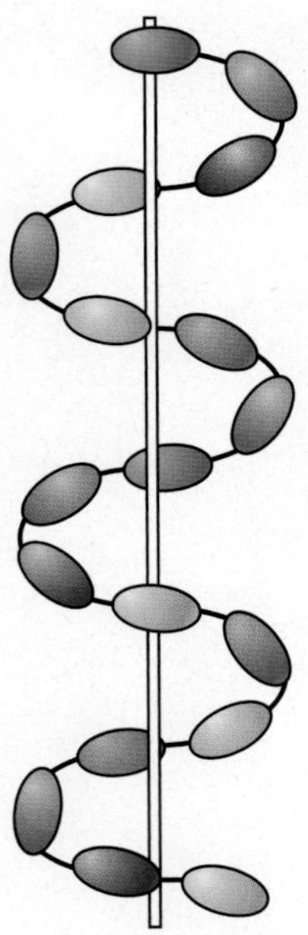

Figure 18-7 Keratin proteins are long, coiled polypeptide chains.

- **Amino acids** are compounds made up of carbon, oxygen, hydrogen, and nitrogen.
- **Peptide** (PEP-tide) **bonds (end bonds)** link amino acids together end to end in long chains, like beads, to form a polypeptide chain.
- **Polypeptide chains** are long chains of amino acids linked together by peptide bonds or end bonds.
- **Keratin** proteins are long, coiled polypeptide chains.
- **Side bonds** (disulfide, salt, and hydrogen bonds) cross-link polypeptide chains together (see Side Bonds section).

CAUTION

Peptide bonds should never be broken during any chemical texture service. Breaking the hair's peptide bonds causes the polypeptide chains to come apart and dramatically weakens the hair. When used incorrectly, chemical texturizers can break peptide bonds and cause hair breakage.

SIDE BONDS

The cortex is made up of millions of polypeptide chains cross-linked by three types of side bonds: disulfide, salt, and hydrogen. Side bonds are responsible for the elasticity and incredible strength of the hair. Altering these three types of side bonds is what makes wet setting, thermal styling, permanent waving, curl re-forming, and chemical hair relaxing possible (Figure 18-9).

DISULFIDE BONDS

Disulfide bonds are strong chemical side bonds formed when the sulfur atoms in two adjacent protein chains are joined together. Disulfide bonds can only be broken by chemicals and cannot be broken by heat or water. The chemical and physical changes in disulfide bonds make permanent waving, curl re-forming and chemical hair relaxing possible. Although there are far fewer disulfide bonds than hydrogen or salt bonds, they are the strongest of the three side bonds, and account for about one-third of the hair's overall strength.

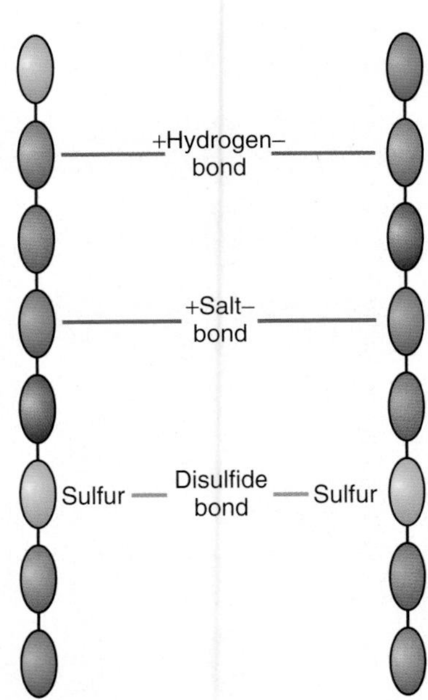

Figure 18-8 Side bonds cross-link polypeptide chains together.

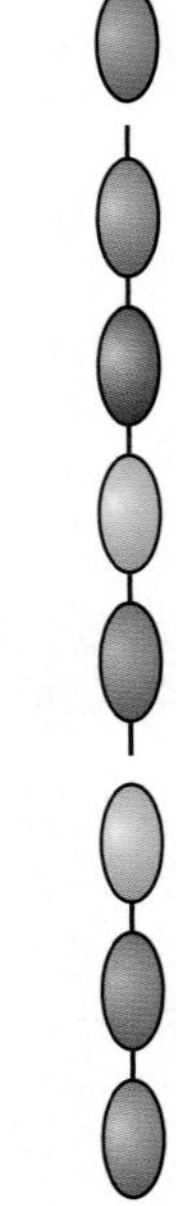

Figure 18-9 A correct permanent wave service only alters the side bonds.

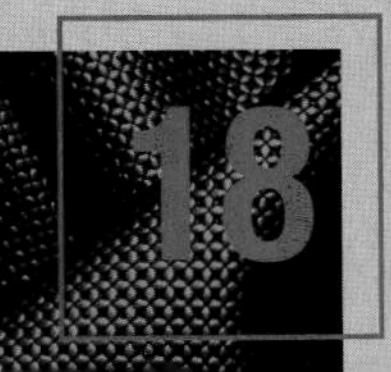

SALT BONDS

Salt bonds are weak physical side bonds that are the result of an attraction between negative and positive electrical charges. Salt bonds are easily broken by changes in pH, and re-form when the pH has returned to normal. Hydrogen bonds can be broken by water, whereas salt bonds are broken by changes in pH. Even though salt bonds are far weaker than disulfide bonds, the hair has so many salt bonds that they account for about one-third of the hair's total strength.

HYDROGEN BONDS

Hydrogen bonds are weak physical side bonds that are also the result of an attraction between opposite electrical charges. They are easily broken by water (wet setting), or heat (thermal styling), and re-form as the hair dries or cools. Although individual hydrogen bonds are very weak, there are so many of them that they, too, account for about one-third of the hair's total strength.

THE CLIENT CONSULTATION

The client consultation is one of the most important parts of any successful texture service. Before proceeding with any service, you must first determine exactly what the client expects, and what is possible. No matter how advanced your technical skills may be, nothing will compensate for a lack of communication between you and your client.

To accurately communicate with your client you must:

- Ask open-ended questions (questions that require more than a "yes" or "no" answer) that allow you to find out why the client wants the texture service, and what results are expected.
- Find out what type of coloring product (if any) is currently being used by the client. This is essential since certain types of haircolor agents—especially those containing metallic salts—should not be used on permed hair. (See Metallic Salts section.)
- Look at pictures with your client to determine the desired style.
- Ask about previous texture services. What did the client like and dislike about the services?
- Ask how the client currently styles her hair and discuss any changes that would result from the texture service.
- Determine the finished hairstyle that the client wants, considering the haircut and the degree of curl or relaxing that is needed.
- Evaluate the condition, texture, and wave pattern of the hair to ensure that the desired style is possible.
- Fill out a chemical texture service record to document the condition of the hair, and the desired outcome (Figure 18-10).

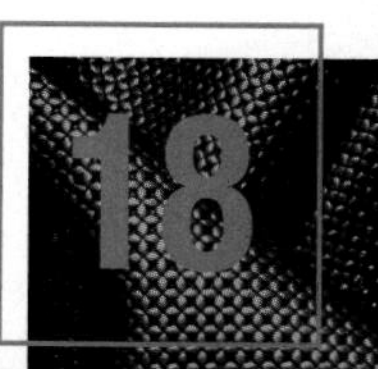

CHEMICAL TEXTURE SERVICE RECORD

Name____________________ Tel__________

Address____________________________

City______________ State______ Zip__________

DESCRIPTION OF HAIR

Length	Texture	Type	Porosity	
☐ short	☐ coarse	☐ normal	☐ very porous	☐ slightly porous
☐ medium	☐ medium	☐ resistant	☐ moderately porous	☐ resistant
☐ long	☐ fine	☐ tinted	☐ normal	
		☐ highlighted		
		☐ bleached		

CONDITION

☐ very good ☐ good ☐ fair ☐ poor ☐ dry ☐ oily

Tinted with____________________________

Previously permed with________________________

TYPE OF PERM

☐ alkaline ☐ acid ☐ body wave ☐ Other______________

No. of rods__________ Lotion________ Strength________

RESULTS

☐ good ☐ poor ☐ too tight ☐ too loose

Date	Perm used	Stylist	Date	Perm used	Stylist

Figure 18–10 Example of a chemical texture service record that you must keep on every client who receives this type of service.

METALLIC SALTS

Some home haircoloring products contain metallic salts that are not compatible with permanent waving. Metallic salts leave a coating on the hair that may cause uneven curls, severe discoloration, or hair breakage.

Metallic salts are more commonly found in men's haircolors that are sold for home use. Haircolor restorers and progressive haircolors that darken the hair gradually with repeated applications are the most likely to contain metallic salts. If you suspect that metallic salts may be present on the hair, perform the following test.

In a glass or plastic bowl, mix 1 ounce of 20-volume peroxide with 20 drops of 28-percent ammonia. Immerse at least 20 strands of hair in the solution for 30 minutes. If metallic salts are not present, the hair will lighten slightly and you may proceed with the service. If metallic salts are present, the hair will lighten rapidly. The solution may get hot and give off an unpleasant odor, indicating that you should not proceed with the service.

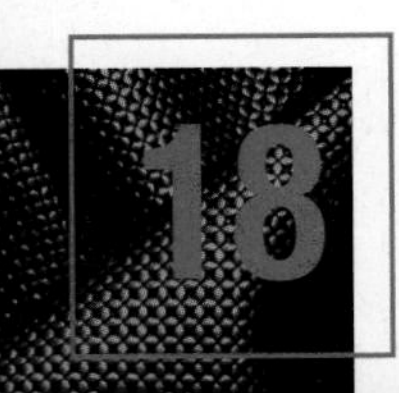

CLIENT RECORDS

Client records should include a complete evaluation of the length, texture, color, and condition of the hair prior to the service, and expected results. Extra caution should be used to determine any previous problems or adverse reactions the client may have had in the past. This information must be re-evaluated prior to each service, since there may have been changes in the client's history or in the formulation of the product since it was last used.

Also include in your records the type of perm, the type and size of perm rods, base direction, base control, wrapping technique, wrapping pattern, processing time, and the results achieved. Always remember to update your records and note any changes.

CLIENT RELEASE FORM

Some schools and salons may require a client to sign a release form prior to receiving any chemical service. Although most release forms state that the school or salon is not responsible for any damages that may occur, they do not release the school or salon from all responsibility. Release forms do indicate that the client knew, before the chemical service was given, that there was a possibility of damage to the hair or an unexpected adverse reaction.

SCALP ANALYSIS

An analysis of the scalp should always be performed prior to any chemical service. Look for cuts, scratches, open sores, redness, or flaking. Do not proceed with the service if there are any skin abrasions or signs of scalp disease. Refer the client to a physician as necessary.

HAIR ANALYSIS

Hair analysis is an essential part of any successful chemical hair service. A complete analysis will help you determine how the hair will react to the service, and will help avoid most problems. The condition, texture, and wave pattern of the hair must be considered when selecting the type of relaxer, perm, type and size of perm rod, and wrapping method.

The five most important factors to consider in a hair analysis follow:

Texture—diameter of a single hair strand

Density—thickness or number of hairs per square inch on the head

Porosity—the ability of the hair to absorb moisture

Elasticity—how far the hair stretches before breaking, and how well it returns to its original shape when stretched

Growth direction—how the hair naturally lays (forward, circular, and so on)

HAIR TEXTURE

Hair texture describes the diameter of a single strand of hair and is classified as coarse, medium, or fine. Hair density differs not only from one individual to another, but also from strand to strand on the same

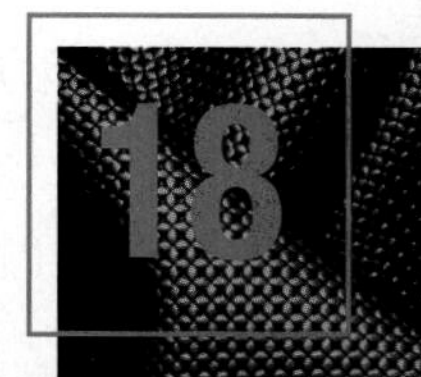

CAUTION

If the hair has poor elasticity, or is overly porous, a conditioning program should be suggested to improve the overall strength and quality of the hair. A chemical service should only be done once the hair has become healthy enough to produce satisfactory results.

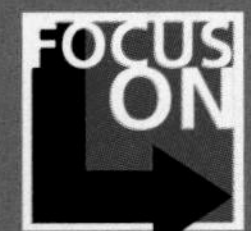

Focus on . . . Building Your Client Base

Accurate, detailed, systematic record keeping is an essential part of successful chemical services. The importance of accurate records cannot be over-emphasized. If you neglect to update your records, you may find yourself repeating past mistakes and losing clients. If you make a habit of keeping good records, however, you will not only improve your technical skills, you will also build your client's trust and loyalty.

person's head. It is best determined by feeling a single, dry strand between the fingers, from the top, sides, and back of the head.

The three types of hair texture have the following characteristics when undergoing a chemical texture service:

- *Coarse hair* usually requires more processing than medium or fine hair, and is usually more resistant to that processing. Coarse hair requires a thorough and careful chemical application to ensure success.
- *Medium hair* is the most common hair texture. It is considered normal, and does not pose any special problems or concerns.
- *Fine hair* is more fragile, easier to process, and more susceptible to damage from chemical services than coarse or medium hair. As a general rule, fine hair will process faster and easier than medium or coarse hair. Treating fine hair gently during the entire chemical process is essential for healthy, beautiful results.

HAIR DENSITY

Hair density measures the number of hairs per square inch on the head to determine whether a client has thin, medium, or thick hair. Individuals with the same hair texture can have different densities. Some individuals with fine hair, for instance, may have high density with many hairs per square inch, while others may have low density with fewer hairs per square inch. Coarse hair naturally looks thicker and fuller, even when there are fewer hairs per square inch. This often causes confusion among clients who believe they have thick or thin hair, when the opposite may be true.

HAIR POROSITY

Hair porosity is the ability of the hair to absorb moisture. The degree of porosity is directly related to the condition of the cuticle layer. Hair porosity is classified as resistant, normal, or porous.

- *Resistant hair* has a tight, compact cuticle layer that resists penetration. Chemical services performed on resistant hair requires a (more alkaline) texturizer than porous hair. Resistant hair requires a thorough and careful chemical application to ensure successful service.
- *Hair with normal porosity* is neither resistant nor overly porous. Texture services performed on this type of hair will usually process as expected.
- *Overly porous hair* has a raised cuticle layer that easily absorbs moisture/chemicals.

Chemical texture services performed on overly porous hair require a less alkaline texturizer than those performed on normal or resistant hair. A lower pH minimizes swelling and helps prevent excessive damage to the hair.

HAIR ELASTICITY

Hair elasticity is an indication of the strength of the side bonds that hold the individual fibers of the hair in place. More than any other single factor, the elasticity of the hair determines its ability to hold curl. Hair elasticity is usually classified as normal or low (Figure 18-11).

- Wet hair with normal elasticity can stretch up to 50 percent of its original length, and then return to that same length without breaking. Hair with normal elasticity usually holds the curl from wet sets, thermal styling, and permanent waves.
- Wet hair with low elasticity does not return to its original length when stretched. Hair with low elasticity may not be able to hold the curl from wet sets, thermal styling, and permanent waves.

DIRECTION OF HAIR GROWTH

The individual growth direction of the hair causes hair streams, whorls, and cowlicks that influence the finished hairstyle, and must be considered when selecting the base direction and wrapping pattern for each permanent wave.

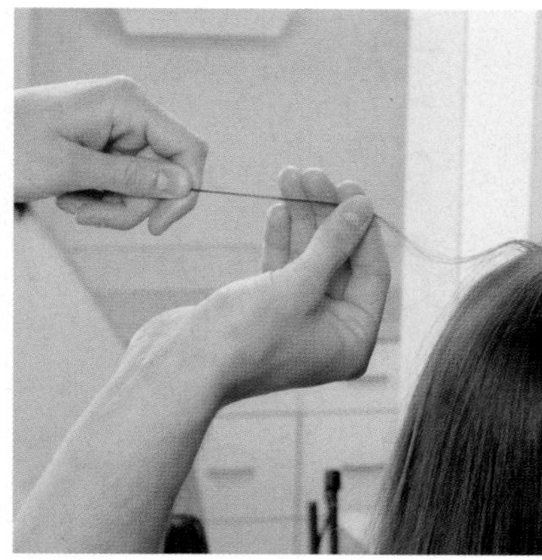

Figure 18-11 Elasticity test.

PERMANENT WAVING

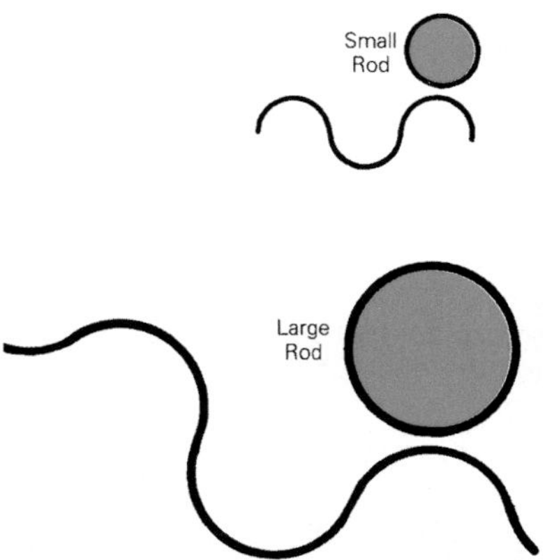

Figure 18-12 The diameter of the rod determines the size of the curl.

Permanent waving is a two-step process. The first part of any perm is the physical change caused by wrapping the hair on the perm rods. The second part involves the chemical changes caused by the permanent waving solution and the neutralizer.

PERM WRAP

A perm wrap is essentially a wet set on perm rods instead of rollers. The major difference between a wet set and a permanent wave is the type of side bonds that are broken. A wet set breaks hydrogen bonds, whereas a permanent wave breaks disulfide bonds that are much stronger and more resistant.

In permanent waving, the size of the rod determines the size of the curl. The shape and type of curl are determined by the shape and type of rod and the wrapping method (Figure 18-12). Selecting the correct perm rod and wrapping method is key to creating a successful permanent. Perm rods come in a wide variety of sizes and shapes that can be combined with different wrapping methods to provide an exciting range of styling options.

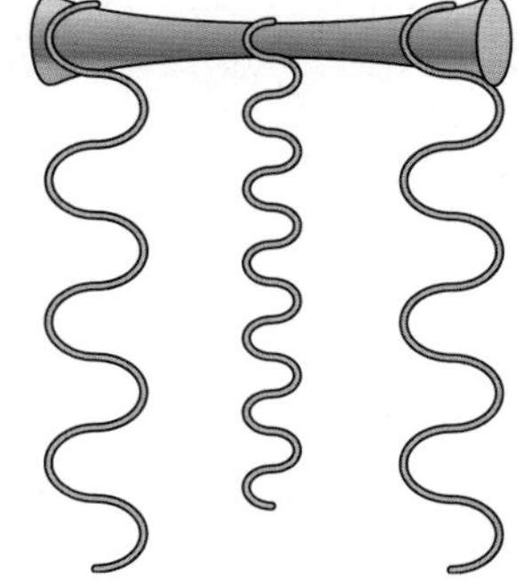

Figure 18-13 Concave rod and resulting curl.

TYPES OF RODS

Concave rods are the most common type of perm rod. They have a smaller diameter in the center that increases to a larger diameter on the ends. Concave rods produce a tighter curl in the center, and a looser curl on either side of the strand (Figure 18-13).

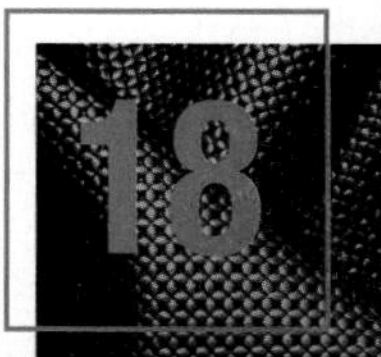

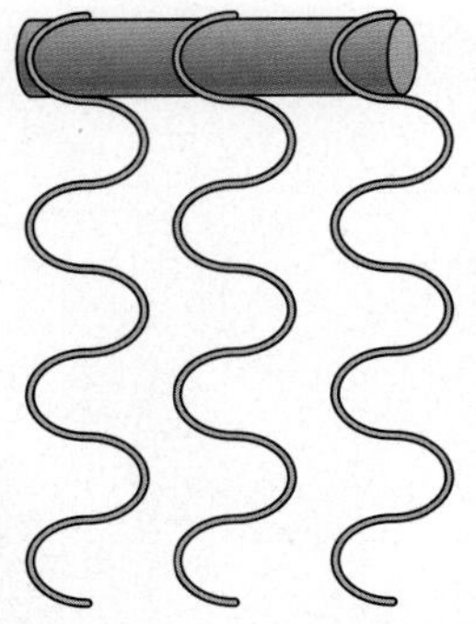

Figure 18–14 Straight rod and resulting curl.

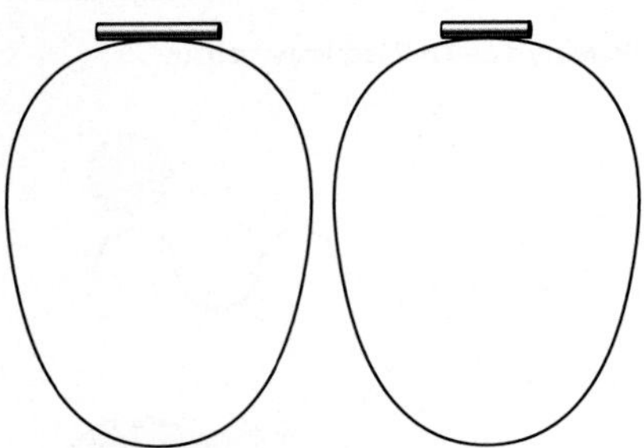

Figure 18–15 Long and short rods and the contours of the head.

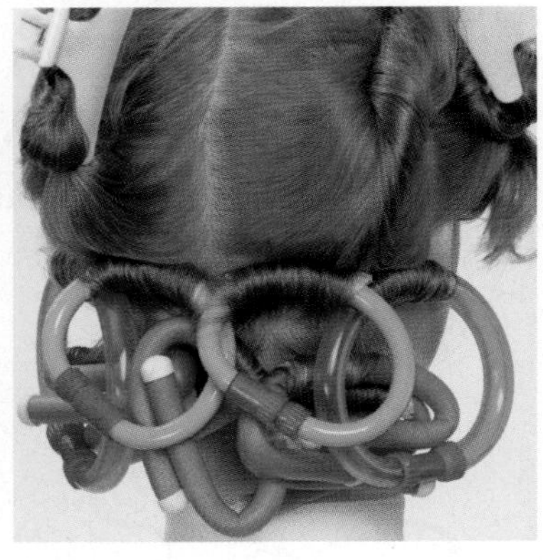

Figure 18–16 Soft bender rods.

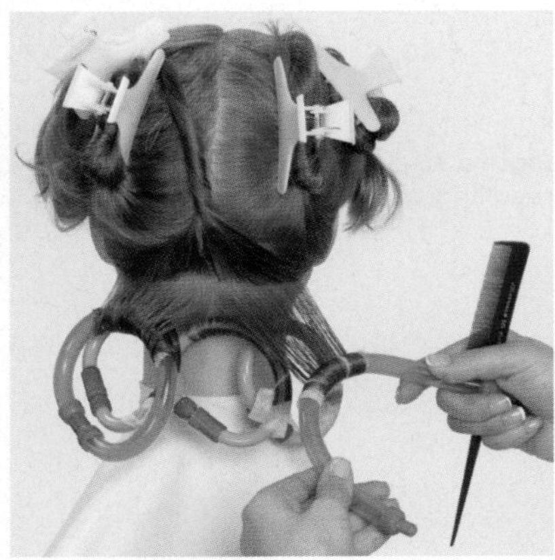

Figure 18–17 Loop rods.

Straight rods are equal in diameter along their entire length. This produces a uniform curl along the entire width of the strand (Figure 18-14).

Both concave and straight rods come in different lengths to accommodate different sections on the head. Short rods, for instance, can be used for wrapping small and awkward sections where long rods would not fit (Figure 18-15).

OTHER PERM RODS

Soft bender rods are usually about 12 inches long with a uniform diameter along the entire length. These soft foam rods have a stiff wire inside that permits them to be bent into almost any shape (Figure 18-16).

The **loop** or **circle rod** is usually about 12 inches long with a uniform diameter along the entire length of the rod. After the hair is wrapped, the rod is secured by fastening the ends together to form a loop (Figure 18-17).

END PAPERS

End papers or **end wraps** are absorbent papers used to control the ends of the hair when wrapping and winding hair on the perm rods. End papers should extend beyond the ends of the hair to keep them smooth and straight and prevent "fishhooks." The most common end paper techniques are the double flat wrap, single flat wrap, and bookend single paper wrap.

- The **double flat wrap** uses two end papers, one placed under and one over the strand of hair being wrapped. Both papers extend past the hair ends. This wrap provides the most control over the hair ends and also helps keep them evenly distributed over the entire length of the rod (Figure 18-18).
- The **single flat wrap** is similar to the double flat wrap, but uses only one end paper, placed over the top of the strand of hair being wrapped (Figure 18-19).
- The **bookend wrap** uses one end paper folded in half over the hair ends like an envelope. The bookend wrap eliminates excess paper and

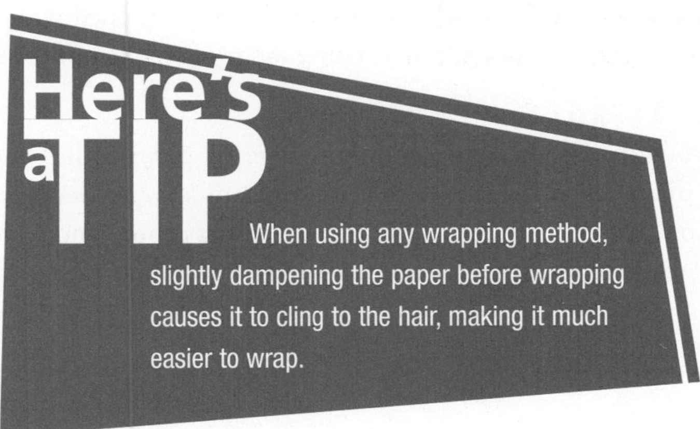

When using any wrapping method, slightly dampening the paper before wrapping causes it to cling to the hair, making it much easier to wrap.

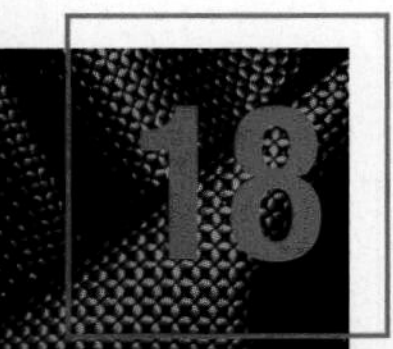

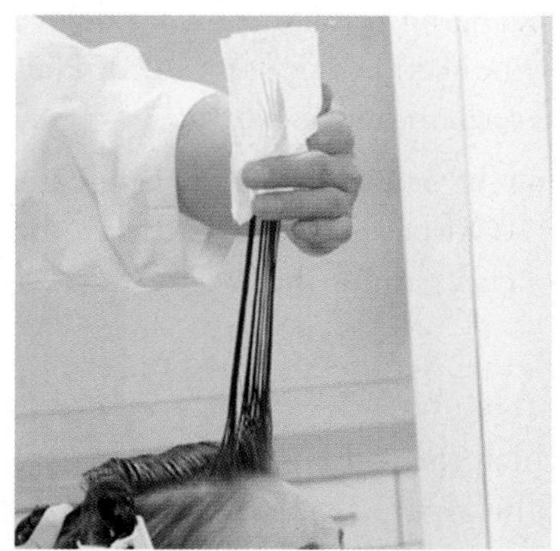
Figure 18–18 Double flat wrap.

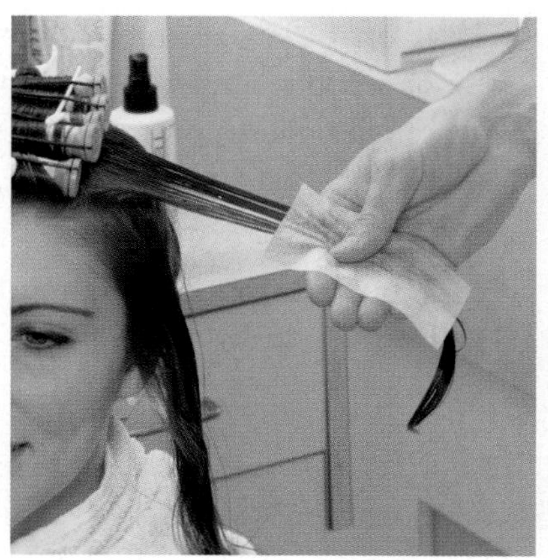
Figure 18–19 Single flat wrap.

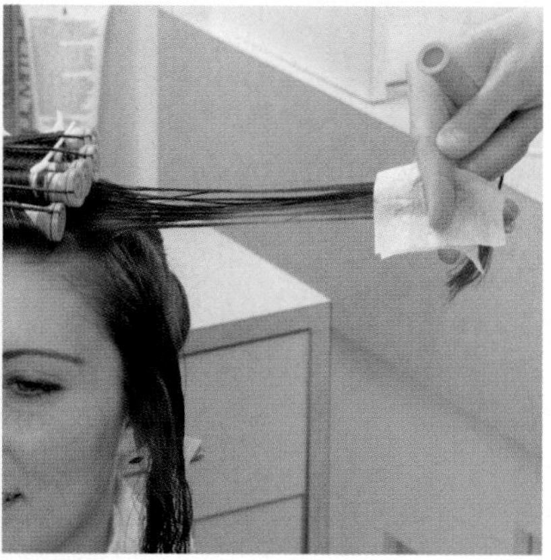
Figure 18–20 Bookend wrap.

can be used with short rods or with very short lengths of hair. When using this wrap method, be careful to distribute the hair evenly over the entire length of the rod. Avoid bunching the hair in the fold of the paper—hair should be in the center—to produce an even curl (Figure 18-20).

SECTIONING A PERM

All perm wraps begin by sectioning the hair into panels. The size, shape, and direction of these panels vary, based on the wrapping pattern and the type and size of the rod being used. Each panel is further divided into subsections called **base sections** (Figure 18-21). One rod is normally placed on each base section. The size of each base section is usually the length and width of the rod being used.

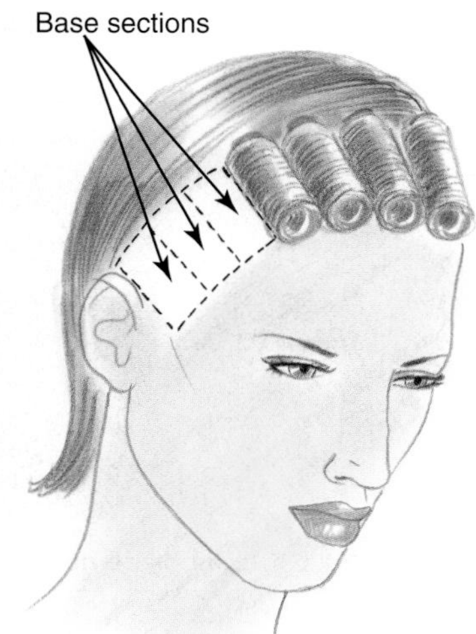

Figure 18–21 All perm wraps section the hair into panels. These panels are then divided into base sections.

BASE PLACEMENT

Base placement refers to the position of the rod in relation to its base section, and is determined by the angle at which the hair is wrapped. Rods can be wrapped on base, half off base, or off base.

For **on-base placement,** the hair is wrapped 45 degrees beyond perpendicular to its base section (Figure 18-22). Although on-base placement may result in greater volume at the scalp area, any increase in volume will be lost as soon as the hair begins to grow out. Caution should be used with on-base placement because the additional stress and tension can mark or break the hair.

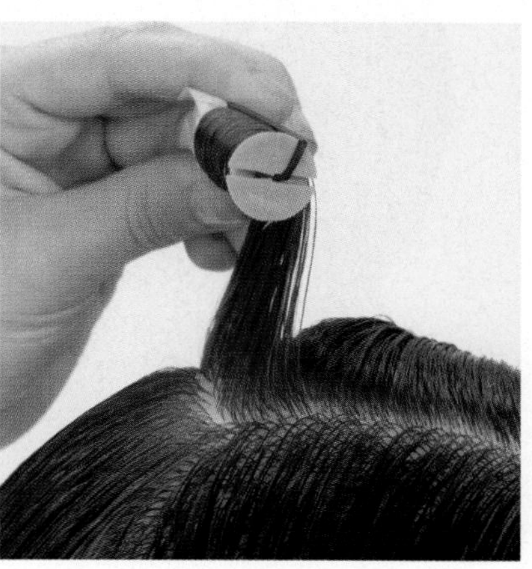
Figure 18–22 On-base placement.

CAUTION

Using a base section that is wider than the perm rod can create an uneven curl pattern and undue tension on the hair.

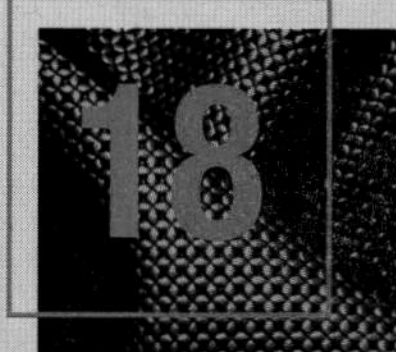

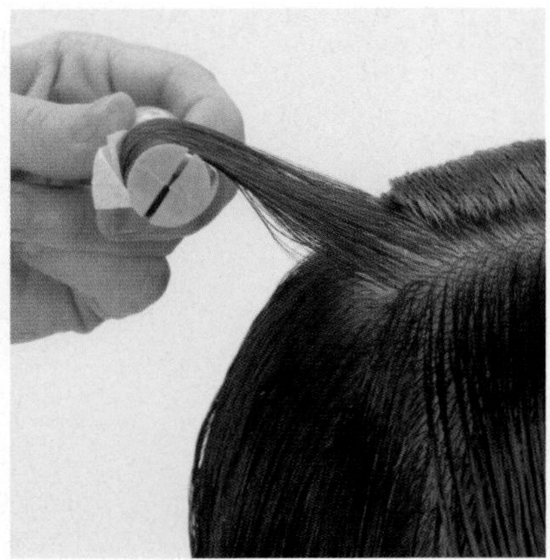

Figure 18-23 Half off-base placement.

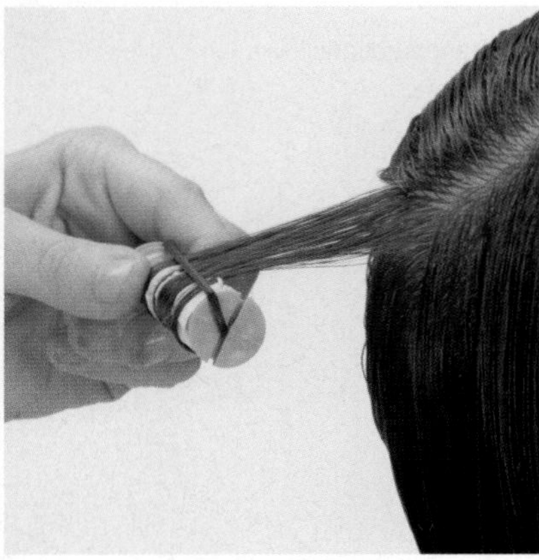

Figure 18-24 Off-base placement.

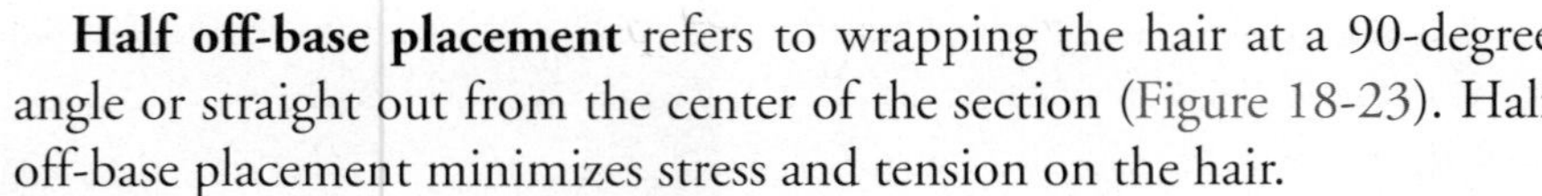

Half off-base placement refers to wrapping the hair at a 90-degree angle or straight out from the center of the section (Figure 18-23). Half off-base placement minimizes stress and tension on the hair.

Off-base placement refers to wrapping the hair at 45 degrees below the center of the base section (Figure 18-24). Off-base placement creates the least amount of volume, and results in a curl pattern that begins farthest away from the scalp.

BASE DIRECTION

Base direction refers to the angle at which the rod is positioned on the head: horizontally, vertically, or diagonally (Figure 18-25). Base direction also refers to the directional pattern in which the hair is wrapped. Although directional wraps can be wrapped backward, forward, or to one side, it is important to remember that wrapping with the natural direction of hair growth causes the least amount of stress to the hair. Wrapping against the natural growth pattern can produce a "band" mark or breakage at the base of the curl.

WRAPPING TECHNIQUES

There are two basic methods of wrapping the hair around the perm rod: croquignole and spiral.

Croquignole perms (KROH-ken-ohl) are wrapped from the ends to the scalp in overlapping concentric layers (Figure 18-26). Because the hair is wrapped perpendicular to the length of the rod, each new layer of hair is wrapped on top of the previous layer. This increases the size (diameter) of the rod with each new overlapping layer. This produces a tighter curl at the ends, and a larger curl at the scalp. Longer, thicker hair increases this effect.

In a **spiral perm wrap,** the hair is wrapped at an angle other than perpendicular to the length of the rod (Figure 18-27). The angle at which the hair is wrapped causes the hair to spiral along the length of the rod, like the grip on a tennis racket.

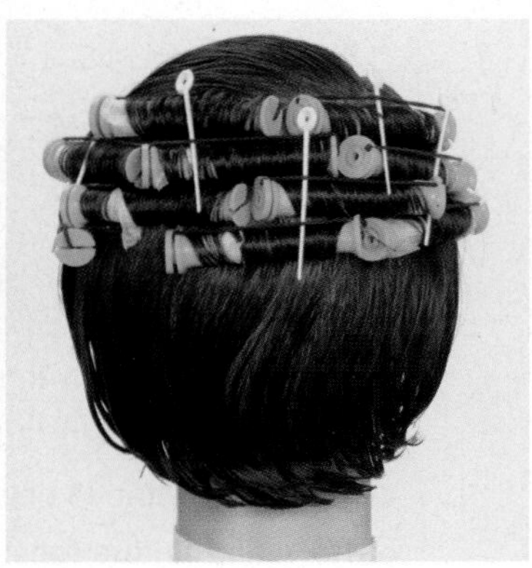

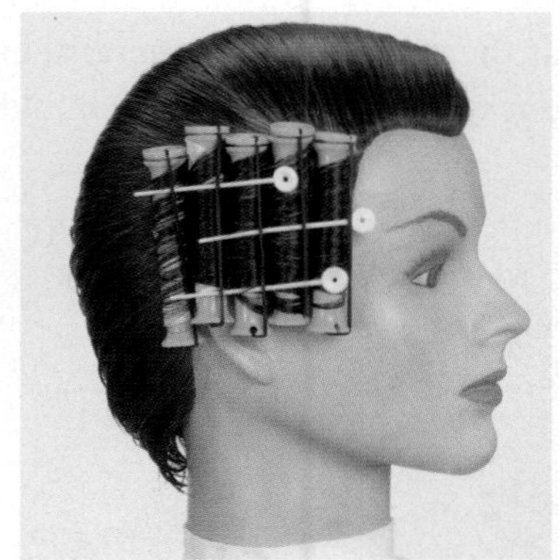

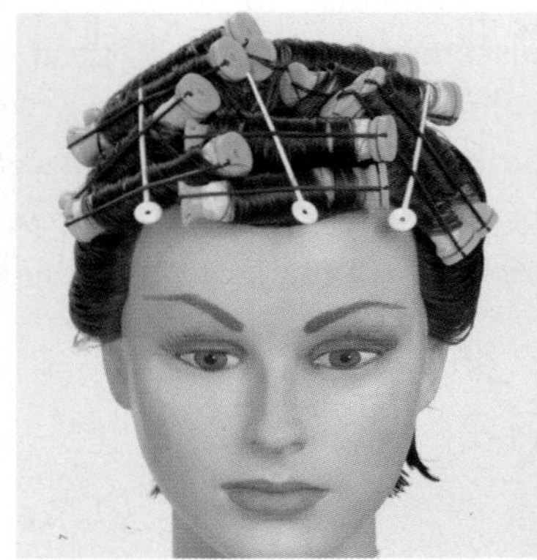

Figure 18-25 Base direction.

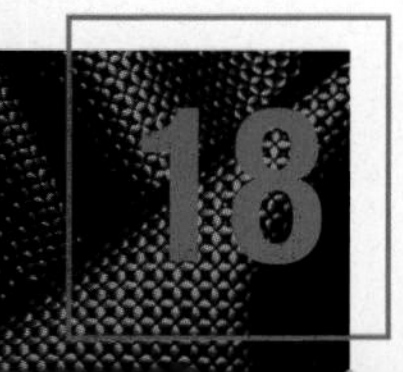

A spiral perm wrap may partially overlap the preceding layers. As long as the angle remains constant, any overlap will be uniform along the length of the rod and the strand of hair (Figure 18-28). This wrapping technique causes the size (diameter) of the rod to remain constant along the entire length of the strand and produces a uniform curl from the scalp to the ends.

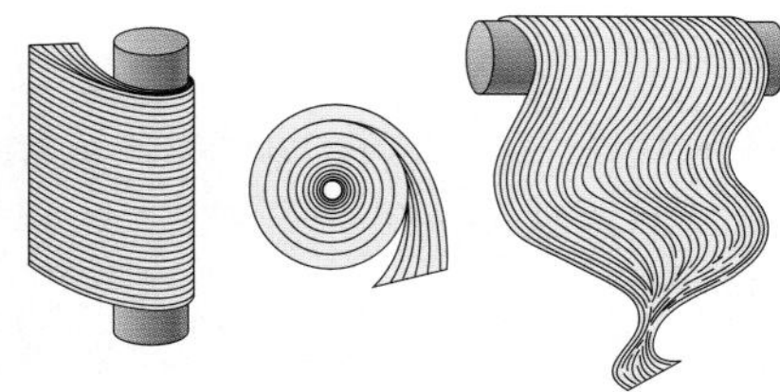

Figure 18-26 Croquignole perm wrap.

For extra-long hair, a double rod wrap (or piggyback wrap) may be indicated. With this technique, the hair is wrapped on one rod from the scalp to midway down the hair shaft (Figure 18-29). Another rod is then used to wrap the remaining hair strand in the same direction. This allows for better penetration of the processing solution and a tighter curl near the scalp than in a conventional croquignole wrap.

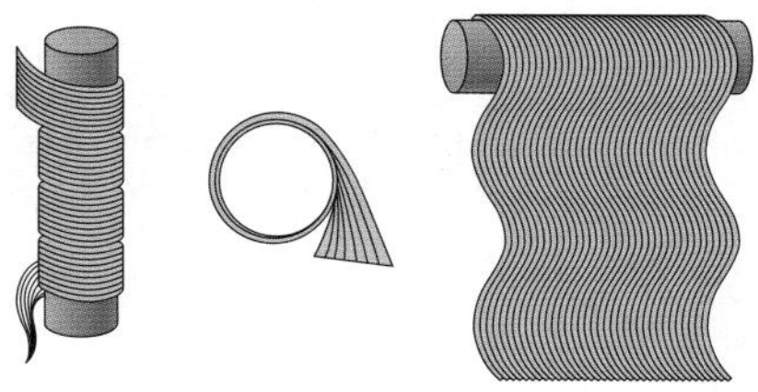

Figure 18-27 Spiral perm wrap.

THE CHEMISTRY OF PERMANENT WAVING

Alkaline permanent waving solutions soften and swell the hair, thus raising the cuticle, which permits the solution to penetrate into the cortex. Figure 18-30 illustrates hair saturated with alkaline permanent waving solution (pH 9.4) for 5 minutes. Note the swelling of the cuticle layer. In Figure 18-31, hair from the same sample has been saturated with acid-balanced permanent waving solution (pH 7.5) for 5 minutes. Note that there is far less swelling of the cuticle layer.

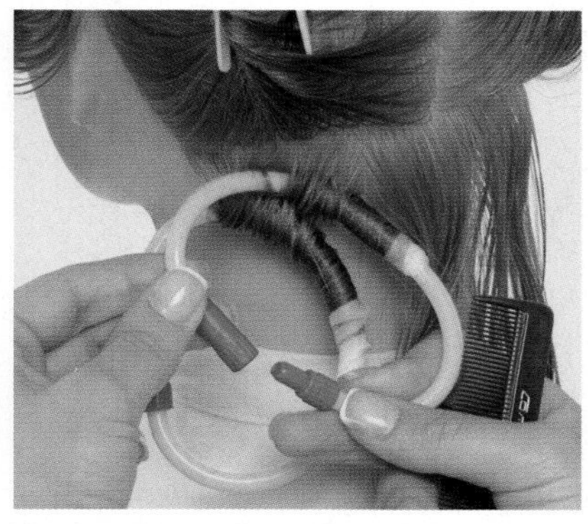

Figure 18-28 Spiral wrap on loop rods.

REDUCTION REACTION

Once in the cortex, the waving solution breaks the disulfide bonds through a chemical reaction called reduction. A reduction reaction involves either the addition of hydrogen, or the removal of oxygen. The reduction reaction in permanent waving is due to the addition of hydrogen.

The chemical process of permanent waving involves the following reactions:

- A disulfide bond joins the sulfur atoms in two adjacent polypeptide chains.
- Permanent wave solution breaks a disulfide bond by adding a hydrogen atom to each of its sulfur atoms.
- The sulfur atoms attach to the hydrogen from the permanent waving solution, breaking their attachment to each other.
- Once the disulfide bond is broken, the polypeptide chains can form into their new curled shape. Reduction breaks disulfide bonds (Figure 18-32) and oxidation reforms them (Figure 18-33).

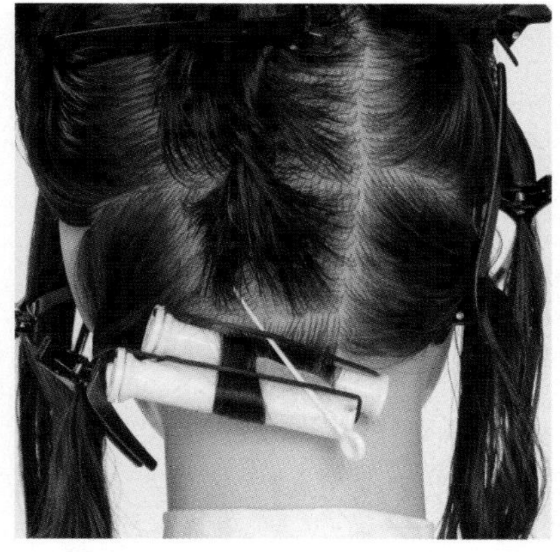

Figure 18-29 Piggyback wrap.

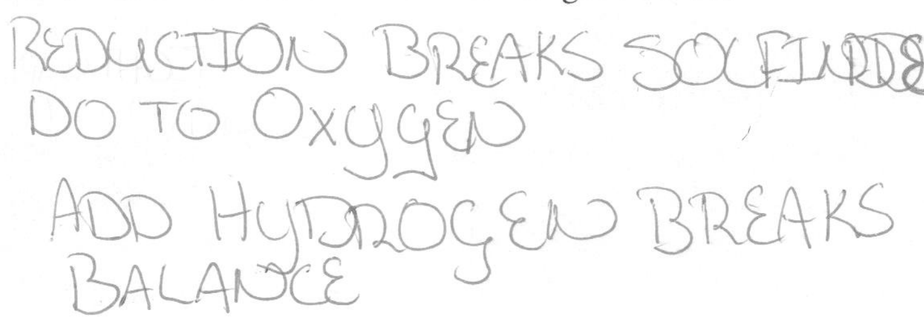

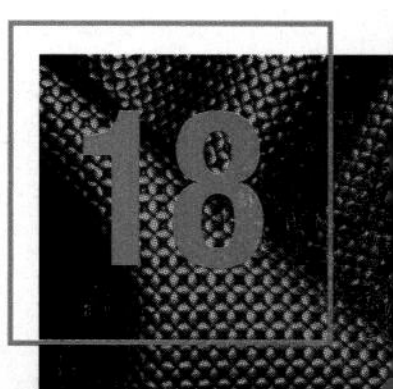

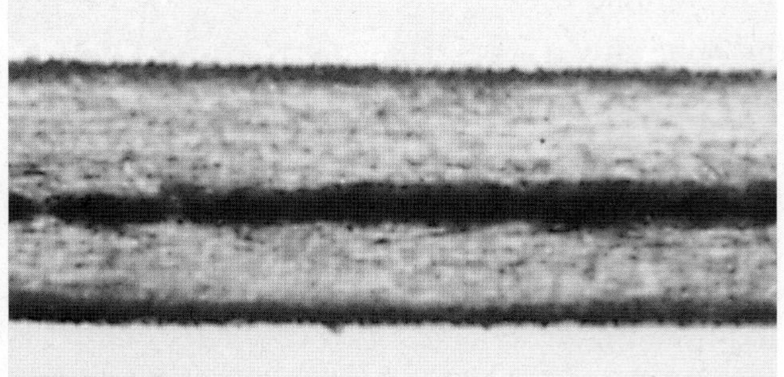

Figure 18–30 Hair that has been saturated with alkaline waving solution (9.4 pH) for 5 minutes.

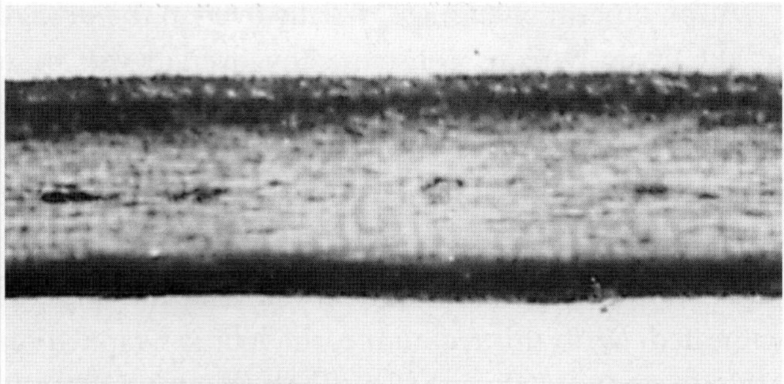

Figure 18–31 Hair that has been saturated with acid-balanced waving solution (7.5 pH) for 5 minutes.

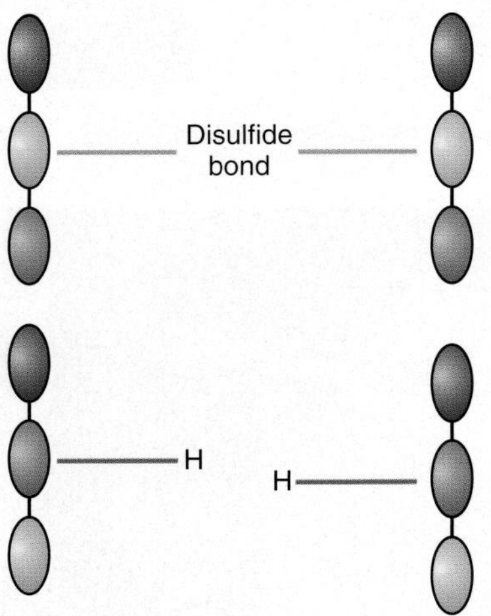

Figure 18–32 A reduction reaction breaks disulfide bonds during the permanent waving process.

All permanent wave solutions contain a "reducing agent." The reducing agents used in permanent waving solutions are thiol (THY-ohl) compounds, commonly referred to as thio (THY-oh) (Figure 18-33).

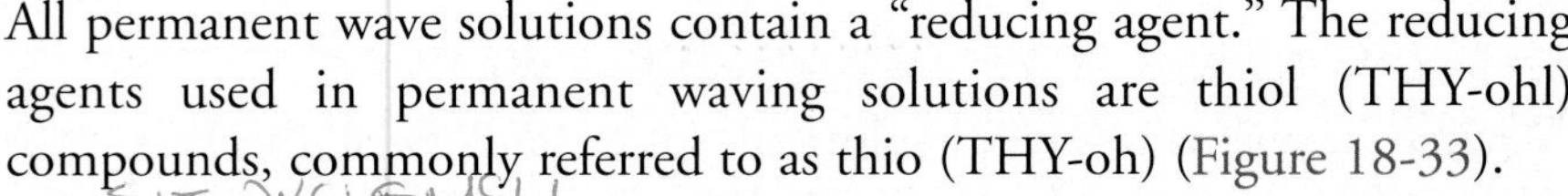

Thioglycolic acid (thy-oh-GLY-kuh-lik), a colorless liquid with a strong, unpleasant odor, is the most common reducing agent. The strength of the permanent waving solution is determined primarily by the concentration of thio. Stronger perms have a higher concentration of thio, which means that more disulfide bonds are broken compared to "weaker" perms.

Because acids do not swell the hair nor penetrate into the cortex, it is necessary for manufacturers to add an alkalizing agent to permanent wave solutions. The addition of ammonia to thioglycolic acid produces a new chemical called **ammonium thioglycolate** (uh-MOH-nee-um thy-oh-GLY-kuh-layt) or **ATG,** which is alkaline. ATG is the active ingredient or reducing agent in alkaline permanents.

The degree of alkalinity (pH) is a second factor in the overall strength of the waving solution. Coarse hair with a strong, resistant cuticle layer needs the additional swelling and penetration that is provided by a more alkaline waving solution.

By contrast, porous hair, or hair with a damaged cuticle layer, is easily penetrated and could be damaged by a highly alkaline permanent waving solution. The alkalinity of the perm solution should correspond to the resistance, strength, and porosity of the cuticle layer.

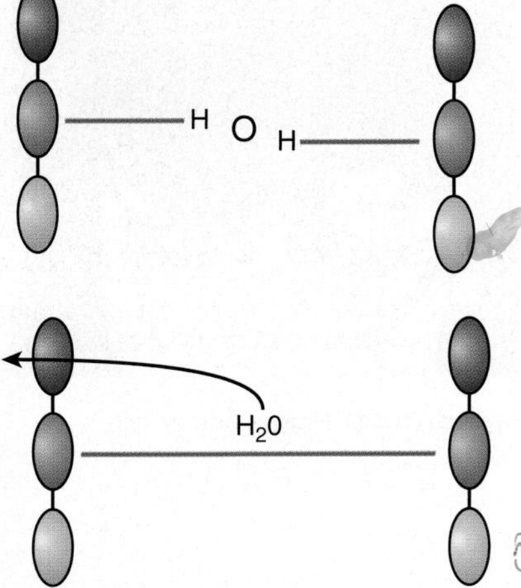

Figure 18–33 Reduction reaction of thio perms and relaxers.

TYPES OF PERMANENT WAVES

A variety of permanent waves are available in salons today (Figure 18-34). Brief descriptions of the most commonly used perms follow.

ALKALINE WAVES OR COLD WAVES

The first **alkaline waves** were developed in 1941, and relied on the same ATG that is still used in alkaline waves today. Since alkaline waves process at room temperature without the addition of heat, they are also called **cold waves.** Most alkaline waves have a pH between 9.0 and 9.6.

ACID WAVES

Glyceryl monothioglycolate (GLIS-ur-il mon-oh-thy-oh-GLY-koh-layt), or **GMTG,** is an acid with a low pH. Although GMTG is the

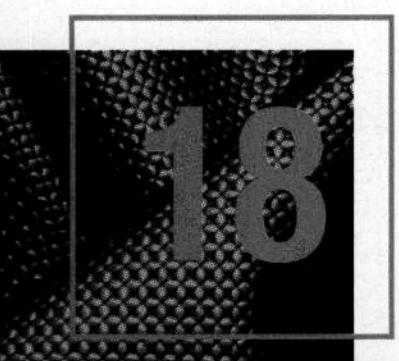

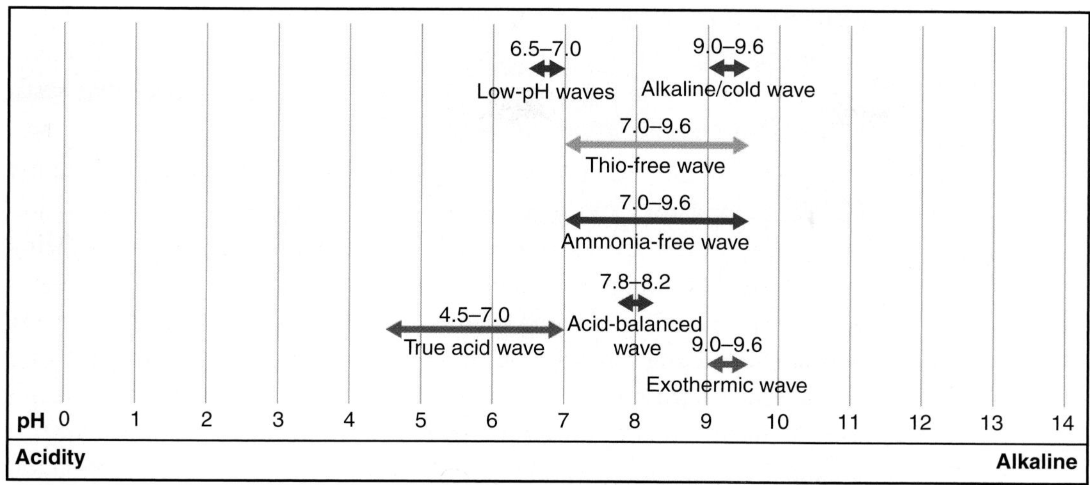

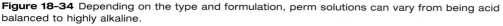

Figure 18-34 Depending on the type and formulation, perm solutions can vary from being acid balanced to highly alkaline.

primary reducing agent in all acid waves, it may not be the only reducing agent. Most acid waves also contain ATG, just like a cold wave. Although the low pH of acid waves may seem ideal, repeated exposure to GMTG is known to cause allergic sensitivity in both hairstylists and clients.

TRUE ACID WAVES

All acid waves have three separate components: permanent waving solution, activator, and neutralizer. The activator tube contains GMTG, which must be added to the permanent waving solution immediately before using. The first **true acid waves** were introduced in the early 1970s. Most true acid waves have a pH between 4.5 and 7.0, and require heat to speed processing. GMTG, which has a low pH, is the active ingredient. Although a lower pH tends to cause less damage to the hair, acid waves process more slowly, may require the added heat of a hair dryer, and do not usually produce as firm a curl as alkaline waves.

Since acidic solutions contract the hair, you may be wondering how a true acid wave, with a pH below 7.0, can cause the hair to swell. Although a pH of 7.0 is neutral on the pH scale, a pH of 5.0 is neutral for hair. Because every step in the pH scale represents a tenfold change in pH, a pH of 7.0 is 100 times more alkaline than the pH of hair (see Chapter 10). Even pure water with a pH of 7.0 can damage the hair and cause it to swell (Figure 18-35).

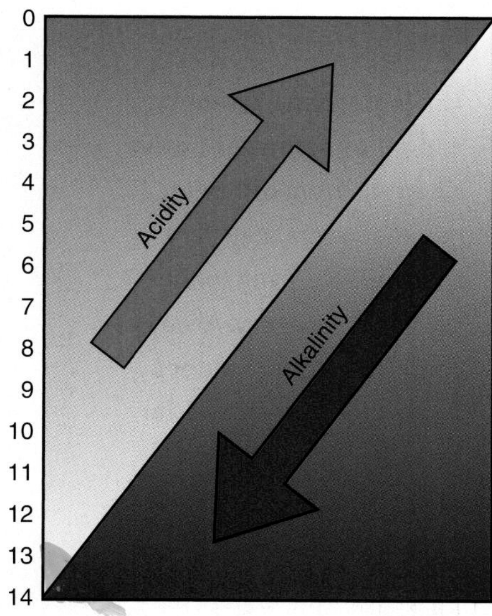

Figure 18-35 Each step on the pH scale represents a tenfold change in pH.

ACID-BALANCED WAVES

In order to permit processing at room temperature and produce a firmer curl, the strength and pH of acid waves have increased steadily over the years. Most of the acid waves found in today's salons have a pH between 7.8 and 8.2. Because 7.0 is neutral, modern acid waves are not true acid waves, but are actually **acid-balanced waves.** Because of their higher pH, they process at room temperature and do not require the added heat of a hair dryer. Acid-balanced waves also process more quickly, and produce firmer curls than true acid waves.

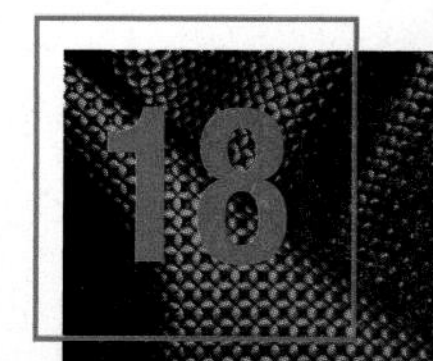

CAUTION

Warning: Accidentally mixing the contents of the activator tube with the neutralizer instead of the permanent waving solution will cause a violent chemical reaction that can cause injury, especially to the eyes.

CAUTION

The ingredients, strength, and pH of permanent wave solutions from different manufacturers may vary considerably, even within the same category. Always check the manufacturer's instructions and MSDS for accurate, detailed information.

EXOTHERMIC WAVES

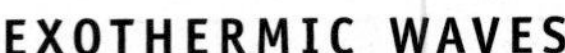

An exothermic chemical reaction produces heat. **Exothermic waves** (Eks-oh-THUR-mik) create an exothermic chemical reaction that heats up the solution and speeds up the processing.

All exothermic waves have three components: permanent waving solution, activator, and neutralizer. The permanent waving solution contains thio, just as in a cold wave. The activator contains an oxidizing agent (usually hydrogen peroxide) that must be added to the permanent waving solution immediately before use. Mixing an oxidizer with the permanent waving solution causes a rapid release of heat and an increase in the temperature of the solution. The increased temperature increases the rate of the chemical reaction, which shortens the processing time.

ENDOTHERMIC WAVES

An endothermic chemical reaction is one that absorbs heat from its surroundings. **Endothermic waves** (en-duh-THUR-mik) are activated by an outside heat source, usually a conventional hood-type hair dryer.

Endothermic waves will not process properly at room temperature. Most true acid waves are endothermic and require the added heat of a hair dryer.

AMMONIA-FREE WAVES

Ammonia-free waves use an ingredient that does not evaporate as readily as ammonia, so there is very little odor associated with their use.

Aminomethylpropanol (uh-MEE-noh-meth-yl-pro-pan-all) or AMP, and monoethanolamine (mahn-oh-ETH-an-all-am-een) or MEA, are examples of alkanolamines that are used in permanent waving solutions as a substitute for ammonia. Even though these solutions may not smell as strong as ammonia, they can still be every bit as alkaline and just as damaging. Remember: Ammonia-free does not necessarily mean damage-free.

THIO-FREE WAVES

Thio-free waves use an ingredient other than ATG as the primary reducing agent. The most common thio-free waves rely on cysteamine (SIS-tee-uhmeen), or mercaptamine (mer-KAPT-uh-meen). Even though these thio substitutes are not technically ATG, they are still thio compounds.

Although thio-free is often marketed as damage-free, that is not necessarily true. At a high concentration, the reducing agents in thio-free waves can be just as damaging as thio.

LOW-PH WAVES

The use of sulfates, sulfites, and bisulfites presents an alternative to ATG known as **low-pH waves.** Sulfites work at a low pH. They have been used in perms for years, but they have never been very popular. Permanents based on sulfites are very weak and do not provide a firm curl, especially on strong or resistant hair. Sulfite permanents are usually marketed as body waves or alternative waves.

SELECTING THE RIGHT TYPE OF PERM

It is extremely important to select the right type of perm for each client. Every client's hair has a distinct texture and condition, so individual

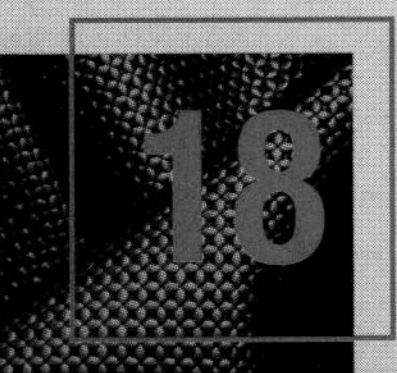

needs must always be addressed. After a thorough consultation, you should be able to determine which type of permanent is best suited to your client's hair type, condition, and desired results. Table 18-1 lists the most common types of permanent waves along with selected advantages and disadvantages for each. These are only general guidelines.

PERMANENT WAVE PROCESSING

The strength of any permanent wave is based on the concentration of its reducing agent. In turn, the amount of processing is determined by the strength of the permanent wave solution. If a weak permanent wave solution is used on coarse hair, there may not be enough hydrogen ions to break the necessary number of disulfide bonds, no matter how long the permanent processes. But the same weak solution may be exactly right for fine hair with fewer disulfide bonds. On the other hand, a strong solution, which releases many hydrogen atoms, may be perfect for coarse hair, but too damaging for fine hair. The amount of processing should be determined by the strength of the solution, and not necessarily how long the perm processes.

In permanent waving, most of the processing takes place as soon as the solution penetrates the hair, within the first 5 to 10 minutes. The

PERM TYPE	PERMANENT WAVE CATEGORIES		
	Active Ingredient	**Process**	**Recommended Hair Type**
alkaline/cold wave pH: 9.0 to 9.6	ammonium thioglycolate (ATG)	room temperature	coarse, thick, or resistant
exothermic wave pH: 9.0 to 9.6	ammonium thioglycolate (ATG)	exothermic	coarse, thick, or resistant
true acid wave pH: 4.5 to 7.0	glyceryl monothioglycolate (GMTG)	endothermic	extremely porous or very damaged hair
acid-balanced wave pH: 7.8 to 8.2	glyceryl monothioglycolate (GMTG)	room temperature	porous or damaged hair
ammonia-free wave pH: 7.0 to 9.6	monoethanolamine (MEA)/ aminomethylpropanol (AMP)	room temperature	porous to normal
thio-free wave pH: 7.0 to 9.6	mercaptamine/cysteamine	room temperature	porous to normal
low-pH waves pH: 6.5 to 7.0	ammonium sulfite/ ammonium bisulfite	endothermic	normal, fine, or damaged

Table 18-1 Permanent Wave Categories

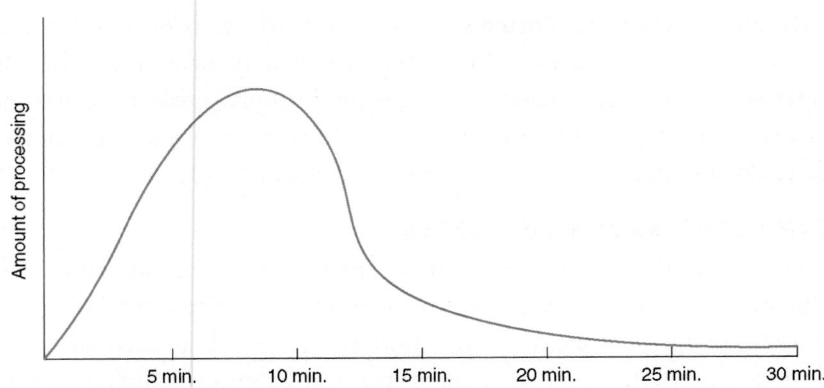

Figure 18-36 Average processing times.

additional processing time allows the polypeptide chains to shift into their new configuration.

If you find that your client's hair has been over-processed, it probably happened within the first 5 to 10 minutes of the service, and a weaker permanent waving solution should have been used. If the hair is not sufficiently processed after 10 minutes, it may require a re-application of waving solution. Resistant hair requires a stronger solution, a higher pH, and a more thorough saturation.

Thorough saturation of the hair is essential to proper processing in all permanent waves, but especially on resistant hair. Regardless of the strength or pH of the solution, resistant hair may not become completely saturated with just one application of waving solution. You may need to apply the solution slowly and repeatedly until the hair looks wet and stays wet!

Remember: A thorough saturation with a stronger (more alkaline) solution will break more disulfide bonds and process the hair more, but processing the hair more does not necessarily translate into more curl. A properly processed permanent wave should break and rebuild approximately 50 percent of the hair's disulfide bonds (Figure 18-36).

If too many disulfide bonds are broken, the hair may not have enough strength left to hold the desired curl. Weak hair equals a weak curl.

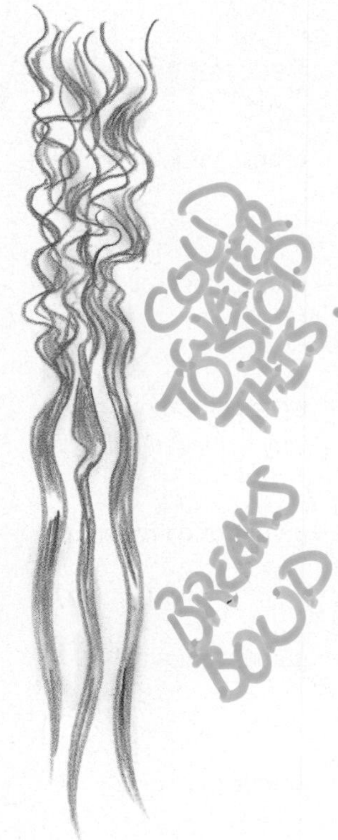

Figure 18-37 Over-processed hair.

Contrary to what many believe, over-processed hair does not necessarily mean hair that is overly curly. If too many disulfide bonds are broken, the hair will be too weak to hold a firm curl. Over-processed hair usually has a weak curl or may even be completely straight. Since the hair at the scalp is usually stronger than the hair at the ends, over-processed hair is usually curlier at the scalp and straighter at the ends (Figure 18-37). If the hair is over-processed, further processing will make it straighter.

UNDER-PROCESSED HAIR

As the title suggests, under-processed hair is the exact opposite of over-processed hair. If too few disulfide bonds are broken, the hair will not be sufficiently softened and will not be able to hold the desired curl.

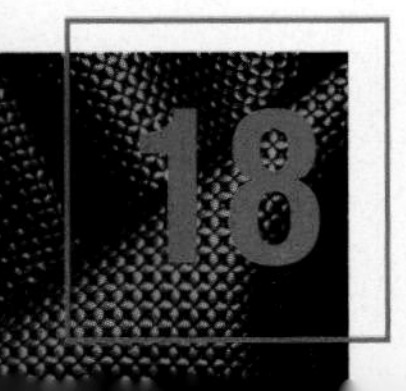

Under-processed hair usually has a very weak curl, but it may also be straight. Since the hair at the scalp is usually stronger than the ends, under-processed hair is usually straighter at the scalp and curlier at the ends (Figure 18-38). If the hair is under processed, processing it more will make it curlier.

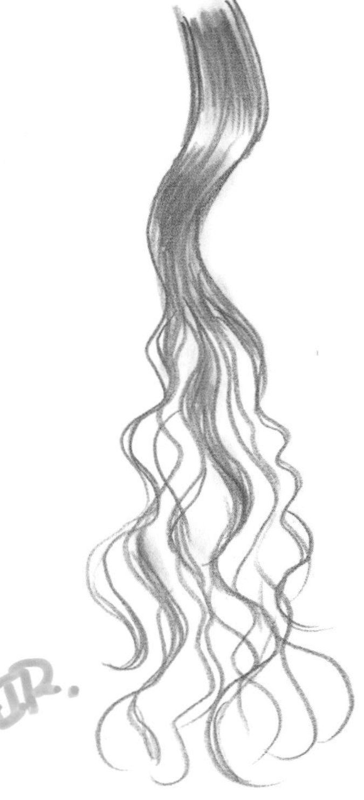

Figure 18–38 Under-processed hair.

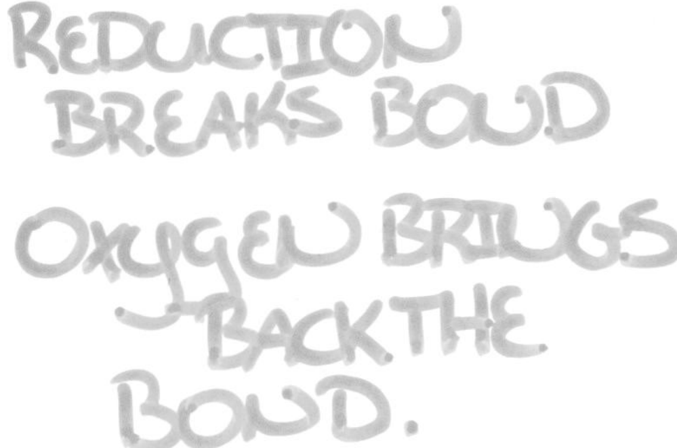

PERMANENT WAVING (THIO) NEUTRALIZATION

Permanent waving **thio neutralization** stops the action of the waving solution, and rebuilds the hair into its new curly form. Neutralization performs two important functions:

1. Any waving solution that remains in the hair is deactivated (neutralized).
2. Disulfide bonds that were broken by the waving solution are rebuilt.

The neutralizers used in permanent waving are oxidizers. In fact, the term neutralizer is not accurate because the chemical reaction involved is actually oxidation. The most common neutralizer is hydrogen peroxide. Concentrations vary between 5 volume (1.5 percent) and 10 volume (3 percent).

Neutralization: Stage One

The first function of permanent waving (thio) neutralization is the deactivation, or (neutralization) of any waving lotion that remains in the hair after processing and rinsing. The chemical reaction involved is called oxidation.

Properly rinsing the hair after the permanent has processed removes any remaining perm solution, prior to applying the neutralizer. Oxidative reactions can also lighten hair color, especially at an alkaline pH. To avoid scalp irritation and unwanted lightening of hair color, always rinse perm solution from the hair for at least 5 minutes, and then blot with towels to remove as much moisture as possible. Excess water left in the hair reduces the effectiveness of the neutralizer.

A successful perm takes time, patience, and expertise. Proper rinsing and blotting are important!

- *Always* rinse the hair with warm water, *never* hot water.
- *Always* use a gentle stream of water, *never* a strong blast of water.
- *Never* apply pressure to the rods while rinsing out the solution.
- *Always* rinse the most fragile areas first (typically the temple area).
- *Always* check the nape area to ensure that you are thoroughly rinsing the bottom rods.
- *Always* rinse for at least the time recommended by the manufacturer.
- *Always* smell the hair after the recommended time has elapsed; if it still smells like perm solution, continue rinsing until the odor is gone.
- *Always* gently blot the hair with a dry towel; *never* firmly or aggressively blot the hair.
- *Always* check for excess moisture, especially at the nape of the neck where water tends to accumulate (pull of gravity), prior to neutralizing the hair.

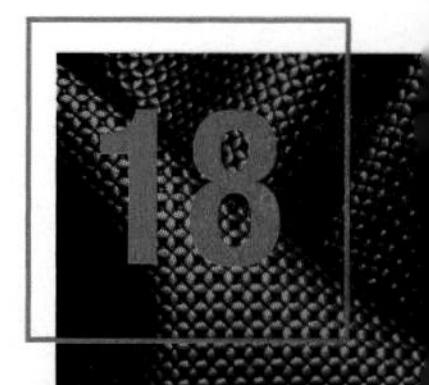

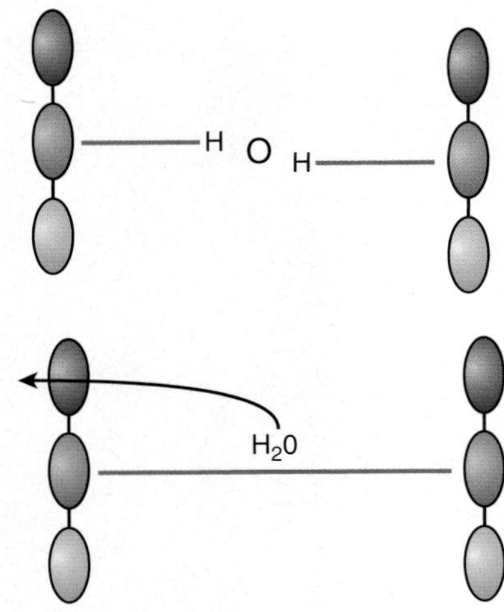

Figure 18-39 Oxidation reaction of thio neutralizers.

- *Always* adjust any rods that have become loose or drifted out of alignment prior to applying the neutralizer.

Some manufacturers recommend the application of a pre-neutralizing conditioner after blotting, and before application of the neutralizer. An acidic liquid protein conditioner can be applied to the hair and dried under a warm hair dryer (hair is uncovered) for 5 minutes or more prior to neutralization. This added step is especially beneficial for very damaged hair because it strengthens the hair prior to neutralization. Always follow the manufacturer's directions, and the procedures approved by your instructor.

Neutralization: Stage Two

As discussed previously, permanent waving solution breaks disulfide bonds. Neutralization rebuilds the disulfide bonds by removing "extra" hydrogen. The hydrogen atoms in the bonds with sulfur are strongly attracted to the oxygen in the neutralizer and release their bond with the sulfur atoms and join with the oxygen (Figure 18-39). Each oxygen atom joins with two hydrogen atoms to rebuild one disulfide bond, and make a water molecule. The water is removed in the final rinse. Side bonds are then reformed into their new shape as different pairs (Figure 18-40).

SAFETY PRECAUTIONS FOR PERMANENT WAVING

- Always protect your client's clothing. Have the client change into a gown, use a waterproof shampoo cape, and double drape with towels to absorb accidental spills.
- Do not give a permanent to any client who has experienced an allergic reaction to a previous permanent.
- Always examine the scalp before the perm service. Do not proceed if there are any skin abrasions, or signs of scalp disease.
- Do not perm hair that is excessively damaged or shows signs of breakage.
- Do not attempt to perm hair that has been previously treated with hydroxide relaxers.

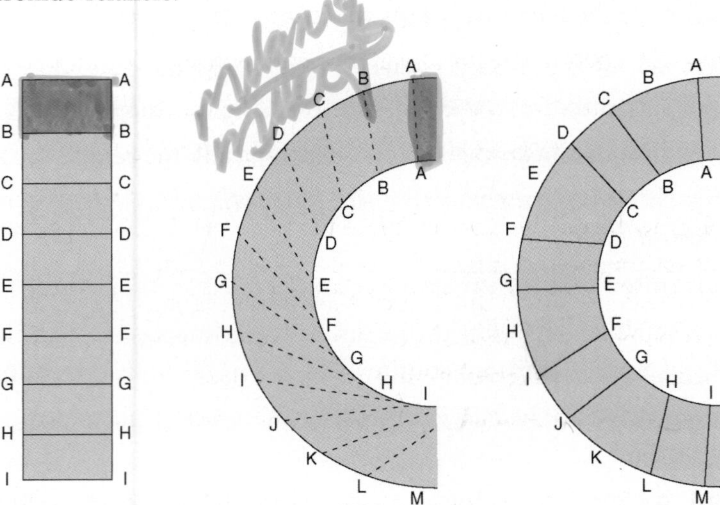

Figure 18-40 New disulfide pairs.

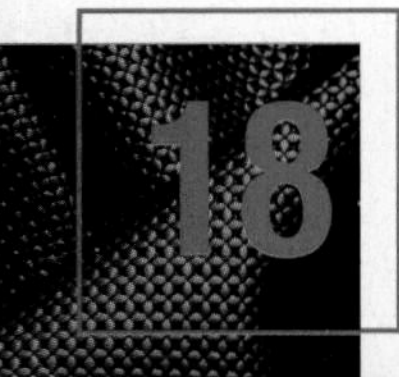

- Always perform a test for metallic salts, if there is a possibility that metallic haircolor was previously used on the hair.
- Always apply protective barrier cream around the client's hairline and ears prior to applying permanent waving solution.
- Do not dilute or add anything to the waving lotion or neutralizer unless specified in the manufacturer's directions.
- Keep waving lotion out of the client's eyes. In case of accidental exposure, rinse thoroughly with cool water.
- Always follow the manufacturer's directions.
- Wear gloves when applying solutions.
- Immediately replace cotton or towels that have become wet with solution.
- Do not save any opened, unused waving solution or neutralizer. When not used promptly, these chemicals may change in strength and effectiveness.

Hair that has been permanently waved should be shampooed and conditioned with products formulated for chemically treated hair.

PERMANENT WAVING PROCEDURES

The following are basic perm procedures. The information presented earlier in the chapter on sectioning, base control, base direction, perm rods, wrapping techniques, and wrapping patterns should be used with the following procedures. These basic wrapping patterns may be combined in different ways to create a wide variety of specialized perm wraps that provide an unlimited number of styling options.

The **basic perm wrap** is also called a straight set wrap. In this wrapping pattern, all the rods within a panel move in the same direction and are positioned on an equal-size basis. All base sections are horizontal, with the same length and width as the perm rod. The **base control** is the position of the tool in relation to its base section, determined by the angle at which the hair is wrapped (Figure 18-41).

In the **curvature perm wrap,** the movement curves within sectioned-out panels. Partings and bases radiate throughout the panels to follow the curvature of the head. This wrapping pattern uses pie-shaped base sections in the curvature areas (Figure 18-42).

The **bricklay perm wrap** is similar to the actual technique of bricklaying. Base sections are offset from each other row by row, to prevent noticeable splits, and to blend the flow of the hair. Different bricklay patterns use different starting points (front hairline, occipital area, and crown), and these starting points affect the directional flow of the hair. The bricklay perm wrap can be used with various combinations of sectioning, base control, base direction, wrapping techniques, and perm rods (Figure 18-43).

The **weave technique** uses zigzag partings to divide base areas. It can be used throughout the entire perm wrap or only in selected areas. This technique is very effective for blending between perm rods with opposite base directions. It can also be used to create a smooth transition from the

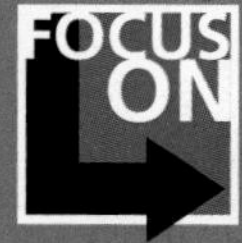

Focus on . . . Retailing

Your client's permanent wave will not be as manageable, or last as long, without a proper at-home maintenance program. Your client depends on you for advice on how to care for the new permanent. Make sure you always explain different styling options, and recommend effective professional retail products to use at home.

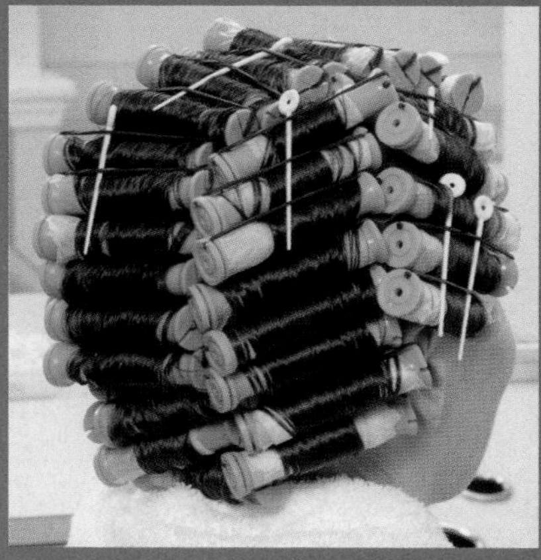

Figure 18-41 Basic perm wrapping pattern.

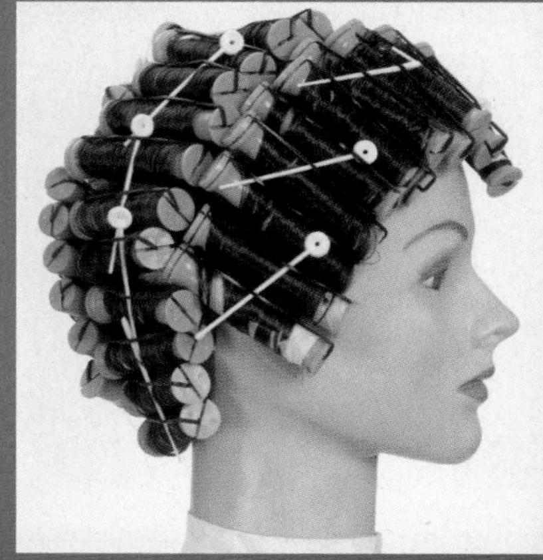

Figure 18-42 Curvature perm wrapping pattern.

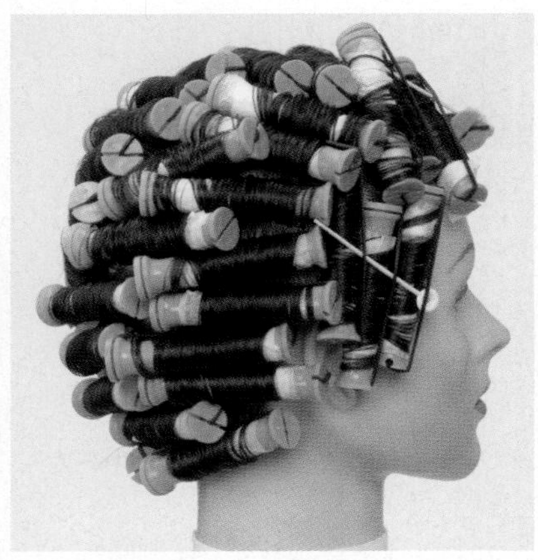

Figure 18-43 Bricklay perm wrapping pattern (drawing).

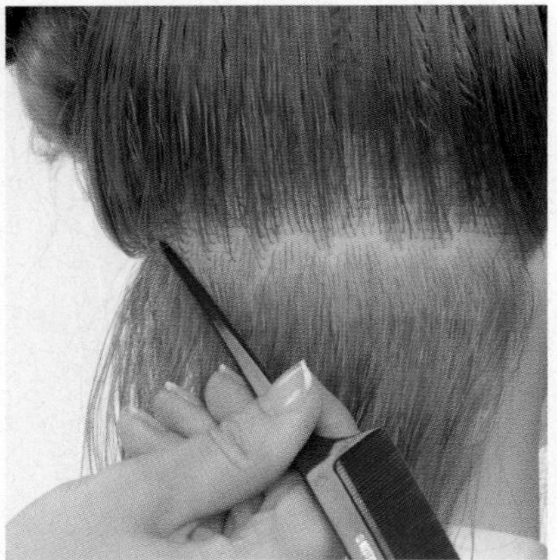

Figure 18-44 Weave technique.

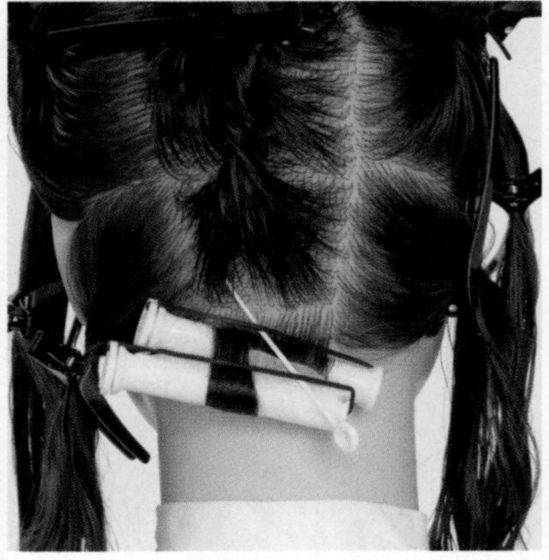

Figure 18-45 Double-rod (piggyback) perm technique.

rolled areas into the unrolled areas of a partial perm. The weave technique can be used with a variety of base directions, wrapping patterns, and perm rods (Figure 18-44).

The **double-rod technique** is also called a **piggyback** wrap because two rods are used for one strand of hair, one on top of the other. The upper half of the strand is wrapped around one rod, and then the lower half of the same strand is wrapped around a second rod in an alternate direction and stacked (piggybacked) on top of the first (Figure 18-45).

The double-rod technique doubles the number of rods used. Using more rods increases the amount of curl in the finished perm, making this technique especially effective on long hair. Rods of various diameters may be used to create different effects. This technique can also be used with a variety of base directions, wrapping patterns, and perm rods.

In a spiral perm wrap, the hair is wrapped at an angle other than perpendicular to the length of the rod, like the grip on a tennis racket. This wrapping technique produces a uniform curl from the scalp to the ends. Longer, thicker hair will benefit most from this effect (Figure 18-46).

The spiral wrapping technique can be used with a variety of base sections, base directions, and wrapping patterns. Base sections may be either horizontal or vertical, and do not affect the finished curl. Conventional rods, bendable soft foam rods, and loop rods can all be used for this technique, depending on the length of the rod and the length of the hair.

PARTIAL PERMS

If your client wants a perm, but does not wish the entire head of hair to be curled, a partial perm may be the answer. Partial perms also allow you to give a perm when some of the hair is too short to roll on rods (Figure 18-47).

Partial perms can be used for:

- Male and female clients who have long hair on the top and crown, but very short hair with tapered sides and nape.

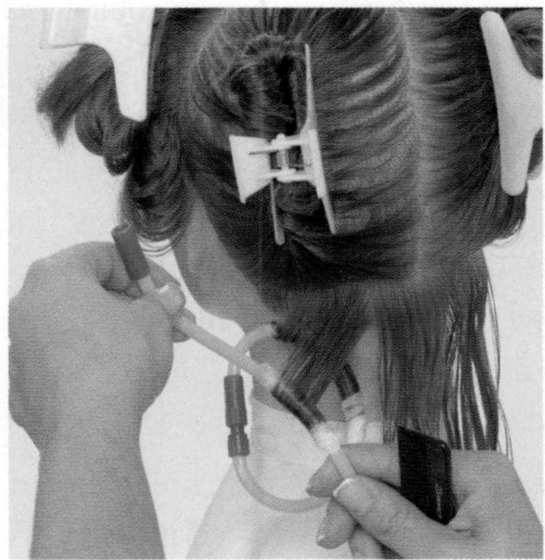

Figure 18-46 Spiral perm wrap.

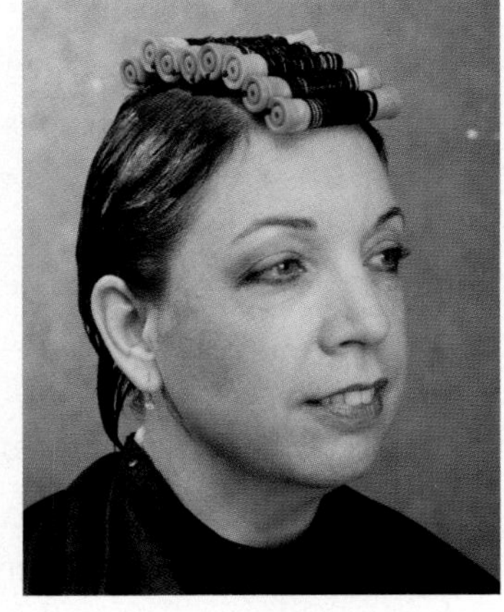

Figure 18-47 Partial perm wrap.

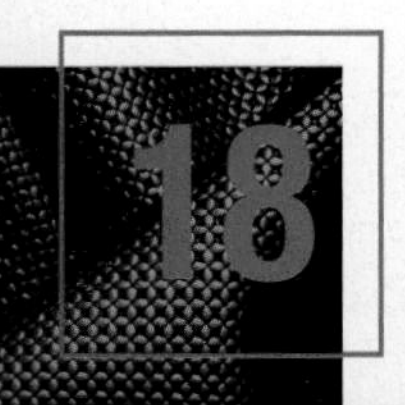

- Clients who only need volume and lift in certain areas.
- Clients who desire a hairstyle with curls along the perimeter but a smooth, sleek crown.

Partial perms rely on the same techniques and wrapping patterns as those used with other perms, but there are additional considerations:

- In order to make a smooth transition from the rolled section to the unrolled section, use a larger rod for the last rod next to an unrolled section.
- Applying waving solution to unrolled hair may straighten it or make it difficult to style. To protect the unrolled hair, apply a protective barrier cream to the unrolled section before applying the waving lotion.

PRELIMINARY TEST CURLS

Preliminary test curls help you determine how your client's hair will react to a perm. It is advisable to take preliminary test curls if the hair is damaged, or if there is any uncertainty about the results. Preliminary test curls provide the following information:

- Correct processing time for the best curl development
- Results you can expect from the type of perm solution you have selected
- Curl results for the rod size and wrapping technique you are planning to use

PROCEDURE 18-1

BASIC PERM

PROCEDURE FOR PRELIMINARY TEST CURLS

IMPLEMENTS AND MATERIALS

- Perm solution
- Neutralizer
- Acid-balanced shampoo (optional)
- Pre-neutralizing conditioner (optional)
- Conditioner (optional)
- Protective barrier cream
- Applicator bottles
- Perm rods
- Shampoo cape
- Towels
- Neutralizing bib
- Cotton coil or rope
- Plastic clips for sectioning
- Styling comb
- Plastic tail comb
- End papers
- Roller picks
- Spray bottle
- Disposable gloves
- Timer

PREPARATION FOR ALL PERMS

1. Wash your hands.
2. Conduct a client consultation and evaluation. Fill out the client's perm record. Note any changes in the client's history.
3. Perform an analysis of the client's hair and scalp.
4. Have the client change into a gown and remove eyeglasses, earrings, and necklace.
5. Drape the client for shampoo.
6. Gently shampoo and towel-dry hair. Avoid irritating the client's scalp.
7. Perform a preliminary test curl procedure.

PROCEDURE

1. Wrap one rod in each different area of the head (top, side, and nape) (Figure 18-48).
2. Wrap a coil of cotton around each rod.
3. **Apply lotion.** Apply waving lotion to the wrapped curls. Do not allow waving lotion to come into contact with unwrapped hair (Figure 18-49).
4. Set a timer, and process according to the manufacturer's directions.

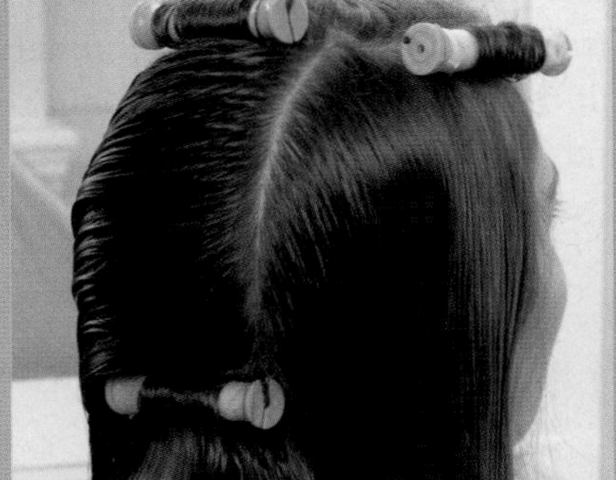

Figure 18-48 Wrap rods in three areas of the head.

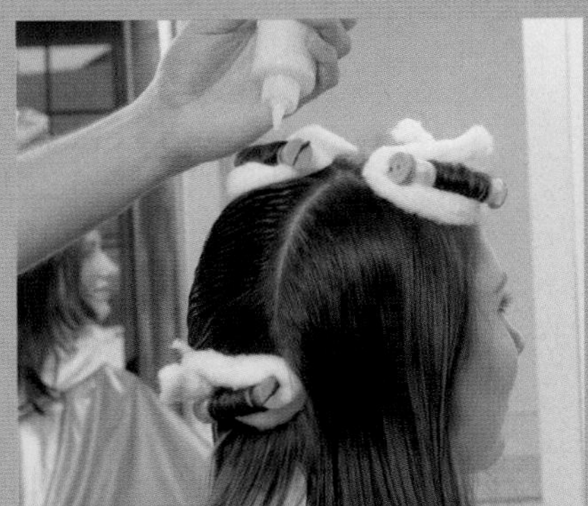

Figure 18-49 Apply waving lotion to test curls.

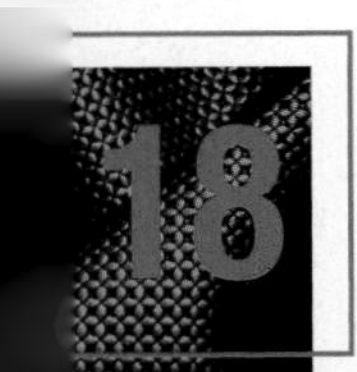

5. **Check test curl.** Check each test curl frequently for proper curl development. Unfasten the rod and unwind the curl about 1-½ turns of the rod. Do not allow the hair to become loose, or completely unwound. Gently move the rod toward the scalp to encourage the hair to fall loosely into the wave pattern.
6. **Check wave development.** Curl development is complete when a firm "S" is formed that reflects the size of the rod used. Different hair textures will have slightly different "S" formations. The wave pattern for fine, thin hair may be weak, with little definition. The wave pattern for coarse, thick hair is usually stronger and better defined (Figure 18-50).
7. **Rinse hair.** When the curl has been formed, rinse thoroughly with warm water for at least 5 minutes, blot thoroughly, apply neutralizer, and process according to the manufacturer's directions. Gently dry the hair and evaluate the results. Do not proceed with the permanent if the test curls are extremely damaged or over-processed. If the test curl results are satisfactory, proceed with the perm, but *do not* re-perm these preliminary test curls. Rinse and process the test rods, but do not remove. Remove them with the rest of the rods after the perm is completed.

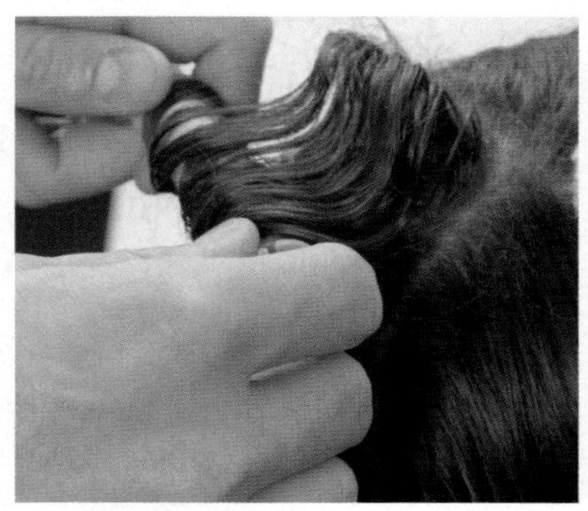

Figure 18-50 S formation.

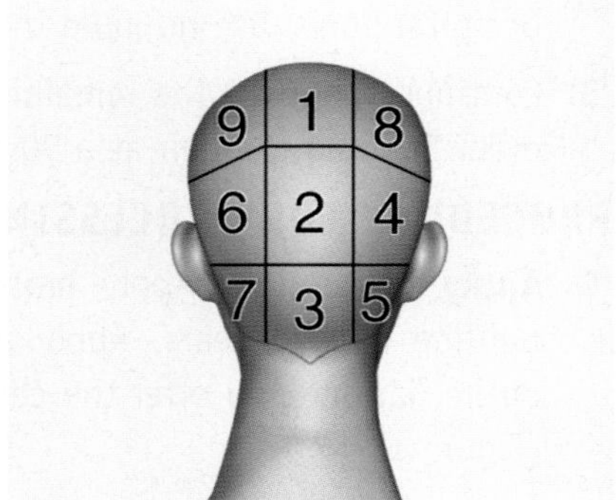

Figure 18-51 Wrapping pattern.

PROCEDURE FOR BASIC PERM WRAP (STRAIGHT SET WRAP)

1. **Section hair.** Divide the hair into nine panels (Figures 18-51 and 18-52). Use the length of the rod to measure the width of the panels.Remember to keep the hair wet as you wrap.
2. **Wrap sections.** Begin wrapping at the front hairline or crown. Make a horizontal parting the same size as the rod. Using two end papers, roll the hair down to the scalp in the direction of hair growth, and position the rod half off base (Figure 18-53). The band should be smooth, not twisted, and should be fastened straight across the top of the rod (Figure 18-54).

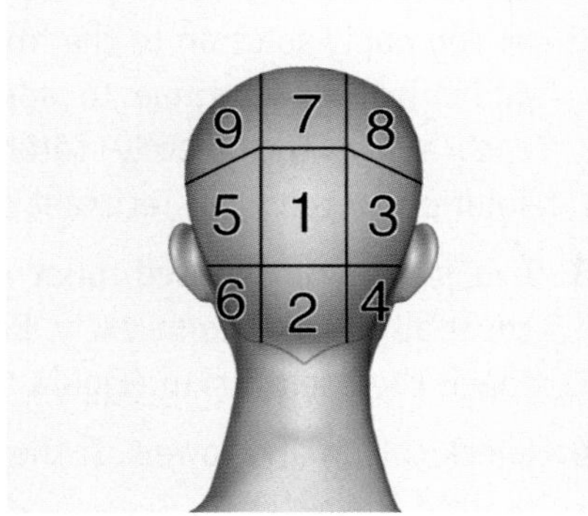

Figure 18-52 Alternate wrapping pattern.

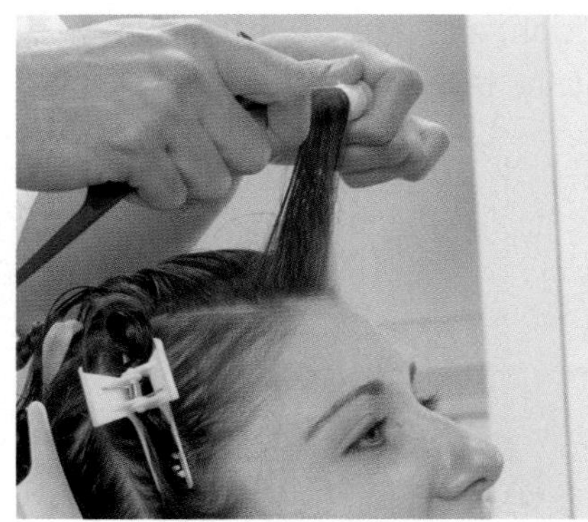

Figure 18-53 Roll the hair down to the scalp.

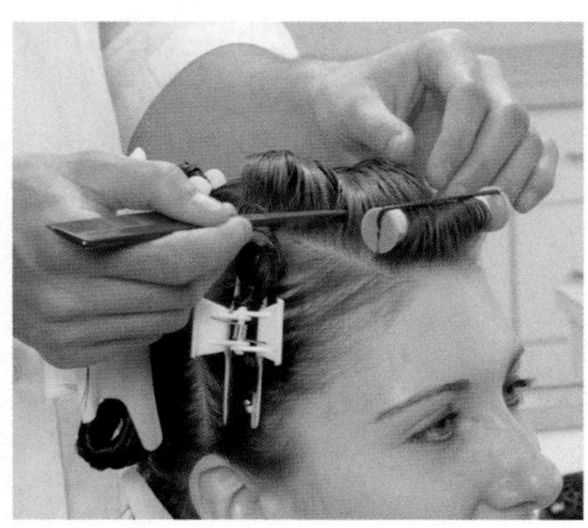

Figure 18-54 Position rod half off-base.

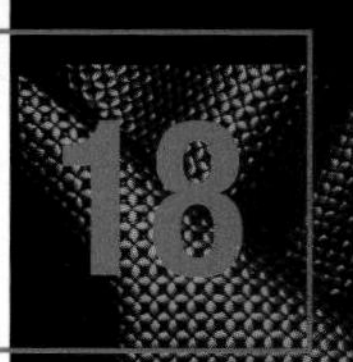

Excessive tension may cause band marks or hair breakage. Continue wrapping the remainder of the first panel using the same technique (Figure 18-55). Insert roller picks to stabilize the rods.

Although roller picks may be used to eliminate any tension caused by the band, they will not compensate for a poorly wrapped perm. If roller picks are not used correctly, they can cause the same or worse damage as the incorrect placement of the rubber band. Hint: Use picks that are no more than 3 inches in length, and use no more than three rods with each pick. To avoid placing undue tension on the hair, in areas where the head curves dramatically (e.g., occipital bone) use no more than two rods with each pick.

3. Continue wrapping the remaining eight panels in numerical order, holding the hair at a 90-degree angle (Figure 18-56).

PROCEDURE FOR PROCESSING PERMS

1. **Apply protection.** Apply protective barrier cream to the hairline and the ears. Apply a coil of cotton around the entire hairline and offer the client a towel to blot any drips (Figure 18-57).
2. **Apply perm solution.** Slowly and carefully apply the perm solution to each rod. Ask the client to lean forward while you apply solution to the back area; ask the client to lean back as you apply solution to the front and sides. Avoid splashing and dripping. Continue to apply the solution slowly until each rod is completely saturated (Figure 18-58). Apply solution to the most resistant area first.
3. If a plastic cap is used, punch a few holes in the cap and cover all the hair completely. Do not allow the plastic cap to touch the client's skin (Figure 18-59).
4. Check cotton and towels. If they are saturated with solution, replace them.
5. **Process perm.** Process according to the manufacturer's directions. Processing time varies according to the strength of the solution, hair type and condition, and desired results. As a general rule, processing usually takes less than 20 minutes at room temperature.

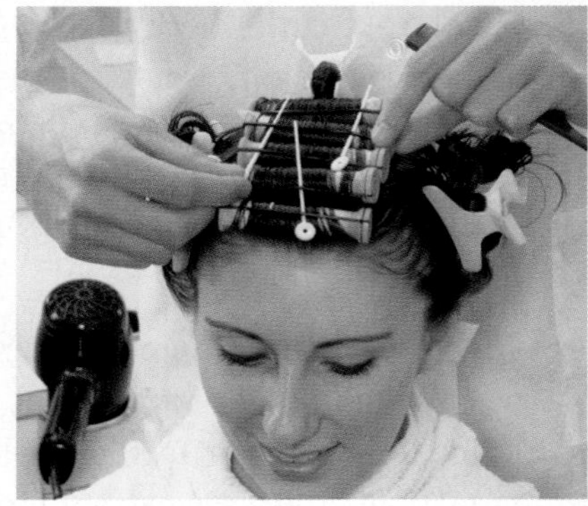
Figure 18-55 Finished first panel.

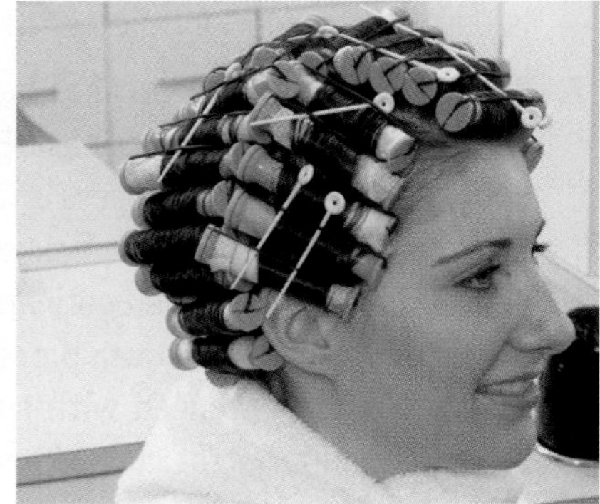
Figure 18-56 Completed basic perm wrap.

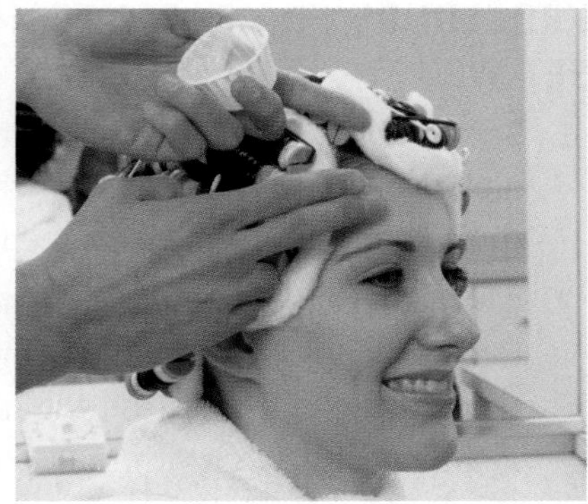
Figure 18-57 Apply protective base cream and cotton.

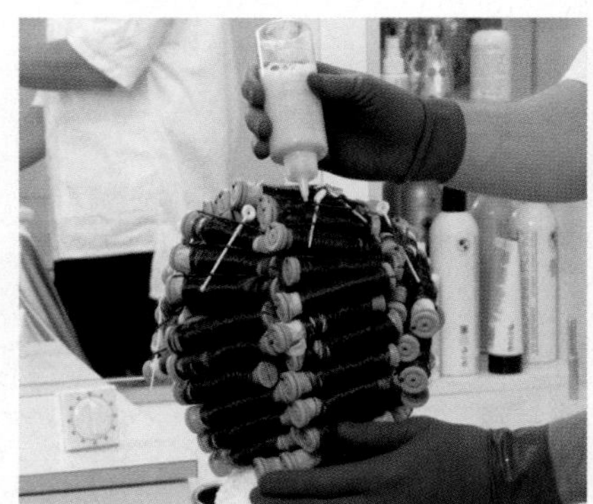
Figure 18-58 Apply perm solution.

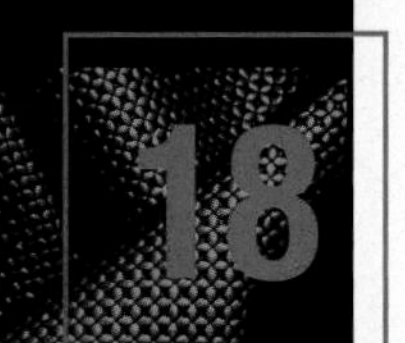

6. **Check curl.** Check frequently for curl development. Unwind the rod and check the "S" pattern formation described in the preliminary test curl procedure (Figure 18-60). Check a different rod each time!
7. **Rinse hair.** When processing is complete, rinse the hair thoroughly for at least 5 minutes, and then towel-blot each rod to remove any excess moisture (Figure 18-61). *Option:* Some manufacturers recommend the application of a pre-neutralizing conditioner after rinsing and blotting, and before applying the neutralizer. Always follow the manufacturer's directions and the procedures approved by your instructor.
8. **Neutralize.** Apply the neutralizer slowly and carefully to the hair on each rod. Ask the client to lean forward while you apply solution to the back area, and then to lean back as you apply solution to the front and sides. Avoid splashing and dripping. Continue to apply the neutralizer until each rod is completely saturated (Figure 18-62).
9. Set a timer for the amount of time specified by the manufacturer.
10. **Rinse thoroughly.** *Option:* Shampoo and condition. Always follow the manufacturer's directions and the procedures approved by your instructor.
11. Style the hair as desired (Figure 18-63).

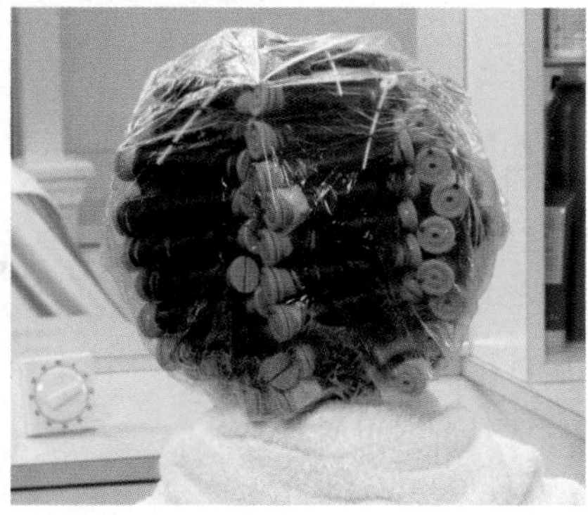

Figure 18-59 Cover head with plastic cap.

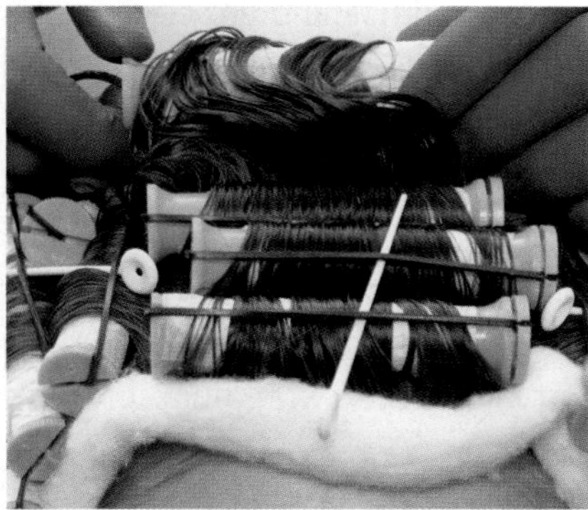

Figure 18-60 Take a test curl.

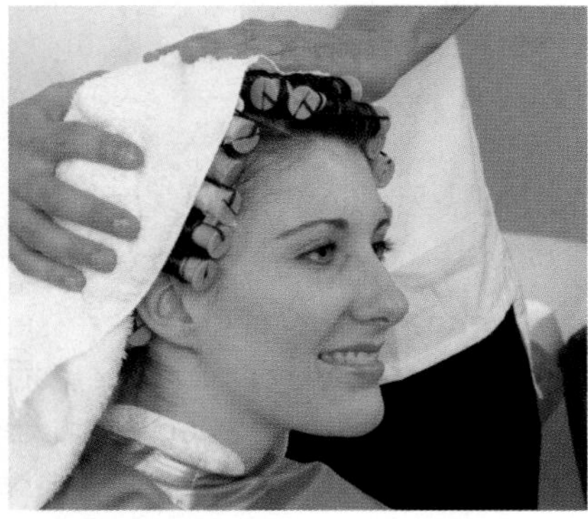

Figure 18-61 Thoroughly and gently towel blot the rods.

CLEANUP AND SANITATION

1. Discard disposable supplies in appropriate receptacles.
2. Sanitize implements and store according to sanitation requirements.
3. Clean, sanitize, and prepare your workstation for the next service.
4. Wash your hands thoroughly with soap and warm water.
5. Complete the client record.

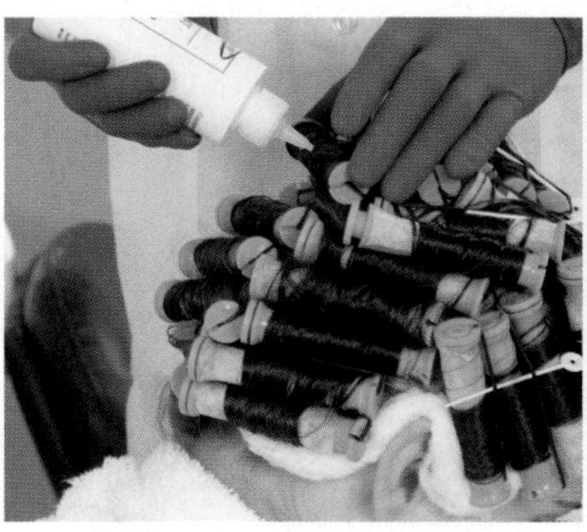

Figure 18-62 Apply neutralizer.

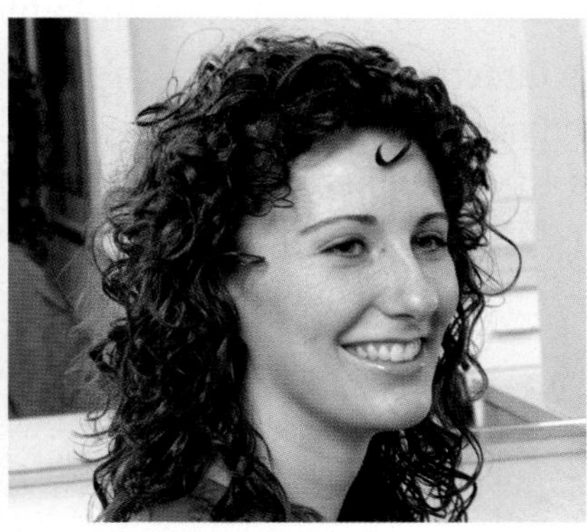

Figure 18-63 Styled basic perm.

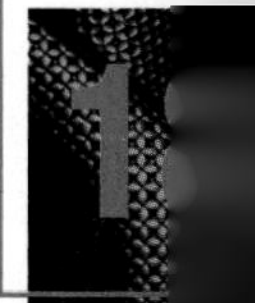

PROCEDURE 18-2

CURVATURE PERM

IMPLEMENTS AND MATERIALS

Same as for basic perm.

PREPARATION

Same as for basic perm.

PROCEDURE

1. **Section hair.** Begin sectioning at the front hairline on one side of the part. Comb the hair in the direction of growth, and then section out individual panels to match the length of the rod (Figure 18-64).
2. **Section panels.** Alternate from side to side as you section out all the curvature panels over the entire head. Sectioning the panels in advance creates a road map that provides direction and gives continuity to the wrapping pattern (Figure 18-65).
3. **Begin wrapping.** Begin wrapping the first panel at the front hairline on one side of the part. Comb out a base section the same width as the diameter of the rod. The base direction should point away from the face. Hold the hair at a 90-degree angle to the head. Using two end papers, roll the hair down to the scalp and position the rod half off base (Figure 18-66).
4. **Complete wrap.** The remaining base sections in the panel should be wider on the outside of the panel (the side farthest away from the face). Continue wrapping the rest of the rods in the panel, alternating rod diameters (Figure 18-67).
5. Insert picks to stabilize the rods and eliminate any tension caused by the band (Figure 18-68).
6. **Change direction.** When you reach the last rod at the hairline, comb the hair flat at the base and change the base direction. Direct the rod up and toward the base, keeping the base area flat (Figure 18-69).

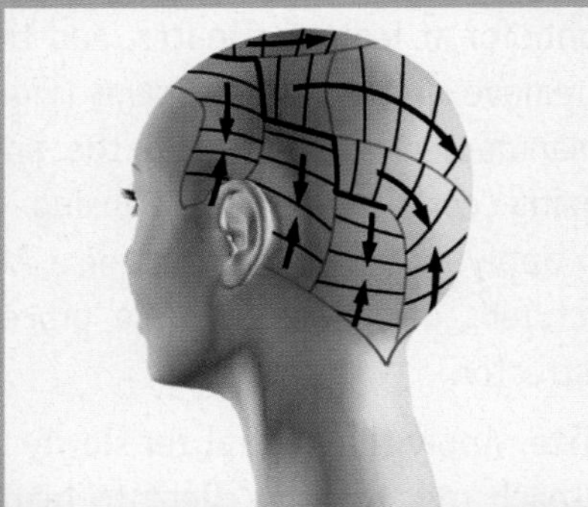

Figure 18-64 Sectioning hair.

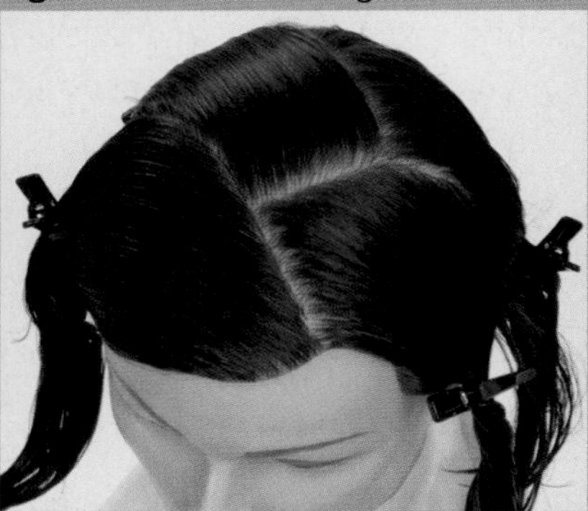

Figure 18-65 Section all panels.

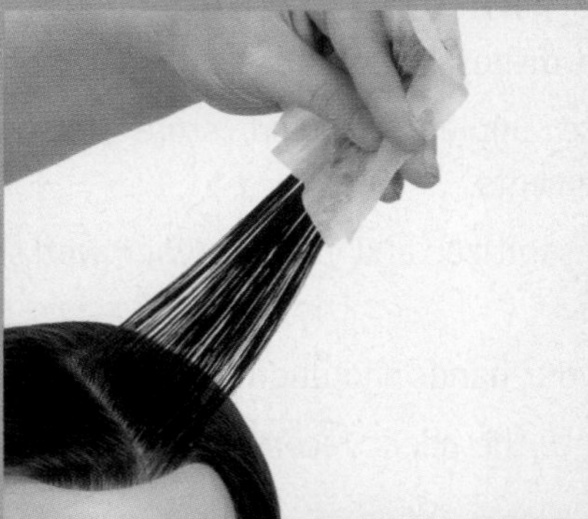

Figure 18-66 Wrap first rod at front hairline.

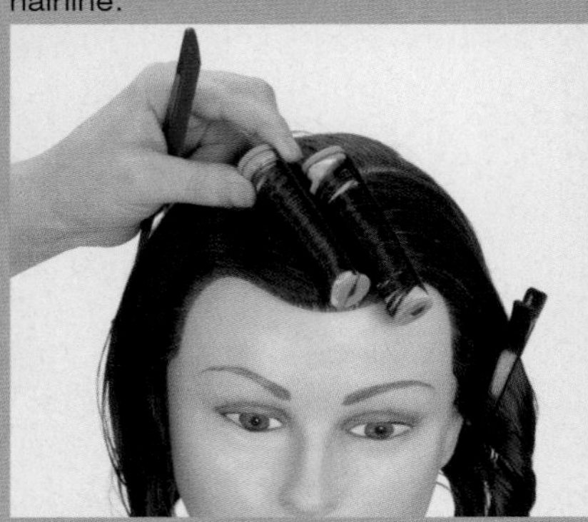

Figure 18-67 Wrap second rod.

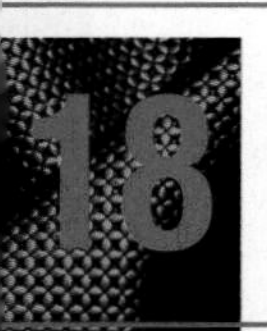

7. **Continue wrapping.** Continue with panel two, which is the front panel on the other side of the part. Repeat the same procedure as on the first panel (Figure 18-70).
8. **Wrap third panel.** Continue with the third panel, which is the panel behind and next to the first panel. Repeat the same procedure until you reach the last two rods at the hairline. Comb the hair flat at the base and change the base direction. Direct the last two rods up and toward the base, keeping the base area flat (Figure 18-71).
9. **Wrap fourth panel.** Continue with the fourth panel, on the opposite side of the head, behind and next to the second panel. Repeat the same procedure you used with the third panel.
10. **Wrap fifth panel.** Follow the same procedure with the fifth panel. The base direction should remain consistent with the pattern already established. The base direction in the back flows around and contours to the perimeter hairline area.
11. All panels should fit the curvature of the head, and should blend into the surrounding panels (Figure 18-72).
12. Process and style the hair (Figure 18-73).

CLEANUP AND SANITATION

Follow cleanup and sanitation procedures for the basic perm.

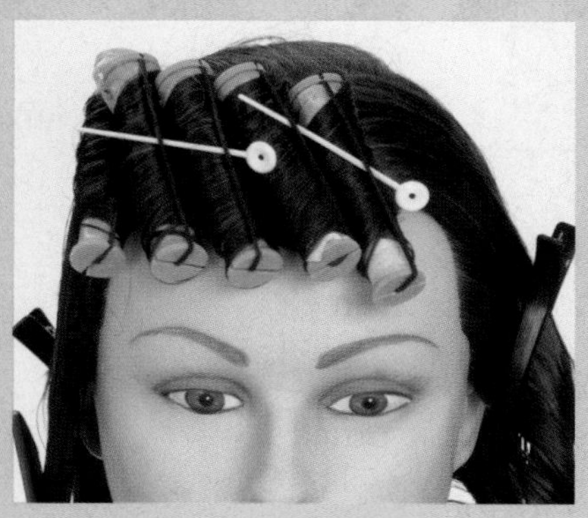

Figure 18-68 Picks are used to stabilize the rods.

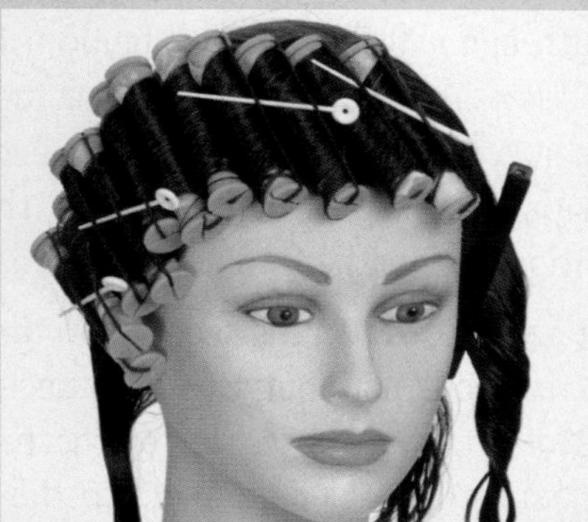

Figure 18-69 Wrap last rod in panel.

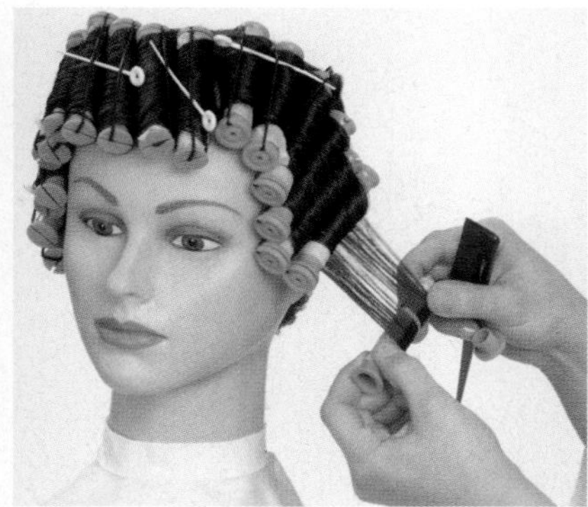

Figure 18-70 The second panel.

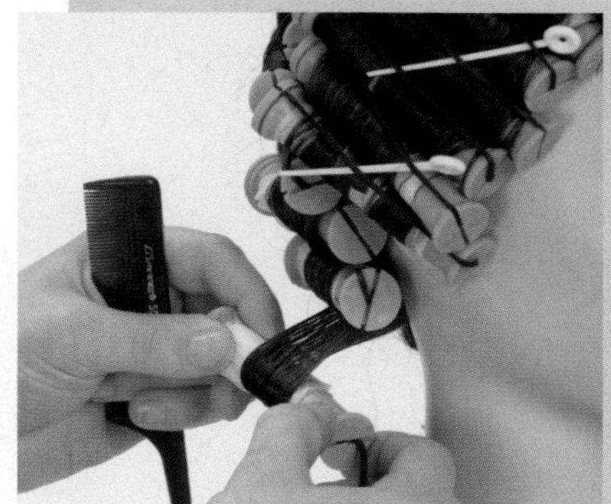

Figure 18-71 The third panel.

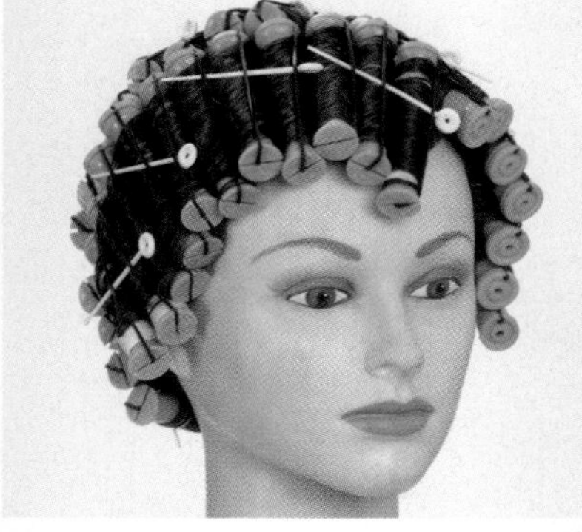

Figure 18-72 Finish wrapping all panels.

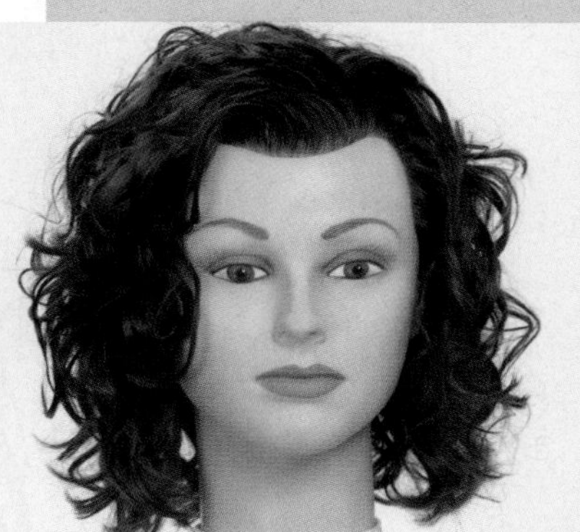

Figure 18-73 Finished and styled curvature perm.

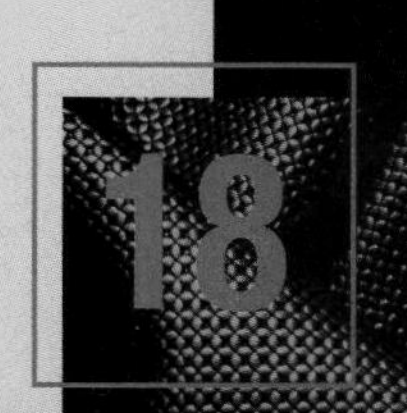

PROCEDURE 18-3

BRICKLAY PERM

IMPLEMENTS AND MATERIALS

Same as for basic perm.

PREPARATION

Same as for basic perm.

PROCEDURE

1. **Part base section.** Begin by parting out a base section parallel to the front hairline that is the length and width of the rod being used. The base direction is back, away from the face. Hold the hair at a 90-degree angle to the head. Using two end papers, roll the hair down to the scalp and position the rod half off base (Figure 18-74).
2. **Part second row.** In the second row directly behind the first rod, part out two base sections for two rods offset from the center of the first rod. Hold the hair at a 90-degree angle to the head. Using two end papers, roll the hair down to the scalp and position the rods half off base (Figure 18-75).
3. Insert picks to stabilize rods and eliminate any tension caused by the band.
4. **Part third row.** Begin the third row by parting out a base section at the point where the two rods meet in the previous row. This same pattern is used throughout the entire wrap (Figure 18-76).

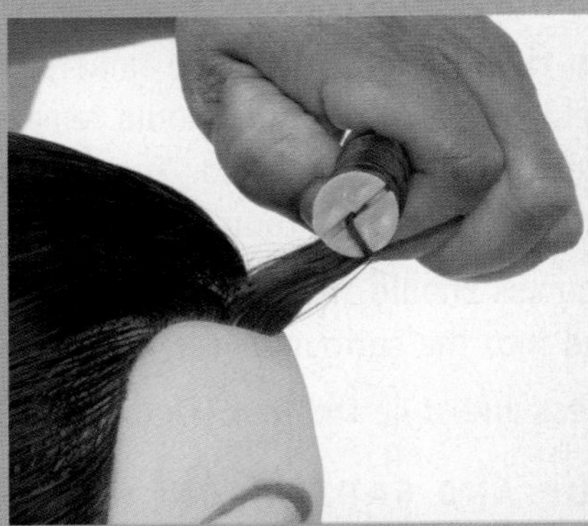

Figure 18-74 Wrap first rod.

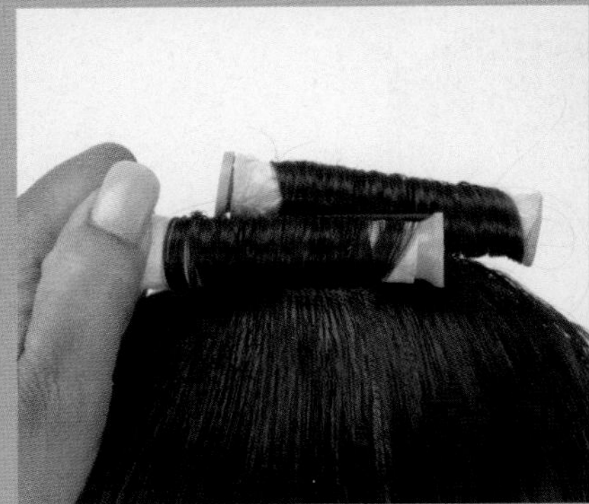

Figure 18-75 Wrap second rod in second row.

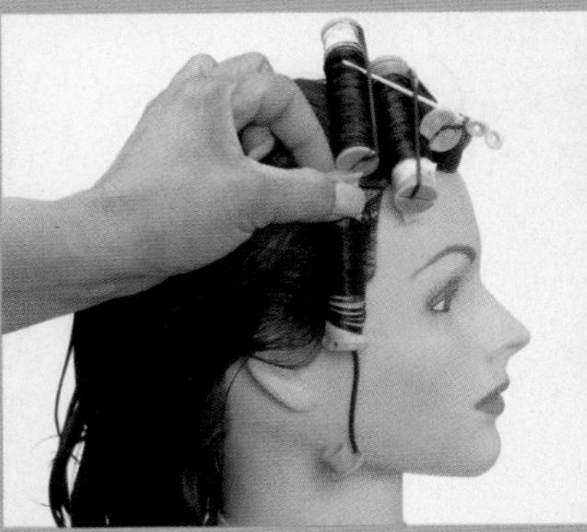

Figure 18-76 Third row.

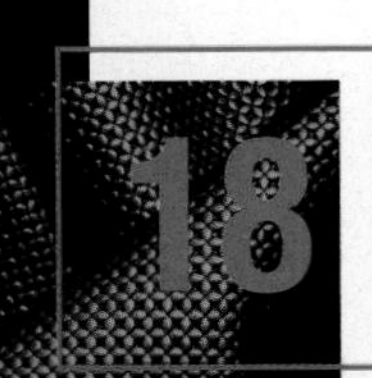

5. **Continue to part.** Continue to part out rows that radiate around the curve of the head through the crown area. Extend rows around and down to the side hairline, parting out base sections at the center of the point where the two rods meet in the previous row (Figure 18-77).
6. **Finish crown.** Stop the curving rows after you have finished wrapping the crown area. Part out horizontal sections throughout the back of the head, and continue with the bricklay pattern. You may need to change the length of the rods from row to row to maintain the pattern (Figure 18-78).
7. Process and style the hair (Figure 18-79).

CLEANUP AND SANITATION

Follow cleanup and sanitation procedures for the basic perm.

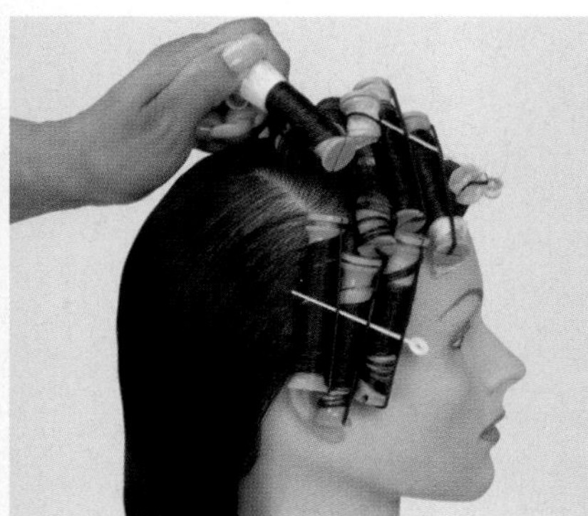

Figure 18-77 Side hairline.

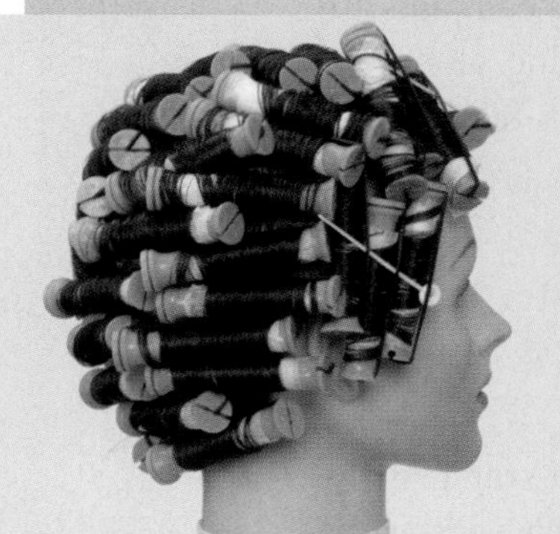

Figure 18-78 Completed bricklay wrap.

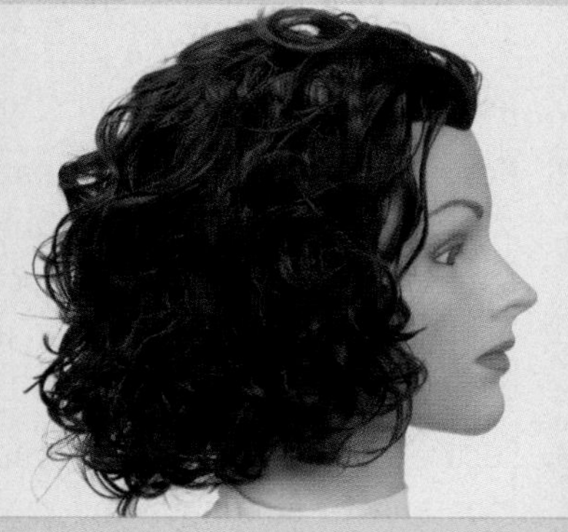

Figure 18-79 Finished style.

PROCEDURE 18-4

WEAVE TECHNIQUE

The weave technique can be used with any of the wrapping patterns in this chapter.

IMPLEMENTS AND MATERIALS

Same as for basic perm.

PREPARATION

Same as for basic perm.

PROCEDURE

1. **Part base section.** Part out one base section the same size as two rods. Comb the entire base section at a 90-degree angle to the head, and use a tail comb to make a zigzag parting along the length of the base section (Figure 18-80).
2. **Roll strand.** Using two end papers, roll half of the strand down to the scalp (Figure 18-81). Comb the remaining half of the base section at a 90-degree angle, use two end papers, and roll the strand down to the scalp (Figure 18-82).
3. Secure the rods and insert picks to stabilize the rods and to eliminate any tension caused by the band.
4. Continue with the same procedure in any sections where the effect is desired (Figure 18-83).
5. Process and style the hair.

CLEANUP AND SANITATION

Follow cleanup and sanitation procedures for the basic perm.

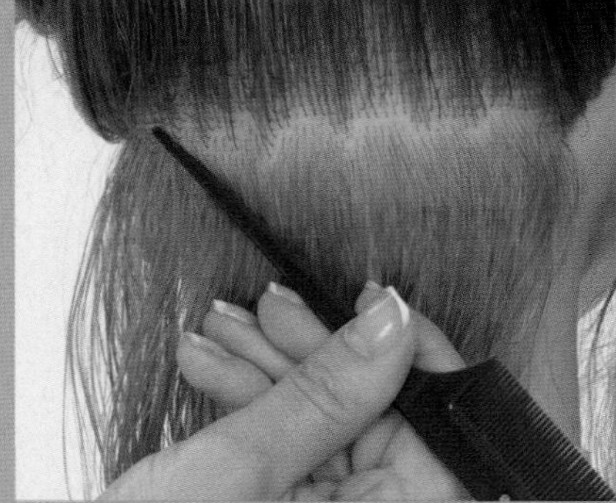

Figure 18-80 Make zigzag parting in base section.

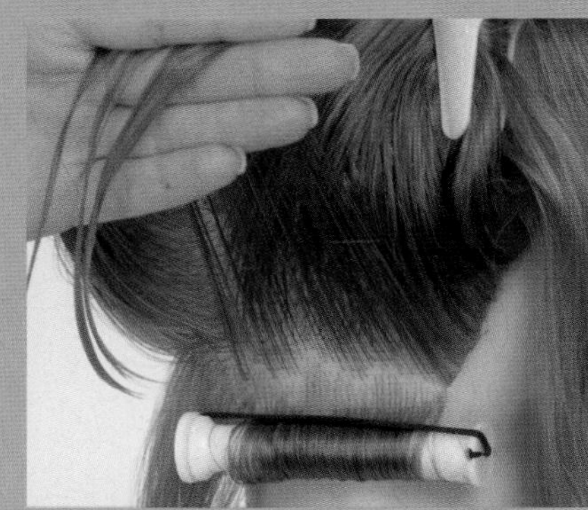

Figure 18-81 Wrap the first rod.

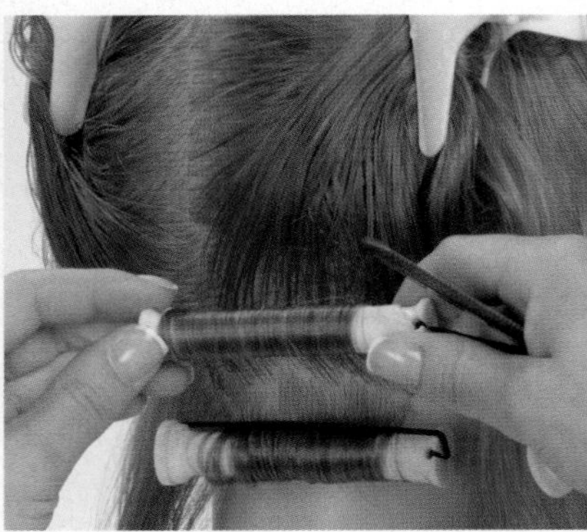

Figure 18-82 Wrap the second rod.

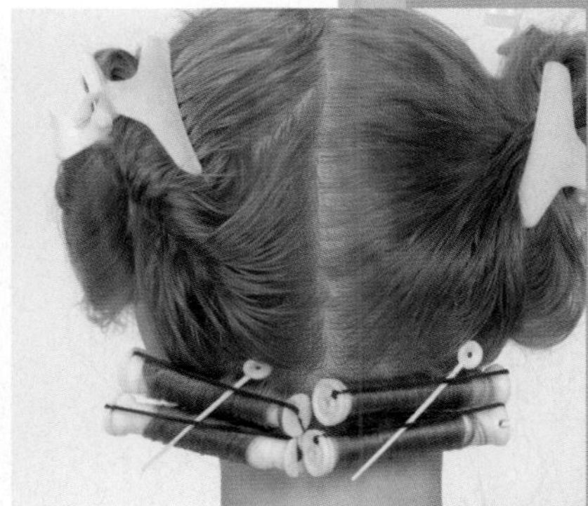

Figure 18-83 Finished weave technique.

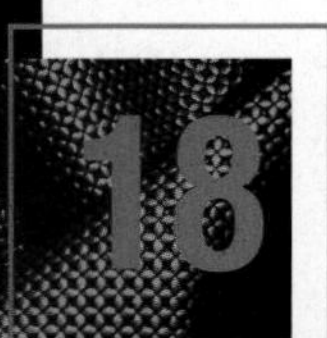

PROCEDURE 18-5

DOUBLE-ROD (PIGGYBACK) TECHNIQUE

The double-rod (piggyback) technique can be used with any of the wrapping patterns in this chapter.

IMPLEMENTS AND MATERIALS

Same as for basic perm.

PREPARATION

Same as for basic perm.

PROCEDURE

1. **Place rod in middle of strand.** Begin by placing the base rod in the middle of the strand. Wrap the end of the strand one revolution around the rod while holding it to one side (Figure 18-84).
2. Roll the rod up to the base area, letting the loose ends follow as you roll (Figure 18-85).
3. Insert picks to stabilize the rods and to eliminate any tension caused by the band.
4. **Use two end papers and roll.** Place two end papers on the ends of the strand and position a rod to roll from the ends toward the base area (Figure 18-86). Secure the end rod on top of the base rod (Figure 18-87).
5. Continue with the same procedure in any sections where the effect is desired (Figure 18-88).
6. Process and style the hair (Figure 18-89).

CLEANUP AND SANITATION

Follow cleanup and sanitation procedures for the basic perm.

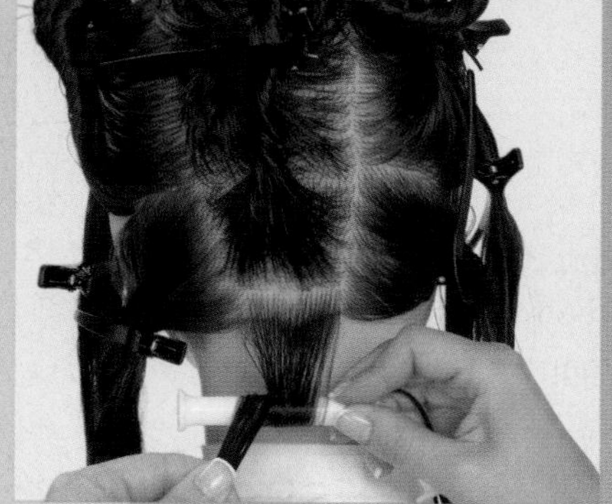

Figure 18-84 Wrap the end of the strand.

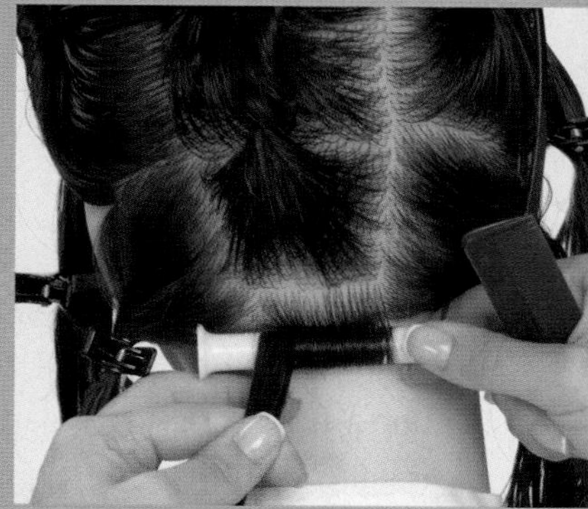

Figure 18-85 Secure rod.

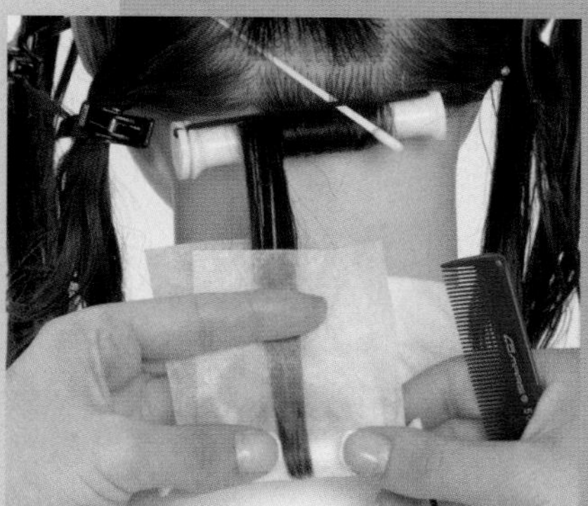

Figure 18-86 Wrap second rod on hair ends.

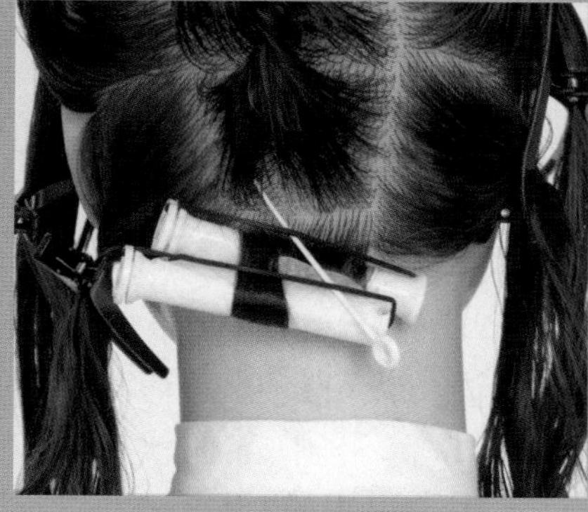

Figure 18-87 Secure end rod on base rod.

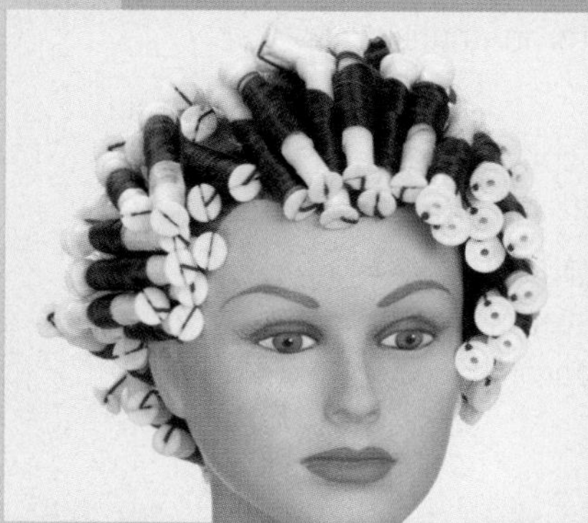

Figure 18-88 Completed double-rod wrap.

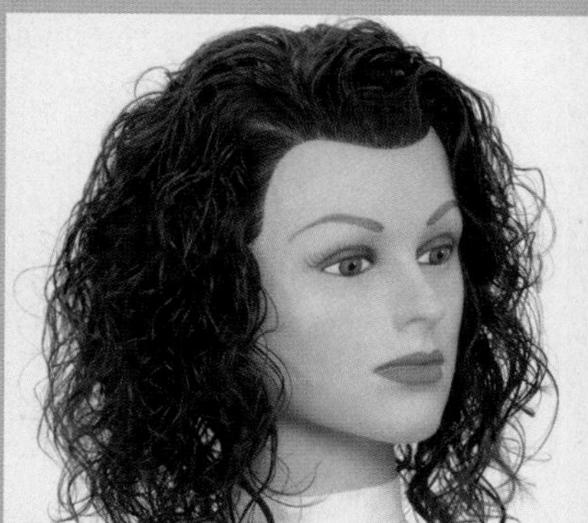

Figure 18-89 Finished and styled double-rod perm.

PROCEDURE 18-6

SPIRAL PERM TECHNIQUE

IMPLEMENTS AND MATERIALS

Same as for basic perm.

PREPARATION

Same as for basic perm.

PROCEDURE

1. **Part off four sections.** Part the hair into four panels, from the center of the front hairline to the center of the nape, and from ear to ear. Section out a fifth panel from ear to ear in the nape area (Figure 18-90).
2. **Comb first section.** Section out the first row along the hairline in the nape area. Comb the remainder of the hair up, and secure it out of the way.
3. **Begin wrapping.** Part out the first base section on one side of the first row. Hold the hair at a 90-degree angle to the head. Using one or two end papers, begin wrapping at one end of the rod. Starting the wrap from the right or left side of the rod will orient the curl in that direction (Figure 18-91).
4. **Spiral the hair.** Roll the first two full turns at a 90-degree angle to the rod to secure the ends of the hair, and then start spiraling the hair on the rod by changing the angle to an angle other than 90 degrees (Figure 18-92).
5. **Roll to scalp.** Continue to spiral the hair toward the other end of the rod. Roll the hair down to the scalp, position the rod half off base, and secure it by fastening the ends of the rod together (Figure 18-93).

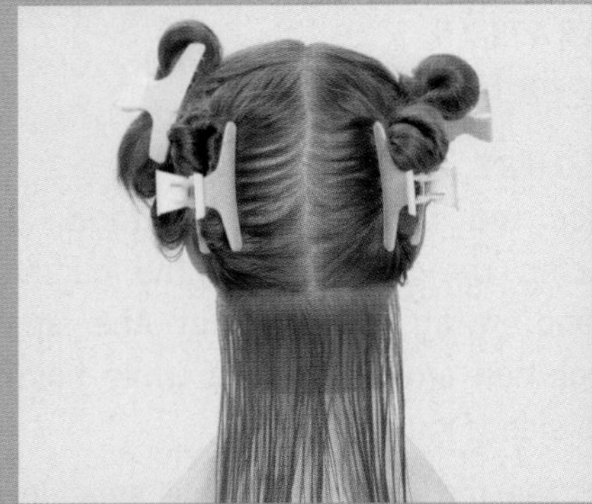

Figure 18-90 Part hair into four sections.

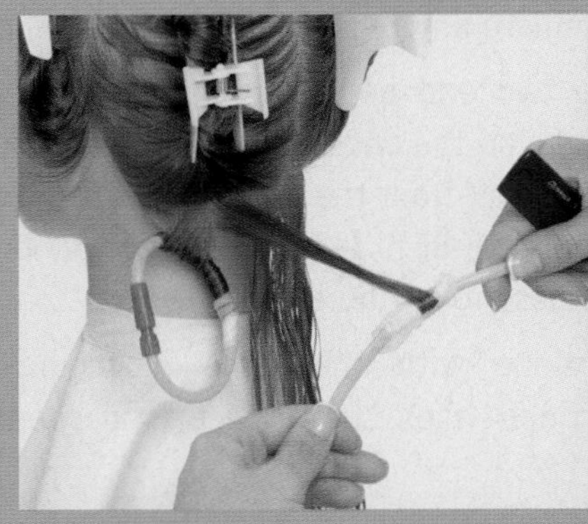

Figure 18-91 Wrap the first two turns.

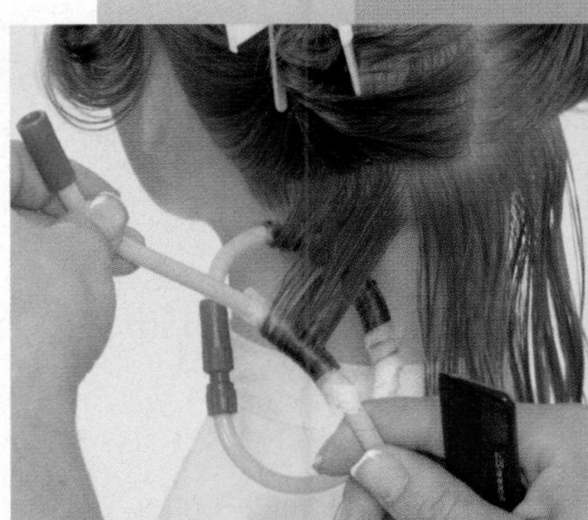

Figure 18-92 Wrap the same rod at an angle.

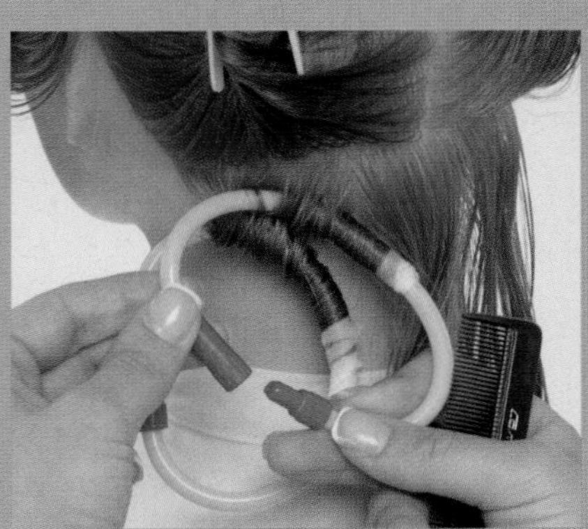

Figure 18-93 Fasten ends of rod together.

6. Continue wrapping with the same technique, in the same direction, until the first row is completed (Figure 18-94).
7. **Section second row.** Section out the second row above and parallel to the first row. Comb the remainder of the hair up, and secure it to keep it out of the way.
8. **Wrap opposite side.** Begin wrapping at the opposite side from the side where the first row began, and move in the direction opposite the direction established in the first row (Figure 18-95).
9. **Complete second row.** Follow the same procedure to wrap the second row but begin wrapping each rod at the opposite end established in the first row. Continue wrapping with the same technique, in the same direction, until the second row is completed (Figure 18-96).
10. **Section third row.** Section out the third row above and parallel to the second row. Follow the same wrapping procedure, alternating the rows from left to right as you move up the head. This will alternate the orientation of the curl throughout the head (Figure 18-97).
11. Process and style the hair (Figure 18-98).

CLEANUP AND SANITATION

Follow cleanup and sanitation procedures for the basic perm.

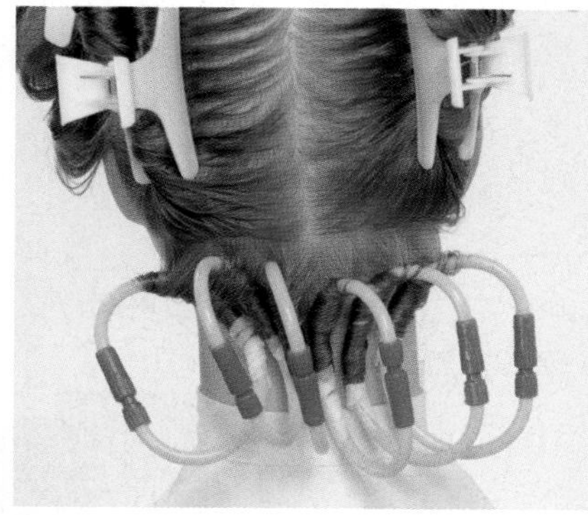

Figure 18-94 Completed first row.

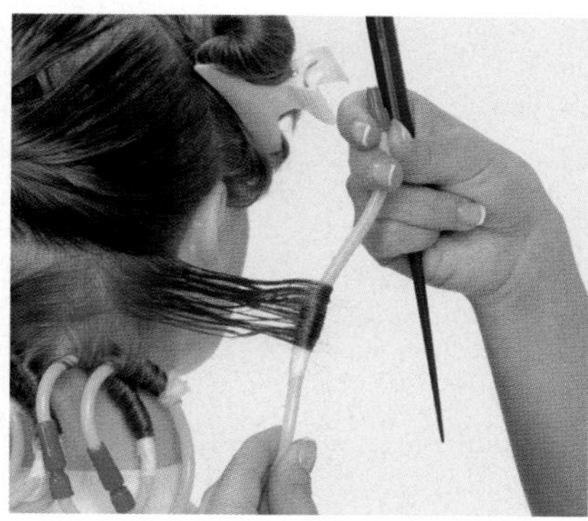

Figure 18-95 Begin second row.

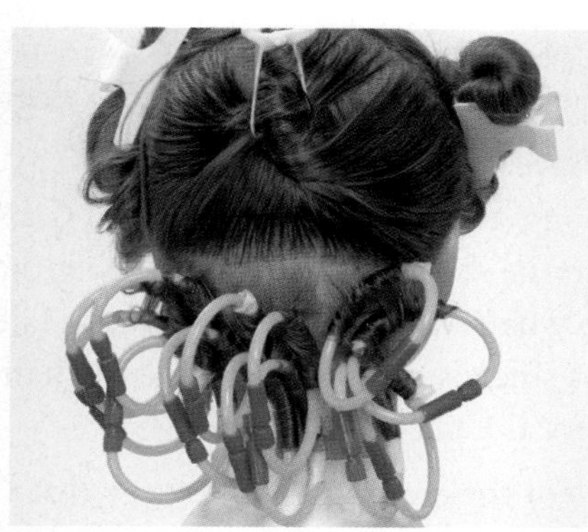

Figure 18-96 Second row.

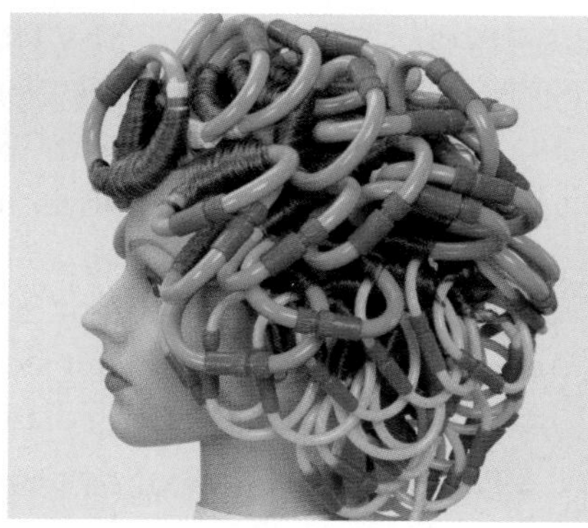

Figure 18-97 Completed spiral wrap.

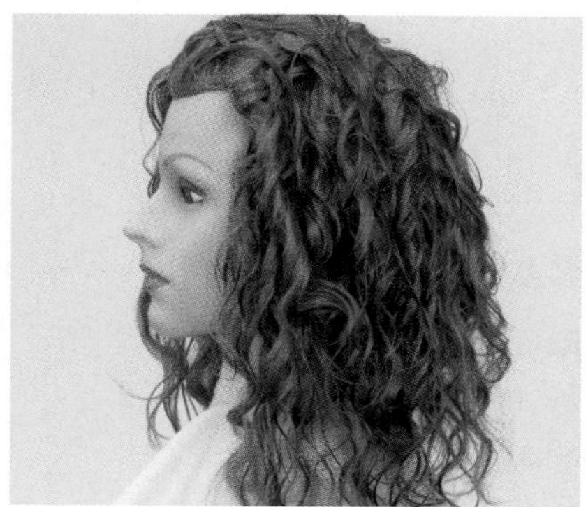

Figure 18-98 Finished styled spiral perm.

PERMS FOR MEN

Do not assume that perms are only for women. Many male clients are looking for the added texture, fullness, style, and low maintenance that only a perm can provide. Perms help thin hair look fuller, make straight or coarse hair more manageable, and help control stubborn cowlicks. Although men's and women's hairstyles may be different, the techniques for permanent waving are essentially the same.

CHEMICAL HAIR RELAXERS

Chemical hair relaxing rearranges the structure of curly hair into a straighter or smoother form. Whereas permanent waving curls straight hair, chemical hair relaxing straightens curly hair (Figure 18-99).

Other than their objectives being quite different, the two services are very similar. In fact, the chemistry of thio relaxers and permanent waving is exactly the same. And even though the chemistry of hydroxide relaxers and permanent waving may be different, all relaxers and all permanents change the shape of the hair by breaking disulfide bonds.

The two most common types of chemical hair relaxers are thio (ammonium thioglycolate) and hydroxide.

CAUTION

Relaxers are characterized by an extremely high alkalinity, and can literally melt or dissolve hair if used incorrectly. Most relaxers contain the same ingredients used in depilatories (products used for temporary hair removal).

EXTREMELY CURLY HAIR

Extremely curly hair exists among all people of all races. This means anyone of any race can have extremely curly hair. Moreover, the degree of curliness varies among individuals within each group.

Extremely curly hair grows in long twisted spirals, or coils. Cross-sections are highly elliptical, and vary in shape and thickness along their lengths. Compared to straight or wavy hair, which tends to possess a fairly regular and uniform diameter along a single strand, extremely curly hair is irregular, exhibiting varying diameters along a single strand.

The thinnest and weakest sections of the hair strands are located at the twists. These sections are also bent at an extremely sharp angle, and will be stretched the most during relaxing. A chain is only as strong as its weakest link, and hair is only as strong as its weakest section. Hair breaks at its weakest point. Extremely curly hair usually breaks at the twists because of the inherent weakness in that section, and the extra physical force that is required to straighten it.

THIO RELAXERS

Ammonium thioglycolate (ATG) is commonly called "thio," and is the same reducing agent that is used in permanent waving. **Thio relaxers** usually have a pH above 10 and a higher concentration of ATG than is used in permanent waving. Thio relaxers are also thicker, with a higher viscosity that is more suitable for application as a relaxer.

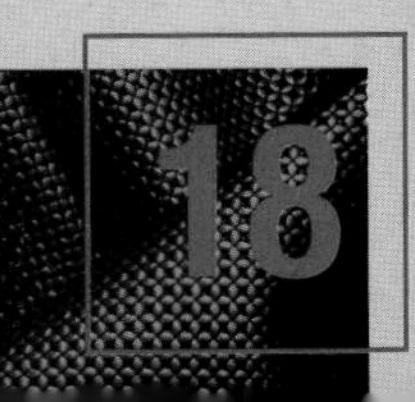

Thio relaxers break disulfide bonds and soften hair, just as in permanents. After enough bonds are broken, the hair is straightened into its new shape and the relaxer is rinsed from the hair. Blotting comes next, followed by a neutralizer. The chemical reactions of thio relaxers are identical to those in permanent waving.

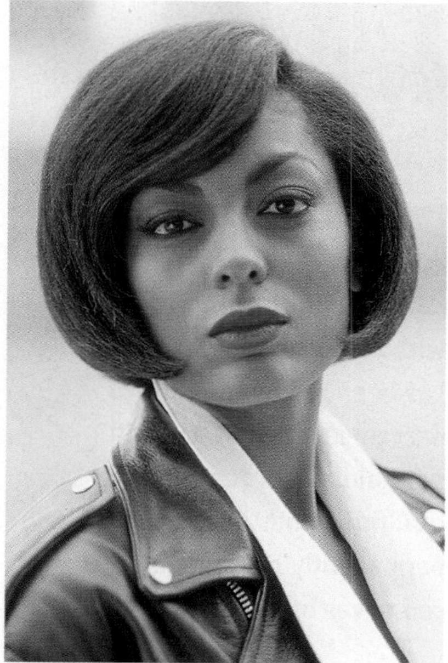

Figure 18–99 Relaxed hair.

THIO NEUTRALIZATION

The neutralizer used with thio relaxers is an oxidizing agent, usually hydrogen peroxide, just as in permanents. The oxidation reaction caused by the neutralizer rebuilds the disulfide bonds that were broken by the thio relaxer.

HYDROXIDE RELAXERS

The hydroxide ion is the active ingredient in all **hydroxide relaxers.** Sodium hydroxide, potassium hydroxide, lithium hydroxide, and guanidine hydroxide are all types of hydroxide relaxers. All hydroxide relaxers are very strong alkalis. Most have a pH over 13 and can swell the hair up to twice its normal diameter.

Hydroxide relaxers are not compatible with thio relaxers, permanent waving, or soft curl perms because they use a different chemistry. Thio relaxers use thio to break the disulfide bonds. The high pH of a thio relaxer is needed to swell the hair but it is the thio that breaks the disulfide bonds.

Hydroxide relaxers have a pH that is so high that the alkalinity alone breaks the disulfide bonds. The average pH of the hair is 5.0, and many hydroxide relaxers have a pH over 13.0. Since each step in the pH scale represents a tenfold change in concentration, a pH of 13.0 is 100 million (100,000,000) times more alkaline than a pH of 5.0 (Figure 18-100).

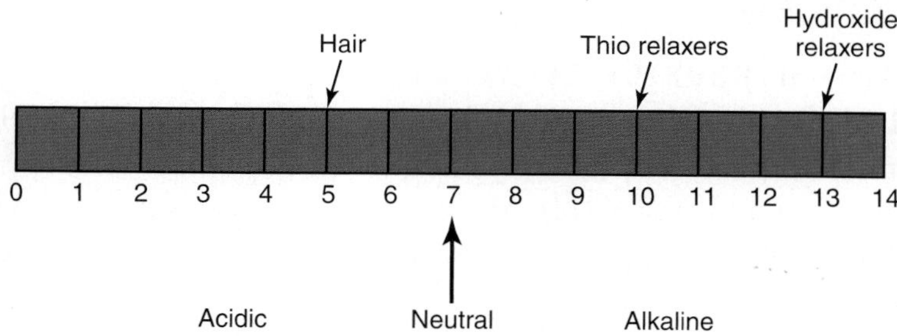

Figure 18–100 pH of thio and hydroxide relaxers.

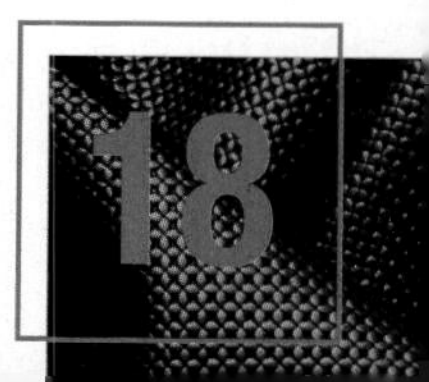

CAUTION

Hair that has been treated with a hydroxide relaxer has been rendered unfit for permanent waving and will not hold a curl. The disulfide bonds have been permanently broken and can never be re-formed.

CAUTION

Application of a thio relaxer or thio permanent on hair that has been treated with a hydroxide relaxer will not properly relax or curl the hair, and may cause extreme damage. Hair that has been treated with hydroxide relaxers is unfit for thio relaxers, or soft curl permanents.

Hydroxide relaxers break disulfide bonds differently than in the reduction reaction of thio relaxers. Hydroxide relaxers remove a sulfur atom from a disulfide bond, converting it into a lanthionine bond by a process called **lanthionization** (lan-thee-oh-ny-ZAY-shun). A disulfide bond consists of two bonded sulfur atoms. Lanthionine bonds contain only one sulfur atom. The disulfide bonds that are broken by hydroxide relaxers are broken permanently, and can never be re-formed. That is why hair that has been treated with a hydroxide relaxer is unfit for permanent waving and will not hold curl.

HYDROXIDE NEUTRALIZATION

Unlike thio neutralization, **hydroxide neutralization** does not involve oxidation or rebuilding disulfide bonds. The neutralization of hydroxide relaxers neutralizes (deactivates) the alkaline residues left in the hair by the relaxer. The pH of hydroxide relaxers is so high that the hair remains at an extremely high pH, even after thorough rinsing. Although rinsing is important, rinsing alone does not neutralize (deactivate) the relaxer, nor restore the normal acidic pH of the hair and scalp.

As suggested in Chapter 10, acids neutralize alkalis. Therefore, the application of an acid-balanced shampoo, or a normalizing lotion, neutralizes any remaining hydroxide ions to lower the pH of the hair and scalp. Some neutralizing shampoos intended for use after hydroxide relaxers have a built-in pH indicator that changes color to show when the pH of the hair has returned to normal.

The neutralization of a hydroxide relaxer does not rebuild the disulfide bonds. Since the disulfide bonds that have been broken by hydroxide relaxers cannot be re-formed by oxidation, application of a neutralizer that contains an oxidizing agent will not be of any benefit and will only damage the hair.

TYPES OF HYDROXIDE RELAXERS

Metal hydroxide relaxers are ionic compounds formed by a metal—sodium (Na), potassium (K), or lithium (Li)—which is combined with oxygen (O) and hydrogen (H). Metal hydroxide relaxers include sodium hydroxide ($NaOH$), potassium hydroxide (KOH), and lithium hydroxide ($LiOH$).

Although calcium hydroxide ($CaOH$) is sometimes added to hydroxide relaxers, it is not used by itself to relax hair.

All metal hydroxide relaxers contain only one component, and are used exactly as they are packaged in the container without mixing. The hydroxide ion is the active ingredient in all hydroxide relaxers. There is no significant difference in the performance of these metal hydroxide relaxers.

Sodium hydroxide ($NaOH$) relaxers are commonly called lye relaxers. Sodium hydroxide is the oldest, and still the most common type of chemical hair relaxer. Sodium hydroxide is also known as lye or caustic soda. Sodium hydroxide is the same chemical that is used in drain cleaners and chemical hair depilatories.

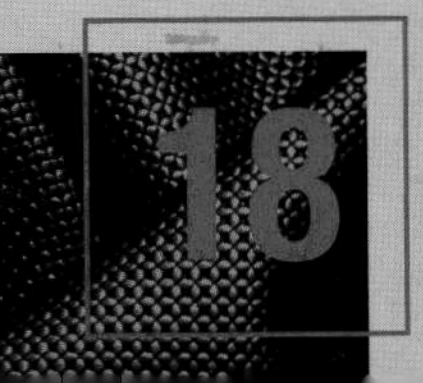

Lithium hydroxide (LiOH) and potassium hydroxide (KOH) relaxers are often advertised and sold as "no mix-no lye" relaxers. Although technically they are not lye, their chemistry is identical, and there is very little difference in their performance.

GUANIDINE HYDROXIDE RELAXERS

Guanidine (GWAN-ih-deen) hydroxide relaxers are usually advertised and sold as "no-lye" relaxers. Although technically they are not lye, the hydroxide ion is still the active ingredient. Guanidine hydroxide relaxers contain two components that must be mixed immediately prior to use.

These relaxers straighten hair completely, with less scalp irritation than other hydroxide relaxers. Most guanidine hydroxide relaxers are recommended for sensitive scalps, and are sold over the counter for home use. Although they reduce scalp irritation, they do not reduce hair damage. They swell the hair slightly more than other hydroxide relaxers, and are also more drying, especially after repeated applications.

LOW-PH RELAXERS

Sulfites and bisulfites are sometimes used as low-pH hair relaxers. The most commonly used are ammonium sulfite and ammonium bisulfite. Sulfites are marketed as mild alternative relaxers. They are compatible with thio relaxers, but not compatible with hydroxide relaxers. They do not completely straighten extremely curly hair. Low-pH relaxers are intended for use on color-treated, damaged, or fine hair. (See Table 18-3 for a summary of the types and uses of relaxers.)

THERMAL IONIC RECONSTRUCTORS

Thermal ionic reconstructors were first manufactured and marketed in Asia. Although they claim to use ions to restructure hair, they are nothing more than a thio relaxer with a double hot blow-dry and a double hot press with flat irons. The added heat while drying and pressing helps make these formulas more effective than standard thio relaxers.

BASE AND NO-BASE RELAXERS

Hydroxide relaxers are usually sold in base and no-base formulas. **Base cream,** also called **protective base cream,** is an oily cream used to protect the skin and scalp during hair relaxing. **Base relaxers** require the application of a protective base cream to the entire scalp prior to the application of the relaxer.

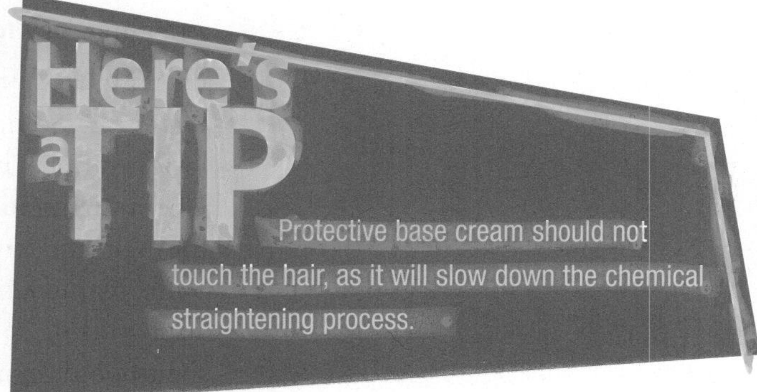

Here's a TIP
Protective base cream should not touch the hair, as it will slow down the chemical straightening process.

No-base relaxers do not require the application of a protective base cream. They contain a protective base cream that is designed to melt at body temperature. As the relaxer is applied, body heat causes the protective base cream to melt and settle out onto the scalp in a thin, oily, protective coating. No-base relaxers are simply an improvement on the protection that is provided by the oils in all hydroxide relaxers. For added protection, protective base cream may be applied to the entire hairline and around the ears, even with no-base relaxers.

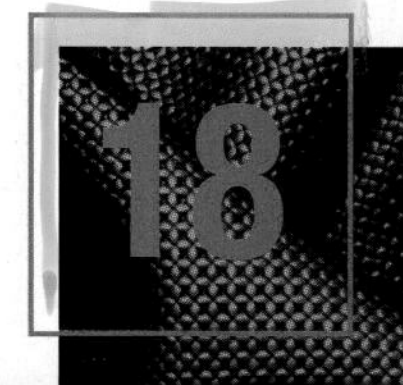

CAUTION

Make sure that the client has not had haircoloring containing metallic salts, such as gradual or progressive haircolors, before applying either thio or hydroxide relaxers to the hair. Extreme damage or breakage can occur.

CAUTION

Before doing any relaxing service, review the Safety Precautions for Hair Relaxing and Curl Re-Forming section at the end of this chapter.

RELAXER STRENGTHS

Most chemical hair relaxers are available in three strengths: mild, regular, and super. The difference in strength of hydroxide relaxers parallels the concentration of hydroxide.

- Mild-strength relaxers are formulated for fine, color-treated, or damaged hair.
- Regular-strength relaxers are intended for normal hair texture with a medium natural curl.
- Super-strength relaxers should be used for maximum straightening on very coarse, extremely curly, and resistant hair. When in doubt, always choose the gentler alternative, that is, mild instead of regular, or regular instead of super.

CHEMICAL HAIR-RELAXING PROCEDURES

Although many steps for applying thio and hydroxide relaxers are the same, there are a few important differences.

HYDROXIDE RELAXER PROCEDURES

Although the same procedure is used for all hydroxide relaxers, application methods vary according to previous use of texture services.

- A *virgin relaxer* application should be used for hair that has not had previous chemical texture services. Since the scalp area and the porous ends will usually process more quickly than the middle of the strand, the application for a virgin relaxer starts ¼ inch (0.6 centimeters) to ½ inch (1.25 centimeters) away from the scalp, and includes the entire strand up to the porous ends. To avoid over-processing and scalp irritation, do not apply relaxer to the hair closest to the scalp or to the ends until the last few minutes of processing.
- A *retouch relaxer* application should be used for hair that has had previous chemical texture services. The application for a retouch relaxer starts ¼ inch to ½ inch away from the scalp and includes only the new growth. To avoid over-processing and scalp irritation, do not apply relaxer to the hair closest to the scalp until the last few minutes of processing. If the previously relaxed hair requires additional straightening, relaxer may be applied during the last few minutes of processing.
- *Option A:* Some manufacturers recommend the use of a normalizing lotion after rinsing out the relaxer and prior to shampooing. **Normalizing lotions** are conditioners with an acidic pH that condition the hair and restore the natural pH prior to shampooing. *Option B:* Some manufacturers include a normalizing shampoo that must be used after rinsing out the relaxer. Normalizing shampoo is an acidic shampoo designed to restore the natural pH of hair and scalp.

After a thorough consultation, you should be able to determine which type of relaxer is best suited to your client's hair type, condition, and desired results. Table 18-2 lists the most common types of relaxers along with selected advantages and disadvantages for each.

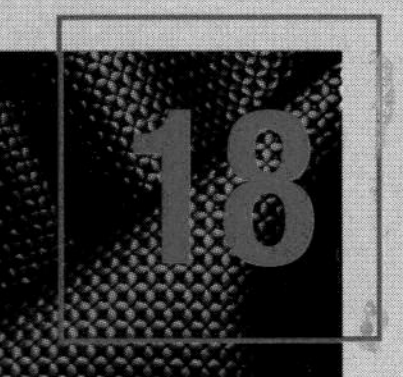

PERIODIC STRAND TESTING

Periodic strand testing during processing will help to tell you when the hair is sufficiently relaxed. After the relaxer is applied, stretch the strands to see how fast the natural curls are being removed. You may also smooth and press the strand to the scalp using the back of the comb, the applicator brush, or your finger. Be gentle! If the strand remains smooth, it is sufficiently relaxed. If the curl returns, continue processing. Processing time will vary according to the strength of the relaxer, hair type and condition, and the desired results (Figures 18-101 and 18-102).

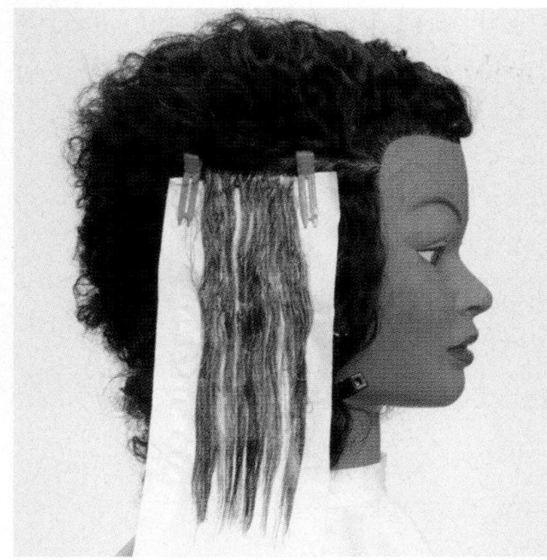

Figure 18–101 Sufficiently relaxed strand.

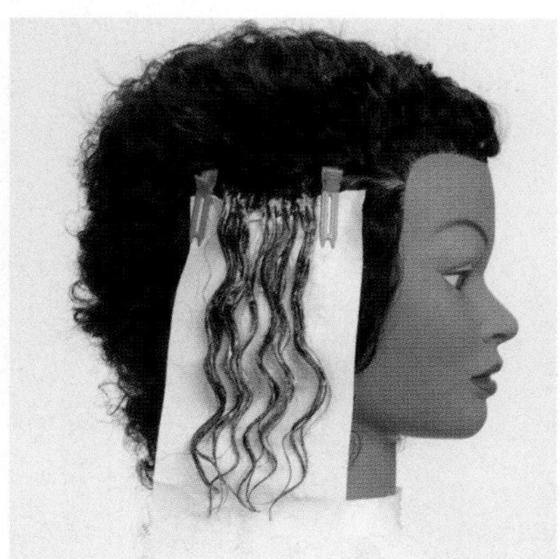

Figure 18–102 Insufficiently relaxed strand.

ACTIVE INGREDIENT	SELECTING THE CORRECT RELAXER			
	pH	**Marketed As**	**Advantages**	**Disadvantages**
sodium hydroxide	12.5–13.5	lye relaxer	very effective for extremely curly hair	may cause scalp irritation and damage the hair
lithium hydroxide and potassium hydroxide	12.5–13.5	no-mix, lye relaxer	very effective for extremely curly hair	may cause scalp irritation and damage the hair
guanidine hydroxide	13–13.5	no-lye relaxer	causes less skin irritation than other hydroxide relaxers	more drying to hair with repeated use
ammonium thioglycolate	9.6–10.0	thio relaxer, no-lye relaxer	compatible with soft curl permanents	strong, unpleasant ammonia smell
ammonium sulfite/ ammonium bisulfite	6.5-8.5	low-pH relaxer, no-lye relaxer	less damaging to hair	does not relax extremely curly hair sufficiently

Table 18-2 Selecting the Correct Relaxer

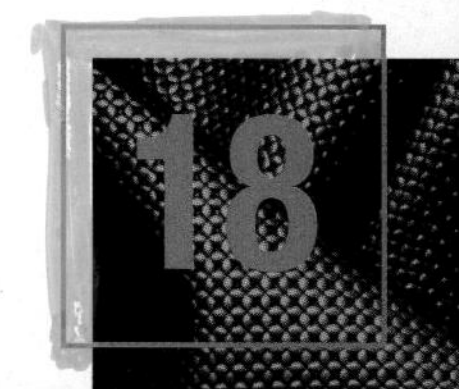

PROCEDURE 18-7

APPLYING VIRGIN HYDROXIDE RELAXERS

IMPLEMENTS AND MATERIALS

- Hydroxide relaxer
- Hydroxide neutralizer
- Protective base cream
- Acid-balanced shampoo
- Conditioner
- Bowl and applicator brush
- Shampoo cape
- Towels
- Plastic clips
- Styling comb
- Plastic tail comb
- Spray bottle
- Disposable gloves
- Timer

PREPARATION

1. Wash your hands.
2. Perform an analysis of the hair and scalp (Figure 18-103). Perform tests for porosity and elasticity.
3. Complete the client consultation. Fill out the client relaxer record. Note any changes in the client's history.
4. Have the client change into a gown and remove eyeglasses, earrings, and necklace.
5. Drape the client with a shampoo cape and two towels. To avoid scalp irritation, do not shampoo the hair prior to a hydroxide relaxer. The hair and scalp must be completely dry prior to the application of a hydroxide relaxer.

PROCEDURE

1. **Section and clip hair.** Part the hair into four sections, from the center of the front hairline to the center of the nape, and from ear to ear. Clip the sections up to keep them out of the way (Figure 18-104).

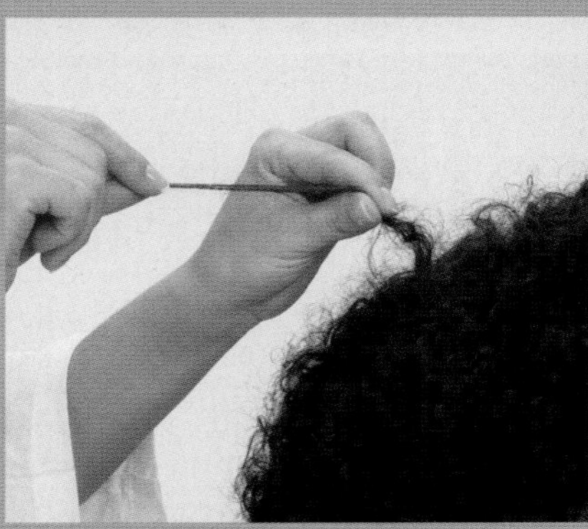

Figure 18-103 Hair analysis.

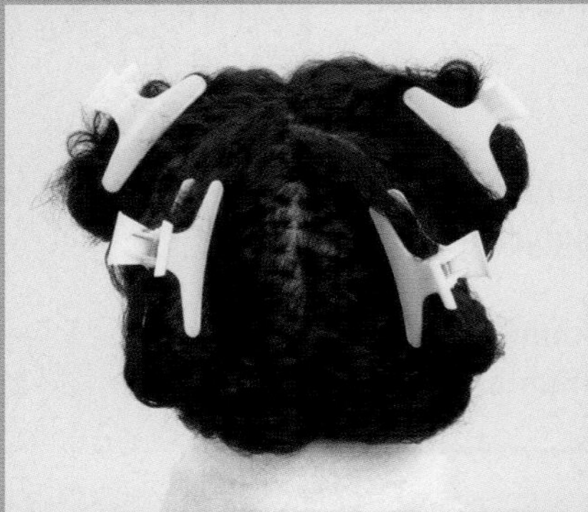

Figure 18-104 Hair sectioning.

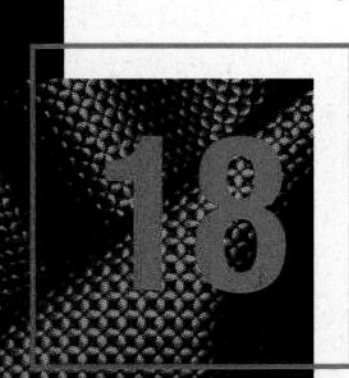

2. **Protect client.** Apply protective base cream to the hairline and ears. *Option:* Take ¼-inch to ½-inch (0.6 to 1.25 centimeters) horizontal partings, and apply a protective base cream to the entire scalp (Figure 18-105). Always follow the manufacturer's directions, and the procedures approved by your instructor.
3. **Begin application.** Wear gloves on both hands. Begin application in the most resistant area, usually at the back of the head. Make ¼-inch to ½-inch horizontal partings, and apply the relaxer to the top of the strand first (Figure 18-106), and then to the underside (Figure 18-107). Apply the relaxer with an applicator brush, or the back of a tail comb or fingers. Apply relaxer ¼ inch to ½ inch away from the scalp, and up to the porous ends. To avoid scalp irritation, do not allow the relaxer to touch the scalp until the last few minutes of processing.
4. Continue applying the relaxer, working your way down the section toward the hairline.
5. Continue the same application procedure with the remaining sections. Finish the most resistant sections first.
6. **Smooth with back of comb.** After the relaxer has been applied to all sections, use the back of the comb or your hands to smooth each section (Figure 18-108). Never comb the relaxer through the hair.
7. **Process and strand test.** Process according to the manufacturer's directions. Perform periodic strand tests. Processing usually takes less than 20 minutes at room temperature. Always follow manufacturer's processing directions.
8. **Work relaxer to scalp.** During the last few minutes of processing, work the relaxer down to the scalp and through the ends of the hair, using additional relaxer as needed (Figure 18-109). Carefully smooth all sections using an applicator brush, fingers, or back of the comb.

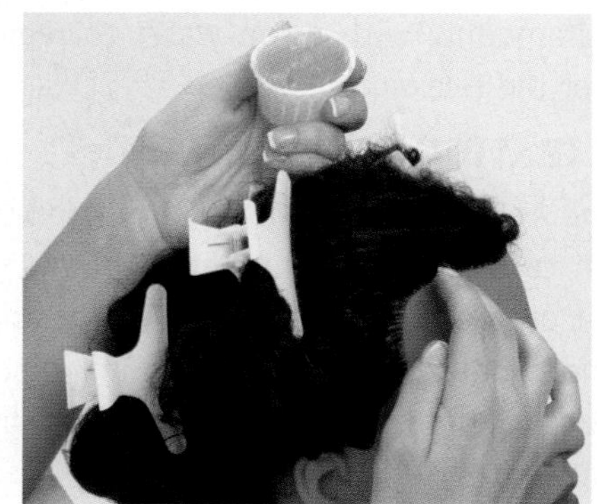

Figure 18–105 Apply protective base cream.

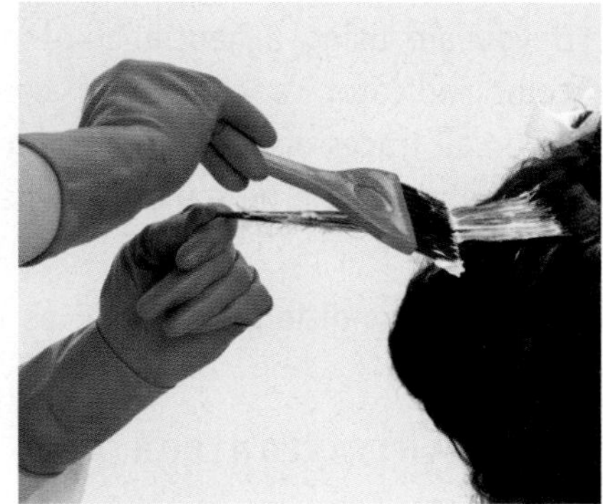

Figure 18–106 Apply relaxer to topside of strand.

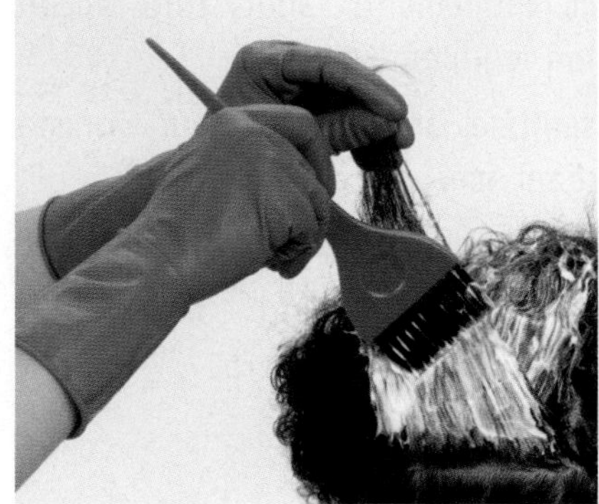

Figure 18–107 Apply relaxer to underside of strand.

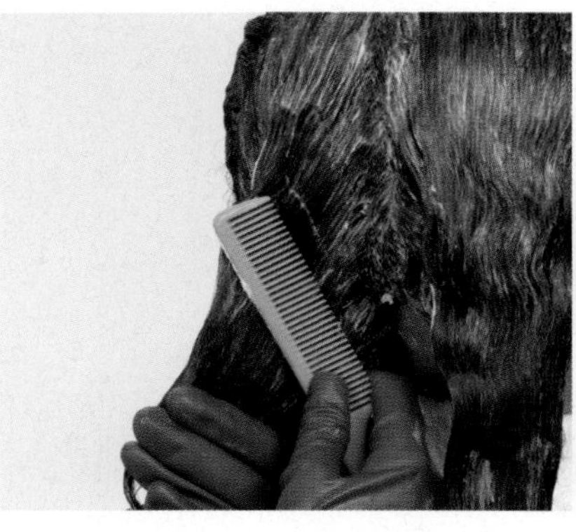

Figure 18–108 Smooth section with back of comb.

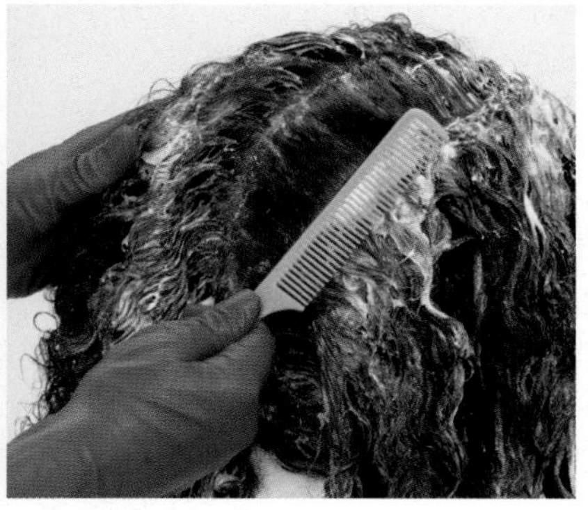

Figure 18–109 Work relaxer down to scalp.

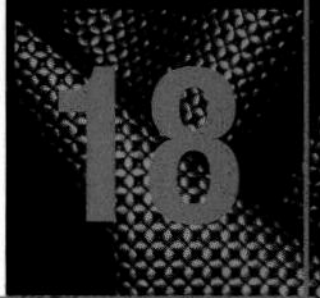

9. Rinse thoroughly with warm water to remove all traces of the relaxer.

NEUTRALIZATION PROCEDURE

1. *Optional:* Apply the normalizing lotion and comb it through to the ends of the hair (Figure 18-110). Leave it on for approximately 5 minutes and then rinse thoroughly. (Always follow the manufacturer's directions, and the procedures approved by your instructor.)
2. Shampoo at least three times with an acid-balanced neutralizing shampoo. It is essential that all traces of the relaxer be removed from the hair. *Option:* If you are using a neutralizing shampoo with a color indicator, a change in color will indicate when all traces of the relaxer are removed and the natural pH of the hair and scalp has been restored.
3. Rinse thoroughly, condition, and style as desired (Figure 18-111).

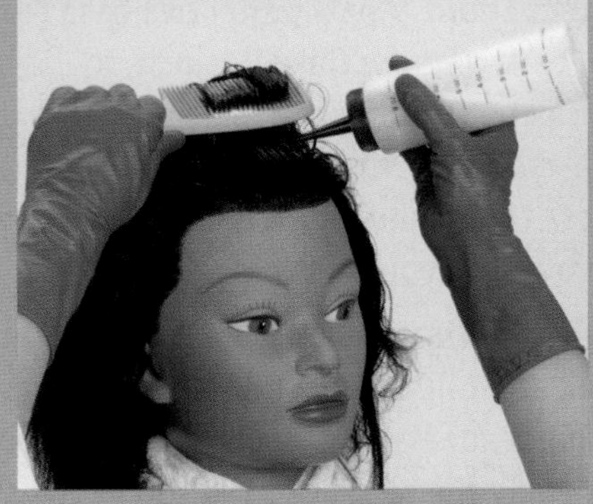

Figure 18–110 Applying normalizing lotion is an optional step.

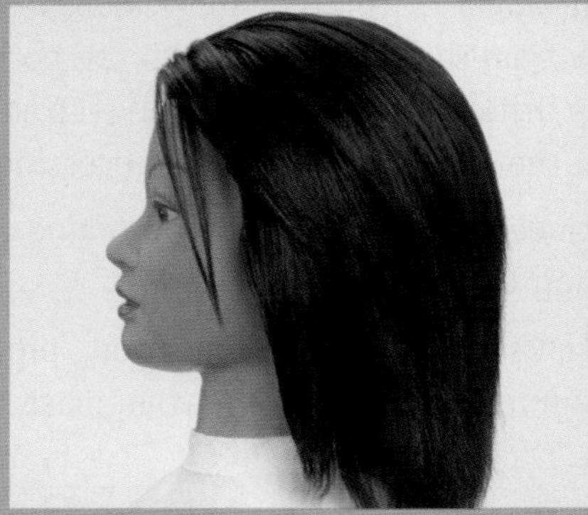

Figure 18–111 Finished relaxed style.

CLEANUP AND SANITATION FOR ALL RELAXERS

1. Discard disposable supplies in appropriate receptacles.
2. Disinfect implements and store according to sanitation requirements.
3. Clean, sanitize, and prepare your workstation for the next service.
4. Wash your hands with warm soap and water.
5. Complete the client record.

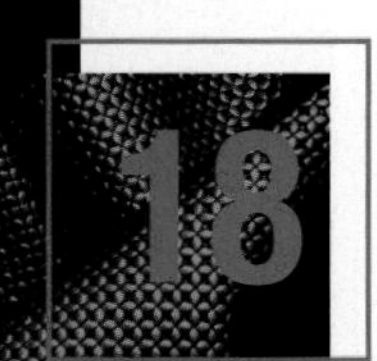

PROCEDURE 18-8

HYDROXIDE RELAXER RETOUCH

IMPLEMENTS AND MATERIALS

Same as for applying virgin hydroxide relaxers.

PREPARATION

Same as for applying virgin hydroxide relaxers.

PROCEDURE

1. **Work on dry hair.** Do not shampoo the hair. Hair and scalp must be completely dry. Divide the hair into four sections, from the center of the front hairline to the center of the nape, and from ear to ear. Clip sections up to keep them out of the way.
2. **Protect hands.** Wear gloves on both hands. Apply a protective base cream to the hairline and ears. *Option:* Take 1/4-inch to 1/2-inch horizontal (0.6 to 1.25 centimeters) partings and apply protective base cream to the entire scalp (Figure 18-112).
3. **Apply relaxer.** Begin application of the relaxer in the most resistant area, usually at the back of the head. Make 1/4-inch to 1/2-inch horizontal partings and apply the relaxer to the top of the strand. Apply the relaxer 1/4 inch to 1/2 inch away from the scalp and only to new growth. Do not allow the relaxer to touch the scalp until the last few minutes of processing. To avoid over-processing or breakage, do not overlap the relaxer onto the previously relaxed hair (Figure 18-113).
4. Continue applying the relaxer, using the same procedure and working your way down the section toward the hairline.

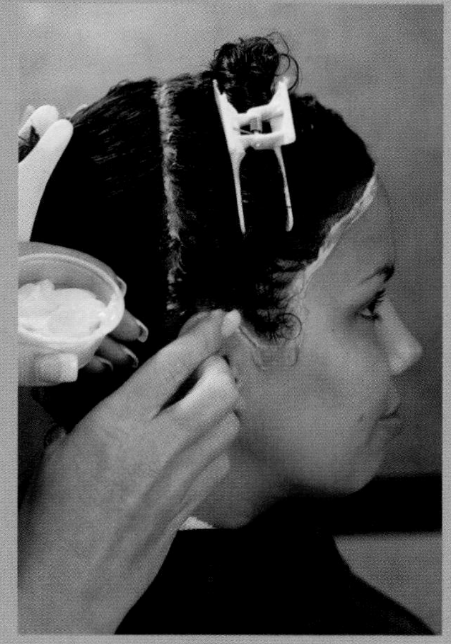

Figure 18–112 Apply protective base cream to the hairline and ears.

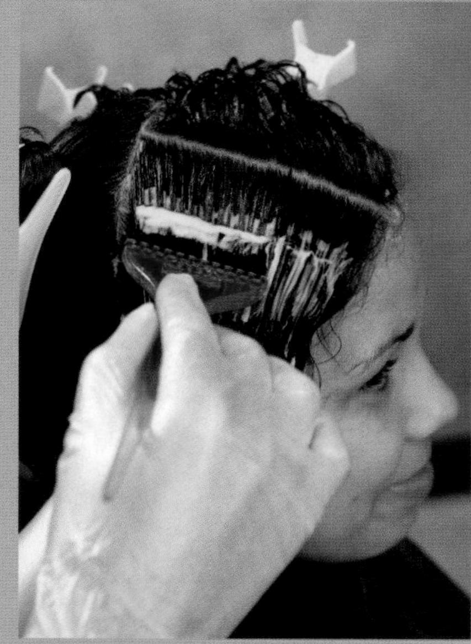

Figure 18–113 Apply relaxer to new growth only.

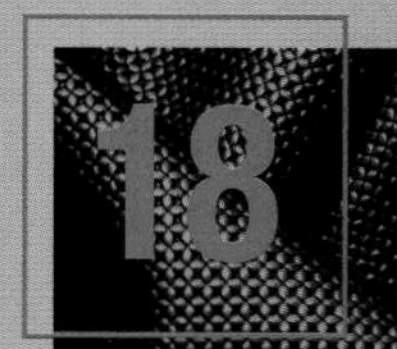

5. Continue the same application procedure with the remaining sections, finishing the most resistant sections first (Figure 18-114).

6. After the relaxer has been applied to all sections, use the back of the comb, the applicator brush, or your hands to smooth each section (Figure 18-115).

7. **Process and strand test.** Process according to the manufacturer's directions. Perform periodic strand tests. Processing usually takes less than 20 minutes at room temperature. Always follow the manufacturer's processing directions.

8. During the last few minutes of processing, gently work the relaxer down to the scalp.

9. **Work relaxer to ends.** If the ends of the hair need additional relaxing, work the relaxer through to the ends for the last few minutes of processing (Figure 18-116). Do not relax ends during each retouch; doing this will cause over-processing. *Option:* A cream conditioner may be applied to relaxed ends to protect from over-processing caused by overlapping.

10. Rinse thoroughly with warm water to remove all traces of the relaxer.

11. Follow virgin hydroxide neutralizing procedure. Style the hair as desired.

CLEANUP AND SANITATION

Same as for applying virgin hydroxide relaxers.

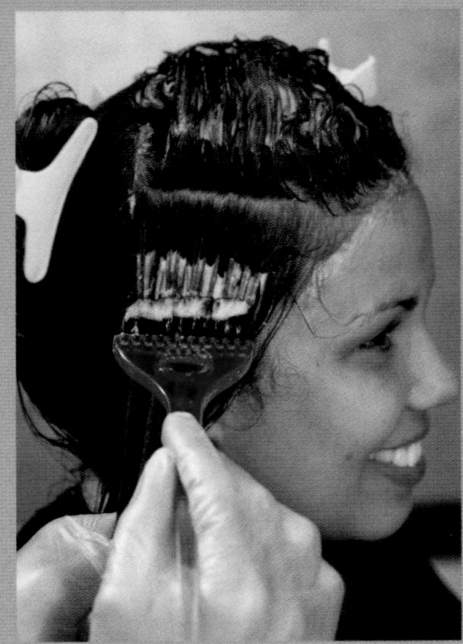

Figure 18–114 Apply relaxer to most resistant sections first.

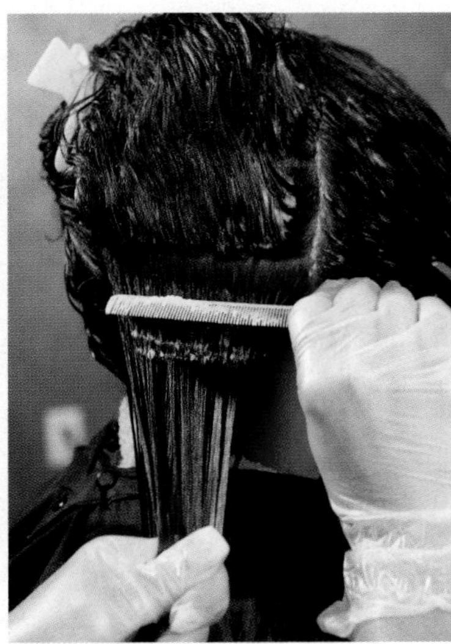

Figure 18–115 Never use the teeth of your comb to distribute the relaxer.

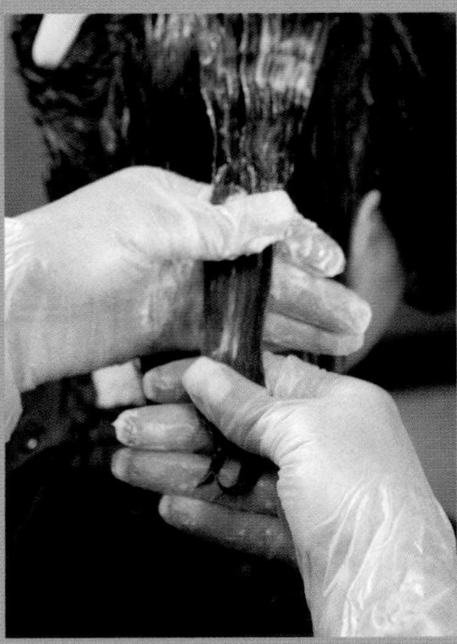

Figure 18–116 If the ends still have a slight amount of curl, work the relaxer through the ends for the last few minutes of processing.

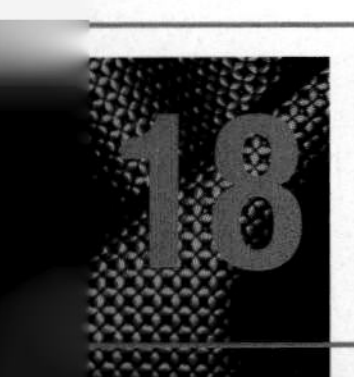

PROCEDURE 18-9

APPLYING THIO RELAXER

VIRGIN THIO RELAXER

The application steps for thio relaxers are the same as those for hydroxide relaxers, although the neutralization procedure is different. Relaxer may be applied with bowl and brush, applicator bottle, or the back of a rattail comb. Although all thio relaxers follow the same procedures, different application methods are used for virgin relaxers and retouch relaxers.

IMPLEMENTS AND MATERIALS

Use the same implements and materials as for virgin hydroxide relaxers, but use thio relaxer, pre-neutralizing conditioner, and thio neutralizer.

PREPARATION

Follow the same preparation steps as for virgin hydroxide relaxers. A light shampoo before a thio relaxer is optional. Do not forget to perform an analysis of the client's hair and scalp. Test the hair for elasticity and porosity on several areas of the head. If the hair has poor elasticity, do not perform a relaxer service.

1. Follow the same application procedure as for Procedure 18-7—virgin hydroxide relaxer.
2. Blot excess water from hair.
3. *Optional:* Apply the pre-neutralizing conditioner and comb it through to the ends of the hair. Leave it on for approximately 5 minutes and then rinse. Always follow the manufacturer's directions, and the procedures approved by your instructor.
4. Apply thio neutralizer in 1/4 to 1/2 inch (0.6 to 1.25 centimeters) sections throughout the hair and smooth with your hands or the back of the comb.
5. Process the neutralizer according to the manufacturer's directions.
6. Rinse thoroughly, shampoo, condition, and style.

PROCEDURE FOR THIO RELAXER RETOUCH

1. Follow the preparation and application procedures for Procedure 18-8—hydroxide relaxer retouch. A light shampoo prior to a thio relaxer is optional.
2. Follow the virgin thio relaxer neutralizing and cleanup procedures.

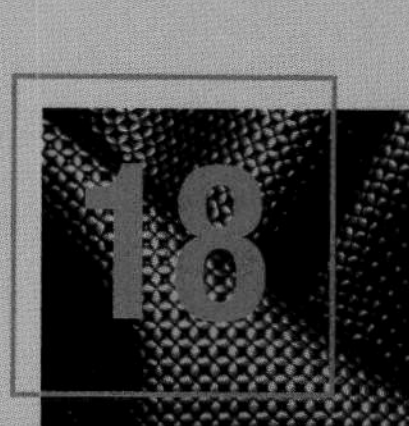

CURL RE-FORMING (SOFT CURL PERMANENTS)

Curl re-forming does not straighten the hair; it simply makes the existing curl larger and looser. A **soft curl permanent** may also be called a Jheri curl (named after beauty pioneer Jheri Redding), or simply a curl. It is a combination of a thio relaxer and a thio permanent that is wrapped on large rods. Soft curl permanents use ATG and oxidation neutralizers, just as thio permanent waves do.

SAFETY PRECAUTIONS FOR HAIR RELAXING AND CURL RE-FORMING

- Perform a thorough hair analysis and client consultation prior to the service.
- Examine the scalp for abrasions. Do not proceed with the service if redness, swelling or skin lesions are present.
- Keep accurate and detailed client records of the services performed and the results achieved.
- Have the client sign a release statement indicating that he/she understands the possible risks involved in the service.
- Do not apply a hydroxide relaxer on hair that has been previously treated with a thio relaxer.
- Do not apply a thio relaxer or soft curl perm on hair that has been previously treated with a hydroxide relaxer.
- Do not chemically relax hair that has been treated with a metallic dye.
- Do not relax overly damaged hair. Suggest instead a series of reconstruction treatments.
- Do not shampoo the client prior to the application of a hydroxide relaxer.
- The client's hair and scalp must be completely dry and free from perspiration prior to the application of a hydroxide relaxer.
- Apply a protective base cream to avoid scalp irritation.
- Wear gloves during the relaxer application.
- Protect the client's eyes.
- If any solution accidentally gets into the client's eye, flush the eye immediately with cool water and refer the client to a doctor.
- Do not allow chemical relaxers to accidentally come into contact with the client's ears, scalp, or skin.
- Perform periodic strand tests to see how fast the natural curls are being removed.
- Avoid scratching the scalp with your comb or fingernails.

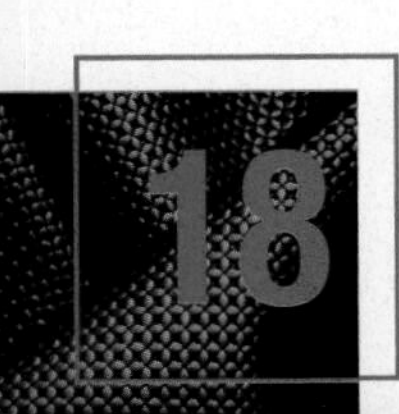

PROCEDURE 18-10

CURL RE-FORMING (SOFT CURL PERM)

IMPLEMENTS AND MATERIALS

- Thio cream relaxer (curl rearranger)
- Thio curl booster
- Pre-neutralizing conditioner (optional)
- Thio neutralizer
- Protective base cream
- Acid-balanced shampoo
- Conditioner
- Plastic or glass bowl
- Applicator brush
- Applicator bottles
- Shampoo cape
- Neutralizing bib
- Disposable gloves
- Cotton coil or rope
- Towels
- Plastic clips
- Styling comb
- Plastic tail comb
- Perm rods
- End papers
- Spray bottle
- Timer

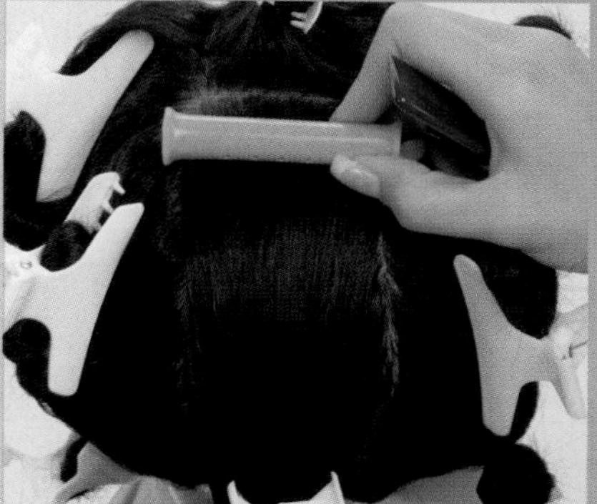

Figure 18-117 Measure panel width.

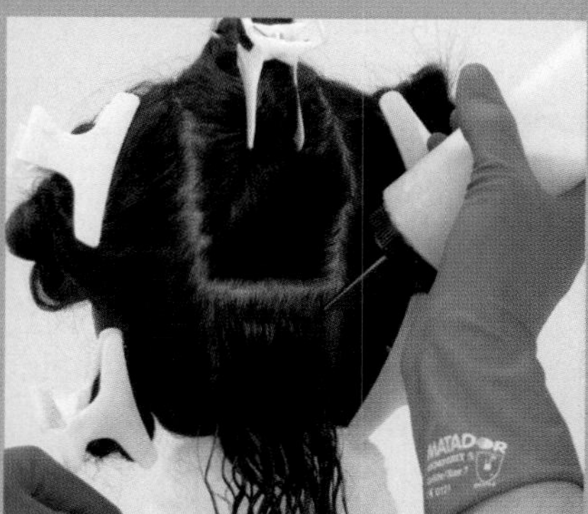

Figure 18-118 Apply thio curl booster.

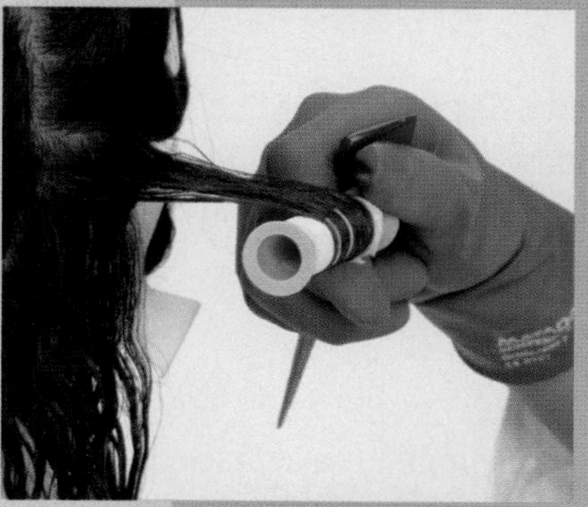

Figure 18-119 Roll hair half off-base.

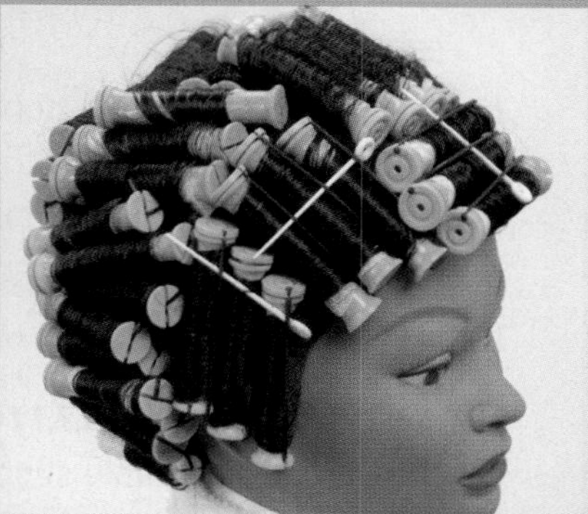

Figure 18-120 Wrap last panel.

PREPARATION

1. Wash your hands.
2. Perform a client consultation, including an analysis of the client's hair and scalp. Note results in the client record.
3. Have the client change into a gown and remove eyeglasses, earrings, and necklace. Drape the client with a shampoo cape, and two towels.
4. *Option:* Shampoo the hair gently and towel-dry. Avoid any irritating scalp manipulations.

PROCEDURE

1. Follow procedure for applying virgin hydroxide relaxer.
2. After rinsing the hair, part it into nine panels. Use the length of the rod to measure the width of the panels (Figure 18-117).
3. **Roll hair.** Wear gloves on both hands and begin wrapping at the most resistant area. Apply and distribute the thio curl booster to each panel as you wrap the hair (Figure 18-118). Make a horizontal parting the same size as the rod. Hold the hair at a 90-degree angle to the head. Using two end papers, roll the hair down to the scalp and position the rod half off base (Figure 18-119). *Option:* Insert roller picks to stabilize the rods and eliminate any tension caused by the band.
4. Continue wrapping the remainder of the first panel using the same technique.
5. Continue wrapping the remaining eight panels in numerical order using the same technique (Figure 18-120).

CAUTION

Hair that has been treated with hydroxide relaxers must not be treated with thio relaxers or soft curl permanents.

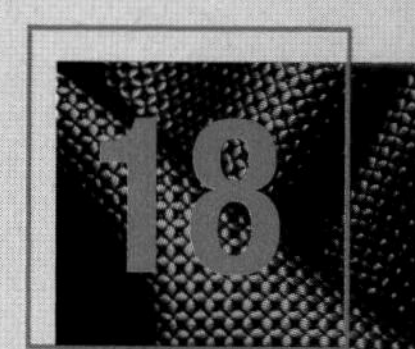

6. Place cotton around the hairline and neck and apply thio curl booster to all the curls until they are completely saturated (Figure 18-121).
7. **Apply plastic cap.** If a plastic cap is used, punch a few holes in the cap and cover all the hair completely. Do not allow the plastic cap to touch the client's skin (Figure 18-122).
8. Check cotton and towels. If they are saturated with solution, replace them.
9. **Process.** Process according to manufacturer's directions. Processing time will vary according to the strength of the product, the hair type and condition, and desired results. Processing usually takes less than 20 minutes at room temperature.
10. Check for proper curl development (Figure 18-123).
11. **Rinse and towel dry hair.** When processing is completed, rinse the hair thoroughly, for at least 5 minutes. Then towel-blot the hair on each rod to remove excess moisture. *Option:* Apply pre-neutralizing conditioner according to the manufacturer's directions.
12. **Neutralize.** Apply the neutralizer slowly and carefully to the hair on each rod. Avoid splashing and dripping. Make sure each rod is completely saturated.
13. **Distribute remaining neutralizer.** Set a timer and neutralize according to the manufacturer's directions. Remove the rods, distribute the remaining neutralizer through the ends of the hair, and rinse thoroughly. *Option:* Shampoo and condition.
14. Style the hair as desired (Figure 18-124).

CLEANUP AND SANITATION

1. Discard all disposable supplies in appropriate receptacles.
2. Disinfect implements and store according to sanitation requirements.
3. Clean, sanitize, and prepare your workstation for the next service.
4. Wash your hands with soap and warm water.
5. Complete the client record.

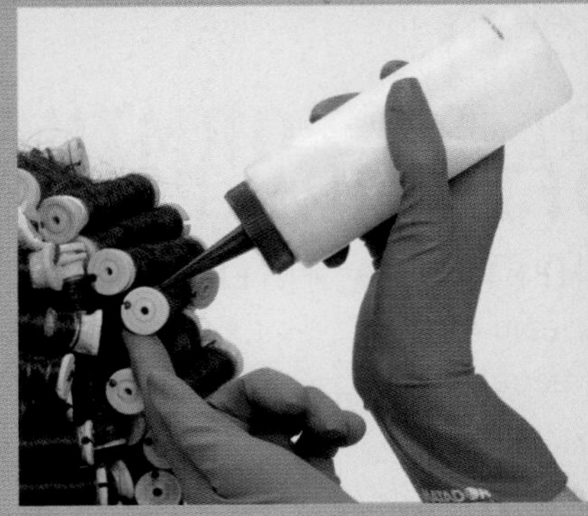

Figure 18-121 Saturate rods with thio booster lotion.

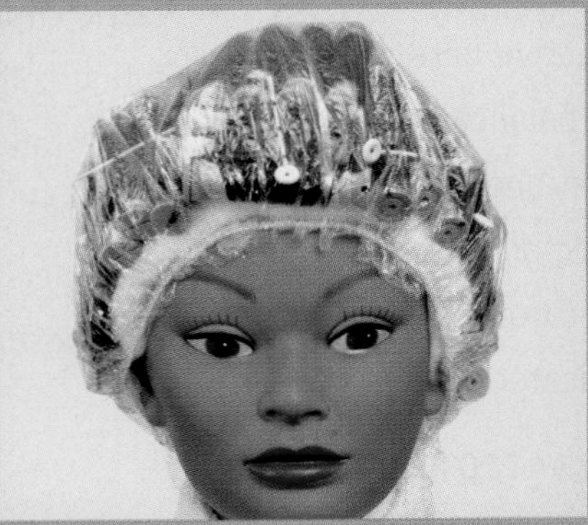

Figure 18-122 Process with plastic cap.

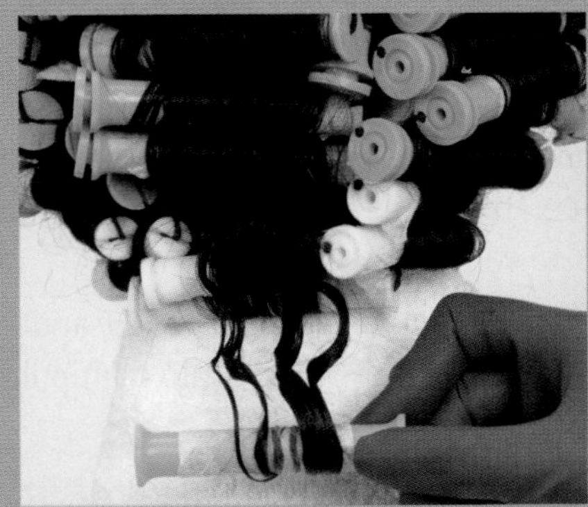

Figure 18-123 Take test curl.

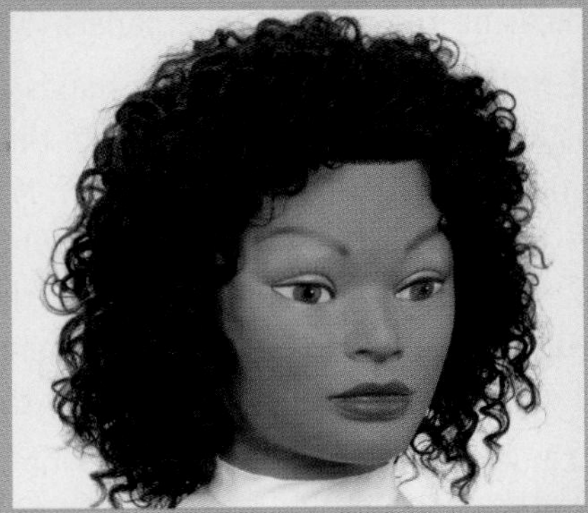

Figure 18-124 Finished soft curl permanent.

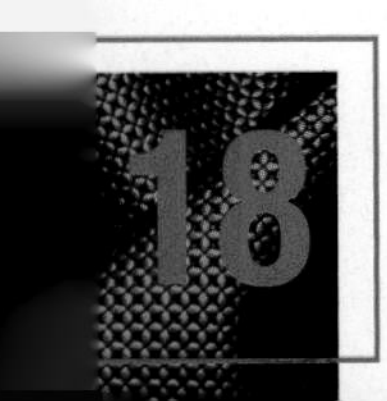

- Do not allow the application of a relaxer retouch to overlap onto previously relaxed hair.
- Never use a strong relaxer on fine or damaged hair. It may cause breakage.
- Do not attempt to remove more than 80 percent of the natural curl.
- Thoroughly rinse the chemical relaxer from the hair. Failure to rinse properly can cause excessive skin irritation and hair breakage.
- Use a normalizing lotion to restore the hair and scalp to their normal acidic pH.
- Use a neutralizing shampoo with a color indicator to guarantee that the hair and scalp have been restored to their normal pH.
- Use a conditioner and wide-tooth comb to eliminate excessive stretching when combing out tangles.
- Do not use hot irons or excessive heat on chemically relaxed hair.

Performing texture services involves using powerful chemicals, which must be handled with the utmost caution. If you act responsibly and perfect your techniques, your services will be in great demand.

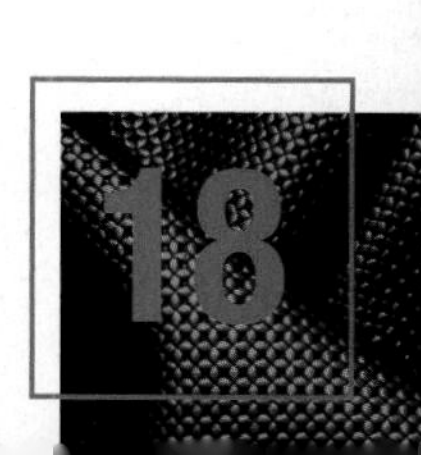

REVIEW QUESTIONS

1. What is the difference between end bonds and side bonds?
2. Describe the three different types of side bonds.
3. How do various hair texture services—wet sets, thermal styling, thio permanents and relaxers, and hydroxide relaxers—change side bonds?
4. What is the difference between a croquignole and a spiral perm wrap?
5. How does the reduction reaction of thio waving solution work?
6. What is the function of thio neutralizer?
7. List and describe the eight major types of permanent waving solutions.
8. Explain the procedure for a soft curl permanent.
9. What is lanthionization?
10. What is the major difference between thio and hydroxide relaxers?
11. What is the difference between thio and hydroxide neutralizers?
12. List at least 10 safety precautions for permanent waving, soft curl permanents, and chemical hair relaxers.

CHAPTER GLOSSARY

acid-balanced waves	Not true acid waves, as they have a pH between 7.8 and 8.2 and use glyceryl monthioglycolate (GMTG) as the primary reducing agent. Acid-balanced waves process at room temperature, do not require the added heat of a hair dryer, process more quickly, and produce firmer curls than true acid waves.
alkaline waves (or cold waves)	Have a pH between 9.0 and 9.6, use ammonium thioglycolate (ATG) as the reducing agent, and process at room temperature.
amino acids	Compounds made up of carbon, oxygen, hydrogen, and nitrogen.
ammonia-free waves	Perms use alkanolamines instead of ammonia, and are popular because of their low odor.
ammonium thioglycolate (ATG)	Active ingredient or reducing agent in alkaline permanents.
base cream or protective base cream	Oily cream used to protect the skin and scalp during hair relaxing.
base control	Position of the rod in relation to its base section, determined by the angle at which the hair is wrapped.
base direction	Angle at which the rod is positioned on the head (horizontally, vertically, or diagonally); also, the directional pattern in which the hair is wrapped.
base placement	The position of the rod in relation to its base section, and is determined by the angle at which the hair is wrapped. Rods can be wrapped on base, half off base, or off base.

CHAPTER GLOSSARY

base relaxers	Relaxers that require the application of protective base cream to the entire scalp prior to the application of the relaxer.
base sections	Subsections of panels into which hair is divided for perm wrapping; one rod is normally placed on each base section.
basic perm wrap	Perm wrap in which all the rods within a panel move in the same direction and are positioned on equal-size bases; all base sections are horizontal, with the same length and width as the perm rod.
bookend wrap	Perm wrap in which one end paper is folded in half over the hair ends like an envelope.
bricklay perm wrap	Perm wrap similar to actual technique of bricklaying; base sections are offset from each other row by row.
chemical hair relaxing	Rearranges the structure of curly hair into a straighter or smoother form.
chemical texture services	Hair services that cause a chemical change that permanently alters the natural wave pattern of the hair.
concave rods	Perm rods that have a smaller diameter in the center that increases to a larger diameter on the ends.
cortex	Middle layer of the hair, located directly beneath the cuticle layer. The cortex is responsible for the incredible strength and elasticity of human hair.
croquignole perms	Perms in which the hair strands are wrapped at an angle perpendicular to the perm rod, in overlapping concentric layers.
curvature perm wrap	Perm wrap in which partings and bases radiate throughout the panels to follow the curvature of the head.
disulfide bonds	Chemical side bonds that are formed when the sulfur atoms in two adjacent protein chains are joined together. Disulfide bonds can only be broken by chemicals and cannot be broken by heat or water.
double flat wrap	Perm wrap in which one end paper is placed under, and one is placed over, the strand of hair being wrapped.
double-rod (piggyback) technique	Perm wrap in which two rods are used for one strand of hair, one on top of the other.
endothermic waves	Perm activated by an outside heat source, usually a conventional hood-type hair dryer.
end papers or end wraps	Absorbent papers used to control the ends of the hair when wrapping and winding hair on perm rods.
exothermic waves	Creates an exothermic chemical reaction that heats up the waving solution and speeds up processing.
glyceryl monothioglycolate (GMTG)	Main active ingredient in true acid and acid-balanced waving lotions.
half off-base placement	Base control in which the hair is wrapped at an angle of 90 degrees (perpendicular) to its base section and the rod is positioned half off its base section.
hydrogen bonds	Weak physical side bonds that are the result of an attraction between opposite electrical charges; easily broken by water, as in wet setting, or heat, as in thermal styling, and re-form as the hair dries or cools.
hydroxide neutralization	The neutralization of hydroxide relaxers is an acid-alkali neutralization reaction that neutralizes (deactivates) the alkaline residues left in the hair by the hydroxide relaxer and lowers the pH of the hair and scalp. Hydroxide relaxer neutralization does not involve oxidation or rebuild disulfide bonds.
hydroxide relaxers	Very strong alkalis with a pH over 13. The hydroxide ion is the active ingredient in all hydroxide relaxers.
lanthionization	Process by which hydroxide relaxers permanently straighten hair; breaks the hair's disulfide bonds during processing and converts them to lanthionine bonds when the relaxer is rinsed from the hair.

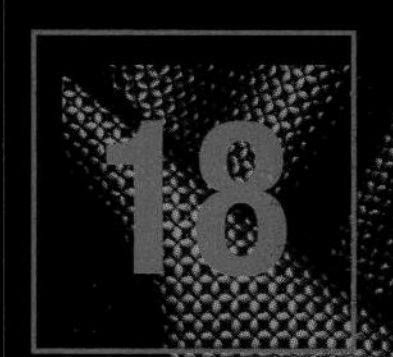

CHAPTER GLOSSARY

loop or circle rod	Tool that is usually about 12 inches long with a uniform diameter along the entire length of the rod.
low-pH waves	Perms that work at a low pH, and use sulfates, sulfites, and bisulfites as an alternative to ammonium thioglycolate.
medulla	Innermost layer of the hair and is often called the pith or core of the hair.
metal hydroxide relaxers	Ionic compounds formed by a metal (sodium, potassium, or lithium) combined with oxygen and hydrogen.
no-base relaxers	Relaxers that do not require application of a protective base cream.
normalizing lotions	Conditioners that restore the hair's natural pH after a hydroxide relaxer and prior to shampooing.
off-base placement	Base control in which the hair is wrapped at a 45-degree angle below perpendicular to its base section, and the rod is positioned completely off its base section.
on-base placement	Base control in which the hair is wrapped at a 45-degree angle beyond perpendicular to its base section and the rod is positioned on its base section.
peptide bonds or end bonds	Chemical bonds that join amino acids together to form polypeptide chains.
polypeptide chains	Long chains of amino acids joined together by peptide bonds.
salt bonds	Relatively weak physical side bonds that are the result of an attraction between opposite electrical charges; easily broken by changes in pH, as in permanent waving, and re-form when the pH returns to normal.
side bonds	Disulfide, salt, and hydrogen bonds that cross-link polypeptide chains together. Side bonds are responsible for the elasticity and incredible strength of the hair.
single flat wrap	Perm wrap that is similar to double flat wrap but uses only one end paper, placed over the top of the strand of hair being wrapped.
soft bender rods	Tool about 12 inches long with a uniform diameter along the entire length. These soft foam rods have a stiff wire inside that permits them to be bent into almost any shape.
soft curl permanent	Combination of a thio relaxer and a thio permanent wrapped on large rods to make existing curl larger and looser.
spiral perm wrap	Hair is wrapped at an angle other than perpendicular to the length of the rod, which causes the hair to spiral along the length of the rod, similar to the grip on a tennis racket.
straight rods	Perm rods that are equal in diameter along their entire length or curling area.
thioglycolic acid	Colorless liquid with a strong unpleasant odor; provides the hydrogen that causes the reduction reaction in permanent waving solutions.
thio neutralization	Stops the action of a permanent wave solution and rebuilds the hair in its new curly form.
thio relaxers	Use the same ammonium thioglycolate (ATG) that is used in permanent waving, but at a higher concentration and a higher pH (above 10).
thio-free waves	Perm that uses cysteamine or mercaptamine instead of ammonium thioglycolate as the primary reducing agent.
true acid waves	Have a pH between 4.5 and 7.0, require heat to process (endothermic), process more slowly than alkaline waves, and do not usually produce as firm a curl as alkaline waves.
weave technique	Wrapping technique that uses zigzag partings to divide base areas.

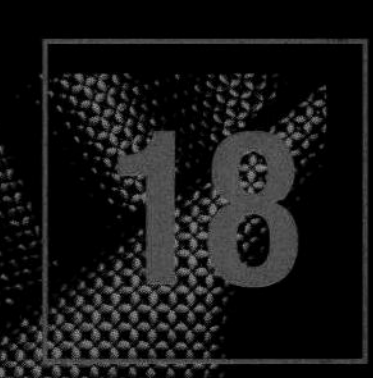

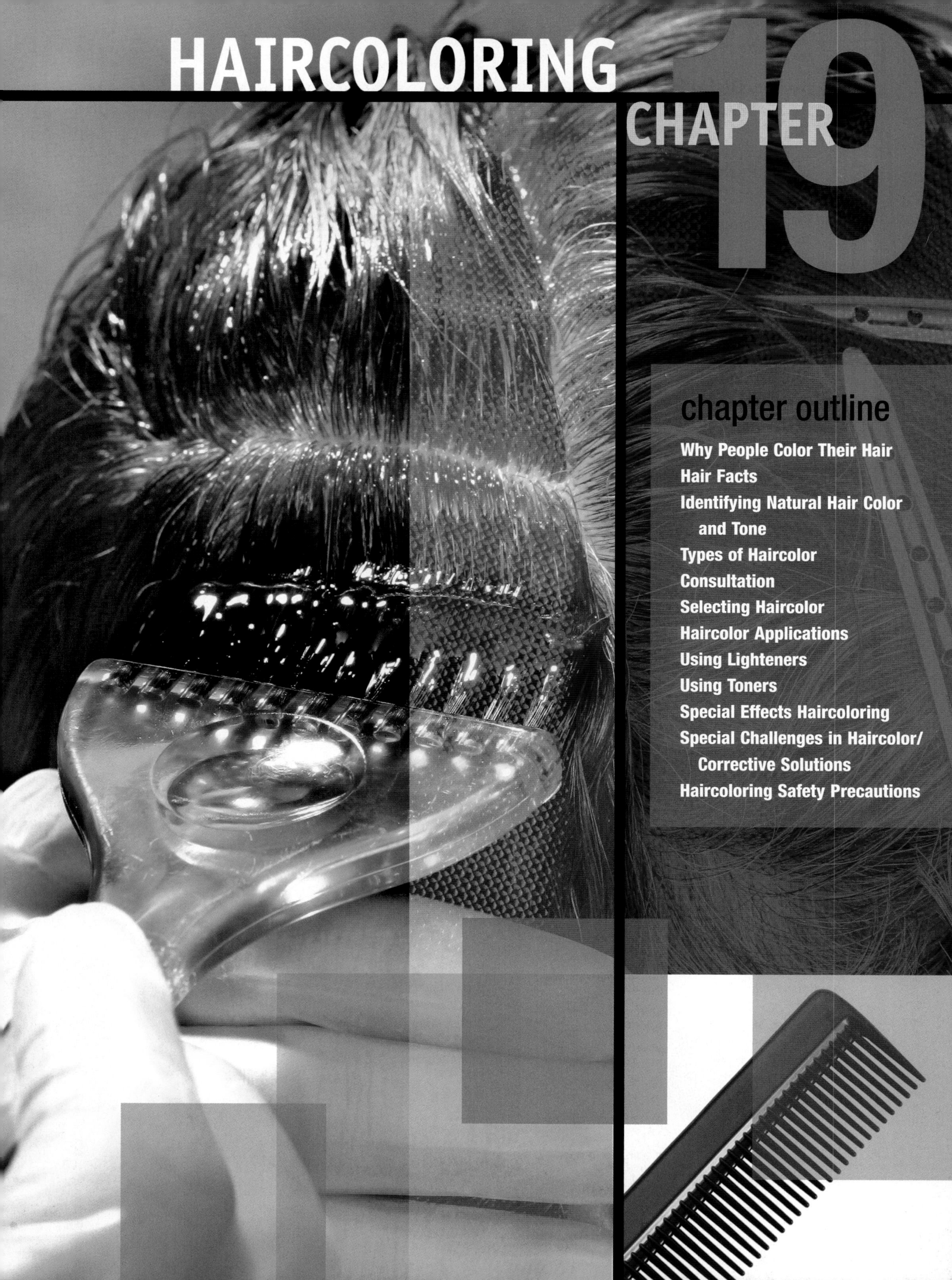

HAIRCOLORING

CHAPTER 19

chapter outline

Learning Objectives

After completing this chapter, you will be able to:

- Identify the principles of color theory and relate them to haircolor.
- Explain level and tone and their role in formulating haircolor.
- List the four basic categories of haircolor, explain their chemical effects on the hair, and give examples of their use.
- Explain the action of hair lighteners.
- Demonstrate application techniques for temporary colors, semipermanent colors, permanent colors, demipermanent colors, and lighteners.
- Demonstrate special-effects haircoloring techniques.

Key Terms

Page number indicates where in the chapter the term is used.

activators pg. 506

aniline derivatives pg. 487

baliage or *free-form technique* pg. 517

base color pg. 483

cap technique pg. 514

color fillers pg. 522

complementary colors pg. 485

conditioner fillers pg. 521

contributing pigment pg. 481

demipermanent haircolor pg. 486

developer pg. 488

double-process application pg. 499

fillers pg. 521

foil techniques pg. 514

glaze pg. 499

hair color pg. 480

haircolor pg. 480

hair lightening pg. 485

highlighting pg. 513

highlighting shampoo pg. 517

law of color pg. 483

level pg. 481

level system pg. 481

lighteners pg. 488

line of demarcation pg. 499

metallic or gradual haircolors pg. 488

natural or vegetable haircolors pg. 487

new growth pg. 507

off-the-scalp lighteners pg. 505

on-the-scalp lighteners pg. 505

oxidation pg. 489

patch test pg. 494

permanent haircolors pg. 487

prelightening pg. 499

presoftening pg. 520

primary colors pg. 483

resistant pg. 481

reverse highlighting or *lowlighting* pg. 513

secondary color pg. 484

semipermanent haircolor pg. 486

single-process haircoloring pg. 499

slicing pg. 514

soap cap pg. 523

special effects haircoloring pg. 513

temporary haircolor pg. 486

tertiary color pg. 484

tone pg. 482

toners pg. 489

virgin application pg. 499

volume pg. 488

weaving pg. 514

One of the most creative, challenging, and popular salon services is haircoloring. It also has the potential for being one of the most lucrative areas in which a stylist can choose to work. You only have to look around a restaurant, or while you are standing in line to see a movie to know this is true. Nearly all adults and many teens now color their hair. You will probably find that most of your clients, at some time or another, will want to enhance or change their hair color, or cover gray. Clients who have their hair colored usually visit the salon every 4 to 12 weeks. These are the kinds of "regulars" you want in your client base (Figure 19-1).

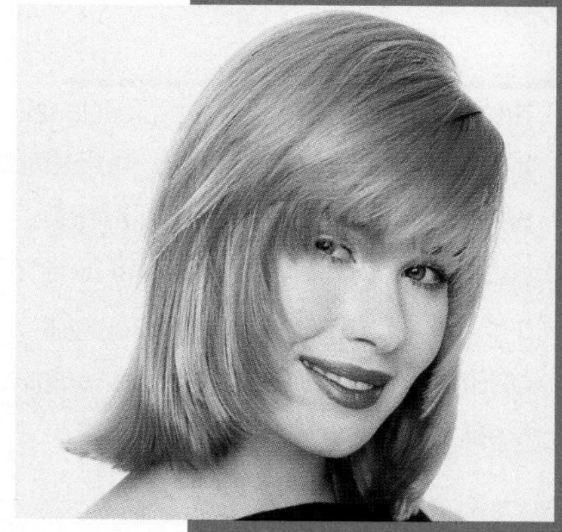

Figure 19–1 Haircoloring is a popular salon service.

Haircoloring is both a science and an art. A skilled haircolorist needs to become an expert in the following services:

- Enhancing natural hair color
- Blending or covering gray
- Lightening natural hair color
- Depositing color on previously colored hair
- Depositing color on hair that has been lightened
- Creating dimensional color

You have reason to be excited about working in the area of haircoloring. It is artistic, adventurous, and in great demand. If you fully understand both the theory and practical aspects of haircolor, you will have the opportunity to build a significant and loyal client base, and earn a higher income. Statistics show that clients who have haircuts only stay with their stylist for an average of 2 years, while clients who receive color services stay with their stylist for 8 years. Once a stylist demonstrates the ability to skillfully color a client's hair, the client will generally remain loyal.

WHY PEOPLE COLOR THEIR HAIR

It is important to have an understanding of what motivates people to color their hair. This information will help you determine which products and haircolor services are appropriate for your client. A few common reasons clients color their hair include the following:

- Cover up or blend gray (unpigmented) hair
- Enhance an existing haircolor
- Create a fashion statement or statement of self-expression

Did You Know

Haircolor (one word) is a professional, industry-coined term referring to artificial haircolor products and services. **Hair color** (two words) is the natural color of hair. For example, you might say of a client, "Mrs. Bailey's natural hair color is brown."

- Correct unwanted tones in hair caused by environmental exposure, such as sun or chlorine
- Accentuate a particular haircut

Many people experiment with haircoloring. When a client turns to you for advice and service, you need to have a thorough understanding of the hair structure, and how haircoloring products affect it. As a trained professional, you will learn which shades of color are most flattering on your clients, and which products and techniques will achieve the desired look.

HAIR FACTS

The structure of the client's hair and the desired results determine which haircolor to use. The hair structure affects the quality and ultimate success of the haircolor service. Some haircolor products may cause a dramatic change in the structure of the hair, while others cause relatively little change. Knowing how products affect the hair will allow you to make the best choices for your client.

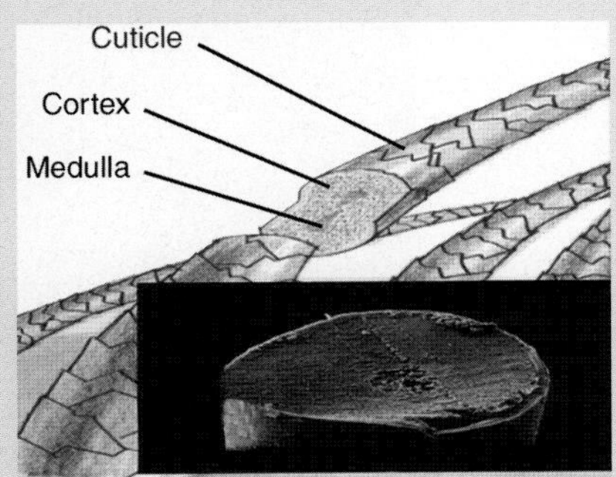

Figure 19-2 A cross-section of the hair shaft.

HAIR STRUCTURE

In this section, the structure of hair is quickly reviewed. For an in-depth discussion, see Chapter 9. Hair is composed of the following three major components (Figure 19-2):

- The cuticle is the outermost layer of the hair. It protects the interior cortex layer and contributes up to 20 percent of the overall strength of the hair.
- The cortex is the middle layer and gives the hair the majority of its strength and elasticity. A healthy cortex contributes about 80 percent to the overall strength of the hair. It contains the natural pigment called melanin that determines hair color. Melanin granules are scattered between the cortex cells like chips in a chocolate chip cookie.
- The medulla is the innermost layer. It is sometimes absent from the hair and does not play a role in the haircoloring process.

TEXTURE

Hair texture is the diameter of an individual hair strand. Large-, medium-, and small-diameter hair strands translate into coarse, medium, and fine hair textures, respectively. Melanin is distributed differently according to texture. The melanin granules in fine hair are grouped more tightly, so the hair takes color faster and can look darker. Medium-textured hair has an average reaction to haircolor. Coarse-textured hair has a larger diameter and can take longer to process (Figure 19-3).

DENSITY

Another aspect of hair that plays a role in haircoloring is density. Hair density, the number of hairs per square inch, can range from thin to

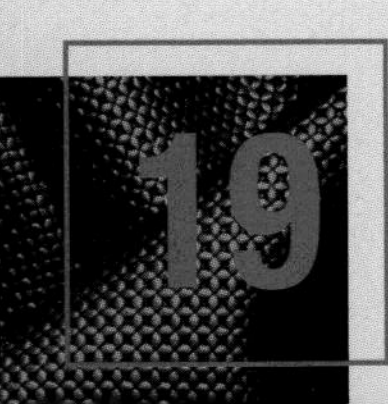

thick. Density must be taken into account when applying haircolor to ensure proper coverage.

POROSITY

Porosity is the hair's ability to absorb moisture. Porous hair accepts haircolor faster, and can result in more color than less porous hair. Degrees of porosity are described below.

- *Low porosity.* The cuticle is tight. The hair is **resistant,** which means it is difficult for moisture or chemicals to penetrate, and thus requires a longer processing time.
- *Average porosity.* The cuticle is slightly raised. The hair is normal and processes in an average amount of time.
- *High porosity.* The cuticle is lifted. The hair is overly porous and takes color quickly; color also tends to fade quickly.

To review the test for porosity, take a strand of several hairs from four different areas of the head: the front hairline, the temple, the crown, and the nape. Hold the strand securely with one hand and slide the thumb and forefinger of the other hand from the ends to the scalp. If the hair feels smooth and the cuticle is compact, dense, and hard, it has low porosity. If you can feel a slight roughness, it has average porosity. If the hair feels very rough, dry, or breaks, it has high porosity.

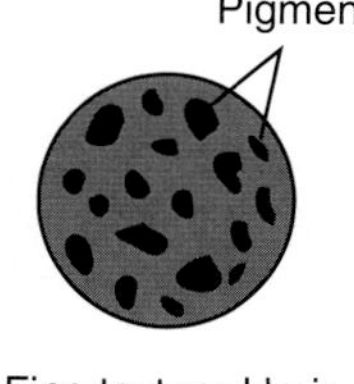

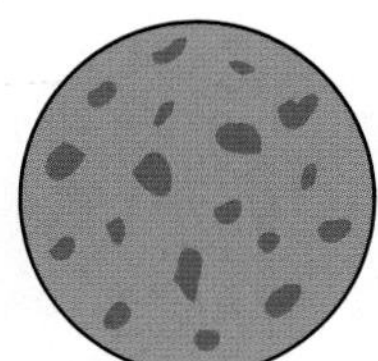

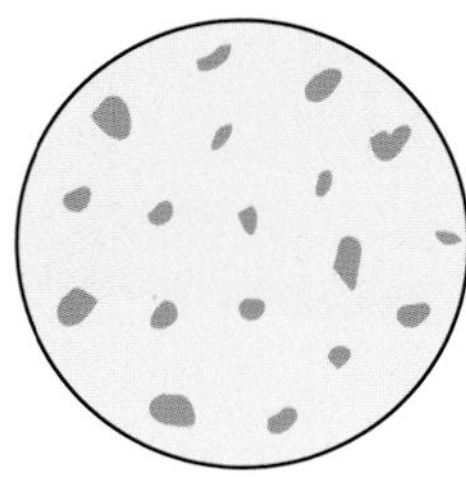

Figure 19–3 Melanin distribution according to hair texture.

IDENTIFYING NATURAL HAIR COLOR AND TONE

Learning to identify a client's natural hair color is the most important step in becoming a good colorist. Natural hair color ranges from black to dark brown to red, and from dark blond to light blond. Hair color is unique to each individual; no two people have exactly the same color. There are two types of melanin in the cortex:

- Eumelanin is the melanin that lends black and brown colors to hair.
- Pheomelanin is the melanin that gives blond and red colors to hair.

Note: Natural hair color contains both pheomelanin and eumelanin.

Contributing pigment (undertone) lies under the natural hair color and must be taken into consideration when you select a haircolor. Generally, when you lighten natural hair color, you expose contributing pigment. Haircoloring modifies this pigment to create new pigment.

THE LEVEL SYSTEM

Level is the unit of measurement used to identify the lightness or darkness of a color. Level is the saturation, density, or concentration of color. The level of color answers the following question: How much color? Colorists use the **level system** to determine the lightness or darkness of colors (Figure 19-4). Haircolor levels are arranged on a scale of 1 to 10, with 1

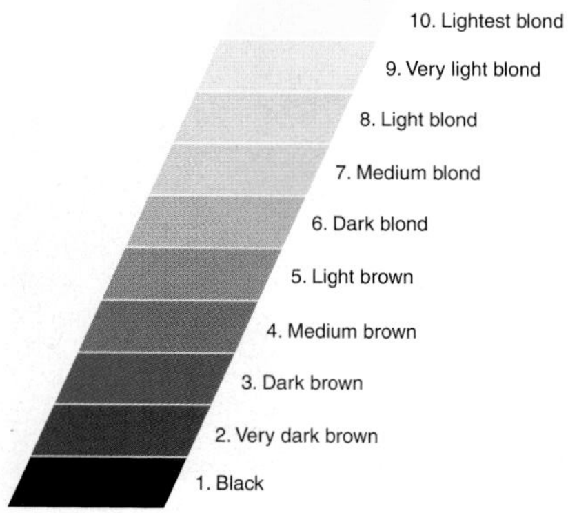

Figure 19–4 Natural hair color levels.

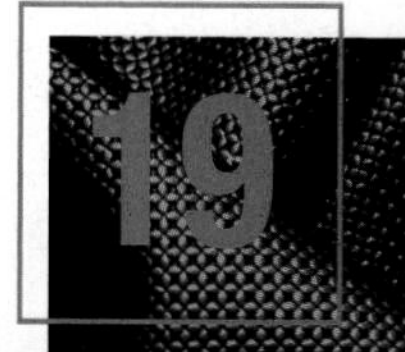

being the darkest, and 10 the lightest. Although the names for the color levels may vary among manufacturers, the important thing is being able to identify the degrees of lightness to darkness in each level.

TONE OR HUE OF COLOR

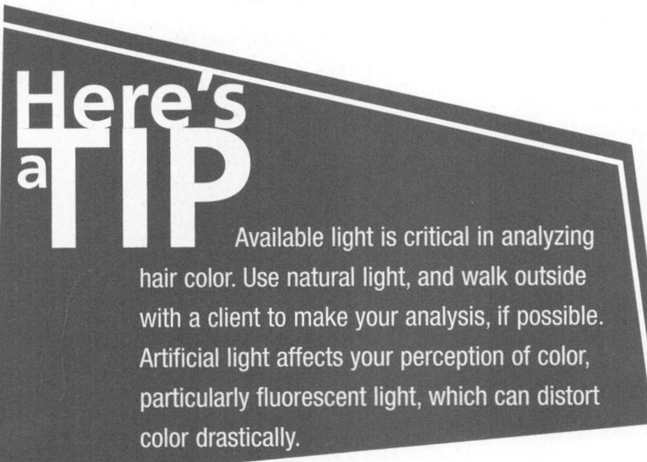

Available light is critical in analyzing hair color. Use natural light, and walk outside with a client to make your analysis, if possible. Artificial light affects your perception of color, particularly fluorescent light, which can distort color drastically.

The **tone** or hue of color is the balance of color. The tone or hue answers the question of which color to use based on the client's desired results. These tones can be described as warm, cool, or neutral.

Warm tones can look lighter than their actual level. These tones are golden, orange, red, and yellow. Some haircolors use words such as auburn, amber, copper, strawberry, and bronze, which may be a better way to discuss haircolor with the client. For example 6RO is a level-6 blond with a red-orange tone, but your client will more easily understand the term "dark strawberry blond."

Cool tones can look deeper than their actual level. These tones are blue, green, and violet. Some describe cool tones as smoky or ash to the client. For example, 4B is a level-4 brown with a blue tone.

Natural tones are warm tones, and are described as sandy or tan. Start by using natural tones in your formulations when you are first learning to color hair. Add ½ ounce of another tone to change the result. As you do this you will begin to see how different tones create different results. Remember, you can make a color as bright or as soft as you like. Color intensifiers serve this purpose.

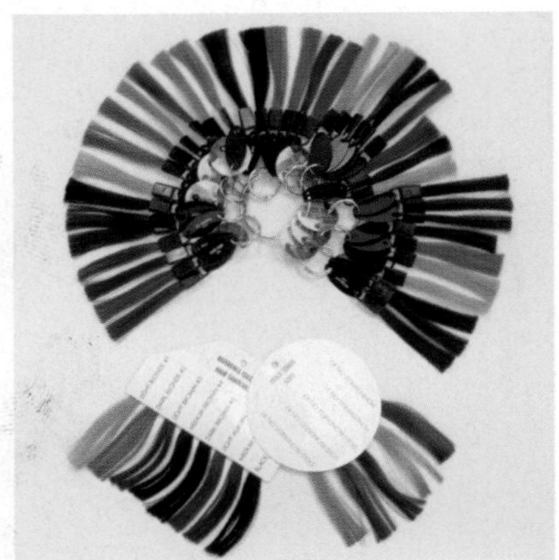

Figure 19-5 Manufacturers' swatches are a useful tool.

IDENTIFYING NATURAL LEVEL AND TONE

Identifying natural levels is the first step in performing a haircolor service. Your most valuable tool is the color wheel. Haircolor swatch books provide a visual representation as well (Figure 19-5).

To determine the natural level, perform the following four steps:

1. Take a ½-inch square section in the crown area and hold it up from the scalp, allowing light to pass through (Figure 19-6).
2. Using the natural level-finder swatches provided by the manufacturer, select a swatch that you think matches the section of hair and place it against the hair. Remember, you are trying to determine depth level (darkness or lightness). Do not part or hold the hair flat against the scalp; that will give you an incorrect reading, as the hair will appear darker (Figure 19-7).
3. Move the swatch from the scalp area along the hair strand.
4. Determine the natural-hair color level.

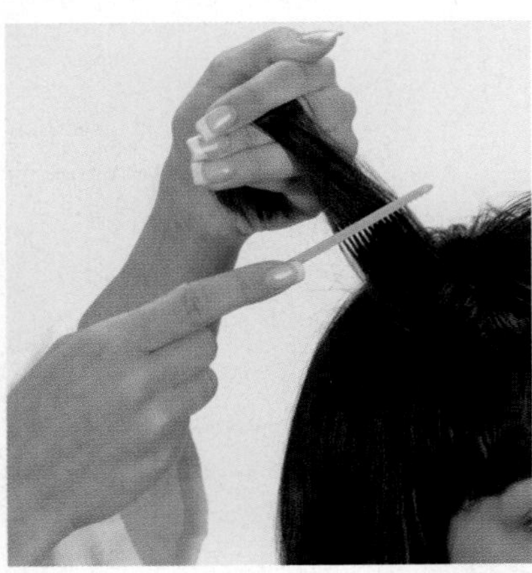

Figure 19-6 Take a ½-inch square section in the crown.

GRAY HAIR

Gray hair is normally associated with aging. Even though the loss of pigment increases as a person ages, few people ever become completely gray haired. Most retain a certain percentage of pigmented hair. The gray can be solid or blended throughout the head as in salt and pepper hair

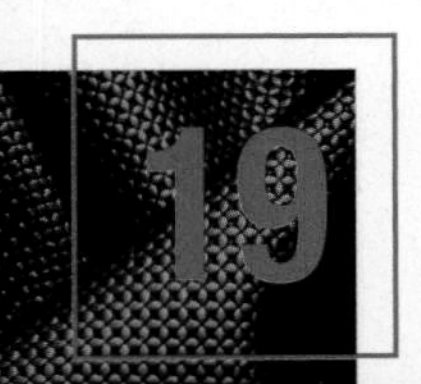

(see Table 19-1). Gray hair requires special attention in formulating haircolor (Figure 19-8). This will be discussed later in the chapter.

COLOR THEORY

Color is described as a property of objects that depends on the *light they reflect* and is perceived (by the human eye) as red, green, blue, or other shades. Thus, colors (the light reflected by objects that is perceivable) by definition is in the visible spectrum of light (see Chapter 11). Before you attempt to apply haircoloring products, it is important to have a general understanding of color. All are developed from primary and secondary colors. A **base color** is the predominant tone of a color. For example, haircolor with a violet base color will deliver cool results and will help minimize unwanted yellow tones. A blue-base haircolor will provide the coolest results and minimize orange tones in the hair. A red-orange base will create the kind of bright, warm results clients are looking for when they wish to be redheads. Gold bases create beautiful golden haircolor, from brunettes to light blonds. These are just a few examples of base colors.

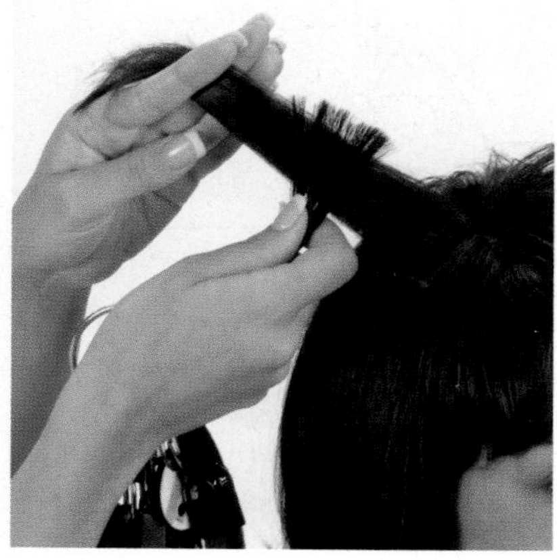

Figure 19-7 Hold the color swatch against the hair strand.

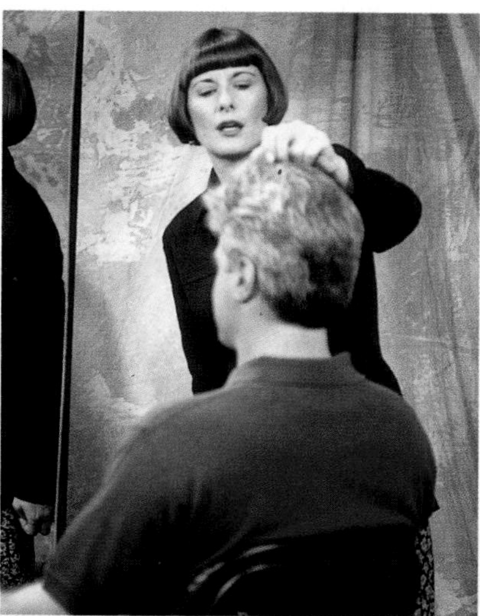

Figure 19-8 Many people choose to cover or blend gray hair.

THE LAW OF COLOR

The **law of color** is a system for understanding color. When combining colors, you will always get the same result from the same combination. Equal parts of red and blue mixed together always make violet. Equal parts of blue and yellow always make green. Equal parts of red and yellow always make orange. The color wheels in Figures 9-9 through 9-11 will help you understand colors.

PRIMARY COLORS

Primary colors are pure colors that cannot be achieved from mixing colors. Primary colors are blue, red, and yellow. All colors are created from these three primaries. Colors with a predominance of blue are cool colors, whereas colors with a predominance of red and/or yellow are warm colors (Figure 19-9).

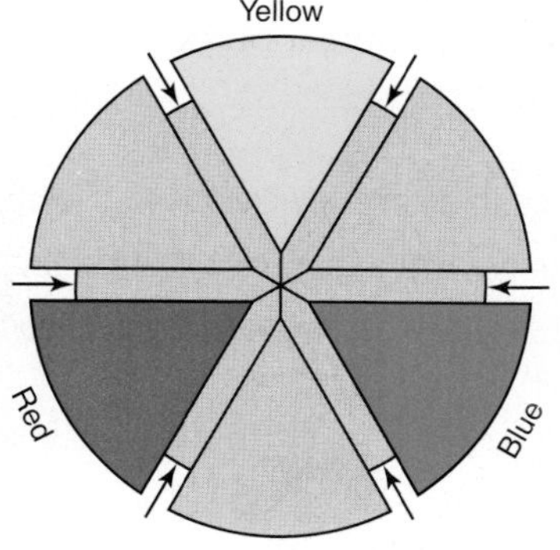

Figure 19-9 Primary colors.

PERCENTAGE OF GRAY HAIR	Characteristics
30%	More pigmented than gray hair
50%	Even mixture of gray and pigmented hair
70 to 90%	More gray than pigmented; most of remaining pigment is located in the back of the head
100%	Virtually no pigmented hair; tends to look white

Table 19-1 Determining the Percentage of Gray Hair

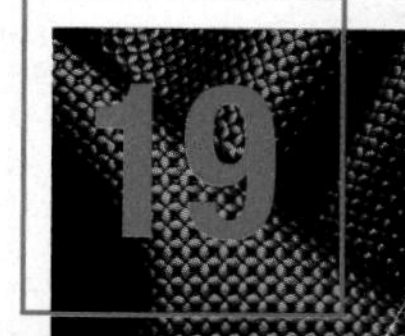

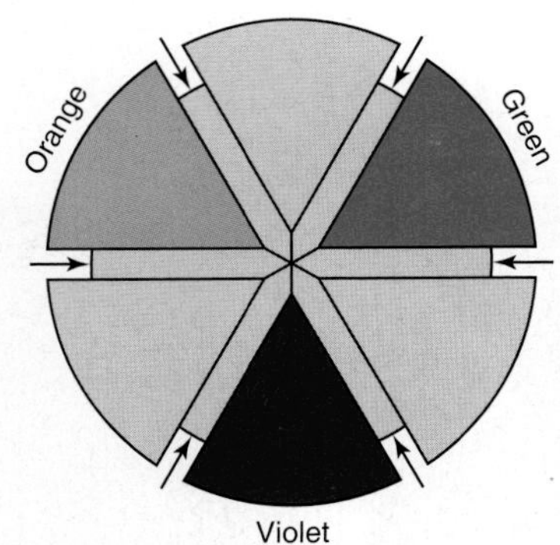

Figure 19-10 Secondary colors.

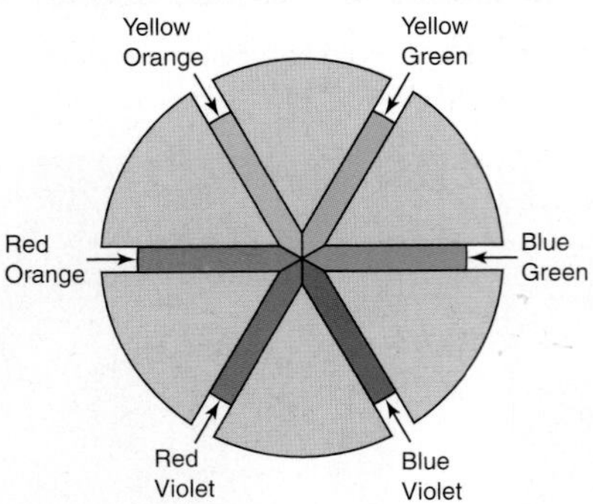

Figure 19-11 Tertiary colors.

Blue is the strongest of the primary colors, and is the only cool primary color. In addition to coolness, blue can also bring depth or darkness to any color.

Red is the medium primary color. Adding red to blue-based colors will make them appear lighter; red added to yellow colors will cause them to become darker.

Yellow is the weakest of the primary colors. When you add yellow to other colors, the resulting color will look lighter and brighter.

When all three primary colors are present in equal proportions, the resulting color is black, white, or gray depending on the level of the color. It is helpful to think of hair colors in terms of their relative proportions of primary colors. Natural brown, for example, has the primary colors in the following proportions: blue-B, red-RR, and yellow-YYY.

SECONDARY COLORS

A **secondary color** is a color obtained by mixing equal parts of two primary colors. The secondary colors are green, orange, and violet. Green is an equal combination of blue and yellow. Orange is an equal combination of red and yellow. Violet is an equal combination of blue and red (Figure 19-10).

TERTIARY COLORS

A **tertiary color** is an intermediate color achieved by mixing a secondary color and its neighboring primary color on the color wheel in equal amounts. The tertiary colors include blue-green, blue-violet, red-violet, red-orange, yellow-orange, and yellow-green. Natural-looking haircolor is made up of a combination of primary and secondary colors (Figure 19-11).

ACTIVITY

Using modeling clay that represents the three primary colors—red, blue, and yellow—create secondary and tertiary colors. You will see that if you mix red clay with yellow clay in equal proportions, you will get orange. If you mix red clay with the orange clay, what is the result? What happens if you change the proportion of each color? The combinations are endless (Figure 19-12).

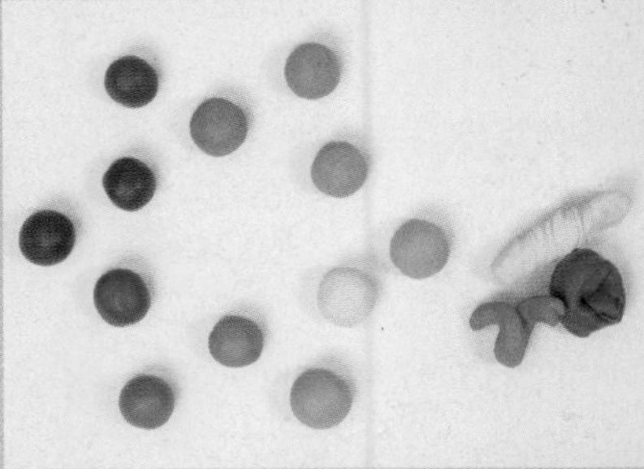
Figure 19-12 Creating the color wheel with clay.

COMPLEMENTARY COLORS

Complementary colors are a primary and secondary color positioned directly opposite each other on the color wheel. Complementary colors include blue and orange, red and green, and yellow and violet.

Complementary colors neutralize each other (Figure 19-13). When formulating haircolor, you will find that it is often your goal to emphasize or distract from skin tones or eye color. You may also want to neutralize or refine unwanted tones in the hair. Understanding complementary colors will help you choose the correct tone to accomplish that goal.

Figure 19-13 Complementary colors neutralize each other.

TYPES OF HAIRCOLOR

Haircoloring products generally fall into two categories: nonoxidative and oxidative. The classifications of nonoxidative haircolor are temporary and semipermanent (traditional). The classifications of oxidative haircolor are demipermanent (deposit-only) and permanent (lift and deposit) (see Table 19-2). All these products, except temporary, require a patch test.

Lighteners, metallic haircolors, and natural colors are also discussed in this chapter. Each of these categories has a unique chemical composition that, in turn, affects the final color result and how long it will last.

First, let us discuss the process of **hair lightening,** often referred to as "bleaching" or "decolorizing," which is a chemical process involving the diffusion of the natural hair color pigment or artificial haircolor from the hair. This process is essential to both permanent haircolor and hair lighteners.

All permanent haircolor products and lighteners contain both a developer, or oxidizing agent, and an alkalizing ingredient (see Chapter 10). The roles of the alkalizing ingredient—ammonia or an ammonia substitute—follow:

- Raise the cuticle of the hair so that the haircolor can penetrate into the cortex.
- Increase the penetration of dye within the hair.
- Trigger the lightening action of peroxide.

When the haircolor containing the alkalizing ingredient is combined with the developer (usually hydrogen peroxide), the peroxide becomes alkaline and decomposes, or breaks up. Lightening occurs when the alkaline peroxide breaks up (decolorizes) the melanin.

CLASSIFICATIONS	Uses
Temporary color	Creates fun, bold results that easily shampoo from the hair Neutralizes yellow hair
Semipermanent color	Introduces a client to haircolor services Adds subtle color results Tones prelightened hair
Demipermanent color	Blends gray hair Enhances natural color Tones prelightened hair Refreshes faded color Filler in color correction
Permanent haircolor	Changes existing haircolor Covers gray Creates bright or natural-looking haircolor changes

Table 19-2 Review of Haircolor Categories and Their Uses

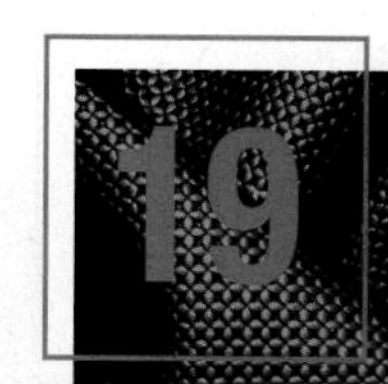

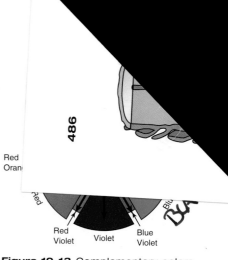

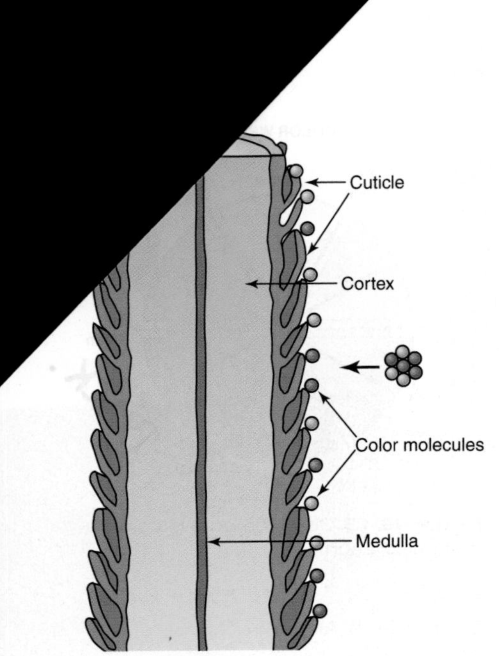

Figure 19-14 Action of temporary haircolor.

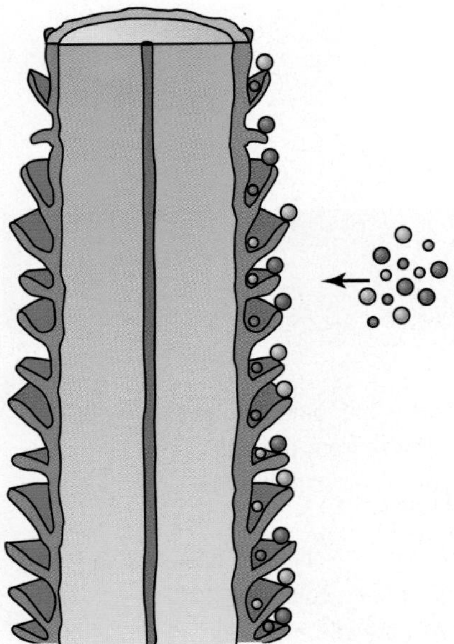
Figure 19-15 Action of semipermanent haircolor.

TEMPORARY HAIRCOLOR

For those who wish to neutralize yellow hair or unwanted tones, **temporary haircolor** is a good choice. The pigments in temporary color are large and do not penetrate the cuticle layer, allowing only a coating action that may be removed by shampooing (Figure 19-14). Temporary haircolors are nonoxidation colors that make only a physical change, not a chemical change, in the hair shaft, and no patch test is required.

Temporary haircolors are available in the following variety of colors and products:

- Color rinses applied weekly to shampooed hair to add color; the hair is styled dry
- Colored mousses and gels used for slight color and for dramatic effects
- Hair mascara used for dramatic effects
- Spray-on haircolor that is easy to apply; used for special effects
- Color-enhancing shampoos used to brighten, impart slight color, and eliminate unwanted tones

SEMIPERMANENT HAIRCOLOR

Traditional **semipermanent haircolor** is formulated to last through several shampoos, depending on the hair's porosity. The pigment molecules are small enough to partially penetrate the hair shaft and stain the cuticle layer, but they are also small enough to diffuse out of the hair during shampooing, thus fading with each shampoo. Traditional semipermanent haircolor only lasts 4 to 6 weeks, depending on how frequently the hair is shampooed. Semipermanent haircolor is a nonoxidation haircolor. It is not mixed with peroxide, and only deposits color. It does not lighten the hair, so it does not require maintenance of new growth. Although it is considered far more gentle than permanent haircolor, it contains some of the same dyes and requires a patch test 24 to 48 hours before application (Figure 19-15). Traditional semipermanent colors are used right out of the bottle.

Demipermanent haircolor (also called deposit-only haircolor by some manufacturers) is formulated to deposit, but not lift (lighten) color and are often called non-lift deposit-only colors. These products are able to deposit without lifting because they are usually less alkaline than permanent colors and are mixed with a low-volume developer. Decolorization requires a high pH and a high concentration of peroxide.

Many demipermanent colors use alkalizing agents other than ammonia, and oxidizing agents other than hydrogen peroxide. It is important to note that these products are not necessarily any less damaging because of the type of alkalizing agent or oxidizer that is used. If they are milder, it is because the concentration of these active ingredients is lower.

No-lift deposit-only haircolors are ideal for the following objectives:

- Introducing a client to a color service, as these products create a change in tone without lightening the natural hair color

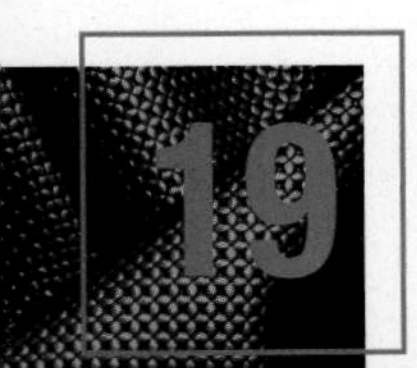

- Blending or covering gray
- Refreshing faded permanent color on the midshaft and ends
- Color corrections and restoring natural color

By their very nature, no-lift deposit-only haircolors deepen or create a change in tone on the natural hair color (Figure 19-16). In recent years, no-lift deposit-only haircolors have been used exclusively on the middle of the hair shaft to the ends after permanent color has been applied to the new growth or scalp area. This reduces the buildup that can occur on previously colored hair, and is also less aggressive, resulting in less fading over time.

No-lift, deposit-only haircolor is available as a gel, cream, or liquid. It requires a patch test 24 to 48 hours before application.

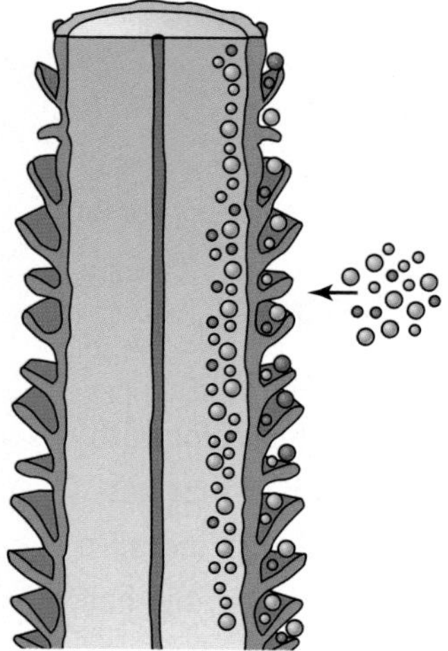

Figure 19-16 Action of demipermanent haircolor.

PERMANENT HAIRCOLOR

Permanent haircolors can lighten and deposit color at the same time and in a single process because they are more alkaline than no-lift deposit-only colors and are usually mixed with a higher-volume developer.

Permanent haircolor is used to match, lighten, and cover gray hair. Permanent haircolor products require a patch test 24 to 48 hours before application.

Permanent haircolors contain uncolored dye precursors, which are very small and can easily penetrate into the hair shaft. These dye precursors, also referred to as **aniline derivatives,** combine with hydrogen peroxide to form larger, permanent dye molecules. These molecules are trapped within the cortex of the hair and cannot be easily shampooed out (Figures 19-17 and 19-18). Permanent haircolors can also lighten (make a permanent change in) the natural hair color, which is why these products are considered permanent.

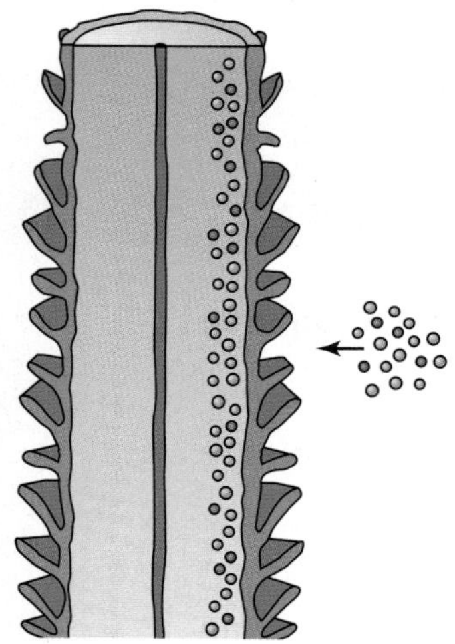

Figure 19-17 Action of permanent haircolors.

Permanent haircoloring products are regarded as the best products for covering gray hair. They remove natural pigment from the hair through lightening; while at the same time add artificial color to the hair. The action of removing and adding color at the same time, blending gray and non-gray hair uniformly, results in a natural-looking color.

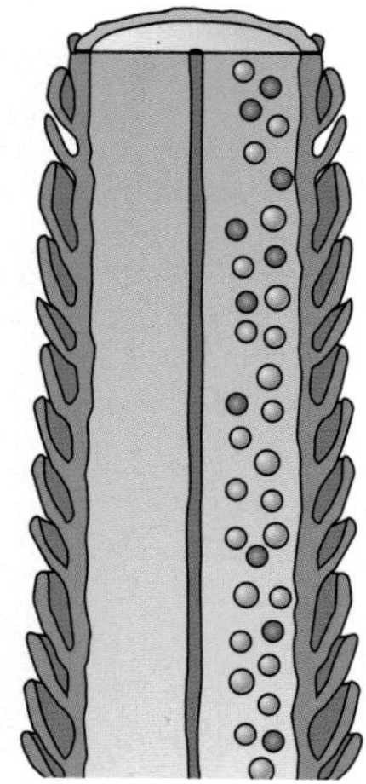

Figure 19-18 Permanent haircolor molecules inside the cortex.

NATURAL AND METALLIC HAIRCOLORS

A group of haircolors that are not generally used in the salon, but you should still be familiar with, are natural or vegetable haircolors and metallic haircolors, also referred to as gradual colors.

NATURAL HAIRCOLORS

Natural or **vegetable haircolors** such as henna are natural colors obtained from the leaves or bark of plants. They do not lighten natural hair color. The color result tends to be weak, and the process tends to be lengthy and messy. Also, shade ranges are limited. For instance, henna is usually available only in clear, black, chestnut, and auburn tones. Finally, when a client who has used natural haircolor comes to the salon for chemical haircoloring services, she may be distressed to find out that many of these chemical products cannot be applied over natural haircolors.

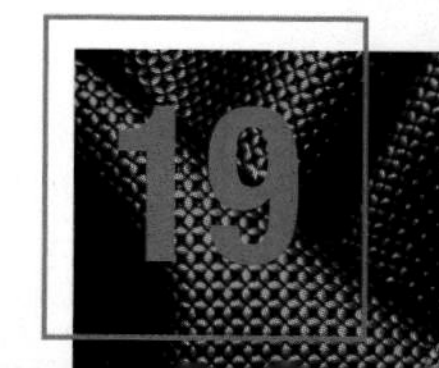

CAUTION

Do not use oxidizing haircolor or haircolor with peroxide on hair that has been treated with metallic hair dye. If you do, the hair will swell and smoke, appearing to be boiling from the inside out.

METALLIC HAIRCOLOR

Metallic haircolors, also called **gradual colors,** contain metal salts and change hair color gradually by progressive buildup and exposure to air, creating a dull, metallic appearance. These products require daily application and historically have been marketed to men. The main problems are unnatural-looking colors and a limited range of available colors.

HYDROGEN PEROXIDE DEVELOPERS

A **developer** is an oxidizing agent that, when mixed with an oxidation haircolor, supplies the necessary oxygen gas to develop the color molecules and create a change in natural hair color. Developers, also called oxidizing agents or catalysts, have a pH between 2.5 and 4.5. Although there are a number of developers on the market, hydrogen peroxide (H_2O_2) is the one most commonly used in haircolor.

Volume measures the concentration and strength of hydrogen peroxide. The lower the volume, the less lift is achieved; the higher the volume, the greater the lifting action (Table 19-3). The majority of permanent haircolor products use 10-, 20-, 30-, or 40-volume hydrogen peroxide for proper lift and color development (see Figure 19-19). Store peroxide in a cool, dark, dry place.

VOLUME	When to Use
10 Volume	When less lightening is desired to enhance a client's natural hair color
20 Volume	The standard volume; used to achieve most results with permanent haircolor and used for complete gray coverage
30 Volume	Used for additional life with permanent haircolor
40 Volume	Used with most high-lift colors to provide maximum lift in a one-step color service

Table 19-3 Hydrogen Peroxide Volume and Uses

VOLUME

Use 10 volume when less lightening is desired. 20 volume is used with permanent haircolor, as well as for complete gray coverage. For additional lift, 30 volume is used, and to provide maximum lift in a one-step color service, 40 volume is commonly used.

LIGHTENERS

Lighteners lighten hair by dispersing, dissolving, and decolorizing the natural hair pigment. As soon as hydrogen peroxide is mixed into the lightener formula, it begins to release oxygen.

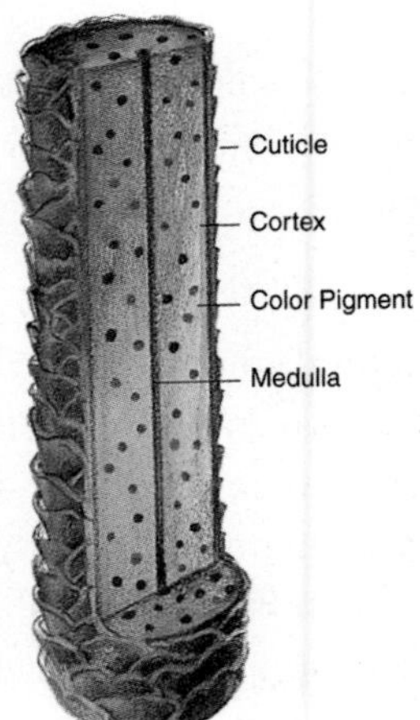

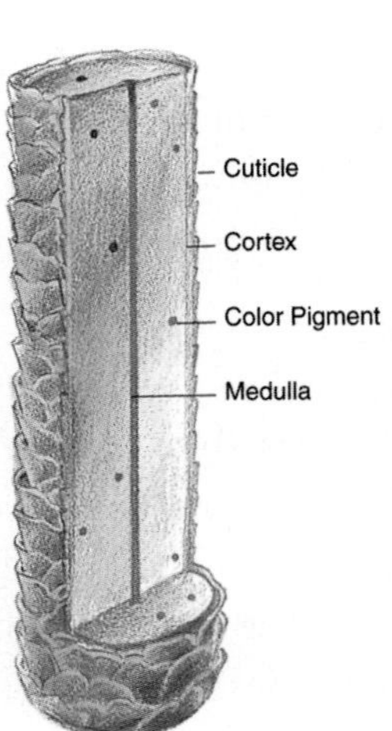

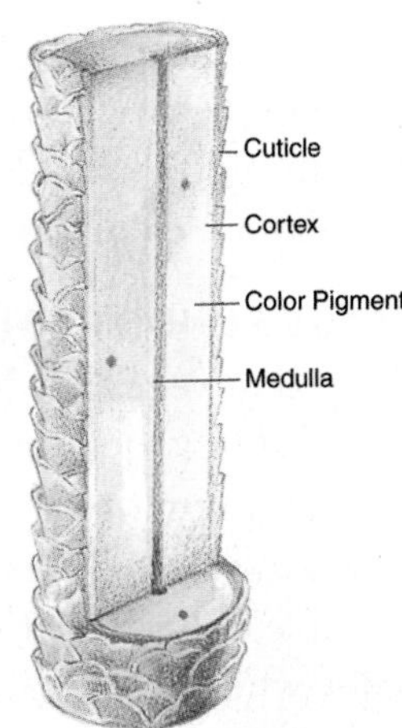

Figure 19-19 Haircolor lighteners diffuse pigments.

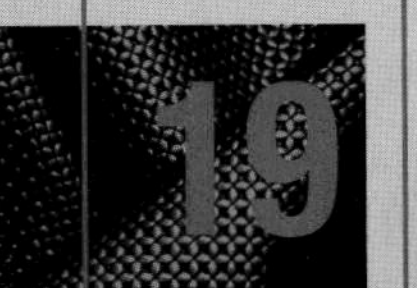

This process, known as **oxidation,** occurs within the cortex of the hair shaft.

Hair lighteners are used to create a light blond shade that is not achievable with permanent haircolor, as well as the following objectives:

- Lighten the hair prior to application of a final color
- Lighten hair to a particular shade
- Brighten and lighten an existing shade
- Lighten only certain parts of the hair
- Lighten dark natural or color-treated levels

THE DECOLORIZING PROCESS

The hair goes through different stages of color as it lightens. The amount of change depends on the amount of pigment in the hair, the strength of the lightening product, and the length of time that the product is processed. During the process of decolorizing, natural hair can go through as many as 10 stages (Figure 19-20).

Decolorizing the hair's natural melanin pigment allows the colorist to create the exact degree of contributing pigment needed for the final result. First, the hair is decolorized to the appropriate level. Then the new color is applied to deposit the desired color. The natural pigment that remains in the hair contributes to the artificial color that is added. Lightening the hair to the correct stage is essential to a beautiful, controlled, final haircoloring result (Figure 19-21).

Toners are traditional semipermanent, demipermanent, and permanent haircolor products that are used on prelightened hair to achieve pale and delicate colors after the decolorizing process.

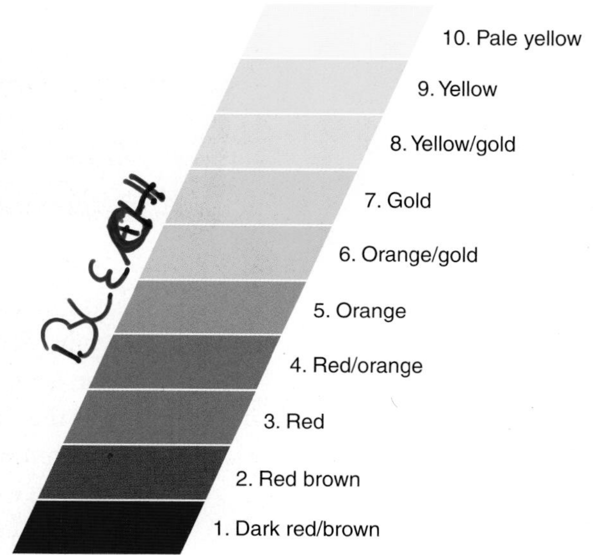

Figure 19-20 Ten degrees of decolorization.

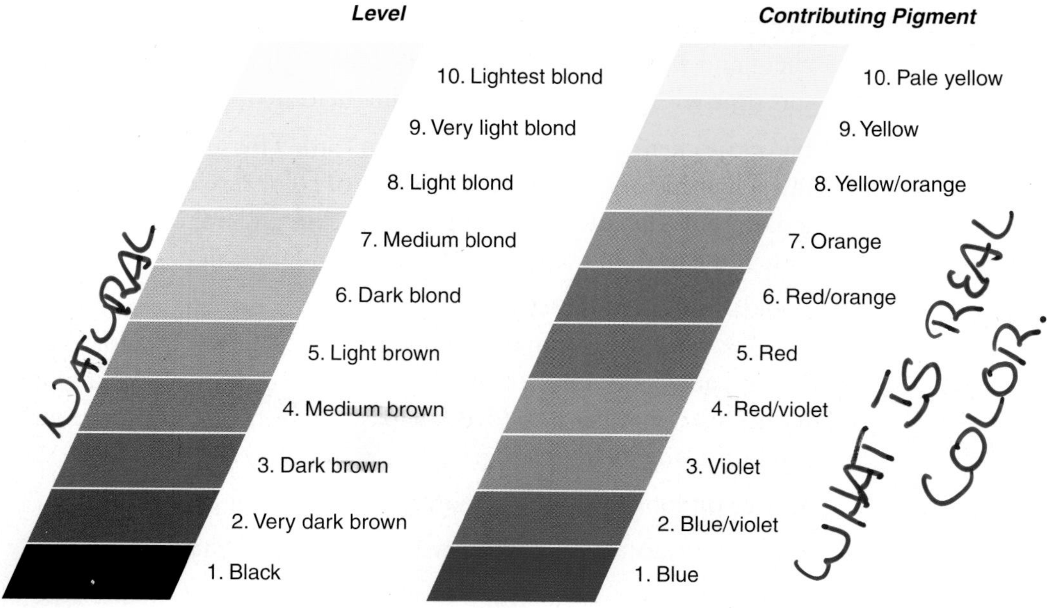

Figure 19-21 Contributing pigment.

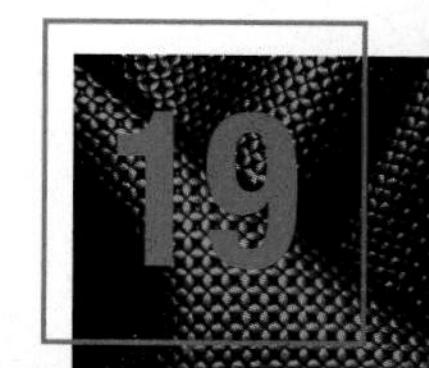

CAUTION

Lightening dark hair to a very pale blond is often difficult without extreme damage to the hair. The client should be alerted to this danger before proceeding with the service.

Not all hair will go through all 10 degrees of decolorization. Each natural hair color starts the decolorization process at a different stage. Remember, the goal is to create the correct degree of contributing pigment as the foundation for the final haircolor.

Hair can not be safely lifted past the pale yellow stage with lightener. The extreme diffusion of color necessary to give hair a white appearance causes excessive damage to the hair. The result is that wet hair feels "mushy" and will stretch without returning to its original length. When dry, the hair is harsh and brittle. Such hair often suffers breakage and will not accept a toner properly. However, this does not mean that only those born with blond hair can be white-blonds. The baby-blond look can be achieved by lightening to pale yellow and neutralizing the unwanted undertone (contributing pigment) with a toner.

CONSULTATION

A haircolor consultation is the most critical part of the color service. The consultation is the first important step in establishing a relationship with your client. During the consultation, your client will communicate what she is looking for in a haircolor service. You will listen carefully, taking in all the information so that you can make an appropriate haircolor recommendation. Allowing sufficient time for the consultation is the single most reliable way to help ensure a client's satisfaction (Figure 19-22).

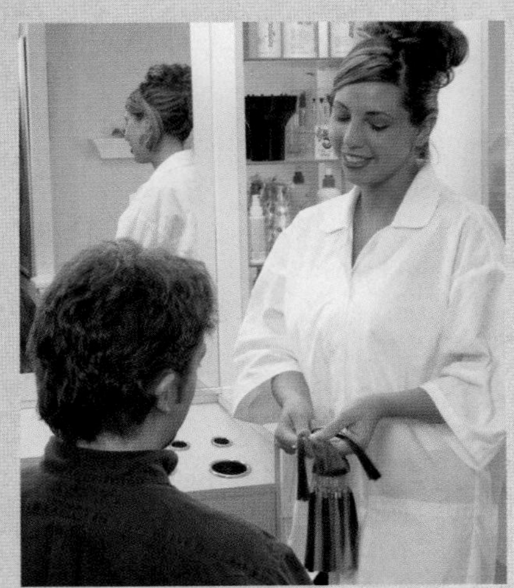

Figure 19-22 A client consultation should precede every haircolor service.

Begin the consultation in an area with proper lighting so that you can accurately determine the client's current hair color. If possible, the walls should be white or neutral. Include the following steps in the consultation.

1. Book 15 minutes extra for the consultation. Introduce yourself to the client and welcome her/him to the salon. Offer a beverage. During this time with a new client, make sure there are no interruptions.
2. Have the client fill out an information card. This allows you to compile a hair history and to note the type of color service the client is looking for. Pay attention to the client's skin and eye color, condition and length of the hair, and amount of gray hair.
3. Look at the client directly. Do not look at her through the mirror. Ask what she is thinking about doing with her hair color. Ask leading questions. Let her talk. Keep her on track by discussing the recent history of her hair (over the past 6 months). Your questions might include the following:
   - Are you looking for a temporary or permanent change?
   - Do you want color all over or just a few highlights?
   - Do you see yourself with a more conservative or dramatic type of color?

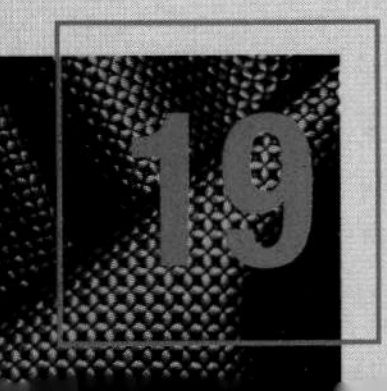

- Have you seen so-and-so's (e.g., a TV celebrity) hair? That color would look great on you.

4. Recommend at least two different haircolor options. Show pictures of different ranges of colors, from brunette to blond, red, and highlighted colors.
5. Review the procedure and application technique, cost of the service, and follow-up maintenance. Sometimes several steps may be necessary to obtain a haircolor result. A client may love a certain haircolor, but may not be able to afford it. Have a more economical backup solution ready.
6. Be honest and do not promise more than you can deliver. If you are faced with a corrective situation, let the client know what you can do today and how many visits it will take to achieve the final results that she wants.
7. Gain approval from the client.
8. Start the haircolor service.
9. Follow through during the service by educating and informing the client about home care, products, and rebooking. Let the client know what type of shampoo and conditioner is needed to maintain the color. Let her know how many weeks it will be before she needs to come back for another service.
10. Fill out the client's haircolor record (Figure 19-23).
    - Use persuasive language in discussing haircolor (e.g., "soft, buttery blond," "rich chocolate brown," "spicy, coppery red").
    - Avoid words that can be interpreted negatively such as "bleached," "frosted," and "roots."
    - Use positive "mood" words to convey the benefits to your client (e.g., "healthy-looking," "richer," "natural-looking," and "subtle").

RELEASE STATEMENT

A release statement is used by schools and many salons when providing chemical services. Its purpose is to explain to clients that there is a risk involved in any chemical service, and if their hair is in questionable condition, the hair may not withstand the requested chemical treatment. It also asks that clients provide more information about any prior chemical services that may affect the current color selection and its end result.

To some degree, the release statement is designed to protect the school or salon from responsibility for accidents or damages, and is required for most malpractice insurance. Take note, however, that a release statement is not a legally binding contract, and will not clear the cosmetologist of responsibility for what may happen to a client's hair (Figure 19-24). If you are unsure about causing excessive damage to the hair, it is wise to decline the service.

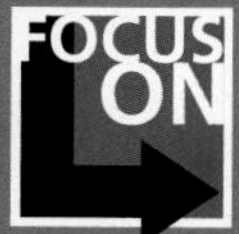

**Focus on . . .
Communication**

Using descriptive language to discuss products and services with your clients is an important part of the communication process. It also helps you sell.

CAUTION

Medications can affect hair color. In the consultation, determine whether the client is taking any medications. Medical treatments for conditions such as diabetes, high blood pressure, and thyroid problems will all affect the outcome of color and most chemical services. Discuss this with your instructor for more information.

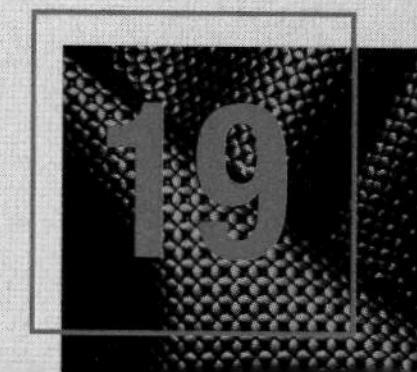

HAIRCOLOR RECORD

Name ______________________________ Tel. ______________________________

Address ______________________________ City ______________________________

Patch Test: ☐ Negative ☐ Positive Date ______________________________

Eye Color ______________________________ Skin Tone ______________________________

DESCRIPTION OF HAIR

Form	**Length**	**Texture**	**Density**	**Porosity**	
☐ straight	☐ short	☐ coarse	☐ low	☐ low	☐ resistant
☐ wavy	☐ medium	☐ medium	☐ medium	☐ average	☐ very resistant
☐ curly	☐ long	☐ fine	☐ high	☐ high	☐ perm. waved

Natural hair color ______________________________

Level (1-10) Tone (Warm, Cool, etc.) Intensity (Mild, Medium, Strong)

Scalp Condition

☐ normal ☐ dry ☐ oily ☐ sensitive

Condition

☐ normal ☐ dry ☐ oily ☐ faded ☐ streaked (uneven)

% unpigmented ______________ Distribution of unpigmented ______________

Previously lightened with ______________ for ______________ (time)

Previously tinted with ______________ for ______________ (time)

☐ original hair sample enclosed ☐ original hair sample not enclosed

Desired hair color ______________________________

Level (1-10) Tone (Warm, Cool, etc.) Intensity (Mild, Medium, Strong)

CORRECTIVE TREATMENTS

Color filler used ______________ Conditioning treatments with ______________

HAIR TINTING PROCESS

whole head ______________ retouch inches (cm) ______________ shade desired ______________

formula: (color/lightener) ______________ application technique ______________

Results: ☐ good ☐ poor ☐ too light ☐ too dark ☐ streaked

Comments: ______________________________

____

____

____

____

Date	**Operator**	**Price**	**Date**	**Operator**	**Price**

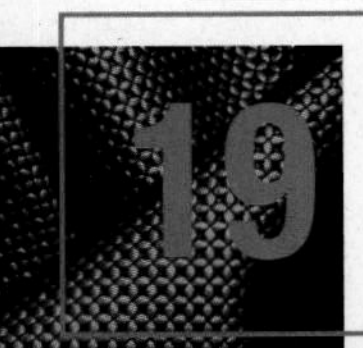

Figure 19-23 Haircolor record.

RELEASE FORM

I, the undersigned, ______________________________
(name)

residing at ______________________________
(street, address)

____
(city, state and zip)

about to receive services in the Clinical Department of

____

and having been advised that the services shall be performed by either students, graduate students, and/or instructors of the school, in consideration of the nominal charge for such services, hereby release the school, its students, graduate students, instructors, agents, representatives, and/or employees, from any and all claims arising out of and in any way connected with the performance of these services.

The Proprietor Is Not Responsible for Personal Property

Signed ______________________________

Date ______________________________

Witnessed ______________________________

THIS RELEASE FORM MUST BE SIGNED BY THE PARENT OR GUARDIAN IF THE CLIENT BEING SERVED IS UNDER 18 YEARS OF AGE.

Figure 19-24 Release form.

SELECTING HAIRCOLOR

FORMULATION

There are four basic questions that must always be asked when formulating a haircolor.

1. What is the natural level and does it include gray hair?
2. What is the client's desired level and tone?
3. Are contributing pigments (undertones) to be revealed?
4. What colors should be mixed to get the desired result?

The combination of the shade selected and the volume of hydrogen peroxide determines the lifting ability of a haircolor. Always remember to formulate with both lift and deposit in mind, in order to achieve the proper balance for the desired end result. A higher-lifting formula, however, may not have enough deposit to cancel the warmth of a client's

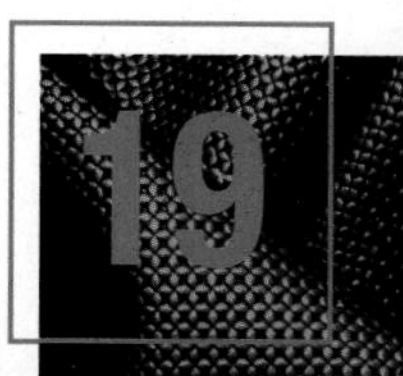

natural contributing pigment. The volume of hydrogen peroxide mixed with the haircolor product will also influence the lift and deposit.

MIXING PERMANENT COLORS

Your method of mixing permanent colors is determined by the type of application you are using. Permanent color is applied by either the applicator bottle or bowl-and-brush method (always follow the manufacturer's directions) (Figure 19-25).

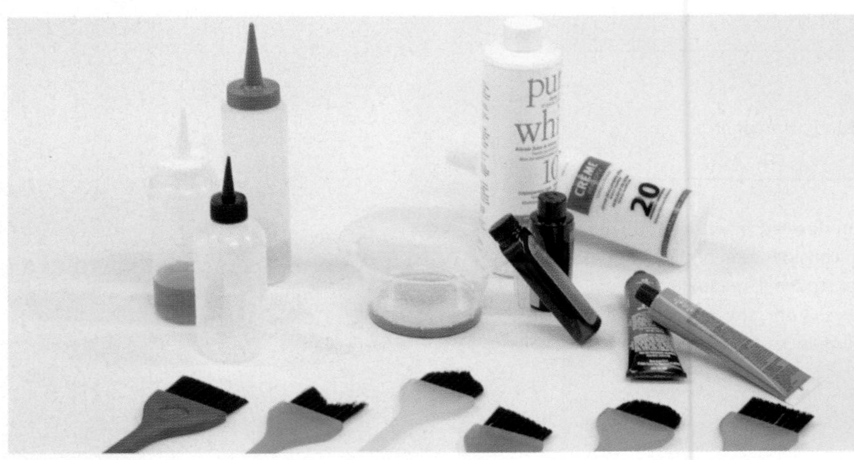

Figure 19-25 Haircolor can be mixed in an application bottle or bowl.

- *Applicator bottle.* Be sure that the applicator bottle is large enough to hold both the color and developer, with enough air space to shake the bottle until the mixture is thoroughly mixed. For a 1:1 ratio, pour 1 ounce of the developer into the bottle, add 1 ounce of the color, put the top on the bottle, and shake gently. For a 2:1 ratio, pour 2 ounces of the developer into the bottle, add 1 ounce of color, and mix. The latter ratio is for most permanent high-lift blond colors (Figure19-26).
- *Brush and bowl.* Use a nonmetallic mixing bowl. Measure the developer into the bowl. Add the color or colors you have selected in the appropriate proportions. Using an applicator brush, stir the mixture until it is blended (Figure 19-27).

CAUTION

A patch test must be given 24 to 48 hours before coloring the hair with an aniline derivative product. Aniline derivative haircolors must never be used on the eyelashes or eyebrows. To do so may cause blindness.

PATCH TEST

When working with haircolor, you will have to determine whether your clients have any allergies or sensitivities to the mixture. To identify an allergy in a client, the U.S. Food, Drug, and Cosmetic Act prescribes that a **patch test,** also called a predisposition test, be given 24 to 48 hours prior to each application of an aniline haircolor. The color used for the patch test must be the same as the color that will be used for the haircolor service (i.e., if a person is having her or his hair colored with 5BR by a particular

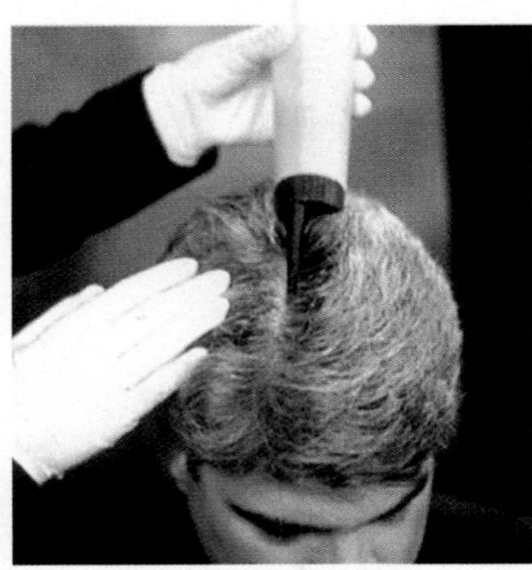

Figure 19-26 Applicator bottle application.

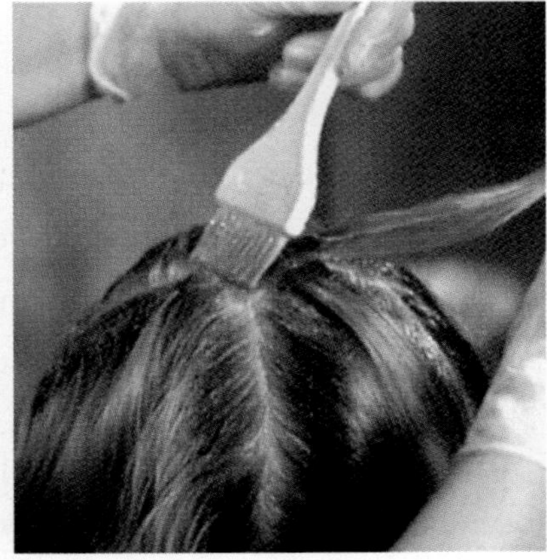

Figure 19-27 Applicator brush application.

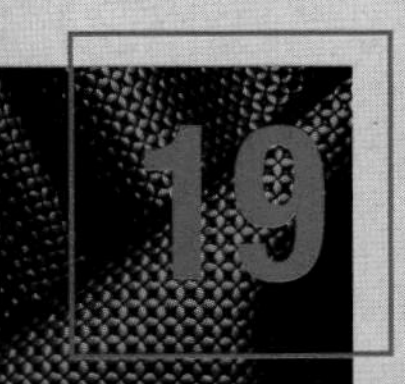

PROCEDURE 19-1

PERFORMING A PATCH TEST

1. Select the test area. Behind the ear or on the inside of the elbow are good choices.
2. Using a mild soap, cleanse and dry an area about the size of a quarter (Figure 19-28).
3. Mix a small amount of product according to the manufacturer's directions (Figure 19-29).
4. Apply to the test area with a sterile cotton swab (Figure 19-30).
5. Leave undisturbed for 24 to 48 hours.
6. Examine the test area. If there are no signs of redness or irritation, the test result is negative, and you can proceed with the color service.
7. Record the results on the client information card.

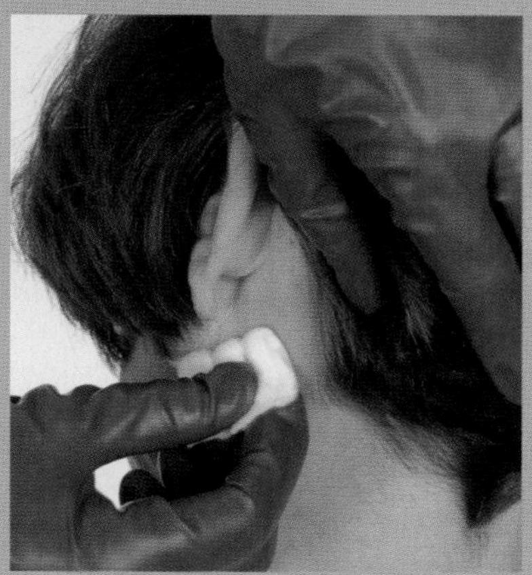

Figure 19-28 Clean patch area.

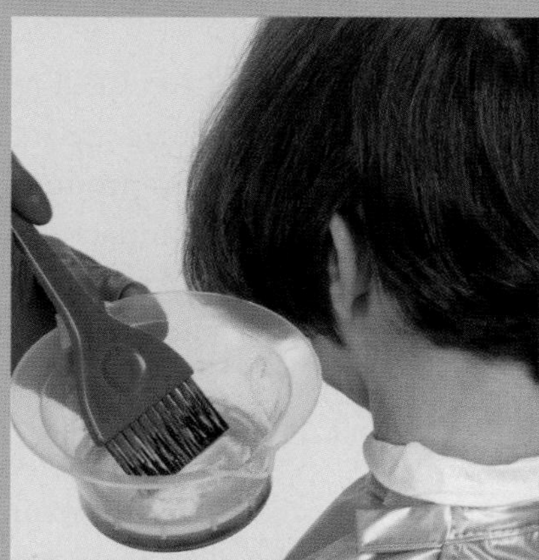

Figure 19-29 Mix haircolor and peroxide.

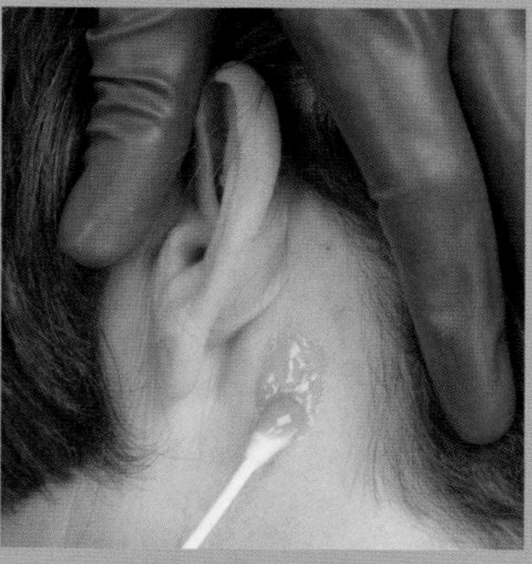

Figure 19-30 Apply haircolor mixture.

CAUTION

Operator dermatitis involves the same types of negative reactions to chemicals as those a client may experience. Since a colorist's hands are in contact with chemical solutions repeatedly during an average day, it is important to take proper precautions. Protect yourself from adverse reactions by wearing gloves until the haircolor product is completely removed from the client's hair.

manufacturer, use the 5BR shade in the patch test). The procedure for patch tests found on page 495 should be closely followed.

A negative skin test will show no sign of inflammation and indicates that the color may be safely applied. A positive result will show redness and a slight rash or welt. A client with these symptoms is allergic, and under no circumstances should she receive a haircolor service with the haircolor tested.

HAIRCOLOR APPLICATIONS

To ensure successful results when performing haircoloring services, the colorist must follow a prescribed procedure. A clearly defined system makes for the greatest efficiency, and the safest and most satisfactory results. Without such a plan, the work will take longer, results will be uneven, and mistakes may be made.

PRELIMINARY STRAND TEST

Once you have created a color formula for your client, try it out first on a small strand of hair. This preliminary strand test will tell you how the hair will react to the formula and how long the formula should be left on the hair. The strand test is performed after the client is prepared for the coloring service. See Procedure 19-2.

TEMPORARY COLORS

There are many methods of applying a temporary color, depending on the product used. Your instructor will help you interpret each manufacturer's directions. One method of applying color rinse is outlined in Procedure 19-3. To apply gels, mousses, foams, or sprays, return the client to your work area after shampooing and apply color according to the manufacturer's directions.

SEMIPERMANENT HAIRCOLORS

Because semipermanent colors do not contain the oxidizers necessary to lift, they only deposit color and do not lighten color. When selecting a semipermanent color, remember that color applied on top of existing color always creates a darker color.

The porosity of the hair will determine how well these products "take." Because they are deposit-only, traditional semipermanent colors can build up on the hair ends with repeated applications. A strand test will help determine the formula and processing time before the service. See Procedure 19-4.

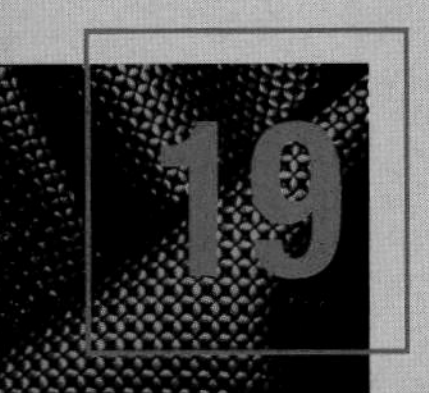

PROCEDURE 19-2

PRELIMINARY STRAND TEST

IMPLEMENTS AND MATERIALS

- Waterproof cape
- Plastic clips
- Glass or plastic mixing bowl
- Spray water bottle
- Shampoo
- Towels
- Color brushes
- Protective gloves
- Aluminum foil or plastic wrap
- Client record card
- Selected haircolor
- Applicator brush or bottle
- Hydrogen peroxide developer

PROCEDURE

1. Client consultation. Perform a scalp and hair analysis.
2. Drape the client to protect her skin and clothing.
3. **Part hair.** Part off a ½-inch (1.25-centimeter) square strand of hair in the lower crown. Using plastic clips as necessary, fasten other hair out of the way.
4. **Apply color.** Place the strand over the foil or plastic wrap and apply the color mixture (Figure 19-31). Follow the application method for the color procedure you will be using.(Figure 19-32).
5. **Check development.** Check the development at 5-minute intervals until the desired color has been achieved (Figure 19-33). Note the timing on the record card.
6. **Shampoo strand.** When satisfactory color has developed, remove the protective foil or plastic wrap. Place a towel under the strand, mist it thoroughly with water, add shampoo, and massage through (Figure 19-34). Rinse by spraying with water. Dry the strand with the towel and observe results.
7. Adjust the formula, timing, or application method as necessary and proceed with the color service.

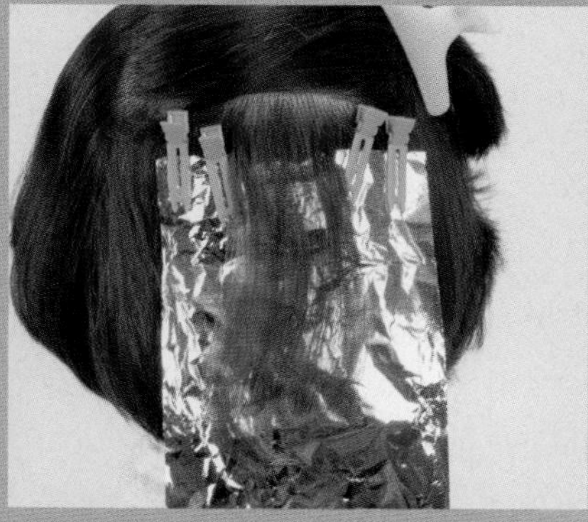

Figure 19-31 Place the test strand over foil.

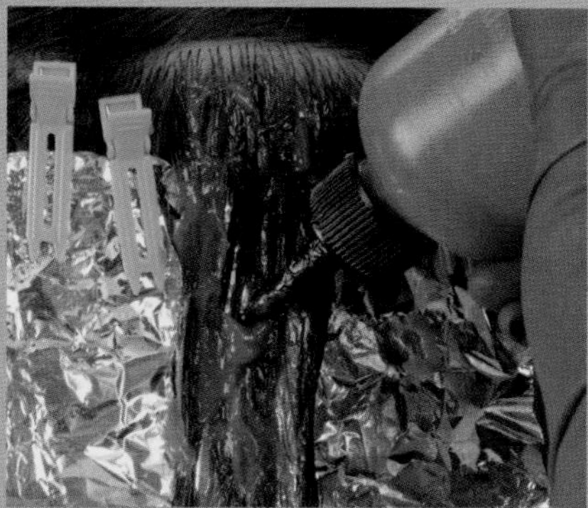

Figure 19-32 Apply tint to strand.

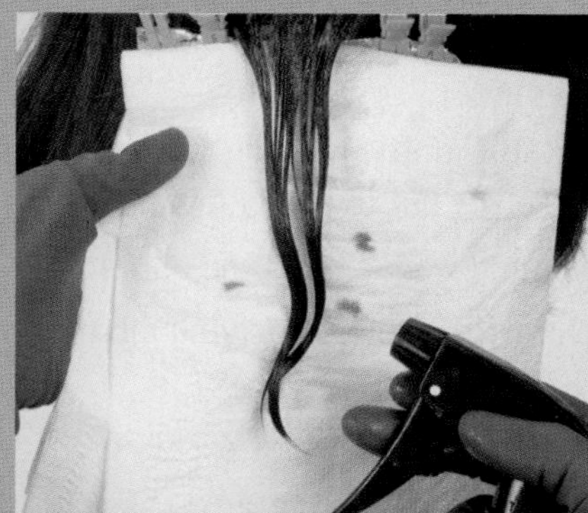

Figure 19-33 Check strand.

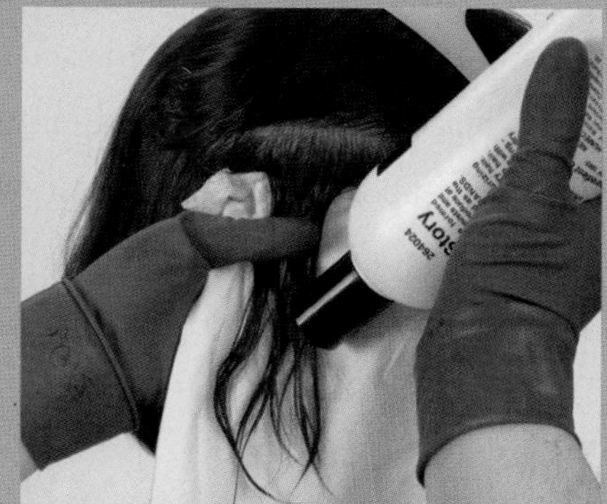

Figure 19-34 Shampoo strand.

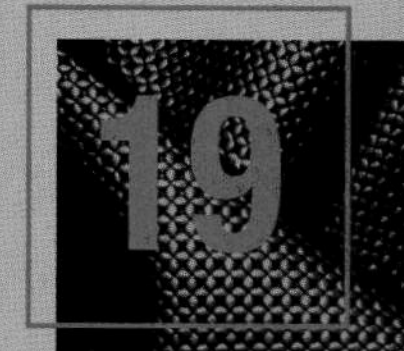

PROCEDURE 19-3

TEMPORARY HAIRCOLOR APPLICATION

IMPLEMENTS AND MATERIALS

- Shampoo cape
- Towels
- Protective gloves
- Comb
- Applicator bottle (optional)
- Temporary haircolor product
- Shampoo
- Record card
- Gloves
- Timer

PREPARATION

1. Perform a client consultation (Figure 19-35).
2. Ask the client to remove any jewelry and keep it in a safe place.

PROCEDURE

1. Drape the client for a haircoloring service. Slide a towel down from the back of the client's head and place lengthwise across the client's shoulders. Cross the ends of the towel beneath the chin and place the cape over the towel. Fasten the cape in the back. Fold the towel over the top of the cape and secure in front.
2. Shampoo and towel-dry the hair.
3. Make sure the client is comfortable reclined at the shampoo bowl.
4. Put on gloves.
5. Use an applicator bottle as directed by your instructor. Shake the bottle gently (Figure 19-36).
6. Apply the color and work around the entire head.
7. Blend the color with a comb, applying more color if necessary (Figure 19-37).
8. Do not rinse the hair. Towel-blot excess product.
9. Proceed with styling (Figure 19-38).

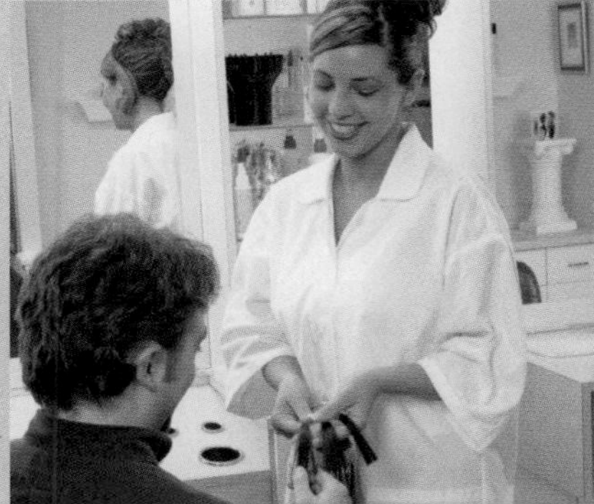
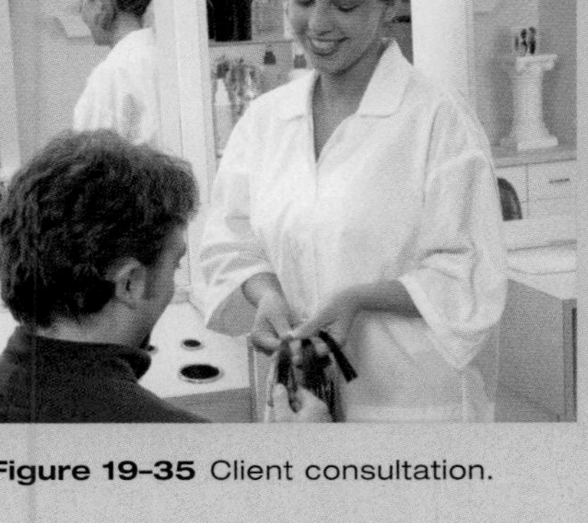

Figure 19-35 Client consultation.

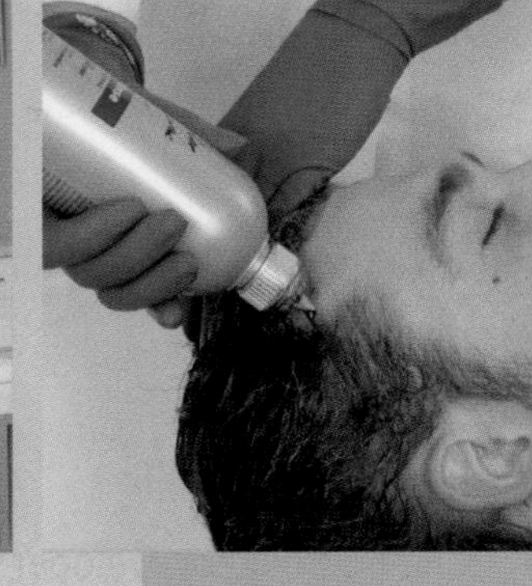

Figure 19-36 Apply color rinse at shampoo bowl.

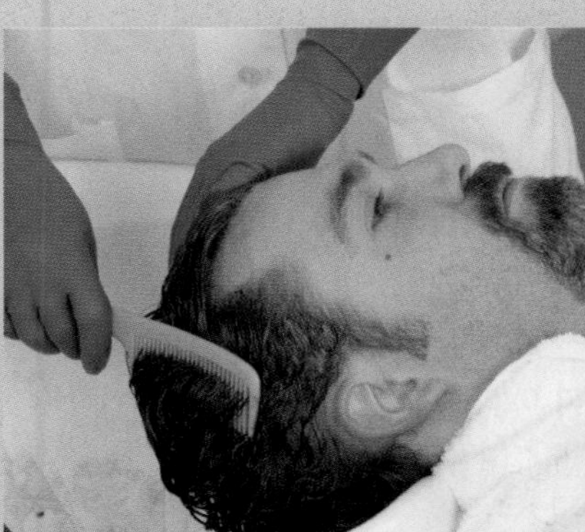

Figure 19-37 Blend color rinse through the hair.

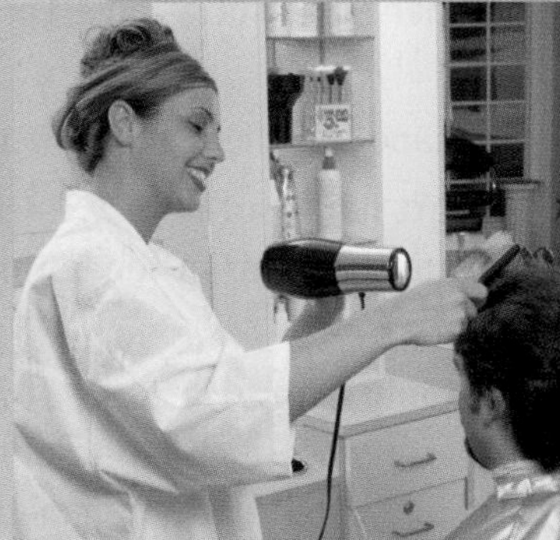

Figure 19-38 Style the hair.

CLEANUP AND SANITATION

1. Discard all disposable supplies and materials.
2. Close containers, wipe them off, and store in the proper place.
3. Sanitize implements, cape, and your workstation.
4. Wash your hands with soap and warm water.
5. Record results on a record card and file for future use.

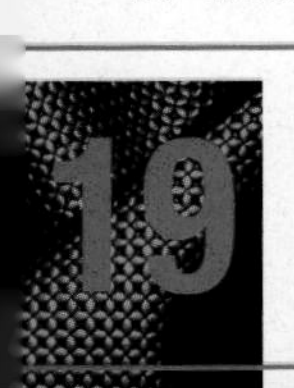

SINGLE-PROCESS PERMANENT COLOR

Single-process haircoloring lightens and deposits color in a single application. Examples of single-process coloring are virgin color applications, and color retouch applications. A **virgin application** refers to the first time the hair is colored. Prelightening or presoftening is not required with these applications.

CAUTION

Do not perform any haircoloring service if the client has abrasions or inflammations on the scalp. Do not brush the hair.

SINGLE-PROCESS COLOR RETOUCH

As the hair grows, you will need to retouch the new growth to keep it looking attractive and to avoid a two-toned effect. Appearing below are steps for applying color to new growth and to refresh faded ends, and a procedure for permanent single-process retouch with a **glaze,** a nonammonia color that adds shine and tone to the hair. For both applications, follow the same preparation steps as for the virgin single-process procedure, including a consultation and patch test.

Steps for applying color to new growth and faded ends follow:

1. Apply color to the new growth only, being careful not to overlap on previously colored hair. Overlapping can cause breakage and a **line of demarcation,** which is the visible line separating colored hair from new growth.
2. Process color according to your analysis and strand test results.
3. To refresh faded ends, formulate a no-lift deposit-only haircolor for the ends to match the new growth, or rinse the color through to the ends. Then shampoo and condition. Remember that the same color formula used with different volumes of peroxide will produce different results.

DOUBLE-PROCESS HIGH-LIFT HAIRCOLOR

If the client asks for a dramatically lighter color, the hair has to be prelightened first. Also, to achieve pale or cool colors, it is sometimes more efficient to use a **double-process application.** By first decolorizing the hair with a lightener and then using a separate product to deposit the desired tone, you will have more control over the coloring process.

Double-process high-lift coloring, also known as two-step blonding is a technique to create light blond hair in two steps. The hair is prelightened first and then toned. **Prelightening** lifts or lightens the natural pigments, before the application of a toner.

Because the lightening action and the deposit of color are independent of each other, a wider range of haircolor is possible.

You may find that the contributing pigment of the hair can help you in a double-process color application. By prelightening the hair to the desired color you can create a perfect foundation for longer-lasting red colors that avoid muddiness and stay true to tone.

The prelightener is applied in the same manner as a regular hair lightening treatment (see the following section). Once the prelightening has reached the desired shade, the hair is lightly shampooed, acidified, and towel-dried. After a strand test has been taken, the color is then applied in the usual manner.

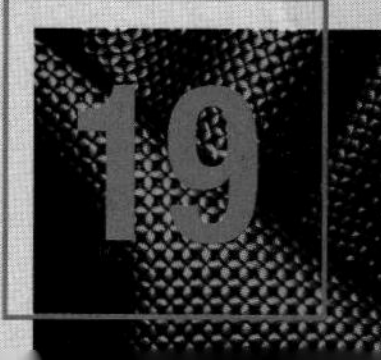

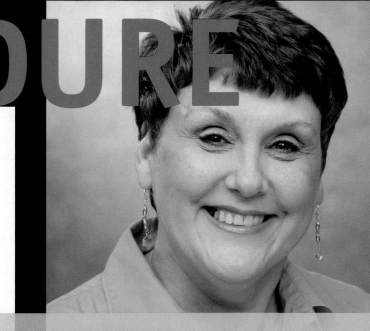

PROCEDURE 19-4

SEMIPERMANENT HAIRCOLOR APPLICATION

IMPLEMENTS AND MATERIALS

- Applicator bottle or brush
- Towels
- Plastic cap (optional)
- Plastic clips
- Waterproof cape
- Comb
- Color chart
- Timer
- Selected color
- Conditioner
- Cotton
- Protective cream
- Protective gloves
- Shampoo
- Record card
- Gloves

PREPARATION

1. **Perform patch test.** Perform a preliminary patch test 24 to 48 hours before the service. Proceed only if the test is negative.
2. **Client consultation.** Thoroughly analyze the hair and scalp. Record the results on the client's record card.
3. Ask the client to remove all jewelry and store it in a safe place. Drape the client for the haircolor service.
4. Perform a strand test. Record the results on the client's card.

PROCEDURE

1. Shampoo the client's hair with mild shampoo and towel-dry.
2. Put on gloves.
3. Apply protective cream around the hairline and over the ears (Figure 19-39).
4. Outline the hair into four sections—from ear to ear and from front center of forehead to center nape (Figure 19-40).

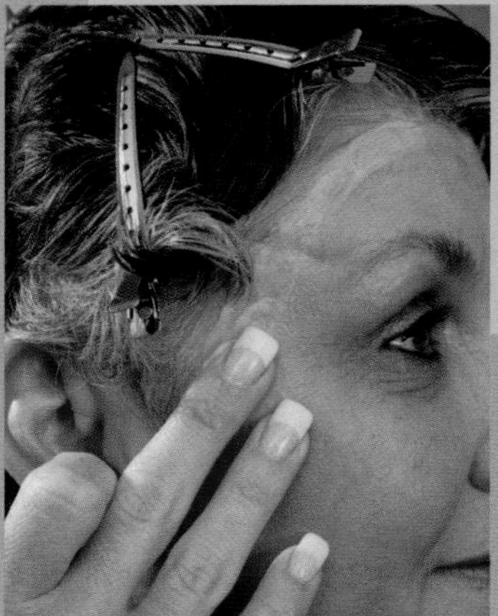

Figure 19-39 Apply protective cream.

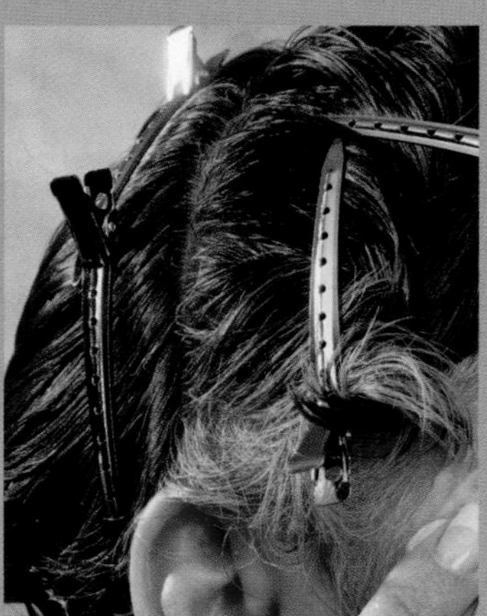

Figure 19-40 Part off from ear to ear.

4. Take ½-inch partings and apply the color to the new growth or scalp area in all four sections (Figure 19-41).
5. After all four sections are completed, work the color through the rest of the hair shaft to the ends until the hair is fully saturated (Figure 19-42).
6. Set timer to process. Follow the manufacturer's directions. Some colors require the use of a plastic cap (Figure 19-43).
7. Rinse, shampoo, condition, and style (Figure 19-44).

CLEANUP AND SANITATION

1. Perform the same cleanup and sanitation as for temporary color rinse.
2. In addition, rinse plastic bottles, bowls, and brushes, and disinfect according to your state's regulations.
3. Complete the record card and file for future use.

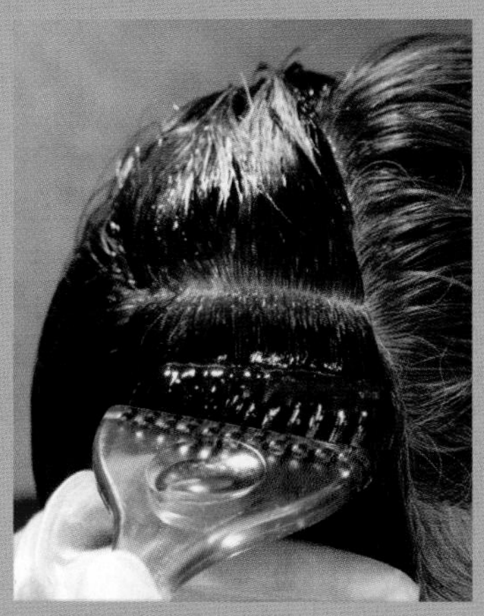

Figure 19-41 Apply in ½-inch sections.

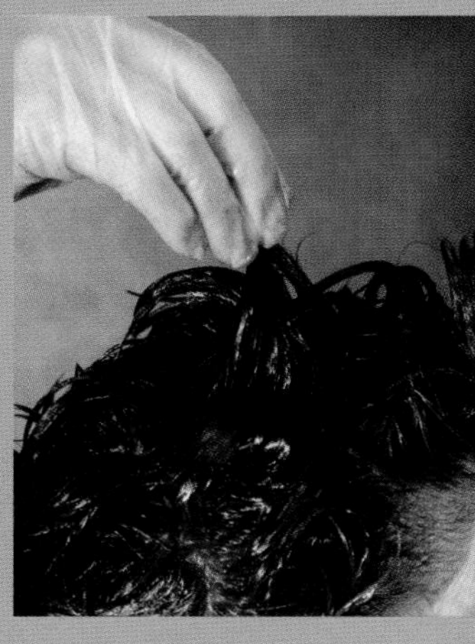

Figure 19-42 Work in remainder of hair.

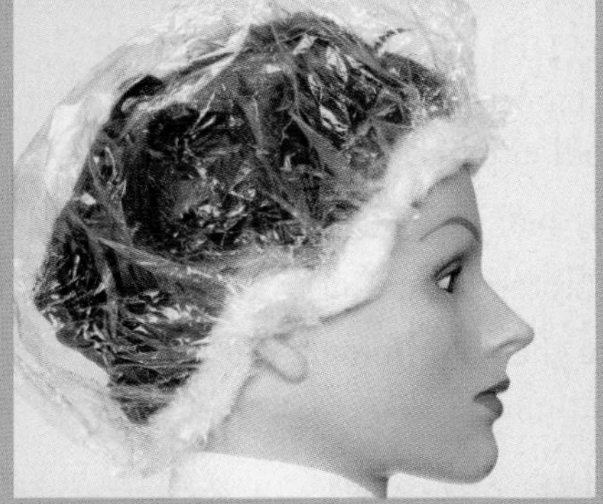

Figure 19-43 Use plastic cap if required.

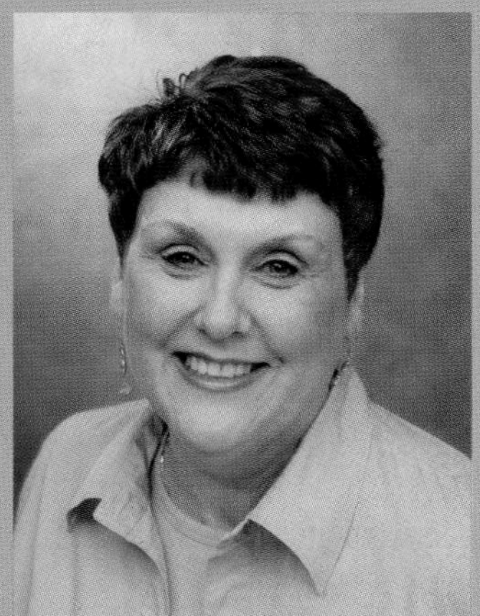

Figure 19-44 Finished result.

PROCEDURE 19-5

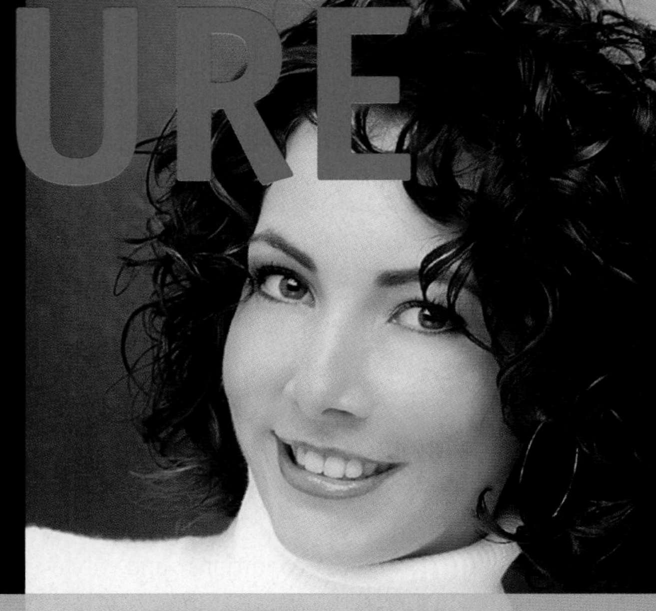

SINGLE-PROCESS COLOR FOR VIRGIN HAIR

IMPLEMENTS AND MATERIALS

Use the list of implements and materials for traditional semipermanent color, and add the following:

- Plastic or glass bowl and applicator brush or applicator bottle
- Selected permanent haircolor
- Hydrogen peroxide

PREPARATION

Same as preparation for traditional semipermanent color, including patch test.

1. Part dry hair into four sections (Figure 19-45).
2. Apply protective cream to the hairline and ears.
3. Prepare the color formula for either bottle or brush application.

PROCEDURE

1. **Apply color.** Begin in the section where the color change will be greatest or where the hair is most resistant, usually the hairline and temple areas. Part off a 1/4-inch (0.6-centimeter) subsection with the applicator (Figure 19-46).
2. **Apply color mid-strand.** Lift the subsection and apply color to the mid-strand area. Stay at least 1/2-inch (1.25 centimeters) from the scalp, and do not apply to the porous ends (Figure 19-47).
3. **Process.** Process according to the strand test results. Check for color development by removing color as described in the strand test procedure.

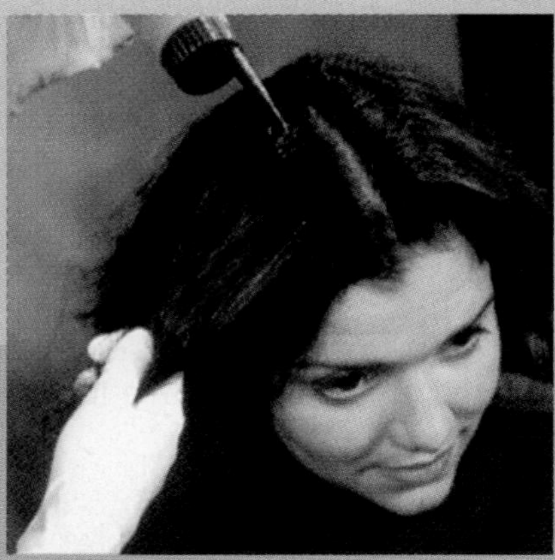

Figure 19-45 Part hair into four sections.

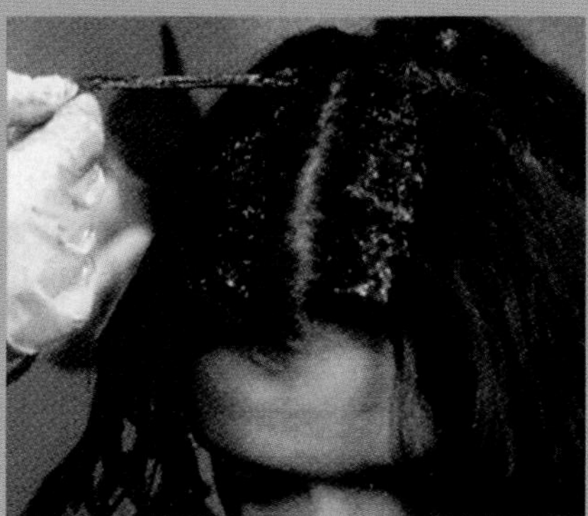

Figure 19-46 Apply 1/4 inch from scalp.

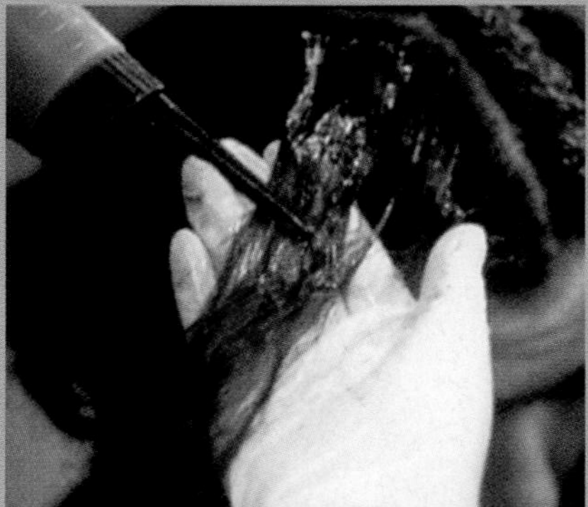

Figure 19-47 Work color down the hair shaft.

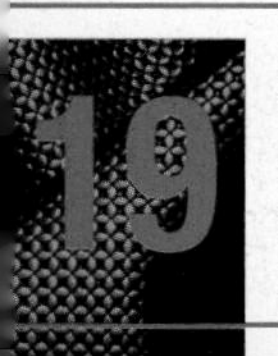

Here's a TIP

The hair at the scalp processes faster due to body heat. For this reason, the color is applied to the mid-strand before being applied to the scalp area. Your strand test will determine the application procedure and timing for even color development.

4. Apply color to the hair at the scalp (Figure 19-48).
5. Pull the color through the ends of the hair (Figure 19-49).
6. Lightly rinse with warm water. Massage color into a lather and rinse thoroughly.
7. Remove any stains around the hairline with shampoo or stain remover. Use a towel to gently remove stains.
8. Shampoo the hair. Condition as needed.
9. Towel-dry and style the hair (Figure 19-50).
10. Complete the client's record card and file for future use.

CLEANUP AND SANITATION

Perform the same cleanup and sanitation as for semipermanent haircolor application.

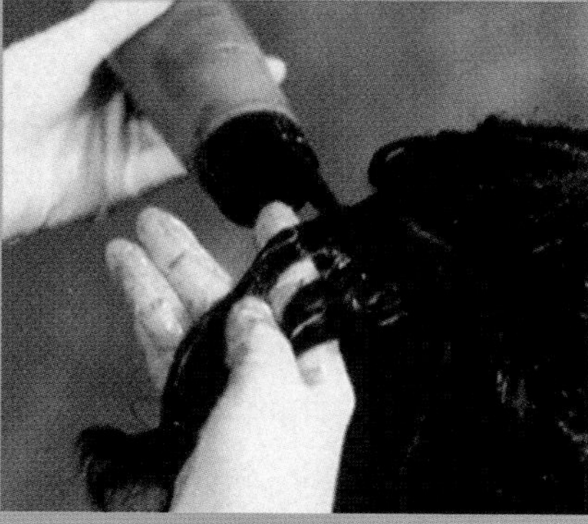

Figure 19-48 Apply to the base area of scalp.

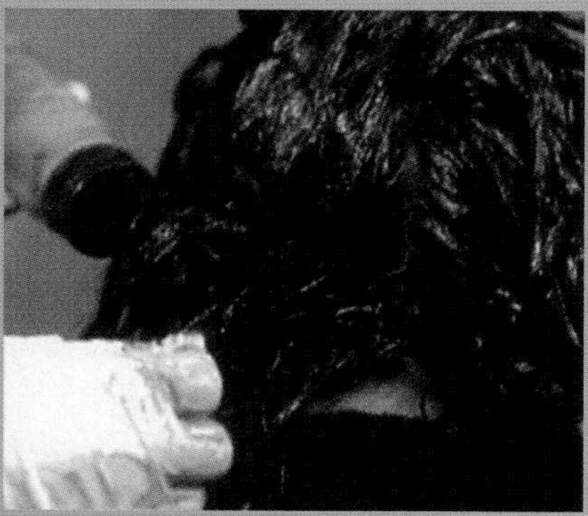

Figure 19-49 Work color through to the ends.

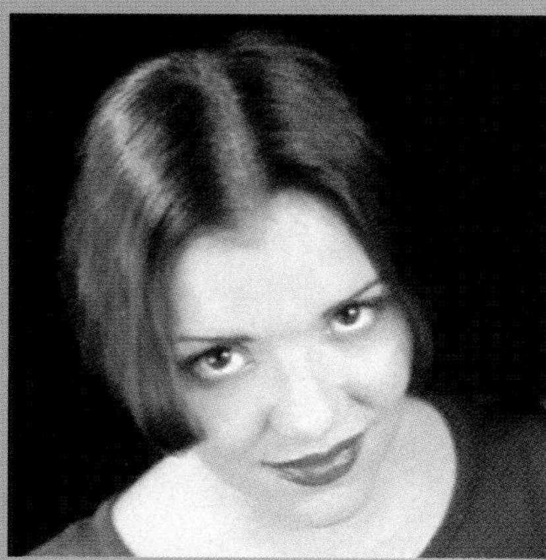

Figure 19-50 Finished color.

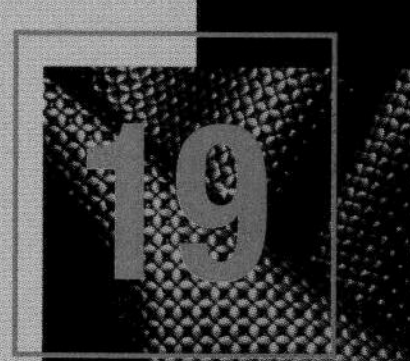

PROCEDURE 19-6

PERMANENT SINGLE-PROCESS RETOUCH WITH A GLAZE

Use the same implements and materials as for single-process haircolor on virgin hair.

1. Part dry hair into four sections (Figure 19-51).
2. Apply the color to the new growth area using 1/4-inch partings (Figure 19-52).
3. Complete all four sides and set timer for 45 minutes. Rinse and towel-dry (Figure 19-53).
4. Prepare a no-lift deposit-only glaze formula to apply to the mid-strand and ends.
5. Apply the no-lift deposit-only glaze and work through the hair (Figures 19-54 and 19-55).
6. Check haircolor results before rinsing.
7. Style the hair (Figure 19-56).
8. Complete the client's record and file it away.

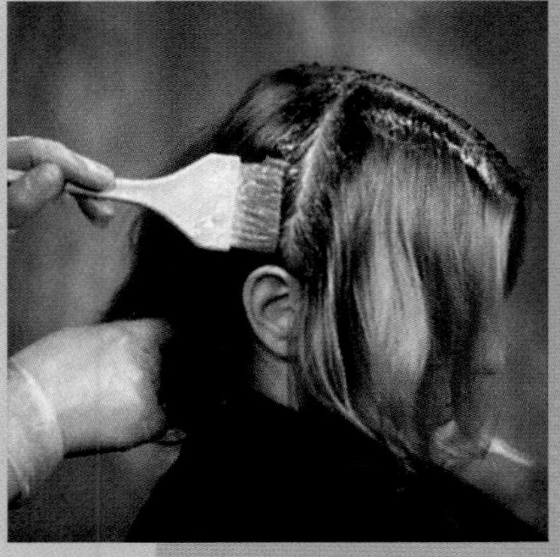

Figure 19-51 Outline four sections.

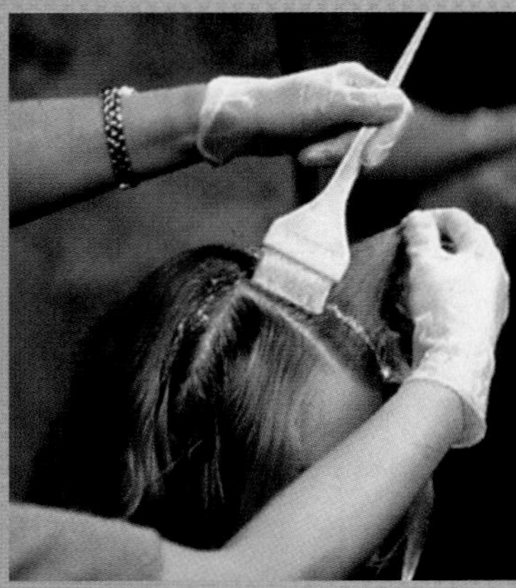

Figure 19-52 Apply color to the new growth.

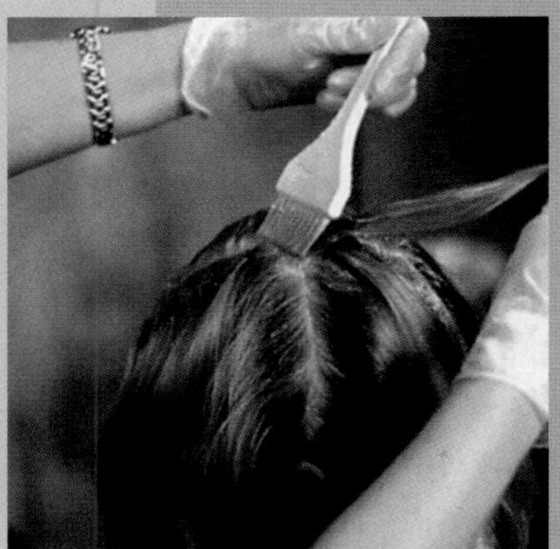

Figure 19-53 Complete all four sides.

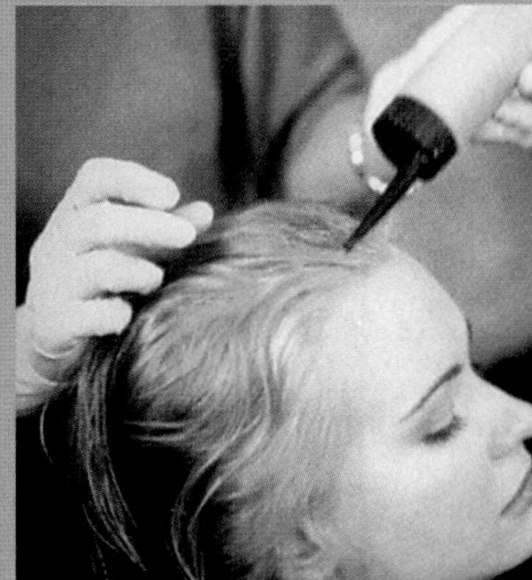

Figure 19-54 Apply glaze.

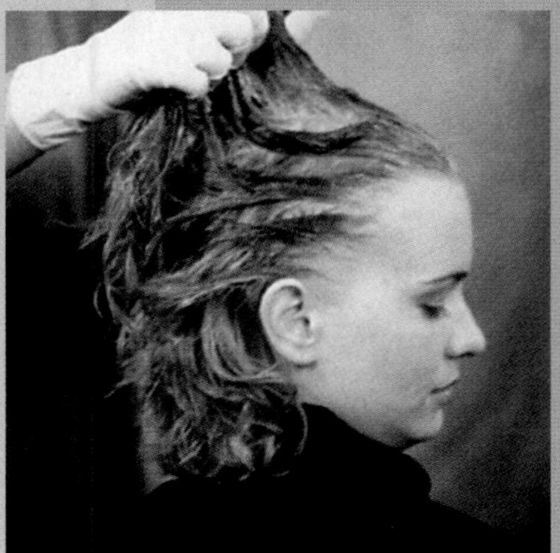

Figure 19-55 Work in the hair.

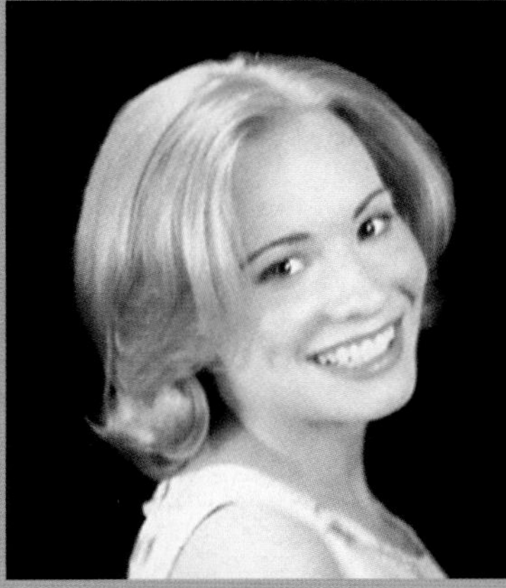

Figure 19-56 Finished result.

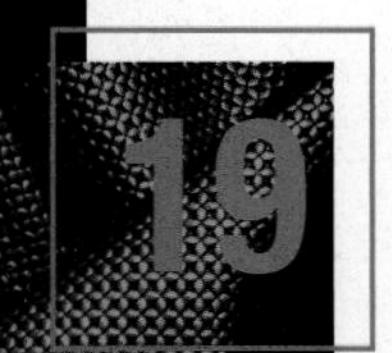

Using an applicator brush, stir the lightener until it is thoroughly mixed. A creamy consistency provides the best for control during application.

DEMIPERMANENT (NO-LIFT DEPOSIT-ONLY) HAIRCOLOR

The application procedure for demipermanent haircolor is similar to that of a traditional semipermanent color, since neither process alters the hair's natural melanin or produces lift. Follow the manufacturer's guidelines for application and processing time for the product you have selected.

Gray (unpigmented) hair presents special challenges when formulating no-lift deposit-only haircolor. Because there is no lift, the resulting depth of color when covering gray hair may appear too harsh unless you allow for some brightness and warmth in your formulation. It is usually not advisable to color gray hair one even shade, since natural hair color has different depths and tones that give it the added warmth that gray hair is lacking.

Hair that has previously received a color service will have a greater degree of porosity, which must also be taken into account when formulating and applying a no-lift deposit-only haircolor.

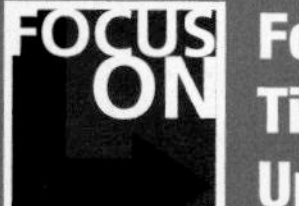

Focus on . . . Ticket Upgrading

Getting your clients interested in haircoloring can be done in indirect as well as direct ways, such as the following:

- Wear color in your hair. As a professional hairstylist, you should be an example of what those services can do.
- Display haircolor-related materials at your workstation. These could be swatches, pictures of great haircoloring you clip out of magazines, and so forth.
- Suggest haircolor to every client, and remember that every client is a potential haircolor client.

USING LIGHTENERS

Colorists can choose from three forms of lighteners: oil, cream, and powder. Oil and cream lighteners are considered **on-the-scalp lighteners,** which can be used directly on the scalp. Powder lighteners are **off-the-scalp lighteners,** which cannot be used directly on the scalp. Each type has its unique chemical characteristics and formulation procedures.

ON-THE-SCALP LIGHTENERS

Cream and oil lighteners are the most popular type of lighteners because they are easy to apply. Oil lighteners are the mildest type, appropriate when only one or two levels of lift are desired. Because they are so mild, they are also used professionally to lighten dark facial and body hair.

Cream lighteners are strong enough for high-lift blonding, but gentle enough to be used on the scalp. They have the following features and benefits:

- Conditioning agents give some protection to the hair and scalp.
- Thickeners give more control during application.
- Because cream lighteners do not run or drip, overlapping is prevented during retouching services. Cream lighteners may be mixed with activators (sometimes called boosters, protinators, or accelerators) in the form of dry crystals.

CAUTION

Powdered off-the-scalp lighteners are used exclusively for off-the-scalp applications and special effects, such as foil-wrapped weaving, highlighting with plastic caps, and hair painting.

CAUTION

When heat is used with hair lighteners, it softens the hair and makes it more fragile. Excessive heat increases the rate of the reaction and swells the hair. Excessive heat can lift and crack the cuticle and break bonds within the cortex. Therefore, extreme caution must always be exercised when using heat.

Activators contain a powdered oxidizer and/or the same persulfate salts that are used in powdered off-the-scalp hair lighteners. They are added to hydrogen peroxide to increase its lifting power. The more activators you use, the lighter the hair will be. Up to three activators can be used for on-the-scalp applications, and up to four for off-the-scalp applications. Activators increase scalp irritation.

POWDERED OFF-THE-SCALP LIGHTENERS

Powdered off-the-scalp lighteners are strong, fast-acting lighteners in powdered form. They are stronger than cream lighteners, and powerful enough for high-lift blonding. However, powdered off-the-scalp lighteners can cause scalp irritation and should not be applied directly to the scalp.

Powdered off-the-scalp lighteners, which are also called quick lighteners, contain (persulfate salts) for quicker and stronger lightening. They may dry out more quickly than other types of lighteners, but they do not run or drip. Most powder lighteners expand and spread out as processing continues and should not be used for retouch services.

TIME FACTORS

Processing time for lightening is affected by the factors listed below.

- The darker the natural hair color, the more melanin it has. The more melanin it has, the longer it takes to lighten the color.
- The amount of time needed to lighten the natural color is also influenced by the porosity. Porous hair of the same color level will lighten faster than hair that is nonporous, because the lightening agent can enter the cortex more rapidly.
- Tone influences the length of time necessary to lighten the natural hair color. The greater the percentage of red reflected in the natural color, the more difficult it is to achieve the delicate shades of a pale blond. Ash blonds are especially difficult to achieve because the melanin must be diffused sufficiently to alter both the level and tone of the hair.
- The strength of the product affects the speed and amount of lightening. Stronger lighteners produce pale shades in the fastest time.
- Heat leads to faster lightening. But the stages of lightening must be carefully observed to avoid excessive lift that could diffuse so much natural pigment that the toner may not produce the desired color. When this occurs, the toner may “grab,” giving the hair an unwanted ashy, cool tone.

PRELIMINARY STRAND TEST

Perform a preliminary strand test prior to lightening to determine the processing time, the condition of the hair after lightening, and the end results. Watch the strand carefully for its reaction to the lightening mixture, and for any discoloration or breakage. Reconditioning may be required prior to toning. If the color and condition are good, you can proceed with the lightening. Carefully record all data on the client’s record card and file for future use.

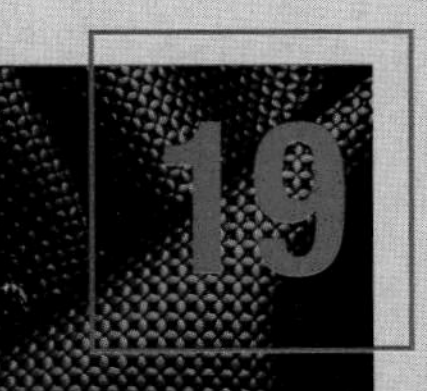

If the test shows the hair is not light enough, increase the strength of the mixture and/or increase the processing time. If the hair strand is too light, decrease the strength of the mixture and/or decrease the processing time.

A patch test must be taken 24 to 48 hours prior to each application of a toner containing aniline derivatives.

CAUTION

In all procedures requiring the use of a towel to check for lightening level, make sure that the towel is damp. Blot—do not rub—the strand. Rubbing could cause a roughening of the cuticle, giving a false reading for the entire process.

LIGHTENER RETOUCH

New growth will become obvious as the hair grows. The new growth is the part of the hair shaft between the scalp and the hair that has previously been colored. On a retouch, always lighten the new growth first. The procedure for a lightener retouch is the same as that for lightening a virgin head of hair, except that the mixture is applied only to the new growth. A cream lightener is generally used for a lightener retouch because it is less irritating to the scalp and its consistency helps prevent overlapping of previously lightened hair. Overlapping can cause severe breakage and lines of demarcation.

Always consult the client's record card for information about which lightener formulas have been used in the past, timing, and other matters.

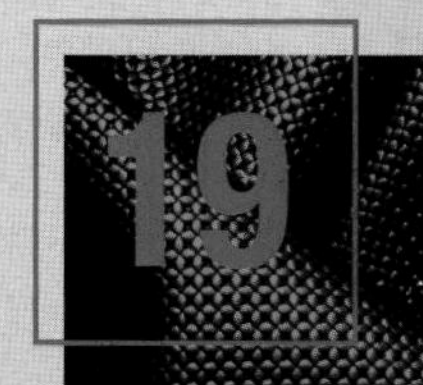

PROCEDURE 19-7

LIGHTENING VIRGIN HAIR

This section is dedicated to procedures used in lightening hair that has not been colored before.

IMPLEMENTS AND MATERIALS

- Towels
- Comb
- Protective gloves
- Plastic clips
- Waterproof cape
- Plastic or glass bowl
- Shampoo
- Hydrogen peroxide developer
- Acid or finishing rinse
- Cotton
- Record card
- Applicator bottle or brush
- Lightener
- Timer
- Protective cream

PREPARATION

Follow the same preparation steps as for traditional semipermanent color application, including a patch test. Carefully analyze the hair and record all information on the client card.

1. Perform a consultation and scalp analysis.
2. Apply a protective cream around the hairline and over the ears.
3. Put on protective gloves.
4. Prepare the lightening formula and use it immediately.

PROCEDURE

1. **Divide the hair into four sections.** Place cotton in all four sections to protect the scalp so the lightener does not contact the scalp (Figures 19-57 and 19-58).
2. **Apply the lightener.** Apply the lightener ½-inch away from the scalp working the lightener through the mid-strand and up to the porous ends (Figure 19-59).
3. Place strips of cotton at the scalp area along the partings to prevent the lightener from touching the base of the hair and complete all four sections in this manner (Figure 19-60).

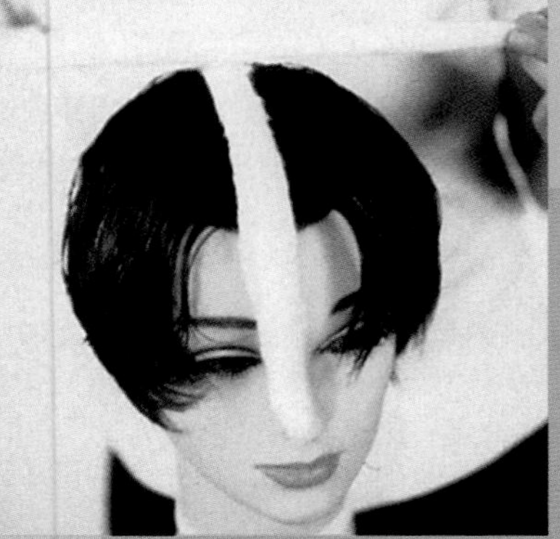

Figure 19-57 Place cotton between sections.

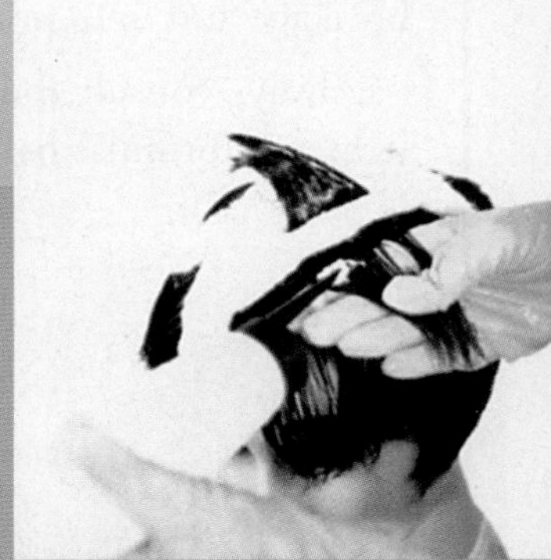

Figure 19-58 Place cotton between each section.

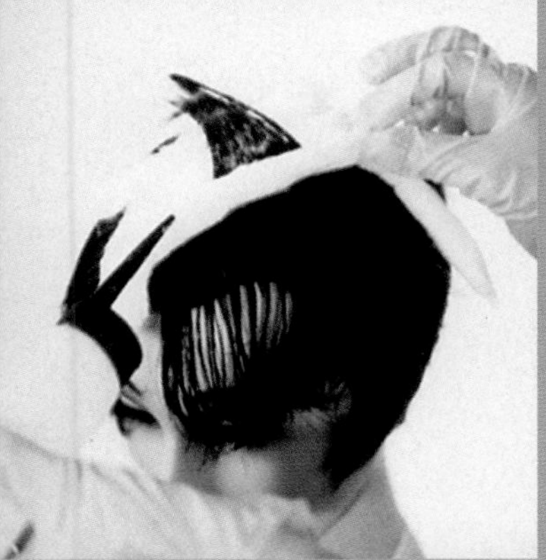

Figure 19-59 Apply lightener starting ½-inch off the scalp.

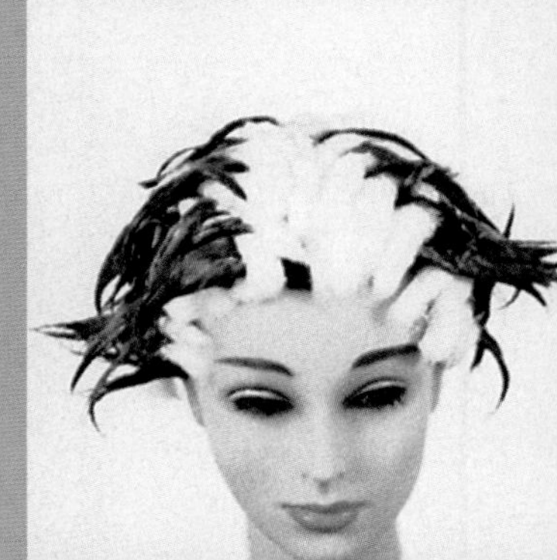

Figure 19-60 Complete all four sections.

4. **Continue applying.** Continue to apply the lightener. Double check the application, adding more lightener if necessary. Do not comb the lightener through the hair. Keep the lightener moist during development by reapplying if the mixture dries on the hair.
5. **Strand test.** Check for lightening action about 15 minutes before the time indicated by the preliminary strand test (Figure 19-61). Spray a hair strand with a water bottle and remove the lightener with a damp towel. Examine the strand. If the strand is not light enough, reapply the mixture and continue testing frequently until the desired level is reached.
6. **Apply lightener to scalp.** Remove the cotton from the scalp area. Apply the lightener to the hair near the scalp with ⅛-inch (0.3-centimeter) partings (Figure 19-62). Apply lightener to the porous ends and process until the entire hair strand (Figure 19-63) has reached the desired stage.
7. **Rinse and shampoo.** Rinse the hair thoroughly with warm water. Shampoo gently and condition as needed, keeping your hands under the hair to avoid tangling.
8. Neutralize the alkalinity of the hair with an acidic conditioner. Recondition if necessary.
9. Towel-dry the hair, or dry it completely under a cool dryer if required by the manufacturer.
10. Examine the scalp for any abrasions. Analyze the condition of the hair.
11. Proceed with a toner application if desired (Procedure 19-8) (Figure 19-64).

CLEANUP AND SANITATION

Perform the same cleanup and sanitation as for semipermanent haircolor application.

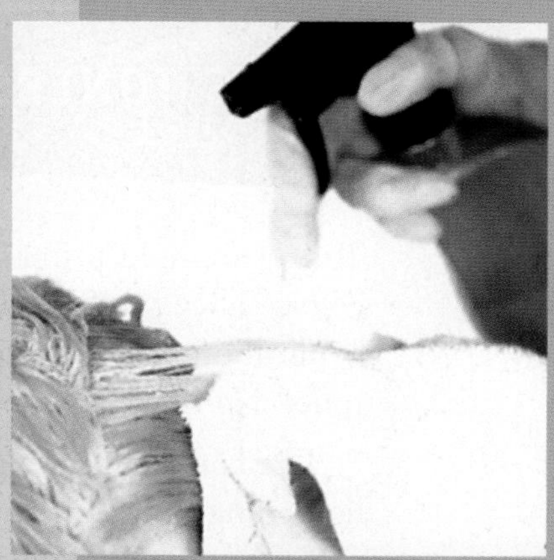

Figure 19-61 Strand test.

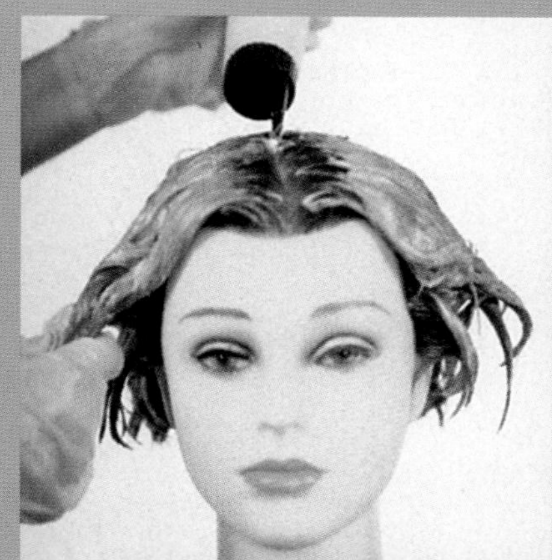

Figure 19-62 Apply lightener to scalp area.

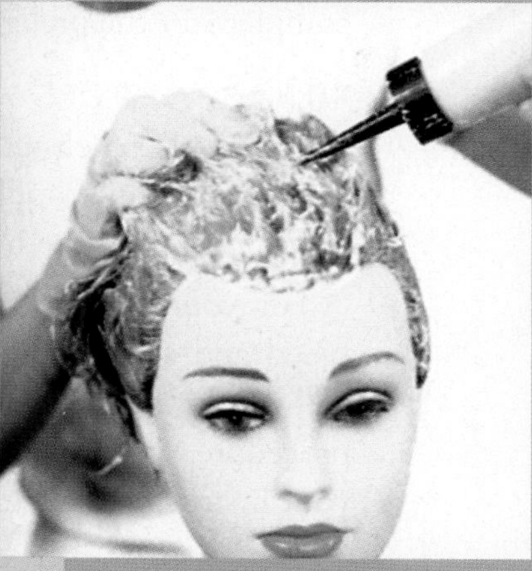

Figure 19-63 Work in lightener.

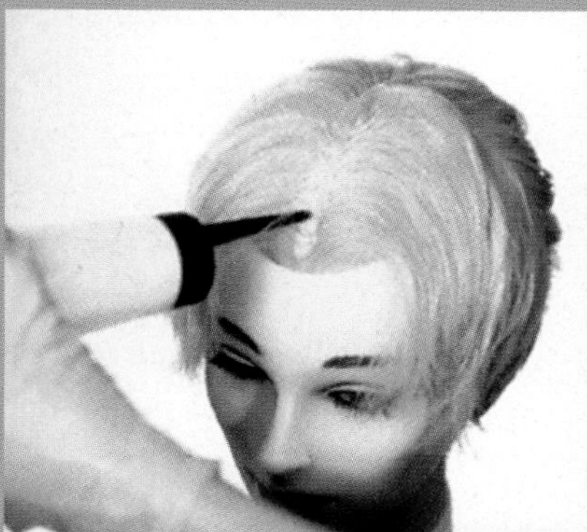

Figure 19-64 Apply toner to prelightened hair.

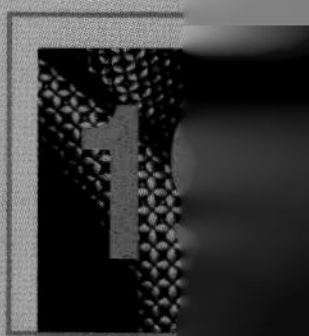

USING TONERS

Toners are used primarily on prelightened hair to achieve pale, delicate colors. They require a double-process application. The first process is the application of the lightener; the second process is the application of the toner. No-lift deposit-only haircolors are often used as toners.

The contributing pigment is the color that remains in the hair after lightening. It is essential that you achieve the correct foundation in order to create the right color and degree of porosity required for proper toner development.

Manufacturers of toners generally include literature with their products that recommend the contributing pigment necessary to achieve the color you desire. As a general rule, the paler the color you are seeking, the lighter the contributing pigment needs to be. It is important to follow the literature closely and to understand that over-lightened hair will "grab" the color of the toner. Under-lightened hair, on the other hand, will appear to have more red, yellow, or orange than the intended color.

It is not advisable to prelighten past the pale yellow stage. This will create overly porous hair that will not have enough natural pigment left. Refer to the law of color to select a toner that will neutralize or complement the prelightened hair and produce the desired color.

TONER APPLICATION

Administer a patch test for allergies or other sensitivities 24 to 48 hours before each toner application. Proceed with the application only if the patch test results are negative and the hair is in good condition.

For your protection, wear gloves throughout the application. Your speed and accuracy are both important factors in the application and will determine, to a large extent, whether you get good color results. The procedure for applying low- or non-peroxide toners may vary. Check with your instructor for directions.

PROCEDURE

19-8 TONER APPLICATION

IMPLEMENTS AND MATERIALS

- Towels
- Tail comb
- Protective gloves
- Plastic clips
- Waterproof cape
- Plastic or glass bowl
- Shampoo
- Hydrogen peroxide developer
- Acid or finishing rinse
- Cotton
- Protective cream
- Record card
- Toner
- Applicator bottle or brush
- Timer

PREPARATION

1. Prelighten the hair to the desired stage of decolorization.
2. Shampoo the hair lightly, rinse and towel-dry. Condition as necessary.
3. Select the desired toner shade.
4. Apply protective cream around the hairline and over the ears.
5. Take a strand test and record the results on the client's record card.
6. **Mix toner.** If using a toner with developer, mix the toner and the developer in a nonmetallic bowl or bottle, following the manufacturer's directions (Figure 19-65).

PROCEDURE

1. **Part hair.** Part the hair into four equal sections, using the end of the tail comb or applicator brush. Avoid scratching the scalp.

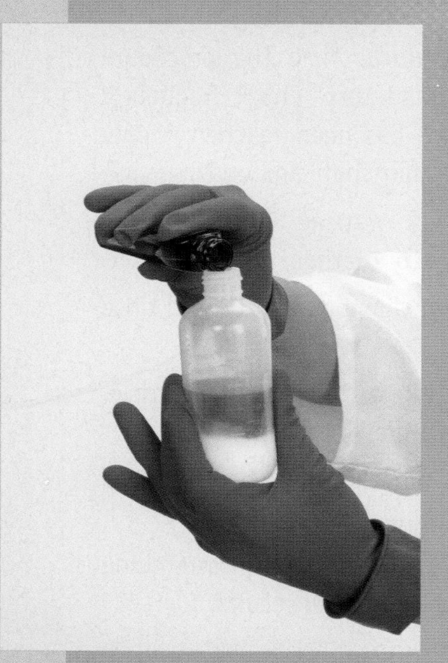

Figure 19-65 Mix toner.

Here's a TIP

Do not apply the toner through to the porous ends of the hair until the end of the procedure, and then only if you are planning to change the tone, or are correcting significant fading. That will only make the ends even more porous and more susceptible to continued fading.

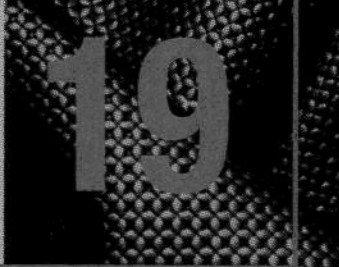

2. **Apply toner.** At the crown of one of the back sections, part off 1/4-inch (0.6-centimeter) partings and apply the toner from the scalp up to, but not including, the porous ends (Figure 19-66).
3. **Strand test.** Take a strand test. If it indicates proper color development, gently work the toner through the ends of the hair, using an applicator brush or your fingers (Figure 19-67).
4. **Apply additional color.** If necessary for coverage, apply additional toner to the hair and distribute evenly. Leave the hair loose or cover with a plastic cap if required.
5. **Check time of procedure.** Time the procedure according to your strand test. Check frequently until the desired color has been reached evenly throughout the entire hair shaft and ends.
6. Remove the toner by wetting the hair and massaging the toner into a lather.
7. Rinse with warm water, shampoo gently, and rinse well again.
8. Apply an acidic conditioner to close the cuticle, lower the pH, and help prevent fading.
9. Remove any stains from the skin, hairline, and neck.
10. Style as desired. Use caution to avoid stretching the hair. Review before and after results.

CLEANUP AND SANITATION

Perform the same cleanup and sanitation as for semipermanent haircolor application.

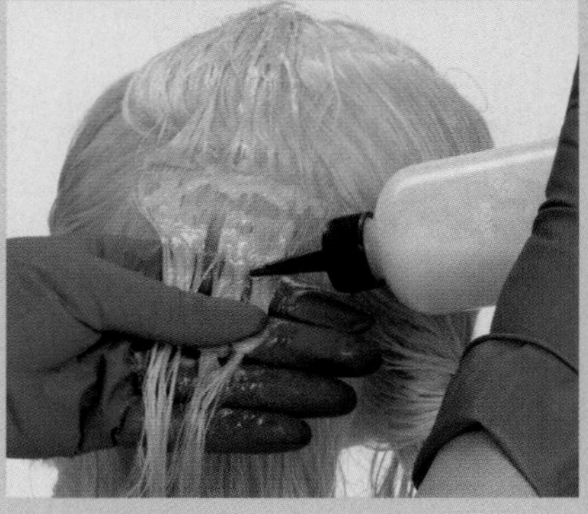

Figure 19-66 Apply toner.

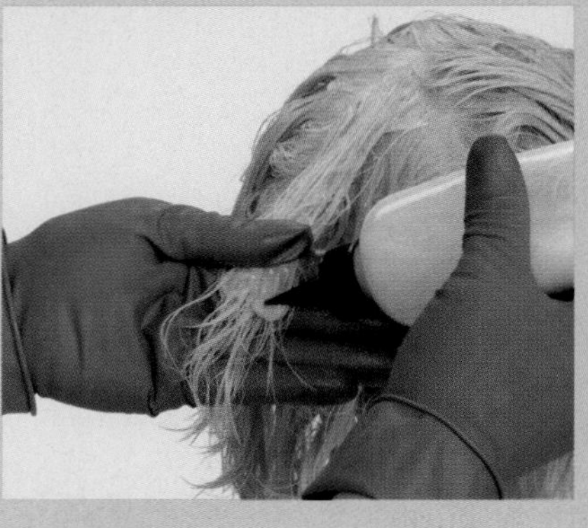

Figure 19-67 Work toner through hair ends.

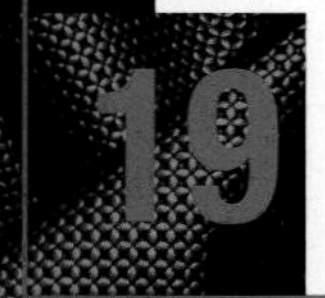

SPECIAL EFFECTS HAIRCOLORING

Special effects haircoloring refers to any technique that involves partial lightening or coloring. Coloring for special effects can be thought of as a pure fashion technique. It is a versatile and exciting haircoloring service.

One way you can create special effects is by strategically placing light and dark colors in the hair. **Highlighting** involves coloring some of the hair strands lighter than the natural color to add a variety of lighter shades and the illusion of depth. Subtle highlights do not contrast strongly with the natural color. Light colors cause an area to advance toward the eye, to appear larger, and to make details more visible. **Reverse highlighting** or **lowlighting** is the technique of coloring strands of hair darker than the natural color. Contrasting dark areas recede, appear smaller, and make detail less visible.

As you begin to expand your knowledge of haircoloring and lightening and develop your technical ability, you will become more creative. Your instructor will help you master the basic techniques, but the rest is up to you.

The possibilities are limited only by your imagination and your ability to create a finished style that meets the needs of your client (Figure 19-68).

There are several methods for achieving highlights. The three most frequently used techniques follow:

- Cap technique
- Foil technique
- Baliage or free-form technique

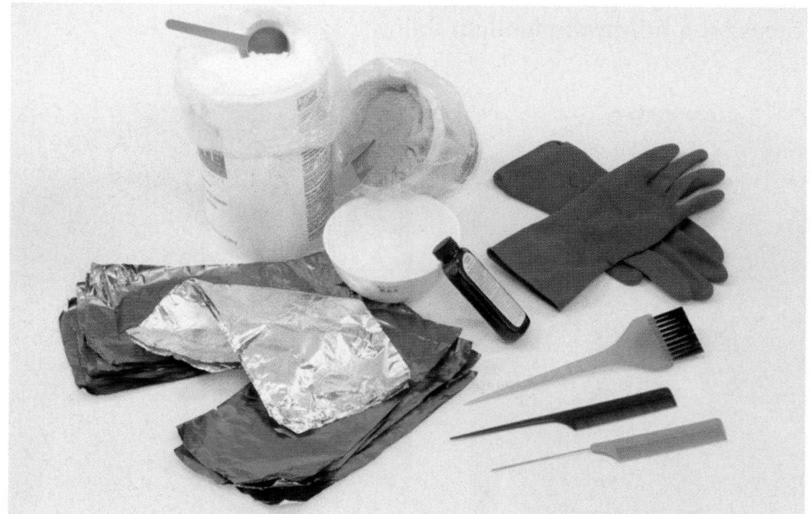

Figure 19-68 Lightening tools.

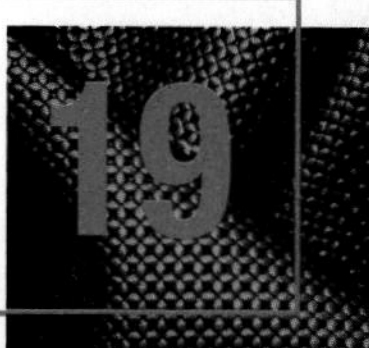

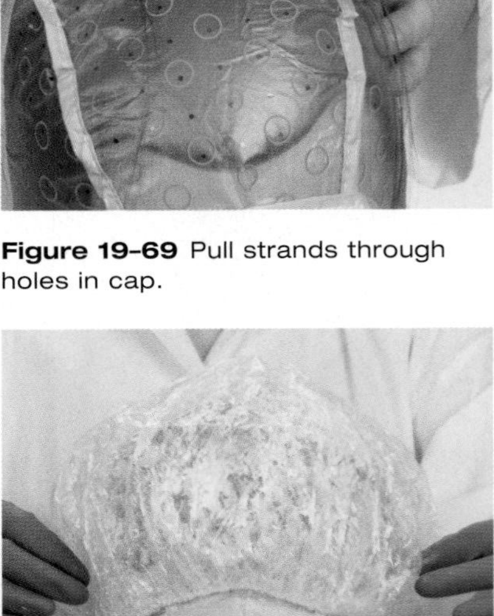

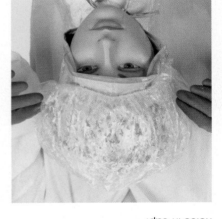

Figure 19-69 Pull strands through holes in cap.

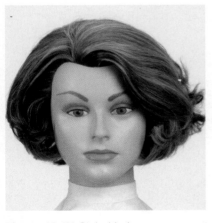

Figure 19-70 Cover loosely with a plastic cap.

Figure 19-71 Styled hair.

CAP TECHNIQUE

The **cap technique** involves pulling clean, dry strands of hair through a perforated cap with a thin plastic or metal hook, then combing them to remove tangles (Figure 19-69). The number of strands pulled through determines the amount of hair that will be highlighted or lowlighted. When only a small number of strands are pulled through, the result will be a subtle look. A more noticeable effect is achieved if many strands are pulled through, and the effect is even more dramatic if larger strands of hair are pulled through.

For highlighting, the hair is usually lightened with a powdered off-the-scalp lightener or high lift color, beginning in the area that is most resistant. The lightener is removed by a thorough rinse and a shampoo. After towel blotting and conditioning (if necessary), the lightened hair can be toned, if desired (Figures 19-70 and 19-71).

FOIL TECHNIQUE

The **foil technique** involves coloring selected strands of hair by slicing or weaving out sections, placing them on foil or plastic wrap, applying lightener or color, and sealing them in the foil or plastic wrap. You can also apply permanent haircolor to the strands to create softer, more natural-looking highlights.

Placing foil in the hair is an art. It takes practice and discipline. To make it easier, start by working to create clean section blocks on the head. Once you have perfected this, you will fully understand the difference between a slice parting and a weave parting. **Slicing** involves taking a narrow, ⅛-inch (0.3-centimeter) section of hair by making a straight part at the scalp, positioning the hair over the foil, and applying lightener or color (Figure 19-72). In **weaving,** selected strands are picked up from a narrow section of hair with a zigzag motion of the comb, and lightener or color is applied only to these strands (Figure 19-73).

There are many patterns in which foil can be placed in the hair. There are face-frame, half-head, three-quarter head, and full-head wrapping patterns that produce different highlights in different portions of the head. Steps for a full-head highlight follow.

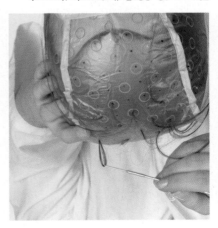

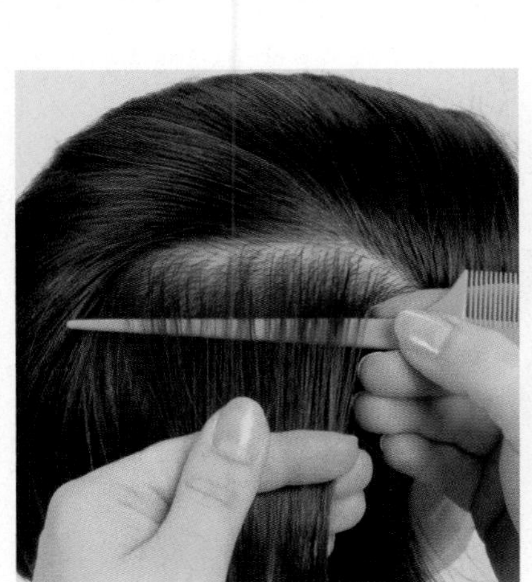

Figure 19-72 Slicing.

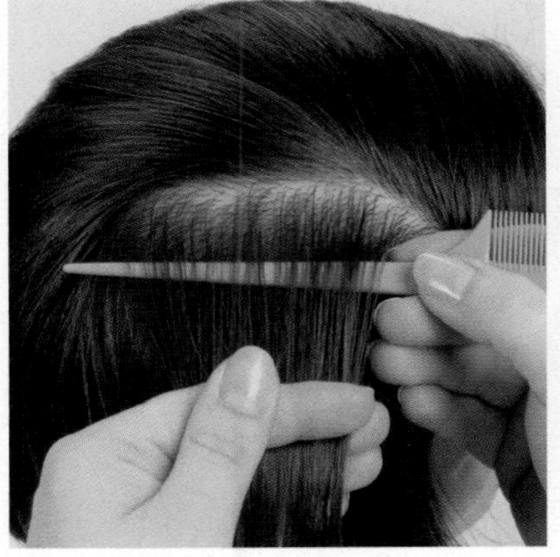

Figure 19-73 Weaving.

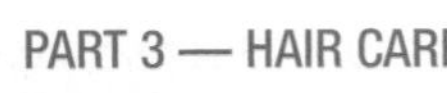

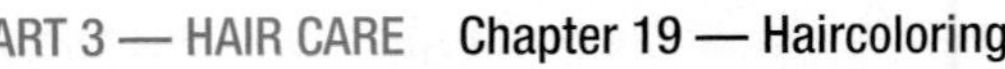

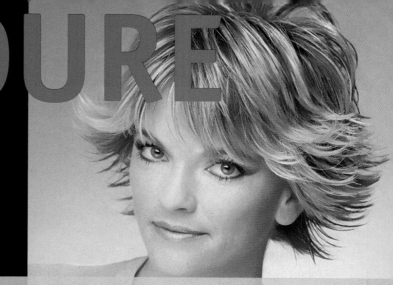

PROCEDURE 19-9

SPECIAL-EFFECTS HAIRCOLORING WITH FOIL, FULL HEAD

IMPLEMENTS AND MATERIALS

- Waterproof cape
- Towel
- Foil
- Gloves
- Plastic clips
- Bowl/brushes
- Tail comb
- Applicator brush
- Lightener
- Record card
- Applicator bottle

PREPARATION

Follow the same preparation steps as for lightening virgin hair, and include a patch test (if toner will be applied) and a strand test. Carefully analyze the hair and record all information on the client's card for future use.

PROCEDURE

1. With a tail comb, take a slice of hair at the lower crown area of the head and place a piece of foil under the slice of hair (Figure 19-74).
2. Holding the hair taut, brush on the lightener, from the upper edge of the foil to the hair ends (Figure 19-75).
3. Fold the foil in half until the ends meet.
4. Fold the foil in half again, using the comb to crease it.
5. Clip the foil upward.
6. Take a 3/4-inch (1.8-centimeter) subsection in between foils. Clip this hair up and out of the way (Figure 19-76). (Note the contrast in size between the foiled and unfoiled subsections.)
7. Continue working down the back center of the head until the section is complete (Figure 19-77).
8. Once the section is complete, release the clipped-up foils.
9. Work around the head into the side area, divide it into two smaller sections.
10. Work down the side, bring fine slices of hair into the foil, and apply lightener to the hair. Clip up the foil.

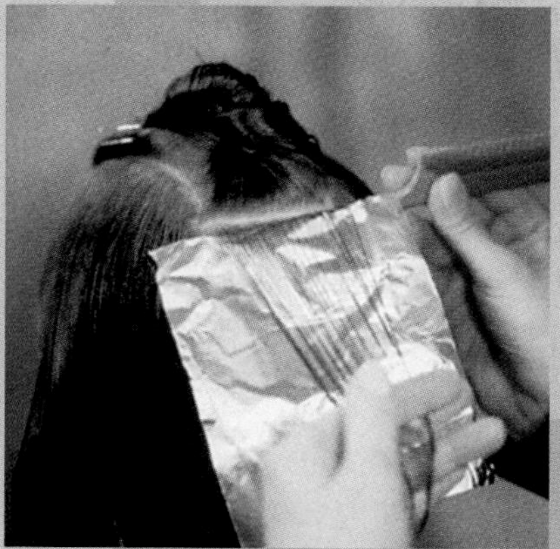

Figure 19-74 Place slice of hair over foil.

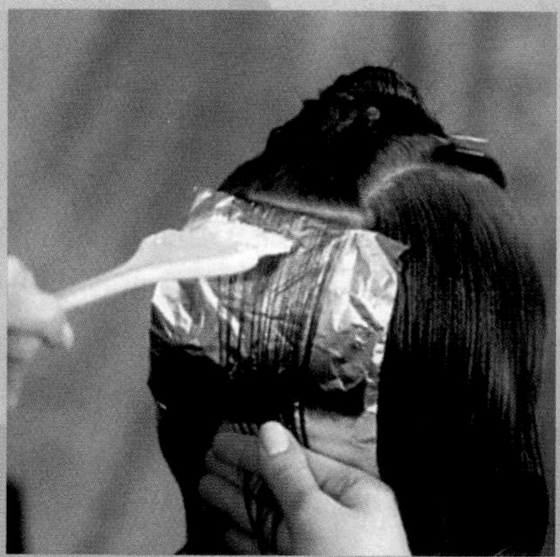

Figure 19-75 Hold taut and paint lightener, working all through the strand.

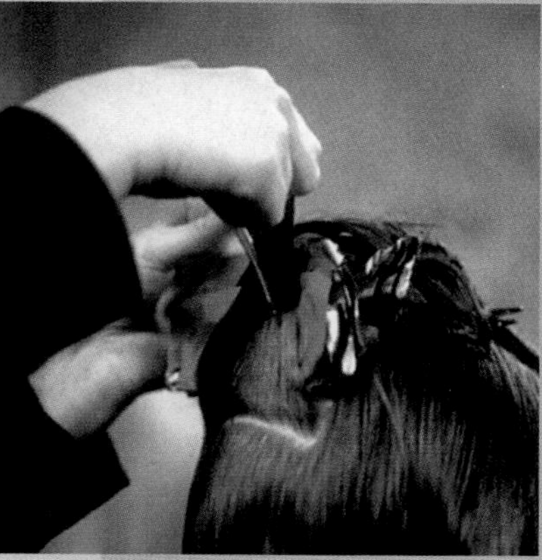

Figure 19-76 Clip foil up and out of the way.

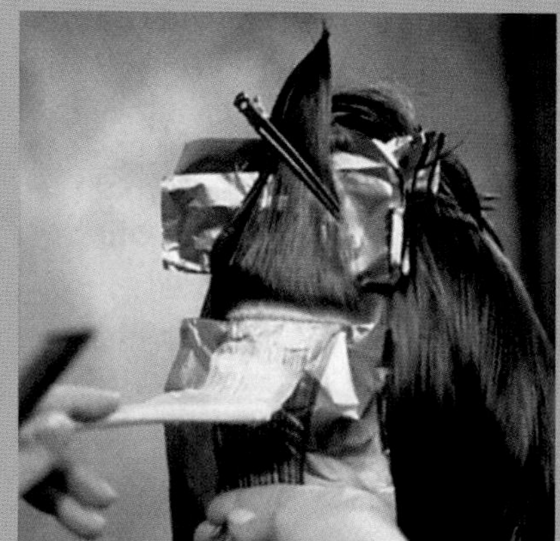

Figure 19-77 Release the foils.

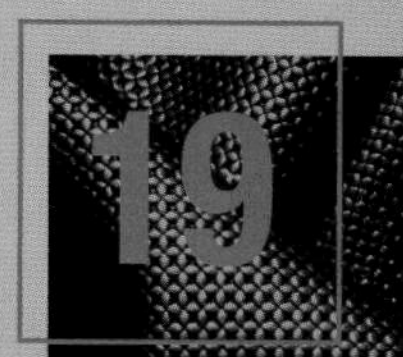

11. Move to the other side of the head and complete the matching sections.
12. Move to the top of the head. Take a fine slice of hair off the top of a large section, place it on the foil, and apply lightener.
13. Part out a larger section, and then take a fine slice from the top of this section. Apply lightener.
14. Continue toward the front until the last foil is placed (Figure 19-78).
15. Allow the lightener to process according to the strand test. Check the foils for the desired lightness.
16. Remove the foils one at a time at the shampoo area. Rinse the hair immediately to prevent the color from affecting the untreated hair.
17. Apply a haircolor glaze to the hair from scalp to ends (Figure 19-79).
18. Work the glaze into the hair to make sure it is completely saturated (Figure 19-80). Process up to 20 minutes.
20. Rinse the hair, shampoo and condition.
21. Style the hair as desired (Figure 19-81).

CLEANUP AND SANITATION

Perform same cleanup and sanitation as for traditional semipermanent color.

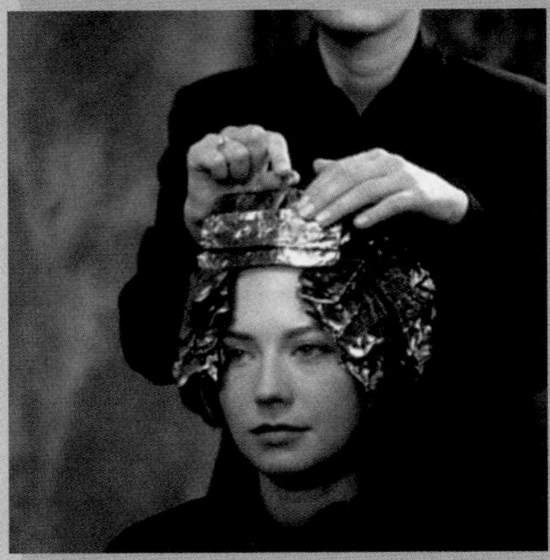

Figure 19-78 Continue working until last foil is placed.

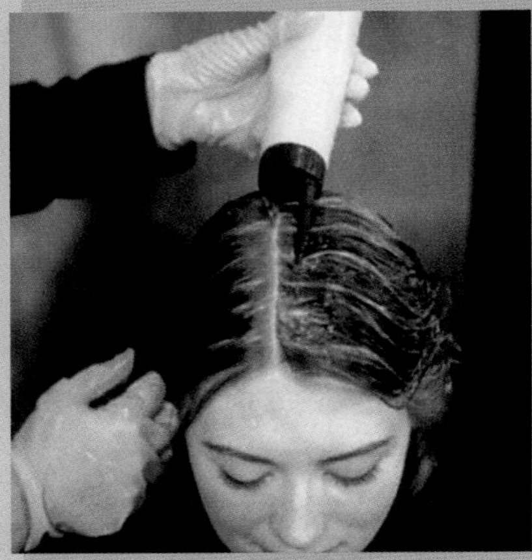

Figure 19-79 Apply glaze over the highlighted hair.

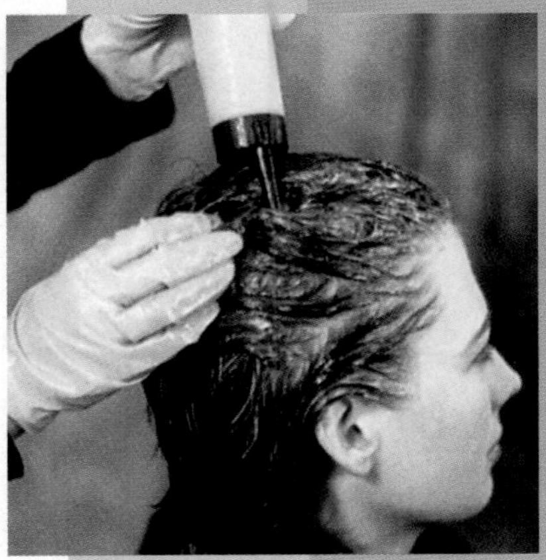

Figure 19-80 Work the glaze through the hair.

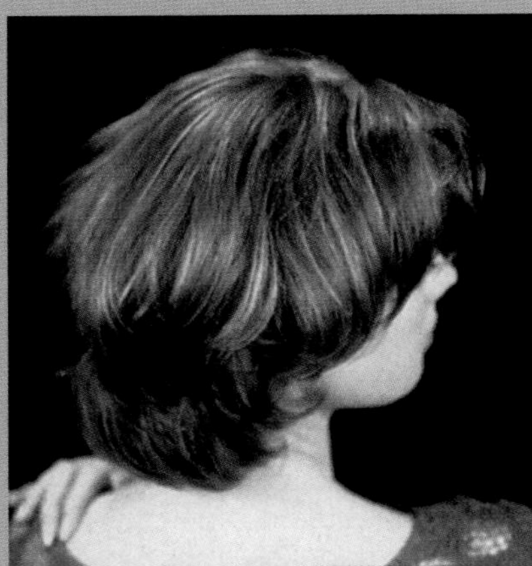

Figure 19-81 The finished look.

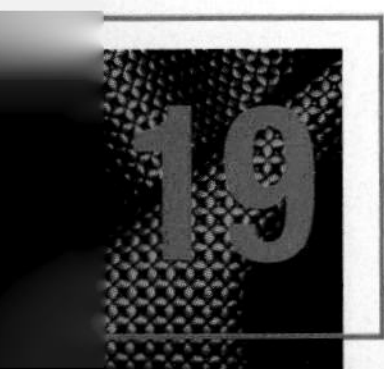

BALIAGE TECHNIQUE

The **baliage** (also spelled balyage) or **free-form technique** involves the painting of a lightener (usually powdered off-the-scalp lightener) directly onto clean styled hair. The lightener is applied with an applicator brush or a tail comb from scalp to ends around the head (Figure 19-82). The effects are extremely subtle and are used to draw attention to the surface of the hair (Figure 19-83).

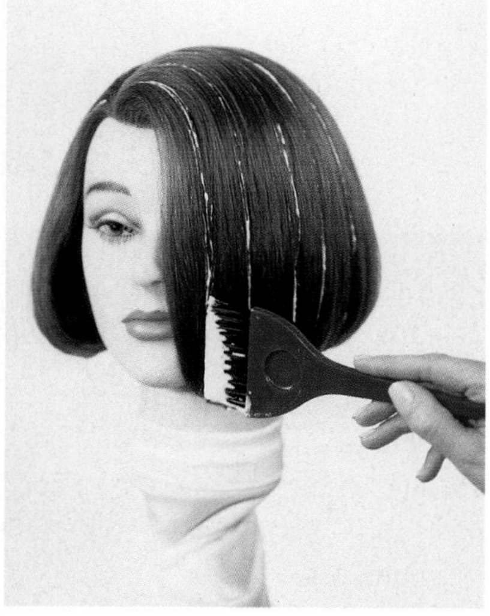

Figure 19-82 Balayage technique.

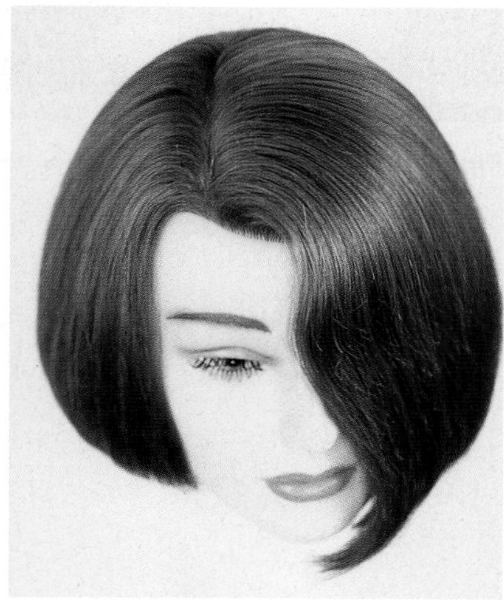

Figure 19-83 Finished hair.

TONING OVERHIGHLIGHTED AND DIMENSIONALLY COLORED HAIR

When the hair is decolorized to the desired level during a highlighting service, the use of a toner may not be necessary. However, if a cool tone is desired, you should use a toner to cancel out any undesirable yellow-contributing pigment.

When using a toner on highlighted hair, it is important to consider not only the varying degrees of porosity in the hair, but also the difference in pigmentation from strand to strand that was created by the lightening process. Although an oxidative toner will add color to the highlighted strands, it might also cause a slight amount of lift to the natural or pigmented hair.

The result may be an uneven tone, with the underlying warmth brought out by the oxidative color. Strand test to ensure best results.

To avoid affecting the untreated hair, choose from the following options:

- A nonoxidative toner, which contains no ammonia, requires no developer (thus producing no lift of the natural hair color), and is gentle on the scalp and hair.
- Semipermanent color may be used to deposit color without lift. Select a color that is delicate enough to avoid overpowering the prelightened hair. Always check the manufacturer's color chart for the color of your chosen toner to make sure that the combination of the toner and the contributing pigment will produce the desired color results.
- A demipermanent haircolor is a no-lift deposit-only color that will not cause additional lightening and lasts longer than temporary or traditional semipermanent colors.

HIGHLIGHTING SHAMPOOS

Highlighting shampoo colors are prepared by combining permanent haircolor, hydrogen peroxide, and shampoo. They are used when a slight change in hair shade is desired, or when the client's hair processes very rapidly. This process highlights the hair's natural color in a single application.

Highlighting shampoos are a mixture of shampoo and hydrogen peroxide. The natural color is slightly lightened. No patch test is required. Follow manufacturer's directions.

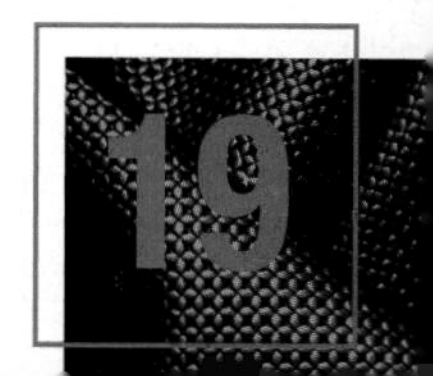

SPECIAL CHALLENGES IN HAIRCOLOR/ CORRECTIVE SOLUTIONS

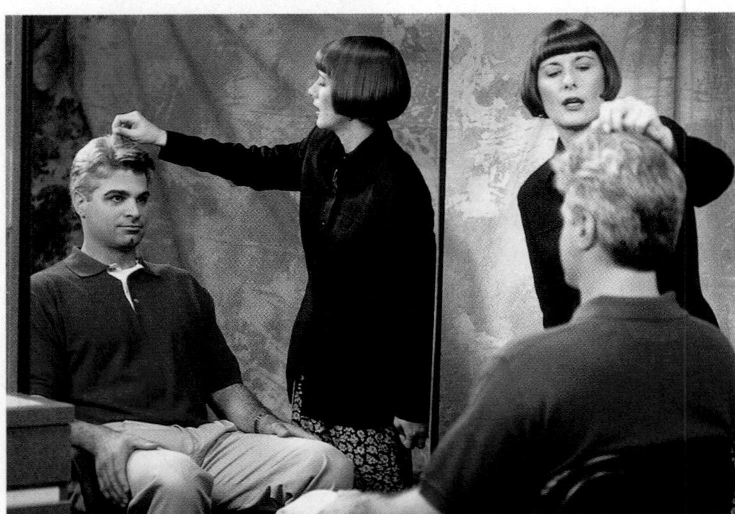

Figure 19-84 Gray hair presents certain challenges.

Each haircoloring service is unique and can present unique challenges. To give each haircoloring service a good start, the colorist must allow enough time for a complete client consultation and analysis of the client' s hair. Strand tests must be taken to ensure satisfactory final results. But even the most skilled colorist will occasionally have a problem that can't be predicted. This may be due to the particular structure or condition of the client's hair. The good news is that most haircoloring problems can be resolved or corrected as long the colorist remains calm.

GRAY HAIR: CHALLENGES AND SOLUTIONS

Gray, white, and salt-and-pepper hair all have characteristics that present unique coloring challenges. For instance, gray hair can turn orange if the lightener used is not processed long enough. A great many salon coloring services, however, will successfully cover or enhance gray hair if used correctly (Figures 19-84 and 19-85).

YELLOWED HAIR

A problem that can occur with gray hair is the yellow cast caused by a variety of factors.

- Smoking
- Medication
- Sun exposure
- Hair sprays and styling aids

Lightener and haircolor removers help remove yellow discoloration. Undesired yellow can often be overpowered by the artificial pigments deposited by violet-based colors of an equal or darker level than the yellow.

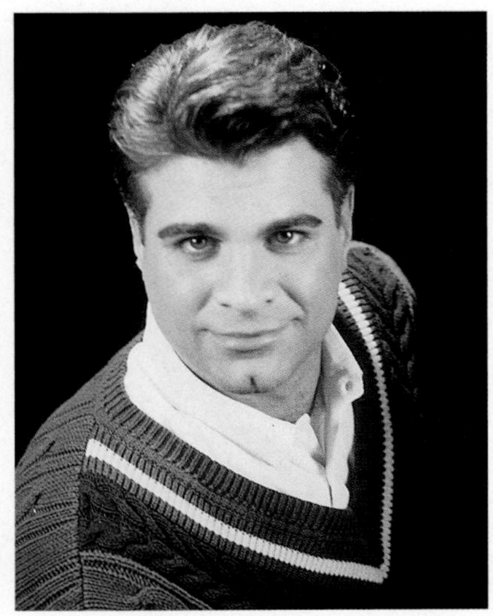

Figure 19-85 Many haircolor options cover gray successfully.

FORMULATING FOR GRAY HAIR

Gray hair accepts the level of the color applied. However, Level 8 or lighter colors may not give complete coverage because of the low concentration of dye found in lighter colors. Formulations from Level 7 and darker will provide better coverage, and can be used to create pastel and blond tones if desired.

For those clients who are 80- to 100-percent gray, a haircolor within the blond range is generally more flattering than a darker shade. This lighter level of artificial color may be selected to give a warm or cool

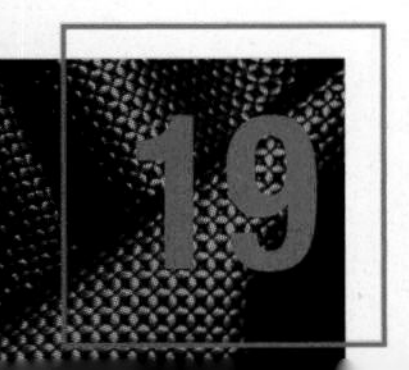

finished color , depending on the client's skin tone, eye color, and personal preference.

Another factor to consider when coloring low percentages of gray or salt-and-pepper hair to a darker level is that color on color will always make a darker color. The addition of dark artificial pigment to the natural pigment results in a color that the eye perceives as darker. For this reason, when attempting to cover the unpigmented hair in a salt-and-pepper head, formulate two levels lighter than the natural level to ensure a natural result.

For the purposes of a strand test, a manufacturer's product color chart can be used in conjunction with the following formulation charts (Tables 19-4 and 19-5) to select a color within the proper level.

PERCENTAGE OF GRAY HAIR	Semipermanent/Demipermanent Color Formulation for Gray Hair
90–100%	Desired level
70–90%	Equal parts desired and one level lighter
50–70%	One level lighter than desired level
30–50%	Equal parts one level lighter and two levels lighter
10–30%	Two levels lighter than desired level

Table 19-4 Semipermanent/Demipermanent Color Formulation for Gray Hair

PERCENTAGE OF GRAY HAIR	Permanent Color Formulation for Gray Hair
90–100%	Desired level
70–90%	Two parts desired level and one part lighter level
50–70%	Equal parts desired and lighter level
30–50%	Two parts lighter level and one part desired level
10–30%	One level lighter

Table 19-5 Permanent Color Formulation for Gray Hair

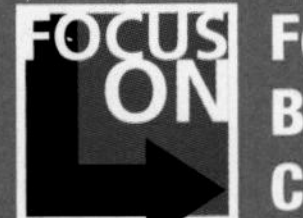

Focus on . . . Building Your Client Base

- Be as knowledgeable about haircolor as you can be. Maintain your skills through continuous education.
- Be honest when recommending color options to your client. That means including information on maintenance, costs, and other issues.
- Keep up to date with celebrity hair trends because your clients will be asking for them.
- Maintain a positive and excited attitude about your work and convey your confidence and enthusiasm to your client.

The gray hair formulation tables provide general guidelines, but there are other considerations to take into account such as the following:

- Client's personality
- Personal preferences
- Amount of gray hair and its location

You will note that in the tables there are no colors given in the formulations, only the levels of haircoloring and various techniques. Also note that the table does not consider the location of the gray hair. The table assumes that the gray hair is equally distributed throughout the entire head. If, for instance, the majority of gray hair is located in the front section of the head, that section would be considered to have more gray hair, with the back portion containing less gray hair. In that instance, you would have to determine what formulation would best suit the client. The gray hair around the face is what the client sees, so it may be wise to formulate based on the percentage of gray hair the client actually sees. The section of hair that surrounds the face is what influences the client's self-image.

There are many techniques to help solve your haircolor challenges. Some tips for working on gray hair follow:

- Use 20-volume developer.
- Process color for a full 45 minutes.
- Add ½ to 1 ounce of a natural/warm tone to the formula for resistant gray hair.
- High-lift blond is not designed for gray coverage. To create a very light result, formulate at a Level 7 and add some highlights.

PRESOFTENING

Occasionally, gray hair is so resistant that even when formulation, application, and time are correct, you will find that the coverage is not satisfactory. In such cases, presoftening becomes necessary. **Presoftening** raises the cuticle layer of gray or resistant hair to allow for better penetration of color. It is a double-application haircoloring service. A presoftener is applied, processed, and removed. Then the haircolor is applied.

Although presoftening is equally effective on pigmented hair, you should leave the presoftening mixture on the hair only long enough to help raise the cuticle, thus making the hair porous enough to accept the color.

To presoften hair, mix the product according to the manufacturer's directions. Apply with an applicator brush or bottle and start in the most resistant areas first. Process at room temperature for 5 to 20 minutes. Wipe the presoftener gently with a cloth or paper towel to remove. Next, apply a haircolor formula of the correct level and tone to achieve your end results.

RULES FOR EFFECTIVE COLOR CORRECTION

Sometimes the color may not turn out as expected. Although this can seem disastrous, for your client and for you, it does not need to be. Problems can always be corrected. Keep the following guidelines in mind.

1. Do not panic. Remain calm.
2. Determine the nature of the problem.
3. Determine what caused the problem.
4. Develop a solution.
5. Always take one step at a time.
6. Never guarantee an exact result.
7. Always strand test for accuracy.

DAMAGED HAIR

Blow-drying, wind, harsh shampoos, and chemical services all take their toll on the condition of the hair. Coating compounds such as hair sprays, styling agents, and some conditioners can block/interfere with color penetration. Hair is considered damaged when it has one or more of the following characteristics:

- Rough texture
- Overporous condition
- Brittle and dry to the touch
- Susceptible to breakage
- No elasticity
- Becomes spongy and matted when wet
- Color fades too quickly or grabs too dark

Any of these hair conditions will create problems during a haircoloring, lightening, permanent waving, or hair relaxing treatment. Therefore, damaged hair should receive reconditioning treatments prior to, and after the application of, these chemical services. Tips for dealing with damaged hair appear below.

- Use a penetrating conditioner that can deposit protein, oils, and moisture-rich ingredients.
- Complete each chemical service by normalizing the pH with an acidic finishing rinse. This will restore the ability of the cuticle to protect the hair.
- Postpone any further chemical service until the hair is reconditioned.
- Schedule the client for between-service conditioning.
- Recommend retail products for use at home to prepare for the next service.

FILLERS

Fillers help equalize porosity. Color fillers equalize porosity and deposit color in one application. Some fillers are ready to use as they come from the manufacturer, while others are a mixture of haircolor and conditioner that your instructor can help you prepare. There are two types of fillers: conditioner fillers and color fillers.

Conditioner fillers are used to recondition damaged, overly porous hair, and equalize porosity so that the hair accepts the color evenly, from

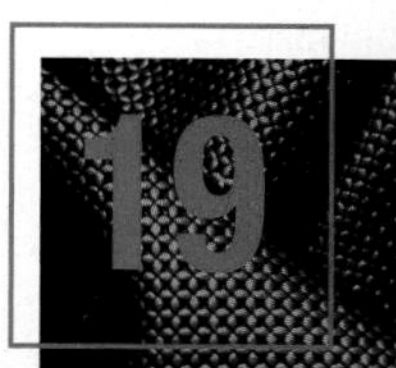

strand to strand and scalp to ends. They can be applied in a separate procedure or immediately prior to the color application.

Color fillers equalize porosity and deposit color in one application. Color fillers are used on overly porous, prelightened hair to equalize porosity and provide a uniform contributing pigment that complements the desired finished color. No-lift deposit-only haircolor products are commonly used as color fillers. Advantages of color fillers are listed below.

- Deposit color to faded ends and hair shaft
- Help hair to hold color
- Prevent streaking and dull appearance
- Prevent off-color results
- Produce more uniform, natural-looking color in a tint
- Produce uniform color when coloring prelightened hair back to its natural color

SELECTING THE CORRECT COLOR FILLER

All three primary colors must be present to produce a haircolor that looks natural. To correct an unwanted haircolor, always use the primary or secondary color that is missing in the hair. That color is called the complementary color. Complementary colors are directly opposite each other on the color wheel.

Yellow blond hair can be corrected to a natural blond by adding the two missing primary colors, red and blue, that is, the secondary color violet. Violet cancels yellow. Orange blond hair can be corrected to a natural blond by adding the missing primary color, blue. Blue cancels orange. Adding blue color to yellow hair would make the hair green. Remember that a primary color always cancels a secondary color and a secondary color always cancels a primary color.

Color fillers may be applied directly from their containers to damaged hair prior to coloring. They may also be added to the haircolor and applied to damaged ends.

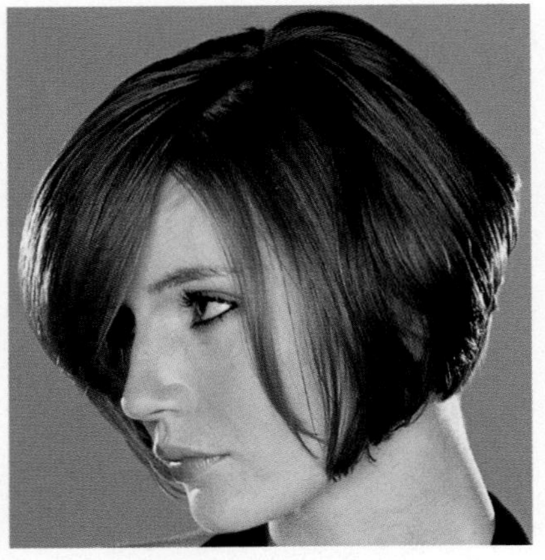

Figure 19-86 Vibrant red hair.

HAIRCOLOR TIPS FOR REDHEADS

Red haircolor is exciting and fun, but fading is a common problem with color-treated red hair (Figure 19-86). A daily shampoo and blow-dry, with an occasional permanent wave, and a few days in the pool or at the beach cause the artificial pigment within the hair to oxidize and fade. It is important to recommend the proper products to maintain the finished haircolor. Tips are summarized below.

- To create warm coppery reds, use a red orange base color.
- To create hot fiery reds, use red-violet or true red colors.
- After the hair has been colored with a permanent color, always use a no-lift deposit-only color to refresh the shaft and ends.
- If gray hair is present, always add ½ to 1 ounce of a natural color to the desired red.

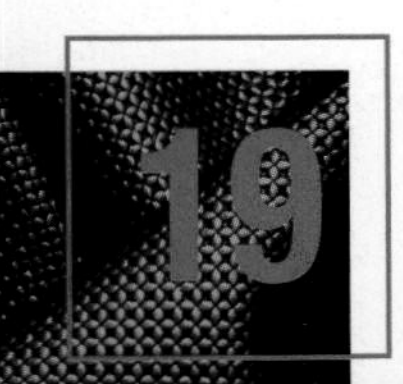

- To brighten haircolor, refresh reds with a **soap cap** of equal parts shampoo and the remaining color formula before rinsing.

HAIRCOLOR TIPS FOR BRUNETTES

- To avoid orange or brassy tones when lifting brown hair with permanent color, always use a cool blue base.
- To avoid unwanted brassy tones, do not lighten more than two levels above the natural color.
- Add 1 ounce of a natural color to cover gray in brunette hair.
- Natural highlights in brunette hair should be deep or caramel colored. Blond highlights have too much contrast with brunette hair. Blond highlights do not look natural and require frequent service.

HAIRCOLOR TIPS FOR BLONDS

- Blond haircolor is popular, profitable, and fun. From single-process blond to highlighting, the possibilities are endless.
- When lightening brown hair to blond, remember that there may be underlying unwanted warm tones.
- When covering gray hair with a blond color, use a Level 7 or darker for the best coverage.
- Double-process blonding is the best way to obtain pale blond results.
- If high-lift blonds that lift only 5 levels, are used on Levels 4 and below, the result may be a color that is too warm or brassy.
- If highlights become too blond or all one color, lowlights or deeper strands can be foiled into the hair to create a more natural color, or you can glaze the hair with a light blond color containing a red-orange base to add missing warmth to the hair.

COMMON HAIRCOLOR SOLUTIONS

GREEN CAST

If the hair has a buildup of minerals from well water or chlorine, you may want to purify the hair with a product designed to remove the mineral buildup. You can apply a no-lift deposit-only color to neutralize any unwanted color that remains in the hair.

OVERALL HAIRCOLOR IS TOO LIGHT

This is a result of incorrect formulation. To correct, apply a no-lift deposit-only color that is one to two levels darker than the previous formula.

OVERALL COLOR IS TOO DARK

Determine how much of the color needs to be removed. Use a haircolor remover in cases where the hair is too dark because of buildup or formulation. Apply haircolor remover to the areas that need to be lightened. Process for 10 minutes and check development. These removers are designed to remove artificial pigment from the hair. Once you have achieved the desired color, rinse and shampoo.

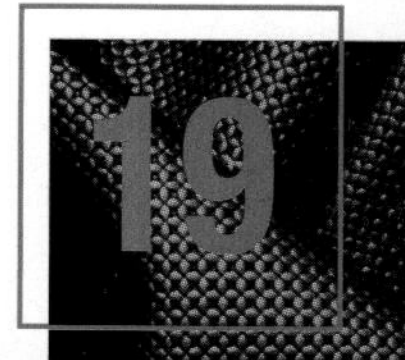

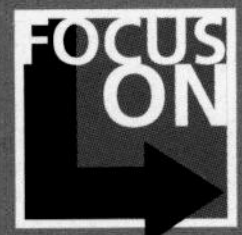

Focus on . . . Retailing

Your color client needs to use high-quality salon products at home to help prevent her haircolor from fading. Using the right products increases the longevity of the hair color, preserves the natural integrity (health) of the hair, and makes your client more likely to return to you for more services. Recommending the right professional products increases your client's satisfaction, and your income.

CAUTION

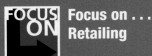

Sometimes the hair is so damaged and overly porous that there may be insufficient structure left within the cortex for the artificial pigment to attach to. Hair that looks "gun-metal gray" is a real danger sign. Hair that is this porous is very fragile, and may be close to the breaking point.

RESTORING BLOND TO NATURAL HAIRCOLOR

Restoring a client's blond hair back to its natural darker color can be tricky. Even if the client says that she wants to go back to her natural color, she may not like it. She is used to seeing light hair and going too dark could be disastrous. A few tips on how to accomplish this objective are listed below.

First, soften the new growth with a level 6-violet base color with 20 volume. Apply to the scalp area, process for 30 minutes, and rinse.

Next, apply a no-lift deposit-only glaze with 1 ounce of a Level-8 light natural blond and 1 ounce of a Level-9 red-orange. Apply to all the lightened hair. Do not apply to the scalp area. Process for 20 minutes. Rinse and towel-dry.

Finally, mix a no-lift deposit-only glaze with 2 ounces of a Level-6 natural blond. Apply the color all over from scalp to ends. Process up to 20 minutes, checking it every 5 minutes.

Reevaluate the haircolor at the client's next visit, and determine what is needed to make the color deeper. Apply a separate color to the scalp area and on the remainder of the hair strand for the best results.

Haircoloring offers you the opportunity to exercise your creative talents and bring great pleasure to your clients (Figure 19-87). Enjoy your work, but most of all, enjoy and appreciate learning now and in the future. Haircolor techniques, fashions, and formulations are constantly changing. Professionals who specialize in haircolor must constantly learn new techniques to keep up with those changes.

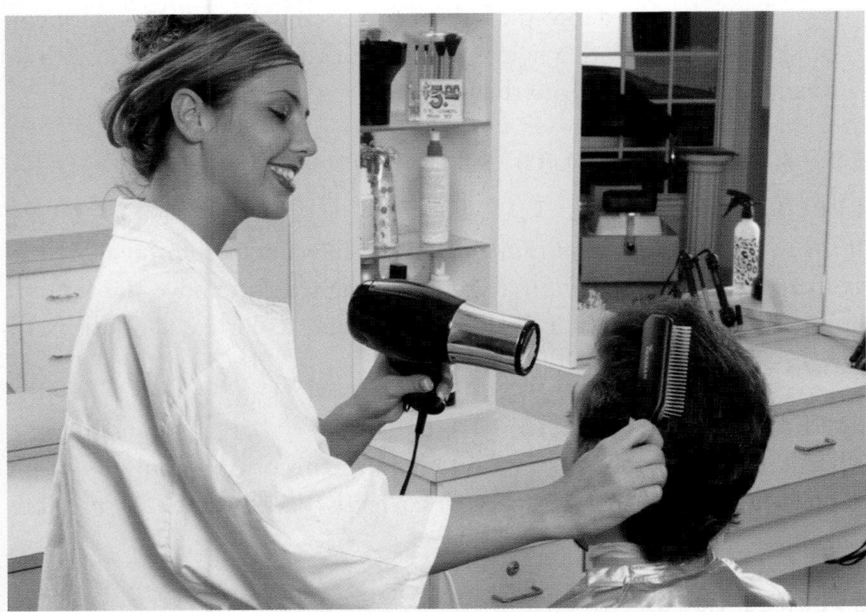

Figure 19-87 A haircolor specialist has both skill and creativity.

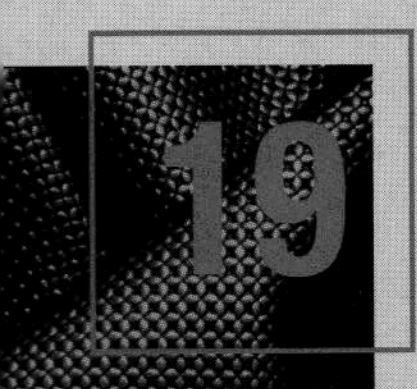

HAIRCOLORING SAFETY PRECAUTIONS

- Perform a patch test 24 to 48 hours prior to each application of aniline-derivative haircolor. Apply haircolor only if the patch test is negative.
- Do not apply haircolor if abrasions are present.
- Do not apply haircolor if a metallic or compound haircolor is present.
- Do not brush the hair prior to applying color.
- Always read and follow the manufacturer's directions.
- Use sanitized applicator bottles, brushes, combs, and towels.
- Protect your client's clothing with proper draping.
- Perform a strand test for color, breakage, and/or discoloration.
- Use an applicator bottle or bowl (glass or plastic) for mixing the haircolor.
- Do not mix haircolor until you are ready to use it; discard leftover haircolor.
- Wear gloves to protect your hands.
- Do not permit the color to come in contact with the client's eyes.
- Do not overlap during a haircolor retouch.
- Use a mild shampoo. An alkaline or harsh shampoo will strip color.
- Always wash hands before and after serving a client.

REVIEW QUESTIONS

1. List the primary, secondary, and tertiary colors.
2. Name the two types of melanin.
3. Define level and tone.
4. What are the classifications of haircolor? Briefly describe each one.
5. Why is a patch test important?
6. What is a strand test?
7. What is the role of ammonia in a haircolor formula?
8. What is the role of hydrogen peroxide in a haircolor formula?
9. What are the four key questions you ask when formulating a haircolor?
10. Explain the procedure for a single-process tint.
11. Explain the procedure for a single-process tint with a glaze.
12. What are the two processes involved in double-process haircoloring?
13. What are three forms of hair lightener?
14. What are the three most commonly used methods for highlighting?
15. What are fillers, and for what purpose are they used?
16. List at least 10 safety precautions to follow during the haircolor process.

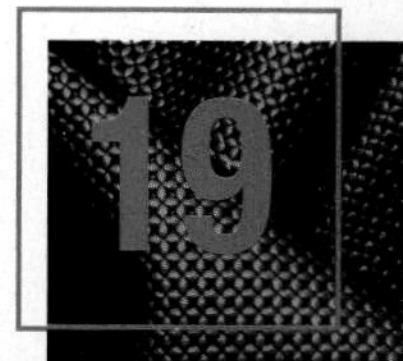

CHAPTER GLOSSARY

activators	Powdered persulfate salts added to haircolor to increase its lightening ability.
aniline derivatives	Contain small, uncolored dyes that combine with hydrogen peroxide to form larger, permanent dye molecules within the cortex.
baliage or free-form technique	Painting a lightener (usually a powdered off-the-scalp lightener) directly onto clean, styled hair.
base color	Predominant tone of a color.
cap technique	Lightening technique that involves pulling clean strands of hair through a perforated cap with a thin plastic or metal hook.
color fillers	Equalize porosity and deposit color in one application to provide a uniform contributing pigment on prelightened hair.
complementary colors	Primary and secondary color combinations that are directly opposite from each other on the color wheel.
conditioner fillers	Used to recondition damaged, overly porous hair, and equalize porosity so that the hair accepts the color evenly from strand to strand and scalp to ends.
contributing pigment	Natural hair color that remains in the hair when the natural color is lightened; must be taken into consideration when haircolor is selected. Also called undertone.
demipermanent haircolor	Also called no-lift, deposit-only color. Formulated to deposit, but not lift (lighten) natural hair color. Demipermanent colors are able to deposit without lifting because they are less alkaline than permanent colors and are mixed with a low-volume developer.
developer	Oxidizing agent that, when mixed with an oxidation haircolor, supplies the necessary oxygen gas to develop color molecules and create a change in hair color.
double-process application	Coloring technique requiring two separate procedures in which the hair is prelightened before the depositing color is applied; also called two-step coloring.
fillers	Used to equalize porosity.
foil technique	Highlighting technique that involves coloring selected strands of hair by slicing or weaving out sections, placing them on foil or plastic wrap, applying lightener or permanent haircolor, and sealing them in the foil or plastic wrap.
glaze	A nonammonia color that adds shine and tone to the hair.
hair color	The natural color of hair.
haircolor	Professional, salon industry term referring to artificial haircolor products and services.

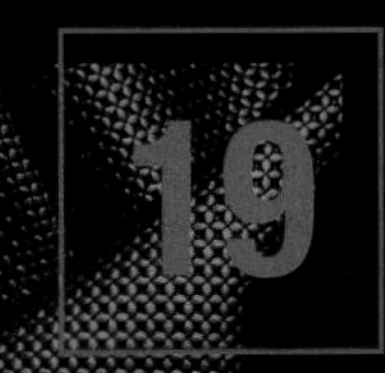

CHAPTER GLOSSARY

hair lightening	Chemical process involving the diffusion of the natural color pigment or artificial color from the hair; often called "bleaching" or "decolorizing."
highlighting	Coloring some of the hair strands lighter than the natural color to add the illusion of sheen and depth; highlights do not generally contrast strongly with the natural color.
highlighting shampoo	Mixture of shampoo and hydrogen peroxide; used to slightly lighten natural hair color.
law of color	System for understanding color relationships.
level	Lightness or darkness of a color. Refers to the saturation, concentration, or density of a color. Answers the question, how much color?
level system	System that colorists use to determine the lightness or darkness of a hair color.
lighteners	Chemical compounds that lighten hair by dispersing, dissolving, and decolorizing the natural hair pigment.
line of demarcation	Visible line separating colored hair from new growth.
metallic or gradual colors	Haircolors containing metal salts that change hair color gradually by progressive buildup and exposure to air, creating a dull, metallic appearance.
natural* or *vegetable haircolors	Colors, such as henna, obtained from the leaves or bark of plants.
new growth	Part of the hair shaft between the scalp and the hair that has been previously colored.
off-the-scalp lighteners	Powdered lighteners that cannot be used directly on the scalp.
on-the-scalp lighteners	Oil and cream lighteners that can be used directly on the scalp.
oxidation	A process by which oxygen is released, occurs within the cortex of the hair shaft.
patch test	Test for identifying a possible allergy in a client, required by Federal Food, Drug, and Cosmetic Act. Also called predisposition test.
permanent haircolors	Lighten and deposit color at the same time and in one application. They are more alkaline than no lift deposit only haircolors and mixed with a higher volume developer.
prelightening	First step of double-process haircoloring, used to lift or lighten the natural pigment before the application of toner.
presoftening	Process of treating gray or very resistant hair to allow for better penetration of color.
primary colors	Pure or fundamental colors (red, yellow, and blue) that cannot be created by combining other colors.
resistant	Characteristic of some hair types that makes penetration by moisture or chemicals difficult.

CHAPTER GLOSSARY

reverse highlighting* or *lowlighting	Technique of coloring strands of hair darker than the natural color.
secondary color	Color obtained by mixing equal parts of two primary colors.
semipermanent haircolor	No-lift, deposit-only, nonoxidation haircolor that is not mixed with peroxide and is formulated to last through several shampoos.
single-process haircoloring	Process that lightens and deposits color in the hair in a single application.
slicing	Coloring technique that involves taking a narrow, ⅛-inch (0.3-centimeter) section of hair by making a straight part at the scalp, positioning the hair over the foil, and applying lightener or color.
soap cap	Combination of equal parts of prepared tint and shampoo applied to the hair like a regular shampoo.
special effects haircoloring	Any technique that involves partial lightening or coloring.
temporary haircolor	Nonpermanent color whose large pigment molecules prevent penetration of the cuticle layer, allowing only a coating action that may be removed by shampooing.
tertiary color	Intermediate color achieved by mixing a secondary color and its neighboring primary color on the color wheel in equal amounts.
tone	Also called hue of color; the balance of color.
toners	Semipermanent, demipermanent, and permanent haircolor products that are used primarily on prelightened hair to achieve pale and delicate colors.
virgin application	First time the hair is colored.
volume	Measure of varying strengths (concentration) of hydrogen peroxide; the higher the volume, the greater the lifting action.
weaving	Coloring technique in which selected strands are picked up from a narrow section of hair with a zigzag motion of the comb, and lightener or color is applied only to these strands.

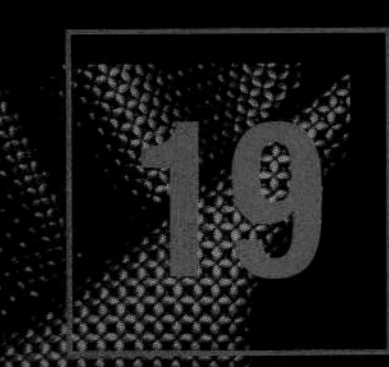

SKIN CARE

PART 4

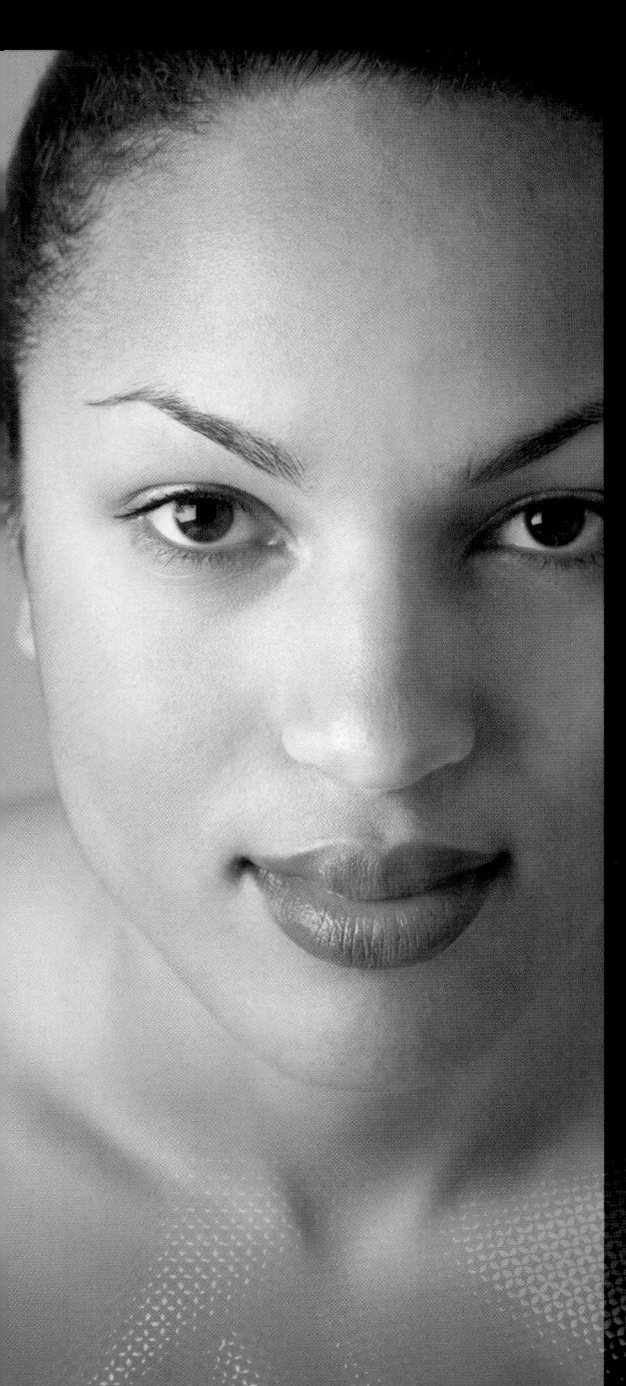

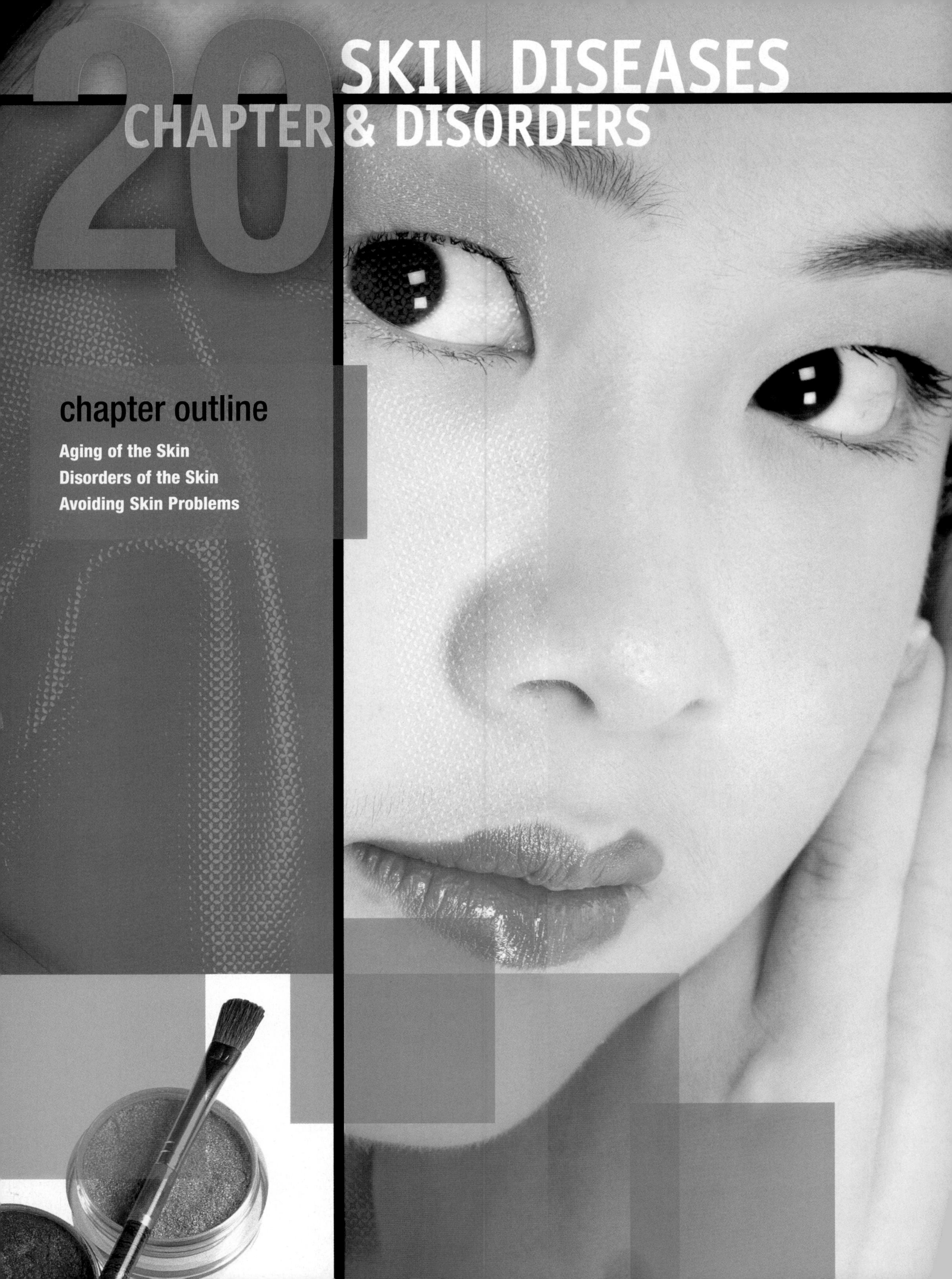

CHAPTER 20 SKIN DISEASES & DISORDERS

chapter outline

Learning Objectives

After completing this chapter, you will be able to:

- **Describe the aging process and the factors that influence aging of the skin.**
- **Define important terms relating to skin disorders.**
- **Discuss which skin disorders may be handled in the salon, and which should be referred to a physician.**

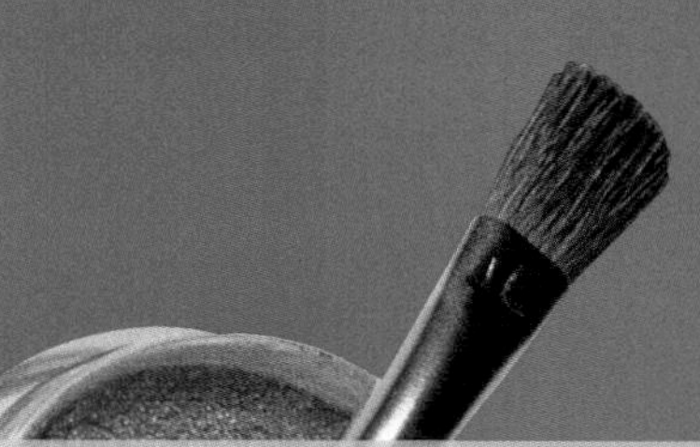

Key Terms

Page number indicates where in the chapter the term is used.

acne
pg. 537

albinism
pg. 539

anhidrosis
pg. 538

asteatosis
pg. 538

basal cell carcinoma
pg. 540

bromhidrosis
pg. 538

bulla (plural: bullae)
pg. 536

chloasma
pg. 539

comedo (plural: comedones)
pg. 537

crust
pg. 537

cyst
pg. 536

dermatitis
pg. 538

dermatitis venenata
pg. 541

eczema
pg. 538

excoriation
pg. 537

fissure
pg. 537

herpes simplex
pg. 538

hyperhidrosis
pg. 538

hypertrophy
pg. 540

keloid
pg. 537

keratoma
pg. 540

lentigines (singular: lentigo)
pg. 539

lesion
pg. 535

leukoderma
pg. 539

macule (plural: maculae)
pg. 536

malignant melanoma
pg. 540

milia
pg. 537

miliaria rubra
pg. 538

mole
pg. 540

nevus
pg. 539

papule
pg. 536

psoriasis
pg. 538

pustule
pg. 536

rosacea
pg. 538

scale
pg. 537

scar or cicatrix
pg. 537

seborrheic dermatitis
pg. 537

sensitization
pg. 541

skin tag
pg. 540

squamous cell carcinoma
pg. 540

stain
pg. 539

steatoma
pg. 538

tan
pg. 539

telangiectasias
pg. 534

tubercle
pg. 536

tumor
pg. 536

ulcer
pg. 537

verruca
pg. 540

vesicle
pg. 536

vitiligo
pg. 539

wheal
pg. 536

20

No matter how advanced the latest skin-care technology may be, knowing how to care for someone's skin begins with understanding its underlying structure and basic needs. As a licensed service provider, you also must recognize adverse conditions, including inflamed skin conditions, diseases, and infectious skin disorders.

Having a good working knowledge of skin care is essential to passing your state board exams. It also may provide you with an exciting new career. Skin care specialists are in high demand in high-end salons and spas, and earn excellent salaries. Some find the work less arduous and physically demanding than doing hair and choose to balance their day by scheduling services in both areas.

AGING OF THE SKIN

Aging of the skin is a process that takes many years and can be influenced by various factors. One does not necessarily age as one's parents have.

Many outside factors like the sun, the environment, health habits, and general lifestyle greatly influence the signs of skin aging to such a great extent that it has been estimated that heredity may only be responsible for 15% of the factors that determine how skin ages.

THE SUN AND ITS EFFECTS

The sun and its ultraviolet (UV) rays have the greatest impact on how skin ages. Approximately 80 to 85 percent of aging is caused by the rays of the sun. As we age, the collagen and elastin fibers of the skin naturally weaken. This weakening happens at a much faster rate when the skin is frequently exposed to UV rays without proper protection. The UV rays of the sun reach the skin in two different forms, UVA and UVB. Each of these forms influences the skin at a different level.

UVA rays, also called the "aging rays," are deep-penetrating rays that can even go through a glass window. These rays weaken the collagen and elastin fibers, causing wrinkling and sagging of the tissues.

UVB rays, also referred to as the "burning rays," cause sunburns and tanning of the skin by affecting the melanocytes, the cells of the epidermis that are responsible for producing melanin, the skin pigment. Melanin is designed to help protect the skin from the sun's UV rays, but can be altered or destroyed when large, frequent doses of UV light are allowed to penetrate the skin. Although UVB penetration is not as deep as UVA, these rays are equally damaging to the skin and can damage the eyes as well. On a positive note, UVB rays contribute to the body's synthesis of Vitamin D and other important minerals. However, the amount of sun exposure necessary for vitamin D synthesis is very minimal, not to mention the fact that you can get vitamin D from fortified milk or orange juice.

As a consultant to your clients, it is appropriate that you advise them about the necessary precautions to take when they are exposed to the sun. Consider offering the following recommendations:

- On a daily basis, wear a moisturizer or protective lotion with a sunscreen of at least SPF 15 on all areas of potential exposure.
- Avoid prolonged exposure to the sun during peak hours, when UV exposure is highest. This is usually between 10 AM and 3 PM.
- Sunscreen should be applied at least 30 minutes before sun exposure to allow time for absorption. Many people make the mistake of applying sunscreen after they have been exposed to the heat and sun's rays for 30 minutes or more. The already inflamed skin is more likely to react to the sunscreen chemicals when applied after sun exposure.
- Apply sunscreen liberally after swimming or any activities that result in heavy perspiration. If the skin is exposed to hours of sun, such as during a boat trip or day at the beach, sunscreen should be applied periodically throughout the day as a precaution.
- All sunscreen used for protection should be full or broad spectrum to filter out UVA and UVB rays of the sun. Check expiration dates printed on the bottle to make sure that the sunscreen has not expired.
- Avoid exposing children younger than 6 months of age to the sun.
- If prone to burning frequently and easily, wear a hat and protective clothing when participating in outdoor activities. Redheads and blue-eyed blonds are particularly susceptible to sun damage.

In addition to following the above precautions, clients should be advised to regularly see a physician specializing in dermatology for checkups of the skin, especially if any changes in coloration, size, or shape of a mole are detected, the skin bleeds unexpectedly, or a lesion or scrape does not heal quickly.

Home self-examinations can also be an effective way to check for signs of potential skin cancer between scheduled doctor visits. When performing a self-care exam, clients should be advised to check for any changes in existing moles and pay attention to any new visible growths on the skin.

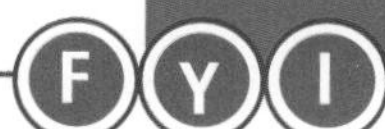

The American Cancer Society recommends using the ABCD Cancer Checklist to help make potential skin cancer easier to recognize. When checking existing moles, look for changes in any of the following: A, asymmetry; B, border; C, color; and D, diameter. Changes to any of these should be examined by a physician. For more information, contact the American Cancer Society at www.cancer.org or (800) ACS-2345.

SKIN AGING AND THE ENVIRONMENT

While the sun may play the major role in how the skin ages, changes in the environment also greatly influence this aging process. Pollutants in the air from factories, automobile exhaust, and even secondhand smoke can all influence the appearance and overall health of skin. While these pollutants affect the surface appearance of the skin, they can also change the health of the underlying cells and tissues, thereby speeding up the aging process.

The best defense against these pollutants is the simplest one: follow a good daily skin-care routine. Routine washing and exfoliating (removing dead surface skin cells) at night helps to remove the buildup of pollutants that have settled on the skin's surface throughout the day. The application of daily moisturizers, protective lotions, and even foundation products all help to protect the skin from airborne pollutants.

AGING AND LIFESTYLE

Aging of the skin cannot be blamed entirely on the outside influences of the sun and other environmental factors. What we choose to put into our bodies also has a profound effect on the overall aging process. The impact of poor choices can be seen most visibly on the skin. Smoking, drinking, drug abuse, and poor dietary choices all greatly influence the aging process. It is the responsibility of the cosmetologist to be aware of how these habits affect the skin and to tactfully point out these effects to clients.

Smoking and tobacco use not only cause cancer, but have also been linked to premature aging and wrinkling of the skin. Nicotine in tobacco causes contraction and weakening of the blood vessels and small capillaries that supply blood to the tissues. In turn, this contraction and weakening cause decreased circulation to the tissues. Eventually, the tissues are deprived of essential oxygen, and the effect of this becomes evident on the skin's surface. The skin may appear yellowish or gray in color and can have a dull appearance.

The use of illegal drugs affects the skin as much as smoking does. Some drugs have been shown to interfere with the body's intake of oxygen, thus affecting healthy cell growth. Some drugs can even aggravate serious skin conditions, such as acne. Others can cause dryness and allergic reactions on the skin's surface.

The overuse of alcohol has an opposite, yet equally damaging effect on the skin. Heavy or excessive intake of alcohol overdilates the blood vessels and capillaries. Over time, this constant overdilation and weakening of the fragile capillary walls will cause them to become distended. These dilated capillaries, called **telangiectasias** (te-lanj-ec-tay-jas), may also be caused by tobacco use, sun exposure, or other environmental factors. Alcohol can also dehydrate the skin by drawing essential water out of the tissues, which causes the skin to appear dull and dry.

Both smoking and drinking contribute to the aging process on their own, but the combination of the two can be devastating to the tissues. The constant dilation and contraction that occur on the tiny capillaries and blood vessels, as well as the constant deprivation of oxygen and water to the tissues, quickly make the skin appear lifeless and dull. It is very difficult for the skin to adjust and repair itself. The damage done by these lifestyle habits is typically hard to reverse or diminish.

DISORDERS OF THE SKIN

Like any other organ of the body, the skin is susceptible to a variety of diseases, disorders, and ailments. In your work as a practitioner, you will often see skin and scalp disorders, so you must be prepared to recognize

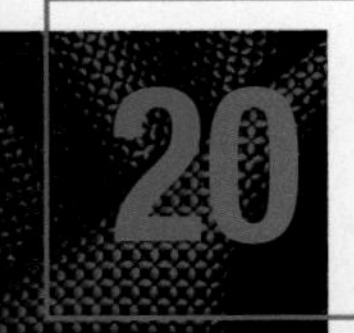

certain common skin conditions and know what you can and cannot do with them. Some skin and scalp disorders can be treated in cooperation with, and under the supervision of, a physician. Medicinal preparations, available only by prescription, must be applied in accordance with a physician's directions. If a client has a skin condition that you do not recognize as a simple disorder, refer the client to a physician.

It is very important that a beauty salon does not serve a client who is suffering from an inflamed skin disorder, infectious or not. The cosmetologist should be able to recognize these conditions, and sensitively suggest that proper measures be taken to prevent more serious consequences.

Numerous important terms relating to skin, scalp, and hair disorders that you should be familiar with are described in subsequent sections.

LESIONS OF THE SKIN

A **lesion** (LEE-zhun) is a mark on the skin. Certain lesions could indicate an injury or damage that changes the structure of tissues or organs. There are three types of lesions: primary, secondary, and tertiary. The cosmetologist is concerned with primary and secondary lesions only. If you are familiar with the principal skin lesions, you will be able to distinguish between conditions that may and may not be treated in a beauty salon (Figure 20-1).

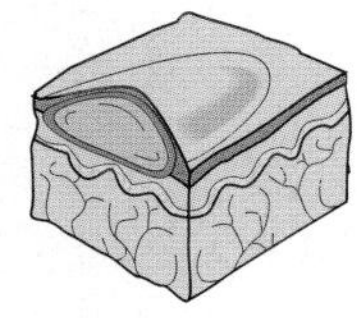

Bulla: Same as a vesicle only greater than 0.5 cm
Example: Contact dermatitis, large second-degree burns, bulbous impetigo, pemphigus

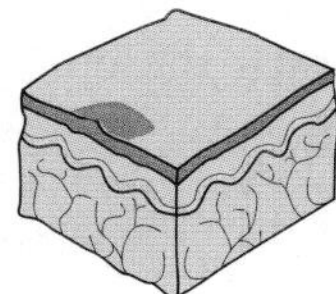

Macule: Localized changes in skin color of less than 1 cm in diameter
Example: Freckle

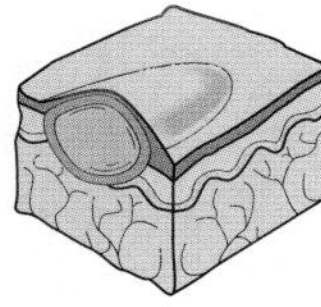

Tubercle: Solid and elevated; however, it extends deeper than papules into the dermis or subcutaneous tissues, 0.5-2 cm
Example: Lipoma, erythema, nodosum, cyst

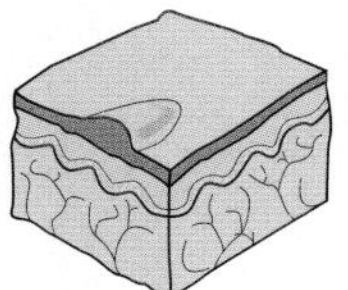

Papule: Solid, elevated lesion less than 0.5 cm in diameter
Example: Warts, elevated nevi

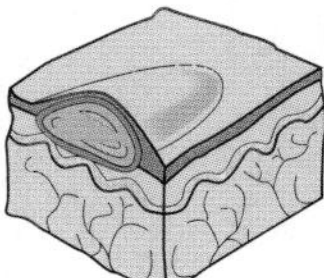

Pustule: Vesicles or bullae that become filled with pus, usually described as less than 0.5 cm in diameter
Example: Acne, impetigo, furuncles, carbuncles, folliculitis

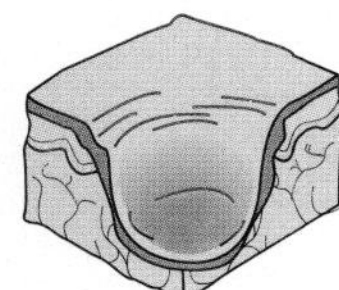

Ulcer: A depressed lesion of the epidermis and upper papillary layer of the dermis
Example: Stage 2 pressure ulcer

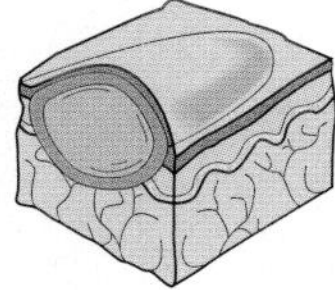

Tumor: The same as a nodule only greater than 2 cm
Example: Carcinoma (such as advanced breast carcinoma); **not** basal cell or squamous cell of the skin

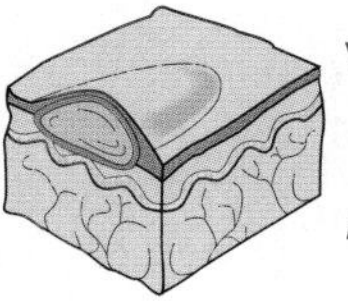

Vesicle: Accumulation of fluid between the upper layers of the skin; elevated mass containing serous fluid; less than 0.5 cm
Example: Herpes simplex, herpes zoster, chickenpox

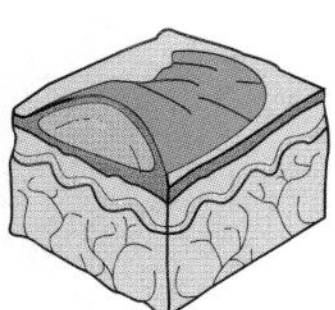

Wheal: Localized edema in the epidermis causing irregular elevation that may be red or pale
Example: Insect bite or a hive

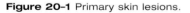

Figure 20-1 Primary skin lesions.

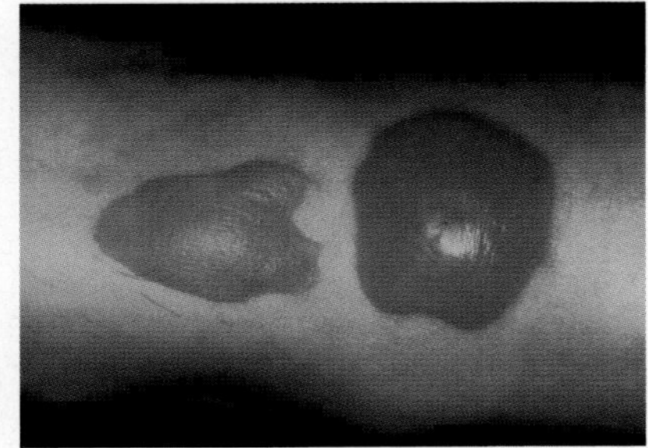

Figure 20-2 Bullae.

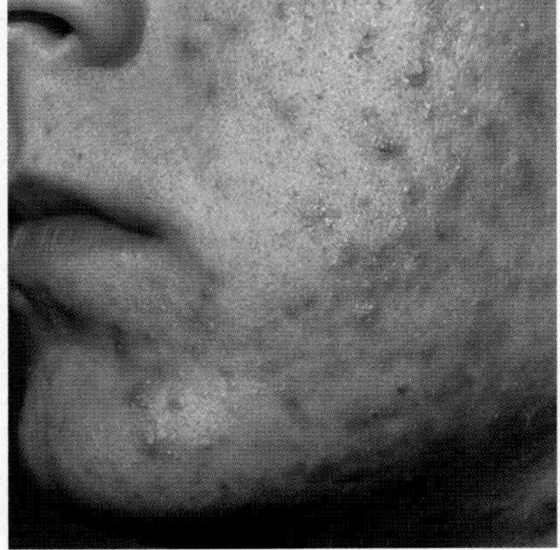

Figure 20-3 Papules and pustules.

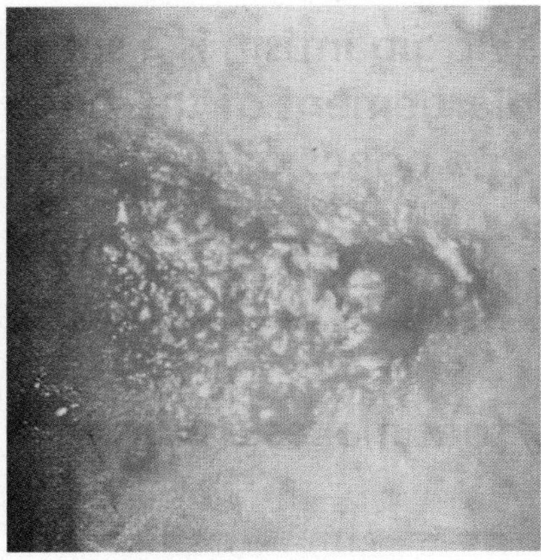

Figure 20-4 Poison oak vesicles.

The terms for different lesions listed below often indicate differences in the area of the skin layers affected and the size of the lesion.

PRIMARY LESIONS

Bulla (BULL-uh) **(plural: bullae)**—A large blister containing a watery fluid; similar to a vesicle but larger (Figure 20-2).

Cyst (SIST)—A closed, abnormally developed sac that contains fluid, pus, semifluid, or morbid matter, above or below the skin.

Macule (MAK-yool) **(plural: maculae)** (MAK-yuh-ly)—A spot or discoloration on the skin, such as a freckle. Macules are neither raised nor sunken.

Papule (PAP-yool)—A pimple; small circumscribed elevation on the skin that contains no fluid but may develop pus.

Pustule (PUS-chool)—An inflamed pimple containing pus (Figure 20-3).

Tubercle (TOO-bur-kul)—An abnormal rounded, solid lump above, within, or under the skin; larger than a papule.

Tumor (TOO-mur)—A swelling; an abnormal cell mass resulting from excessive multiplication of cells, varying in size, shape, and color. Nodules are also referred to as tumors, but are smaller.

Vesicle (VES-ih-kel)—A small blister or sac containing clear fluid, lying within or just beneath the epidermis. Poison ivy and poison oak, for example, produce vesicles (Figure 20-4).

Wheal (WHEEL)—An itchy, swollen lesion that lasts only a few hours; caused by a blow, the bite of an insect, urticaria (skin allergy), or the sting of a nettle. Examples include hives and mosquito bites.

SECONDARY LESIONS

Secondary skin lesions develop in the later stages of disease (Figure 20-5).

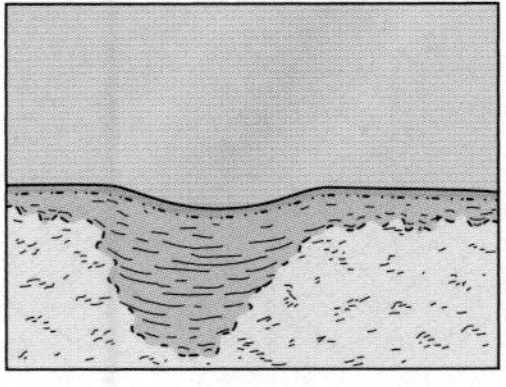

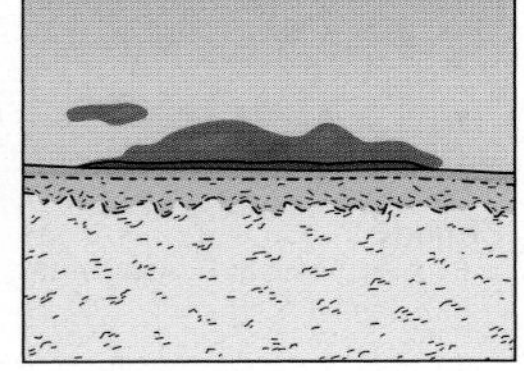

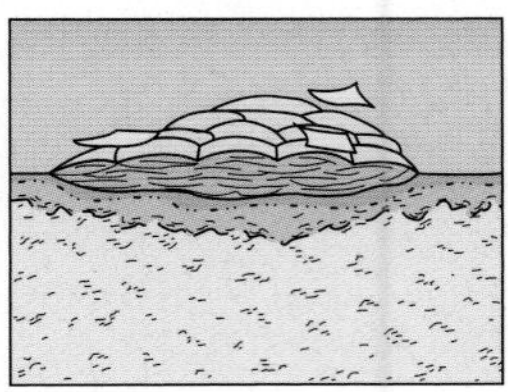

Fissure

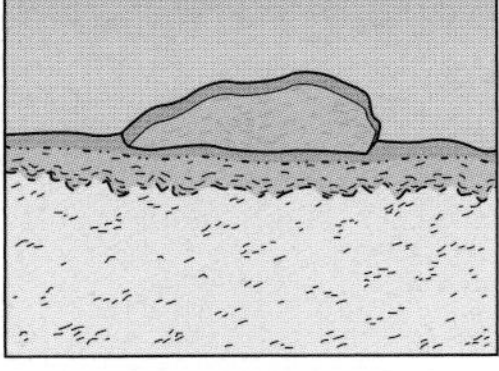

Figure 20-5 Secondary skin lesions.

Crust—Dead cells that form over a wound or blemish while it is healing; an accumulation of sebum and pus, sometimes mixed with epidermal material. An example is the scab on a sore.

Excoriation (ek-skor-ee-AY-shun)—A skin sore or abrasion produced by scratching or scraping.

Fissure (FISH-ur)—A crack in the skin that penetrates the dermis. Examples are chapped hands or lips.

Keloid (KEE-loyd)—A thick scar resulting from excessive growth of fibrous tissue (Figure 20-6).

Scale—Any thin dry or oily plate of epidermal flakes. An example is abnormal or excessive dandruff.

Scar or **cicatrix** (SIK-uh-triks)—Light-colored, slightly raised mark on the skin formed after an injury or lesion of the skin has healed.

Ulcer (UL-sur)—An open lesion on the skin or mucous membrane of the body, accompanied by pus and loss of skin depth.

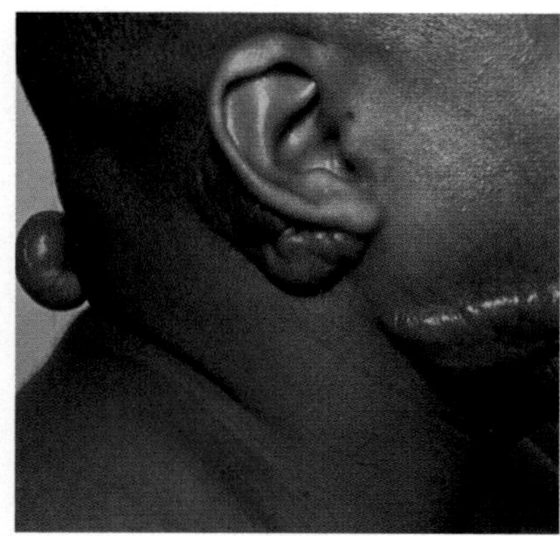

Figure 20-6 Keloids.

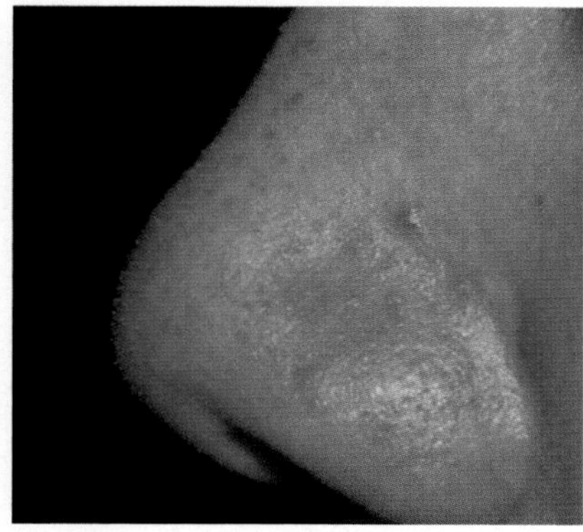

Figure 20-7 Comedones.

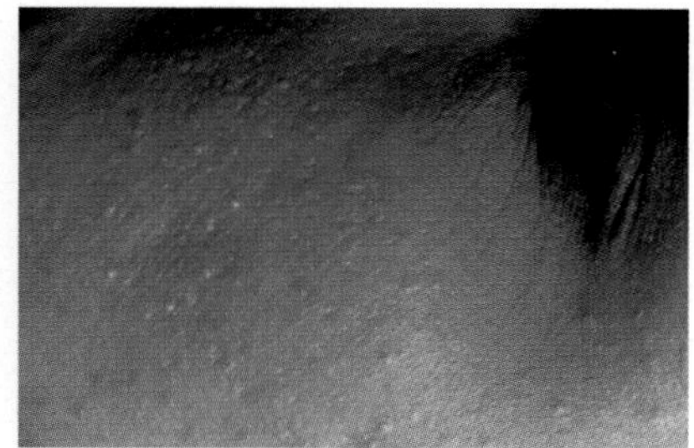

Figure 20-8 Milia.

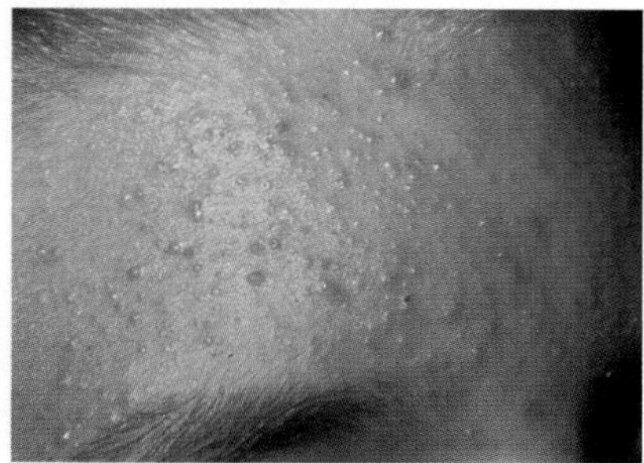

Figure 20-9 Acne.

DISORDERS OF THE SEBACEOUS (OIL) GLANDS

There are several common disorders of the sebaceous (oil) glands that the cosmetologist should be able to understand and identify.

A **comedo** (KAHM-uh-doh) (plural: comedones) is a hair follicle filled with keratin and sebum. Comedones appear most frequently on the face, especially in the T-zone (Figure 20-7). When the sebum of the comedo is exposed to the environment, it oxidizes and turns black (blackheads, also known as open comedones). When the follicle is closed and not exposed to the environment, the sebum remains a white or cream color (whiteheads or closed comedones). Comedones should be removed under aseptic conditions using proper extraction procedures. Should the condition become severe, medical attention is necessary.

Milia (MIL-ee-uh) are benign, keratin-filled cysts that appear just under the epidermis and have no visible opening. They resemble small sesame seeds, and are almost always perfectly round. They are commonly associated with newborn babies, but can appear on the skin of people of all ages. They are usually found around the eyes, cheeks, and forehead, and appear as small, whitish masses (Figure 20-8).

Acne (AK-nee) is a skin disorder characterized by chronic inflammation of the sebaceous glands from retained secretions, and bacteria known as *Propionibacterium acnes.* It occurs most frequently on the face, back, and chest. Acne, or common pimples, is also known as acne vulgaris (Figure 20-9). The seriousness of acne is rated by grades, ranging from 1 to 4. Grade 1 is common pimples with comedones, typically considered minor acne. Cosmetologists and estheticians often treat clients with comedones. Grade 4 is cystic acne with large nodules and pustular cysts. The higher grades of acne should be referred to a dermatologist for medical treatment.

Seborrheic dermatitis (seb-oh-REE-ick derm-ah-TIE-tus) is a skin condition caused by an inflammation of the sebaceous glands. It is often

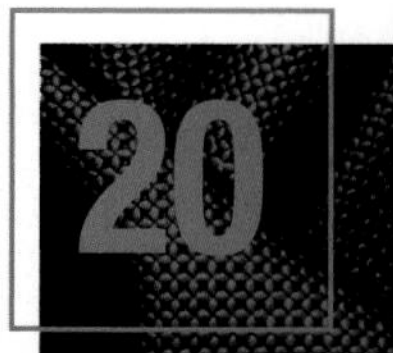

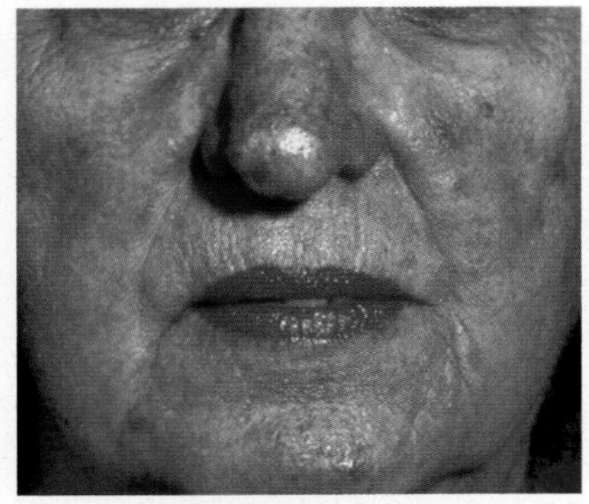
Figure 20-10 Rosacea.

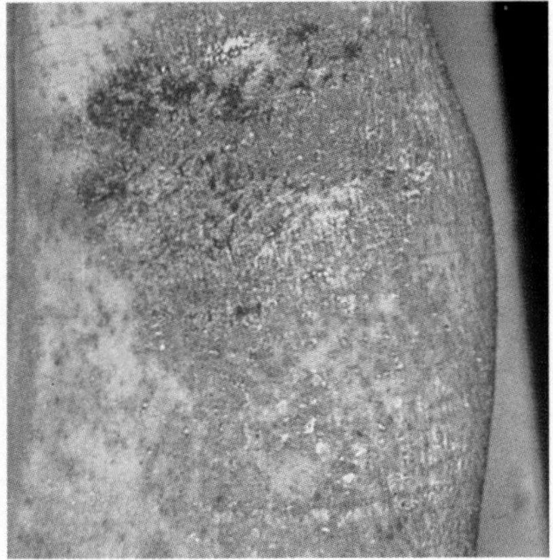
Figure 20-11 Eczema.

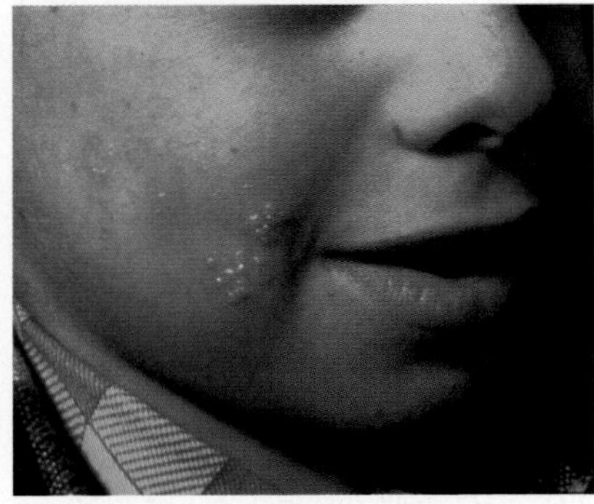
Figure 20-12 Herpes simplex.

characterized by inflammation, dry or oily scaling or crusting, and/or itchiness. The red, flaky skin often appears in the eyebrows, in the scalp and hairline, the middle of the forehead, and along the sides of the nose. This condition is sometimes treated with cortisone creams. Severe cases should be referred to the dermatologist.

Asteatosis (as-tee-ah-TOH-sis) is a condition of dry, scaly skin due to a deficiency or absence of sebum, caused by old age and exposure to cold.

Rosacea (roh-ZAY-shee-uh), formerly called acne rosacea, is a chronic condition appearing primarily on the cheeks and nose, characterized by flushing (redness), telangiectasia (dilation of the surface blood vessels), and the formation of papules (small, solid bumps) and pustules (raised lesions containing pus). The cause of rosacea is unknown, but certain factors are known to aggravate the condition in some individuals. These include spicy foods, caffeine, alcohol, exposure to extremes of heat and cold or sunlight, and stress (Figure 20-10).

A **steatoma** (stee-ah-TOH-muh) is a sebaceous cyst or fatty tumor. It is filled with sebum and ranges in size from a pea to an orange. It usually appears on the scalp, neck, and back. A steatoma is sometimes called a wen.

DISORDERS OF THE SUDORIFEROUS (SWEAT) GLANDS

Anhidrosis (an-hih-DROH-sis)—Deficiency in perspiration, often a result of fever or certain skin diseases. It requires medical treatment.

Bromhidrosis (broh-mih-DROH-sis)—Foul-smelling perspiration, usually noticeable in the armpits or on the feet.

Hyperhidrosis (hy-per-hy-DROH-sis)—Excessive sweating, caused by heat or general body weakness. Medical treatment is required.

Miliaria rubra (mil-ee-AIR-ee-ah ROOB-rah)—Prickly heat; acute inflammatory disorder of the sweat glands, characterized by the eruption of small red vesicles and accompanied by burning, itching skin. It is caused by exposure to excessive heat.

INFLAMMATIONS OF THE SKIN

Dermatitis (dur-muh-TY-tis)—Inflammatory condition of the skin. The lesions come in various forms, including vesicles or papules.

Eczema (EG-zuh-muh)—An inflammatory, painful itching disease of the skin, acute or chronic in nature, presenting many forms of dry or moist lesions. There are several different types of eczema. All cases of eczema should be referred to a physician for treatment. Eczema is not contagious (Figure 20-11).

Herpes simplex (HER-peez SIM-pleks)—Fever blister or cold sore; recurring viral infection. It is characterized by the eruption of a single vesicle or group of vesicles on a red swollen base. The blisters usually appear on the lips, nostrils, or other part of the face, and can last up to 3 weeks. Herpes simplex is contagious (Figure 20-12).

Psoriasis (suh-RY-uh-sis)—A skin disease characterized by red patches, covered with silver-white scales usually found on the scalp, elbows,

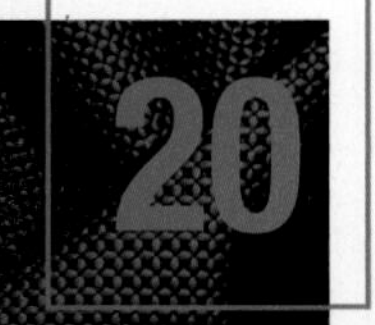

knees, chest, and lower back. Psoriasis is caused by the skin cells turning over faster than normal. It rarely occurs on the face. If irritated, bleeding points occur. Psoriasis is not contagious (Figure 20-13).

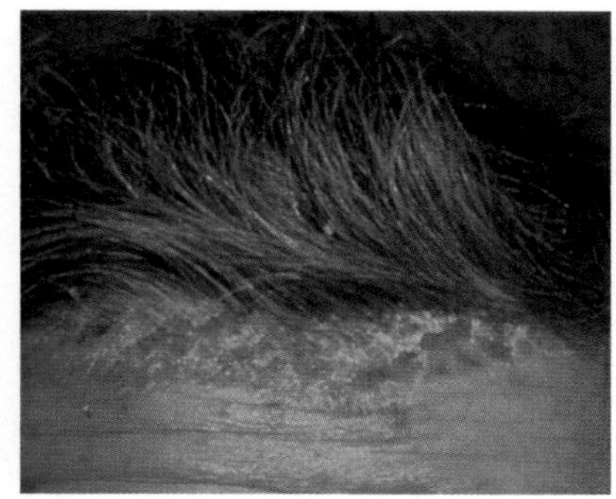

Figure 20-13 Psoriasis.

PIGMENTATIONS OF THE SKIN

Pigment can be affected by internal factors such as heredity or hormonal fluctuations, or by outside factors such as prolonged exposure to the sun. Abnormal coloration accompanies every skin disorder and many systemic disorders. A change in pigmentation can also be observed when certain drugs are being taken internally. The following terms relate to changes in the pigmentation of the skin.

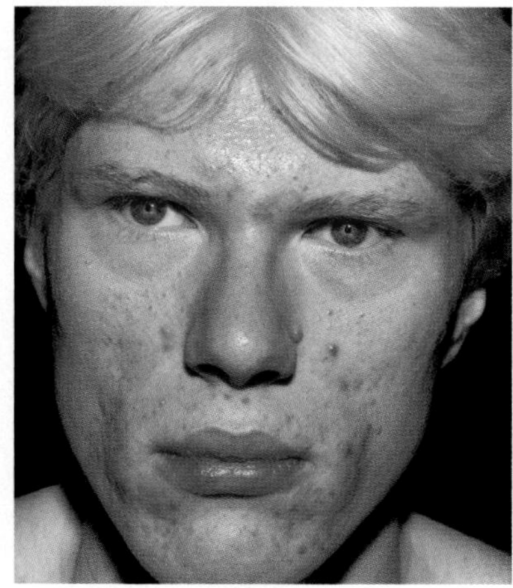

Figure 20-14 Albinism.

Albinism (AL-bi-niz-em)—Congenital leukoderma, or absence of melanin pigment of the body, including the skin, hair, and eyes (Figure 20-14). Hair is silky white. The skin is pinkish white and will not tan. The eyes are pink, and the skin is sensitive to light and ages early.

Chloasma (kloh-AZ-mah)—Condition characterized by increased pigmentation on the skin in spots that are not elevated. Chloasma is also called liver spots, although they have nothing to do with the liver. They are generally caused by cumulative sun exposure.

Lentigines (len-TIJ-e-neez) (singular: lentigo) (len-TY-goh)—Technical term for freckles. Small yellow- to brown-colored spots on skin exposed to sunlight and air.

Leukoderma (loo-koh-DUR-muh)—Skin disorder characterized by light abnormal patches; caused by a burn or congenital disease that destroys the pigment-producing cells. It is classified as vitiligo and albinism.

Nevus (NEE-vus)—Small or large malformation of the skin due to abnormal pigmentation or dilated capillaries; commonly known as a birthmark.

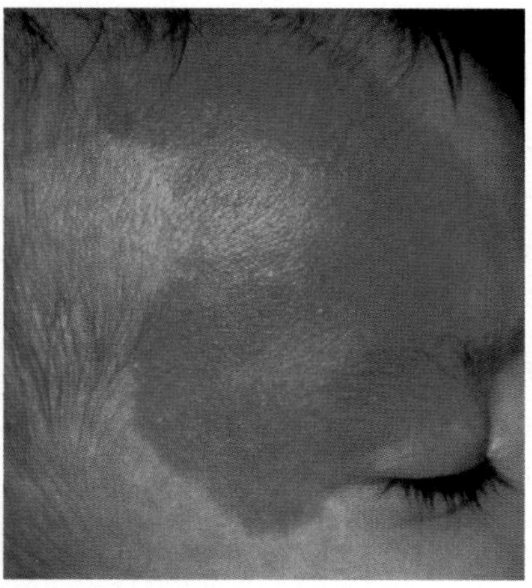

Figure 20-15 Port wine stain.

Stain—Abnormal brown or wine-colored skin discoloration with a circular and irregular shape (Figure 20-15). Its permanent color is due to the presence of darker pigment. Stains occur during aging, after certain diseases, and after the disappearance of moles, freckles, and liver spots. The cause is unknown.

Tan—Change in pigmentation of skin caused by exposure to the sun or ultraviolet rays.

Vitiligo (vih-til-EYE-goh)—Milky-white spots (leukoderma) of the skin. Vitiligo is hereditary, and may be related to thyroid conditions (Figure 20-16). Skin with vitiligo must be protected from overexposure to the sun.

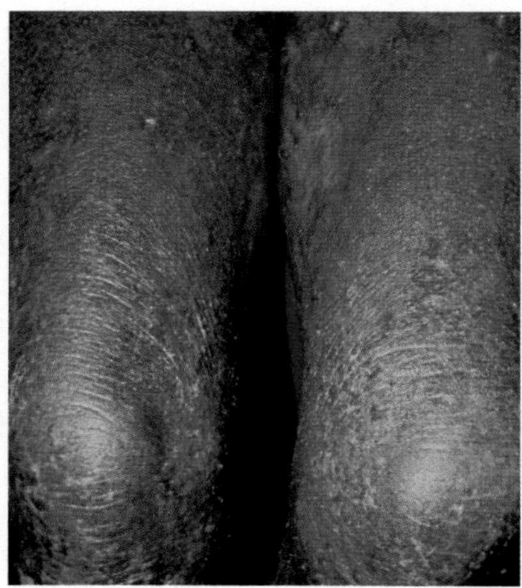

Figure 20-16 Vitiligo.

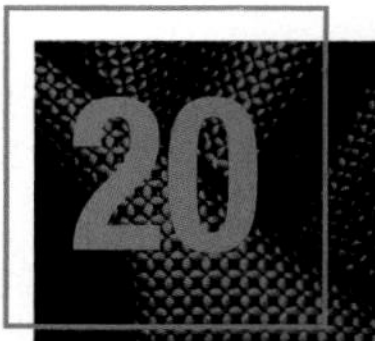

CAUTION

Do not treat or remove hair from moles.

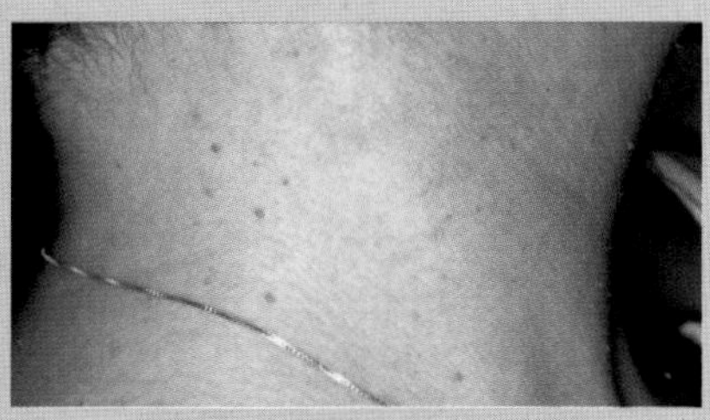

Figure 20-17 Skin tags.

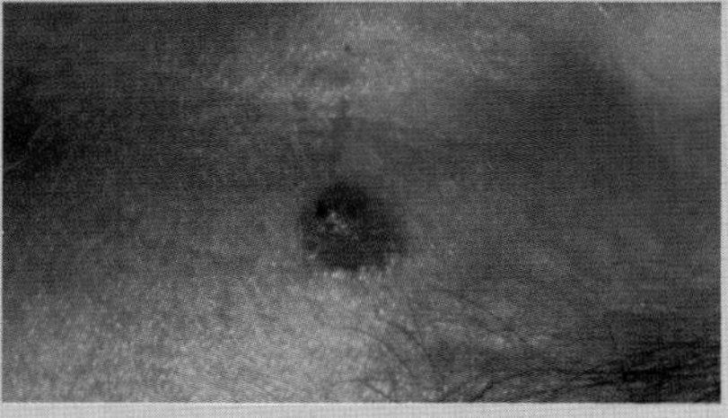

Figure 20-18 Basal cell carcinoma.

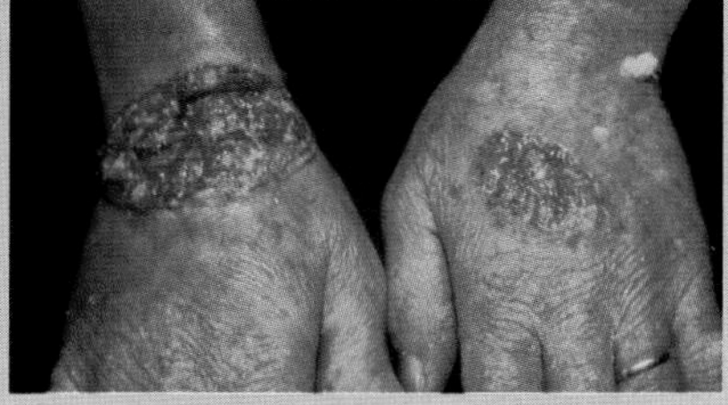

Figure 20-19 Squamous cell carcinoma.

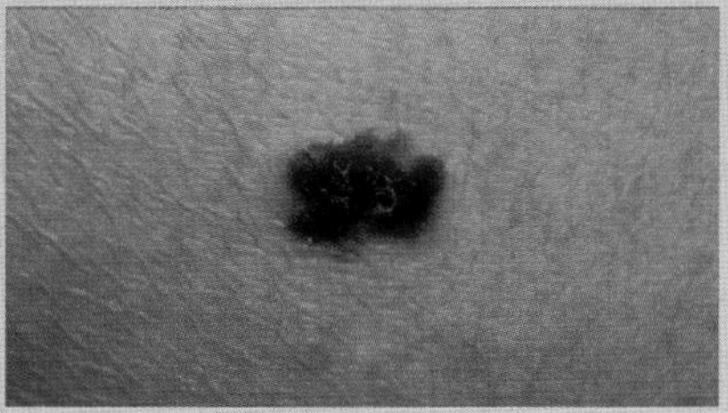

Figure 20-20 Malignant melanoma.

HYPERTROPHIES OF THE SKIN

A **hypertrophy** (hy-PUR-truh-fee) of the skin is an abnormal growth of the skin. Many hypertrophies are benign, or harmless.

Keratoma (kair-uh-TOH-muh)—An acquired, superficial, thickened patch of epidermis commonly known as callus, caused by pressure or friction on the hands and feet. If the thickening grows inward, it is called a corn.

Mole—A small, brownish spot or blemish on the skin, ranging in color from pale tan to brown or bluish black. Some moles are small and flat, resembling freckles; others are raised and darker in color. Large, dark hairs often occur in moles. Any change in a mole requires medical attention.

Skin tag—Small brown or flesh-colored outgrowth of the skin (Figure 20-17). Skin tags occur most frequently on the neck of an older person. They can be easily removed by a dermatologist.

Verruca (vuh-ROO-kuh)—Technical term for wart; hypertrophy of the papillae and epidermis. It is caused by a virus and is infectious. Verruca can spread from one location to another, particularly along a scratch in the skin.

SKIN CANCER

Skin cancer—primarily caused from overexposure to the sun—comes in three distinct forms that vary in severity. Each is named for the type of cells that it affects.

Basal cell carcinoma (BAY-zul SEL kar-sin-OH-muh) is the most common type and the least severe. It is often characterized by light or pearly nodules (Figure 20-18). **Squamous** (SKWAY-mus) **cell carcinoma** is more serious than basal cell carcinoma, and often is characterized by scaly red papules or nodules (Figure 20-19). The third and most serious form of skin cancer is **malignant melanoma** (muh-LIG-nent mel-uh-NOH-muh), which is often characterized by black or dark brown patches on the skin that may appear uneven in texture, jagged, or raised (Figure 20-20).

Malignant melanomas often appear on individuals who do not receive regular sun exposure, and are most commonly located on areas of the body that are not regularly exposed. It is often nicknamed the "city person's cancer." Malignant melanoma is the least common, but also the most dangerous type of skin cancer.

If detected early, anyone with any of these three forms of skin cancer has a good chance for survival. It is important for a cosmetologist to be able to recognize the appearance of serious skin disorders in order to better serve clients. It also important to remember that a cosmetologist should not attempt to diagnose a skin disorder, but should sensitively suggest that the client seek the advice of a dermatologist.

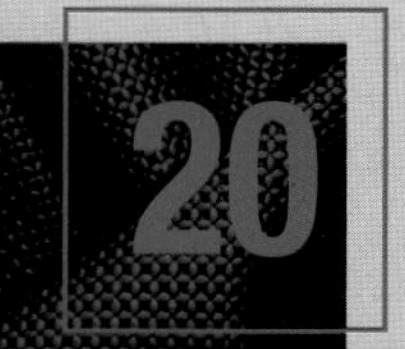

AVOIDING SKIN PROBLEMS

Skin problems are common in every facet of the professional salon industry. Nail, skin, and hair services can cause problems for the sensitive client. Fortunately, the vast majority of skin-related problems can be easily avoided—if you understand how!

DERMATITIS

Dermatitis is a medical term for abnormal skin inflammation. There are many kinds of dermatitis, but only one is important in the salon. **Dermatitis venenata,** also known as contact dermatitis is the most common skin disease for nail practitioners. Contact dermatitis is caused by touching certain substances to the skin. This type of dermatitis can be short term or long term. Contact dermatitis can have several causes. The skin may be irritated by a substance, and is called irritant contact dermatitis. It is also possible to become allergic to an ingredient in a product. This is called allergic contact dermatitis.

PROLONGED OR REPEATED CONTACT

Allergic reactions are caused by prolonged or repeated direct skin contact. This type of skin problem does not occur overnight. Acrylic (methacrylate) liquids, haircolor, and chemical texture solutions are all capable of causing allergic reactions. In general, a reaction takes from 4 to 6 months. As a professional service provider, you may also be at risk. Prolonged, repeated, or long-term exposures can cause anyone to become sensitive. This is usually caused by overexposure. Simply touching products or solutions does not cause sensitivities. These typically require months of improper handling and overexposure. Some likely places for allergies to occur are listed below.

1. On practitioner's fingers, palms, or on the back of the hand
2. On practitioner's face, especially the cheeks
3. On client's scalp, hairline, forehead, or neckline

If you examine the area where the problem occurs, you can usually determine the cause. For example, haircolorists often strand test color with their bare fingers and hands. This is both prolonged and repeated contact!

Sensitization is a greatly increased or exaggerated sensitivity to products.

IRRITANT CONTACT DERMATITIS

Irritating substances will temporarily damage the epidermis. Corrosive substances are examples of irritants. When the skin is damaged by irritating substances, the immune system springs into action. It floods the tissue with water, trying to dilute the irritant. This is why swelling occurs.

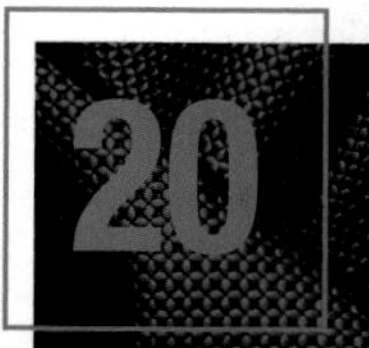

The immune system also tells the blood to release histamines, which enlarge the vessels around the injury. Blood can then rush to the scene more quickly and help remove the irritating substance.

You can see and feel all the extra blood under the skin. The entire area becomes red, warm, and may throb. Histamines cause the itchy feeling that often accompanies contact dermatitis. After everything calms down, the swelling will go away. The surrounding skin is often left damaged, scaly, cracked, and dry. Fortunately, irritations are not permanent. If you avoid repeated and/or prolonged contact with the irritating substance, the skin will usually quickly repair itself. However, continued or repeated exposure may lead to permanent allergic reactions.

Surprisingly, tap water is a very common salon irritant. Hands that remain damp for long periods often become sore, cracked, and chapped. Avoiding the problem is simple. Always completely dry the hands. Regularly use moisturizing hand creams to compensate for loss of skin oils.

Frequent hand washing, especially in hard water, can further damage the skin. Do not wash your hands excessively. Washing your hands more than 10 or 15 times a day can cause them to become irritated and damaged. Cleansers and detergents worsen the problem. They increase damage by stripping away sebum and other natural skin chemicals that protect the skin. Prolonged or repeated contact with many solvents will strip away skin oils, leaving the skin dry or damaged. Sometimes it is difficult to determine the cause of the irritation. One way to identify the irritant is by observing the location of the reaction. Symptoms are always isolated to the contact area. The cause will be something that you are doing to this part of the skin.

Once a client becomes allergic, things will only get worse if you continue using the same products and techniques. It is best to discontinue use until you figure out what you are doing wrong. Otherwise, more clients will eventually be affected.

PROTECT YOURSELF

Take extreme care to keep brush handles, containers, and table tops clean and free from product, dusts, and residues. Repeatedly handling these items will cause overexposure if the items are not kept clean. If you avoid contact, neither you nor your client will ever develop an allergic reaction.

Many serious problems can be related to contact dermatitis. Do not fall into the trap of developing bad habits.

REVIEW QUESTIONS

1. List the factors that contribute to the aging of the skin.
2. Explain the effect of overexposure to the sun on the skin.
3. What is a skin lesion?
4. Name and describe at least five disorders of the sebaceous glands.
5. Name and describe at least five changes in skin pigmentation.
6. List at least six skin conditions and disorders that should be referred to a physician.
7. Name and describe the three forms of skin cancer.

CHAPTER GLOSSARY

acne	Skin disorder characterized by chronic inflammation of the sebaceous glands from retained secretions and *Propionibacterium acnes* (*P. acnes*) bacteria.
albinism	Congenital leukoderma or absence of melanin pigment of the body, including the hair, skin, and eyes
anhidrosis	Deficiency in perspiration, often a result of fever or certain skin diseases.
asteatosis	Condition of dry, scaly skin due to a deficiency or absence of sebum that is caused by old age and by exposure to cold.
basal cell carcinoma	Most common and least severe type of skin cancer; often characterized by light or pearly nodules.
bromhidrosis	Foul-smelling perspiration, usually noticeable in the armpits or on the feet.
bulla (plural: bullae)	Large blister containing a watery fluid; similar to a vesicle but larger.
chloasma	Condition characterized by increased pigmentation on the skin in spots that are not elevated.
comedo (plural: comedones)	Hair follicle filled with keratin and sebum. When the sebum of the comedone is exposed to the environment, it oxidizes and turns black (blackheads). When the follicle is closed and not exposed to the environment, comedones are a white or cream color (whiteheads).
crust	Dead cells that form over a wound or blemish while it is healing; an accumulation of sebum and pus, sometimes mixed with epidermal material.
cyst	Closed, abnormally developed sac containing fluid, semifluid, or morbid matter, above or below the skin.

CHAPTER GLOSSARY

dermatitis	Inflammatory condition of the skin.
dermatitis venenata	Also known as contact dermatitis. An eruptive skin infection caused by contact with irritating substances such as chemicals or tints.
eczema	Inflammatory, painful itching disease of the skin, acute or chronic in nature, presenting many forms of dry or moist lesions.
excoriation	Skin sore or abrasion produced by scratching or scraping.
fissure	Crack in the skin that penetrates the epidermis, such as chapped hands or lips.
herpes simplex	Fever blister or cold sore; recurring viral infection.
hyperhidrosis	Excessive sweating, caused by heat or general body weakness.
hypertrophy	Abnormal growth of the skin.
keloid	Thick scar resulting from excessive growth of fibrous tissue.
keratoma	Acquired, superficial, thickened patch of epidermis commonly known as callus, caused by pressure or friction on the hands and feet.
lentigines (singular: lentigo)	Technical term for freckles. Small yellow- to brown-colored spots on skin exposed to sunlight and air.
lesion	Mark on the skin. May indicate an injury or damage that changes the structure of tissues or organs.
leukoderma	Skin disorder characterized by light abnormal patches; caused by a burn or congenital disease that destroys the pigment-producing cells.
macule (plural: maculae)	Spot or discoloration on the skin, such as a freckle.
malignant melanoma	Most serious form of skin cancer; often characterized by black or dark brown patches on the skin that may appear uneven in texture, jagged, or raised.
milia	Benign, keratin-filled cysts that can appear just under the epidermis and have no visible opening.
miliaria rubra	Acute inflammatory disorder of the sweat glands, characterized by the eruption of small red vesicles and accompanied by burning, itching skin.
mole	Small, brownish spot or blemish on the skin, ranging in color from pale tan to brown or bluish black.
nevus	Small or large malformation of the skin due to abnormal pigmentation or dilated capillaries; commonly known as birthmark.
papule	Pimple; small circumscribed elevation on the skin that contains no fluid but may develop pus.

CHAPTER GLOSSARY

psoriasis	Skin disease characterized by red patches, covered with silver-white scales usually found on the scalp, elbows, knees, chest, and lower back, but rarely on the face.
pustule	Inflamed pimple containing pus.
rosacea	Chronic congestion appearing primarily on the cheeks and nose, characterized by redness, dilation of the blood vessels, and formation of papules and pustules.
scale	Any thin plate of epidermal flakes, dry or oily, such as abnormal or excessive dandruff.
scar or cicatrix	Light-colored, slightly raised mark on the skin formed after an injury or lesion of the skin has healed.
seborrheic dermatitis	Skin condition caused by an inflammation of the sebaceous glands. Often characterized by inflammation, dry or oily scaling, or crusting and/or itchiness.
sensitization	A greatly increased or exaggerated sensitivity to products.
skin tag	A small brown or flesh-colored outgrowth of the skin.
squamous cell carcinoma	Type of skin cancer more serious than basal cell carcinoma; often characterized by scaly red papules or nodules.
stain	Abnormal brown or wine-colored skin discoloration with a circular and irregular shape.
steatoma	Sebaceous cyst or fatty tumor.
tan	Change in pigmentation of skin caused by exposure to the sun or ultraviolet rays.
telangiectasias	Dilation of the surface blood vessels.
tubercle	Abnormal rounded, solid lump above, within, or under the skin; larger than a papule.
tumor	A swelling; an abnormal cell mass resulting from excessive multiplication of cells, varying in size, shape, and color.
ulcer	Open lesion on the skin or mucous membrane of the body, accompanied by pus and loss of skin depth.
verruca	Technical term for wart; hypertrophy of the papillae and epidermis.
vesicle	Small blister or sac containing clear fluid, lying within or just beneath the epidermis.
vitiligo	Milky-white spots (leukoderma) of the skin. Vitiligo is hereditary and may be related to thyroid conditions.
wheal	Itchy, swollen lesion that lasts only a few hours; caused by a blow, the bite of an insect, urticaria, or the sting of a nettle.

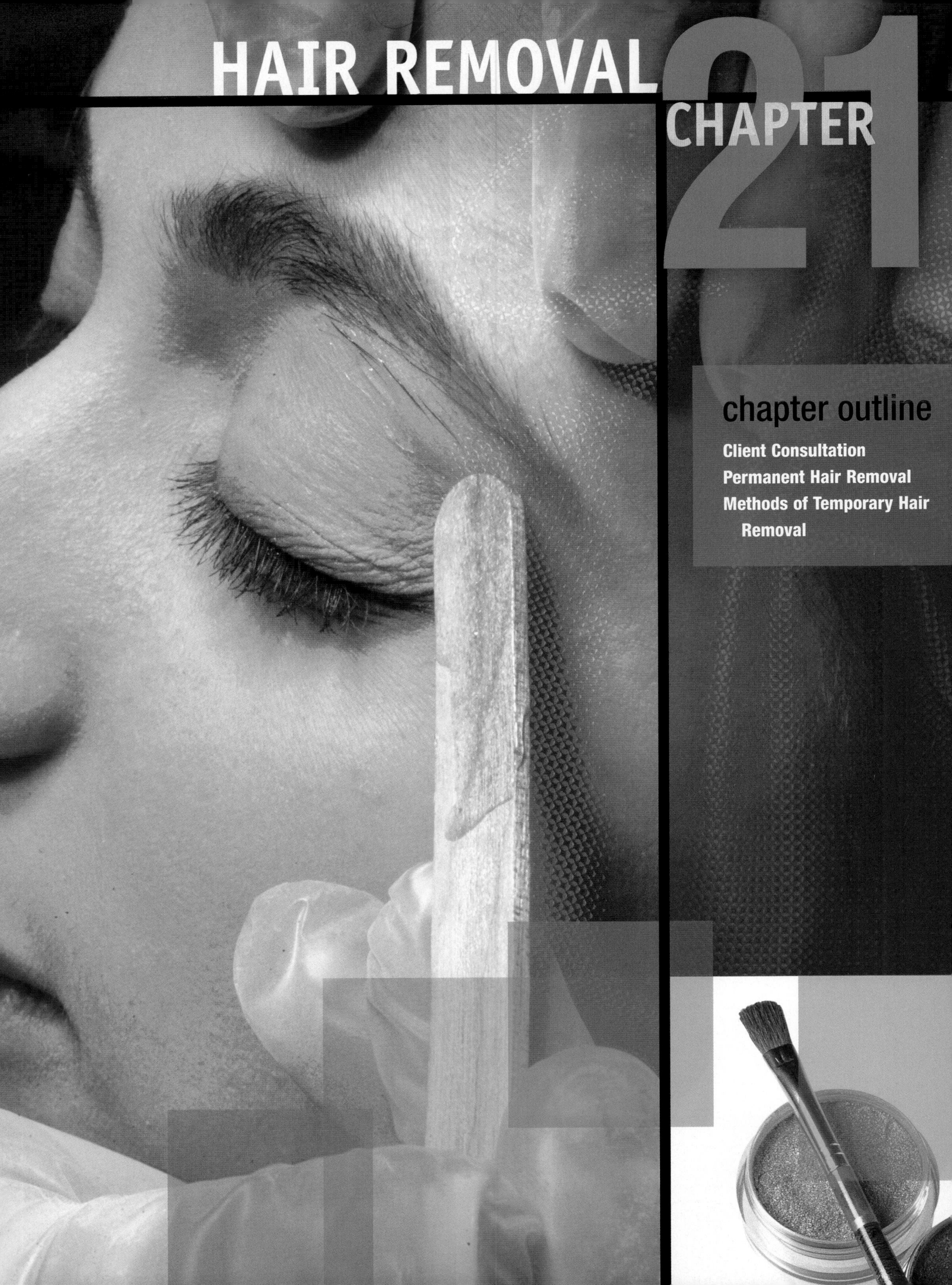

HAIR REMOVAL

CHAPTER 21

chapter outline

Client Consultation
Permanent Hair Removal
Methods of Temporary Hair Removal

Learning Objectives

After completing this chapter, you will be able to:

- **Describe the elements of a client consultation for hair removal.**
- **Name the conditions that contraindicate hair removal in the salon.**
- **Identify and describe three methods of permanent hair removal.**
- **Demonstrate the techniques involved in temporary hair removal.**

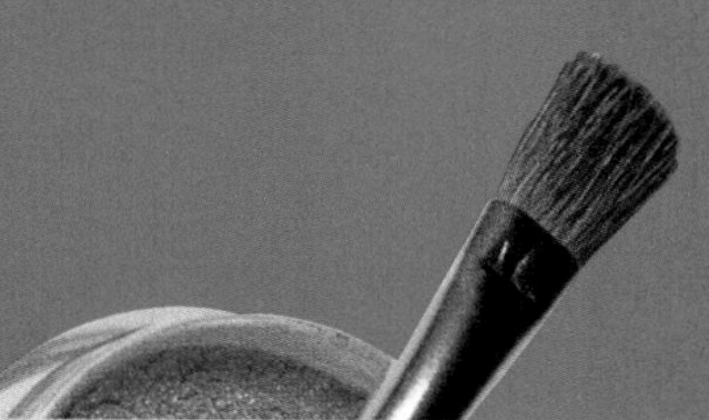

Key Terms

Page number indicates where in the chapter the term is used.

depilatory
pg. 552

electrolysis
pg. 551

epilator
pg. 555

hirsuties or *hypertrichosis*
pg. 548

laser hair removal
pg. 551

photoepilation
pg. 551

sugaring
pg. 559

threading
pg. 559

One of the fastest growing services in the salon and spa businesses is hair removal. Once restricted to an occasional lip or brow service, a growing number of clients want to have their entire face, arms, and legs bare of hair. Bikini hair removal has also evolved into its own art form, with different designs becoming sought-after services by many clients. Men are also jumping on the bandwagon, with the nape of the neck, chest, and back being frequent removal requests. The most common form of hair removal in salons and spas is waxing, although with the popularity of these services on the rise, many different methods are now coming into play.

Hirsuties (hur-SOO-shee-eez) or **hypertrichosis** (hy-pur-trih-KOH-sis) are terms that refer to the growth of an unusual amount of hair on parts of the body normally bearing only downy hair, such as the faces of women and the backs of men. Clients with an overabundance of hair are certainly the best candidates for hair removal, although many clients with even just a few unwanted hairs on their arms or legs are now requesting these services.

Unwanted hair has been treated throughout the ages by a variety of methods. Excavations of early Egyptian tombs indicate that abrasive materials, such as pumice stone, were used to rub away hair. Ancient Greek and Roman women were known to remove most of their body hair by similar methods. Native Americans used sharpened stones and seashells to rub off and pluck out hair.

History also records chemical means of removing excess hair. For example, the ancient Turks used *rusma,* a combination of yellow sulfide of arsenic, quicklime, and rose water, as a crude hair removal agent.

Facial and body hair removal has become increasingly popular as evolving technology makes it easier to perform with more effective results. All of the various approaches to hair removal, though, fall into two major categories: permanent and temporary. Salon techniques are generally limited to temporary methods.

CLIENT CONSULTATION

Before performing any hair removal service, a consultation is always necessary. Ask the client to complete a questionnaire that discloses all medications, both topical (applied to the skin) and oral (taken by mouth), along with any known skin disorders or allergies (Figure 21-1). Allergies or sensitivities must be noted and documented. Keep in mind that many changes can occur between client visits. Since the last time you saw them, clients may have been placed on medications such as antidepressants, hormones, cortisone, medicine for blood pressure or diabetes, or such topical prescriptions as Retin-A®, Renova®, and hydroquinone. A client taking any one of these prescriptions may not be a candidate for hair removal. See Figure 21-2 or a sample client assessment form.

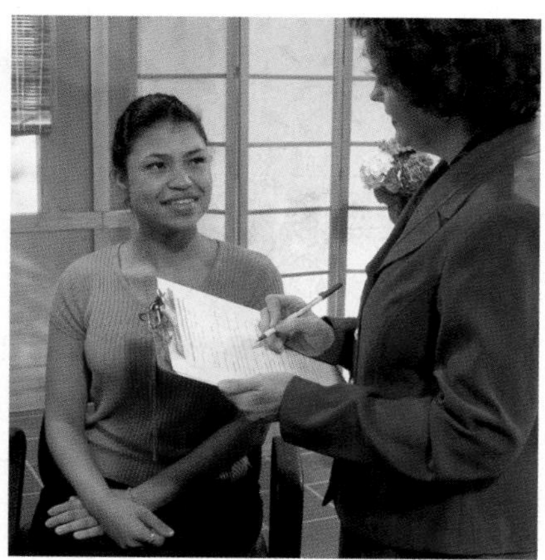

Figure 21-1 Filling out a client questionnaire.

CLIENT ASSESSMENT FORM

Date______________

Name____ Sex______________

Address____

City______________________________________ State______________ Zip______________

1. Have you been seen by a dermatologist? Yes____ No____ If yes, for what reason?______________

   ____

2. Please list all medications that you take regularly. Include hormones, vitamins, and the like.

   ____

   Have you ever used Accutane®? Yes____ No____ If yes, when did you stop taking Accutane®?_____

   Do you use or have you recently used Retin-A®, Renova®, Tazorac®, Differin®, Azelex®, or other medical peeling agent? Yes____ No____ If yes, for how long?______________

3. Do you have any allergies? Are you allergic to any medications? Yes____ No____

   If yes, please list allergies:______________________________

4. Are you pregnant or lactating? Yes____ No____
5. Have you had any of the following procedures?

   Laser resurfacing Yes____ Date_______ No____

   Light chemical peel Yes____ Date_______ No____

   Medium/heavy chemical peel Yes____ Date_______ No____

   Have you had any microdermabrasion? Yes____ Date_______ No____

6. Do you ever experience tightness or flaking of your skin? Yes____ No____
7. Do you frequent tanning booths? Yes____ No____
8. Do you have a history of fever blisters or cold sores? Yes____ No____

Figure 21-2 Client assessment form.

RELEASE FORM FOR HAIR REMOVAL

I,________________________________, am_____ am not_____ presently using:

____ Retin-A, or any other topical prescription medication

____ Accutane

____ any alphahydroxy-based products

____ any medications such as cortisone, blood thinners, or diabetic medication

____ I understand that if I begin using any of the above products and do not inform my esthetician/cosmetologist prior to hair removal, I am accepting full responsibility for any skin reactions.

____ The hair removal process has been thoroughly explained to me, and I have had an opportunity to ask questions and receive satisfactory answers.

Client's Signature______________________________ Date_______________

Technician's Signature____________________________ Date_______________

Figure 21-3 Sample release form.

It is imperative that every client fill out a release form for the hair removal service you are going to provide. This should be completed prior to every service. It serves as a reminder to the client to really think about any topical or oral medication they might have started since their last visit. See Figure 21-3 for a sample release form.

CONTRAINDICATIONS FOR HAIR REMOVAL

One of the main purposes of client consultation is to determine the presence of any contraindications for hair removal. Clients should not have *any* waxing or hair removal performed *anywhere on the body* if they have one or more of the following conditions, without first obtaining written permission from their physician.

- Accutane use in the last 6 months
- Blood-thinning medications
- Drugs for autoimmune diseases including lupus
- Psoriasis, eczema, or other chronic skin diseases
- Sunburn
- Presence of pustules or papules in area to be waxed
- Recent cosmetic or reconstructive surgery
- Any other questionable medical condition

Facial waxing should not be performed on clients with any of the following conditions, without first obtaining permission from their physician.

- Rosacea or very sensitive skin
- History of fever blisters or cold sores
- Recent chemical peel using glycolic, alpha hydroxy, salicylic acid, or other acid-based products
- Recent microdermabrasion

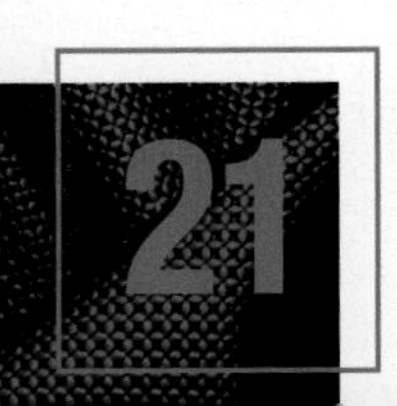

- Use of any exfoliating topical medication including Retin-A®, Renova®, Tazorac®, Differin®, Azelex®, or other medical peeling agent
- Use of hydroquinone for skin lightening

PERMANENT HAIR REMOVAL

Although permanent hair removal services are not often offered in salons, it is useful to know the options that exist. Permanent hair removal methods include electrolysis, photoepilation (light-based hair removal), and laser hair removal.

ELECTROLYSIS

Electrolysis is the removal of hair by means of an electric current that destroys the growth cells of the hair. The current is applied with a very fine, needle-shaped electrode that is inserted into each hair follicle. This technique must only be performed by a licensed electrologist.

PHOTOEPILATION

Photoepilation uses intense light to destroy the growth cells of the hair follicles. This treatment has minimal side effects, requires no needles, and thus minimizes the risk of infection. Clinical studies have shown that photoepilation can provide 50 to 60 percent clearance of hair in 12 weeks. This method can be administered in some salons by cosmetologists and estheticians, depending on state law. Manufacturers of photoepilation equipment generally provide the special training necessary for administering this procedure.

LASER HAIR REMOVAL

Lasers are another method for the rapid removal of unwanted hair. In **laser hair removal,** a laser beam is pulsed on the skin, impairing hair growth. It is most effective when used on follicles that are in the growth or anagen phase.

The laser method was discovered by chance when it was noted that birthmarks treated with certain types of lasers became permanently devoid of hair. Lasers are not for everyone; an absolute requirement is that one's hair must be darker than the surrounding skin. Coarse, dark hair responds best to laser treatment. For some clients, this method produces permanent hair removal. For other clients, laser hair removal treatments simply slow down regrowth.

In certain states and provinces, cosmetologists or estheticians are allowed to perform laser hair removal under a doctor's supervision. This method requires specialized training, most commonly offered by laser equipment manufacturers.

Laws regarding photoepilation and laser hair removal services vary by state and province. Be sure to check with your regulatory agency for guidelines.

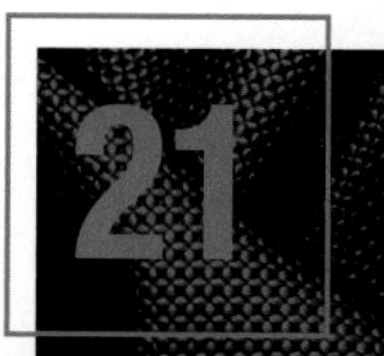

METHODS OF TEMPORARY HAIR REMOVAL

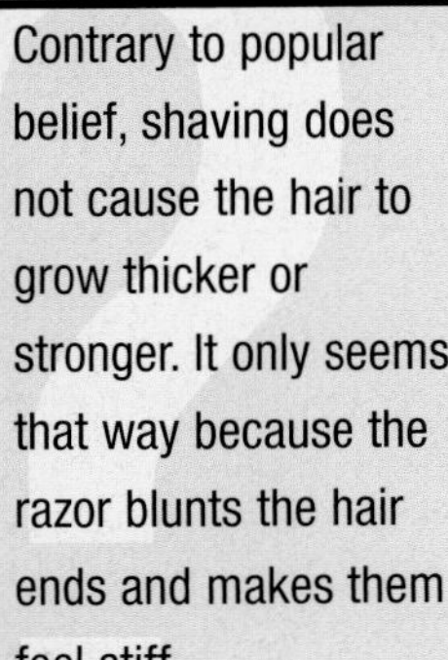

Contrary to popular belief, shaving does not cause the hair to grow thicker or stronger. It only seems that way because the razor blunts the hair ends and makes them feel stiff.

Temporary methods of hair removal, some of which may be offered in your salon or spa, are discussed below.

SHAVING

The most common form of temporary hair removal, particularly of men's facial hair, is shaving. The targeted area should be softened by applying a warm, moist towel, and then applying a shaving cream or lotion that has excellent lubrication qualities and calms the skin. An electric clipper may also be used, particularly to remove unwanted hair at the nape of the neck. The application of a preshaving lotion helps to reduce any irritation. An electric trimmer can also make short work of unwanted hair at the nape of the neck.

TWEEZING

Tweezing is commonly used to shape the eyebrows, and can also be used to remove undesirable hairs from around the mouth and chin. Eyebrow arching is often done as part of a professional makeup service. Correctly shaped eyebrows have a strong, positive impact on the overall attractiveness of the face. The natural arch of the eyebrow follows the orbital bone, or the curved line of the eye socket. Clients can have hair growth both above and below the natural line. These hairs should be removed to give a clean and attractive appearance.

ELECTRONIC TWEEZERS

Another method for the removal of superfluous hair used in salons and spas is electronically charged tweezers. This method transmits radio frequency energy down the hair shaft into the follicle area. The papilla is thus dehydrated and eventually destroyed.

The tweezers are used to grasp a single strand of hair. The energy is then applied, first at a low level to pre-warm and then at a higher level for up to 2 minutes to remove the hair. Most manufacturers suggest that the area be steamed first in order to increase efficiency.

Electronic tweezers are not a method of permanent hair removal. Furthermore, the process of clearing any area of hair by this method is slow.

DEPILATORIES

A **depilatory** is a substance, usually a caustic alkali preparation, used for the temporary removal of superfluous hair by dissolving it at the skin surface level. It contains detergents to strip the sebum from the hair and adhesives to hold the chemicals to the hair shaft for the 5 to 10 minutes necessary to remove the hair. During the application time, the hair expands and the disulfide bonds break. Finally, such chemicals as sodium hydroxide, potassium hydroxide, thioglycolic acid, or calcium thioglycolate

PROCEDURE 21-1

TWEEZING EYEBROWS

IMPLEMENTS AND MATERIALS

- Towels
- Tweezers
- Cotton balls
- Eyebrow brush
- Emollient cream
- Antiseptic lotion
- Gentle eye makeup remover
- Astringent
- Disposable gloves

PREPARATION

1. Seat the client in a facial chair in a reclining position, as for a facial massage. Or, if you prefer, seat the client in a half-upright position and work from the side.
2. Discuss with the client the type of eyebrow arch suitable for her facial characteristics.
3. Drape a towel over the client's chest.
4. Wash and dry your hands and put on disposable gloves.

Before tweezing or waxing brows, discuss with the client her desires to improve the eyebrow appearance. Some clients prefer a more natural line, leaving a few hairs in the edge of the brow. Removing every single hair outside the brow can create a hard look, especially on aging clients.

PROCEDURE

1. Cleanse the eyelid area with cotton balls moistened with gentle eye makeup remover.
2. Brush the eyebrows with a small brush to remove any powder or scaliness (Figure 21-4).
3. Soften brows. Saturate two pledgets (tufts) of cotton or a towel with warm water and place over the brows. Allow them to remain on the brows 1 to 2 minutes to soften and relax the eyebrow tissue (Figure 21-5). You may soften the brows and surrounding skin by rubbing emollient cream into them.
4. Use a mild antiseptic on a cotton ball prior to tweezing.

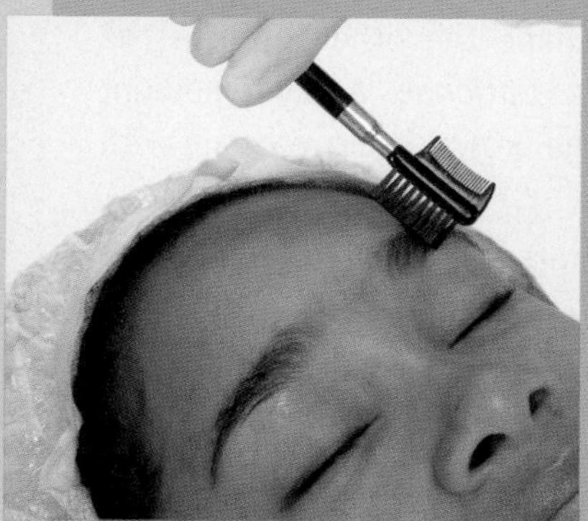

Figure 21-4 Brush the eyebrows with a small brush.

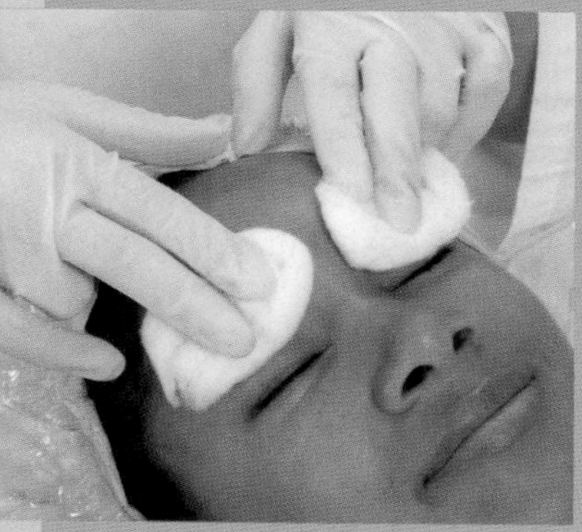

Figure 21-5 Hold a wet cotton pledget over each eyebrow.

5. Remove the hairs between the brows. When tweezing, stretch the skin taut with the index finger and thumb (or index and middle fingers) of your nondominant hand. Grasp each hair individually with tweezers and pull with a quick motion in the direction of growth (Figure 21-6). Tweeze between the brows and above the brow line first, because the area under the brow line is much more sensitive.
6. Sponge the tweezed area frequently with cotton moistened with an antiseptic lotion to avoid infection.
7. Brush the hair downward. Remove excessive hairs from above the eyebrow line. Shape the upper section of one eyebrow, and then shape the other (Figure 21-7). Frequently sponge the area with antiseptic.
8. Brush the hairs upward. Remove hairs from under the eyebrow line. Shape the lower section of one eyebrow, and then shape the other. Sponge the area with antiseptic. *Optional:* Apply emollient cream and massage the brows. Remove cream with tissues.
9. After tweezing is completed, sponge the eyebrows and surrounding skin with astringent to contract the skin.
10. Brush the eyebrow hair to its normal position.

CLEANUP AND SANITATION

1. If eyebrow tweezing is part of a makeup service, continue the makeup procedure. If not, complete the next steps.
2. Remove the towel from the client and place in a closed hamper.
3. Accompany the client to the reception area and suggest rebooking (the eyebrows should be treated about once a month).
4. Discard disposable materials in a closed receptacle and disinfect implements.
5. Wash your hands with soap and warm water.

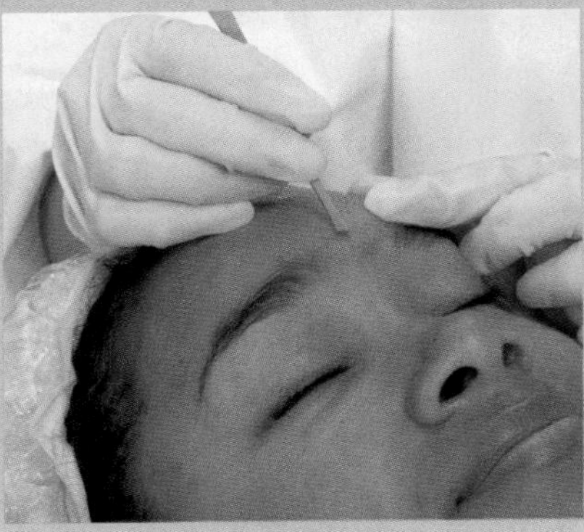

Figure 21-6 Tweeze hair from between eyebrows.

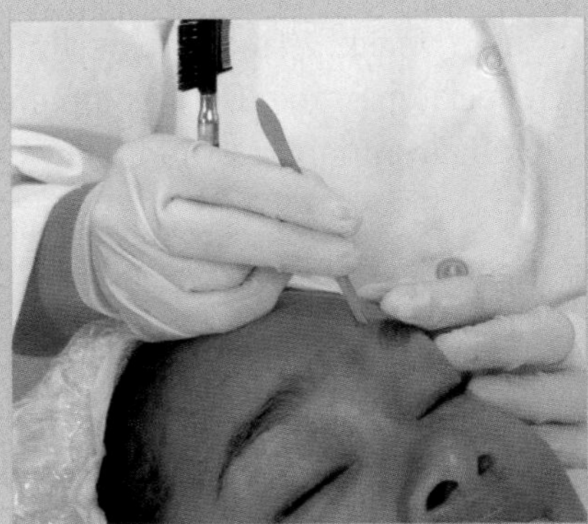

Figure 21-7 Tweeze hair along the upper edge of the eyebrow.

CAUTION

Washing your hands thoroughly with soap and warm water is critical before and after every client procedure you perform. The importance of proper sanitation in these procedures cannot be overemphasized.

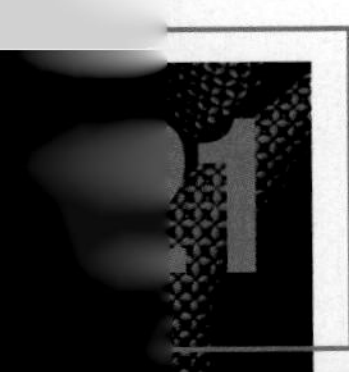

destroy the disulfide bonds. These chemicals turn the hair into a soft, jelly-like mass that can be scraped from the skin. Although depilatories are not commonly used in salons, you should be familiar with them in the event that your clients have used them.

If a client requests a chemical depilatory, you should perform a patch test to determine whether the individual is sensitive to the action of the depilatory. Select a hairless part of the arm, apply a small amount according to the manufacturer's directions, and leave it on the skin for 7 to 10 minutes. If there are no signs of redness, swelling, or rash, the depilatory can probably be used with safety over a larger area of the skin. Follow the manufacturer's directions for application.

EPILATORS

An **epilator** removes the hair from the bottom of the follicle. Wax is a commonly used epilator, applied in either hot or cold form as recommended by the manufacturer. Both products are made primarily of resins and beeswax. Cold wax is somewhat thicker and does not require fabric strips for removal. Because waxing removes the hair from the follicle, the hair takes longer to grow back. The time between waxings is generally 4 to 6 weeks.

Wax may be applied to various parts of the face and body, such as the eyebrows, cheeks, chin, upper lip, arms, and legs. On male clients, wax may be used to remove hair on the back and nape of the neck. The hair should be at least ¼ inch (0.6 centimeter) to ½ inch (1.25 centimeters) long for waxing to be effective. If hair is more than ¼ inch long, it should be trimmed before waxing.

Do not remove vellus (lanugo) hair; doing so may cause the skin to lose its softness. When waxing is done properly, the hair will not feel like beard stubble as it grows out.

Before beginning a wax treatment, be sure to complete a client consultation card and have the client sign a release form. Wear disposable gloves to prevent contact with bloodborne pathogens.

SAFETY PRECAUTIONS

- To prevent burns, always test the temperature of the heated wax before applying to the client's skin. Use a professional wax heater for warming wax. *Never* heat wax in a microwave or on a stovetop. Wax can become overheated and burn the client's skin.
- Use caution so that the wax does not come in contact with the eyes.
- Do not apply wax over warts, moles, abrasions, or irritated or inflamed skin. Do not remove hair protruding from a mole, as the wax could cause trauma to the mole.
- The skin under the arms is sometimes very sensitive. If so, use cold wax.
- Redness and swelling sometimes occur on sensitive skin. Apply an aloe gel to calm and soothe the skin.

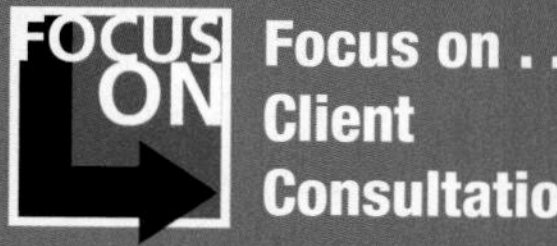

Focus on . . . Client Consultation

As with any procedure, always perform a client consultation prior to tweezing or waxing the eyebrows. Determine the client's wishes for final eyebrow shape. If you remove too much hair, it will generally grow back, but the process takes a long time. You will also end up with an unhappy client who is not likely to return for your services. Conducting a thorough consultation beforehand will help you avoid such mistakes.

PROCEDURE 21-2

HOT WAXING EYEBROWS

WAXING EYEBROWS

EQUIPMENT, IMPLEMENTS, AND MATERIALS

- Facial chair
- Roll of disposable paper
- Wax
- Single or double wax heater
- Wax remover
- Small disposable spatula or small wooden applicators
- Fabric strips for hair removal
- Hair cap or headband
- Towels for draping
- Disposable gloves
- Mild skin cleanser
- Emollient or antiseptic lotion

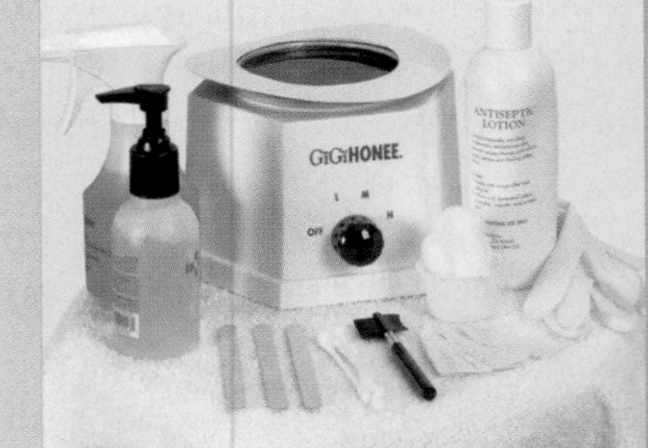

Figure 21-8 Melt the wax.

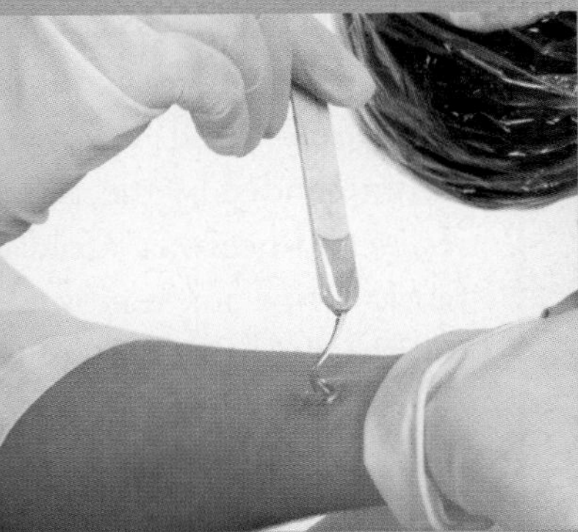

Figure 21-9 Test the temperature of the melted wax.

PREPARATION

1. **Melt the wax in the heater.** The length of time it takes to melt the wax depends on how full the wax holder is—15 to 25 minutes if it is full, and 10 minutes if it is a quarter to half full. Be sure it is not too hot (Figure 21-8).
2. Complete client consultation.
3. Lay a clean towel over the top of the facial chair, and then a layer of disposable paper.
4. Place a hair cap or headband on the client's head to keep hair out of the face.
5. Drape a towel over the client's chest.
6. Wash and dry your hands, and put on disposable gloves.

PROCEDURE

1. Remove makeup, cleanse the area thoroughly with a mild astringent cleanser, and dry.
2. Test the temperature and consistency of the heated wax by applying a small drop on your inner wrist. It should be warm but not hot, and it should run smoothly off the spatula (Figure 21-9).

CAUTION

Be sure not to use an excessive amount of wax, as it will spread when the fabric is pressed and may spread to hair you do not wish to remove.

3. **Spread wax.** With the spatula or wooden applicator, spread a thin coat of the warm wax evenly over the area to be treated, going in the same direction as the hair growth (Figure 21-10). Be sure not to put the spatula in the wax more than once. No double-dips!
4. **Apply fabric.** Apply a sterile fabric strip over the waxed area. Press gently in the direction of hair growth, running your finger over the surface of the fabric three to five times (Figure 21-11).
5. **Apply pressure and pull fabric.** Gently applying pressure to hold the skin taut with one hand, quickly remove the fabric strip and the wax that sticks to it by pulling it in the direction opposite the hair growth. Do not pull straight up on the strip (Figure 21-12).
6. Lightly massage the treated area.
7. Remove any remaining wax residue from the skin with a gentle wax remover.
8. Repeat procedure on the area around the other eyebrow.
9. Cleanse the skin with a mild emollient cleanser and apply an emollient or antiseptic lotion (Figure 21-13).

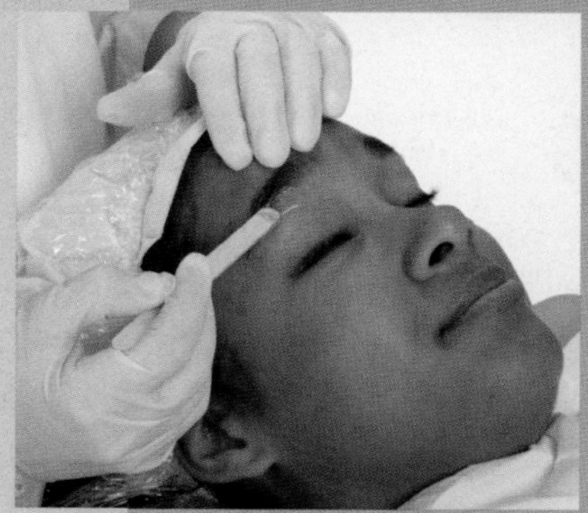

Figure 21-10 Spread warm wax over the eyebrow area.

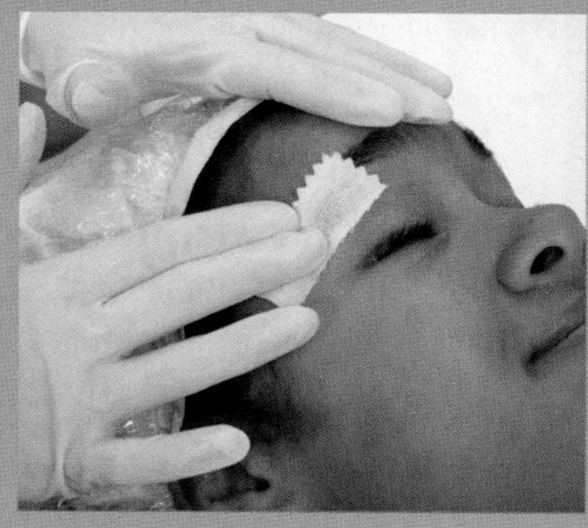

Figure 21-11 Press a fabric strip over the waxed eyebrow.

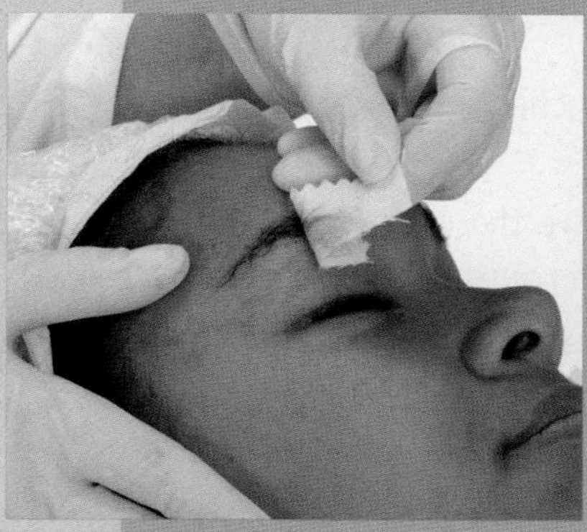

Figure 21-12 Pull off the fabric strip in the direction opposite hair growth.

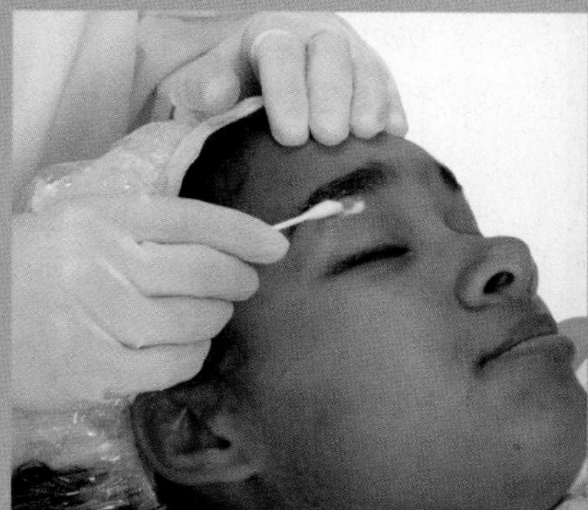

Figure 21-13 Apply emollient or antiseptic lotion to the eyebrow area.

CLEANUP AND SANITATION

Some states or provinces require sanitizing the area prior to tweezing or waxing and applying an antiseptic at the end of the procedure. Always check with your regulatory agency.

1. Remove headband and towel drape from the client and place in a closed hamper.
2. Discard all used disposable materials in a closed hazardous waste container. Never reuse wax. Do not lay used spatula, muslin strips, wax, or any other materials used in waxing on the counter.
3. Sanitize the treatment area. This includes counter surfaces, facial chair, wax heater and container, floor, bottle caps, and lids.
4. Wash your hands with soap and warm water.

CAUTION

Beeswax has a relatively high incidence of allergic reaction. Always give a small patch test of the product to be used prior to the service.

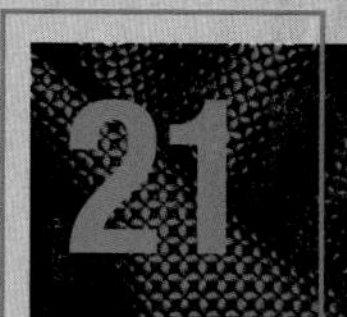

PROCEDURE 21-3

BODY WAXING

EQUIPMENT, IMPLEMENTS, AND MATERIALS

Use the same equipment as for eyebrow waxing, with the addition of a metal or disposable wooden spatula. A metal spatula holds the heat longer, but it must not touch the client's skin as you apply the wax. You may find disposable spatulas more convenient.

PREPARATION

1. Melt the wax in the heater.
2. Complete your client consultation.
3. Drape the treatment bed with disposable paper or a bed sheet with paper over the top.
4. If bikini waxing, offer the client disposable panties or a small sanitized towel.
5. If waxing the underarms, have the client remove her bra and put on a terry wrap. Offer a terry wrap when waxing the legs as well.
6. Assist the client onto the treatment bed and drape with towels.
7. Wash your hands.

PROCEDURE

1. Thoroughly cleanse the area to be waxed with a mild astringent cleanser and dry.
2. Apply a light covering of powder (Figure 21-14).
3. Test the temperature and consistency of the heated wax by applying a small drop to your inner wrist.
4. **Spread wax.** Using a metal or disposable spatula, spread a thin coat of the warm wax evenly over the skin surface in the same direction as the hair growth (Figure 21-15). Be sure not to put the spatula in the wax more than once. If the wax strings and lands in an area you do not wish to treat, remove it with lotion designed to dissolve and remove wax.
5. **Apply fabric.** Apply a fabric strip in the same direction as the hair growth. Press gently, running your hand over the surface of the fabric three to five times (Figure 21-16).
6. **Apply pressure and remove fabric.** Gently apply pressure to hold the skin taut with one hand and quickly remove the adhering wax in the opposite direction of the hair growth (Figure 21-17).

CAUTION

Never leave the wax heate on overnight, as it is a fire hazard and can damage th wax.

CAUTION

When waxing sensitive areas such as underarms o bikini lines, be sure the wa is not too hot. Trim the ha with scissors if it is more than ½-inch (1.25 centimeters) long.

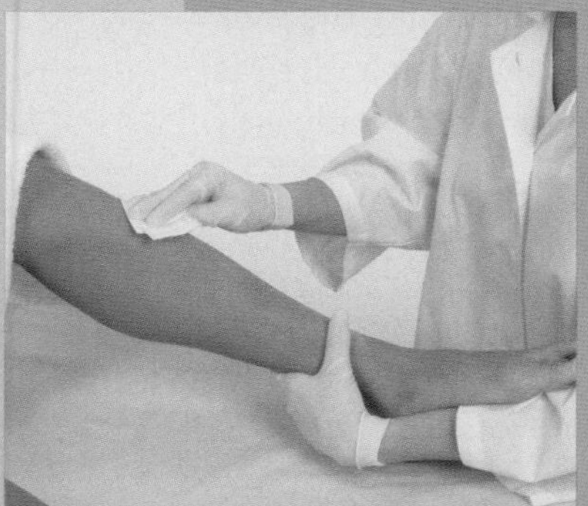

Figure 21-14 Apply a light coating of powder.

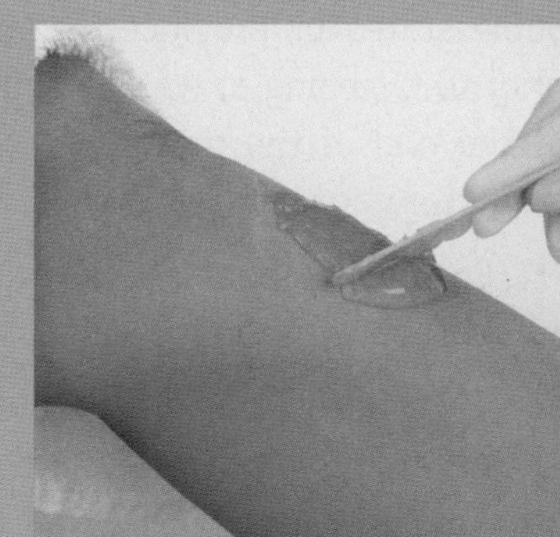

Figure 21-15 Spread warm wax over the top of the leg.

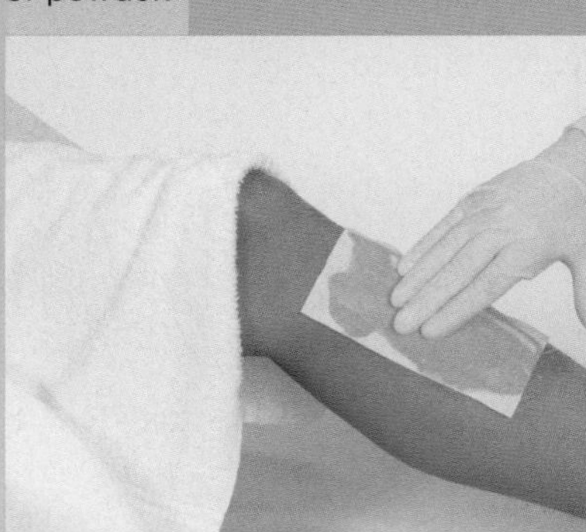

Figure 21-16 Press a fabric strip over the waxed area.

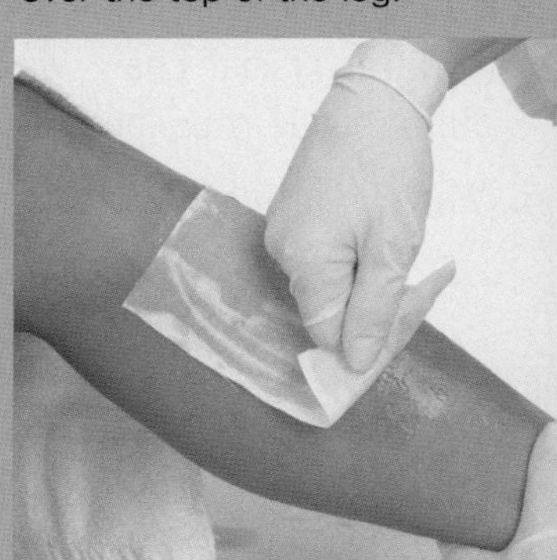

Figure 21-17 Pull off the fabric st in the direction opposite hair grow

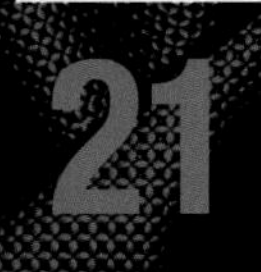

7. Apply gentle pressure and lightly massage the treated area.
8. Repeat, taking a fresh fabric strip as each strip becomes covered with wax.
9. Have the client turn over, and repeat the procedure on the backs of the legs (Figure 21-18).
10. Remove any remaining residue of powder from the skin.
11. Cleanse the area with a mild emollient cleanser and apply an emollient or antiseptic lotion.
12. Undrape the client and escort her to the dressing room.

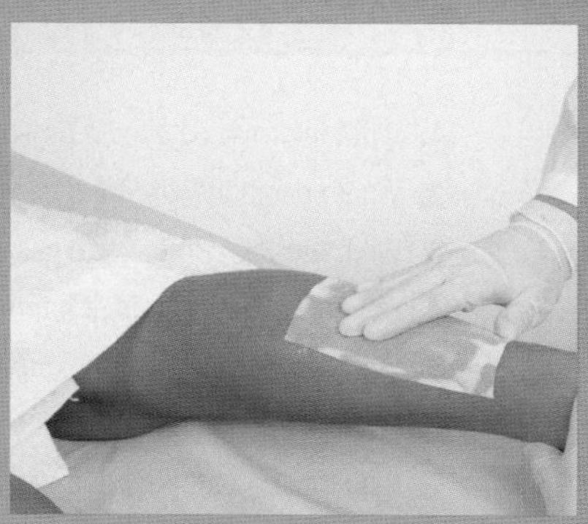

Figure 21-18 Pull the fabric strip from the back of the leg.

CLEANUP AND SANITATION

1. Discard used disposable materials in a closed hazardous waste container.
2. Place linens and robe in a closed hamper.
3. Remove any wax from the metal spatula (if you used one) with wax removal solution. Disinfect the spatula and store in a clean, covered container.
4. Sanitize the treatment bed and counter.

THREADING

Threading is a temporary hair removal method that is still practiced in many Eastern cultures today. It involves the manipulation of cotton thread, which is twisted and rolled along the surface of the skin, entwining the hair in the thread and lifting it from the follicle. Threading has become increasingly popular in the United States as an alternative to other methods. It requires specialized training.

SUGARING

Sugaring, another epilator treatment, is also becoming more popular and produces the same results as hot or cold wax. It involves the use of a thick, sugar-based paste and is especially appropriate for more sensitive skin types. One advantage with sugar waxing is the hair can be removed even if it is only ⅛-inch long.

Removing the residue from the skin is simple, as it dissolves with warm water. (See Table 21-1 for a list of the hair removal procedures described in this chapter and their uses.)

BODY AREA	Waxing	Tweezing	Depilatories
Face/upper lips/eyebrows	X	X	
Underarms	X		
Arms	X		X
Bikini line	X	X (after waxing or sugaring)	
Legs	X		X
Tops of feet/toes	X		X

Table 21-1 Appropriate Hair Removal Procedures

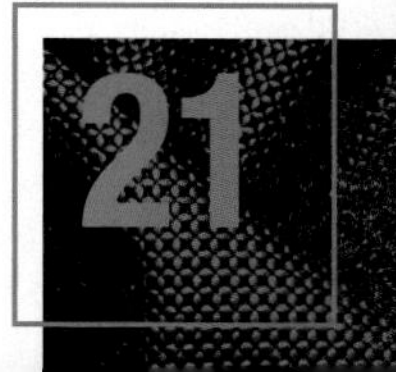

REVIEW QUESTIONS

1. What information should be entered in the client record during the consultation?
2. What conditions, treatments, and medications contraindicate hair removal in the salon?
3. What are the two major types of hair removal? Give examples of each.
4. Define these methods of hair removal: electrolysis, photoepilation, and laser removal.
5. Which hair removal techniques should not be performed in the salon without special training?
6. What is the difference between a depilatory and an epilator?
7. Why must a patch test be given before waxing?
8. List safety precautions that must be followed for hot and cold waxing.
9. Define threading and sugaring.

CHAPTER GLOSSARY

depilatory	Substance, usually a caustic alkali preparation, used for the temporary removal of superfluous hair by dissolving it at the skin surface level.
electrolysis	Removal of hair by means of an electric current that destroys the root of the hair.
epilator	Substance used to remove hair by pulling it out of the follicle.
hirsuties or *hypertrichosis*	Growth of an unusual amount of hair on parts of the body normally bearing only downy hair, such as the faces of women or the backs of men.
laser hair removal	Permanent hair removal treatment in which a laser beam is pulsed on the skin, impairing the hair growth.
photoepilation	Permanent hair removal treatment that uses intense light to destroy the hair follicles.
sugaring	Temporary hair removal method that involves the use of a thick, sugar-based paste.
threading	Temporary hair removal method that involves twisting and rolling cotton thread along the surface of the skin, entwining the hair in the thread, and lifting it from the follicle.

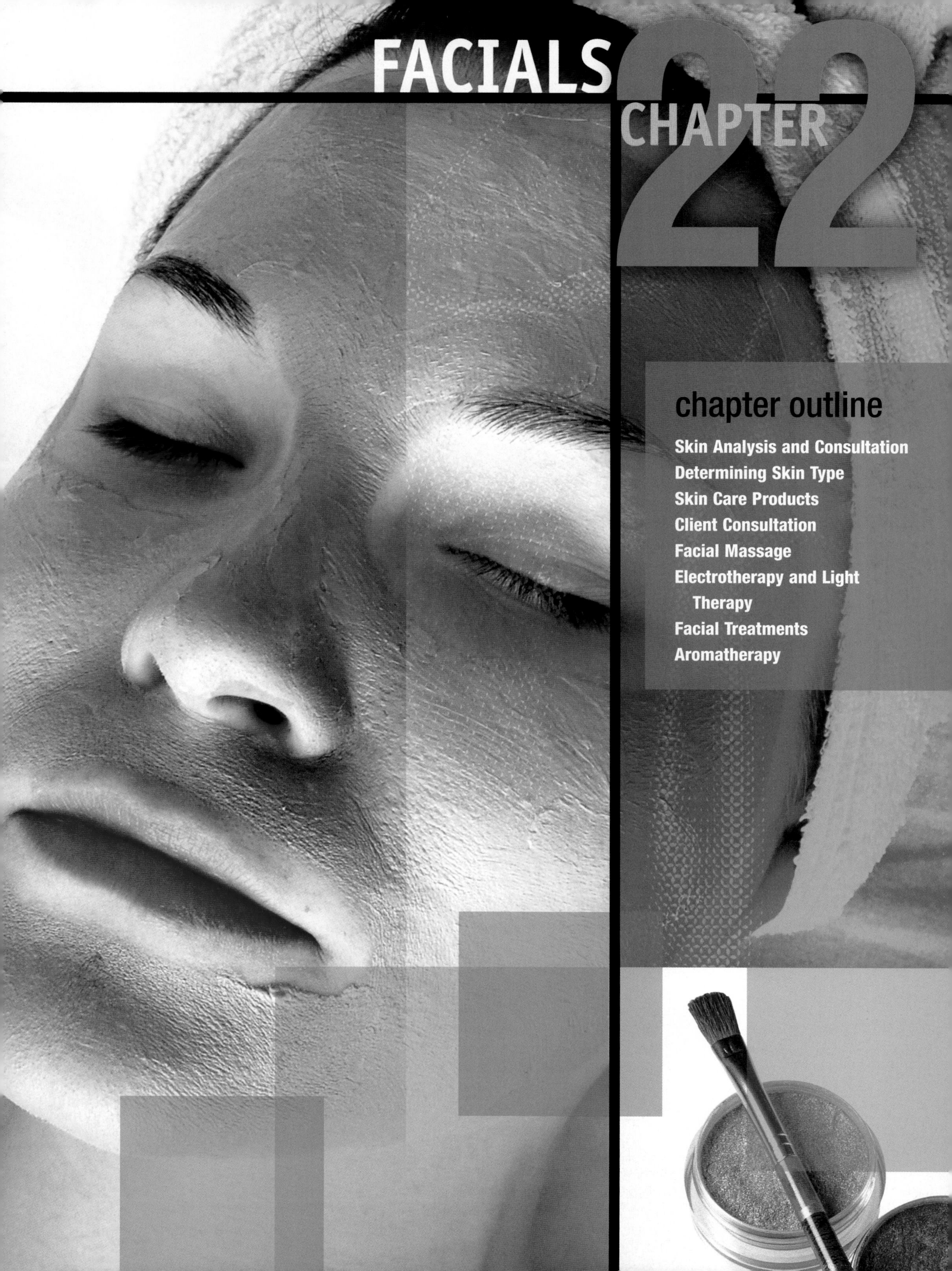

FACIALS

CHAPTER 22

chapter outline

Learning Objectives

After completing this chapter, you will be able to:

- **List and describe various skin types and conditions.**
- **Understand contraindications and the use of health screening forms to safely perform facial treatments.**
- **Identify the various types of massage movements and their physiological effects.**
- **Be able to describe different types of products used in facial treatments.**
- **Understand the basic types of electrical equipment used in facial treatments.**
- **Demonstrate the procedure for a basic facial.**

Key Terms

Page number indicates where in the chapter the term is used.

alipidic
pg. 567

alpha hydroxy acids
pg. 571

ampoules
pg. 573

anode
pg. 584

aromatherapy
pg. 599

astringents
pg. 570

brushing machine
pg. 584

cathode
pg. 584

chemical exfoliants
pg. 571

chucking
pg. 578

clay-based masks
pg. 573

cleansing milks
pg. 570

closed comedones
pg. 568

contraindication
pg. 563

couperose
pg. 569

cream masks
pg. 573

effleurage
pg. 577

electrode
pg. 584

electrotherapy
pg. 584

emollients
pg. 572

enzyme peels
pg. 571

exfoliants
pg. 570

exfoliation
pg. 570

foaming cleansers
pg. 570

fresheners
pg. 570

friction
pg. 578

fulling
pg. 578

gommages
pg. 570

hacking
pg. 579

humectants
pg. 572

keratolytic enzymes
pg. 571

light therapy
pg. 587

masks
pg. 573

massage
pg. 577

massage creams
pg. 573

mechanical exfoliants
pg. 570

microcurrent
pg. 586

microdermabrasion
pg. 570

modelage masks
pg. 574

moisturizers
pg. 572

motor point
pg. 579

open comedones
pg. 568

ostium
pg. 568

paraffin wax masks
pg. 573

petrissage
pg. 578

rolling
pg. 578

steamer
pg. 583

tapotement or percussion
pg. 578

telangiectasias
pg. 569

toners
pg. 570

treatment cream
pg. 573

vibration
pg. 579

wringing
pg. 578

Good skin care can make a big difference in the way skin looks, and the way the client feels about his or her appearance. Besides being very relaxing, facial treatments can offer many improvements to the appearance of the skin.

Proper skin care can make oily skin look cleaner and healthier, dry skin look and feel more moist and supple, and aging skin look smoother, firmer, and less wrinkled. A combination of good salon facial treatments and helping the client plan an effective home care program individualized for their skin will show visible results.

It is extremely rewarding to be able to help people relax, improve their appearance, and feel better about themselves (Figure 22-1).

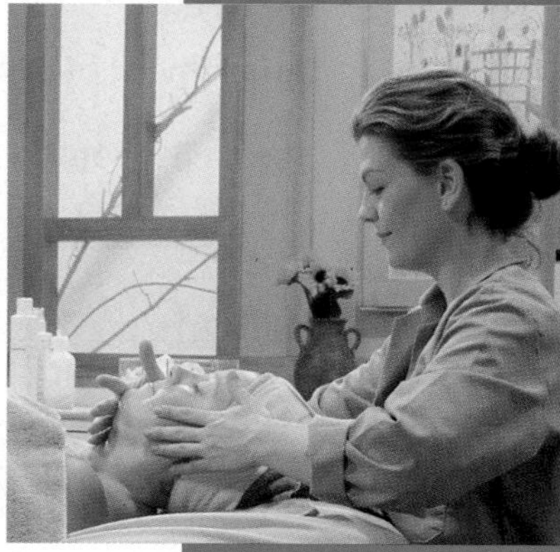

Figure 22-1 A facial is a soothing, pleasurable experience for the client.

SKIN ANALYSIS AND CONSULTATION

Skin analysis is a very important part of the facial treatment because it determines what type of skin the client has, the condition of the skin, and what type of treatment the client's skin needs. *Consultation* allows you the opportunity to ask the client questions about his or her health, skin care history, and to advise the client about appropriate home care products and treatments.

HEALTH SCREENING

Before beginning the analysis, you must have the client fill out a health-screening questionnaire (Figure 22-2). Similar to the form used for waxing, the main purpose of the health-screening form is to determine any *contraindications* the client might have that might indicate avoiding certain types of treatment on that particular client's skin. A **contraindication** is a condition the client has, or a treatment the client is undergoing, that might cause a negative side effect during the facial treatment. For example, if the client is allergic to fragrance, using a fragranced product would be *contraindicated.* If a client is using a prescription drug, such as Retin-A® or Tazorac® (both topical drugs that cause skin exfoliation), using other exfoliants in the facial treatment is contraindicated. Accutane, an oral medication for cystic acne, causes thinning of the skin all over the body. Waxing, stimulating treatments, or exfoliation procedures should never be performed on the skin of someone using Accutane, or someone who has used the drug in the last 6 months. Because Accutane is an oral drug, it stays in the body for several months after the client stops using the drug.

CAUTION

As a cosmetology student, you should always receive hands-on training from your instructor before attempting any of the procedures discussed in this chapter.

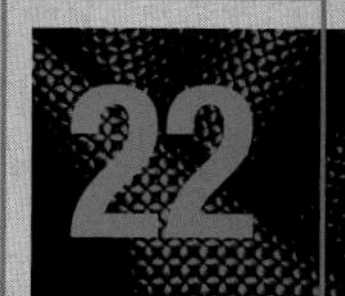

Department of Skin Care

Health Screening Form

Client History

Name____

Address____

City______________________State____________ Zip Code____________________

Home phone____________________ Work Phone______________________________

Occupation_______________Referred by_______________Date of Birth__________

Is this your first facial treatment? YES___ NO___

Have you ever used:

Retin-A®? YES___ NO___

Accutane®? YES___ NO___

Are you using glycolic or alphahydroxy acids? YES___ NO___

Do you smoke? YES___ NO___

Are you pregnant? YES___ NO___

Do you have acne or frequent blemishes? YES___ NO___

Are you nursing? YES___ NO___

Taking birth control pills? YES___ NO___ If so, how long?____________________

Have you had skin cancer? YES___ NO___

Do you experience stress? YES___ NO___ If so, how often?____________________

Do you wear contact lenses? YES___ NO___

Are you under a physician's care? YES___ NO___

Physician's Name____________________________

Do you have any allergies to cosmetics, foods, or drugs? YES___ NO___

Please list____

Are you presently on any medications - oral or topical-dermatological? YES___ NO___

Please list____

Figure 22-2 Health Screening Form.

What products do you use presently?________________________________

Please circle: Soap Cleansing Milk Toner Daily Sunscreen Creams

Other____

Please circle if you are affected by or have any of the following:

Have had hysterectomy	Pacemaker/Cardiac Problems	Immune Disorders
Psychological	Herpes	Urinary or Kidney Problems
Taking Depression/Mood	Chronic Headaches	Hepatitis
Altering Medications	Fever Blisters	Lupus
Seborrhea/Psoriasis/Eczema	Metal Bone Pins or Plates	Epilepsy
Asthma	Sinus Problems	Other Skin Diseases
High Blood Pressure		

Please explain above problems or list any significant others:

____

____

I understand that the services offered are not a substitute for medical care, and any information provided by the therapist is for educational purposes only and not diagnostically prescriptive in nature. I understand that the information herein is to aid the therapist in giving better service and is completely confidential.

SALON POLICIES

1. Professional consultation is required before initial dispensing of products.
2. Our active discount rate is only effective for clients visiting every 4 weeks.
3. We do not give cash refunds.

I fully understand and agree to the above salon policies.

________________________________ ______________

Client Signature Date

Figure 22-2 Health Screening Form (cont'd).

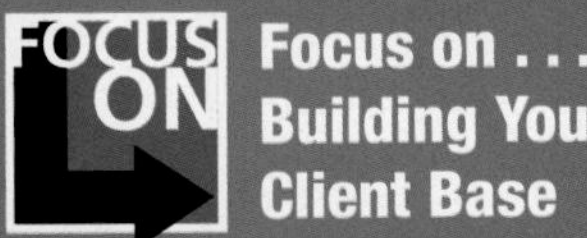

Focus on . . . Building Your Client Base

It is useful to note on the consultation card how the client was referred to the salon. This helps you determine the type of advertising that draws your clients. If the referral has come from another salon client, you will want to make a point of thanking that client. This small courtesy can well lead to other valuable referrals.

CAUTION

The cosmetologist does not treat skin diseases or disorders. However, as a professional, you must be able to recognize the presence of various skin ailments in order to suggest that the client seek medical advice from a physician.

The main contraindications to look for are summarized below.

- Use of Accutane or any skin-thinning or exfoliating drug, including Retin-A®, Renova®, Tazorac®, Differin®, and so on. Avoid waxing, any exfoliation or peeling treatment, or stimulating treatments.
- Pregnancy—The client should not have any electrical treatments, or any questionable treatment without her physician's written permission. Some pregnant clients also experience sensitivities from waxing.
- Metal bone pins or plates in the body—Avoid all electrical treatment.
- Pacemakers or heart irregularities—Avoid all electrical treatment.
- Allergies—Any allergic substances listed should be strictly avoided. Clients with multiple allergies should always use nonfragranced products designed for sensitive skin.
- Seizures or epilepsy—Avoid all electrical and light treatments.
- Use of oral steroids like Prednisone—Avoid any stimulating or exfoliating treatment or waxing.
- Autoimmune diseases such as lupus—Avoid any harsh or stimulating treatments.
- Diabetes—Be aware that many diabetics heal very slowly. If you have questions, you should get approval from the client's physician before treatment.
- Blood thinners—No extraction or waxing.

Clients who have obvious skin abnormalities, such as open sores, fever blisters (herpes simplex), or other abnormal-looking signs should be referred to a physician for treatment or written approval of facial services.

Should you ever have any questions regarding a client's treatment and his or her health conditions, *always* check with the client's doctor first! Remember one simple rule: When in doubt, don't!

When the client completes the health-screening form, you can obtain other important information such as the following:

- Client's name, address, and phone number(s).
- Client's occupation
- Medical conditions that might affect your treatment
- Any medications the client is using, including topical drugs for the skin
- Home skin care program that the client is using presently, or if the client has had facial treatments before
- How did the client hear about you?

TREATMENT RECORDS

You should record and highlight with a color pen any important observations or contraindications in the client's treatment record. Keep the health forms filed separately in a secure filing cabinet, as the client may have revealed information that is private. The client treatment record should include the client's name, address, and phone numbers, and have space for the results of the analysis, areas for recording each treatment performed on the client's skin, your observations on each visit, any home care products purchased by the client, and the date of the treatment or product purchase. Recording product purchases helps to find a product a client wants to re-purchase in case the client has forgotten the product name.

ANALYSIS PROCEDURE

After carefully reading the client's health-screening form and discussing any questions you have with the client, have the client change into a smock, seat the client in the facial chair, and drape the client using a hair cap, headband, or towels. The hair should be covered and any jewelry should be removed by the client and put away in a safe place. Jewelry can get in the way during treatment or might be soiled or damaged.

Recline the client in the chair. Warm some cleansing milk in your hands and apply the cleanser to the face in upward circular movements. When cleansing the eye area, use a special cleanser made for eye makeup removal. Apply a small amount to the eye areas, being careful not to use so much that it gets in the eyes. Gently remove the cleanser with warm damp facial sponges or cotton pads. Remember to remove the cleanser using upward and outward movements. When working around the eyes, move outward on the upper lid, and inwards on the lower lid.

After thoroughly cleansing the face, apply a cotton eye pad to the client's eyes to avoid extreme brightness when using the magnifying lamp.

DETERMINING SKIN TYPE

Look through the magnifying lamp at the client's skin. *Skin type* is determined by how oily or dry the skin is. Skin type is hereditary and cannot be permanently changed with treatments, although the skin may look considerably better after treatment. *Skin conditions* are characteristics of the skin associated with a particular skin type (Table 22-1).

The first thing you should look for is the presence or absence of visible pores (follicles). The amount of sebum produced by the sebaceous glands determines the size of the pores, and is hereditary. Obvious pores indicate oily skin areas, and lack of pores indicates dry (alipidic) skin.

SKIN TYPES

The term **alipidic** means "lack of lipids," that is, the skin is not producing enough sebum. This skin type is also referred to as *dry skin.* Alipidic skin becomes dehydrated because it does not produce enough sebum to prevent the evaporation of cell moisture. Dehydration indicates a lack of moisture in the skin. Dehydrated skin may be flaky or dry looking, with small fine lines and wrinkles. It may look like it has a piece of cellophane

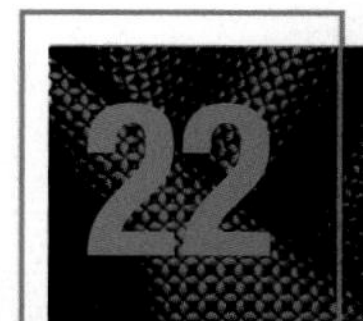

SKIN	Signs of Skin Type	Conditions Associated with Skin Type
Oily	Obvious, large pores.	Open and closed comedones, clogged pores. Shiny, thick appearance. Yellowish color. Orange peel texture.
Dry	Pores very small or not visible.	Tight, poreless-looking skin. May be dehydrated with fine lines and wrinkles, dry and rough to the touch.
Normal	Even pore distribution throughout the skin. Very soft smooth surface. Lack of wrinkles.	Normal skin is actually very unusual. Most clients have combination skin.
Combination dry	Obvious pores down center of face. Pores not visible or becoming smaller toward the outer edges of the face.	May have clogged pores in the nose, chin, and center of the forehead. Dry, poreless toward outside edges of the face.
Combination oily	Wider distribution of obvious or large pores down the center of the face extending to the outer cheeks. Pores become smaller towards edges of the face.	Comedones, clogged pores, or obvious pores in the center of the face.
Acne	Very large pores in all areas. Acne is considered a skin type because it is hereditary.	Presence of numerous open and closed comedones, clogged pores, and red papules and pustules (pimples).

Table 22-1 Signs and Conditions Associated with Skin Types

on top of it. Dehydrated skin also may feel itchy or tight. Dehydration can occur on almost any skin type. The key to truly alipidic skin is the absence of visible pores.

Oily skin that produces too much sebum will have large pores, and the skin may appear shiny or greasy. Pores may be clogged from dead cells building up in the hair follicle, or there may be **open comedones** (blackheads) present. Open comedones are a mixture of solidified sebum and dead cell buildup stuck in the follicles. **Closed comedones** are small bumps just underneath the skin surface. The difference between closed and open comedones is the size of the follicle opening or **ostium.**

ACNE

The presence of pimples in oily areas indicates *acne.* Acne is considered a skin type because the tendency to develop acne is hereditary. Acne is a disorder in which the follicles become clogged, resulting in infection of the follicle with redness and inflammation. Acne bacteria are *anaerobic,* which means they cannot survive in the presence of oxygen. When follicles are blocked with solidified sebum and dead-cell buildup, oxygen cannot readily get to the bottom of the follicle where acne bacteria live.

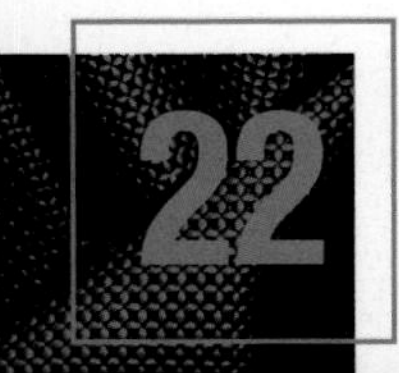

Acne bacteria survive from breaking down sebum into fatty acids, which is their only food source. A blocked follicle is an ideal environment for acne bacteria. When acne bacteria flourish from the lack of oxygen and a food source like a blocked follicle, they multiply quickly, eventually causing a break in the follicle wall. This rupture allows blood to come into the follicle causing redness. *Acne papules* are red pimples that do not have a pus head. Pimples with a pus head are called *pustules. Pus* is a fluid inside a pustule, largely made up of dead white blood cells that tried to fight the infection (Table 22-1).

CAUTION

Severe or unresponsive cases of acne should be referred to a dermatologist for treatment. If you are ever unsure about treating a client who has acne, always refer that client to a dermatologist!

ANALYSIS OF SKIN CONDITIONS

Conditions of the skin are generally treatable. They are generally not hereditary, but may be associated with a particular skin type.

Dehydration is indicated by flaky areas or skin that wrinkles easily on the surface. Very gently pinching the skin surface will result in the formation of lines. This is an indication of dehydration. Dehydrated skin can be caused from lack of care, improper or overdrying skin care products, sun exposure, and other causes. Dehydrated skin is treated by using hydrators that help to bind water to the skin surface. These hydrating products should be chosen based on skin type. Hydrators for alipidic skin are generally heavier in texture. Hydrators for oilier skin are lighter weight. Proper hydration of the skin can result in smoother-looking and softer skin.

Most types of *hyperpigmentation,* or dark blotches of color, are caused by sun exposure or hormone imbalances. Clients who have spent a lot of time in the sun will often have hyperpigmentation. Hyperpigmentation is treated with mild exfoliation and home care products that discourage pigmentation. Daily use of sunscreen and avoidance of sun exposure are very important for this skin type.

Sensitive skin has a thin, red-pink look. Skin will turn red easily, and is easily inflamed by some skin care products. You should avoid strong products or cleansers, fragranced products, and strong exfoliants when treating sensitive skin. *Rosacea* is a chronic hereditary disorder that can be indicated by constant or frequent facial blushing. *Dilated capillaries* (ca-pill-larrys), also known as **telangiectasias** (te-lang-ec-tasias) or **couperose** (coo-per-ros) are often present. Rosacea is considered a medical disorder, and should be diagnosed by a dermatologist. You should treat a client who has rosacea with very gentle products and treatments, avoiding any treatment that releases heat or stimulates the skin.

Aging skin has loss of elasticity, and the skin tends to sag in areas around the eyes and jawline. Wrinkles may be apparent in areas of normal facial expression. Treatments that hydrate and exfoliate improve the appearance of this skin.

Sun-damaged skin is skin that has been chronically exposed to sun frequently over the client's lifetime. Sun-damaged skin will have many areas of hyperpigmentation, lots of wrinkled areas including areas not in the normal facial expression, and sagging skin from damage to the elastic fibers. The skin looks older than it should for the age of the client. It is often confused with aging skin.

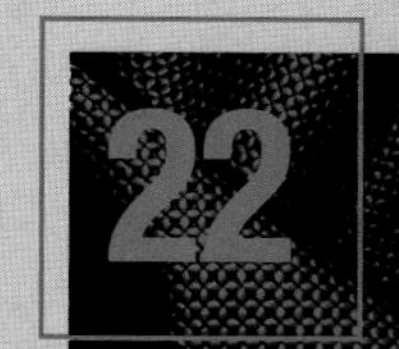

SKIN CARE PRODUCTS

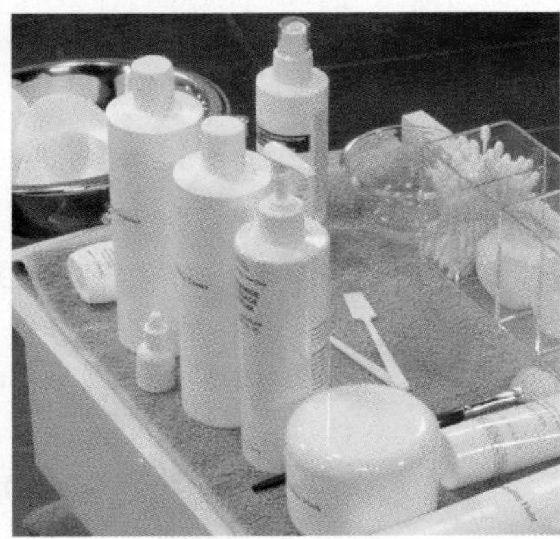

Figure 22-3 There is a wide variety of skin care products for every skin type.

There are many, many types of skin care products available for salon use and home care for the client to use. Most skin care products are designed for specific skin types or conditions. Major categories of skin care products are described below (Figure 22-3).

Cleansers are designed to clean the surface of the skin and to remove makeup. There are basically two types of cleansers: cleansing milks and foaming cleansers.

Cleansing milks are nonfoaming lotions. They are designed to cleanse dry and sensitive skin types and to remove makeup. They can be applied with the hands or an implement, but must be removed with a dampened facial sponge, soft cloth, or cotton pad. Ingredients are sometimes added to cleansing milks to make them more specific to a given skin type.

Foaming cleansers are wash-off types of products. These products contain *surfactants,* also known as *detergents,* that cause the product to foam and rinse easily. These products are generally for combination or oilier skin types, although there are some rinse-off cleansers for dry and sensitive skin. Clients love using these products as they may be used quickly and easily in the shower. They have varying amounts of detergent ingredients to treat specific levels of oiliness. Foaming cleansers, like cleansing milks, may have special ingredients to make them more specific for certain skin types. Some have antibacterial ingredients for acne-prone skin.

CAUTION

It is important to note that the cosmetology professional's domain is the hair and superficial epidermis. Cosmetology professionals must not perform treatments that remove cells beyond the stratum corneum of the epidermis.

Toners, also sometimes known as **fresheners** or **astringents,** are designed to lower the pH of the skin after cleansing, and to help remove excess cleansing milk. They may also contain ingredients that help to hydrate or soothe, and may sometimes contain an exfoliating ingredient to help remove dead cells. Fresheners and astringents are usually stronger products, often with higher alcohol content, and are used to treat oilier skin types. Toning products are applied with cotton pads after cleansing. Some alcohol-free toners can be sprayed onto the face.

Exfoliants are products that help bring about **exfoliation** or removal of excess dead cells from the skin surface. By removing dead cells from the surface of the skin, it looks smoother and clearer. Exfoliants help clear the skin of clogged pores and can improve the appearance of wrinkles, aging, and hyperpigmentation. Cosmetology professionals may use products that remove dead surface cells from the stratum corneum. Deeper, surgical level peels must only be administered by dermatologists and plastic surgeons.

Mechanical exfoliants work by physically "bumping off" dead cell buildup. Examples are granular scrubs, roll-off masks (**gommages**), and the use of **microdermabrasion** scrub products that have small crystals to remove dead cell buildup on the surface. Microdermabrasion can also be used as a machine treatment, which is briefly discussed later (Figure 22-4). Skin brushing machines are another example of mechanical exfoliation (Figures 22-5 and 22-6).

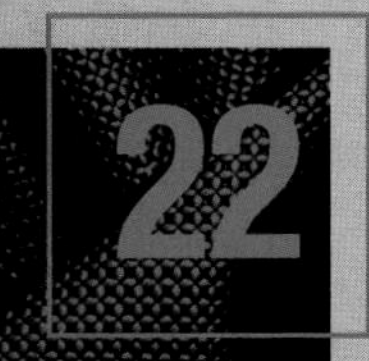

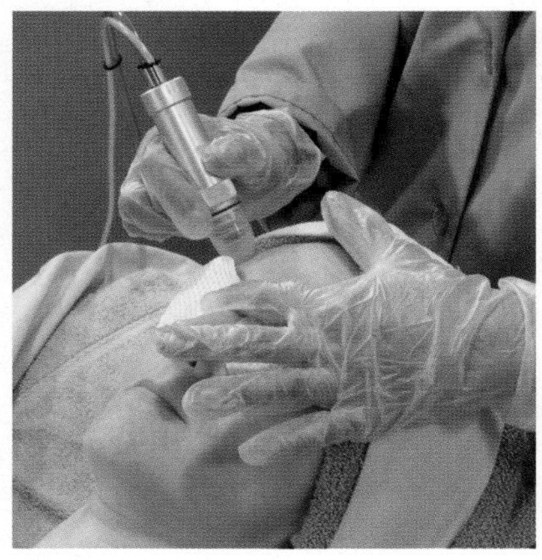
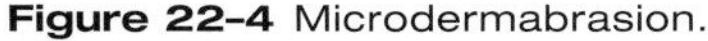

Figure 22-4 Microdermabrasion.

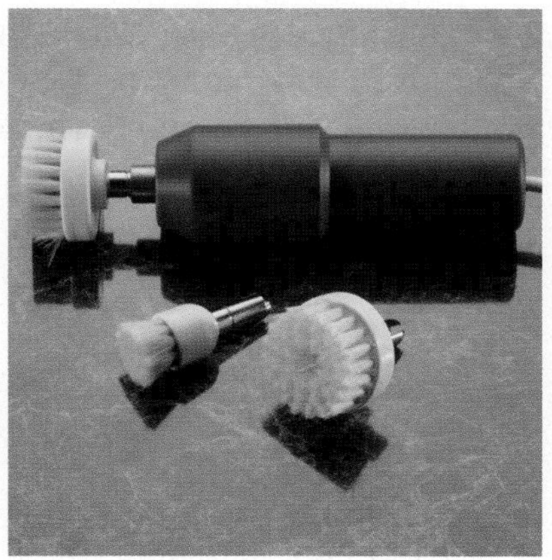

Figure 22-5 Skin-brushing machine.

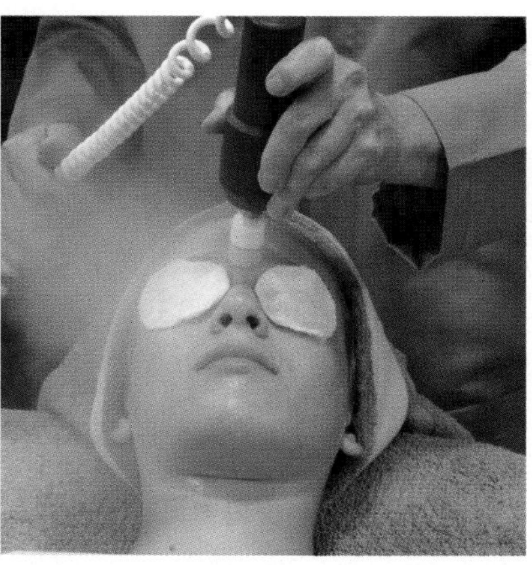

Figure 22-6 Using a skin-brushing machine on a client's face.

Chemical exfoliants contain chemicals that either loosen or dissolve dead cell buildup. They are either used for a short time, although some may be worn as a day or night treatment, or combined in a moisturizer. Popular exfoliating chemicals are **alpha hydroxy acids** or *beta hydroxy acids.* These gentle acids help dissolve the bonds and "intercellular cement" between cells. As dead cells are removed from the surface over time, wrinkles appear less deep, skin discolorations may fade, clogged pores are loosened and reduced, new clogged pores are prevented, and skin is smoother and more hydrated. These acids encourage cell renewal, resulting in firmer and healthier-looking skin.

Salon alpha hydroxy acid exfoliants, often referred to as *peels,* contain larger concentrations of alpha hydroxy acids, usually around 20 to 30 percent. They should never be used unless the client has been using 10-percent alpha hydroxy acid products at home for at least 2 weeks prior to the higher concentration salon treatment.

Enzyme peels are another type of chemical exfoliant. Enzyme peels work by dissolving keratin protein in the surface cells. They are known as **keratolytic** (kair-uh-tuh-LIT-ik) **enzymes** or protein-dissolving agents. Enzyme products are usually made from plant-extracted enzymes from papaya, *papain* (pa-PAIN) or pineapple, *bromelain* (bro-ma-LAIN), or *pancreatin* (pan-cree-at-tin), which is derived from beef by-products. Enzymes sometimes are blended into scrubs or wearable products, but they are most often designed for use in the salon.

There are two basic types of keratolytic enzyme peels. Cream-type enzyme peels usually contain papain. They are applied to the skin and allowed to dry for a few minutes. They form a crust, which is then "rolled" off the skin. This type of product rolled off the skin is known as a *gommage* (go-mahj) (Figure 22-7). The most

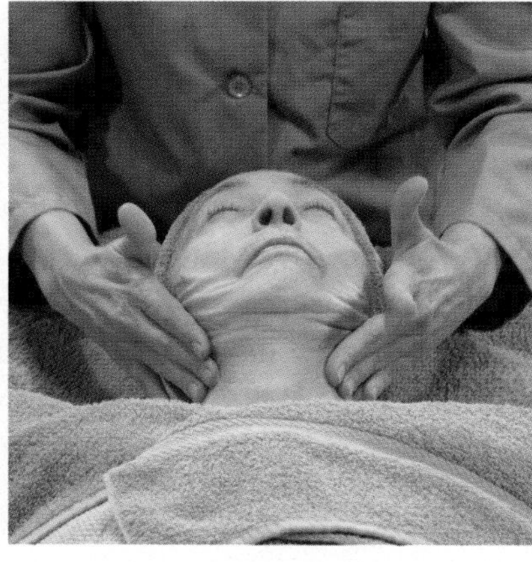

Figure 22-7 Rolling a gommage mask off the face.

CAUTION

Do not use brushing machines, scrubs, or any harsh mechanical peeling techniques on the following skin types and conditions:

- **Skin with many visible capillaries**
- **Thin skin that reddens easily**
- **Older skin that is thin and bruises easily**
- **Skin being medically treated with tretinoin (retinoic acid or Retin-A), Accutane, azelaic acid, adapalene (Differin), alpha hydroxy acid (AHA), or salicylic acid (found in many common skin products)**
- **Acne-prone skin with inflamed papules and pustules**

CAUTION

You should always receive hands-on training from your instructor before attempting chemical exfoliation treatments!

CAUTION

Overexfoliation of the skin can result in ultrasensitive and inflamed skin. Never use an exfoliant more often than recommended by the manufacturer. Combining more than one type of exfoliation may lead to irritation. Always carefully advise your client on the proper use of a home care exfoliant, including the need for the use of a daily sunscreen with an SPF of at least 15.

popular type of enzyme peel is likely a powder form that is mixed with water in the treatment room and applied to the face. This type of enzyme treatment does not dry, and can even be used during a steam treatment.

Proper exfoliation may improve the appearance of the skin in the following ways:

- Reduces clogged and oily skin
- Promotes skin smoothness
- Increases moisture content and hydration
- Reduces hyperpigmentation
- Decreases uneven skin color
- Eliminates or softens wrinkles and fine lines
- Increases elasticity

In addition, proper exfoliation speeds up cell turnover, and allows for better penetration of treatment creams and serums. Makeup applies more evenly on an exfoliated skin.

MOISTURIZERS

Moisturizers are products that help increase the moisture content of the skin surface. Moisturizers help the appearance of fine lines and wrinkles. They are basically mixtures of **humectants** (hew-mec-tunts) also known as *hydrators* or water-binding agents and **emollients,** which are oily or fatty ingredients that prevent moisture from leaving the skin.

Moisturizers for oily skin are most often in lotion form and generally contain smaller amounts of emollient. They are intended for oilier skin that does not need as much emollient since the skin produces more than adequate amounts of protective sebum.

Moisturizers for dry skin are often in the form of a heavier cream, and contain more emollients needed by alipidic skin.

All moisturizers may have other ingredients that will perform additional functions. These ingredients may include soothing agents for sensitive skin, alpha hydroxy acids or peptides for aging skin, or sunscreens.

SUNSCREENS AND DAY PROTECTION PRODUCTS

Shielding the skin from sun exposure is probably the most important habit to benefit the skin. Cumulative sun exposure causes the majority of skin cancers, and prematurely ages the skin.

Most sun exposure over a lifetime is from casual sun exposure. Therefore, every client should be instructed to use a daily sunscreen. Look for daily moisturizers that contain broad-spectrum sunscreens, which means that they protect against both UVA and UVB sunrays. An SPF-15 or higher is considered to be adequate strength.

Sunscreens are made in lotion, fluid, and cream forms, and are easily adaptable to combination, oilier, or dry skin types.

Night treatment products are usually more intensive products designed for use at night to treat specific skin problems. These products are generally heavier than day-use products, and theoretically contain higher levels of conditioning ingredients.

Serums and **ampoules** (am-pyools) are concentrated products that generally contain higher amounts of ingredients that have an effect on skin appearance (Figure 22-8). They are typically used at home, and are applied under a moisturizer or sunscreen.

Massage creams are lubricants to make the skin slippery during massage. They often contain oils or petrolatum. If a massage cream is used during a facial treatment, it must be thoroughly removed before any other product can penetrate the skin.

There is a trend towards using treatment products that penetrate during massage. One of the biggest benefits of massage is that it increases absorption of the skin.

Did You Know

A valuable ingredient in moisturizers is sunscreen; its presence is particularly important in day creams. Not only does sunscreen guard against premature aging of the skin, but when used consistently, it is one of the best ways to help prevent skin cancer.

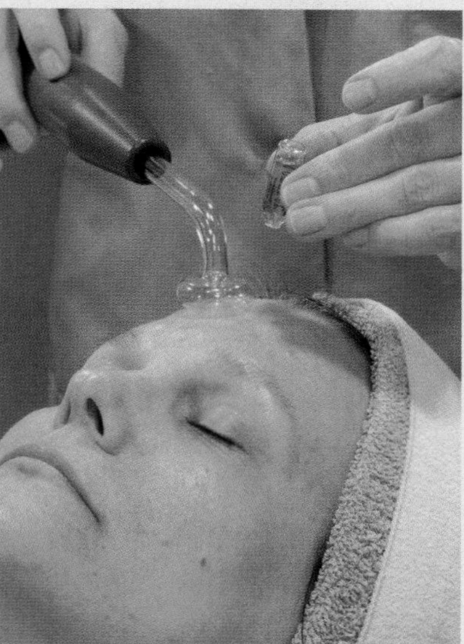

Figure 22-8 Skin treatment in an ampoule.

MASKS

Masks are products that are applied to the skin for a short time, but have more immediate effects. **Clay-based masks** are often used for oily and combination skin. They are generally oil-absorbing cleansing masks, and have an exfoliating effect and an astringent effect, making large pores temporarily appear smaller. They may have additional beneficial ingredients for soothing, or antibacterial ingredients like *sulfur,* which is helpful for acne-prone skin.

Cream masks do not dry on the skin like clay masks, and are often used for dry skin. They often contain oils and emollients as well as humectants, and have a strong moisturizing effect.

Gel masks can be used for sensitive or dehydrated skin, and do not dry hard. They often contain hydrators and soothing ingredients, and thus help plump surface cells with moisture, making the skin look more supple and more hydrated.

Alginate masks (al-gin-ate) are often seaweed based. They come in a powder form, and are mixed with water or sometimes serums. After mixing, they are quickly applied to the face, and dry to form a rubberized texture. A **treatment cream** or serum is generally applied under them. The alginate mask forms a seal that encourages the skin's absorption of the serum or treatment cream underneath. They are generally used only in the salon.

Paraffin wax masks are specially prepared facial masks containing paraffin and other beneficial ingredients. They are melted at a little more than body temperature before application. The paraffin quickly cools to a lukewarm temperature and hardens to a candle-like consistency. Paraffin masks are used with a treatment cream because the paraffin, which has no treatment properties of its own, allows for deeper penetration of the cream's ingredients into the surface layers of the skin. Eye pads and gauze are also used in a paraffin mask application, as facial hair could stick to the wax if not covered, making it difficult and painful to remove.

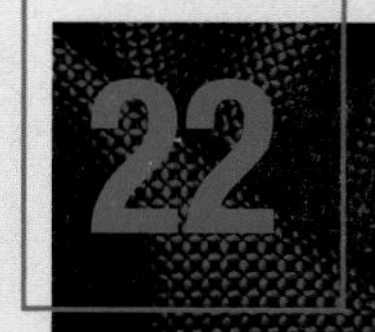

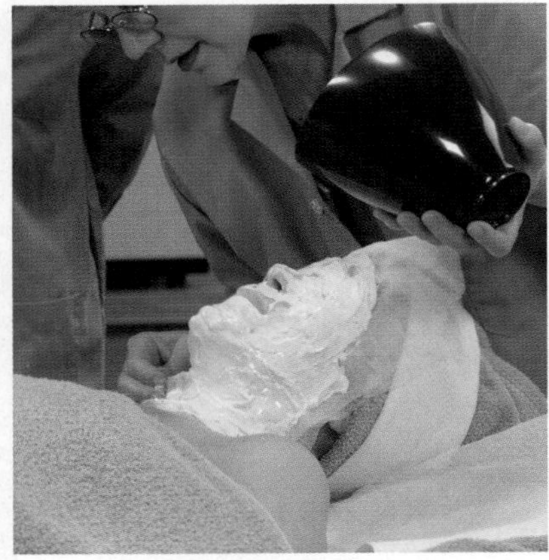

Figure 22-9 Modelage mask.

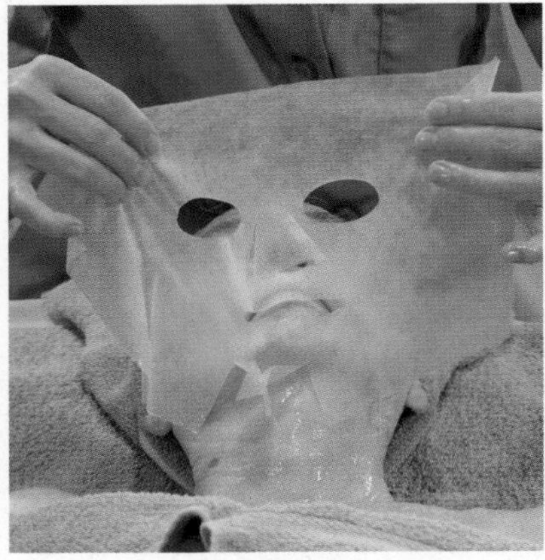

Figure 22-10 Placing gauze on the client's face.

Modelage masks (MAHD-lahzh) contain special crystals of gypsum, a plaster-like ingredient (Figure 22-9). As with paraffin masks, modelage masks are used with a treatment cream. When mixed with cold water immediately before application, and applied about ¼-inch (0.6 centimeter) thick, the modelage mask hardens. The chemical reaction that occurs when the plaster and the crystals mix with water produces a gradual increase in temperature that reaches approximately 105° F. As the mask is left on the skin, the temperature gradually cools, until it has cooled down completely. The setting time for modelage masks is approximately 20 minutes.

The heat increases blood circulation, and is very beneficial for dry, mature skin, or skin that looks dull and lifeless. This type of mask is not recommended for use on sensitive skin, skin with capillary problems, oily skin, or skin with blemishes. Modelage masks can become quite heavy on the face and should not be applied to the lower neck, or to clients who suffer from claustrophobia, a fear of being closed in or confined.

THE USE OF GAUZE FOR MASK APPLICATION

Gauze is a thin, open-meshed fabric of loosely woven cotton. Masks that have a tendency to run can be applied over a layer of gauze. The gauze holds the mask on the face, while allowing the ingredients to seep through to benefit the skin. Cheesecloth is sometimes used as well. In some cases, it is necessary to apply a second layer of gauze over the mask to keep the ingredients from sliding off. Gauze is also used to keep paraffin and gypsum/plaster masks from sticking to the skin, and the tiny hairs on the skin.

To prepare gauze, cut a piece large enough to cover the entire face and neck. Cut out spaces for the eyes, nose, and mouth. Although the client is able to breathe through the gauze, the cut-out spaces will make it more comfortable (Figure 22-10 and 22-11).

CLIENT CONSULTATION

The salon should designate a quiet area for facial treatments. Not only does the relaxing nature of a facial call for a quiet spot, but the area also needs to be quiet enough that you can conduct a thorough consultation with your client. All facial treatments should begin with a consultation.

RECORD-KEEPING

During the consultation, keep client record cards at hand so that you can write down all necessary information (Figure 22-12). The record card should contain the following information:

- Client's name, home address, and home telephone number
- Client's occupation and date of birth (this is useful so that you can determine if any signs of aging are premature)

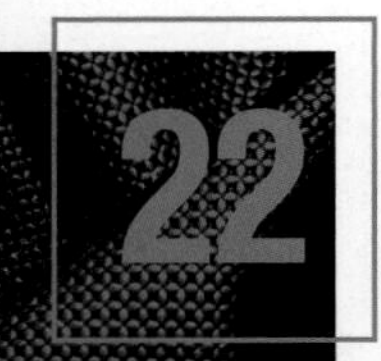

- Client's medical history, and whether the client is presently taking or using any kind of medication. It should also be noted whether the client is under the care of a physician or dermatologist.
- Contraindications—a pacemaker, metal implants, pregnancy, diabetes, epilepsy, allergies, high blood pressure—that call for alternative methods of treatment
- Information as to whether the client has had facials before, and what kind of treatments were performed
- Information on any skincare products the client is currently using
- Notation of how the client was referred to the salon
- Observations on the client's skin type, skin condition, and any abnormalities of the skin

Use the back of the consultation card to record the date and type of service and/or treatment being performed, the products that are being used, and products purchased by the client for home care. Often, a client will want to purchase a product that she has used before, but has lost or discarded the container and cannot remember the product name (Figure 22-13).

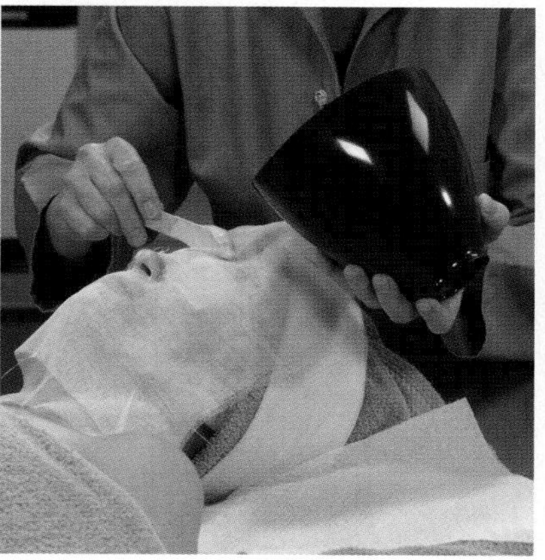

Figure 22-11 Applying a mask over the gauze.

CONSULTATION CARD				
Name			Date of Consultation	
Address			D.O.B.	
City	State	Zip	Occupation	
Tel. (Home)	(Business)		Ref. by	
			Contraindications	
Medical History				
Current Medication				
Previous treatments				
Home Care Products used				
SKIN TYPE	Oily	Normal	Dry (alipidic)	Combination
SKIN CONDITION	Clogged pores	Sensitive	Dehydrated	Mature
Skin Abnormalities				
Remarks				

Figure 22-12 Client consultation card (front).

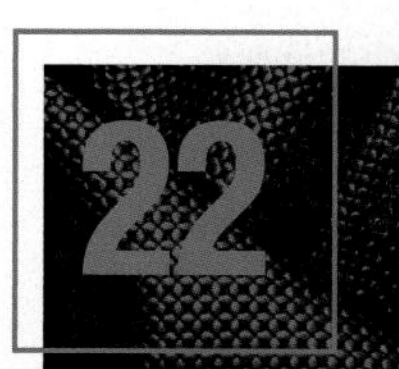

FACIAL RECORD			
Date	Type of treatment	By	Products purchased
2/14	Cleansing, Peel- Relaxing Massage	Mary	Moisturizer with sunscreen
3/16	Cleansing, Peel Modelage Mask	Mary	Cleanser, Toner
4/5	Cleansing, Peel High Frequency indirect	Mary	Moisturizer, Foundation #7
4/26	Cleansing, Peel Massage Alginate Mask	John	
5/13	Cleansing, Peel Iontophoresis Paraffin Mask Skin is showing marked improvement.	Mary	Night cream for dry skin Lipstick #43
6/1	Cleansing, Peel Relaxing Massage	Mary	Eye contour mask

Figure 22-13 Client consultation card (back).

As part of the consultation, do not hesitate to recommend services and products that will be beneficial to the client (Figure 22-14). Since the client has taken the initiative to come into the salon, she will feel disappointed if you neglect to discuss treatments and products, as well as proper home care for the skin. Also, if you do not recommend professional products, your client may go elsewhere for advice, such as a department store or drugstore. She might not get the kind of product you would have advised, and you and the salon will not get the retail income.

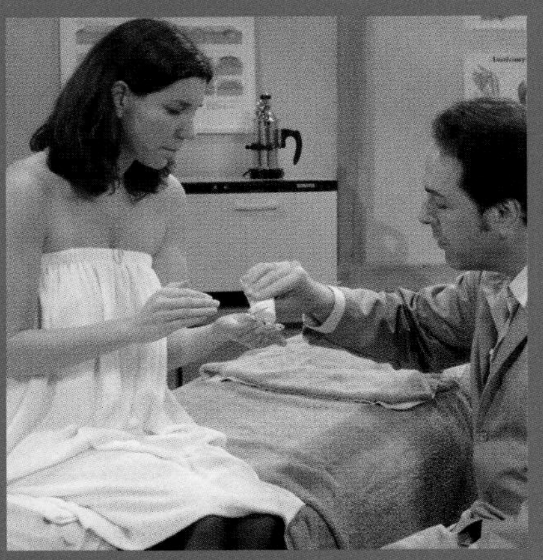

Figure 22-14 Recommend skin care products to the client.

Make it clear to your client that if she wishes to achieve the best results from a treatment, she must follow a proven routine of skin care at home with products that reinforce the salon treatments. Be careful, however, not to make the client feel that the sole purpose of the consultation is to sell products. Review appropriate and discreet retailing techniques with your instructor to make sure you achieve the right tone with your client.

CLASSIFICATION OF SKIN TYPES

During the first consultation, and before every subsequent facial treatment, it is important to perform a thorough analysis of the client's skin prior to cleansing. If the skin is oily, it will often look shiny or greasy. If the skin is dry, it may look flaky. Table 22-1 lists brief descriptions of basic skin types.

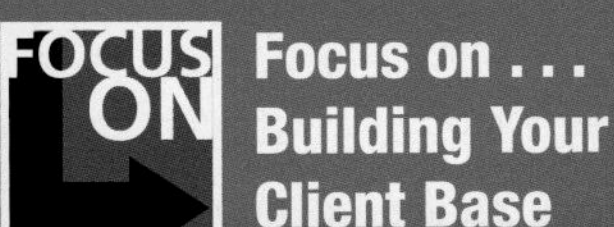

Focus on . . . Building Your Client Base

Send your client a birthday card. This form of advertisement is not expensive, and is always greatly appreciated. Ask for your clients' e-mail addresses for this purpose, and for other kinds of communications. E-mail is now the preferred mode of communication for many people, who may also like to book their appointments this way.

FACIAL MASSAGE

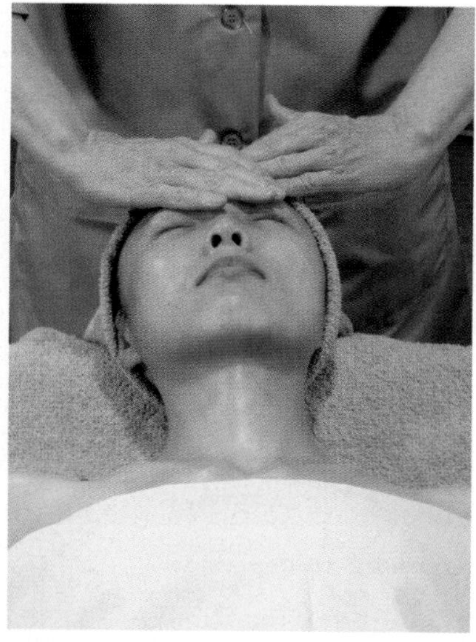

Figure 22-15 Palmar stroking of the face.

Massage is the manual or mechanical manipulation of the body by rubbing, gently pinching, kneading, tapping, and other movements to increase metabolism and circulation, promote absorption, and relieve pain. Cosmetologists massage their clients to help keep the facial skin healthy and their muscles firm.

To master massage techniques, you must have a basic knowledge of anatomy and physiology, as well as considerable practice in performing the various movements. It is important that you use a firm, sure touch when giving a massage. To do this, you must develop flexible hands, a quiet temperament, and self-control.

Keep your hands soft by using creams, oils, and lotions. File and shape your nails to avoid scratching your client's skin. Your wrists and fingers should be flexible, and your palms firm and warm. Cream or oil should be applied to your hands to permit smoother and gentler hand movements, and to prevent drag or damage to the client's skin.

BASIC MASSAGE MANIPULATIONS

All massage treatments combine one or more basic movements or manipulations. Each manipulation is applied to the superficial muscles in a certain way to achieve a certain end. The impact of a massage treatment depends on the amount of pressure, the direction of movement, and the duration of each type of manipulation involved.

The direction of movement is always from the insertion of the muscle toward its origin. The insertion is the portion of the muscle at the more movable attachment (where it is attached to another muscle, or to a movable bone or joint). The origin is the portion of the muscle at the fixed attachment (to an immovable section of the skeleton). Massaging a muscle in the wrong direction could result in a loss of resiliency and sagging of the skin and muscles.

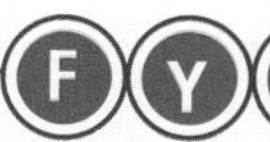

As a cosmetologist, your services are limited to certain areas of the body: scalp, face, neck, and shoulders; the upper chest and back; the hands and arms; and the feet and lower legs. Therapeutic massage, such as deep muscle and tissue massage and lymph drainage, should only be performed by therapists specialized in working on various kinds of tissues. Therapeutic massage requires special training and, in many cases, licensure.

EFFLEURAGE

Effleurage (EF-loo-rahzh) is a light, continuous stroking movement applied with the fingers (digital) or the palms (palmar) in a slow, rhythmic manner. No pressure is used. The palms work the large surfaces, while the cushions of the fingertips work the small surfaces, such as those around the eyes (Figure 22-15). Effleurage is frequently used on the forehead, face, scalp, back, shoulder, neck, chest, arms, and hands for its soothing and relaxing effects. Every massage should begin and end with effleurage.

When performing effleurage, hold your whole hand loosely, and keep your wrist and fingers flexible. Curve your fingers slightly to conform to the shape of the area being massaged, with just the cushions of the fingertips touching the skin. Do not use the ends of the fingertips. They are pointier than the cushions, and will cause the effleurage to be less

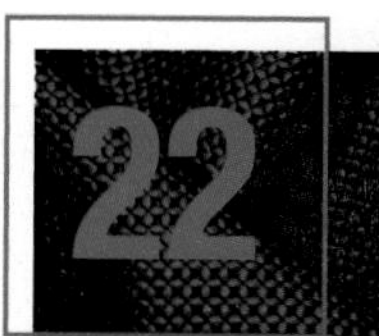

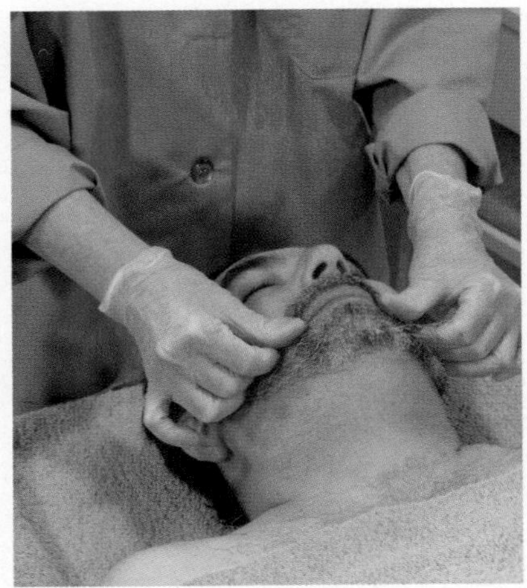
Figure 22-16 Petrissage.

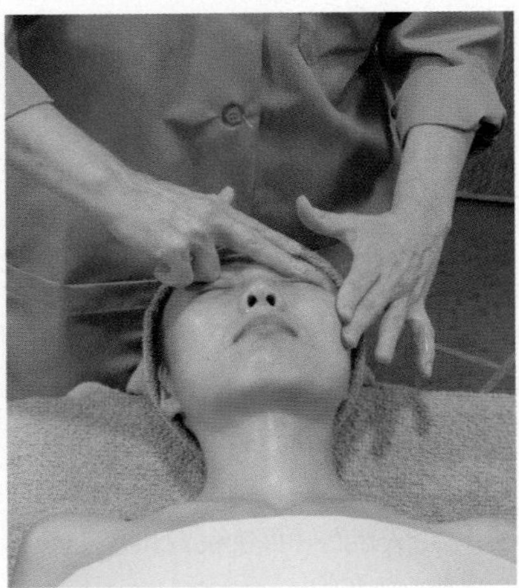
Figure 22-17 Friction.

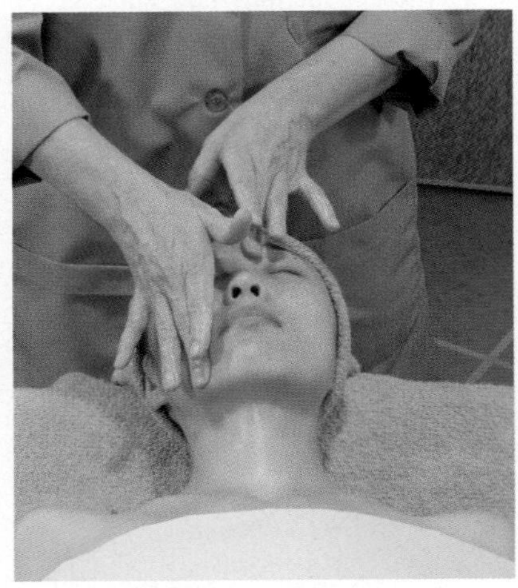
Figure 22-18 Tapotement.

smooth. Also, the free edges of your fingernails may scratch the client's skin.

PETRISSAGE

Petrissage (PEH-treh-sahzh) is a kneading movement performed by lifting, squeezing, and pressing the tissue with a light, firm pressure. Petrissage offers deeper stimulation to the muscles, nerves, and skin glands, and improves circulation. These kneading movements are usually limited to the back, shoulders, and arms.

Although typically used on larger surface areas such as the arms and shoulders, digital kneading can also be used on the cheeks with light pinching movements (Figure 22-16). The pressure should be light but firm. When grasping and releasing the fleshy parts, the movements must be rhythmic and never jerky.

Fulling is a form of petrissage in which the tissue is grasped, gently lifted, and spread out, used mainly for massaging the arms. With the fingers of both hands grasping the arm, apply a kneading movement across the flesh, with light pressure on the underside of the client's forearm and between the shoulder and elbow.

FRICTION

Friction (FRIK-shun) is a deep rubbing movement in which you apply pressure on the skin with your fingers or palm while moving it over an underlying structure. Friction has been known to have a significant benefit on the circulation and glandular activity of the skin. Circular friction movements are typically used on the scalp, arms, and hands. Light circular friction is used on the face and neck (Figure 22-17).

Chucking, rolling, and wringing are variations of friction, and are used mainly to massage the arms and legs, as follows:

- **Chucking.** Grasping the flesh firmly in one hand and moving the hand up and down along the bone while the other hand keeps the arm or leg in a steady position.
- **Rolling.** Pressing and twisting the tissues with a fast back-and-forth movement.
- **Wringing.** Vigorous movement in which the hands, placed a little distance apart on both sides of the client's arm or leg and working downward, apply a twisting motion against the bones in the opposite direction.

TAPOTEMENT

Tapotement (tah-POHT-mant) or **percussion** (per-KUSH-un) consists of short, quick tapping, slapping, and hacking movements. This form of massage is the most stimulating and should be applied with care and discretion. Tapotement movements tone the muscles and impart a healthy glow to the area being massaged.

In facial massage, use only light digital tapping. Bring the fingertips down against the skin in rapid succession. Your fingers must be flexible enough to create an even force over the area being massaged (Figure 22-18).

In slapping movements, keeping your wrists flexible allows your palms to come in contact with the skin in light, firm, and rapid slapping movements. One hand follows the other. With each slapping stroke, lift the flesh slightly.

Hacking is a chopping movement performed with the edges of the hands. Both the wrists and hands move alternately in fast, light, firm, and flexible motions against the skin. Hacking and slapping movements are used only to massage the back, shoulders, and arms.

VIBRATION

Vibration (vy-BRAY-shun) is a rapid shaking of the body part while the balls of the fingertips are pressed firmly on the point of application. The movement is accomplished by rapid muscular contractions in your arms. It is a highly relaxing movement, and should be applied at the end of the massage (Figure 22-19). Deep vibration in combination with other classical massage movements can also be produced by the use of a mechanical vibrator to stimulate blood circulation and increase muscle tone in muscles of the body.

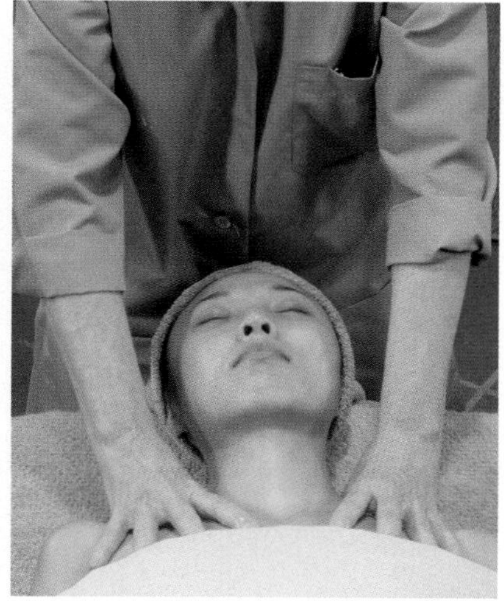

Figure 22-19 Vibration on the shoulders.

PHYSIOLOGICAL EFFECTS OF MASSAGE

To obtain proper results from a scalp or facial massage, you must have a thorough knowledge of the structures involved, including muscles, nerves, connective tissues, and blood vessels. Every muscle has a **motor point,** which is a point on the skin over the muscle where pressure or stimulation will cause contraction of that muscle. Some examples are illustrated in Figures 22-20 and 22-21. In order to obtain the maximum benefits from a facial massage, you must consider the motor points that affect the underlying muscles of the face and neck. The location of motor points varies among individuals due to differences in body structure. However, a few manipulations on the proper motor points will relax the client early in the massage treatment.

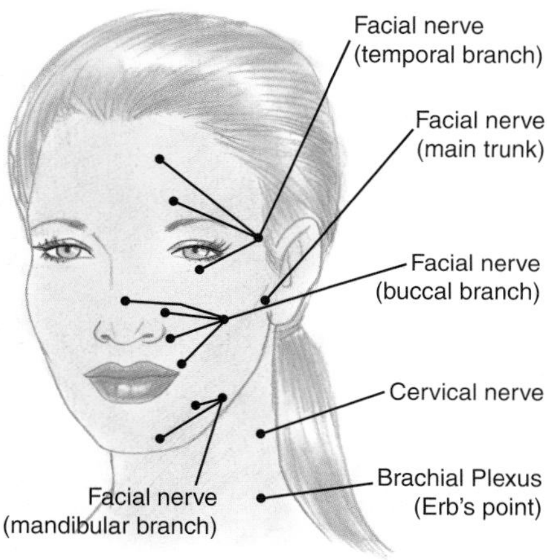

Figure 22-20 Motor nerve points of the face.

Relaxation is achieved through light but firm, slow, rhythmic movements, or very slow, light hand vibrations over the motor points for a short time. Another technique is to pause briefly over the motor points, using light pressure.

Skillfully applied massage directly or indirectly influences the structures and functions of the body. The immediate effects of massage are first noticed on the skin. The area being massaged shows increased circulation, secretion, nutrition, and excretion. The following benefits may be obtained by proper facial and scalp massage:

- Skin and all structures are nourished
- Skin becomes softer and more pliable
- Circulation of blood is increased
- Activity of skin glands is stimulated
- Muscle fibers are stimulated and strengthened
- Nerves are soothed and rested
- Pain is sometimes relieved

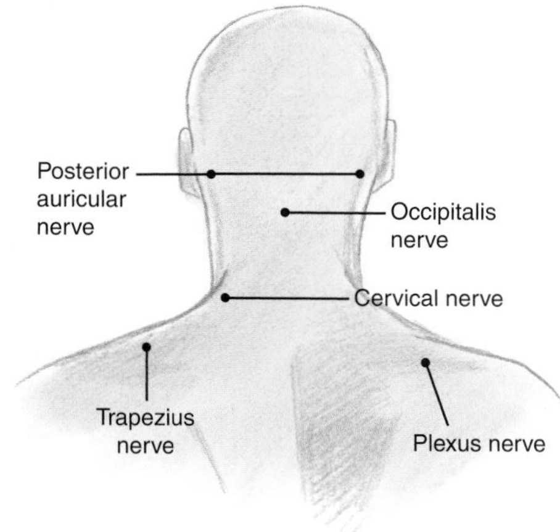

Figure 22-21 Motor nerve points of the neck.

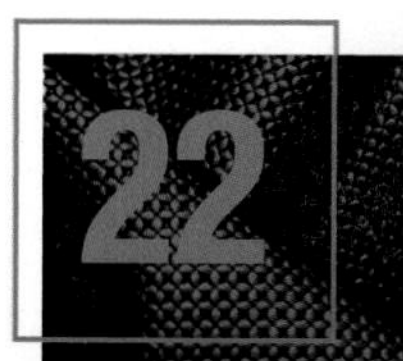

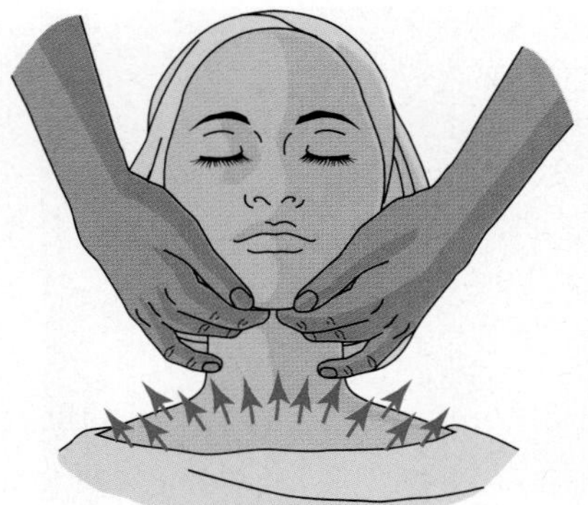
Figure 22-22 Chin movement.

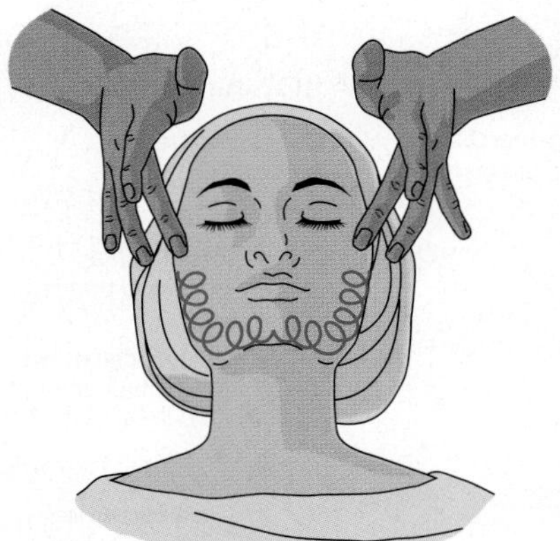
Figure 22-23 Circular movement of lower cheeks.

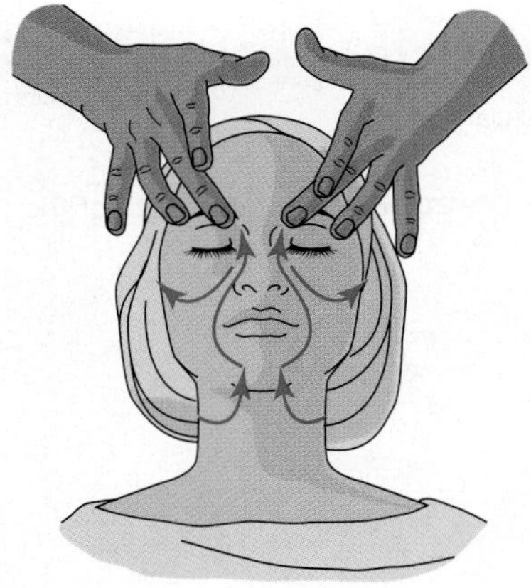
Figure 22-24 Mouth, nose, and cheek movements.

The frequency of facial or scalp massage depends on the condition of the skin or scalp, the age of the client, and the condition being treated. As a general rule, normal skin or scalp can be kept in excellent condition with the help of a weekly massage, accompanied by proper home care.

FACIAL MANIPULATIONS

Now that we have had an overview of basic massage/manipulation techniques and guidelines, the best manipulations to use on the face are discussed here. When performing facial manipulations, keep in mind that an even tempo, or rhythm, brings on relaxation. Do not remove your hands from the client's face once you have started the manipulations.

Should it become necessary to remove your hands, feather them off, then gently replace them with feather-like movements. Remember that massage movements are generally directed from the insertion toward the origin of a muscle, in order to avoid damage to muscle tissues.

The following illustrations show the different movements that may be used on the various parts of the face, chest, and back. Each instructor may have developed her own routine, however. For example, some instructors and practitioners prefer to start massage manipulations at the chin, while others prefer to start at the forehead. Both are correct. Be guided by your instructor.

- *Chin movement.* Lift the chin, using a slight pressure (Figure 22-22).
- *Lower cheeks.* Using a circular movement, rotate from chin to ears (Figure 22-23).
- *Mouth, nose, and cheek movements.* Follow the diagram (Figure 22-24).
- *Linear movement over the forehead.* Slide fingers to the temples and then stroke up to hairline, gradually moving your hands across the forehead to the right eyebrow (Figure 22-25).

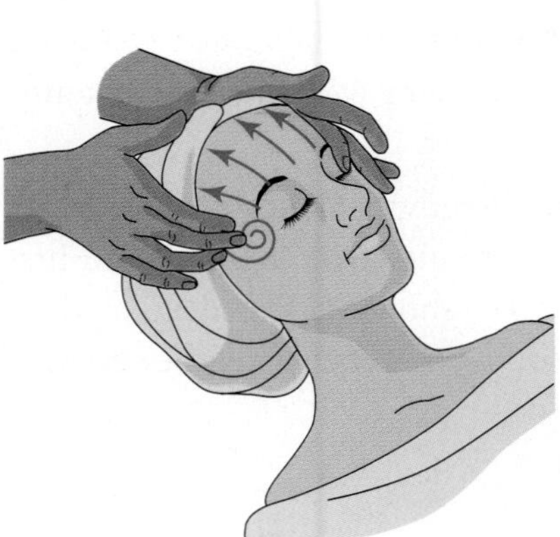
Figure 22-25 Linear movement over forehead.

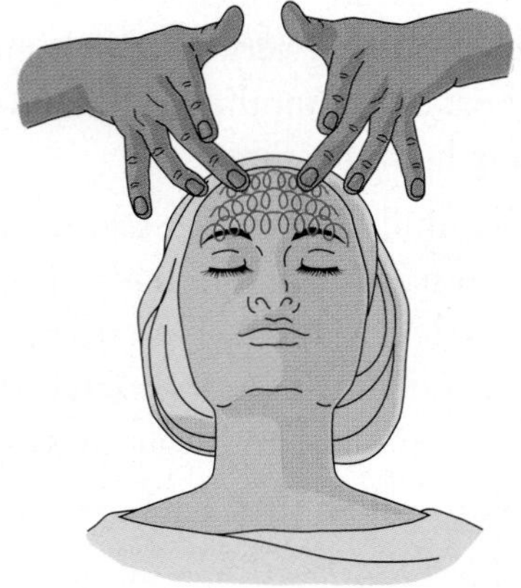
Figure 22-26 Circular movement over forehead.

- *Circular movement over the forehead.* Starting at the eyebrow line, work across the middle of the forehead and then toward the hairline (Figure 22-26).
- *Crisscross movement.* Start at one side of forehead and work back (Figure 22-27).
- *Stroking (headache) movement.* Slide your fingers toward the center of the forehead and then draw your fingers, with slight pressure, toward the temples and rotate (Figure 22-28).
- *Brow and eye movement.* Place your middle fingers at the inner corners of the eyes and your index fingers over the brows. Slide them toward the outer corners of the eyes, under the eyes, and then back to the inner corners (Figure 22-29).
- *Nose and upper cheek movement.* Slide your fingers down the nose. Apply a rotary movement across the cheeks to the temples and rotate gently. Slide your fingers under the eyes and then back to the bridge of the nose (Figure 22-30).
- *Mouth and nose movement.* Apply a circular movement from the corners of the mouth up to the sides of the nose. Slide your fingers over the

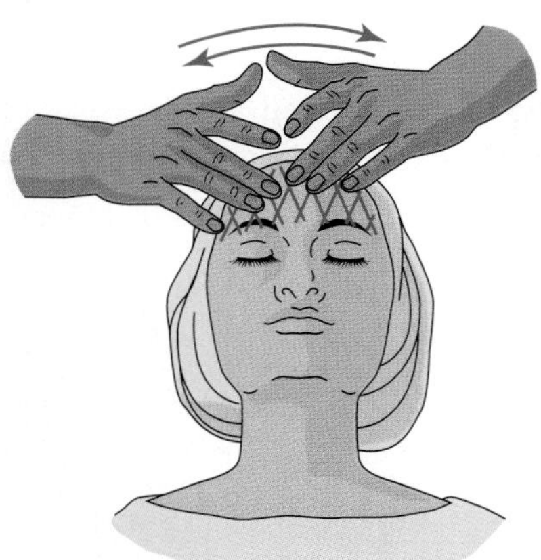

Figure 22-27 Crisscross movement.

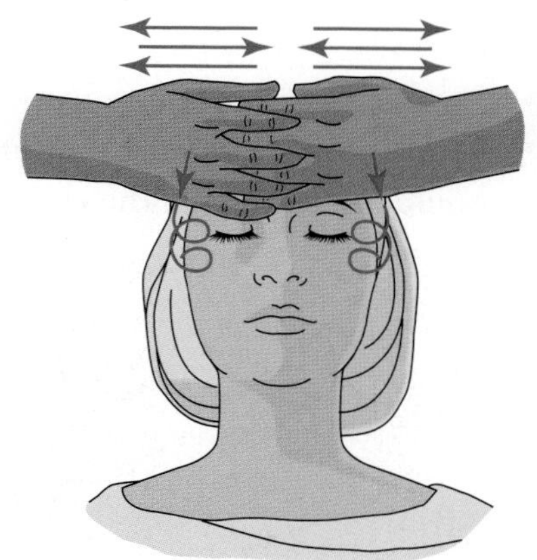

Figure 22-28 Stroking (headache) movement.

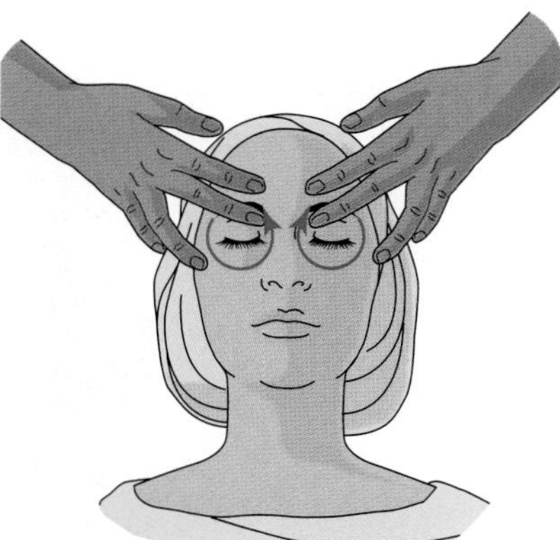

Figure 22-29 Brow and eye movement.

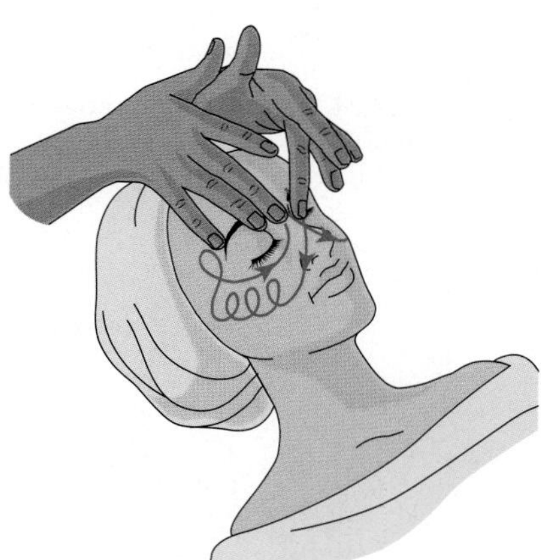

Figure 22-30 Nose and upper cheek movement.

CAUTION

Do not massage a client who has high blood pressure, a heart condition, or has had a stroke. Massage increases circulation and may be harmful to such a client. Have the client consult a physician first. If a client has arthritis, be very careful to avoid vigorous massage of the joints. Communicate with your client throughout the massage and adjust your touch according to the needs that she expresses.

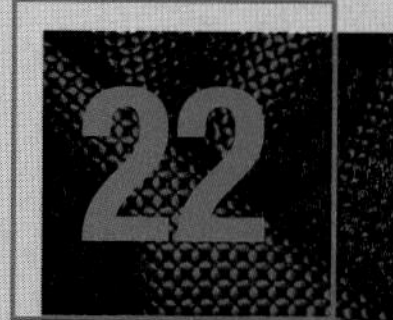

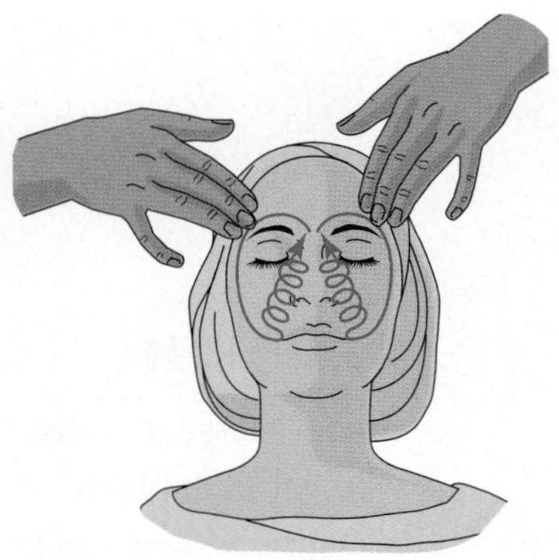
Figure 22-31 Mouth and nose movement.

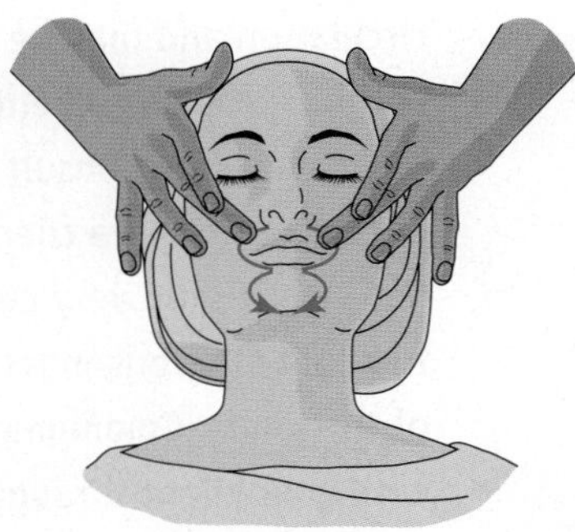
Figure 22-32 Lip and chin movement.

brows and then down to the corners of the mouth up to the sides of nose. Follow by sliding your fingers over the brows and down to the corners of the mouth again (Figure 22-31).

- *Lip and chin movement.* From the center of the upper lip, draw your fingers around the mouth, going under the lower lip and chin (Figure 22-32).
- *Optional movement.* Hold the head with your left hand, and draw the fingers of your right hand from under the lower lip and around mouth, moving to the center of the upper lip (Figure 22-33).
- *Lifting movement of the cheeks.* Proceed from the mouth to the ears, and then from the nose to the top part of the ears (Figure 22-34).
- *Rotary movement of the cheeks.* Massage from the chin to the ear lobes, from the mouth to the middle of the ears, and from the nose to the top of the ears (Figure 22-35).
- *Light tapping movement.* Work from the chin to the earlobe, from the mouth to the ear, from the nose to the top of the ear, and then across the forehead. Repeat on the other side (Figure 22-36).
- *Stroking movement of the neck.* Apply light upward strokes over the front of the neck. Use heavier pressure on the sides of neck in downward strokes (Figure 22-37).
- *Circular movement over the neck and chest.* Starting at the back of the ears, apply a circular movement down the side of the neck, over the shoulders, and across the chest (Figure 22-38).

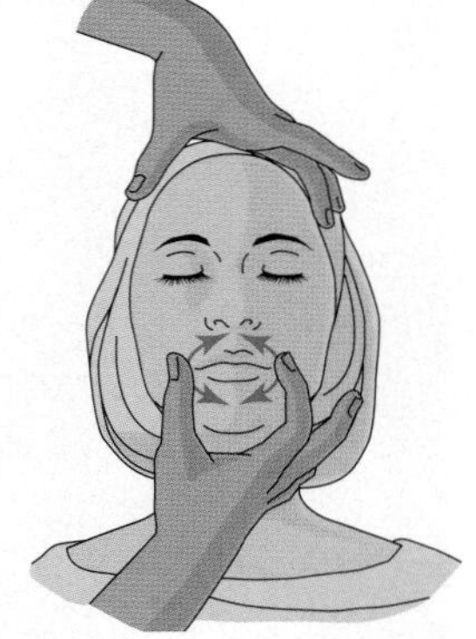
Figure 22-33 Optional movement.

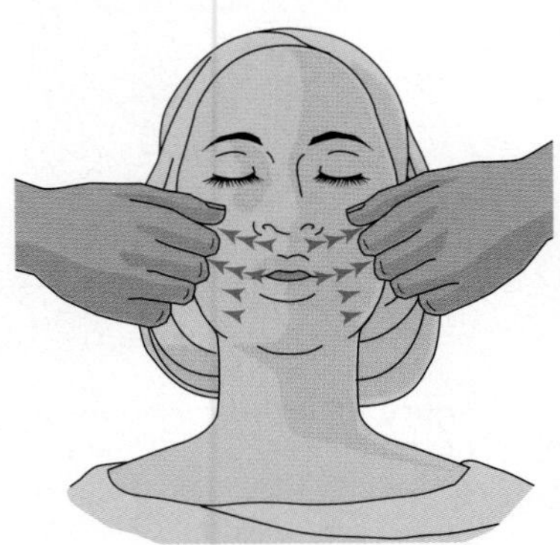
Figure 22-34 Lifting movement of cheeks.

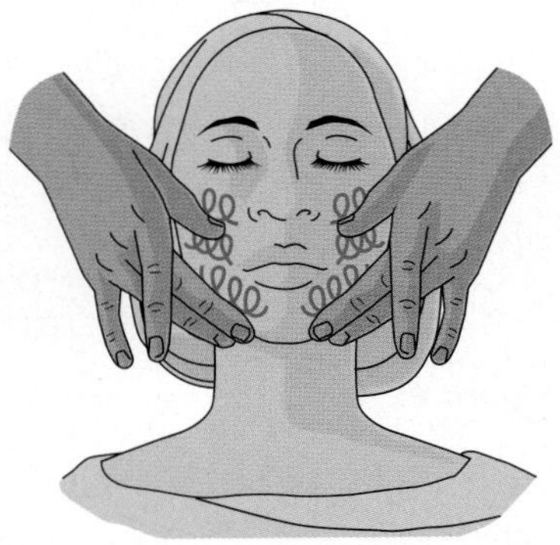
Figure 22-35 Rotary movement of cheeks.

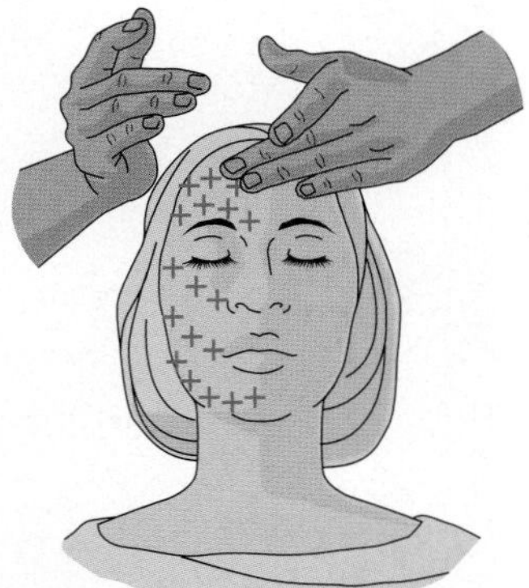
Figure 22-36 Light tapping movement.

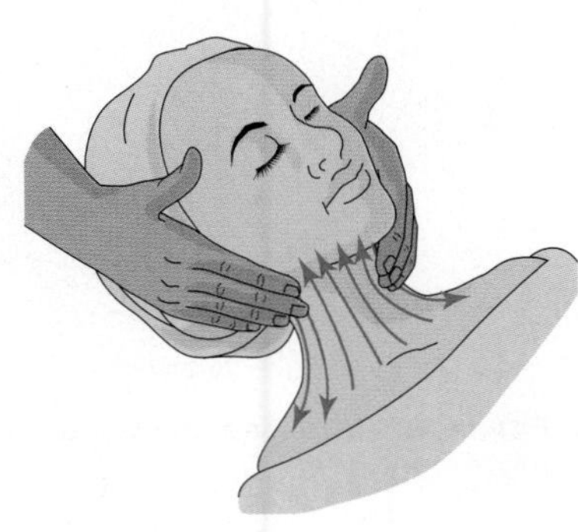
Figure 22-37 Stroking movement of neck.

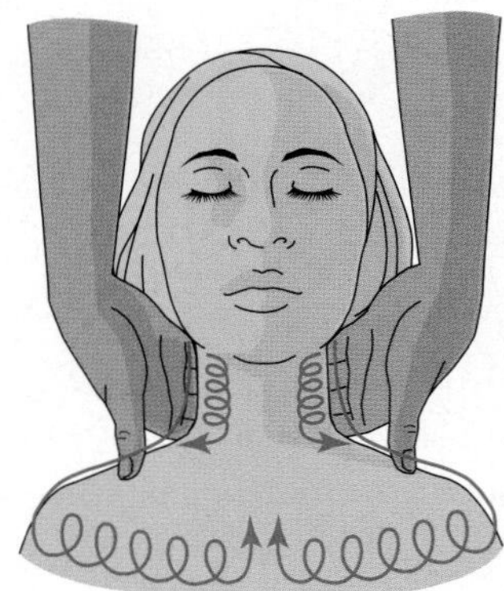
Figure 22-38 Circular movement over neck and chest.

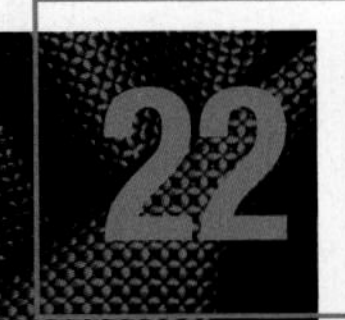

Male skin is not all that different from female skin. However, it needs more attention in the areas of the face where there is hair growth. For your male clients, use downward movements in the area of beard growth. Massaging against hair growth causes great discomfort. Pressure point massage in the beard area is much appreciated by male clients.

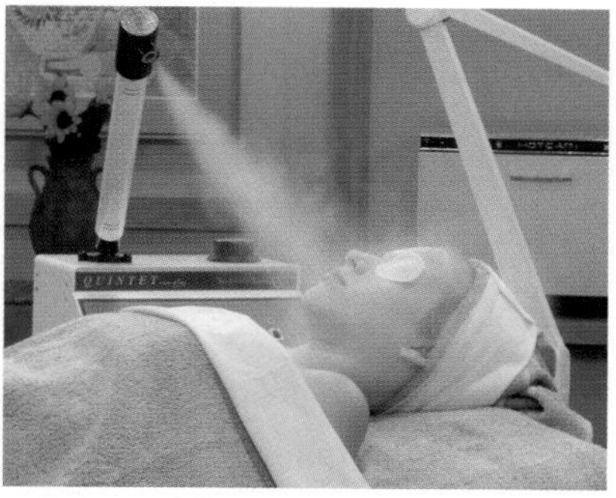

Figure 22-39 Facial steamer being used during a facial treatment.

CHEST, BACK, AND NECK MANIPULATIONS (OPTIONAL)

Some instructors prefer to treat these areas first before starting the regular facial. Apply cleanser, and remove with a tissue or a warm moist towel. Then apply massage cream and perform the following manipulations:

- *Chest and back movement.* Use a rotary movement across the chest and shoulders, and then down to the spine. Slide your fingers to the base of the neck. Rotate three times.
- *Shoulders and back movement.* Rotate the shoulders three times. Glide your fingers to the spine and then to the base of the neck. Apply circular movement up to the back of the ear, and then slide your fingers to the front of the earlobe. Rotate three times.
- *Back massage.* To stimulate and relax the client, use your thumbs and bent index fingers to grasp the tissue at the back of the neck. Rotate six times. Repeat over the shoulders and back to the spine. Remove cream with tissues or a warm, moist towel. Dust the back lightly with talcum powder and smooth.

CAUTION

This section is intended as an overview. You should receive hands-on experience from your instructor before using any facial equipment! Machine models differ, and thus precautions vary as well. Consult with your instructor and the specific machine manual for safe operation. In some states, use of certain equipment may not be permissible for cosmetologists. Again, check with your instructor to find out what is allowed in your state.

FACIAL EQUIPMENT

There are many types of facial equipment that can enhance your abilities to perform an outstanding facial treatment. These machines help to increase the efficacy of your products, increase product penetration, and provide for a more complete and relaxing treatment.

A facial **steamer** heats and produces a stream of warm steam that can be focused on the client's face or other areas of skin. Steaming the skin helps to soften the tissues, making it more accepting of moisturizers and other treatment products. Steam also helps to relax and soften follicle accumulations such as comedones and clogged follicles, making them easier to extract (Figure 22-39).

Most steamers work by having a heating coil that boils water. The steam from the boiling water flows through a pipe that can be focused on the area to be treated, normally the face. Steam is usually administered at the beginning of the facial treatment.

Most clients enjoy steam, but precautions should be taken with clients who have asthma or other breathing disorders.

It is strongly recommended that a professional steamer be used, but if one is not available, a warm steamed towel may be gently wrapped around the face, leaving the nose exposed so the client can breathe comfortably. The towel should be comfortably warm, but not hot. Do not use steamed towels on clients with sensitive skin, redness-prone skin, rosacea, or on clients who are claustrophobic.

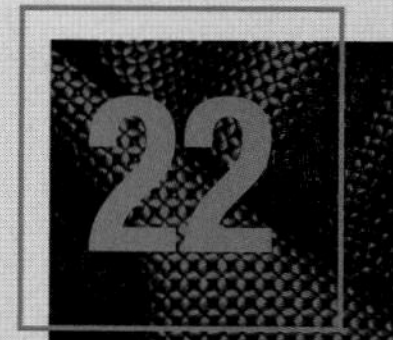

CAUTION

Do not use the galvanic current on the following clients:

- **With metal implants, a pacemaker, or any heart insufficiency**
- **With epilepsy**
- **Who are pregnant**
- **With high blood pressure, fever, or any infection**
- **With insufficient nerve sensibility**
- **With open or broken skin (wounds, new scars) or a pustular acne condition**
- **Who are afraid of electrical current**

A **brushing machine** is a rotating electric appliance with interchangeable brushes that can be attached to the rotating head. Brushes of various sizes as well as textures are common. Larger and stiffer brushes are used for back treatment, and smaller and softer brushes are used for the face.

Brushing is a form of exfoliation, and is usually administered after or during steam. A fairly thick layer of cleanser or moisturizer should be applied to the face before using the brushing machine. This applied product provides a buffer for the brushes so that they do not scratch the face, as they might if the face was completely dry.

Brushing helps remove dead cells from the skin surface, making the skin look smoother and more even in coloration, and helps to stimulate blood circulation.

Brushing should never be used on clients using keratolytic drugs such as Retin-A®, Differin®, Tazorac®, or other drugs that thin or exfoliate the skin. Clients who have rosacea, sensitive skin, pustular acne, or other forms of skin inflammation or reddening should not have brushing administered. Never use a brushing machine at the same time as another exfoliation technique, such as an alpha hydroxy acid treatment or microdermabrasion.

Brushes must be thoroughly cleansed and disinfected between clients.

The skin suction and cold spray machine is used to increase circulation, and to jet-spray lotions and toners onto the skin. Skin suction should only be used on nonsensitive, and noninflamed skin.

Spray can be used on almost any skin type. Spray is often used to hydrate the skin and to help clean off mask treatments.

ELECTROTHERAPY AND LIGHT THERAPY

Galvanic and *high-frequency* treatment are types of **electrotherapy,** that is, the use of electrical currents to treat the skin.

There are several contraindications for electrotherapy. Electrotherapy should never be administered on heart patients, clients with pacemakers, metal implants, pregnant clients, clients with epilepsy or seizure disorders, clients who are afraid of electric current, or those with open or broken skin. Further, if you ever have any doubts if the client can have electrotherapy safely, request that the client get a note from her physician approving her for electrotherapy.

An **electrode** is an applicator for directing the electric current from the machine to the client's skin (Figure 22-40). High-frequency machines have only one electrode. Galvanic machines have two positive electrodes called an **anode,** which has a red plug and cord, and a negative electrode called a **cathode,** which has a black plug and cord (Figure 22-41).

Galvanic current accomplishes two basic tasks. *Desincrustation* is the process of softening and emulsifying hardened sebum stuck in the follicles. It is very helpful when treating oily areas with multiple comedones and most acne-prone skin. Desincrustation products are alkaline fluids or gels that act as solvents for the solidified sebum. This makes extraction of the impactions and comedones much easier. When the negative pole is applied to the face over a desincrustation product, the current forces the product deeper into the follicle. The current also produces a chemical reaction that helps to loosen the impacted sebum (Figure 22-42).

Both electrodes are wrapped in wet cotton. The *active electrode* is the electrode applied to the skin. The active electrode, in the case of desincrustation, the negative electrode, is applied to the oily areas of the face for 3 to 5 minutes. The positive electrode is held by the client in her right hand or attached to a pad that is placed in contact with the client's right shoulder (Figure 22-43). After the desincrustation process has taken place, sebum deposits can easily be extracted with gentle pressure.

Iontophoresis is the process of using galvanic current to penetrate water-soluble products that contain ions into the skin. Products suitable for iontophoresis will be labeled as such by manufacturers. When the negative current is applied to the face, products with negative ions are penetrated, and when the positive current is applied to the face, products with positive ions are penetrated. Many ampoules and serums are prepared for iontophoresis.

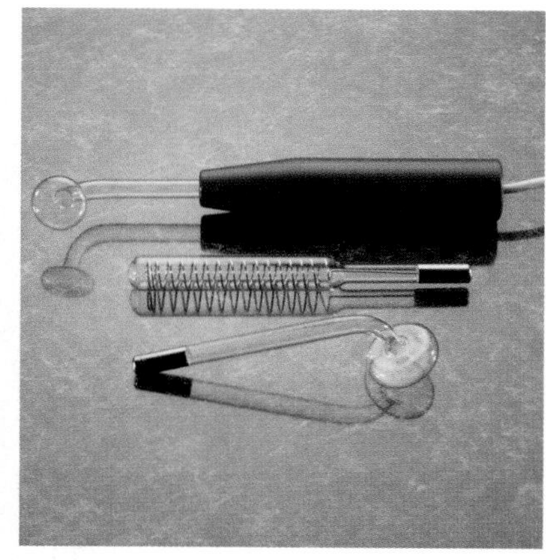

Figure 22-40 Various electrodes.

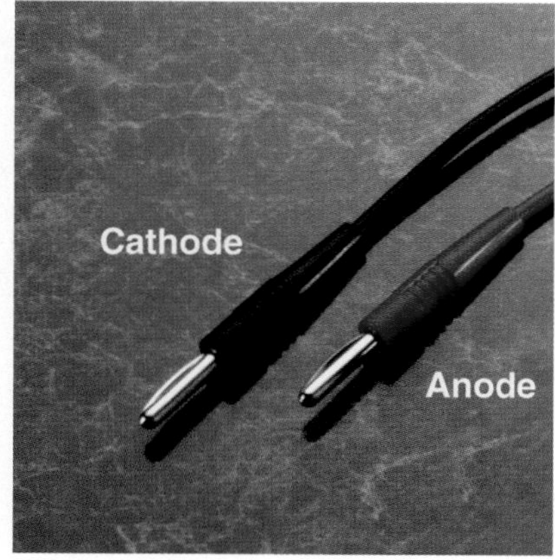

Figure 22-41 Cathodes.

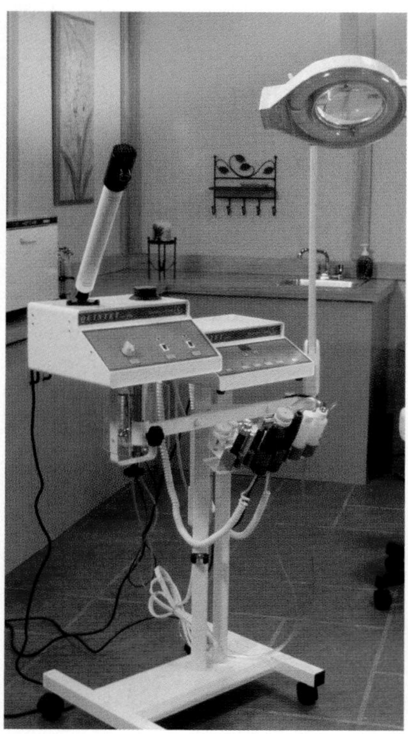

Figure 22-42 "Five-in-one" machine, including galvanic electrodes.

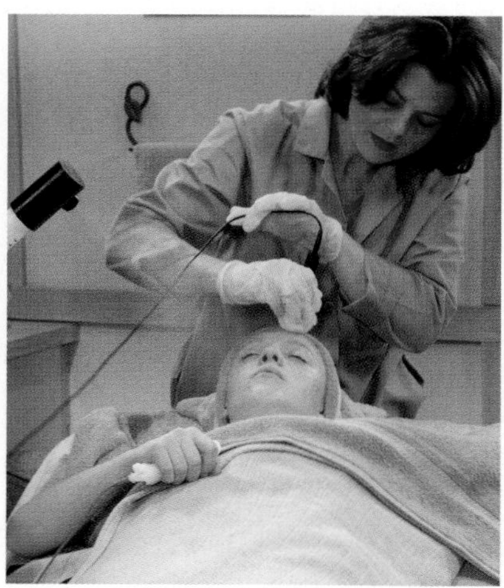

Figure 22-43 Client holding passive electrode.

CAUTION

Place the passive electrode on the right side of the client's body only (never on the left side) to avoid current flow through the heart.

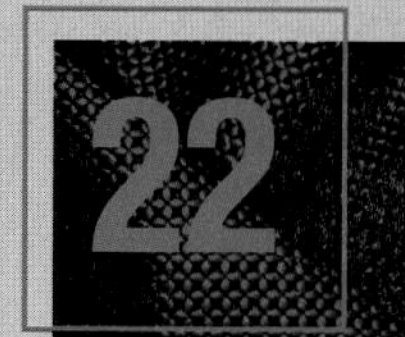

Again, you must receive thorough hands-on instruction from your teacher before attempting this procedure.

MICROCURRENT

Microcurrent is a type of galvanic treatment that is a computerized device that has many applications in skin care. Microcurrent is best known for helping to tone the skin, producing a "lifting" effect for aging skin with lack of elasticity.

HIGH-FREQUENCY CURRENT

High-frequency current, discovered by Nikolas Tesla, can be used to stimulate blood flow and help products penetrate. It works by warming tissues, which allows better absorption of moisturizers and other treatment products. High-frequency current can also be applied after extraction or during treatments for acne-prone skin because it has a germicidal effect.

Electrodes for the high-frequency machine are made of glass, and contain different types of gas, such as neon, which lights up as a color when current is flowing through the electrode. Unlike the galvanic machine, it is only necessary to use one electrode when performing high-frequency treatment. There are several different types of electrodes used with high frequency. The most common is shaped like a mushroom, and referred to as a mushroom electrode (Figure 22-44).

High frequency can be applied either directly to the skin known as *direct* application, or the electrode can be held by the client during treatment creating an electrical stimulating massage, known as *indirect massage* or *Viennese* massage (Figure 22-45).

High frequency is applied to the skin as part of the treatment phase of the facial treatment. Because machines vary, you should, again, check with your instructor and manufacturer's manual for instructions for the specific machine you are using.

CAUTION

For high-frequency current, either direct or indirect, the same contraindications apply as for galvanic current. In addition, to prevent burns, the client should avoid any contact with metal, such as chair arms, stools, jewelry, and metal bobby pins during the treatment.

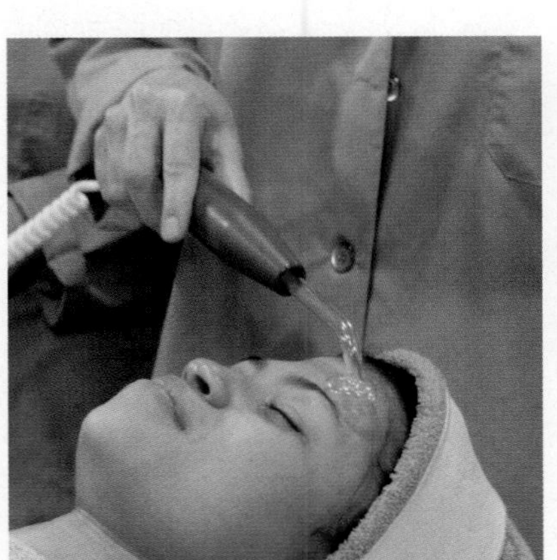

Figure 22-44 Direct application of high frequency.

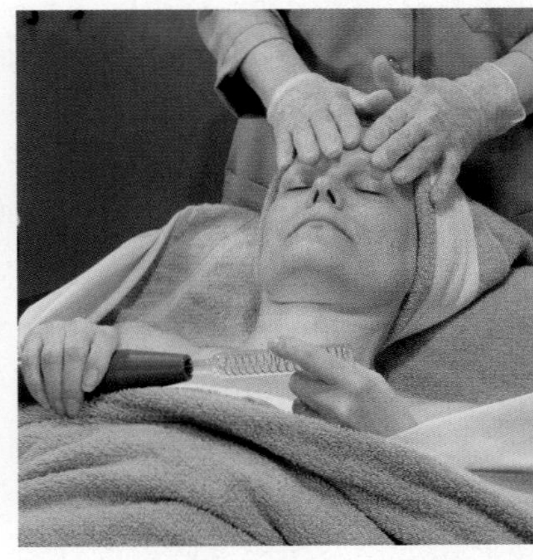

Figure 22-45 Client holding electrode as stylist massages the face.

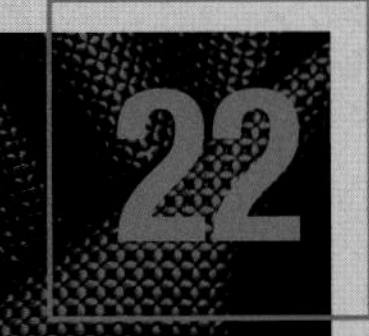

LIGHT THERAPY

Several types of light are used in **light therapy.** Traditionally, *infrared* lamps have been used to heat the skin and increase blood flow. Infrared lights have also been used for hair and scalp treatments.

The newest type of light therapy is called *light-emitting diode* or *LED* treatment (Figure 22-46). This treatment uses concentrated light that flashes very rapidly. LEDs were originally developed to help with wound healing. However, in cosmetology, LED machines are used cosmetically to minimize redness, warm lower-level tissues, stimulate blood flow, and improve skin smoothness, and are applied to improve acne-prone skin. The type and color of the light varies according to treatment objective. Red lights are used to treat aging and redness, and blue light is used for acne-prone skin.

LEDs are a very safe treatment for most clients, but should be avoided on clients who have seizure disorders. Clients who have questionable health conditions should receive written approval from their physician before having an LED treatment.

CAUTION

The client's eyes always should be protected during any light ray treatment. Use cotton pads saturated with alcohol-free freshener or distilled water. The eye pads protect the eyes from the glare of the reflecting rays.

MICRODERMABRASION

Microdermabrasion, a type of mechanical exfoliation, uses a closed vacuum to shoot crystals onto the skin, bumping off cell buildup that is then vacuumed up by suction. Microdermabrasion is a popular treatment because it produces fast visible results. It is used primarily to treat surface wrinkles and aging skin. Microdermabrasion requires extensive training to provide safe and effective treatment.

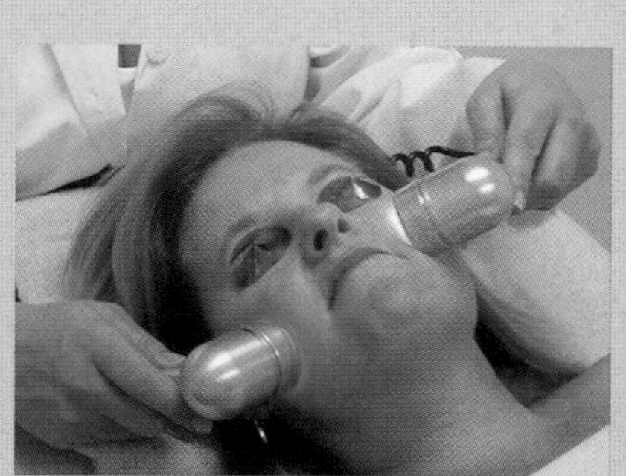

Figure 22-46 LED machine.

FACIAL TREATMENTS

A professional facial is one of the most enjoyable and relaxing services available to the salon client. Clients who have experienced this very restful, yet stimulating experience, do not hesitate to return for more. When received on a regular basis, facials result in a noticeable improvement in the client's skin tone, texture, and appearance.

Facial treatments fall into one of the following categories:

1. **Preservative.** Maintains the health of the facial skin by cleansing correctly, increasing circulation, relaxing the nerves, and activating the skin glands and metabolism through massage.
2. **Corrective.** Correct certain facial skin conditions, such as dryness, oiliness, comedones, aging lines, and minor conditions of acne.

As with other forms of massage, facial treatments help to increase circulation, activate glandular activity, relax the nerves, maintain muscle tone, and strengthen weak muscle tissues.

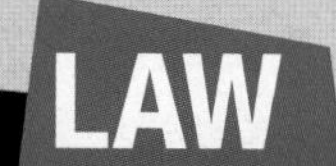

LAW

Please check with your state regulatory agency to determine if electrical machines are approved for use in your state.

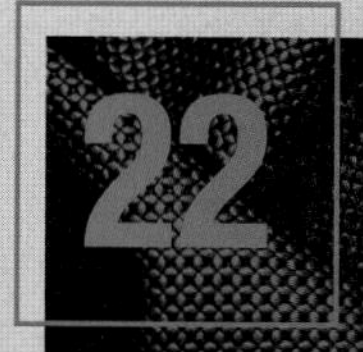

CAUTION

For sanitary reasons, never remove products from containers with your fingers. Always use a spatula.

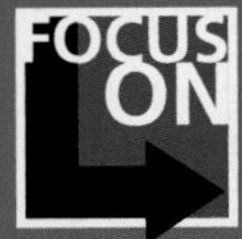

Focus on . . . Sharpening Your Personal Skills

If a client seems dissatisfied with a facial treatment, check to see if you have been guilty of any of the following:

- Offensive breath or body odor
- Rough, cold hands or ragged nails that may have scratched the client's skin
- Allowing cream or other substances to get into the client's eyes, mouth, nostrils, or hairline
- Towels that were too hot or too cold
- Talking too much
- Manipulating the skin roughly or in the wrong direction
- Being disorganized and interrupting the facial to get supplies

GUIDELINES FOR FACIAL TREATMENTS

Your facial treatments are bound to be successful and to inspire return visits if you follow the simple guidelines summarized below.

- Help the client to relax by speaking in a quiet and professional manner.
- Explain the benefits of the products and service, and answer any questions the client may have.
- Provide a quiet atmosphere, and work quietly and efficiently.
- Maintain neat, clean, sanitary conditions in the facial work area with an orderly arrangement of supplies.
- Follow systematic procedures.
- If your hands are cold, warm them before touching the client's face.
- Keep your nails smooth and short to prevent scratching the client's skin.

Another guideline you must always be sure to follow is to perform an analysis of your client's skin. After the client is draped and seated on the facial table (also called bed), you should inspect the skin to determine the following:

- Is the skin dry, normal, or oily?
- Are there fine lines or creases?
- Are comedones or acne present?
- Are dilated capillaries visible?
- Is skin texture smooth or rough?
- Is skin color even?

The results of your analysis will determine the products to use for the massage, what areas of the face need special attention, how much pressure to use when massaging, and what equipment should be used.

BASIC FACIAL APPLICATION

The steps for performing a basic facial are listed in Procedure 22-1. Some procedures may vary, however, so be guided by your instructor.

A note on the implements and materials you will need; the list found on page 590 includes items for a basic facial. You can add other items if you wish. There are several types of head coverings on the market. Some are a turban design; others are designed with elastic, like a shower cap. They are generally made of either cloth or paper towels. For the paper towel procedure, be guided by your instructor.

SPECIAL PROBLEMS

There are a number of special problems that must be considered when you are performing a facial. These include dry skin, oily skin and blackheads, and acne.

Dry skin is caused by an insufficient flow of sebum (oil) from the sebaceous glands. The facial for dry skin helps correct this condition. Although it can be given with or without an electrical current, the use of electrical current provides better results.

Oily skin is often characterized by comedones, which are caused by hardened masses of sebum formed in the ducts of the sebaceous glands. Oily skin can benefit from the facial procedure described below.

Acne is a disorder of the sebaceous glands that requires thorough and sometimes ongoing medical attention. If the client is under medical care, the role of the cosmetologist is to work closely with the client's physician, following the physician's instructions for the kind and frequency of facial treatments. Generally, medical direction limits the cosmetologist to the following measures in the treatment of acne:

- Cleansing the skin
- Reducing the oiliness of the skin by local applications
- Removing comedones, using proper procedures
- Using special medicated preparations

Because acne skin contains infectious matter, you must wear protective gloves and use disposable materials such as cotton cleansing pads.

SPECIAL NOTES FOR ACNE-PRONE SKIN

Minor problem and oily skin should respond well to facial treatments as described above. Unresponsive or severe cases of acne need medical treatment, and should be referred to a dermatologist.

Cosmetologists can work with a dermatologist to help the client with extraction treatments, proper choices of home care products and makeup, and helping the client understand how to coordinate medications with her home skin care program.

There are numerous topical prescription medications that can make the skin more sensitive and more reactive to skin care products. Always check with the client's dermatologist if you are performing treatments to clients under dermatological care.

CONSULTATION AND HOME CARE

Home care is probably the most important factor in a successful skin care program. The key word here is "program." Clients' participation is essential to achieve results. A program consists of a long-range plan involving home care, salon treatments, and client education.

Every new client should be thoroughly consulted about home care for his or her skin conditions. After the first treatment, block out about 30 minutes to explain proper home care for the client.

After the treatment is finished, sit the client up in the facial chair, or invite her or him to move to a well-lighted consultation area. A mirror should be provided for the client, so that he or she can see conditions you will be discussing.

PROCEDURE 22-1

BASIC FACIAL

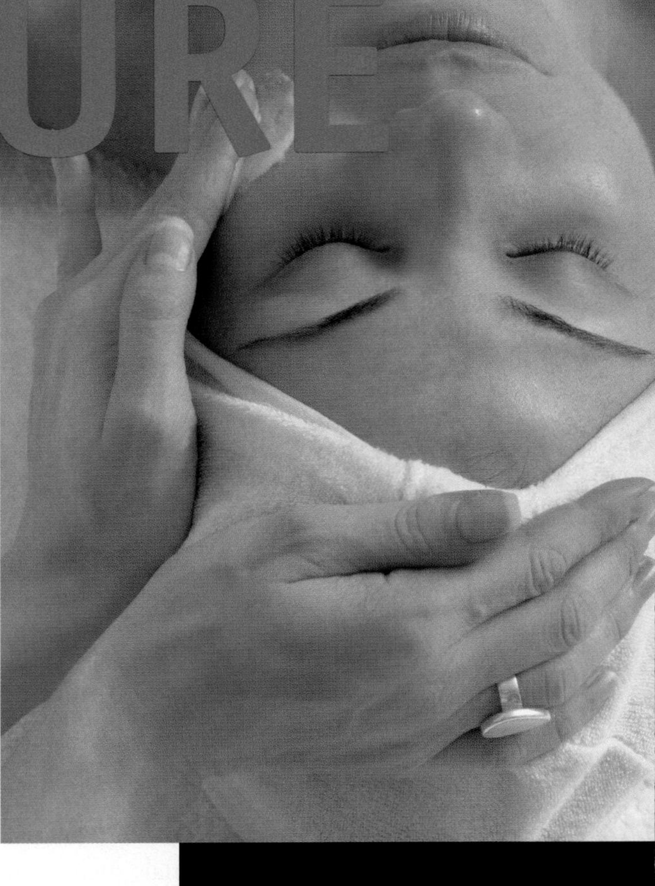

EQUIPMENT, IMPLEMENTS, AND MATERIALS

- Facial table or chair
- Facial steamer
- Garbage can
- Magnifying lamp
- Makeup tray
- Trolley for products and implements
- Clean sheet or other covering (blanket if necessary)
- Cotton (roll)
- Cotton pads
- Cotton swabs and pledgets
- Gauze
- Headband or head covering
- Salon gown
- Towels
- Plastic bobby pins/safety pins
- Spatulas
- Sponges
- Tissues
- Antiseptic lotion
- Toner
- Cleansers and makeup removers
- Hand sanitizer
- Massage cream or lubricating oil
- Masks
- Moisturizers
- Sun-protection products
- Tonic lotions

OPTIONAL ITEMS

- Specialty or intensive care products
- Infrared lamp
- Other electrical equipment

PREPARATION

1. Wash your hands with soap and warm water before each client.
2. Greet the client in a friendly and professional way. This helps to put the client at ease.
3. Ask the client to remove any jewelry such as a necklace or earrings, and store it in a safe place. Clients may wish to keep their handbags nearby during the facial.
4. Show the client to the dressing room and offer assistance if needed.
5. Place a clean towel across the back of the facial table to prevent the client's bare shoulders from coming into contact with the bed (Figure 22-47).
6. **Assist the client onto the facial table.** Offer assistance to your client if needed and place a towel across the client's chest. Next, place a coverlet or sheet over the client's body and fold the top edge of the towel over it. Remove the client's shoes and tuck the coverlet around the feet (Figure 22-48). Some salons provide disposable slippers that can be worn to and from the dressing room.

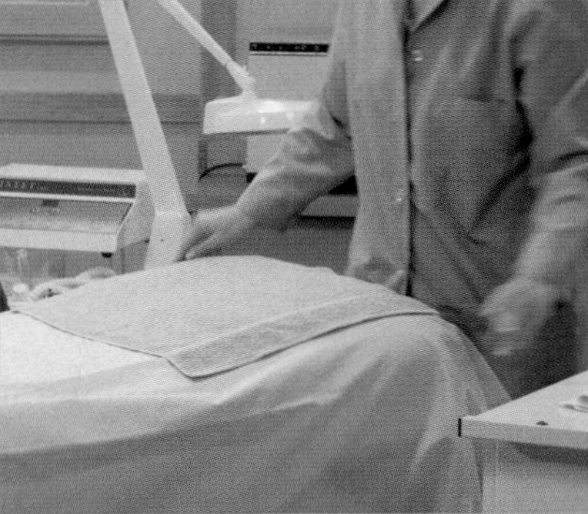

Figure 22-47 Place a towel across the back of the facial bed.

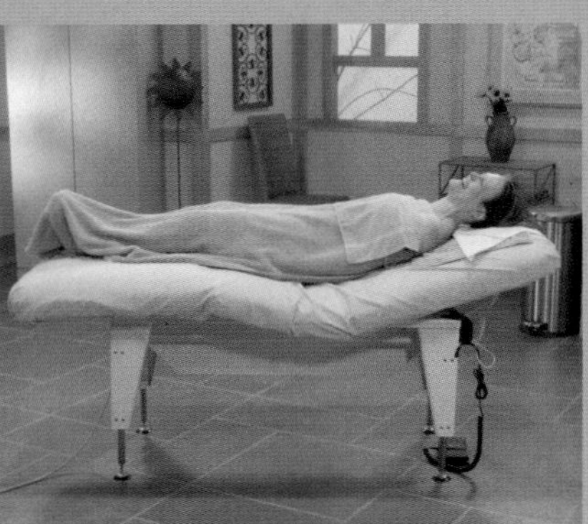

Figure 22-48 Client in facial bed.

7. **Drape client's head.** Fasten a headband lined with tissue, a towel, or other head covering around the client's head to protect the hair. To drape the head with a towel, follow these steps:
   a. Fold the towel lengthwise from one of the top corners to the opposite lower corner, and place it over the headrest with the fold facing down. Place the towel on the headrest before the client enters the facial area.
   b. When the client is in a reclined position, the back of the head should rest on the towel, so that the sides of the towel can be brought up to the center of the forehead to cover the hairline (Figures 22-49 and 22-50).
   c. Use a headband with a Velcro closure or a pin to hold the towel in place (Figure 22-51). Make sure that all strands of hair are tucked under the towel, that the earlobes are not bent, and that the towel is not wrapped too tightly (Figure 22-52).
8. Remove lingerie straps from a female client's shoulders. *Alternative method:* If client is given a strapless gown to wear, tuck the straps into the top of the gown.
9. Wash your hands with soap and warm water.
10. Perform a client consultation.

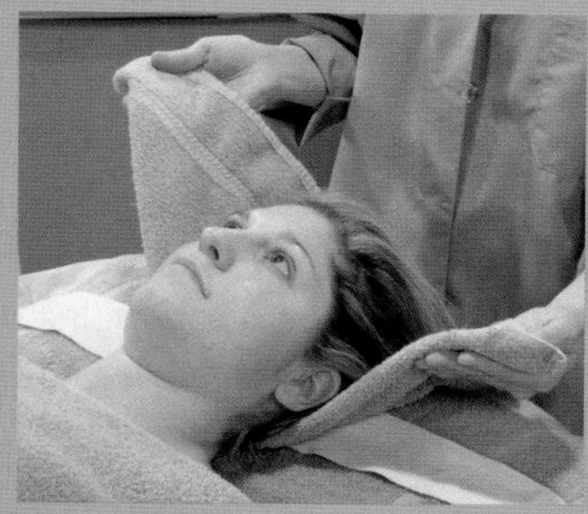
Figure 22-49 Bring the sides of the towel around the client's head.

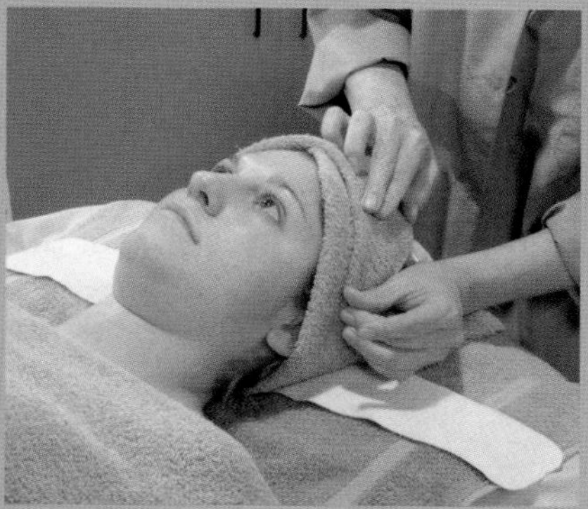
Figure 22-50 Bring one side of the towel over the other.

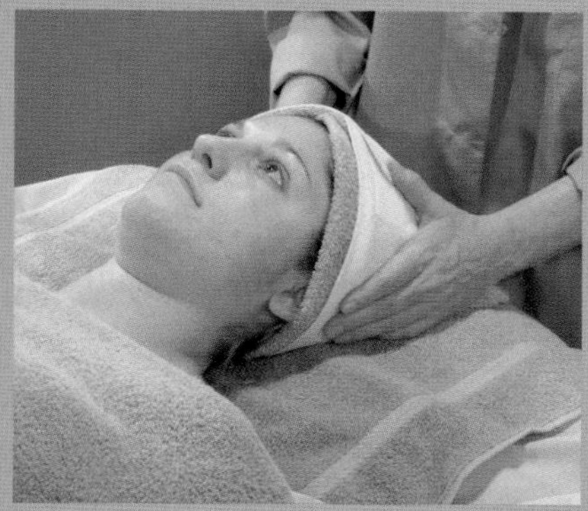
Figure 22-51 Secure the towel with a terrycloth headband.

PROCEDURE

1. If your client wears makeup, use the following steps to remove it. If your client has no makeup, skip this part and proceed to Step 2.
   a. Apply a pea-sized amount of eye makeup remover to each of two damp cotton pads and place them on the client's closed eyes. Leave them in place for 1 minute (Figure 22-53).
   b. Meanwhile, apply another pea-sized amount of eye makeup remover to a damp cotton pad and gently remove the client's lipstick with even strokes from the corners of the lips toward the center. Repeat the procedure until the lips are clean.
   c. Now, remove the eye makeup in the same way, gently stroking down and outward with the cotton pad. Do one eye first, and then the other. Repeat the procedure until the eyelids and lashes are clean (Figure 22-54).

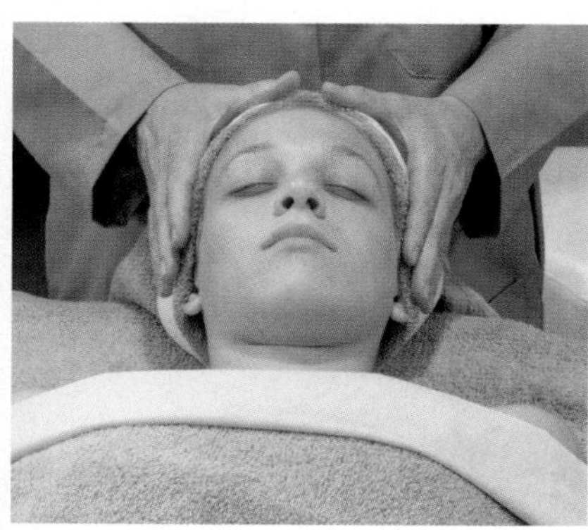
Figure 22-52 The client is prepared for the facial.

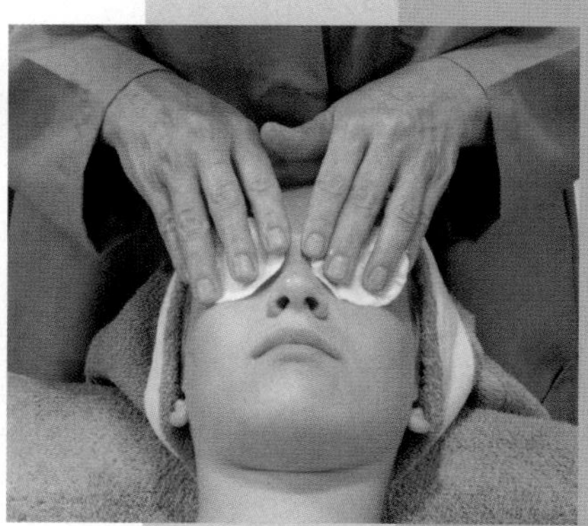
Figure 22-53 Leave cotton pads on the client's eyes.

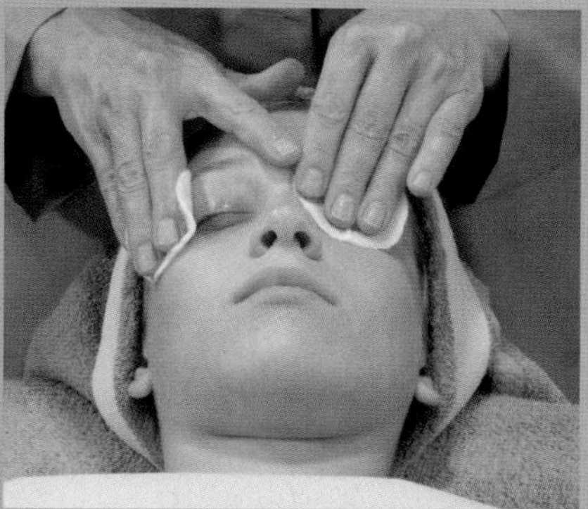
Figure 22-54 Stroke down and outward with the pads.

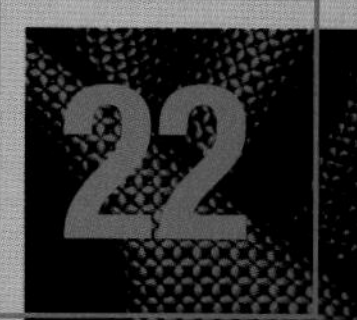

d. Ask the client to look up, and then remove any makeup underneath the eyes. Always be gentle around the eyes. Never rub or stretch the skin, as it is very delicate and thin.

2. **Apply cleanser.** Remove about a teaspoon of cleanser from the container with a clean spatula. Blend with your fingers to soften it.

   a. Starting at the neck with a sweeping movement, use both hands to spread the cleanser upward on the chin, jaws, cheeks, and the base of the nose to the temples and along the sides and the bridge of the nose (Figure 22-55). Make small circular movements with your fingertips around the nostrils and sides of the nose. Continue the upward sweeping movements between the brows and across the forehead to the temples.

   b. Take additional cleanser from the container with a clean spatula and blend. Smooth down the neck, chest, and back with long, even strokes.

   c. Starting at the center of the forehead, move your fingertips lightly in a circle around the eyes to the temples, and then back to the center of the forehead (Figure 22-56).

   d. Slide your fingers down the nose to the upper lip, from the temples through the forehead, lightly down to the chin, and then firmly up the jaw line back toward the temples and forehead.

3. **Remove cleanser.** Remove the cleanser with facial sponges, tissues, moist cotton pads, or warm, moist towels. Start at the forehead and follow the contours of the face. Remove all the cleanser from one area of the face before proceeding to the next. Finish with the neck, chest, and back (Figure 22-57).

4. Analyze the skin to determine the products and procedures to be used (Figure 22-58). *Optional:* If eyebrow arching is to be done, it should be done at this time.

5. **Steam the face.** Use warm, moist towels, or a facial steamer to open the pores of the face so that they can be cleansed of oil and comedones. If you use a steamer, cover the client's eyes with cotton pads moistened with distilled water or alcohol-free freshener. Steam helps to soften superficial lines and increases blood circulation to the surface of the skin (Figures 22-59 and 22-60).

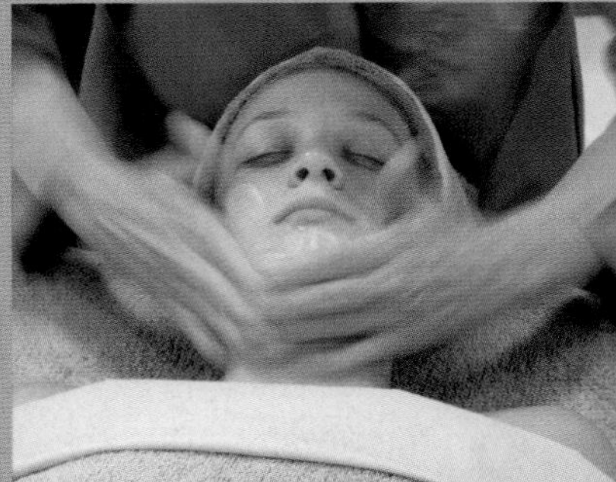

Figure 22-55 Spread cleanser over the neck.

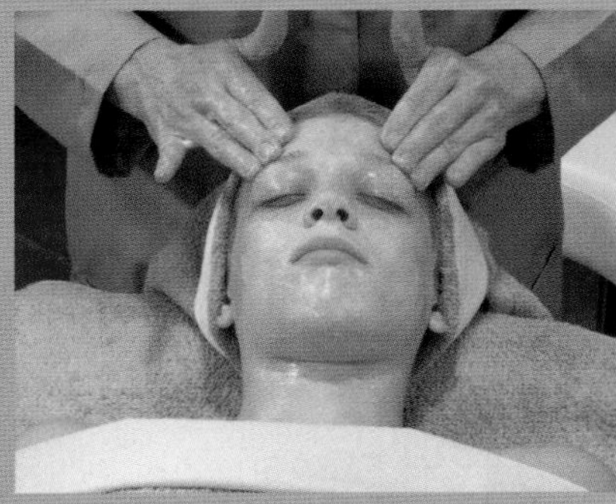

Figure 22-56 Spread cleanser over the forehead.

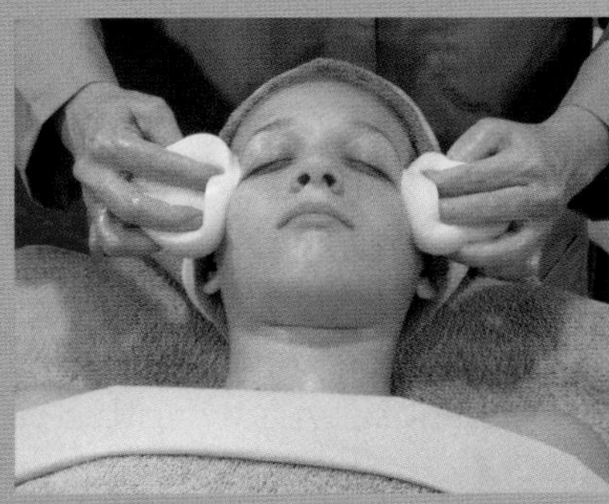

Figure 22-57 Remove cleanser with facial sponges.

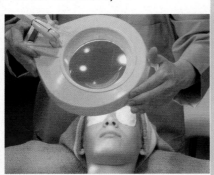

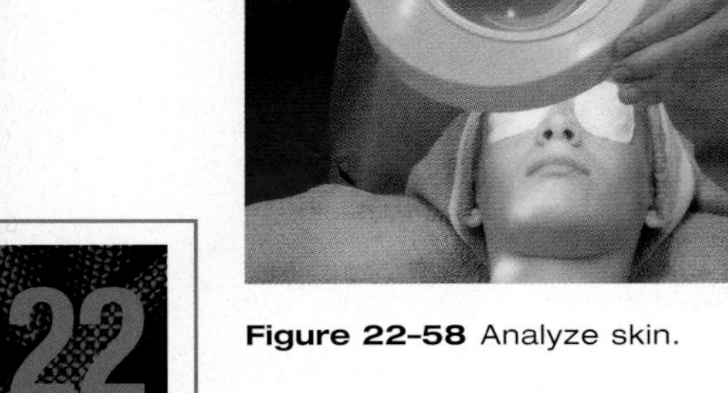

Figure 22-58 Analyze skin.

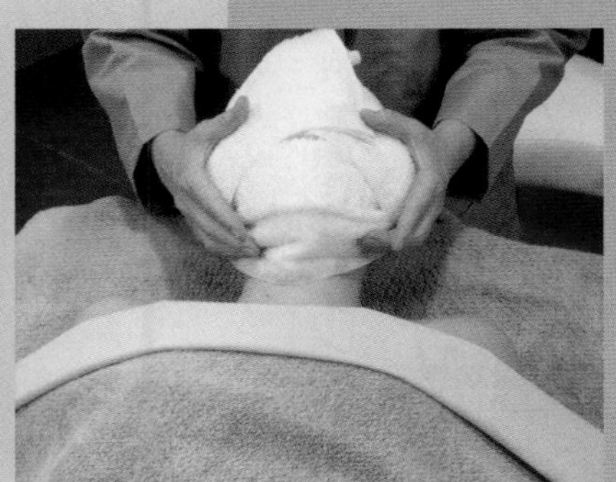

Figure 22-59 Steam face with warm moist towels.

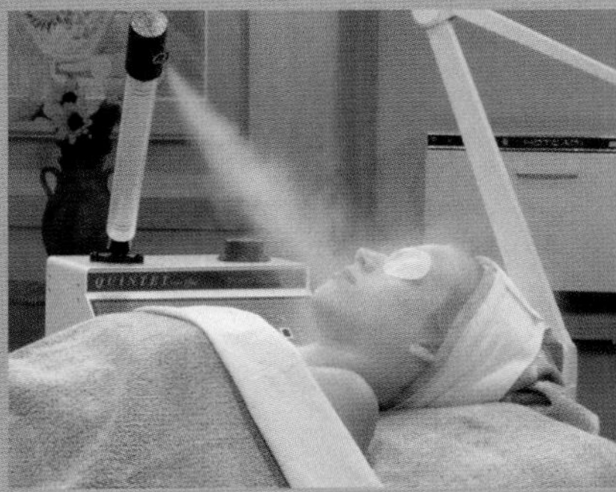

Figure 22-60 You may also use a steamer to steam the face.

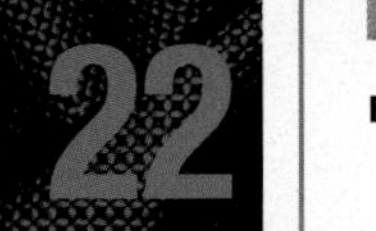

6. **Exfoliate.** Assuming that the client's skin is nonsensitive, apply a granular scrub to the face and gently massage the scrub in small circular movements. Do not use this near the eye area to prevent granules accidentally getting into the eye. This procedure should take about 2 minutes. If you like, this granular scrub can be used during exposure to the facial steamer. Remove the scrub carefully with damp sponges or cotton pads. A brushing machine can be used here instead of the granular scrub. Remember to apply cleansing milk before using the machine. Check with your instructor to have her show you the correct way to use the brushing machine. Choose a treatment cream, lotion, or massage cream appropriate for the skin type. Using the same procedure as for the cleanser, apply the cream to the face, neck, shoulders, chest, and back (Figure 22-61). If needed, apply lubrication oil or cream around the eyes and on the neck.
7. Massage the face, using the facial manipulations described in the Facial Massage section.
8. Remove massage cream with warm, moist towels, moist cleansing pads, or sponges. Follow the same procedure as for removing cleanser.
9. Sponge the face with cotton pledgets moistened with toner or freshener (Figure 22-62).
10. Apply a treatment mask formulated for the client's skin condition.
    a. Remove the mask from its container with a clean spatula and place it in a little cup.
    b. Apply the mask with a natural bristle brush, starting at the neck. Use long slow strokes from the center outward.
    c. Proceed to the jawline and apply the mask on the face from the center outward on half of the face, and then the other (Figure 22-63).
    d. Allow it to remain on the face for 7 to 10 minutes.
11. Remove the mask with wet cotton pledgets, sponges, or towels (Figure 22-64).
12. Apply toner, astringent, or freshener.
13. Apply a moisturizer or sunscreen.

CLEANUP AND SANITATION

1. Remove the head covering and show the client to the dressing room, offering assistance if needed.
2. Discard all disposable supplies and materials.
3. Close product containers tightly, clean them, and put them away in their proper places. Return unused cosmetics and other items to the dispensary.
4. Place used towels, coverlets, head covers, and other linens in hamper.
5. Sanitize your workstation, including the facial table.
6. Wash your hands with soap and warm water.

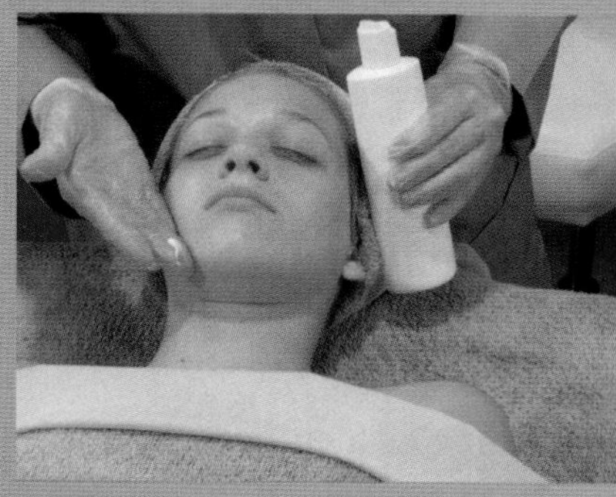

Figure 22-61 Apply massage cream.

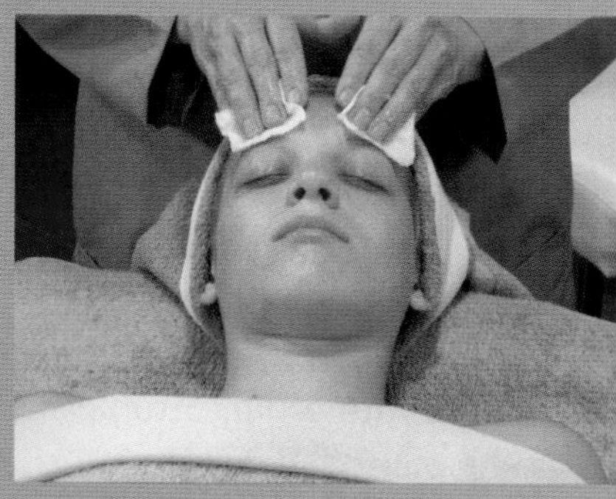

Figure 22-62 Apply tonic lotion or freshener.

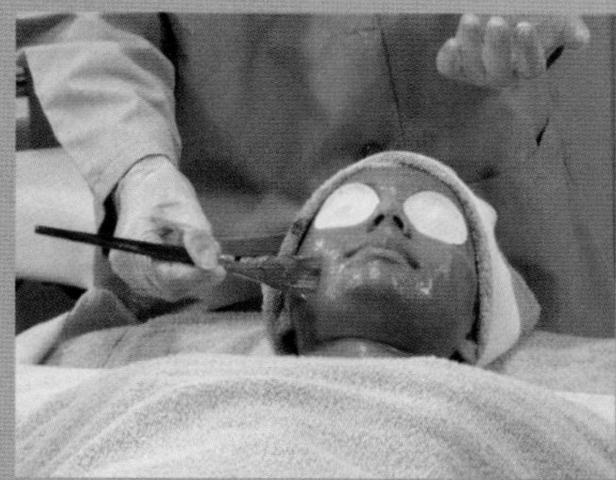

Figure 22-63 Apply a mask, starting at the neck.

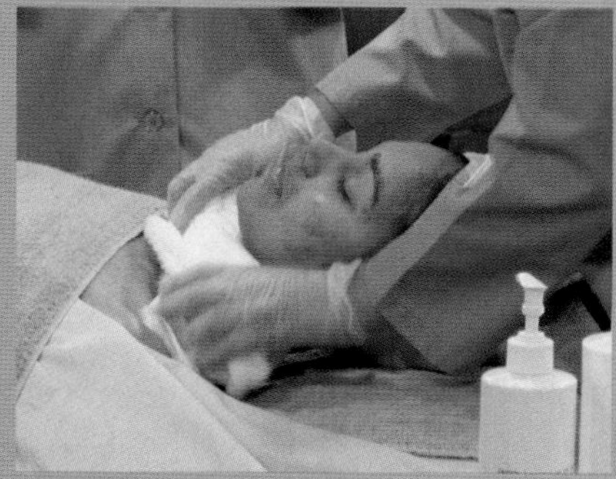

Figure 22-64 Remove the mask.

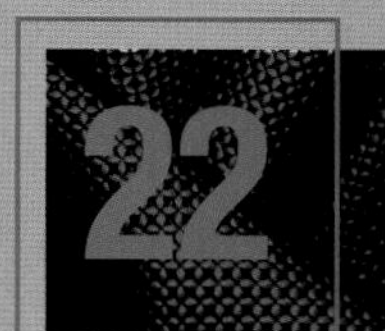

PROCEDURE 22-2

FACIAL FOR DRY SKIN

EQUIPMENT, IMPLEMENTS, AND MATERIALS

This list is the same as for the basic facial, with the following additions:

- Galvanic or high-frequency machine, depending on treatment
- Specialized creams, serums, and toners for dry skin
- Eye cream

PREPARATION

Prepare the client in the same way as for the basic facial.

PROCEDURE

1. Apply cleanser, gently massage to apply, and then remove with damp cotton pads, soft sponges, or a warm moist soft towel.
2. Remove residue with toner on damp cotton pad or soft sponge.
3. Focus steam on the face and allow steaming for 5 minutes.
4. **Exfoliate.** During or after steaming, apply a mild granular exfoliating product designed for dry skin. Gently massage with light circular movements. Remove with damp cotton pads, soft sponges, or a warm moist soft towel.
5. Apply eye cream under the eyes.
6. Apply a moisturizing lotion, cream, or massage product designed for dry skin.
7. Massage the skin with manipulations.
8. If massage cream is used, remove with damp cotton pads, soft sponges, or a warm moist soft towel.
9. If you are not using electrotherapy, proceed to Step 12.

CAUTION

For dry skin, avoid using lotions that contain a high percentage of alcohol. Read the manufacturer's directions.

10. Electrotherapy option 1, galvanic treatment: Apply ionized specialized serum, gel, or lotion. Apply galvanic current as directed by manufacturer's or instructor's directions (Figure 22-65). Electrotherapy option 2, high-frequency indirect current treatment: Use high-frequency machine as directed by manufacturer or instructor. Have the client hold the electrode in his or her hand. Perform manipulations, using the indirect method of high frequency, for 7 to 10 minutes. Do not lift your hands from the client's face. Turn off high-frequency machine (Figure 22-66).
11. Apply additional moisturizing or specialty product for dry skin with slow massage movements.
12. **Apply a mask.** Starting at the neck using a soft mask brush, apply a soft-setting cream or hydrating gel mask. Make sure you remove the mask from its container with a sanitized spatula. Mask should be applied from the center outward.
13. Apply cold cotton eye pads. Allow client to rest mask to process for 7 to 10 minutes. Make sure client is comfortable and warm enough.
14. Remove the mask with warm wet cotton pads, sponges, or warm moist soft towels.
15. Apply toner for dry skin with cotton pads.
16. Apply moisturizer or sunscreen designed for dry skin.

CLEANUP AND SANITATION

Use the same techniques as listed for basic facial. Make sure that all equipment is cleaned and sanitized as directed by manufacturer's instructions.

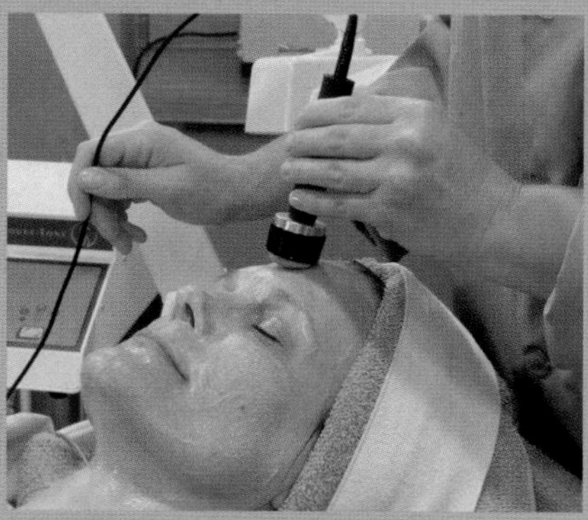

Figure 22-65 Apply galvanic current.

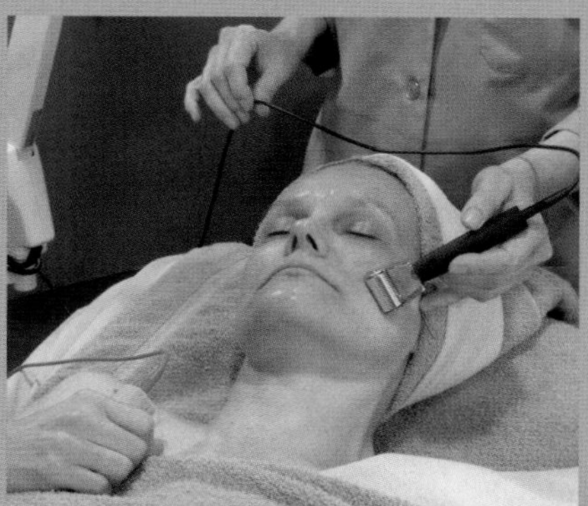

Figure 22-66 Apply indirect high-frequency current.

PROCEDURE 22-3

FACIAL FOR OILY SKIN WITH OPEN COMEDONES (BLACKHEADS)

EQUIPMENT, IMPLEMENTS, AND MATERIALS

This list is the same as for the basic facial, with the following additions:

- Galvanic or high-frequency machine, depending on treatment
- Specialized fluids, serums, mask, and toner for oily skin
- Desincrustation gel or lotion
- Gloves

PREPARATION

Prepare the client in the same way as for the basic facial.

PROCEDURE

1. Apply cleanser designed for oily skin, gently massage to apply, and then remove with damp cotton pads, soft sponges, or a warm moist soft towel.
2. Remove residue with damp cotton pad or soft sponge. Do *not* tone at this time.
3. Focus steam on the face and allow steaming for 5 minutes.
4. **Exfoliate.** During or after steaming, apply a mild granular exfoliating product designed for oily or combination skin. Gently massage with light circular movements. Remove with damp cotton pads, soft sponges, or a warm, moist soft towel.
5. **Apply a desincrustation lotion or gel to any area with clogged pores.** Negative galvanic current may be applied over this lotion, depending on the manufacturer's instructions. The lotion should generally remain on the skin for 5 to 8 minutes, again, depending on the manufacturer's instructions. Remove the preparation with damp cotton pads, soft sponges, or a warm, moist soft towel.
6. **Extraction.** Apply latex gloves prior to extraction. Apply damp cotton pads to the client's eyes to avoid glaring light from the magnifying lamp. Cover your fingertips with cotton, and using the magnifying lamp, gently pressing out open comedones. Place your middle fingers on either side of the comedone or clogged pore, stretching the skin. Push your fingers down to reach underneath the follicle, and then *gently* squeeze. Apply the same technique to all sides of the follicle. Do not extract for more than 5 minutes for the entire face. *Never squeeze with bare fingers or fingernails!* See Figure 22-67. If galvanic desincrustation

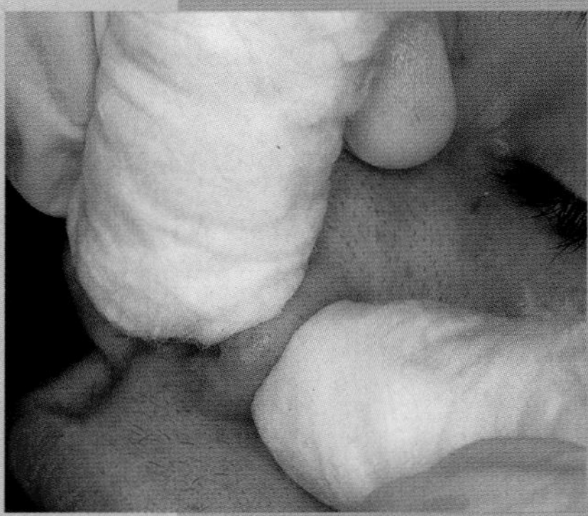

Figure 22-67 Press out comedones.

CAUTION

You must receive hands-on instruction to properly perform extraction of clogged pores and comedones. *Do not attempt this procedure without first obtaining instruction!*

was performed prior to extraction, apply *positive* galvanic current to the face after extractions are complete. This will help to re-establish the proper pH of the skin surface.

7. **Apply astringent.** After extraction is complete, apply an astringent lotion, toner for oily skin, or specialized serum designed for after extraction. Allow to dry.
8. **Apply high-frequency current.** Unfold gauze across the face and apply direct high frequency using the mushroom-shaped electrode, according to the machine manufacturer's directions.
9. **Extremely oily or clogged skin should not be massaged.** If the skin is very clogged, proceed to mask step. If skin is not extremely clogged, apply a hydration fluid or massage fluid designed for oily and combination skin, and perform massage manipulations.
10. **Apply mask.** Using a mask brush, apply a clay-based mask to all oily areas. To dry areas, such as the eye and neck areas, you may choose to apply a gel mask for dehydrated skin. Allow the mask to process for about 10 minutes. Do not allow the mask to overdry so that it cracks.
11. Remove the mask with damp cotton pads, soft sponges, or a warm moist soft towel.
12. Apply toner for oily skin with cotton pads.
13. Apply moisturizer or sunscreen designed for oily or combination skin.

CLEANUP AND SANITATION

Use same techniques as listed for the basic facial. Make sure that all equipment is cleaned and sanitized as directed by manufacturer's instructions.

CAUTION

Some people are allergic to latex or rubber. Check with your client to determine whether such an allergy exists and, if so, make a note of this on the client card. Then proceed, using vinyl gloves.

CAUTION

When treating acne-prone skin, disposable gloves should be worn throughout the treatment.

PROCEDURE 22-4

FACIAL FOR ACNE-PRONE AND PROBLEM SKIN

EQUIPMENT, IMPLEMENTS, AND MATERIALS

This list is the same as for the basic facial, with the following additions:

- Galvanic or high-frequency machine, depending on treatment
- Specialized fluids, serums, and toners for acne-prone skin
- Desincrustation gel or lotion
- Antibacterial clay or sulfur mask
- Gloves

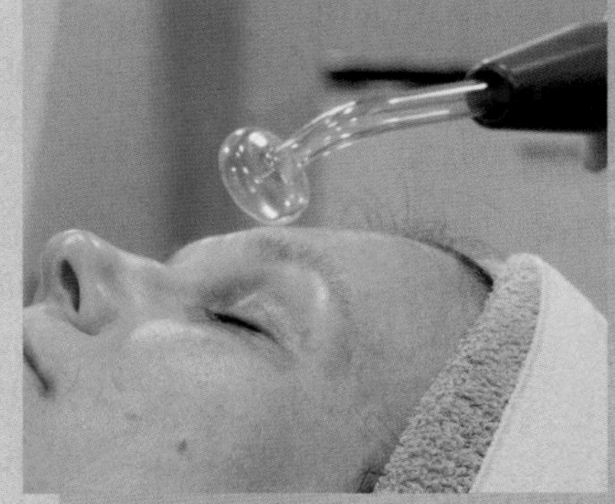

Figure 22-68 Apply high-frequency current with a facial electrode.

PREPARATION

Prepare the client in the same way as for the basic facial.

PROCEDURE

1. Apply cleanser designed for oily/acne-prone skin, gently massage to apply, and then remove with damp cotton pads, soft sponges, or a warm, moist soft towel.
2. Remove residue with damp cotton pad or soft sponge. Do not tone at this time.
3. Focus steam on the face and allow steaming for 5 minutes.
4. **Apply a desincrustation lotion or gel to any area with pimples or clogged pores.** Negative galvanic current may be applied over this lotion, depending on the manufacturer's instructions. The lotion should generally remain on the skin for 5 to 8 minutes, again, depending on the manufacturer's instructions. Remove the preparation with damp cotton pads, soft sponges, or a warm, moist soft towel.
5. Extract comedones as in Procedure 22-3.
6. After extraction is complete, apply an astringent lotion, toner for oily skin, or specialized serum designed for after extraction. Allow to dry. Unfold gauze across the face and apply direct high-frequency using the mushroom-shaped electrode, according to machine manufacturer's and your instructor's directions (Figure 22-68).
7. If galvanic desincrustation was performed prior to extraction, apply *positive* galvanic current to the face after extractions are complete. This will help to re-establish the proper pH of the skin surface.
8. Acne-prone skin should *not* be massaged.
9. **Apply mask.** Using a mask brush, apply an antibacterial or sulfur-based mask to all oily and acne-prone areas. To dry skin, such as the eye and neck areas, you may choose to apply a gel mask for dehydrated skin. Allow the mask to process for about 10 minutes. Do not allow the mask to overdry so that it cracks (Figure 22-69).
10. Remove the mask with damp cotton pads, soft sponges, or a warm, moist soft towel.
11. Apply toner for oily skin with cotton pads.
12. Apply specialized lotion or sunscreen designed for oily or acne-prone skin.

CLEANUP AND SANITATION

Use the same techniques as listed for the basic facial. Make sure that all equipment is cleaned and sanitized as directed by manufacturer's instructions.

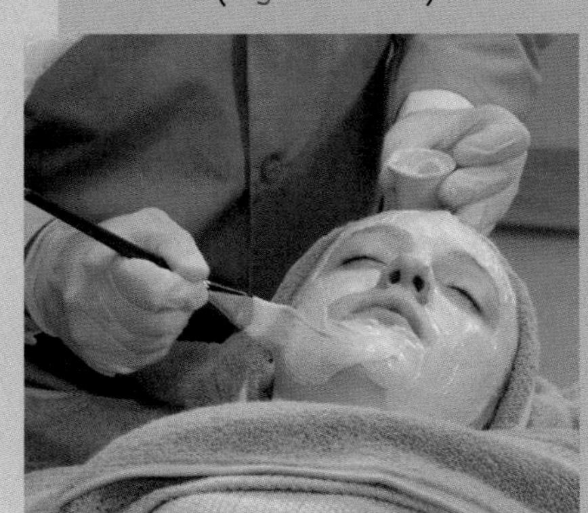

Figure 22-69 Apply a facial mask for acne skin.

Explain, in simple terms, the client's skin conditions, informing the client of how you propose to treat the conditions. Inform the client about how often treatments should be administered in the salon, and very specifically what he or she should be doing at home.

You should organize the products you want the client to purchase and use. Explain the use of each one at a time, in the order of use. Make sure to have written instructions for the client to take home.

It is very important to have products available for the client that you believe in and that produce results. Retailing products for clients to use at home is very important for success in treatment and in your business.

CAUTION

Aromatherapy is sometimes used as a healing modality by natural healers who have received extensive training in the properties and uses of essential oils and their aromatherapy benefits. Cosmetologists should never attempt to perform healing treatments with aromatherapy.

AROMATHERAPY

The therapeutic use of essential oils such as lemon verbena, rosemary, and rose has greatly improved the efficacy of many skin care preparations. Many essential oils are also used for their **aromatherapy** benefits to enhance a person's physical, emotional, mental, and spiritual well-being. Using various oils and oil blends for specific benefits is believed to create positive effects on the body, mind, and spirit (Figure 22-70).

Essential oils can be used in a variety of ways. Lighting a cinnamon candle in the winter can give the salon a cozy feeling, and cheer up both clients and service givers. You can use a spray bottle to diffuse well-diluted essential oils in the treatment room, or on the sheets. For a more balanced massage, you can create your own aromatherapy massage oil by adding a few drops of essential oil to a massage oil, cream, or lotion.

Always be careful to use essential oils lightly, however, as they sometimes have a tendency to be overpowering.

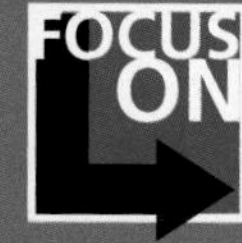

Focus on . . . Sharpening Your Personal Skills

The importance of following proper hygiene and sanitation guidelines when giving facials cannot be overemphasized. As much as possible, perform your sanitation procedures in the presence of your clients. When they see you doing this, they will feel more confidence in you as a professional.

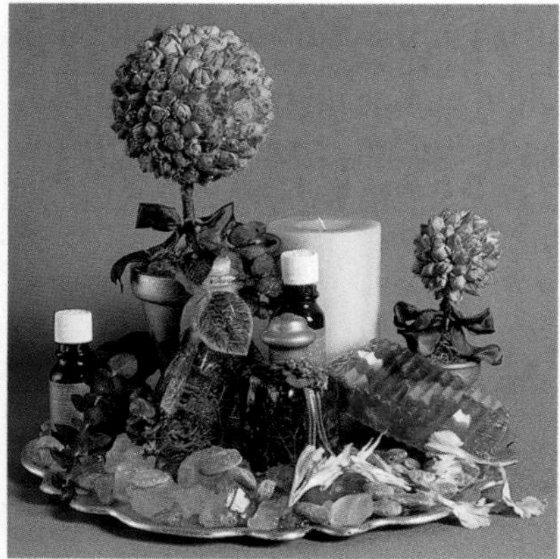

Figure 22-70 Some ingredients for aromatherapy.

REVIEW QUESTIONS

1. Explain skin analysis techniques. Why is skin analysis important?
2. What is a contraindication? List five examples.
3. Why is it important to have every client complete a health-screening questionnaire?
4. Describe the differences between alipidic and oily skin.
5. What is the difference between skin type and skin condition?
6. Discuss the different types of skin care products.
7. How does a chemical exfoliant work?
8. Explain the purpose of massage.
9. Name and briefly describe the five categories of massage manipulations.
10. Who is not a good candidate for electrical current treatment?
11. Name and define the two basic categories of facial treatments.
12. Why is home care so important for clients?
13. List the steps in giving a basic facial treatment.

CHAPTER GLOSSARY

alipidic	Skin that does not produce enough sebum, indicated by absence of visible pores.
alpha hydroxy acids	Acids derived from plants, mostly fruit, and used to exfoliate the skin.
ampoules	Sealed glass vials containing highly concentrated extract in a water or oil base.
anode	Positive electrode.
aromatherapy	Therapeutic use of essential oils.
astringents	Liquid that helps remove the excess oil in the skin.
brushing machine	A rotating electric appliance with interchangeable brushes that can be attached to the rotating head.
cathode	Negative electrode.
chemical exfoliants	Chemical agent that dissolves dead skin cells.
chucking	Massage movement accomplished by grasping the flesh firmly in one hand and moving the hand up and down along the bone while the other hand keeps the arm or leg in a steady position.
clay-based masks	Clay preparations used to stimulate circulation and temporarily contract the pores of the skin.

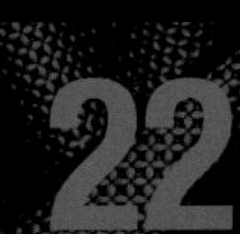

CHAPTER GLOSSARY

cleansing milks	Nonfoaming lotion cleansers for the face.
closed comedones	Clogged follicles just under the skin surface.
contraindication	Procedure or condition that requires avoiding certain treatment to prevent undesirable side effects.
couperose	European term describing areas of diffuse redness and dilated red capillaries.
cream masks	Mask treatments for dry skin that do not harden or dry on the face.
effleurage	Light, continuous stroking movement applied with the fingers (digital) or the palms (palmar) in a slow, rhythmic manner.
electrode	Applicator for directing the electric current from the machine to the client's skin.
electrotherapy	Electrical facial treatments.
emollients	Oil or fatty ingredients that prevent moisture from leaving the skin.
enzyme peels	Chemical exfoliants that involve the use of enzymes that help speed up the breakdown of keratin, the protein in skin.
exfoliants	Ingredient that assists in the process of exfoliation.
exfoliation	Removal of excess dead cells from the skin surface.
foaming cleansers	Wash-off product that contains a surfactant.
fresheners	Liquid that helps remove excess oil in the skin.
friction	Deep rubbing movement requiring pressure on the skin with the fingers or palm while moving them over an underlying structure.
fulling	Form of petrissage in which the tissue is grasped, gently lifted, and spread out; used mainly for massaging the arms.
gommages	Enzyme peels in which a cream is applied to the skin before steaming and forms a hardened crust that is then massaged or "rolled" off the skin.
hacking	Chopping movement performed with the edges of the hands in massage.
humectants	Substances that absorb moisture or promote the retention of moisture.
keratolytic enzymes	Substances that help speed up the breakdown of keratin, the protein in skin.
light therapy	Application of light rays to the skin for treating disorders.
masks	Special cosmetic preparations applied to the face to tighten, tone, hydrate, and nourish the skin.

CHAPTER GLOSSARY

massage	Manual or mechanical manipulation of the body by rubbing, pinching, kneading, tapping, and other movements to increase metabolism and circulation, promote absorption, and relieve pain.
massage creams	Lubricants designed to give the practitioner a good slip (slippery quality) during massage.
mechanical exfoliants	Methods of physical contact used to scrape or bump cells off the skin.
microcurrent	A galvanic treatment that is a computerized device with many skin care applications, namely, toning.
microdermabrasion	Mechanical exfoliation that involves "shooting" aluminum oxide or other crystals at the skin with a hand-held device that exfoliates dead cells.
modelage masks	Facial masks containing special crystals of gypsum, a plaster-like ingredient.
moisturizers	Products formulated to add moisture to the skin.
motor point	Point on the skin over the muscle where pressure or stimulation will cause contraction of that muscle.
open comedones	Also known as blackheads; follicles impacted with solidified sebum and dead cell buildup.
ostium	Follicle opening.
paraffin wax masks	Specially prepared facial masks containing paraffin and other beneficial ingredients; typically used with treatment cream.
petrissage	Kneading movement performed by lifting, squeezing, and pressing the tissue with a light, firm pressure.
rolling	Massage movement in which the tissues are pressed and twisted using a fast back-and-forth movement.
steamer	Heats and produces a stream of warm steam that can be focused on various areas of the skin.
tapotement or percussion	Most stimulating massage movement, consisting of short, quick tapping, slapping, and hacking movements.
telangiectasias	Dilated red capillaries.
toners	Liquid that helps remove excess oil in the skin.
treatment cream	Cream designed to hydrate and condition the skin during the night; heavier in consistency and texture than a moisturizer.
vibration	In massage, the rapid shaking of the body part while the balls of the fingertips are pressed firmly on the point of application.
wringing	Vigorous movement in which the hands, placed a little distance apart on both sides of the client's arm or leg and working downward, apply a twisting motion against the bones in the opposite direction.

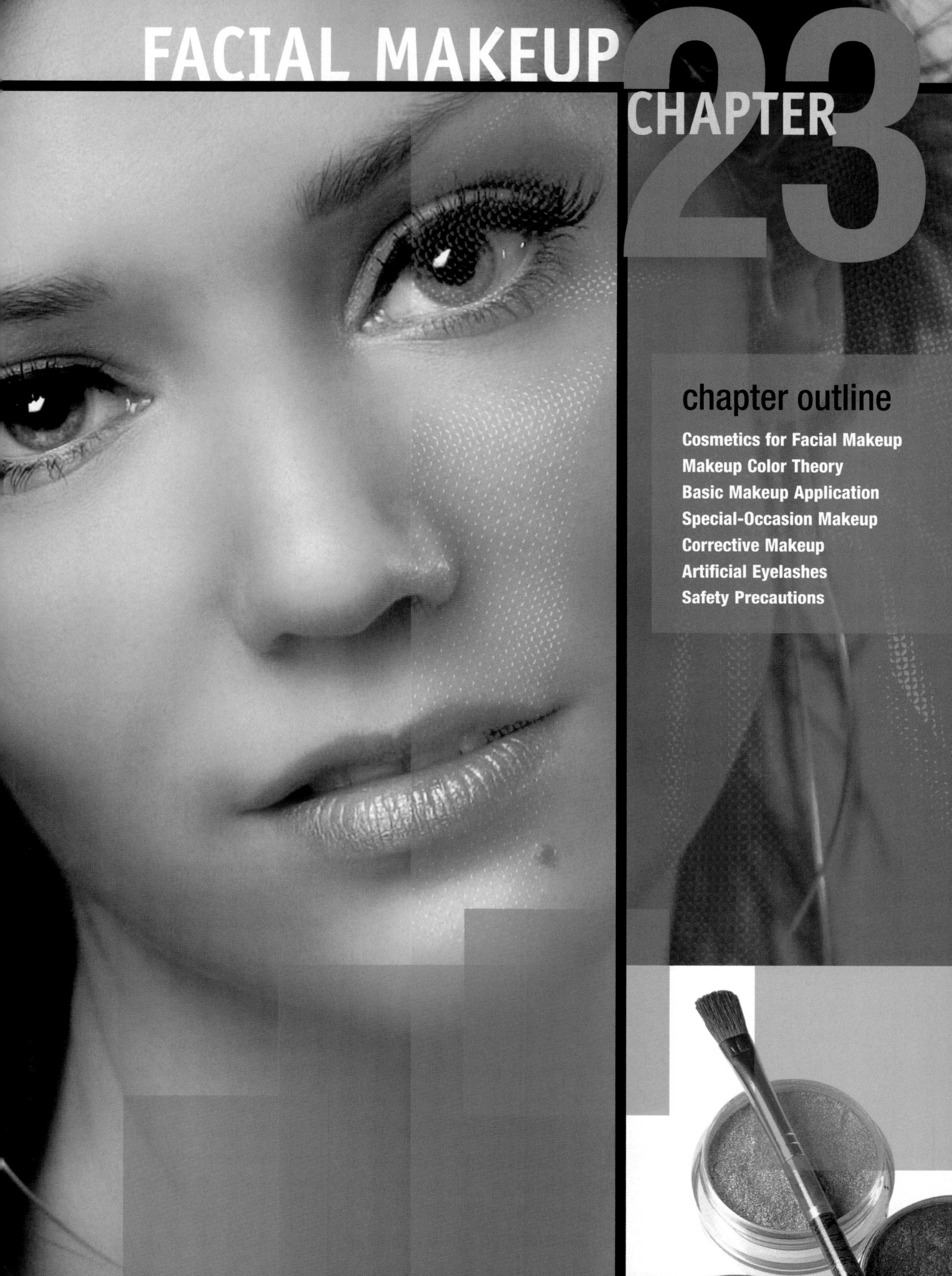

FACIAL MAKEUP

CHAPTER 23

chapter outline

Learning Objectives

After completing this chapter, you will be able to:

- Describe the various types of cosmetics and their uses.
- Demonstrate an understanding of cosmetic color theory.
- Demonstrate a basic makeup procedure for any occasion.
- Identify different facial types and demonstrate procedures for basic corrective makeup.
- Demonstrate the application and removal of artificial lashes.
- List safety measures to be followed during makeup application.

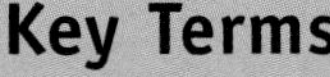

Key Terms

Page number indicates where in the chapter the term is used.

band lashes pg. 634

cake (pancake) makeup pg. 611

cheek color pg. 608

concealers pg. 607

cool colors pg. 614

eyebrow pencils pg. 610

eyelash adhesive pg. 634

eyeliner pg. 610

eye makeup removers pg. 611

eye shadows pg. 609

eye tabbing pg. 634

face powder pg. 607

foundation pg. 605

greasepaint pg. 611

lip color pg. 608

lip liner pg. 609

mascara pg. 611

matte pg. 606

warm colors pg. 614

Makeup is a part of cosmetology that is very interesting and can produce dramatic and immediate changes in clients' appearance. Most clients prefer a natural look, simply covering or focusing attention away from facial flaws, and accenting good facial features (Figure 23-1). Application of makeup can vary greatly among clients, and the needs of each client can be very different.

In this chapter, you will learn about basic makeup techniques and products, and about how to use color to make your clients look their best. You will also learn about highlighting and contouring, methods that help to accent good features, hide not-so-good features, and change the appearance of facial shapes (Figure 23-2).

When you have learned these techniques, you can imagine the client's face as a blank canvas, using your skills to cover, change, or accentuate features, making your client look her very best. Combining hairstyles, color, and makeup can help your client achieve beautiful changes.

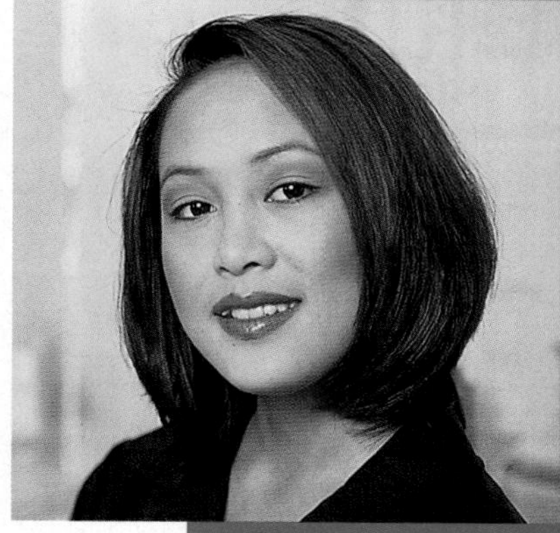

Figure 23-1 Enhancing a client's natural beauty.

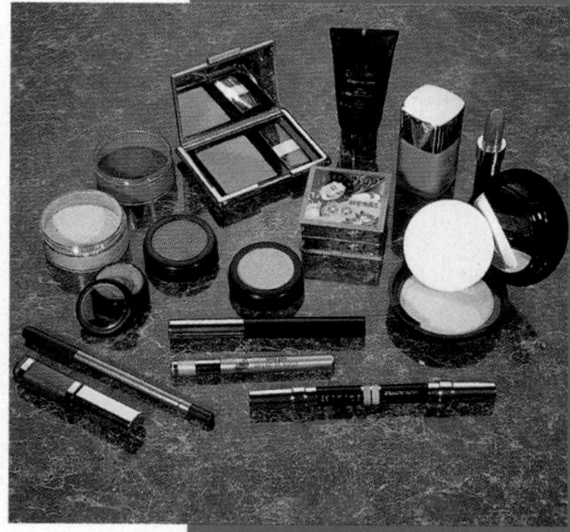

Figure 23-2 A wide variety of cosmetics is available to you and your client.

COSMETICS FOR FACIAL MAKEUP

FOUNDATION

Foundation is a tinted cosmetic, also known as base makeup, and is used to cover or even out the coloring of the skin. It can be used to conceal dark spots, blemishes, and other imperfections. Foundation is usually the first cosmetic used during makeup application (Figure 23-3).

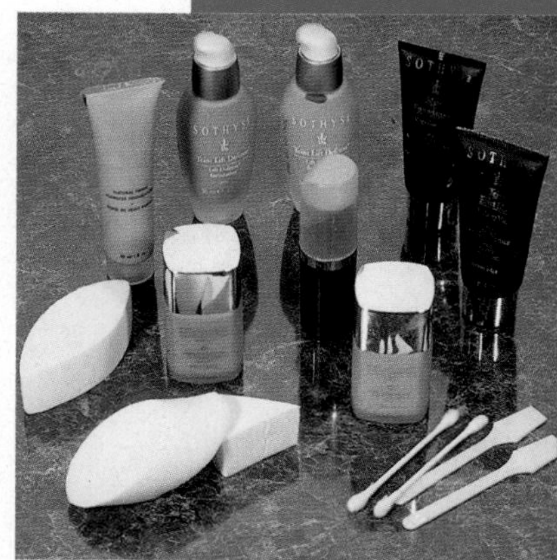

Figure 23-3 Foundations.

Foundation comes in liquid, stick, and cream forms. One of the newest trends, mineral powder makeup, is a powder form of foundation.

FOUNDATION CHEMISTRY

Most liquid and cream forms of makeup are mixtures of water and oil spreading agents as a base that contain a significant amount of talc and various color agents called pigments. Pigments can be natural derived minerals or color agents called lakes.

Liquid foundations, also called water-based foundation, is mostly water, but often contains an emollient such as mineral oil or a silicone such as cyclomethicone. Some may contain alcohols or other drying agents to

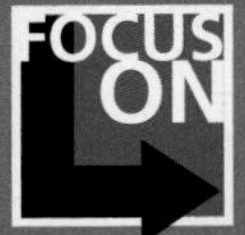

Focus on . . . Retailing

Retailing cosmetics is a great way to increase your income. Most salons will pay you a 5- to 10-percent commission on every product you retail. If you focus on retailing to every client, this amount will add up quickly. It is not unusual for a cosmetologist who is retailing makeup on a daily basis to pay for a long weekend vacation or even make a car payment or two each year using these rewards. And you will be helping your clients by giving them professional advice and allowing them to shop for makeup while receiving other salon services. If you don't take advantage of this opportunity, the department store down the street surely will!

help the product dry quickly on the skin. The mixture of water and oil helps in applying the makeup color agents evenly, and keeps the colors suspended evenly throughout the product. Water-based foundation is most often used for lighter coverage needs, and for oily to combination skin types. They often dry quickly and produce a **matte** finish, meaning they dry to become nonshiny.

Some foundations are marketed as oil-free. These are usually intended for oilier skin types, but some contain oil substitutes that can be equally as oily as a foundation containing oil. Be sure to read the label carefully and to check with the manufacturer to make sure it has been tested for oily and acne-prone skin.

Cream foundation, also known as oil-based foundation, is a considerably thicker product and is often sold in a jar or a tin. It may or may not contain water. The thicker the product, the less likely it is to contain water. Cream foundations provide heavier coverage and are usually intended for dry skin types. They tend to produce a shinier appearance than water-based products.

Using a cream foundation on oily or acneic skin can possibly cause more clogged pores to form. Cosmetic products that cause the formation of clogged pores or comedones are called comedogenic, which means that they produce comedones.

All types of foundation can contain sunscreen ingredients.

USING FOUNDATION

Choosing the correct color of foundation is extremely important in making makeup look natural. The foundation should be as close to the client's natural skin coloring as possible. To choose the correct foundation color, have the client sit in a well-lit area. Apply a small amount of the foundation product to the jawline. It is important that the color chosen matches the skin on both the face and neck. If the color of the foundation is too light, it will look dull and chalky. If the color is too dark, it will look muddy or splotchy.

Makeup should be blended onto the skin with a disposable makeup sponge. After choosing the correct color, remove some makeup from the container with a clean sanitized spatula. The foundation product may be placed in or on a small disposable palette or plastic cup to avoid contamination of the product container. Using the sponge, blend out the foundation across the skin with short strokes. The product should match the color of the skin very closely. A line of demarcation is an obvious line where the foundation starts or stops. These are very unattractive, and should not be obvious if the correct color has been chosen.

Cream foundation is usually applied to the sponge and then blended across the skin. Liquid foundation is often applied to the skin in small dots across the face and then quickly blended with a sponge.

Mineral powder foundation is applied with a large fluffy brush. It contains a lot of pigment for coverage. The pigments stick to the skin, providing natural-looking coverage.

CONCEALERS

Concealers are thicker and heavier types of foundation that contain more talc or pigment for heavier coverage. They are used to hide dark eye circles, dark splotches, and other imperfections. They are also available in a wide range of colors, and should match the skin color very closely. If the color is not matched perfectly, the concealer may draw attention to the area instead of hiding it! Concealers are packaged in tins, jars, or tubes with wands.

Some concealer products may also contain ingredients to add moisture or control oil, and some actually containing anti-acne ingredients to be used on acne blemishes.

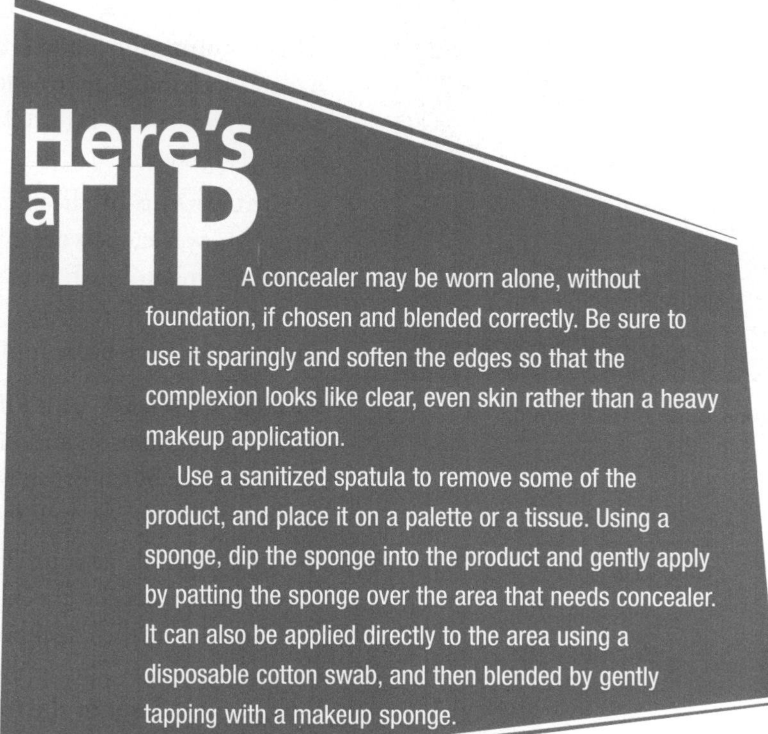

Here's a TIP

A concealer may be worn alone, without foundation, if chosen and blended correctly. Be sure to use it sparingly and soften the edges so that the complexion looks like clear, even skin rather than a heavy makeup application.

Use a sanitized spatula to remove some of the product, and place it on a palette or a tissue. Using a sponge, dip the sponge into the product and gently apply by patting the sponge over the area that needs concealer. It can also be applied directly to the area using a disposable cotton swab, and then blended by gently tapping with a makeup sponge.

FACE POWDERS

Face powder is a cosmetic powder, sometimes tinted or scented, that is used to add a matte or nonshiny finish to the face. It helps to absorb excess oil, and minimizes the shine of oily skin. It is used to "set" the foundation, making it easier to apply other powder, such as blush (Figure 23-4).

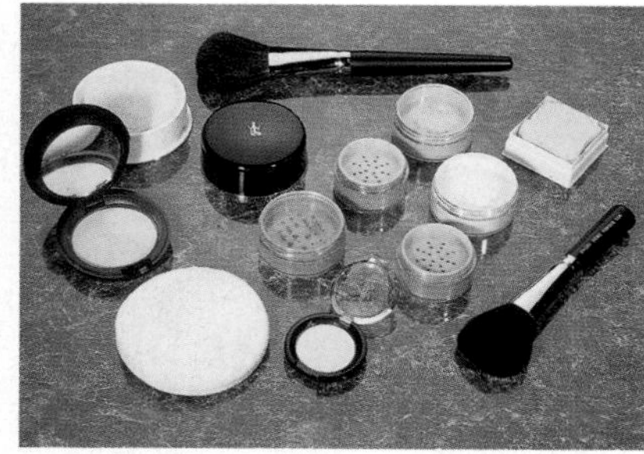

Figure 23-4 Commonly used forms of powder.

Face powder comes in two forms: loose and pressed. Pressed powder is blended with binding agents to keep it in a caked form in the tin. Loose powder does not contain as much binder, and comes in a jar.

Both powders are usually a mixture of talc or cornstarch with color pigments added. Some powders that do not contain much color are called translucent. They are intended not to add color when applied over a foundation. Pressing agents or binders such as zinc stearate are added to press the foundation, and to help it adhere to the skin. If a colored powder is used, it should match the natural skin tone.

APPLYING POWDER

Loose powder is applied with a large powder brush. Remove some loose powder from the container and place it in a disposable cup or tissue. Dip the brush in the powder and fluff it across the face. Make sure all areas of the face are covered, and remove any excess powder. You can also use a disposable cotton ball to apply loose powder.

Powder can also be used to brush out hard edges from blush or eyeshadow application. Powder should never look caked, streaked, or blotchy after application.

Pressed powder in tins is marketed primarily for touchups, as it can easily be carried in a purse. They normally come with a powder puff applicator. Powder puffs should never be used in the salon because they cannot be easily sanitized.

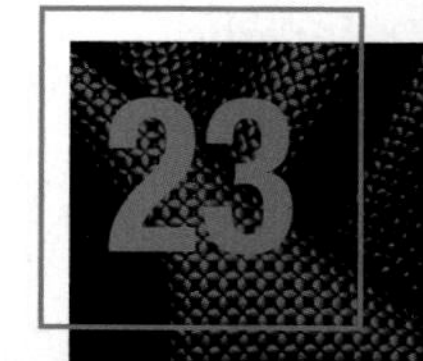

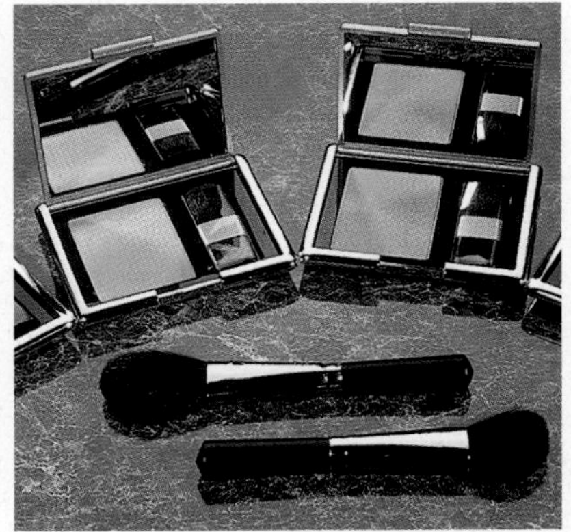

Figure 23-5 Cheek colors.

CHEEK COLOR

Cheek color, also known as blush or rouge, is used primarily to add a natural-looking glow to the cheeks, but can also be used to add a little extra color to the face. Cheek color comes in powder, gel, and cream forms (Figure 23-5).

Cream forms of cheek color have traditionally been used by makeup artists; however, powder blushes are easier to use, and are much more popular. Cream blush is used immediately after the foundation to blend color into the foundation. Powder blush is used after both the foundation and powder have been applied.

USING POWDER BLUSH

After the foundation and face powder have been applied, take a sanitized or disposable blush brush and dip it once into the pressed blush. Do not re-dip the blush! As an alternative, a disposable cotton puff can be used.

Look carefully at your client's face and notice the natural hollow of the cheek, just under the cheekbone. Apply the blush with short strokes to the area just under the cheekbone and to the area where natural color would normally appear. The application should look soft and natural. It should look like it fades into the foundation. It is always better to apply too little blush, instead of too much. You can always add more if necessary.

Never apply blush in a circle on the "apple" of the cheek, beyond the corner of the eye, or inwards between the cheekbone and the nose.

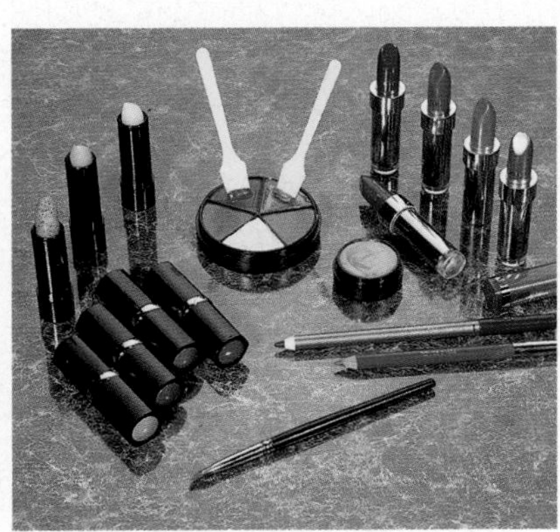

Figure 23-6 Lip colors.

LIP COLOR

Lip color, more commonly called lipstick or gloss, is a paste-like cosmetic, usually in a metal or plastic tube. Lip color comes in a large variety of colors (Figure 23-6). Lip color is used to change or enhance the color of the lips. Some lip color products contain conditioners to moisturize the lips, or sunscreen to protect against sun exposure.

Lip color is available in many forms, including creams, glosses, pencils, gels, and sticks. These products are a mixture of oils and color dyes.

Properly selecting lipstick color takes some talent. You should understand color theory, covered later in this chapter, to properly select a lipstick color. The lip color must blend (not match) with the client's hair and eye color and other makeup used.

Current fashion also dictates both color and application of lipstick. Fashion trends have called for light or dark lip color, shiny versus matte applications, and various application styles.

Lip color must never be applied directly from the container unless it belongs to the client. Lip color must be removed from the container or applied with a one-application disposable lip brush, which must never be re-used! It can also be removed from the container with a spatula, placed on a palette and then can be applied more freely.

After placing the lip color on the brush, begin by applying at the outer corners and work toward the middle. Repeat on the opposite side. Connect the center peaks using rounded strokes, following the natural lip line. Repeat on the bottom lip.

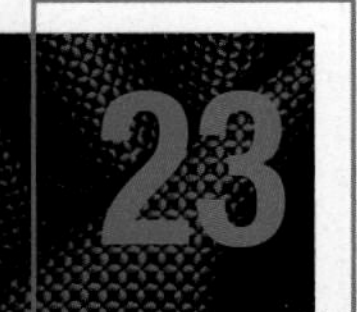

Properly applied lipstick should be even and symmetrical on both sides of the mouth.

Lip liner is a colored pencil used to outline the lips. It also helps to keep the lipstick from "bleeding" into small lines around the mouth. Lip liners are available as thin or thick pencils, sometimes as automatic roll-up pencils. Lip liner is usually applied before the lip color to define the shape of the lip. Choose a color that coordinates with the chosen lipstick. The liner color should not be dramatically different than the natural lip shade.

Before application, sharpen the pencil, and after use, sanitize the pencil. Remember to sanitize your sharpener also!

Beginning at the outer corner of the upper lip and working towards the middle, color the natural lip line. Repeat on the opposite side. Connect the center peaks with rounded strokes, following the natural lip line. Outline the lower lip from the outer corners in, and then apply liner on the lips, staying within the outline.

EYE SHADOW

Eye shadows are cosmetics applied on the eyelids to accentuate or contour them. They are available in almost every color of the rainbow, from warm to cool, neutral to bright, and light to dark. Some powder eye shadows are designed to be used wet or dry. They also come in a variety of finishes, including metallic, matte, frost, shimmer, or dewy.

Eye shadow is available in stick, cream, pressed, and dry powder form, and usually comes with an applicator (Figure 23-7).

USING EYE SHADOW

When applied to the lids, eye color or shadow makes the eyes appear brighter and more expressive. Matching eye shadow to eye color creates a flat field of color and should generally be avoided. Using color other than the actual eye color (i.e., a contrasting or complementary color) can enhance the eyes. Using light and dark can also bring attention to the eyes.

Generally, a darker shade of eye color makes the natural color of the iris appear lighter, while a lighter shade makes the iris appear deeper. However, the only set rules for selection of eye makeup colors are they should enhance the client's eyes, and color choices should be more subtle for daytime. If desired, eye makeup color may match or coordinate with the client's clothing color.

Eye shadow colors are generally referred to as highlight, base, and contour colors. A *highlight color* is lighter than the client's skin tone and may have any finish. Popular choices include matte or iridescent (shiny). As the name suggests, these colors highlight a specific area, such as the brow bone. Remember that a lighter color will make an area appear larger.

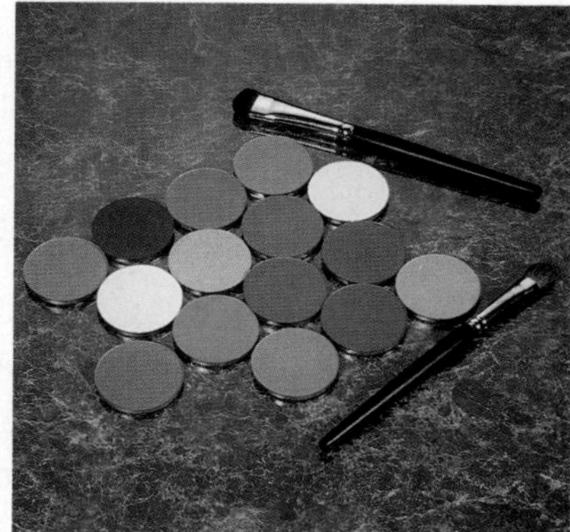

Figure 23-7 Eye shadows.

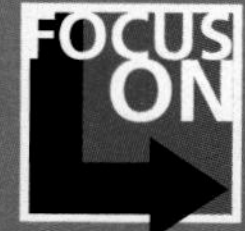

Focus on . . . Retailing

Lip colors create a huge opportunity for retail. Think of how many lipsticks you own. Most women own several lipsticks, glosses, and pencils. Some carry more than five at a time in their purses. Suggest a few colors to a client in a variety of finishes. Lip color is a simple way to change a look, and it provides a great way for your client to give herself a treat and brighten her day.

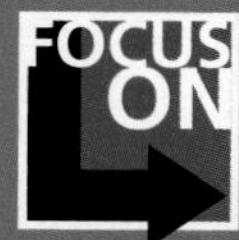

Focus on . . . Retailing

One of the biggest challenges that women face when purchasing cosmetics is finding the correct colors and finishes. When you start to use specific and "colorful" language, you will see a great improvement in your selling technique. Consider persuasive phrases such as the following:

- "This cocoa shadow will really make your green eyes look beautiful."
- "You have a great smile. This new peach lipstick will show it off."
- "What a great dress. This silver eyeliner would look fabulous with it."

Here's a TIP

Eye shadow in pressed powder form may be applied to the eyes with an eyeliner brush to create a softer lined effect. Whether using shadow or pencil liner, it may be helpful to pull the skin taut, from right below the eyebrow up, to ensure smooth application.

A *base color* is generally a medium tone that is close to the client's skin tone. It is available in a variety of finishes. This color is generally used to even skin tone on the eye. It is often applied all over the lid and brow bone from lash to brow before other colors are applied, thus providing a smooth surface for the blending of other colors. If used this way, a matte finish is generally preferred.

A *contour color* is a color, in any finish, that is deeper and darker than the client's skin tone. It is applied to minimize a specific area, to create contour in a crease, or to define the eyelash line.

To apply eye shadow, remove the product from its container with a spatula, and then use a fresh applicator or clean brush. Unless you are doing corrective makeup, apply the eye color close to the lashes on the upper eyelid, sweeping the color slightly upward and outward. Blend to achieve the desired effect. More than one color may be used if a particular effect is desired.

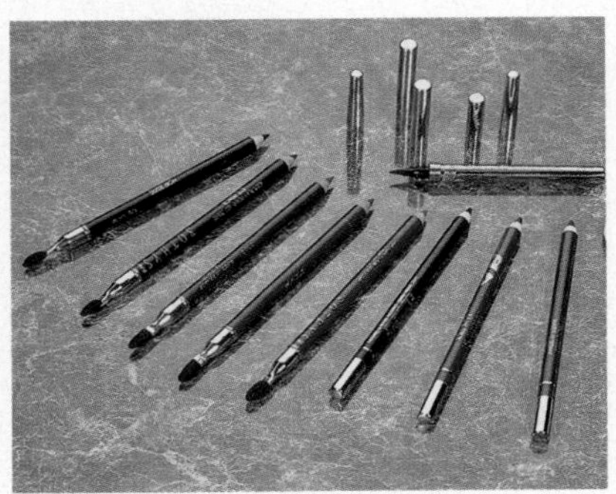

Figure 23-8 Eyeliners.

EYELINERS

Eyeliner is a cosmetic used to outline and emphasize the eyes. It is available in a variety of colors, in pencil, liquid, pressed (cake), or felt tip pen form.

With eyeliner you can create a line on the eyelid close to the lashes to make the eyes appear larger and the lashes fuller (Figure 23-8).

Eyeliner pencils consist of a wax (paraffin) or hardened oil base (petrolatum) with a variety of additives to create color. They are available in both soft and hard form for use on the eyebrow as well as the upper and lower eyelid.

CAUTION

According to the American Medical Association, eye pencils should not be used to color the inner rim of the eyes, because this can lead to infection of the tear duct, causing tearing, blurring of vision, and permanent pigmentation of the mucous membrane lining the inside of the eye.

USING EYELINERS

Most clients prefer eyeliner that is the same color as the lashes or mascara for a more natural look. More dramatic colors may be chosen depending on seasonal color trends.

Be extremely cautious when applying eyeliner. You must have a steady hand and be sure that your client remains still. Sharpen the eyeliner pencil and wipe with a clean tissue before each use. Also, remember to sanitize the sharpener before each use. Apply to the desired area with short strokes and gentle pressure; the most common placement is close to the lash line. For powder shadow liner application, scrape a small amount onto a tissue and apply to the eyes with a disposable applicator or clean brush. If desired, wet the brush before the application for a more dramatic look.

EYEBROW COLOR

Eyebrow pencils or shadows are used to add color and shape to the eyebrows, usually after tweezing or waxing. They can be used to darken the eyebrows, correct their shape, or fill in sparse areas. Brow powders are similar to pressed eye shadows, and are applied to the brows with a brush. Brow powders cling to eyebrow hairs, making the brows appear darker and fuller.

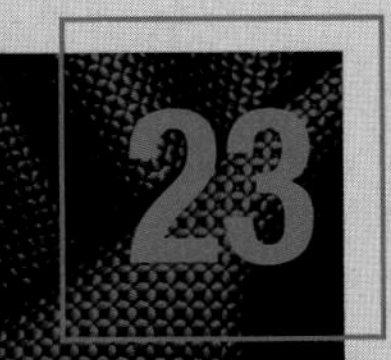

The chemistry of eyebrow pencils is similar to that of eyeliner pencil. The chemical ingredients in eyebrow shadows are also similar to those in eye shadows.

USING EYEBROW COLOR

Sharpen the eyebrow pencil and wipe with clean tissue before each use. Sanitize the sharpener before each use. For powder shadow application, scrape a small amount onto a tissue and use a disposable applicator or clean brush to apply shadow to brows. Avoid harsh contrasts between hair and eyebrow color, such as pale blond or silver hair with black eyebrows.

MASCARA

Mascara is a cosmetic preparation used to darken, define, and thicken the eyelashes. It is available in liquid, cake, and cream form, and in a variety of shades and tints (Figure 23-9). Mascara brushes can be straight or curved, with fine or thick bristles. The most popular mascara colors are shades of brown and black, which enhance the natural lashes, making them appear thicker and longer.

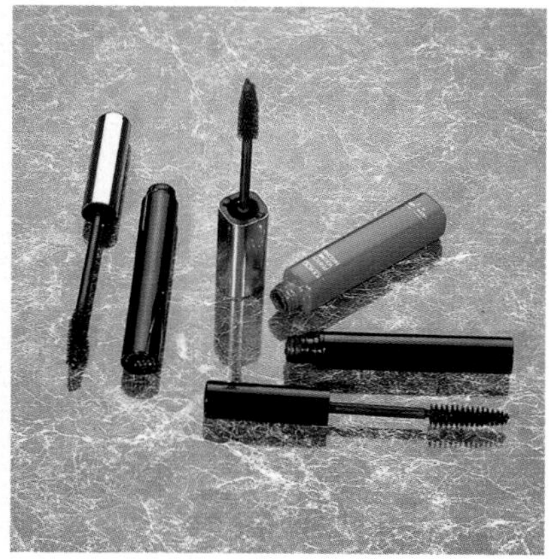

Figure 23-9 Mascara products.

Mascara is available in tube and wand applicators. Both are polymer products that include water, wax, thickeners, film formers, and preservatives. The pigments in mascara must be inert (unable to combine with other elements) and usually are carbon black, carmine, ultramarine, chromium oxide, and iron oxides. Some wand mascaras contain rayon or nylon fibers to lengthen and thicken the hair fibers.

USING MASCARA

Mascara may be used on all the lashes, from the inner to outer corners. Using a disposable wand, dip into a clean tube of mascara and apply from close to the base of the lashes out toward the tips, making sure your client is comfortable throughout the application. Dispose of the wand. Never double-dip!

If you are using an eyelash curler, you must curl the lashes before applying mascara. If lashes are curled after mascara, eyelashes may be broken or pulled out. Use extreme caution whenever using an eyelash curler.

The easiest way to learn how to use this tool is by first observing its use. Ask your instructor to demonstrate before attempting to use an eyelash curler on someone else.

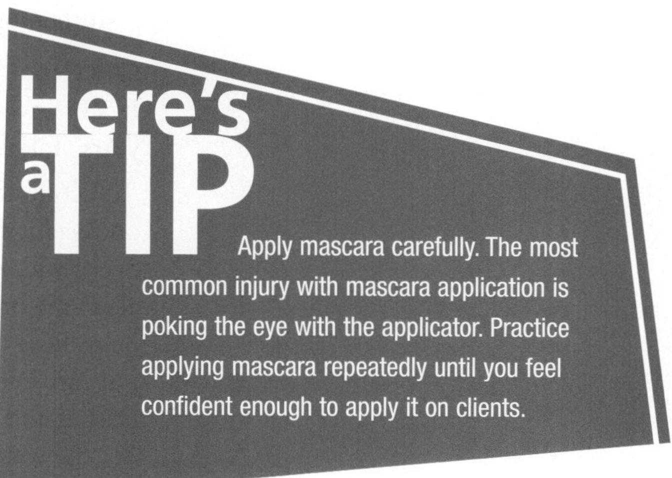

Here's a TIP

Apply mascara carefully. The most common injury with mascara application is poking the eye with the applicator. Practice applying mascara repeatedly until you feel confident enough to apply it on clients.

OTHER COSMETICS

Eye makeup removers do just that: remove eye makeup. Most eye makeup products are water-resistant, so plain soap and water are less effective for removal. Eye makeup removers are either oil-based or water-based. Oil-based removers are generally mineral oil with a small amount of fragrance added. Water-based removers are comprised of a water solution to which other solvents have been added.

Greasepaint is a heavy makeup used for theatrical purposes. **Cake (pancake) makeup** is a shaped, solid mass applied to the face with a

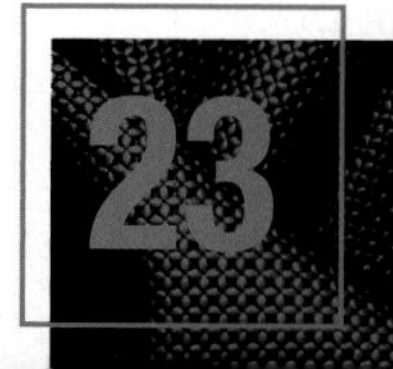

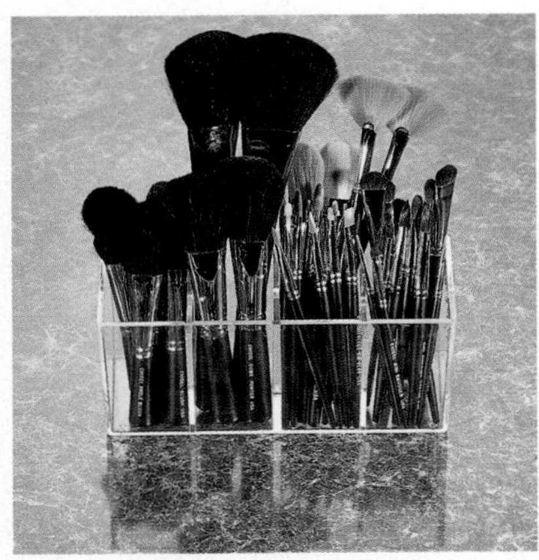

Figure 23–10 Makeup brushes.

moistened cosmetic sponge. It gives good coverage and is generally used to cover scars and pigmentation defects.

MAKEUP BRUSHES AND OTHER TOOLS

Makeup brushes come in a variety of shapes and sizes (Figure 23-10). They may be made of synthetic or animal hair with wooden or metal handles. Commonly used makeup brushes and implements are listed below.

- *Powder brush.* Large, soft brush used to apply powder and for blending edges of color.
- *Blush brush.* Smaller, more tapered version of the powder brush, excellent for applying powder cheek color.
- *Concealer brush.* Usually narrow and firm with a flat edge, used to apply concealer around the eyes or over blemishes.
- *Lip brush.* Similar to the concealer brush, with a more tapered edge; may be used to apply concealer or lip color.
- *Eye shadow brushes.* Available in a variety of sizes, from small to large, and in finishes from soft to firm. The softer and larger the brush, the more diffused and blended the shadow will be. A firm brush is better for depositing dense color than for blending it.
- *Eyeliner brush.* Fine, tapered, firm bristles; used to apply liquid liner or shadow to the eyes.
- *Angle brush.* Firm, thin bristle; angled for ease of application of shadow to the eyebrows or shadow liner to the eyes.
- *Lash and brow brush.* Comb-like brush used to remove excess mascara on lashes or to comb brows into place.
- *Tweezers.* Available in metal or plastic; used to remove excess facial hair.
- *Eyelash curler.* Metal or plastic device used to give lift and upward curl to the upper lashes.

CARING FOR MAKEUP BRUSHES

If you invest in high-quality makeup brushes, you will have them for years. Take good care of your brushes by cleaning them gently.

A commercial sanitizer can be used for quick cleaning, although spray-on instant sanitizers contain a high level of alcohol and will dry brushes over time. A gentle shampoo or brush solvent should be used to truly clean the brushes. These products will not hurt brushes and may actually help them last longer. One cautionary note: the brush should always be put into running or still water with the ferrule (the metal ring that keeps bristles and handle together) pointing downward. If the brush is pointed up, the water may remove the glue that keeps the bristles in place. Rinse brushes thoroughly after cleansing. Because they will dry in the shape they are left in, reshape the wet bristles and lay the brushes flat to dry.

DISPOSABLE IMPLEMENTS

Disposable implements include the following items:

- *Sponges.* Available in a variety of sizes and shapes, including wedges and circles, and work well to apply and blend foundation, cream or powder blush, powder, or concealer.

- *Powder or cotton puffs.* May be made of velour or cotton and are used to apply and blend powder, powder foundation, or powder blush.
- *Mascara wands.* Usually plastic and are used to apply mascara on a client; generally disposable, so as to ensure proper hygiene.
- *Spatulas.* Wooden or plastic, with a wide, flat base; used to remove makeup such as lipstick, foundation, concealer, powder, blush, and shadow from their containers.
- *Disposable lip brushes.* May be plastic or another synthetic; used to hygienically apply lip color to a client.
- *Sponge-tipped shadow applicators.* Used to apply shadow and lip color or to blend eyeliner; may be used to remove unwanted makeup from eyes or lips.
- *Cotton swabs.* May be used to apply shadow, blend eyeliner, or remove unwanted makeup from the eyes or lips.
- *Cotton pads or puffs.* May be used with astringents or makeup removers; also used to apply powder products.
- *Pencil sharpener.* Used before each application of eye or lip liner pencil to ensure hygienic application.

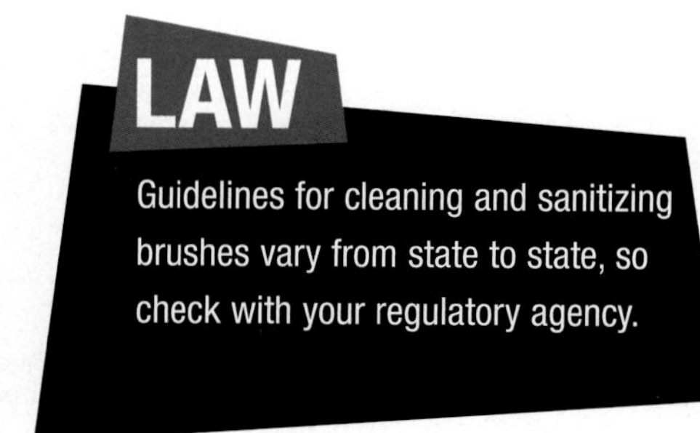
LAW
Guidelines for cleaning and sanitizing brushes vary from state to state, so check with your regulatory agency.

MAKEUP COLOR THEORY

A strong understanding of how color works is vital to effective makeup application. Everyone sees color a little differently, and it may take a while to learn to see color naturally and easily. The following guide will help you to identify primary, secondary, and tertiary colors, as well as warm, cool, and complementary colors. Once you understand these basics of color theory, you can use your creative instincts to invent any color palette you desire.

Primary colors are fundamental colors that cannot be obtained from a mixture. The primary colors are yellow, red, and blue (Figure 23-11).

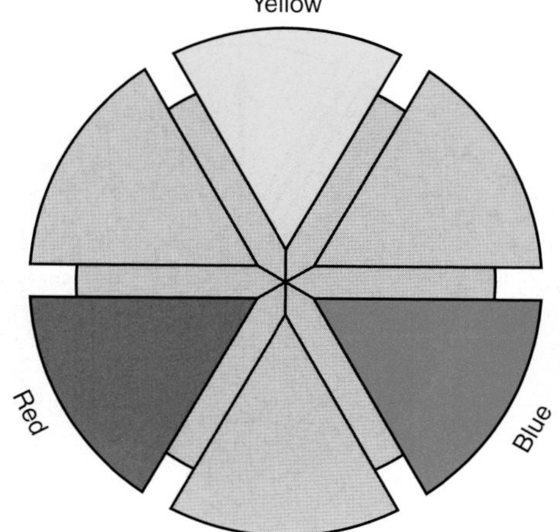

Figure 23–11 Primary colors.

Secondary colors are obtained by mixing equal parts of two primary colors. Yellow mixed with red makes orange. Red mixed with blue makes violet. Yellow mixed with blue makes green (Figure 23-12).

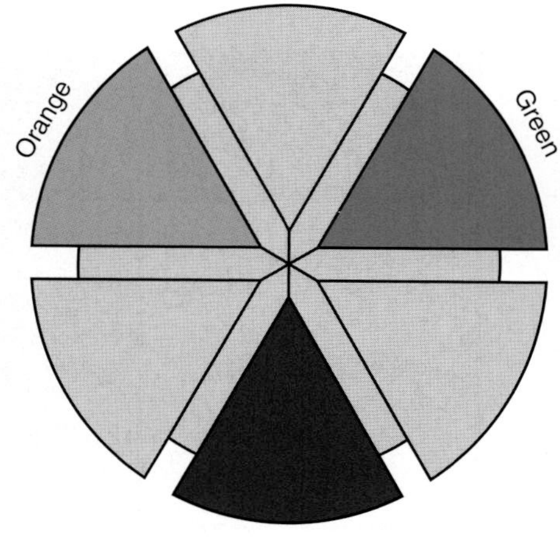

Figure 23–12 Secondary colors.

Tertiary colors are formed by mixing equal amounts of a secondary color and its neighboring primary color on the color wheel. These colors are named by primary color first, and secondary color second. For example, when we mix blue (a primary) with violet (a neighboring secondary), we call the resulting color blue-violet (Figure 23-13).

Primary and secondary colors directly opposite each other on the color wheel are called complementary colors. When mixed, these colors cancel each other out to create a neutral brown or gray color. When complementary colors are placed next to each other, each color makes the

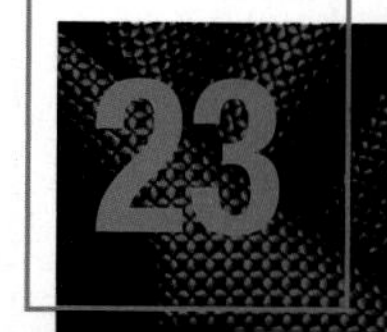

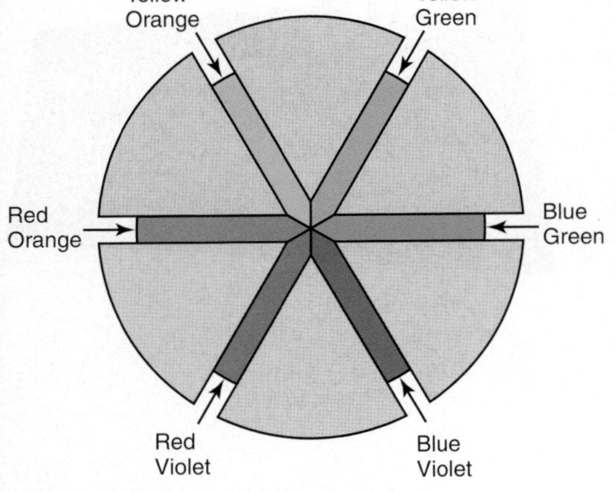

Figure 23-13 Tertiary colors.

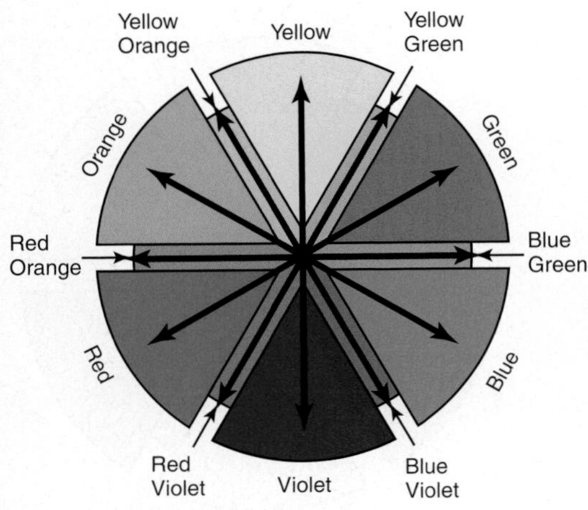

Figure 23-14 Complementary colors.

other look brighter, resulting in greater contrast. For example, if you place blue next to orange, the blue seems bluer, the orange brighter. Try this with markers or colored paper to compare. The concept of complementary colors is useful when determining color choice. For example, the use of complementary colors will emphasize eye color, making the eyes appear brighter (Figure 23-14).

WARM AND COOL COLORS

Learning the difference between warm and cool colors is essential to your success as a makeup artist. This is the basis of all color selection, and understanding the difference will enable you to properly enhance your client's coloring.

As you look at the color wheel, think of it as a tool in determining color choice. There are three main factors to consider when choosing colors for a client: skin color, eye color, and hair color.

DETERMINING SKIN COLOR

When determining skin color, you must first decide if the skin is light, medium, or dark in level. Then determine whether the tone of the skin is warm or cool (use Table 23-1 as a guide). You may not see skin colors truly in the beginning. Give yourself time and practice to develop your eye.

Warm colors are the range from yellow and gold through the oranges, red-oranges, most reds, and even some yellow-greens. **Cool colors** suggest coolness and are dominated by blues, greens, violets, and blue-reds (Figure 23-15). You will notice that reds can be both warm and cool. If the red is orange-based, it is warm. If it is blue-based, it is cool. Green is similar: if a green contains more gold, it is warm; if it contains more blue, it is cool.

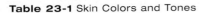

SKIN COLORS	Warm	Cool
Light skin	yellow, gold, pale peach	pink or slightly ruddy (reddish); florid undertones
Medium skin	yellow, yellow-orange, red	olive (yellow-green)
Dark skin	red, orange-brown, red-brown	dark olive, blue, blue-black, ebony

Table 23-1 Skin Colors and Tones

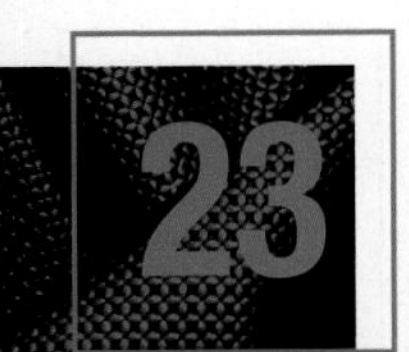

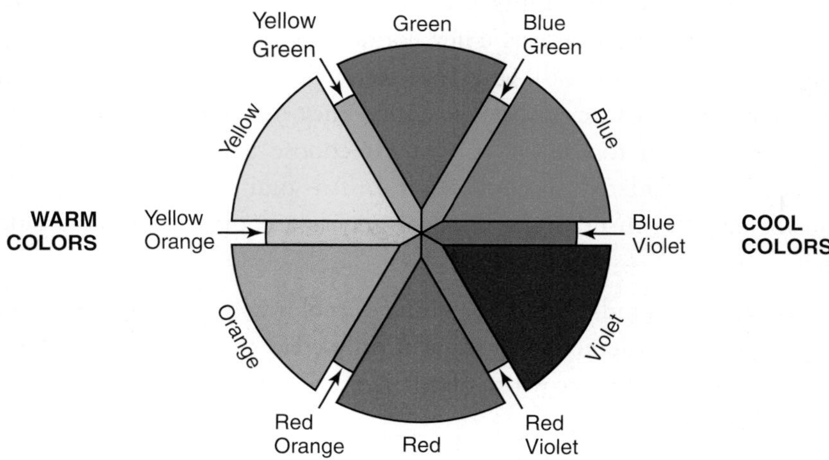

Figure 23-15 Warm and cool colors.

You may hear people refer to a color as having a lot of blue in it. For example: "This lipstick has a blue base" or "That blush is very blue." This does not mean that the color is truly blue. Rather, it means that when the pigments were mixed to create that cosmetic, more blue color was added. What you are seeing might look primarily violet or magenta.

SELECTING MAKEUP COLORS

Now that we have defined warms and cools, it is time to learn a system that will help you feel more comfortable when choosing colors for your clients. Keep in mind that this is simply one way of choosing colors. The art of makeup application allows for more than one way to achieve the result you want.

A neutral skin tone contains equal elements of warm and cool, no matter how light or dark the skin is. Remember to always match your foundation color to the color of the skin, or use the corrective techniques discussed later in this chapter.

Once you have determined if the skin is light, medium, or dark, you may choose eye, cheek, and lip colors to match the skin color in level, or try contrast for more impact. Most skin tones and levels can wear a surprisingly wide range of eye, cheek, and lip colors.

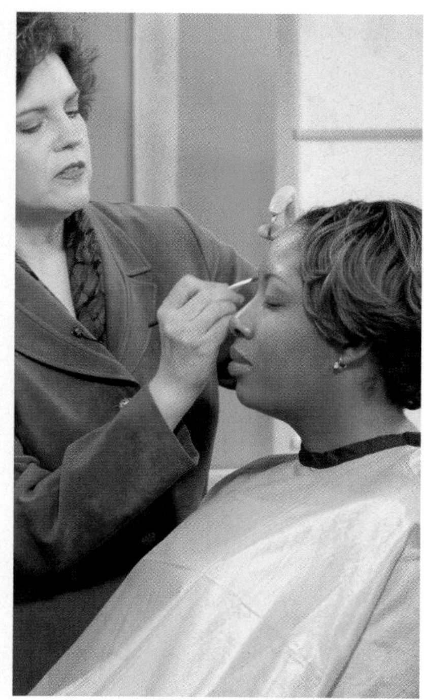

Figure 23-16 Choose cosmetics to enhance your client's skin color and hair color.

- If skin color is light, you may use light colors for a soft, natural look. Medium to dark colors will create a more dramatic look.
- If skin color is medium, medium tones will create an understated look. Light or dark tones will provide more contrast and will appear bolder.
- If skin color is dark, dark tones will be most subtle. Medium to medium-light or bright tones will be striking and vivid (Figure 23-16).

Be cautious when choosing tones lighter than the skin. If the color is too light, it will turn gray or chalky on the skin. Look for translucent, shimmery colors if you are choosing these tones.

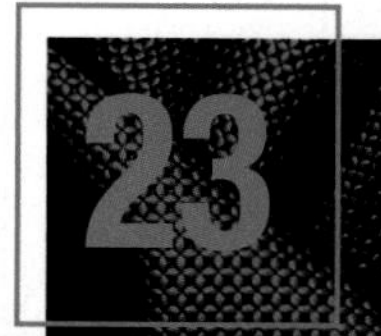

COMPLEMENTARY COLORS FOR EYES

As you begin recommending eye, cheek, and lip colors, neutrals will always be your safest choice. They contain elements of warm and cool and work well on any skin tone, eye color, or hair color. They come in variations of brown or gray. For instance, they may have a warm or cool base with brown tones. Or you might choose a plum-brown, which would be considered a cool neutral. An orange-brown would be considered a warm neutral. Charcoal gray is a cool neutral, as is blue-gray.

Contrary to popular belief, matching eye color with shadow color is not the best way to enhance this area as it only creates a flat region of color. By contrasting eye color with complementary colors, you emphasize the color most effectively.

The following is a guideline for eye color selection. You may refer back to the color wheel for additional help in determining complementary colors.

REVIEWING COLOR SELECTION STEPS

1. Determine skin level: light, medium, or dark.
2. Determine skin undertone: warm, cool, or neutral.
3. Determine eye color: blue, green, brown, and so forth.
4. Determine complementary colors.
5. Determine hair color: warm or cool.
6. Choose eye makeup colors based on complementary or contrasting colors.
7. Coordinate cheek and lip colors within the same color family: warm, cool, or neutral.
8. Apply makeup.

The best thing about choosing colors is the unlimited number of choices you have. Try one or all methods of choosing color. Complementary color choices for eye colors are summarized below.

- *Complementary colors for blue eyes.* Orange is the complementary color to blue. Because orange contains yellow and red, shadows with any of these colors in them will make eyes look bluer. Common choices include gold, warm orange-browns like peach and copper, red-browns like mauves and plum, and neutrals like taupe or camel.
- *Complementary colors for green eyes.* Red is the complementary color to green. Because red shadows tend to make the eyes look tired or bloodshot, pure red tones are not recommended. Instead, use brown-based reds or other color options next to red on the color wheel. These include red-orange, red-violet, and violet. Popular choices are coppers, rusts, pinks, plums, mauves, and purples.
- *Complementary colors for brown eyes.* Brown eyes are neutral and can wear any color. Recommended choices include contrasting colors such as greens, blues, grays, and silvers.

ADDING CHEEK AND LIP COLOR

After you have chosen eye makeup, use the color wheel to determine whether your choices are warm or cool and then coordinate cheek and lip makeup in the same color family as the eye makeup. For example, if your client has green eyes, you recommended plums for her, which are cool. Now you should stay with cool colors for the cheeks and lips in order to coordinate with the eye makeup. You may also choose neutrals, as these contain both warm and cool elements and coordinate with any makeup colors.

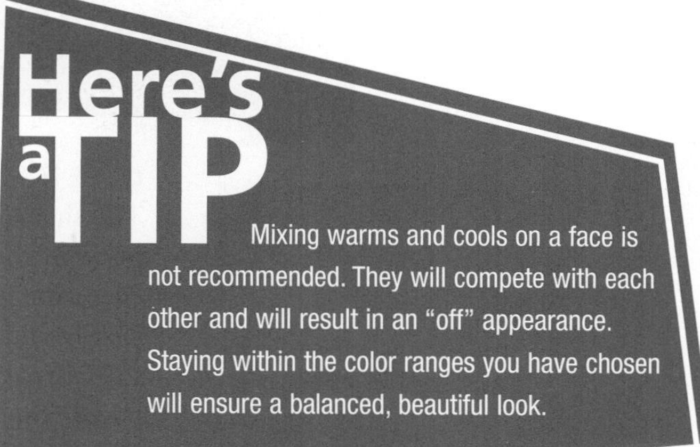

Mixing warms and cools on a face is not recommended. They will compete with each other and will result in an "off" appearance. Staying within the color ranges you have chosen will ensure a balanced, beautiful look.

HAIR COLOR AND EYE COLOR

Hair color needs to be taken into account when determining eye makeup color. For example, if a woman has blue eyes, your instinct might be to select orange-based eye makeup as the complementary choice. But if she has cool blue-black hair, the orange will not be flattering. In this case, you would choose cool colors to coordinate with the hair color. Red-violets (plums) would be a more flattering choice. Look at orange on the color wheel: it is warm. Go around the wheel toward the cool end. Red-violets are the closest to orange on the color wheel while still remaining cool. As stated earlier, there is a range of colors to choose from for any client. Use Table 23-2 as a general guide.

HAIR COLOR	Warm	Cool
Blond hair	yellow, orange	white-blond, ash
Red hair	gold, copper, orange, red	red-violet, violet
Brown hair	yellow, gold, orange	ash
Dark brown/black hair	copper, red	violet, blue

Table 23-2 Determining Hair Color Tones

ACTIVITY

Apply makeup to a partner, using color theory to choose and coordinate makeup colors. Have fun and experiment. Keep track of which colors enhance her appearance and coordinate with her wardrobe, and which ones do not. And remember, while a haircut or haircolor may represent a big commitment, makeup does not. If you do not like it, you can simply wash it off and try again!

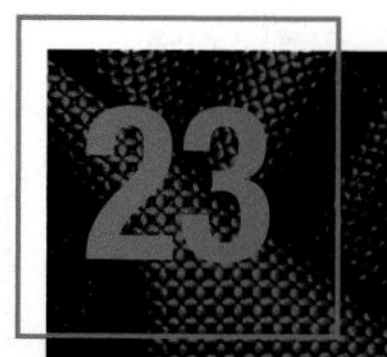

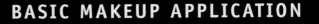

BASIC MAKEUP APPLICATION

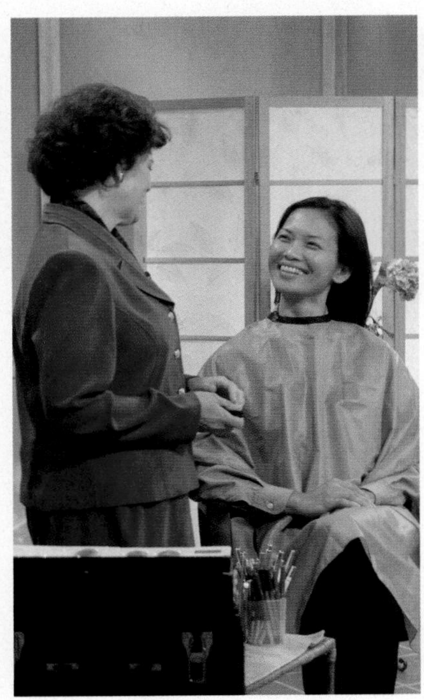

Figure 23-17 Client consultation.

CLIENT CONSULTATION

The first step in the makeup process, as with all other services that take place in the salon, is the client consultation. This is where you ask the client the questions that will bring out her wishes and concerns. Listen closely and try not to impose your own opinions too much. Your role is to listen to what your client is saying, and only then make recommendations based on your knowledge. If she chooses not to act on your recommendations, do not take it personally. In time, perhaps she will.

CONSULTATION AREA

The area that you use for consultations must be clean and tidy. No one wants to see a messy makeup unit or dirty brushes lying about. Clean your brushes after each use and tidy your makeup area daily. Also, keep a portfolio in the consultation area that includes photographs of your own work, or pictures from magazines. The client can go through your portfolio to find styles and colors that appeal to her.

LIGHTING

Adequate and flattering lighting is essential for both the consultation and application parts of the makeup process. Be sure your client's face is evenly lit and without dark shadows. Natural light is the best choice, but if it is necessary to use artificial light, it should be a combination of incandescent light (warm bulb light) and fluorescent light (cool industrial tube light). If you must choose between the two, incandescent light will be more flattering.

Make sure that the light always shines directly and evenly on the face. And remember, good lighting makes a client look good, and clients who look good are more likely to purchase the products you recommend. When this happens, everyone comes out a winner.

MAKEUP CONSULTATION

A makeup service should always begin with a warm introduction to your client. Visually assess her to understand her personal style. This will give you cues as you continue your consultation (Figure 23-17).

Engaging the client in conversation will help you to determine her needs. Gather whatever information you can on her skin condition, how much or how little makeup she wears, daily versus special occasion makeup, the amount of time she spends applying makeup, colors she likes or dislikes, and any makeup areas she is having trouble with.

Record this information on a client consultation card. Also, write down your recommendations so that you may refer back to them at the end of the makeup application. Reviewing and restating your written advice with the client at the end of the service will also help you sell the retail products you hope she will purchase (Figure 23-18). Escort your client to the reception area where you can assist her in gathering the products that

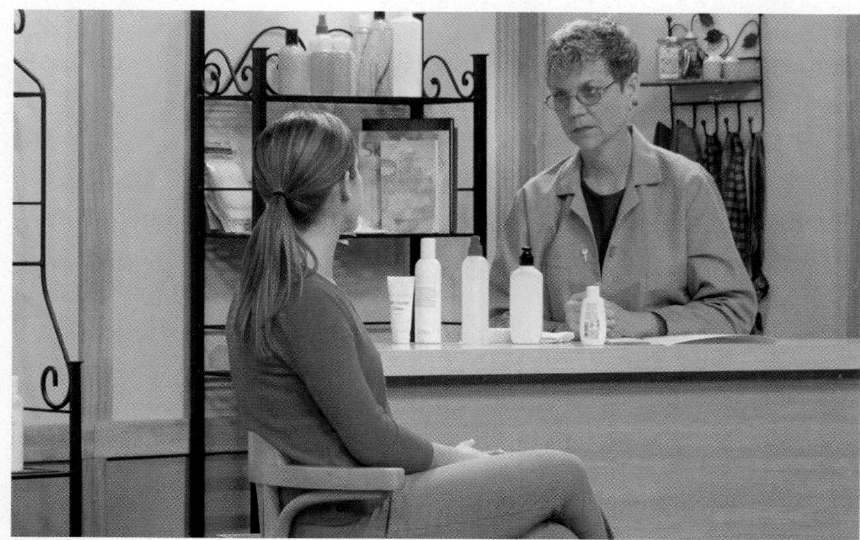

Figure 23–18 Retailing cosmetic products.

you have recommended. Ask her if she has any other questions and, if so, give clear answers. If possible, set up a time for her next appointment. Then give her a business card with your name on it and shake her hand as you turn her over to the receptionist who will check her out.

PROCEDURE 23-1

PROFESSIONAL MAKEUP APPLICATION

EQUIPMENT, IMPLEMENTS, AND MATERIALS

Skin Care

- Cleansers
- Astringent and skin freshening lotion
- Moisturizers

Makeup

- Foundations
- Concealers
- Face powders
- Lip liners
- Cheek colors
- Lip colors
- Eye shadows
- Eyeliner pencils
- Mascara

Procedure accessories

- Towels and draping sheets, if desired
- Makeup cape
- Headband or hair clip
- Eyelash curler
- Assorted makeup brushes (for eye shadow, eyeliner, lip color, concealer, blush, powder, and flat or slanted brush for brows or eyeliner)
- Small makeup palette

Disposables

- Mascara wands
- Shadow applicators
- Sponge wedges
- Tissues
- Pencil sharpener
- Disposable lip brushes
- Cotton swabs
- Spatulas
- Cotton pads or puffs

PREPARATION

1. **Client consultation.** Determine the client's needs and choose products and colors accordingly.
2. Wash your hands.
3. Drape the client and use a headband or hair clip to keep the hair out of the face (Figure 23-19).

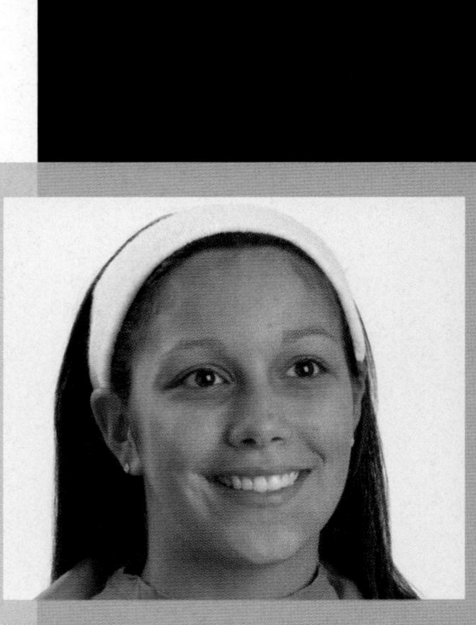

Figure 23-19 Use a headband to keep the client's hair off her face.

4. **Apply cleansing cream or lotion.** Remove a small quantity of cleanser from the container with a spatula and place it in the palm of the left hand, or apply a dab of lotion to an applicator. With the fingertips of the right hand, place dabs of cleanser on the forehead, nose, cheeks, chin, and neck. Spread the cleanser over the face and neck with light upward and outward circular movements (Figure 23-20).
5. **Remove cleanser.** Use tissue mitts or moistened cotton pads to remove the cleanser, using an upward and outward motion (Figure 23-21). Be especially gentle around the eyes. If makeup or color is particularly heavy on the eyes and lips, apply the cleanser a second time, as needed.
6. **Apply astringent lotion or toner.** For oily skin, apply astringent lotion; for dry skin, apply a skin toner. Moisten a cotton pad with the lotion and pat it lightly over the entire face and under the chin and neck. Blot off excess moisture with tissues or a cotton pad (Figure 23-22).
7. **Apply moisturizer.** When necessary, as in the case of dry and delicate skin, apply a moisturizing lotion. Dab a small amount of the moisturizer on the forehead, cheeks, and chin. Blend upward over the face. Remove excess with a tissue, cotton pad, or facial sponge.
8. **Groom eyebrows.** Eyebrow arching (tweezing) is a complete service in itself (see Chapter 21.) You may, however, choose to remove a few stray hairs before a facial makeup by tweezing the hair in the same direction in which it grows.

PROCEDURE

1. **Apply foundation.** Test the color by blending the foundation on the client's jawline. When you are satisfied with your choice, place a small amount of the foundation on a palette, in the palm, or on the back of your hand and, using the tips of your fingers or a cosmetic sponge, apply sparingly and evenly over the entire face and around the neckline.

   Starting at the center of the face, blend with outward and downward motions (Figure 23-23). Blend near the hairline, and remove excess foundation with a cosmetic sponge or cotton pledget.

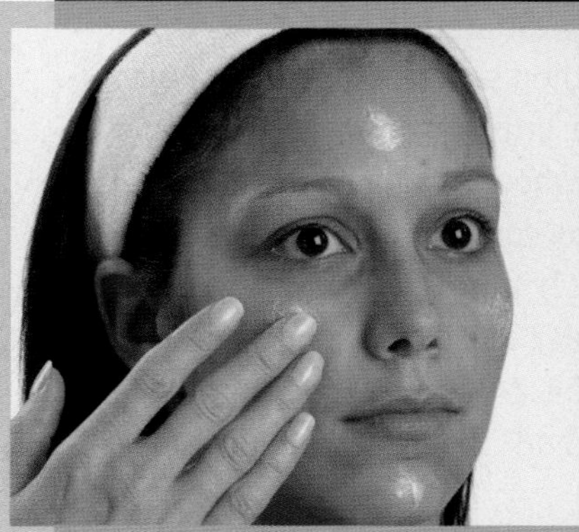

Figure 23-20 Apply cleansing cream or lotion.

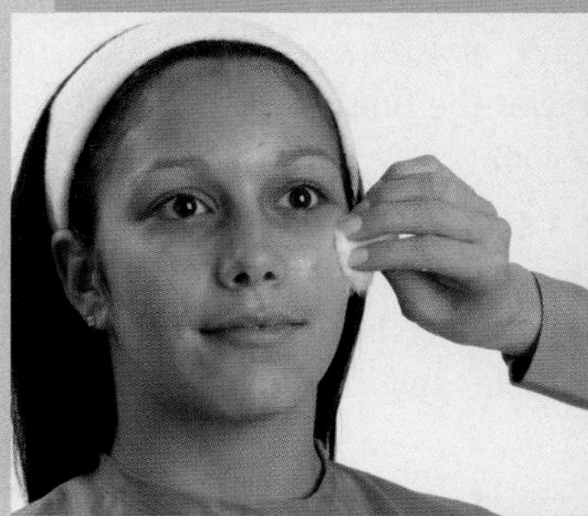

Figure 23-21 Remove the cleanser.

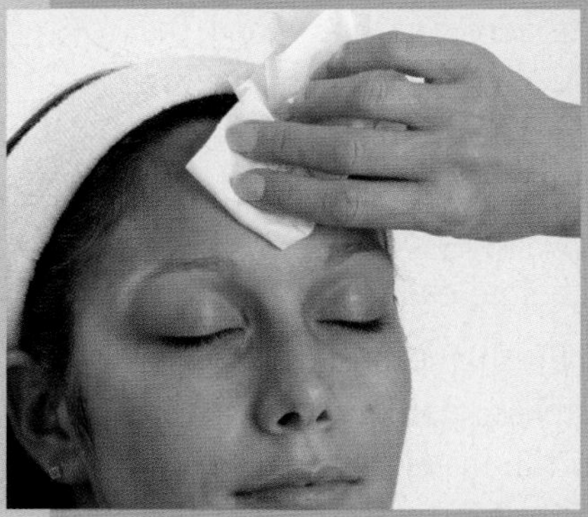

Figure 23-22 Blot excess moisture.

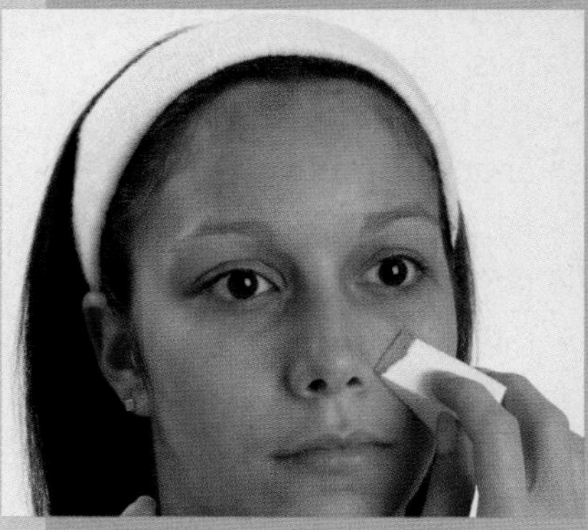

Figure 23-23 Apply foundation.

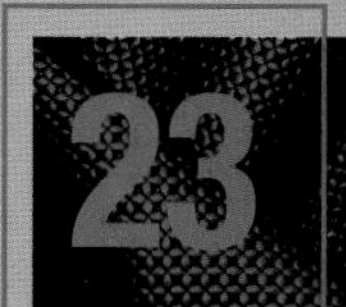

2. **Apply concealer.** Select the appropriate type and color of concealer and then scrape a small amount onto a spatula. Using a brush or fingertips, apply the concealer lightly where needed (under the eyes, over blemishes, to cover redness). Blend in with a patting motion. If a powder foundation is being used, the concealer must be applied before the foundation (Figure 23-24). Your instructor may prefer a different method that may be equally correct.
3. **Apply powder.** Apply the powder with a sanitary puff or cosmetic sponge, pressing it over the face and whisking off the excess with a puff or powder brush (Figure 23-25). A moistened cosmetic sponge may be pressed over the finished makeup to give the face a matte look.
4. **Apply eye color.** Select a complementary color in a medium tone and then, beginning at the lash line or crease, apply lightly and blend outward with a brush or disposable applicator (Figure 23-26).
5. **Apply eyeliner.** Select pencil, pressed, or liquid liner in a color to harmonize with the mascara you will be applying. Pull the eyelid taut as the client looks down, and draw a very fine line along the entire lid (Figure 23-27). You may apply to the top lash line and/or bottom lash line. If eyeliner pencil is used, the point should be fine and care should be taken to avoid injury or discomfort. Be sure to trim the pencil before each use.
6. **Apply eyebrow color.** Brush the brows in place. With light feathery strokes, apply color with a fine-pointed pencil or fill in with a brush and shadow (Figure 23-28). Excess color can be removed with a cotton-tipped swab.
7. **Apply mascara.** Apply mascara to the top and underside of the upper lashes with careful, gentle strokes until the desired effect is achieved (Figure 23-29). Use a fresh brush or applicator to separate the lashes. Mascara may be applied to the lower lashes if desired, but the effect should be subtle.
8. **Apply cheek color.** Have the client smile, to raise the cheeks, and then apply powder cheek color,

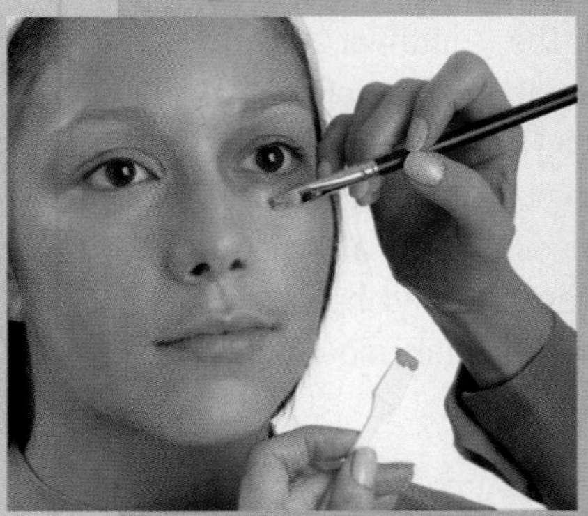

Figure 23-24 Apply concealer.

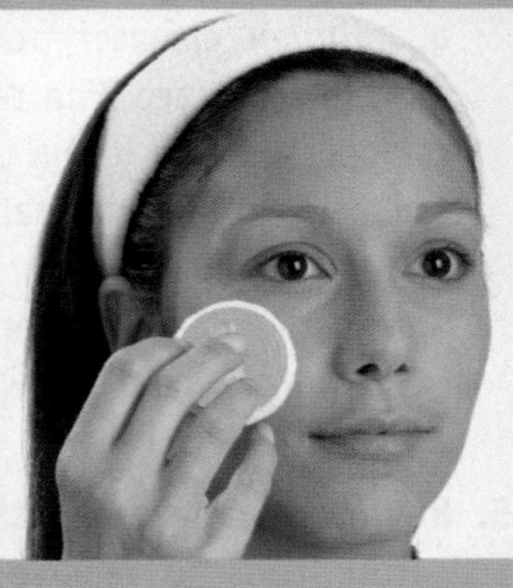

Figure 23-25 Apply powder.

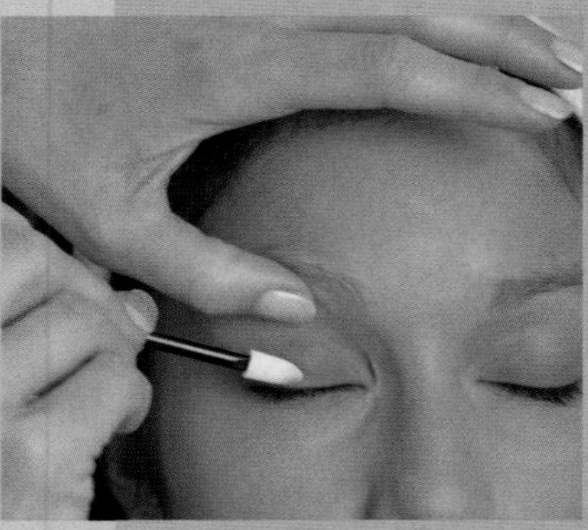

Figure 23-26 Apply eye color.

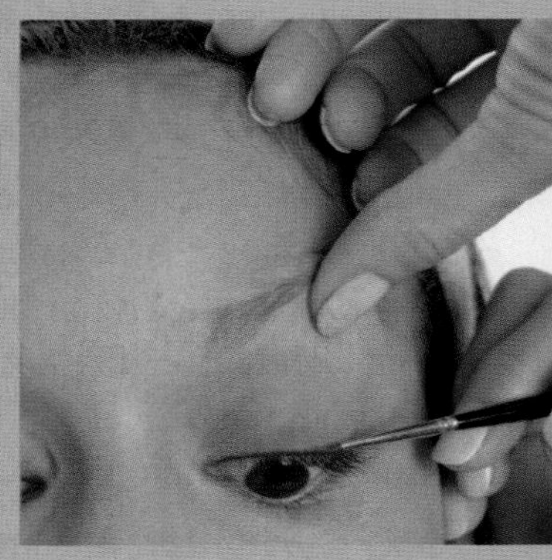

Figure 23-27 Apply eyeliner.

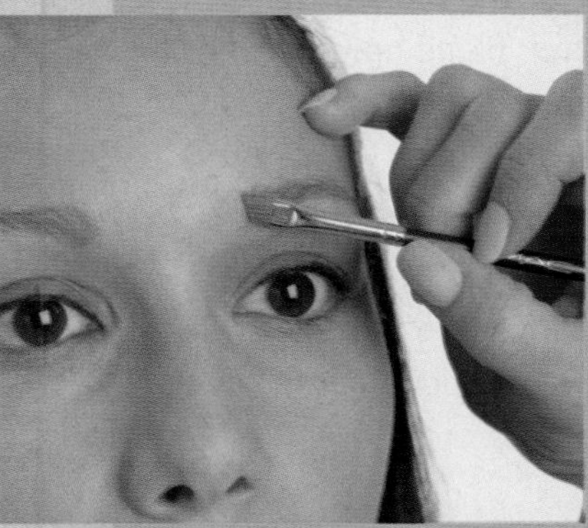

Figure 23-28 Apply eyebrow color.

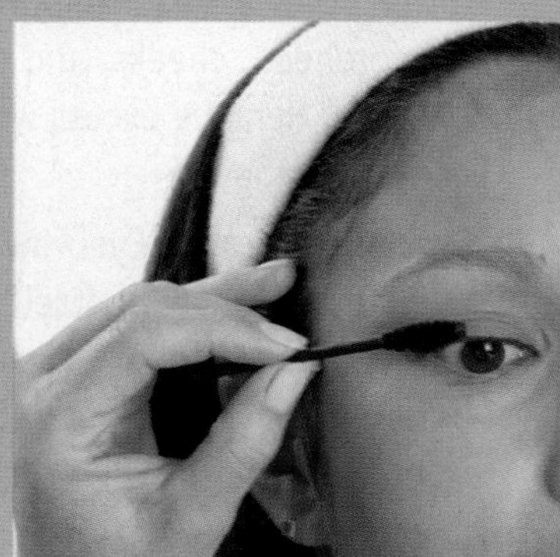

Figure 23-29 Apply mascara.

blending outward and upward toward the temples (Figure 23-30). Liquid or cream cheek color is applied with a sanitized applicator before powder, and sometimes on bare skin.

9. **Apply lip color.** Use a freshly sharpened pencil to line the lips, beginning at the outer corner of the upper lip and working toward the middle (Figure 23-31). Repeat on the opposite side. Connect the center peaks using rounded strokes, following the natural line of the lip.

   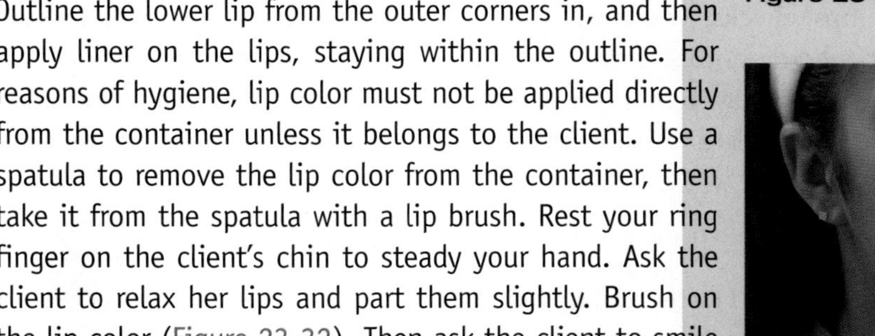

   Outline the lower lip from the outer corners in, and then apply liner on the lips, staying within the outline. For reasons of hygiene, lip color must not be applied directly from the container unless it belongs to the client. Use a spatula to remove the lip color from the container, then take it from the spatula with a lip brush. Rest your ring finger on the client's chin to steady your hand. Ask the client to relax her lips and part them slightly. Brush on the lip color (Figure 23-32). Then ask the client to smile slightly so that you can smooth the lip color into any small crevices. Blot the lips with tissue to remove excess product and set the lip color. Powdering is not recommended, as a moist look is more desirable for lips (Figure 23-33).

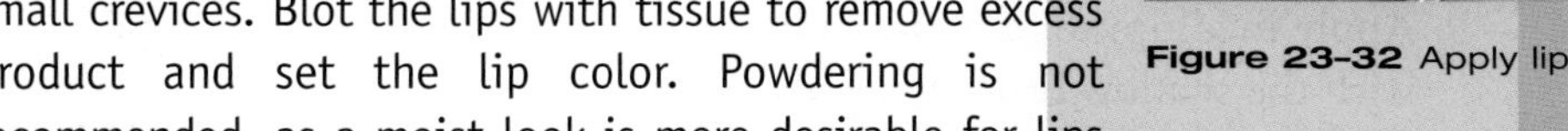

CLEANUP AND SANITATION

1. Discard all disposable items, such as sponges, pads, spatulas, and applicators, after each use.
2. Disinfect implements such as eyelash curlers.
3. Clean and sanitize brushes using a commercial brush sanitizer.
4. Place towels, linens, makeup cape, and other washable items in a hamper.
5. Sanitize your workstation.
6. Wash your hands with soap and warm water.

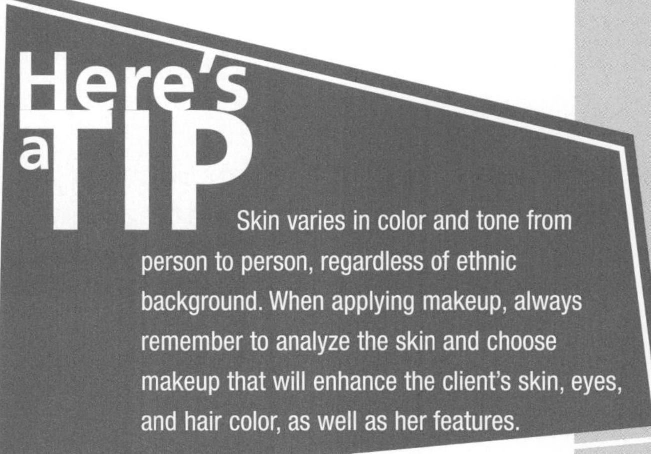

Skin varies in color and tone from person to person, regardless of ethnic background. When applying makeup, always remember to analyze the skin and choose makeup that will enhance the client's skin, eyes, and hair color, as well as her features.

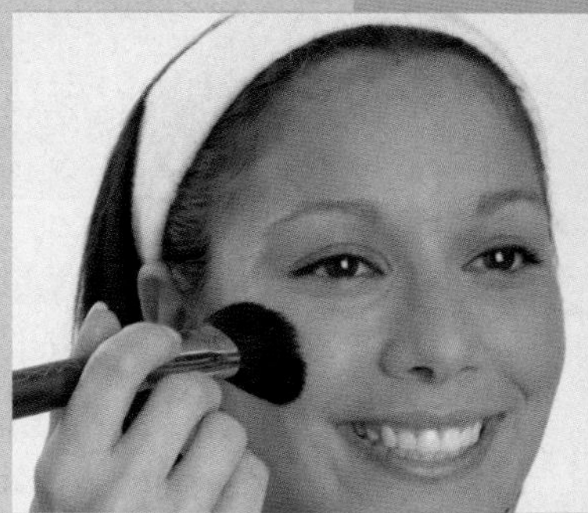

Figure 23-30 Apply cheek color.

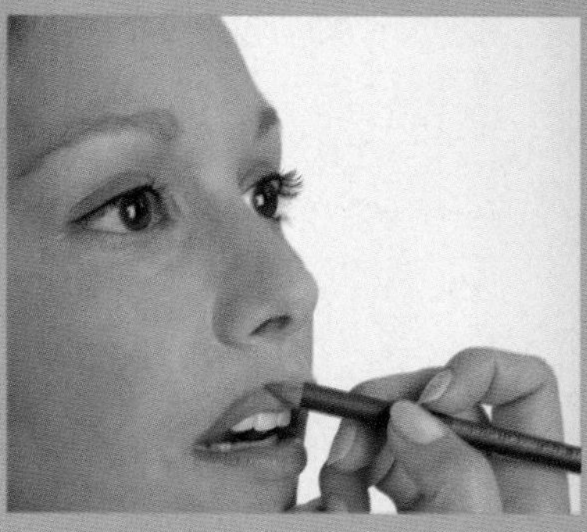

Figure 23-31 Outline the lips with lip liner.

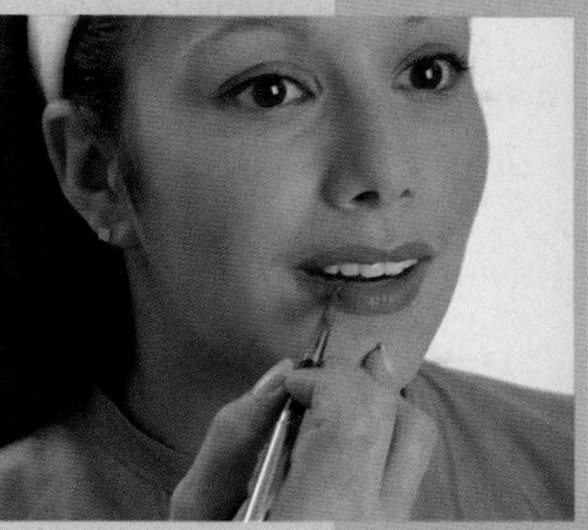

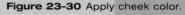

Figure 23-32 Apply lip color.

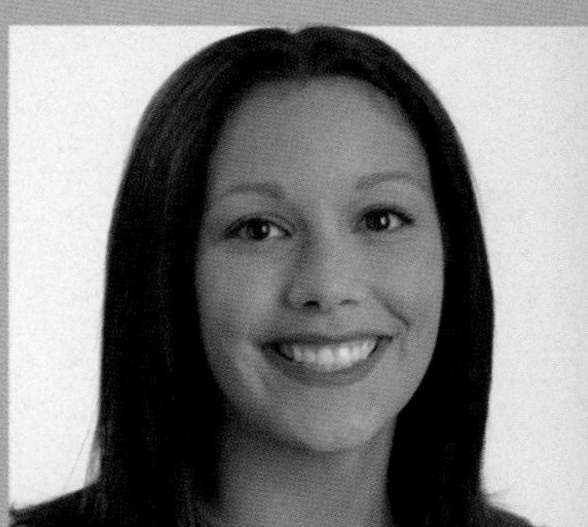

Figure 23-33 Finished makeup application.

CAUTION

Remember, when applying mascara, use a disposable mascara wand and dip into a clean tube of mascara. Then dispose of the wand. Never "double dip."

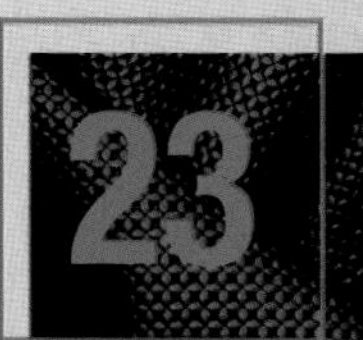

SPECIAL-OCCASION MAKEUP

When a client asks for makeup for a special occasion, the time is right to work your magic. Special occasions often come with special conditions.

For instance, many are evening events, when lighting is subdued. That means more definition is required for the eyes, cheeks, and lips. You may also add drama by applying false lashes and using shimmery colors on the eyes, lips, cheeks, or complexion. If the special occasion is a wedding, however, where photography is an issue, matte colors are recommended, since shimmer may reflect light too much. Follow the basic makeup procedure above but consider the pointers discussed in the following subsections.

SPECIAL-OCCASION MAKEUP FOR EYES

OPTION 1: STRIKING CONTOUR EYES

1. Apply the base color from the lashes to the brow with a shadow brush or applicator.
2. Apply medium tone on the lid, blending from lash line to crease with the shadow brush or applicator.
3. Apply medium to deep color in the crease, blending up toward the eyebrow, but ending below it.
4. Apply highlight shadow under the brow bone with the shadow brush or applicator.

Here's a TIP

It is not recommended that you intensify every feature, as this will tend to look overdone and garish. For example, you can intensify the eyes and lips, or the cheeks and lips, but not the eyes, cheeks, and lips.

ACTIVITY

Using a model (or yourself) and two different color applications, divide the face in half. Try different foundations, colors, and intensity on each side. This will give you a visual example of how makeup will work on a face. Actually applying makeup is the best way to learn how to use it.

5. Apply eyeliner on the upper lash line from the outside corner in, tapering as you reach the inner corner. Blend with the small brush or applicator.
6. Apply shadow in the same color as the liner, directly over the liner. This will give longevity and intensity to the liner. Repeat on the bottom lash line, if desired.
7. Apply mascara with a disposable wand.

OPTION 2: DRAMATIC SMOKY EYES

1. Encircle the eye with dark gray, dark brown, or black eyeliner.
2. Smudge with a small shadow brush or disposable applicator.
3. Using the shadow brush or applicator, apply dark shadow from the upper lash line to the crease, softening and blending as you approach the crease. The shadow should be dark from outer to inner corner. You may choose shimmering or matte finish eye shadows.
4. Repeat on the lower lash line, carefully blending any hard edges.
5. If desired, add a highlight color in a shimmering or matte finish to the upper brow area with the shadow brush or applicator.
6. Apply mascara with a disposable wand (Figure 23-34).
7. Add individual or band lashes if desired (Figure 23-35).

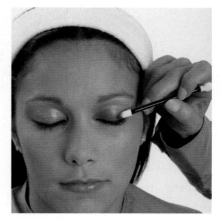

Figure 23-34 Striking contour eyes.

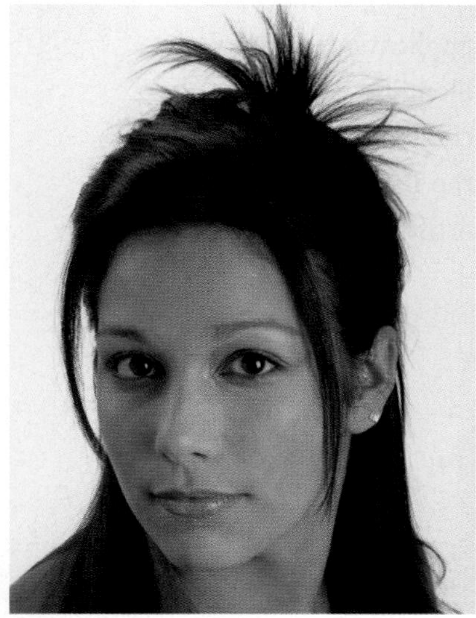

Figure 23-35 Dramatic smoky eyes.

SPECIAL-OCCASION MAKEUP FOR CHEEKS

Refer to the "Corrective Makeup" section on techniques you can use to remedy less attractive aspects of the cheeks. You can also try one of the following steps:

- Use a darker blush color under the cheekbones to add definition. Apply with a blush brush or applicator and blend carefully. Add a brighter, lighter cheek color to the apples of the cheeks and blend.
- Use a cheek color with shimmer or glitter over the cheekbones for highlight. You may use cream or powder colors.

SPECIAL-OCCASION MAKEUP FOR LIPS

Most clients prefer brighter or darker colors for special occasions. You may use shimmer colors or matte colors, if desired.

1. Apply liner color to the lips. Fill in the lip line with pencil and blot.
2. Add similar color in lipstick over the entire mouth with a lip brush or applicator.
3. Apply gloss to the center of the lips with a lip brush or applicator.

CORRECTIVE MAKEUP

All faces are interesting in their own special ways, but few are perfect. When you analyze a client's face, you might see that the nose, cheeks, lips, or jawline are not the same on both sides, one eye might be larger

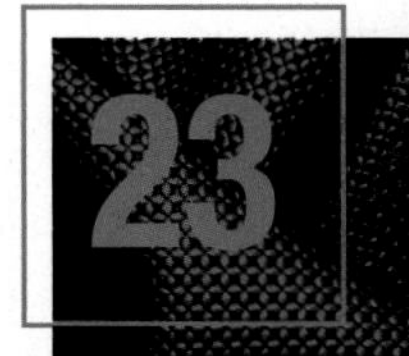

CAUTION

Corrective makeup can be very effective if applied properly. However, a less-experienced cosmetologist should proceed with caution, as improper application, insufficient blending, or the wrong choice of colors can make the face look dirty and artificial.

than the other, or the eyebrows might not match. In fact, these tiny imperfections can make the face more interesting if treated artfully. In any case, facial makeup can create the illusion of better balance and proportion when so desired.

Facial features can be accented with proper highlighting, subdued with correct shadowing or shading, and balanced with the proper hairstyle. A basic rule for the application of makeup is that highlighting emphasizes a feature, while shadowing minimizes it. A highlight is produced when a cosmetic, usually foundation that is lighter than the original foundation, is used on a particular part of the face. A shadow is formed when the foundation is darker than the original color. The use of shadows (dark colors and shades) minimizes prominent features so they are less noticeable.

Before you undertake any kind of corrective makeup application, you should have a clear sense of how to analyze the shape of the faces you will be working with.

ANALYZING FEATURES AND FACE SHAPE

The basic rule of makeup application is to emphasize the client's attractive features, while minimizing features that are less appealing. Learning to see the face and its features as a whole and determining the best makeup for an individual takes practice. While the oval face with well-proportioned features has long been considered the ideal, other face shapes are just as attractive in their own way. The goal of effective makeup application is to enhance the client's individuality, not to "remake" her image according to some ideal standard.

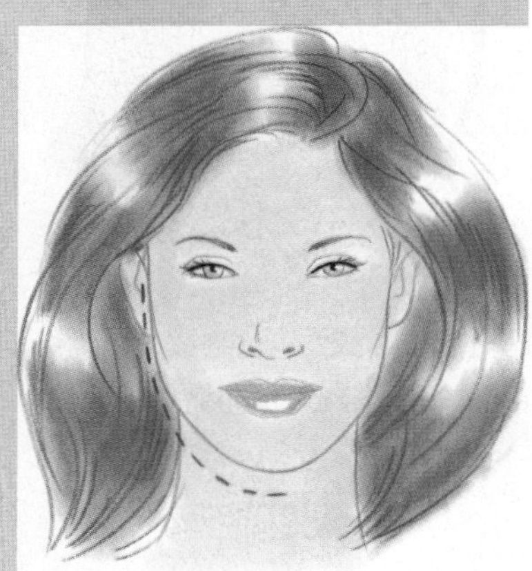

Figure 23-36 Oval face.

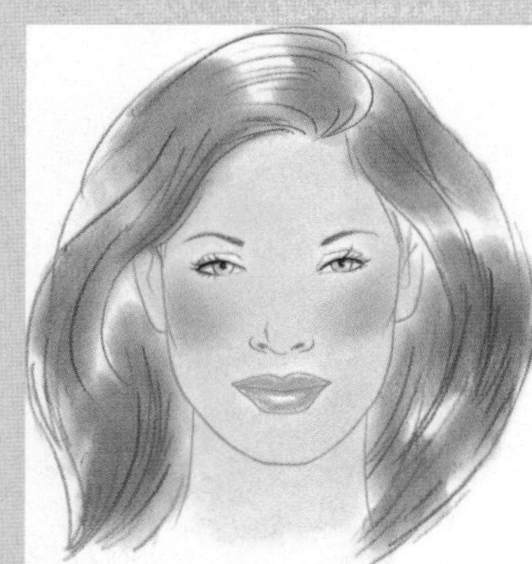

Figure 23-37 Oval face with makeup.

OVAL-SHAPED FACE

The artistically ideal proportions and features of the oval face are the standard to which you will refer when learning the techniques of corrective makeup application. The face is divided into three equal horizontal sections.

The first third is measured from the hairline to the top of the eyebrows. The second third is measured from the top of the eyebrows to the end of the nose. The last third is measured from the end of the nose to the bottom of the chin.

The ideal oval face is approximately three-fourths as wide as it is long. The distance between the eyes is the width of one eye (Figures 23-36 and 23-37).

ROUND FACE

The round face is usually broader in proportion to its length than the oval face. It has a rounded chin and hairline. Corrective makeup can be applied to slenderize and lengthen the face (Figures 23-38 and 23-39).

SQUARE-SHAPED FACE

The square face is composed of comparatively straight lines with a wide forehead and square jawline. Corrective makeup can be applied to offset the squareness and soften the hard lines around the face (Figures 23-40 and 23-41).

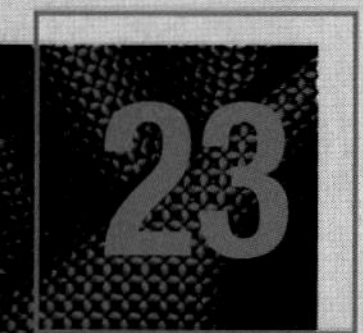

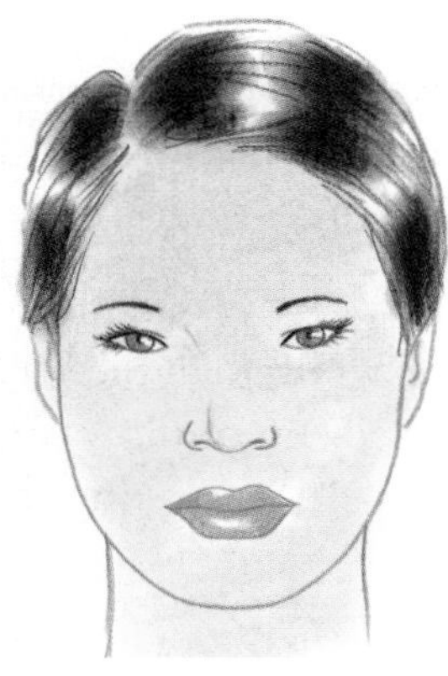
Figure 23-38 Round face.

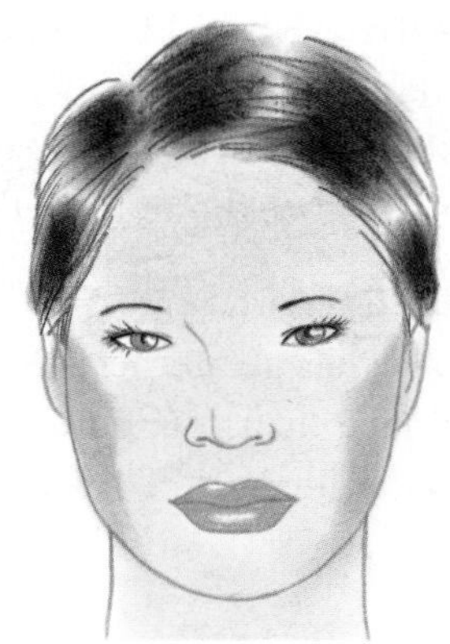
Figure 23-39 Round face with corrective makeup.

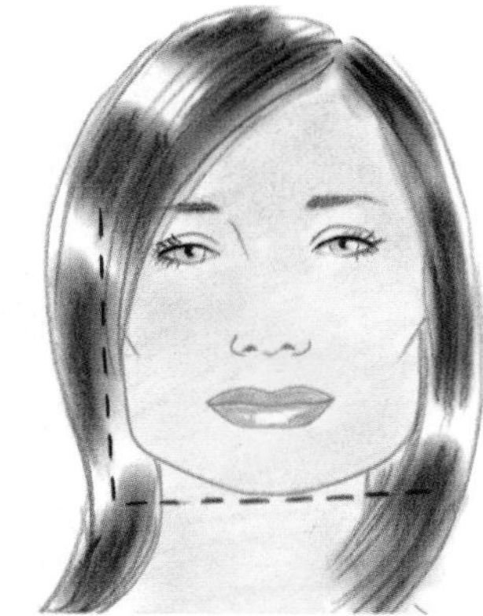
Figure 23-40 Square face.

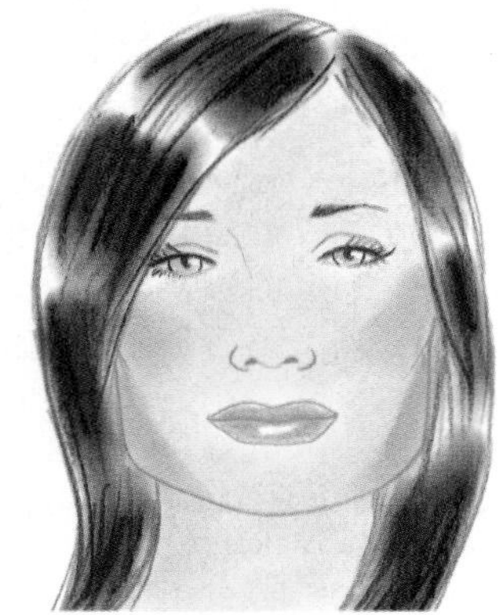
Figure 23-41 Square face with corrective makeup.

TRIANGULAR (PEAR-SHAPED) FACE

A jaw that is wider than the forehead characterizes the pear-shaped face. Corrective makeup can be applied to create width at the forehead, slenderize the jawline, and add length to the face (Figures 23-42 and 23-43).

INVERTED TRIANGLE (HEART-SHAPED) FACE

The inverted triangle or heart-shaped face has a wide forehead and narrow, pointed chin. Corrective makeup can be applied to minimize the width of the forehead and increase the width of the jawline (Figures 23-44 and 23-45).

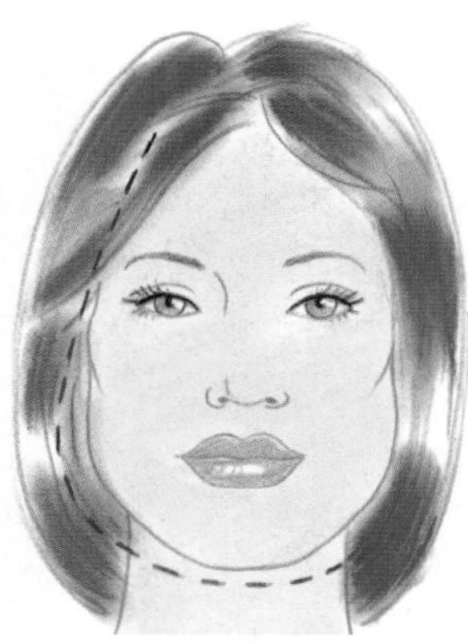
Figure 23-42 Triangular face.

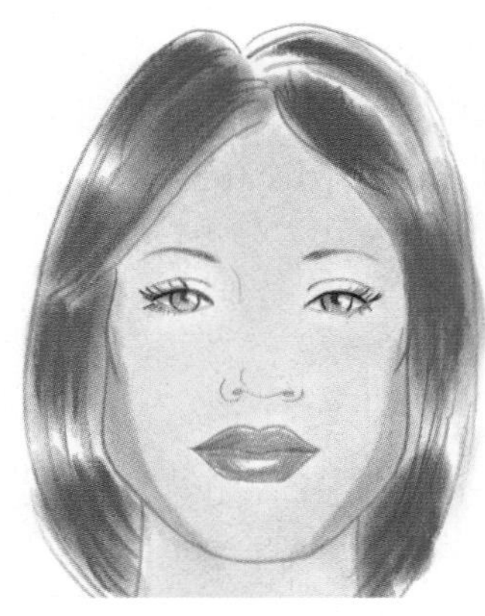
Figure 23-43 Triangular face with corrective makeup.

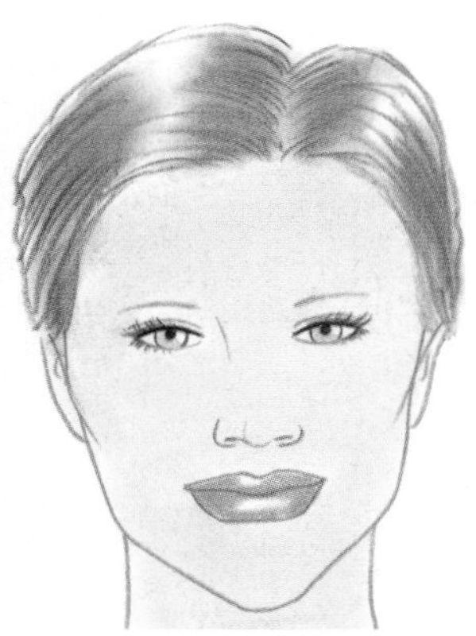
Figure 23-44 Inverted triangle-shaped face.

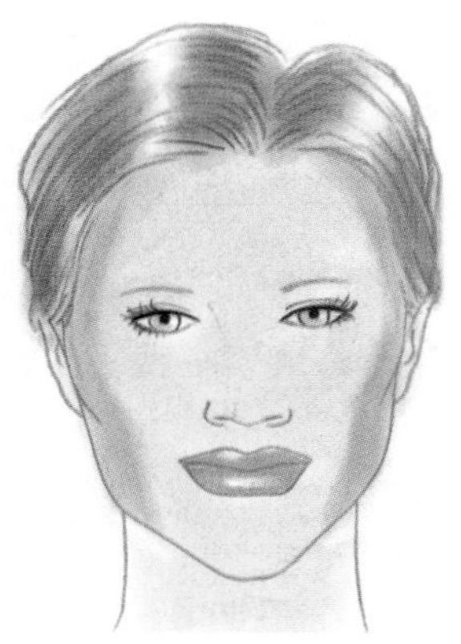
Figure 23-45 Inverted triangle-shaped face with corrective makeup.

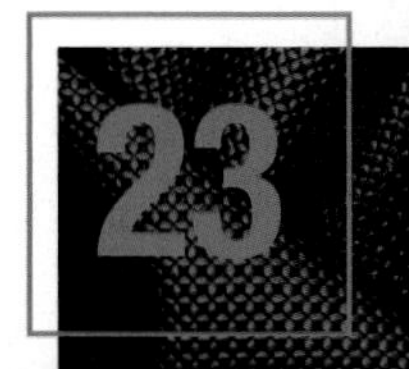

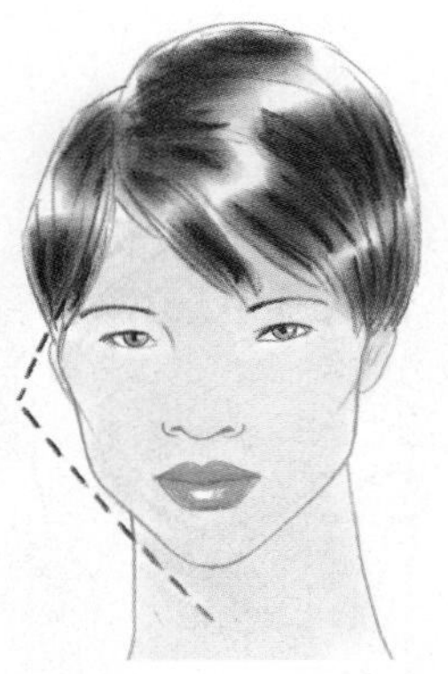

Figure 23-46 Diamond-shaped face.

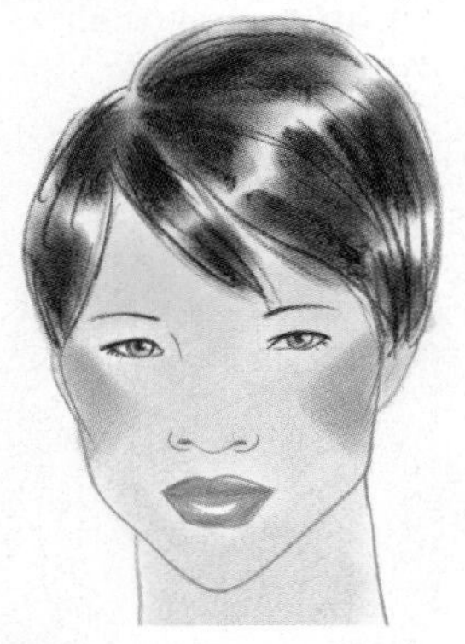

Figure 23-47 Diamond-shaped face with corrective makeup.

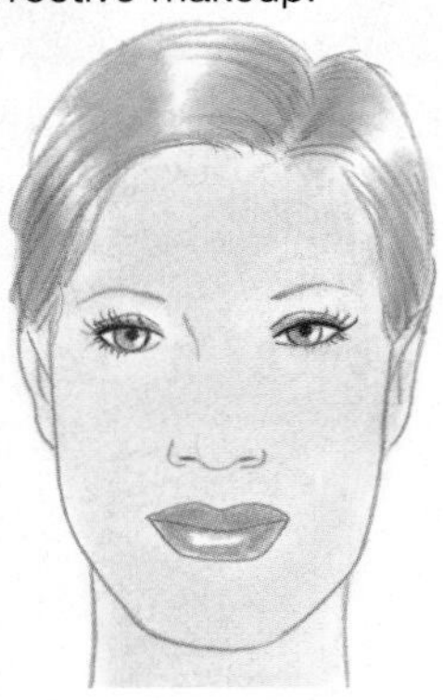

Figure 23-48 Oblong face.

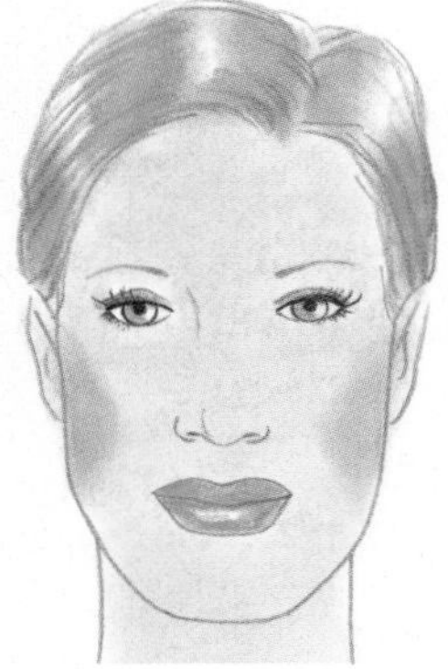

Figure 23-49 Oblong face with corrective makeup.

DIAMOND-SHAPED FACE

This face has a narrow forehead. The greatest width is across the cheekbones. Corrective makeup can be applied to reduce the width across the cheekbone line (Figures 23-46 and 23-47).

OBLONG FACE

This face has greater length in proportion to its width than the square or round face. It is long and narrow. Corrective makeup can be applied to create the illusion of width across the cheekbone line, making the face appear shorter (Figures 23-48 and 23-49).

FOREHEAD AREA

For a low forehead, the application of a lighter foundation lends a broader appearance between the brows and hairline. For a protruding forehead, applying a darker foundation over the prominent area gives an illusion of fullness to the rest of the face and minimizes the bulging forehead. A suitable hairstyle also goes a long way toward drawing attention away from the forehead (Figure 23-50).

NOSE AND CHIN AREAS

For a large or protruding nose, apply a darker foundation on the nose and a lighter foundation on the cheeks at the sides of the nose. This will create fullness in the cheeks and will make the nose appear smaller. Avoid placing cheek color close to the nose.

For a short and flat nose, apply a lighter foundation down the center of the nose, ending at the tip. This will make the nose appear longer and larger.

If the nostrils are wide, apply a darker foundation to both sides of the nostrils (Figure 23-51).

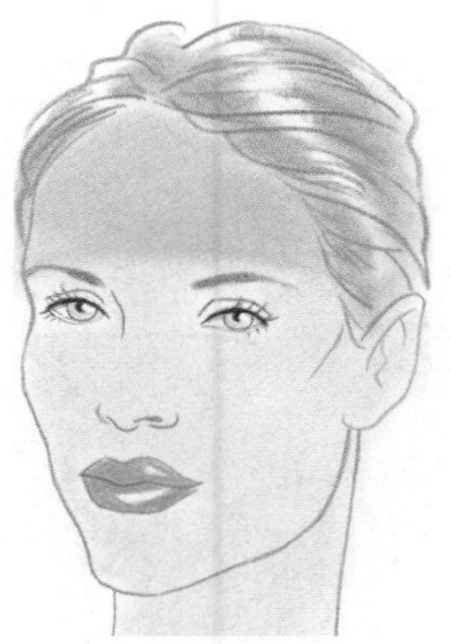

Figure 23-50 Protruding forehead with corrective makeup.

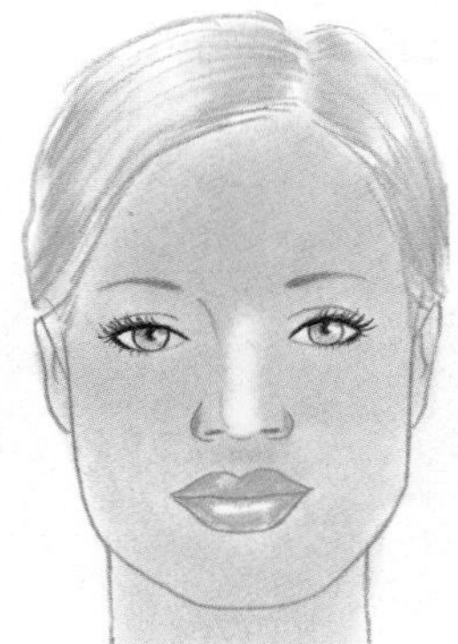

Figure 23-51 Short flat nose with corrective makeup.

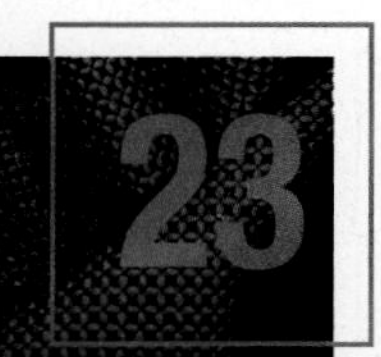

For a broad nose, use a darker foundation on the sides of the nose and nostrils. Avoid carrying this dark tone into the laugh lines because it will accentuate them. The foundation must be carefully blended to avoid visible lines (Figure 23-52).

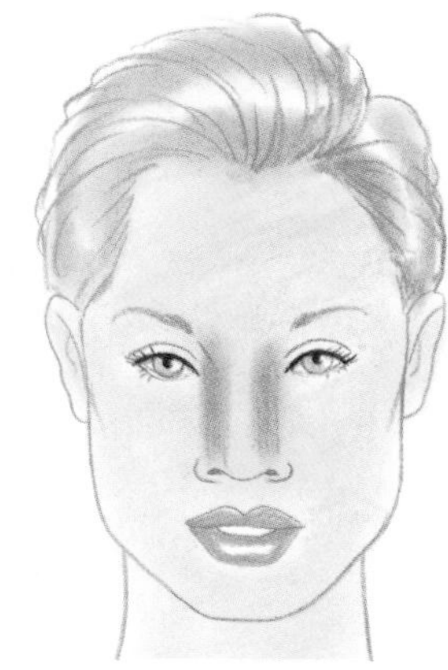

Figure 23-52 Broad nose with corrective makeup.

For a protruding chin and receding nose, shadow the chin with a darker foundation and highlight the nose with a lighter foundation. For a receding chin, highlight the chin by using a lighter foundation than the one used on the face.

For a sagging double chin, use a darker foundation on the sagging portion, and use a natural skin tone foundation on the face (Figure 23-53).

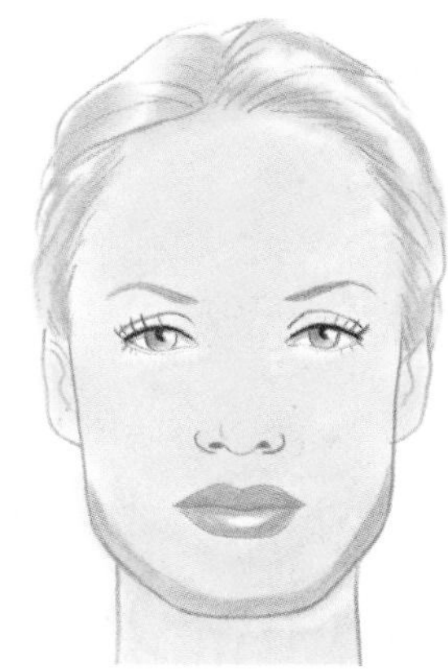

Figure 23-53 Double chin with corrective makeup.

JAWLINE AND NECK AREA

The neck and jaw are just as important as the eyes, cheeks, and lips. When applying makeup, blend the foundation onto the neck so that the client's color is consistent from face to neck. Always set with a translucent powder to avoid transfer onto the client's clothing.

To correct a broad jawline, apply a darker shade of foundation over the heavy area of the jaw, starting at the temples. This will minimize the lower part of the face and create an illusion of width in the upper part of the face (Figure 23-54).

To correct a narrow jawline, highlight by using a lighter foundation shade (Figure 23-55).

For a round, square, or triangular face, apply a darker shade of foundation over the prominent part of the jawline. By creating a shadow over this area, the prominent part of the jaw will appear softer and more oval.

For a small face and a short, thick neck, use a darker foundation on the neck than the one used on the face. This will make the neck appear thinner.

For a long, thin neck, apply a lighter shade of foundation on the neck than the one used on the face. This will create fullness and counteract the long, thin appearance of the neck (Figure 23-56).

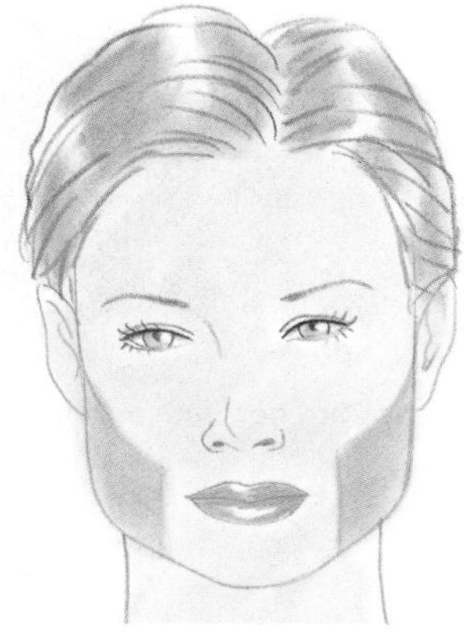

Figure 23-54 Broad jawline with corrective makeup.

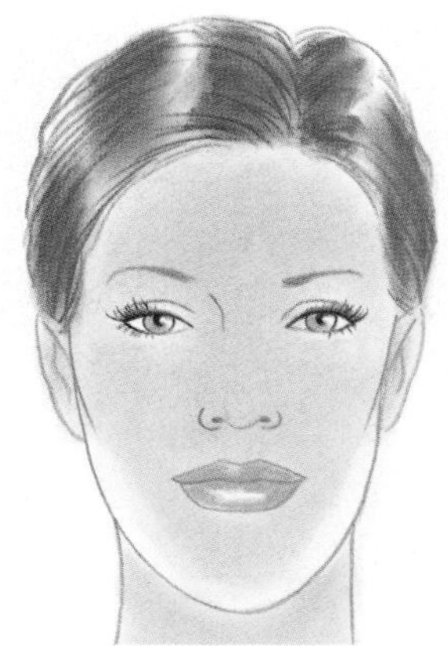

Figure 23-55 Narrow jawline with corrective makeup.

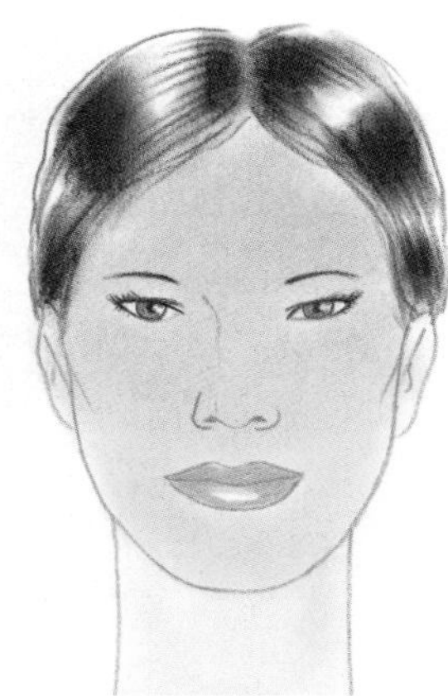

Figure 23-56 Long, thin neck with corrective makeup.

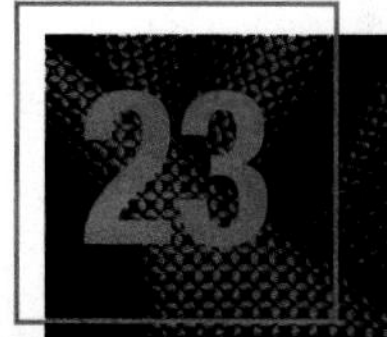

CORRECTIVE MAKEUP FOR THE EYES

The eyes are very important in balancing facial features. The proper application of eye colors and shadow can create the illusion of the eyes being larger or smaller, and will enhance the overall attractiveness of the face.

Round eyes can be lengthened by extending the shadow beyond the outer corner of the eyes (Figure 23-57 and 23-58).

Close-set eyes are closer together than the length of one eye. For eyes that are too close together, lightly apply shadow up from the outer edge of the eyes (Figure 23-59 and 23-60).

Protruding or bulging eyes can be minimized by blending the shadow carefully over the prominent part of the upper lid, carrying it lightly toward the eyebrow. Use a medium to deep shadow color (Figures 23-61 and 23-62).

Heavy-lidded eyes. Shadow evenly and lightly across the lid from the edge of the eyelash line to the small crease in the eye socket (Figures 23-63 and 23-64).

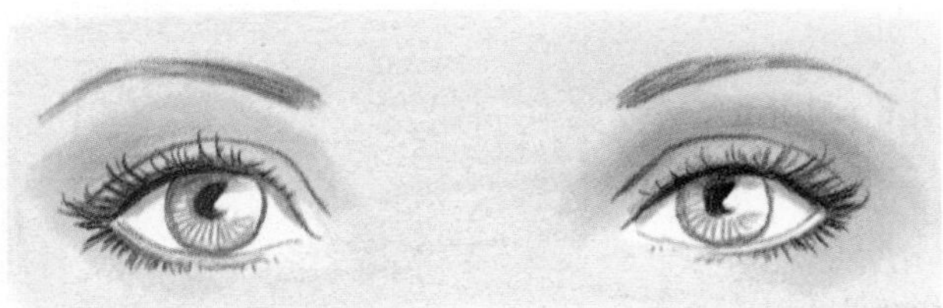

Figure 23-57 Round eyes.

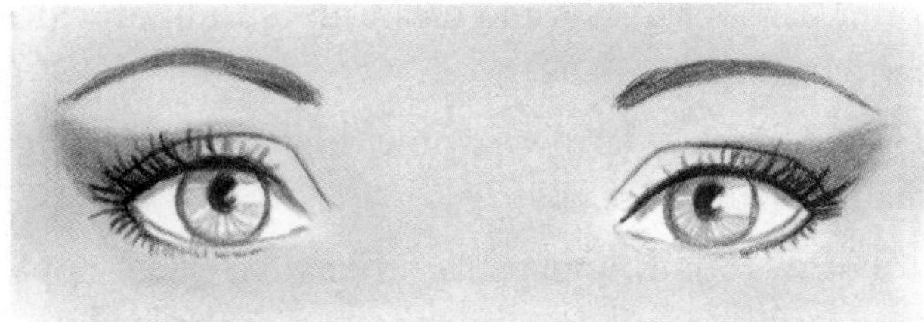

Figure 23-58 Round eyes with corrective makeup.

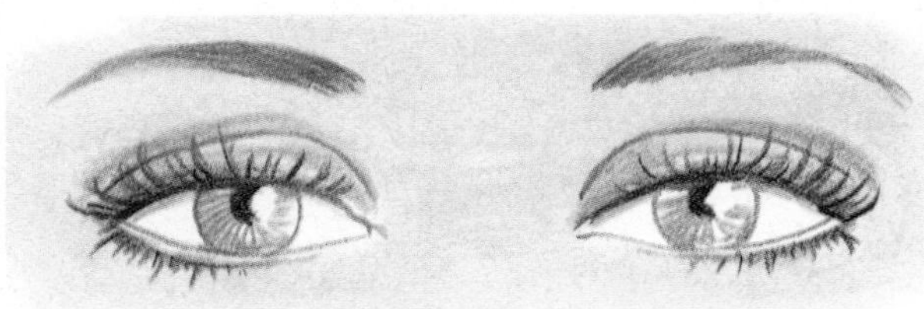

Figure 23-59 Close-set eyes.

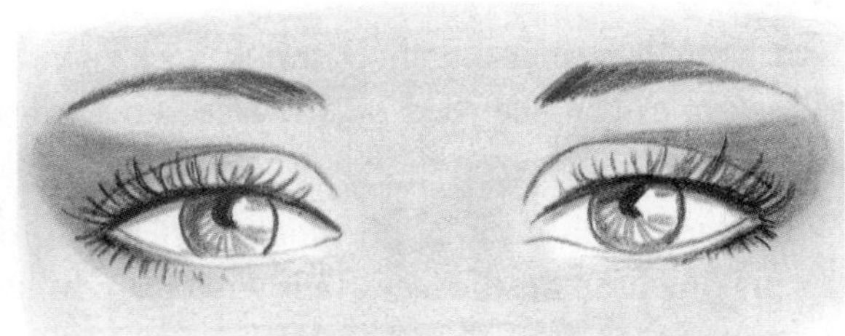

Figure 23-60 Close-set eyes with corrective makeup.

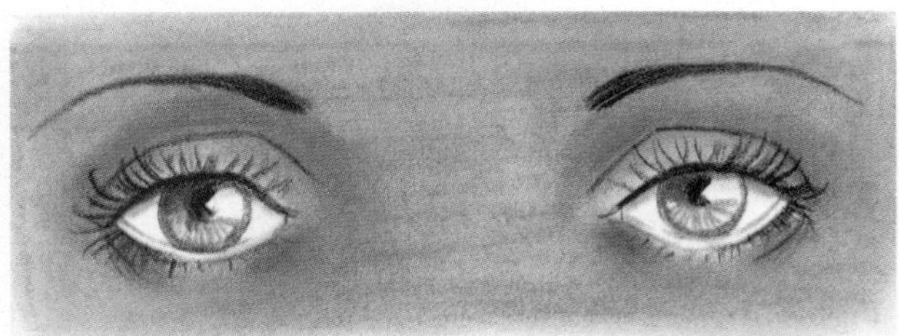

Figure 23-61 Protruding eyes.

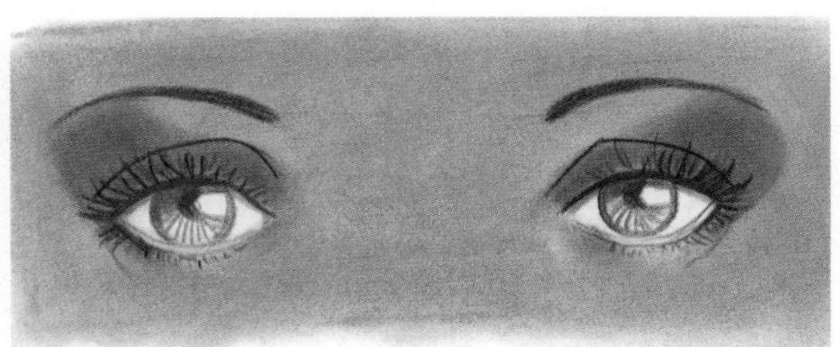

Figure 23-62 Protruding eyes with corrective makeup.

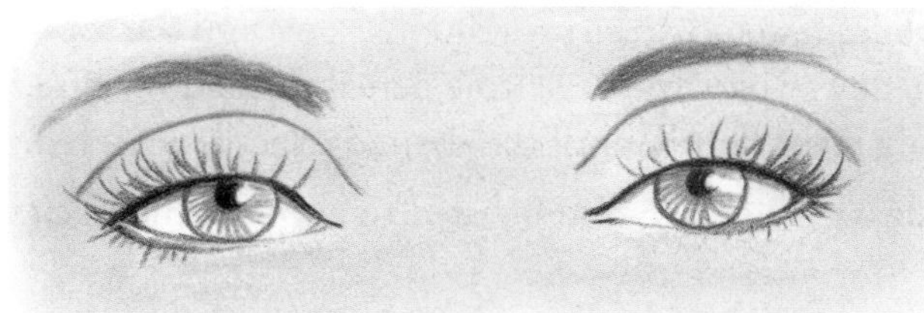
Figure 23-63 Heavy-lidded eyes.

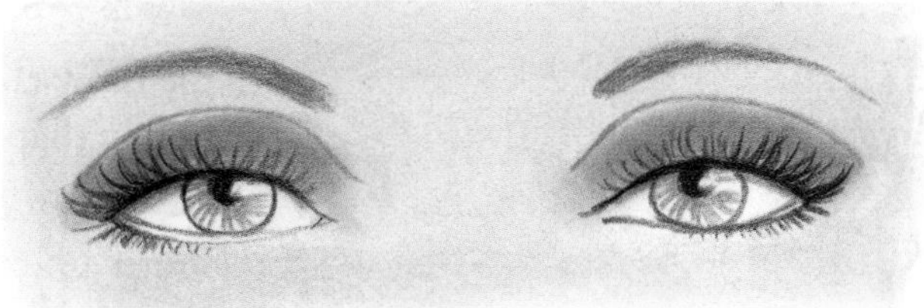
Figure 23-64 Heavy-lidded eyes with corrective makeup.

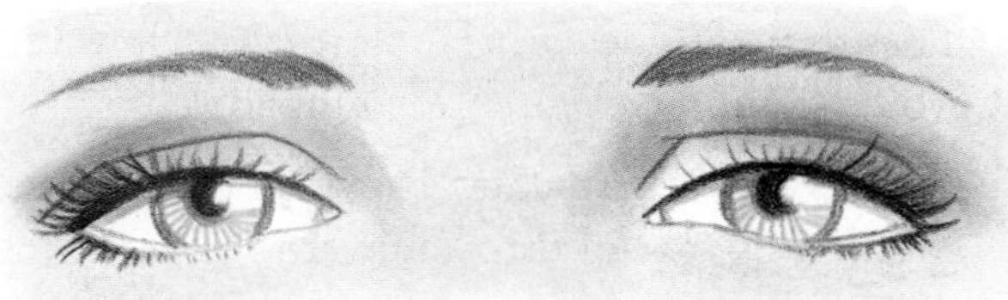
Figure 23-65 Deep-set eyes.

Small eyes. To make small eyes appear larger, extend the shadow slightly above, beyond, and below the eyes.

Wide-set eyes. Apply the shadow on the upper inner side of the eyelid, toward the nose, and blend carefully.

Deep-set eyes. Use bright, light, reflective colors. Use the lightest color in the crease, and a light-to-medium color sparingly on the lid and brow bone (Figure 23-65).

Dark circles under eyes. Apply concealer over the dark area, blending and smoothing it into the surrounding area. Set lightly with translucent powder (Figure 23-66).

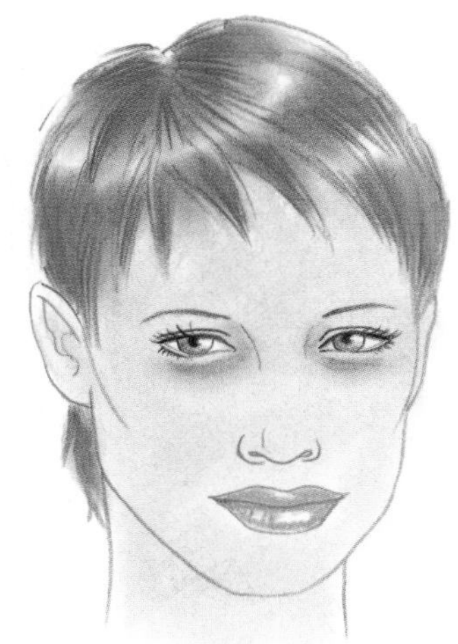
Figure 23-66 Dark circles under eyes.

EYEBROWS

Reshaping and defining eyebrows can be an art unto itself. Well-groomed eyebrows are part of a complete and effective makeup application. The eyebrow is the frame for the eye. Overgrown eyebrows can cast a shadow on the brow bone or between the two eyebrows. Over-tweezed eyebrows can make the face look puffy or protruding, or may give the eyes a surprised look.

When a client wants to correct eyebrow shape, begin by removing all unnecessary hairs and then demonstrate how to use the eyebrow pencil or shadow to fill in until the natural hairs have grown in again. When there are spaces in the eyebrow hair, they can be filled in with hair-like strokes of an eyebrow pencil or shadow, applied with an angled brush. Use an eyebrow brush to soften the pencil or shadow marks.

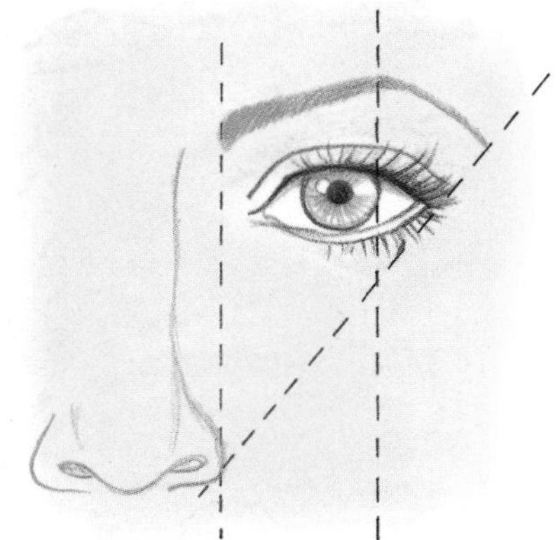
Figure 23-67 Ideal eyebrow shape.

The ideal eyebrow shape can be drawn in three lines (Figure 23-67). The first line is vertical, from the inner corner of the eye upward. This is where the eyebrow should begin. The second line is drawn at an angle from the outer corner of the nose to the outer corner of the eye. This is where the eyebrow should end. The third line is vertical, from the outer circle of the iris of the eye upward. The client should be looking straight ahead as you determine this line. This is where the highest part of the arch would ideally be. Of course, not everyone's eyebrows fit exactly within these measurements, so use them only as guidelines.

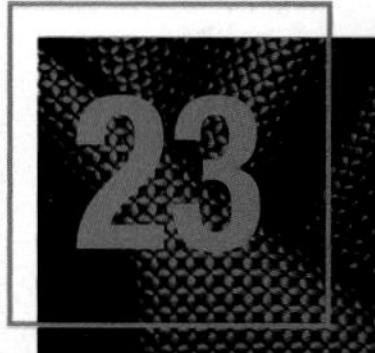

When the arch is too high, remove the superfluous hair from the top of the brow and fill in the lower part with eyebrow pencil or shadow. Build up the shape by layering color lightly until the desired effect is achieved.

Adjustments to eyebrow shape can also be used to correct other facial shortcomings listed below.

- *Low forehead.* A low arch gives more height to a very low forehead.
- *Wide-set eyes.* The eyes can be made to appear closer together by extending the eyebrow lines to the inside corners of the eyes. However, care must be taken to avoid giving the client a frowning look.
- *Close-set eyes.* To make the eyes appear farther apart, widen the distance between the eyebrows and slightly extend them outward.
- *Round face.* Arch the brows high to make the face appear narrower. Start on a line directly above the inside corner of the eye and extend to the end of the cheekbone.
- *Long face.* Making the eyebrows almost straight can create the illusion of a shorter face. Do not extend the eyebrow lines farther than the outside corners of the eyes.
- *Square face.* The face will appear more oval if there is a high arch on the ends of the eyebrows. Begin the lines directly above the corners of the eyes and extend them outward.

THE LIPS

Lips are usually proportioned so that the curves or peaks of the upper lip fall directly in line with the nostrils. In some cases, one side of the lips may differ from the other. Lips can be very full, very thin, or uneven. Figures 23-68 to 23-76 show various lip lines and how lip color can be used to create the illusion of better proportions.

SKIN TONES

For whatever reason, some clients may wish to alter their skin tone. In terms of corrective makeup, you will be dealing with two basic skin tones.

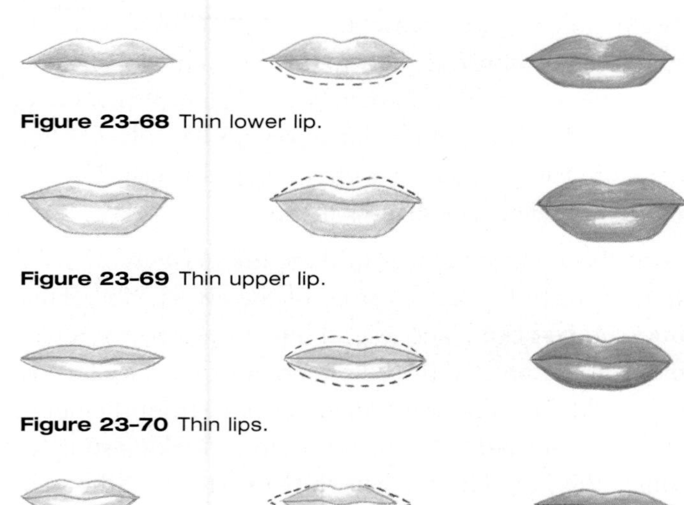

Figure 23-68 Thin lower lip.

Figure 23-69 Thin upper lip.

Figure 23-70 Thin lips.

Figure 23-71 Small mouth.

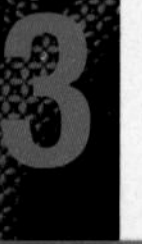

Figure 23-72 Drooping corners.

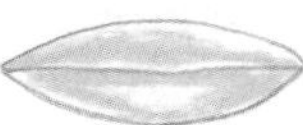  

Figure 23-74 Oval lips.

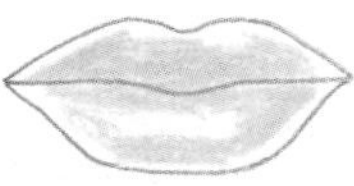 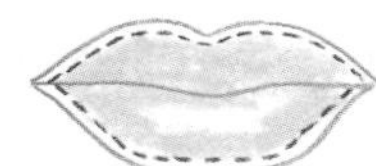 

Figure 23-73 Large, full lips.

Figure 23-75 Sharp peaks.

Figure 23-76 Uneven lips.

For ruddy skin (skin that is red, wind-burned, or affected by rosacea), apply a yellow or green foundation to affected areas, blending carefully. You may then apply a light layer of foundation with a yellow base over the entire complexion. Set it with translucent or yellow-based powder. Avoid red or pink blushes.

For sallow skin (skin that has a yellowish hue), apply a pink-based foundation on the affected areas and blend carefully into the jaw and neck. Set with translucent powder. Avoid yellow-based colors for eyes, cheeks, and lips.

WRINKLES

Age lines and wrinkles due to dry skin can be minimized with a foundation. Apply the foundation sparingly and evenly, in a light, outward, circular motion over the entire surface of the face. Care should be taken to remove any foundation that collects in lines and wrinkles of the face.

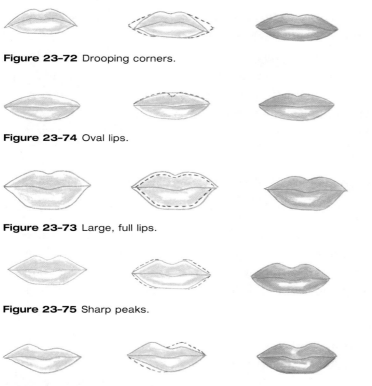

CAUTION

Some clients may be allergic to a particular eyelash adhesive. When in doubt, give the client an allergy test before applying the lashes. This test may be done in one of two ways: (1) put a drop of the adhesive behind one ear, or (2) attach a single individual eyelash to each eyelid. In either case, if there is no reaction over the next 24 hours, it is probably safe to proceed with the application.

ARTIFICIAL EYELASHES

The use of artificial eyelashes has grown enormously, mainly because the technology has improved dramatically, and fashion has become more reliant on these accessories. Clients with sparse lashes and those who wish to enhance their eyes for special occasions are most likely to request this

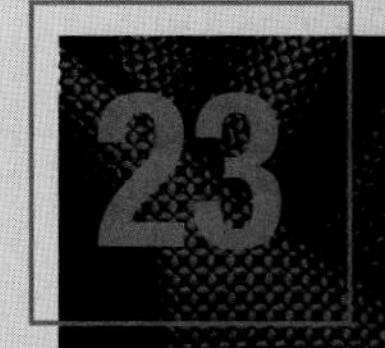

service. The objective is to make the client's own lashes look fuller, longer, and more attractive without appearing unnatural.

Two types of artificial eyelashes are commonly used. **Band lashes** (also called strip lashes) are eyelash hairs on a strip that are applied with adhesive to the natural lash line. Individual lashes are separate artificial eyelashes that are applied to the eyelids one at a time. **Eyelash adhesive** is used to make artificial eyelashes adhere, or stick, to the natural lash line.

APPLYING BAND LASHES

Band lashes (sometimes referred to as strip lashes) are available in a variety of sizes, textures, and colors. They can be made from human hair, certain animal hair such as mink, or synthetic fibers. Synthetic fiber eyelashes are made with a permanent curl and do not react to changes in weather conditions. Artificial eyelashes are available in natural colors ranging from light to dark brown and black or light to dark auburn, as well as bright, trendy colors. Black and dark brown are the most popular choices.

REMOVING BAND EYELASHES

You may use commercial preparations, such as pads saturated with special lotions, to remove band eyelashes. The lash base may also be softened by applying a face cloth or cotton pad saturated with warm water and a gentle facial cleanser. Hold the cloth over the eyes for a few seconds to soften the adhesive. Starting from the outer corner, remove the lashes carefully to avoid pulling out the client's own lashes. Use cotton tips to remove any makeup and adhesive remaining on the eyelid.

INDIVIDUAL LASHES

Individual eyelashes are synthetic and attach directly to a client's own lashes at their base. This procedure is sometimes referred to as **eye tabbing.** Follow the manufacturer's instructions for attaching individual lashes.

PROCEDURE 23-2

BAND LASH APPLICATION

IMPLEMENTS AND MATERIALS

- Wet sanitizer for metal implements
- Headband or hair clip
- Tweezers
- Cotton swabs
- Eyelash brushes
- Eyelash curler
- Hand mirror
- Manicure scissors
- Adjustable light (gooseneck lamp)
- Makeup chair
- Lash adhesive
- Adhesive tray
- Eyelid and eyelash cleanser
- Eyelash remover
- Cotton pads
- Eye makeup remover
- Makeup cape
- Trays of artificial eyelashes
- Pencil sharpener

PREPARATION

1. **Client consultation.** Discuss with the client the desired length of the lashes and the effect she hopes to achieve.
2. **Wash your hands.**
3. **Seat client.** Place the client in the makeup chair with her head at a comfortable working height. The client's face should be well and evenly lit, but avoid shining the light directly into the eyes. Work from behind or to the side of the client. Avoid working directly in front of the client whenever possible.
4. **Drape client.** Properly drape the client to protect her clothing and have her use a hairline strip, headband, or turban during the procedure.
5. **Remove contact lenses.** If the client wears contact lenses, they must be removed before starting the procedure.
6. **Remove eye makeup.** If the client has not already done so, remove all eye makeup so that the lash adhesive will adhere properly. Work carefully and gently. Follow the manufacturer's instructions carefully.

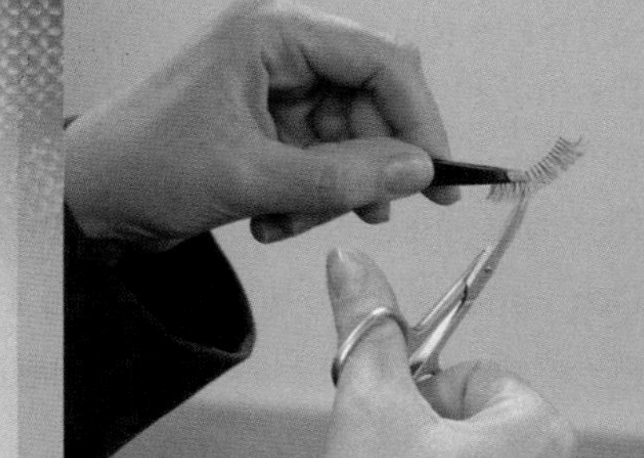

Figure 23-77 Feather the band lashes.

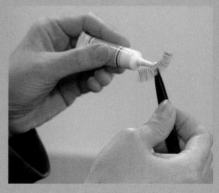

Figure 23-78 Apply lash adhesive to the band lashes.

PROCEDURE

1. **Prepare lashes.** Brush the client's eyelashes to make sure they are clean and free of foreign matter, such as mascara particles. If the client's lashes are straight, they can be curled with an eyelash curler before you apply the artificial lashes.
2. Carefully remove the eyelash band from the package.
3. **Shape eyelash.** Start with the upper lash. If it is too long to fit the curve of the upper eyelid, trim the outside edge. Use your fingers to bend the lash into a horseshoe shape to make it more flexible so that it fits the contour of the eyelid.
4. **Feather lash.** Feather the lash by nipping into it with the points of your scissors. This creates a more natural look (Figure 23-77).
5. **Apply adhesive.** Apply a thin strip of lash adhesive to the base of the lash and allow a few seconds for it to set (Figure 23-78).

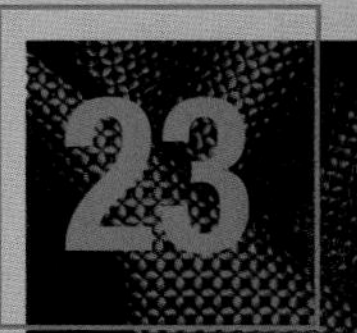

6. **Apply the lash.** Start with the shorter part of the lash and place it on the inner corner of the eye toward the nose. Position the rest of the artificial lash as close to the client's own lash as possible. Use the rounded end of a lash liner brush or tweezers to press the lash on (Figure 23-79). Be very careful and gentle when applying the lashes. If eyeliner is to be used, the line is usually drawn on the eyelid before the lash is applied and retouched when the artificial lash is in place (Figure 23-80).
7. **Apply the lower lash.** Lower lash application is optional, as it tends to look more unnatural. Trim the lash as necessary and apply adhesive in the same way you did for the upper lash. Place the lash on top of the client's lower lash. Place the shorter lash toward the center of the eye and the longer lash toward the outer part of the lid (Figure 23-81).

CLEANUP AND SANITATION

1. Discard all disposable items, such as sponges, pads, spatulas, and applicators.
2. Disinfect implements, such as the eyelash curler.
3. Clean and sanitize brushes using a commercial brush sanitizer.
4. Place all towels, linens, and makeup cape in a hamper.
5. Sanitize your workstation.
6. Wash your hands with soap and warm water.

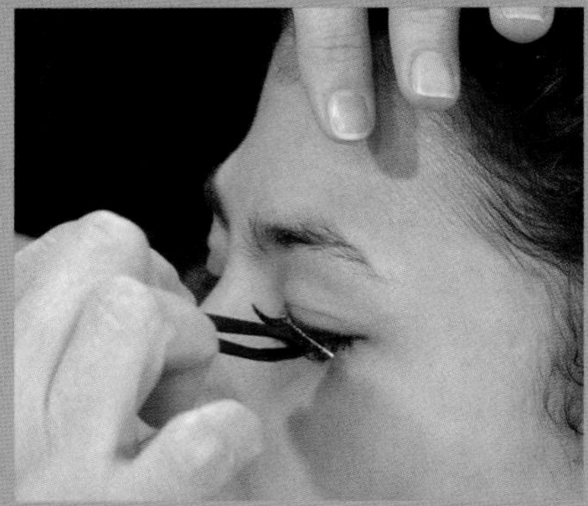

Figure 23-79 Apply the band lashes to the eyelid.

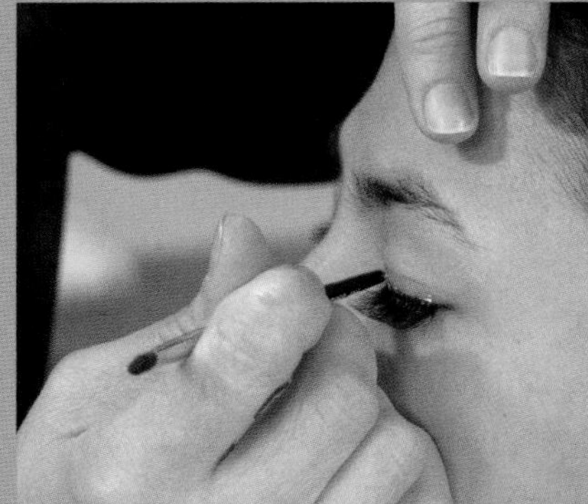

Figure 23-80 Retouch the lash line with eyeliner.

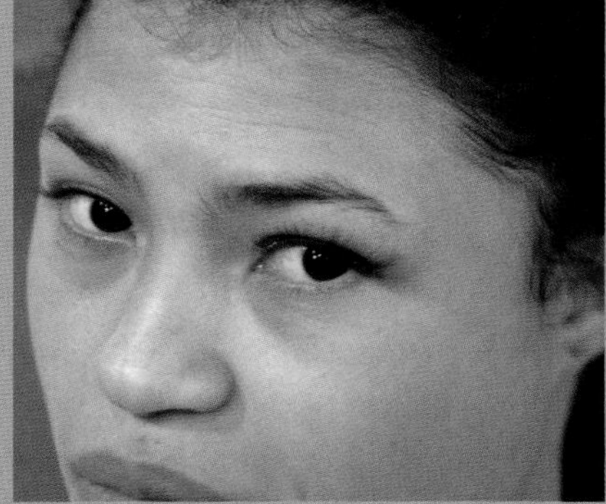

Figure 23-81 Finished band eyelash application.

CAUTION

Remind the client to take special care with artificial lashes when swimming, bathing, or cleansing the face. Water or cleansing products will loosen artificial lashes.

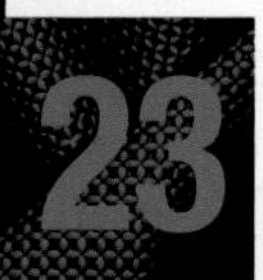

SAFETY PRECAUTIONS

- Wash your hands thoroughly with soap and warm water before and after every makeup application.
- Properly drape the client to protect her clothing, and have her use a headband or hair clip during the makeup procedure.
- Protect the client's hair and skin from direct contact with the facial chair.
- Keep your fingernails smooth to avoid scratching the client's skin.
- Use only sanitized brushes and implements.
- Use a shaker-type container for loose powder.
- Pour all lotions from bottle containers.
- Always use a clean spatula or cosmetic applicator to remove cosmetics from their containers.
- Never apply lip color directly from the container to the client's lips. Use a spatula or disposable applicator to remove the product from the container, and then use a brush to apply.
- Use an antiseptic on tweezed areas of the eyebrow to avoid infection.
- Discard all disposable items, such as sponges, pads, spatulas, and applicators, after use.
- Place all towels, linens, makeup capes, and other items that can be washed and sanitized in the proper containers.
- Keep your workstation sanitary, neat, and well organized.

REVIEW QUESTIONS

1. What is the main objective of makeup application?
2. List eight types of facial cosmetics and how they are used.
3. Name the various types and uses of foundation.
4. Name three types of cheek color.
5. Name the three different types of eye shadow and how they are used.
6. List the primary and secondary colors.
7. Name the colors in the warm range and the cool range.
8. What are complementary colors?
9. List the cosmetics used in a basic makeup procedure in the order in which they are applied.
10. What are the seven facial types?
11. Name and describe the two types of artificial eyelashes.
12. List at least 10 safety measures that should be followed when applying makeup.

CHAPTER GLOSSARY

band lashes	Eyelash hairs on a strip that are applied with adhesive to the natural lash line.
cake (pancake) makeup	Shaped, solid mass applied to the face with a moistened cosmetic sponge; gives good coverage.
cheek color	Use primarily to add a natural looking glow to the cheeks; also known as blush and rouge.
concealers	Cosmetics used to hide dark eye circles, dark splotches, and other imperfections.
cool colors	Colors that suggest coolness and are dominated by blues, greens, violets, and blue-reds.
eyebrow pencils	Pencils used to add color and shape to the eyebrows.
eyelash adhesive	Product used to make artificial eyelashes adhere, or stick, to the natural lash line.
eyeliner	Cosmetic used to outline and emphasize the eyes.
eye makeup removers	Cosmetic preparations for removing eye makeup.
eye shadows	Cosmetics applied on the eyelids to accentuate or contour.

CHAPTER GLOSSARY

eye tabbing	Procedure in which individual synthetic eyelashes are attached directly to a client's own lashes at their base.
face powder	Cosmetic powder, sometimes tinted and scented, that is used to add a matte or nonshiny finish to the face.
foundation	Cosmetic, usually tinted, that is used as a base makeup and is used to cover or even out the coloring of skin.
greasepaint	Heavy makeup used for theatrical purposes.
lip color	Cosmetic in paste form, usually in a metal or plastic tube, manufactured in a variety of colors and used to color the lips; also called lipstick or gloss.
lip liner	Colored pencil or brush used to outline the lips and to help keep lip color from bleeding into the small lines around the mouth.
mascara	Cosmetic preparation used to darken, define, and thicken the eyelashes.
matte	Nonshiny.
warm colors	Range of colors from yellow and gold through oranges, red-oranges, most reds, and even some yellow-greens.

NAIL CARE

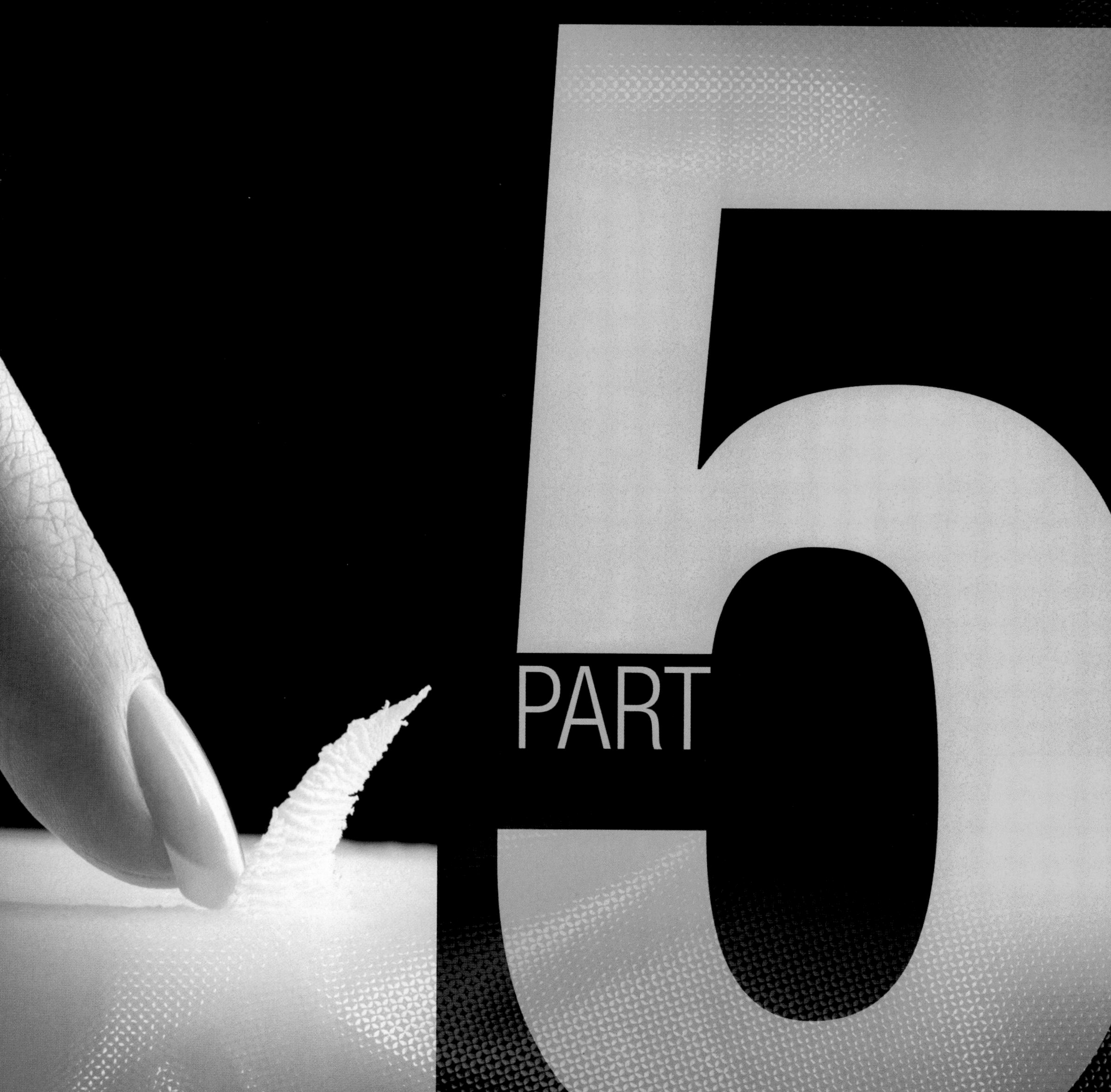

PART 5

CHAPTER 24 NAIL DISEASES & DISORDERS

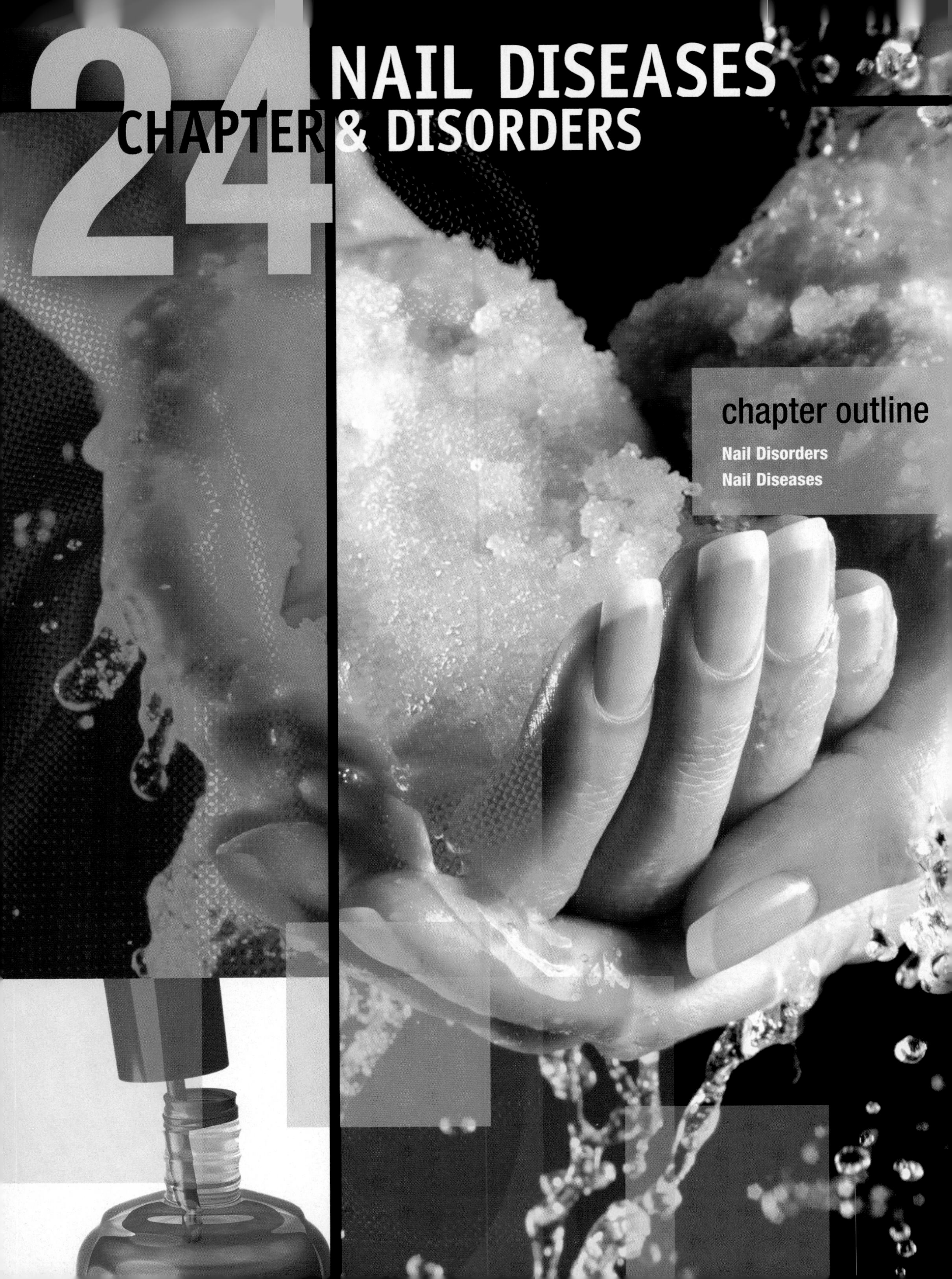

chapter outline

Learning Objectives

After completing this chapter, you will be able to:

- **List and describe the various disorders and irregularities of nails.**
- **Recognize diseases of the nails that should not be treated in the salon.**

Key Terms

Page number indicates where in the chapter the term is used.

Beau's lines **pg. 645**

bruised nails **pg. 644**

corrugations **pg. 648**

eggshell nails **pg. 645**

furrows **pg. 648**

hangnail or *agnail* **pg. 645**

infected finger **pg. 648**

leukonychia spots **pg. 646**

melanonychia **pg. 646**

nail disorder **pg. 644**

nail psoriasis **pg. 651**

nail pterygium **pg. 646**

onychauxis (hypertrophy) **pg. 648**

onychia **pg. 650**

onychocryptosis **pg. 650**

onychogryposis **pg. 650**

onycholysis **pg. 650**

onychomadesis **pg. 651**

onychomycosis **pg. 652**

onychophagy **pg. 646**

onychophosis **pg. 650**

onychoptosis **pg. 650**

onychorrhexis **pg. 646**

onychosis **pg. 650**

paronychia **pg. 650**

plicatured nail **pg. 646**

Pseudomonas aeruginosa **pg. 647**

pterygium **pg. 648**

pyogenic granuloma **pg. 650**

ridges **pg. 645**

tile-shaped nails **pg. 648**

tinea pedis **pg. 652**

tinea (ringworm) **pg. 650**

tinea unguium **pg. 650**

trumpet nails (pincer nails) **pg. 648**

To give clients professional and responsible service and care, you need to know when it is safe to work on a client. Nails are an interesting and surprising part of the human body. They are small mirrors of the general health of the entire body. You must be able to recognize conditions you may encounter while servicing clients. Many of these conditions are easily treated in the salon—hangnails, for instance, or bruising—but others are infectious and should not be treated by salon professionals. A select few may even signal serious health problems that warrant the attention of a doctor. Carefully studying this chapter will vastly improve your expertise in caring for nails. It will also help ensure that you are protecting your clients, rather than promoting the spread of disease.

A normal healthy nail is firm and flexible, and should be shiny and slightly pink in color, with more yellow tones in some races. Its surface should be smooth and unspotted, without any pits or splits. Certain health problems in the body can show up in the nails as visible disorders or poor nail growth.

NAIL DISORDERS

A **nail disorder** is a condition caused by injury or disease. Most, if not all, of your clients have experienced one or more types of common nail disorder at some time in their lives. The technician should recognize normal and abnormal nail conditions, and understand what to do. You may be able to help your clients with nail disorders in one of two ways.

- You can tell clients that they may have a disorder and refer them to a physician, if required.
- You can cosmetically improve certain nail plate conditions if the problem is cosmetic and not a medical disorder.

It is your professional responsibility and a requirement of your license to know which option to choose. A client whose nail or skin is infected, inflamed, broken, or swollen should not receive services. Instead, the client should be referred to a physician, if you feel that is an appropriate recommendation, based on the condition.

Bruised nails are a condition in which a blood clot forms under the nail plate, forming a dark purplish spot. These discolorations are usually due to small injuries to the nail bed. The dried blood absorbs into the bed epithelium on the underside of the nail plate and grows out with it. Treat this injured nail gently and advise your clients to be more careful with their nails if they want to avoid this problem in the future. Advise them to treat their nails like "jewels" and not "tools"!

Ridges running vertically down the length of the natural nail plate are caused by uneven growth of the nails, usually the result of age. Older clients are more likely to have these ridges, and unless they become very deep and weaken the nail plate, they are perfectly normal. When manicuring a client with this condition, carefully buff the nail plate to minimize the appearance of these ridges. This helps to remove or minimize the ridges, but great care must be taken not to overly thin the nail plate, which could lead to nail plate weakness and additional damage. Ridge filler is less damaging to the natural nail plate, and can be used with colored polish to give a smooth appearance to the plate while keeping it strong and healthy.

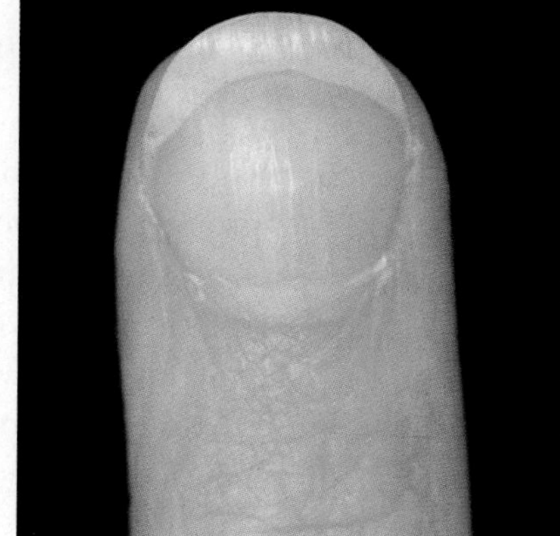
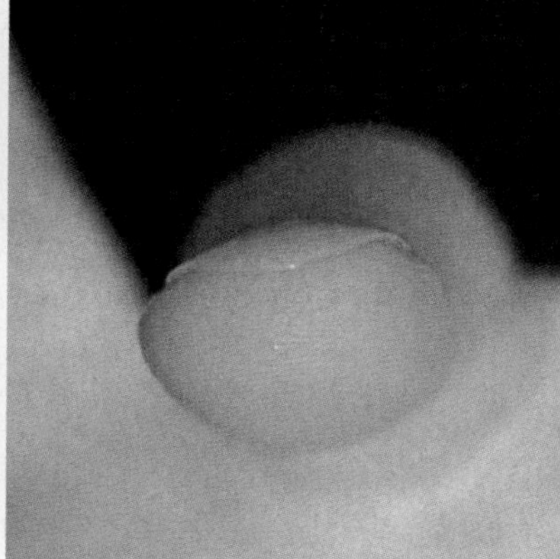

Figure 24-1 A: Eggshell nail, front view. B: Eggshell nail, end view.

Eggshell nails are noticeably thin, white nail plates that are much more flexible than normal. Eggshell nails are normally weaker and can curve over the free edge (Figure 24-1). The condition is usually caused by improper diet, hereditary factors, internal disease, or medication. Be very careful when manicuring these nails because they are fragile and can break easily. Use the fine side of an abrasive board (240 grit or higher) to file them gently and remove as little of the nail plate as possible. Do not use heavy pressure with a pusher at the base of the nail plate, because the nail is thinnest here and most likely to be punctured.

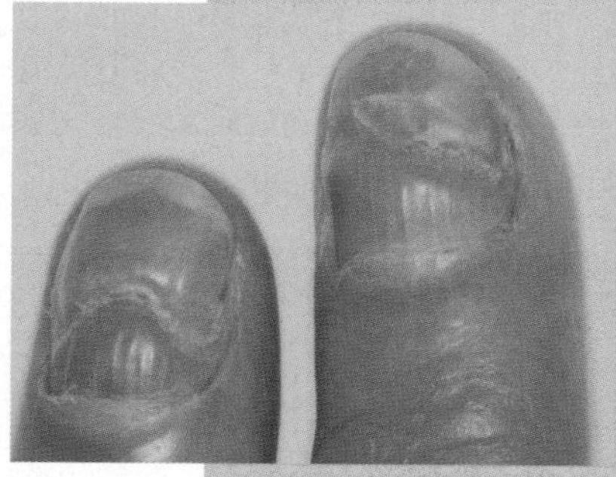

Figure 24-2 Beau's lines.

Beau's lines are visible depressions running across the width of the natural nail plate (Figure 24-2). They usually result from major illness or injury that has traumatized the body, such as pneumonia, adverse drug reaction, surgery, heart failure, massive injury, and high fever. Beau's lines occur because the matrix slows down in producing nail cells for an extended period of time, say a week or a month. This causes the nail plate to grow thinner for a period of time. The nail plate thickness usually returns to normal after the illness or condition is resolved.

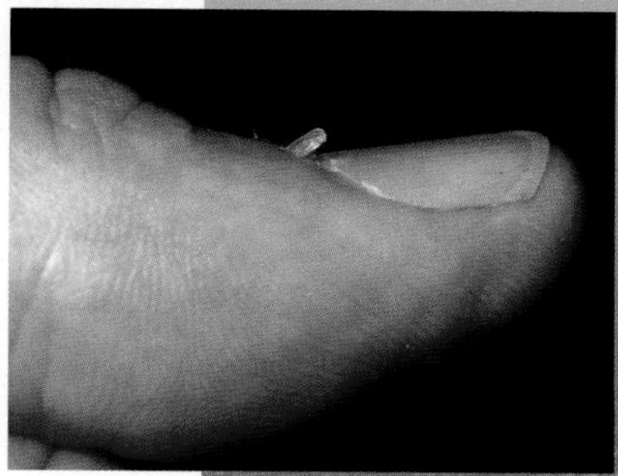

Figure 24-3 Hangnail.

Hangnail or **agnail** (AG-nayl) is a condition in which the living skin splits around the nail (Figure 24-3). Dryness of the skin or cutting this living tissue can result in hangnails. Advise the client that proper nail care, such as hot oil manicures, will aid in correcting the condition. In addition, never cut the living skin around the natural nail plate. It is against state regulatory agency regulations and can lead to serious infections for which you and the salon may be legally liable. If not properly cared for, a hangnail can become infected. Clients with symptoms of infections in their fingers should be referred to a physician. Signs of infection are redness, pain, swelling, or pus.

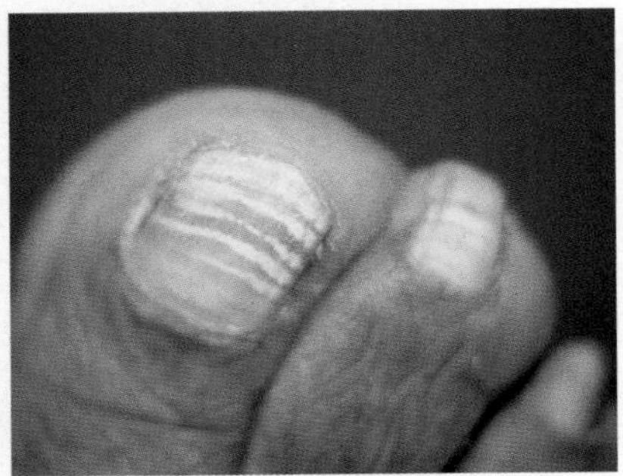
Figure 24-4 Leukonychia spots.

Leukonychia spots (loo-koh-NIK-ee-ah), or white spots, are a whitish discoloration of the nails, usually caused by injury to the nail matrix. They are not a symptom of any vitamin or mineral deficiency. Instead, they are results of minor damage to the matrix. It is a myth that these result from calcium or zinc deficiency (Figure 24-4). They appear frequently in the nails but do not indicate disease. As the nail continues to grow, the white spots eventually disappear.

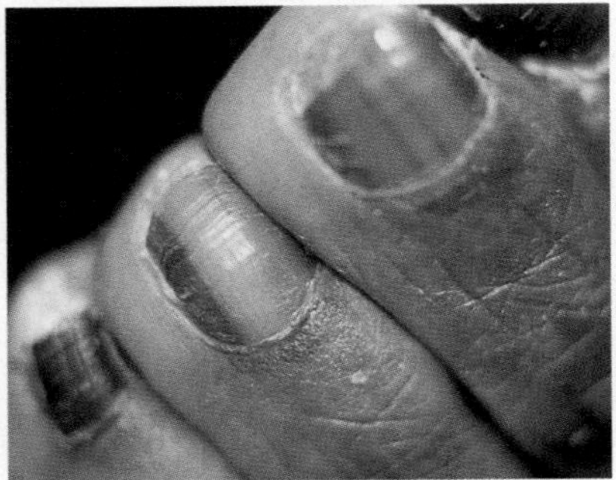
Figure 24-5 Melanonychia.

Melanonychia (mel-uh-nuh-NIK-ee-uh) is darkening of the fingernails or toenails. It may be seen as a black band within the nail plate, extending from the base to the free edge. In some cases, it may affect the entire nail plate. A localized area of increased pigment cells (melanocytes), usually within the matrix bed, is responsible for this condition. As matrix cells form the nail plate, melanin is laid down within the plate by the melanocytes. This is a fairly common occurrence and considered normal in African Americans, but could be indicative of a disease condition in Caucasians (Figure 24-5).

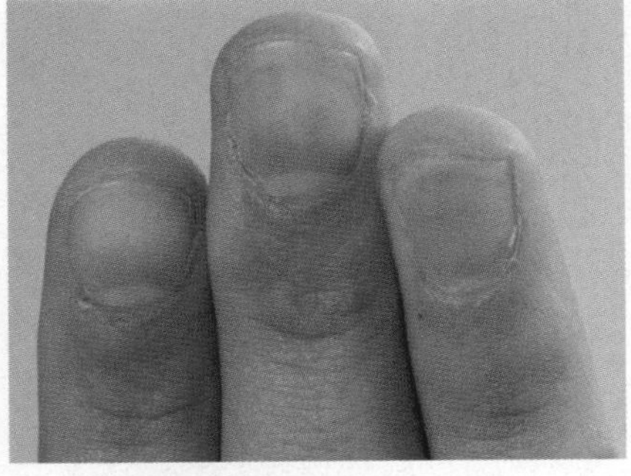
Figure 24-6 Onychophagy.

Onychophagy (ahn-ih-koh-FAY-jee), or bitten nails, is the result of a habit that prompts the individual to chew the nail or the hardened, damaged skin surrounding the nail plate (Figure 24-6). Advise the client that frequent manicures and care of the hardened eponychium can often help to overcome this habit, while improving the health and appearance of the hands. Sometimes, the application of nail enhancements can beautify deformed nails and discourage the client from biting the nails.

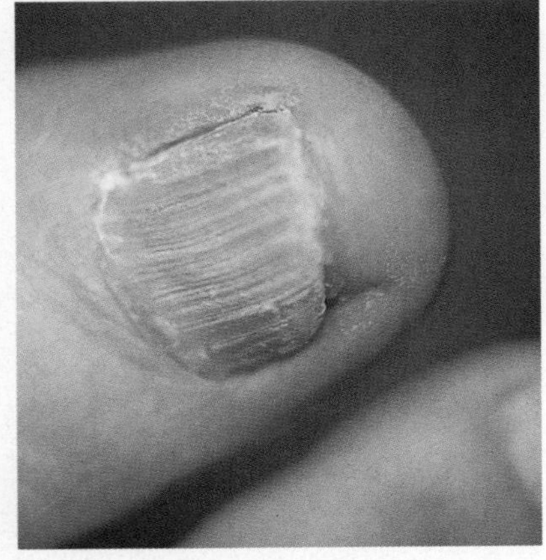
Figure 24-7 Onychorrhexis.

Onychorrhexis (ahn-ih-koh-REK-sis) refers to split or brittle nails that also have a series of lengthwise ridges giving a rough appearance to the surface of the nail plate. This condition is usually caused by injury to the matrix, excessive use of cuticle removers, harsh cleaning agents, nail polish removers, aggressive filing techniques, or hereditary causes. Nail services can be performed only if the nail is not split and exposing the nail bed. This condition may be corrected by softening the nails with a conditioning treatment, that is, hot oil manicures, and discontinuing the use of harsh detergents, cleaners, polish removers, or improper filing (Figure 24-7). These nail plates often lack sufficient moisture, so twice daily treatments with a high-quality, penetrating nail oil can be very beneficial.

Plicatured nail (plik-a-CHOORD) figuratively means "folded nail" (Figure 24-8), and is a type of highly curved nail plate often caused by injury to the matrix, but may be inherited. This condition often leads to ingrown nails.

Nail pterygium (teh-RIJ-ee-um) is an abnormal condition that occurs when skin is stretched by the nail plate. This disorder is usually caused by serious injury, such as burns or an adverse skin reaction to chemical products (Figure 24-9). The terms "cuticle" and "pterygium" are not the same thing, and they should never be used interchangeably. Nail pterygium is abnormal, that is, it denotes damage to the eponychium or hyponychium.

Do not treat nail pterygium by pushing the extension of skin back with an instrument. Doing so will cause more injury to the tissues and will make the condition worse. The gentle massage of conditioning oils or creams into the affected area may be beneficial. Hot oil manicures may be very helpful. If this condition becomes painful or show signs of infection, recommend that the client see a physician.

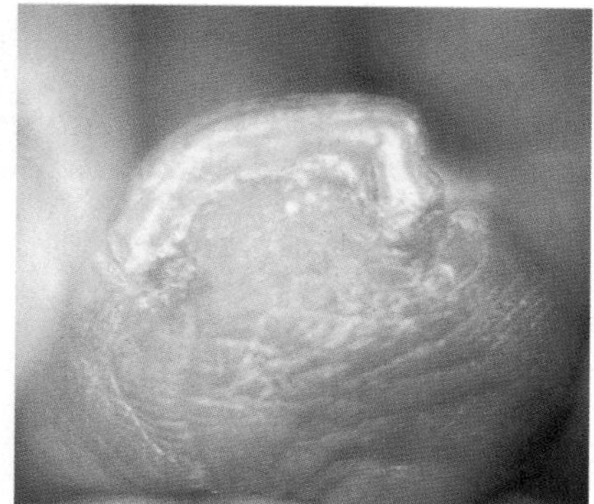

Figure 24-8 Plicatured nail.

INCREASED CURVATURE NAILS

Nail plates with a deep or sharp curvature at the free edge have this shape because of the matrix. The greater the curvature of the matrix, the greater the curvature of the free edge. Increased curvature can range from mild to severe pinching of the soft tissue at the free edge. In some cases, the free edge pinches the sidewalls into a deep curve. This is known as a trumpet or pincer nail. The nail can also curl in upon itself (Figure 24-10) or may only be deformed only on one sidewall. In each of these cases, the natural nail plate should be carefully trimmed and filed. Extreme or unusual cases should be referred to a qualified medical doctor or podiatrist. A brief summary of nail disorders is found in Table 24-1.

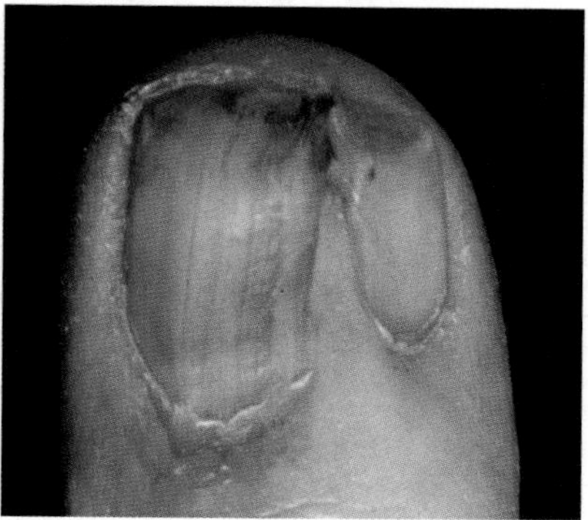

Figure 24-9 Nail pterygium.

NAIL FUNGUS

Fungi (FUN-jy) (singular fungus, FUNG-gus) are parasites, which under some circumstances may cause infections of the feet and hands. Nail fungi are of concern to the salon professional because they are contagious and can be transmitted through unsanitary implements. Fungi can spread from nail to nail on the client's feet, but it is much less likely that these pathogens will cause fingernail infections. Fungi infections prefer to grow in conditions where the skin is warm, moist, and dark, that is, feet inside shoes. It is extremely unlikely that a cosmetologist could become infected from a client, but it is possible to transmit fungal infections from one client's foot or toe to another client.

With proper sanitation and disinfection practices the transmission of fungal infections can be very easily avoided. Clients with suspected nail fungal infection must be referred to a physician.

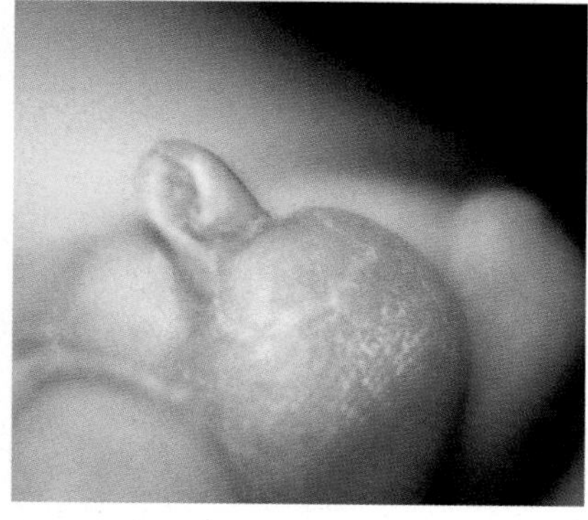

Figure 24-10 Trumpet or pincer nail

IT IS NOT A MOLD!

In the past, discolorations of the nail plate (especially those between the plate and artificial enhancements) were incorrectly referred to as "molds." This term should not be used when referring to infections of the fingernails or toenails. The discoloration is actually a bacterial infection that is caused by several types of ***Pseudomonas aeruginosa*** bacteria. These naturally occurring skin bacteria can grow out of control and cause an infection if conditions are correct for growth (Figure 24-11). Bacterial infections are more often seen on the hands. Bacteria do not need the same growing conditions as fungal organisms, and can thrive on fingernails more easily. Infection can be caused by the use of implements that are contaminated with large numbers of these bacteria. These infections are not a result of moisture trapped between the natural nail and artificial nail enhancements. This is a myth! Water does not cause infections. Infections are caused by large numbers of bacteria or fungal

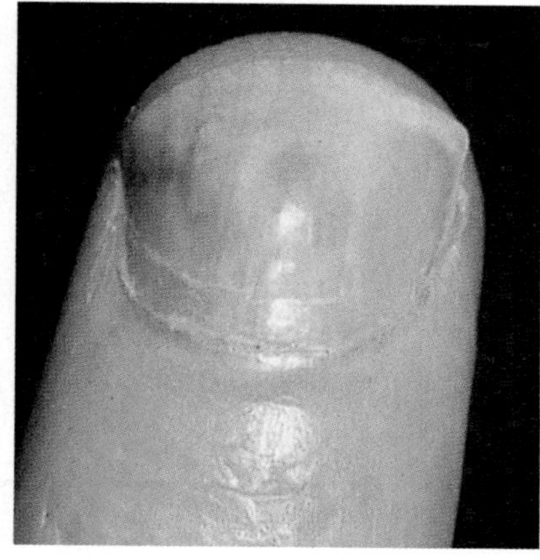

Figure 24-11 Pseudomonas aeruginosa.

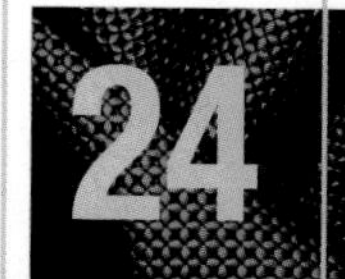

DISORDER	Signs or Symptoms
Blue nails (discolored nails)	Nails turn variety of colors; may indicate systemic disorder
Bruised nails	Dark purplish spots; ususally due to injury
Corrugations	Wavy ridges caused by uneven nail growth; usually result of illness or injury
Eggshell nails	Noticeably thin white nail plate that is more flexible than normal; may be caused by diet, illness, or medication
Furrows	Depressions in the nail that run either lengthwise or across the nail; result from illness or injury, stress, or pregnancy
Hangnail (Agnail)	The cuticle splits around the nail
Infected finger	Redness, pain, swelling, or pus; refer to physician
Leukonychia (white spots)	Whitish discoloration of the nails; usually caused by injury to the base of the nail
Melanonychia	Darkening of the fingernails or toenails
Onychatrophia	Atrophy or wasting away of the nail; caused by injury or disease
Onychauxis (hypertrophy)	Overgrowth in thickness of the nail; caused by local infection, internal imbalance, or may be hereditary
Onychophagy	Bitten nails
Onychorrhexis	Abnormal brittleness with striation (lines) of the nail plate
Plicatured nails	Folded nails
Pterygium	Forward growth of the cuticle
Tile-shaped nails	Increased crosswise curvature throughout the nail plate
Trumpet nails (pincer nails)	Edges of the nail plate curl around to form the shape of a trumpet or cone around the free edge

Table 24-1 Overview of Nail Disorders

organisms on a surface. This is why proper cleansing and preparation of the natural nail plate, as well as sanitation and disinfection of implements, are so important. If these pathogens are not present, infections cannot occur. A typical bacterial infection on the nail plate can be identified in the early stages as a yellow-green spot that becomes darker in its advanced stages. The color usually changes from yellow to green to brown to black.

You should not provide nail services for a client who has a nail fungal or bacterial infection.

CAUTION

Infection by bacteria and fungi can be easily avoided by following state regulatory agency guidelines for proper sanitation and disinfection. Do not take shortcuts or omit any of the sanitation and disinfection procedures when performing an artificial nail service. Do not perform nail services for clients who are suspected of having an infection of any kind on their nails. If you repeatedly encounter nail infections on your clients' nails, you should re-examine your sanitation, disinfection, preparation, and application techniques. Completely disinfect all metal and reusable implements, wash linens or replace with disposable towels, and thoroughly clean the table surface before and after the procedure (Figure 24-12).

NAIL DISEASES

There are several nail diseases that you may come across. A brief summary of nail diseases is found in Table 24-2. Any nail disease that shows signs of infection or inflammation (redness, pain, swelling, or pus) should not be treated in the salon. Medical treatment is required for all nail diseases.

A person's occupation can cause a variety of nail infections. For instance, infections develop more readily in people who regularly place their hands in harsh cleaning solutions. Natural oils are removed from the skin by frequent exposure to soaps, solvents, and many other types of substances. The cosmetologist's hands are exposed daily to professional products. These products should be used according to manufacturer's instructions to ensure that they are being used correctly and safely. If those instructions or warnings tell you to avoid skin contact, you should take heed and follow such advice. If the manufacturer recommends that you wear gloves, make sure that you do so to protect your skin. Contact the product manufacturer if you are not sure how to use the product safely. Product manufacturers can always provide you with additional information and guidance. Call them whenever you have any questions related to safe handling and proper use.

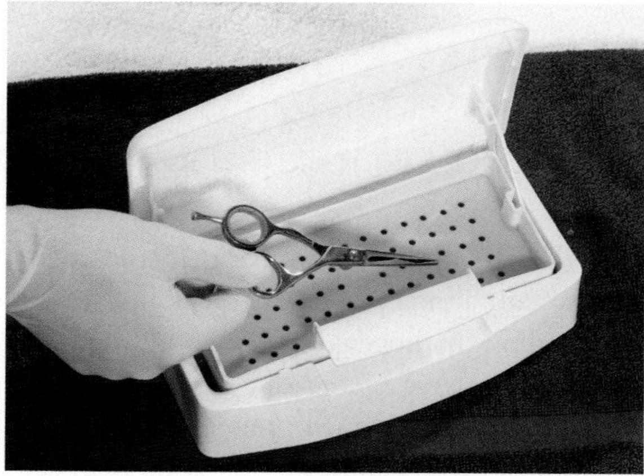

Figure 24-12 Always practice strict sanitation when working with the nails.

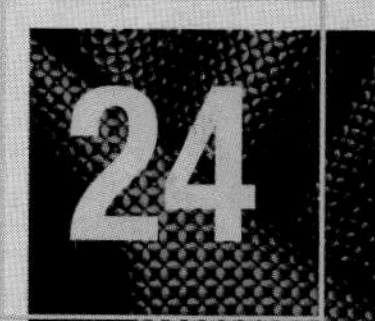

DISEASE	Signs or Symptoms
Onychia	Inflammation of the matrix with pus and shedding of the nail
Onychocryptosis	Ingrown nails
Onychogryposis	Thickening and increased curvature of the nail
Onycholysis	Loosening of the nail without shedding
Onychomadesis	Separation and falling off of a nail from the nail bed
Onychophosis	Growth of horny epithelium in the nail bed
Onychoptosis	Periodic shedding of one or more nail
Paronychia (felon)	Bacterial inflammation of the tissues around the nail; pus, thickening, and brownish discoloration of the nail plate
Pyogenic granuloma	Severe inflammation of the nail in which a lump of red tissue grows up from the nail bed to the nail plate
Tinea (ringworm)	Reddened patches of small blisters; slight or severe itching
Tinea pedis (ringworm of foot or athlete's foot)	Deep, itchy, colorless blisters
Tinea unguium (onychomycosis or ringworm of the nails)	Whitish patches on the nail that can be scraped off or long yellowish streaks within the nail substance

Table 24-2 Overview of Nail Diseases

Onychosis (ahn-ih-KOH-sis) is the term used for any deformity or disease of the nails.

Onychia (uh-NIK-ee-uh) is an inflammation of the nail matrix followed by shedding of the natural nail plate. Any break in the skin surrounding the nail plate can allow pathogens to infect the matrix. Be careful to avoid injuring sensitive tissue, and make sure that all implements are properly sanitized and disinfected. Improperly sanitized and disinfected nail implements can cause this and other diseases, if an accidental injury occurs.

Onychocryptosis (ahn-ih-koh-krip-TOH-sis), or ingrown nails, can affect fingers as well as toes (Figure 24-13). In this condition, the nail grows into the sides of the tissue around the nail. The movements of walking can press the soft tissues up against the nail plate, contributing to the problem. If the tissue around the nail plate is not infected, or if the nail is not deeply imbedded in the flesh, you can carefully trim the corner of the nail in a curved shape to relieve the pressure on the nail groove. You may not work on infected or deeply ingrown nails. Refer the client to a physician.

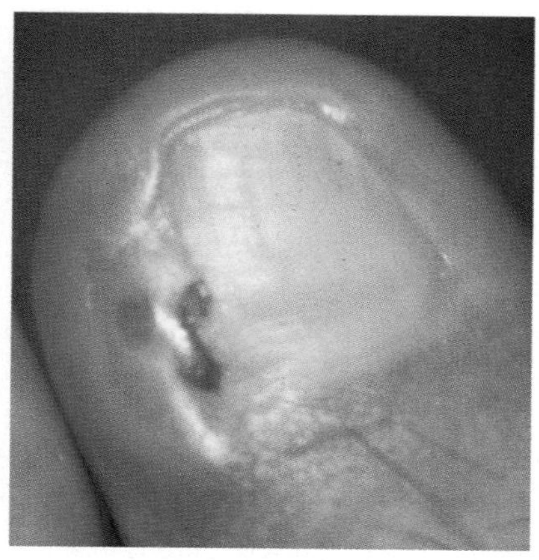

Figure 24-13 Onychocryptosis.

Onycholysis (ahn-ih-KAHL-ih-sis) is the lifting of the nail plate from the bed without shedding, usually beginning at the free edge and continuing toward the lunula area (Figure 24-14). This is usually the result of physical injury, trauma, or allergic reaction of the nail bed, and less often related to a health disorder. It often occurs when the natural nails are filed too aggressively or artificial nails are improperly removed. If there is no indication of an infection or open sores, a basic pedicure or manicure may be given. The nail plate should be short to avoid further injury, and the area underneath the nail plate should be kept clean and dry. If the trauma that caused the onycholysis is removed, the area will begin to slowly heal itself. Eventually, the nail plate will grow off the free edge and the hyponychium will reform the seal that provides a natural barrier against infection (Figure 24-15).

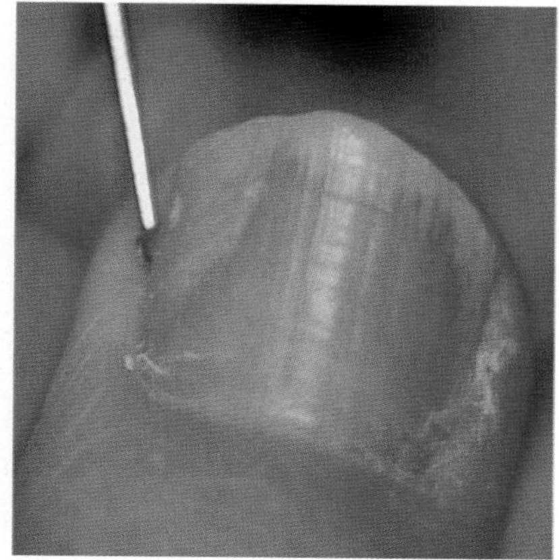

Figure 24-14 Onycholysis.

Onychomadesis (ahn-ih-koh-muh-DEE-sis) is the separation and falling off of a nail plate from the bed. It can affect fingernails and toenails (Figure 24-16). In most cases, the cause can be traced to a localized infection, injuries to the matrix, or a severe systemic illness. Drastic medical procedures such as chemotherapy may also be the cause.

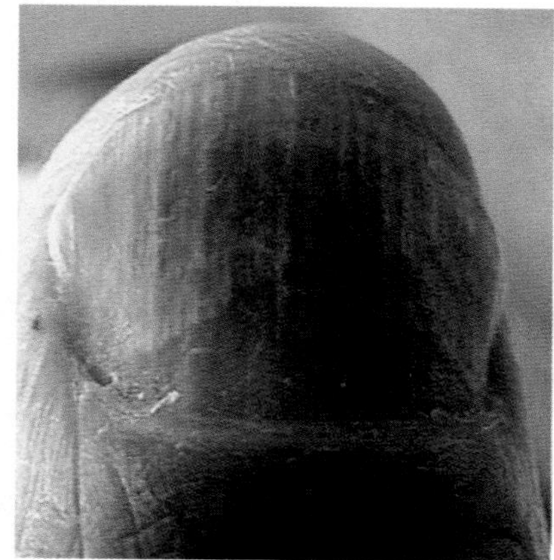

Figure 24-15 Onycholysis caused by trauma.

Whatever the reason, once the problem is resolved, a new nail plate will eventually grow again. If onychomadesis is present, do not apply enhancements to the nail plate. If there is no indication of an infection or open sores, a basic manicure or pedicure service may be given.

Nail psoriasis often causes tiny pits or severe roughness on the surface of the nail plate. Sometimes these pits occur randomly, and sometimes they appear in evenly spaced rows. Nail psoriasis can also cause the surface of the plate to look like it had been filed with a coarse abrasive, or may create a ragged free edge or all of the above (Figure 24-17). People with

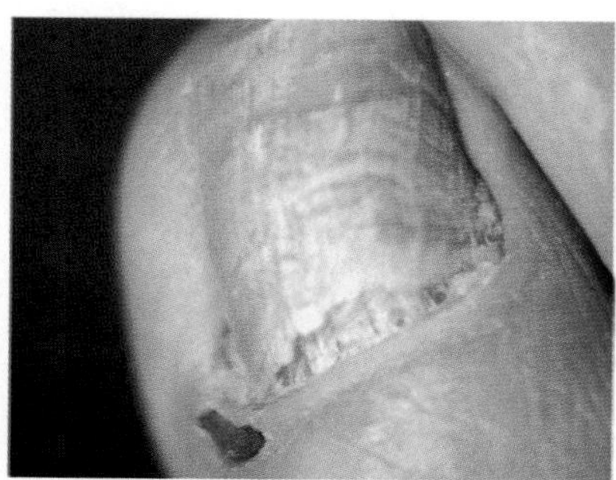

Figure 24-16 Onychomadesis.

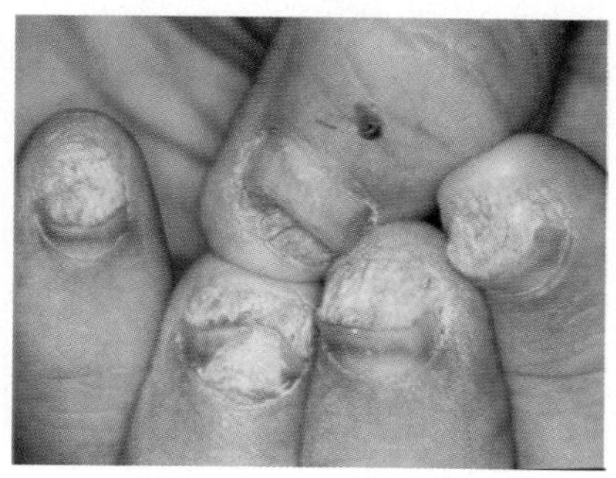

Figure 24-17 Nail psoriasis.

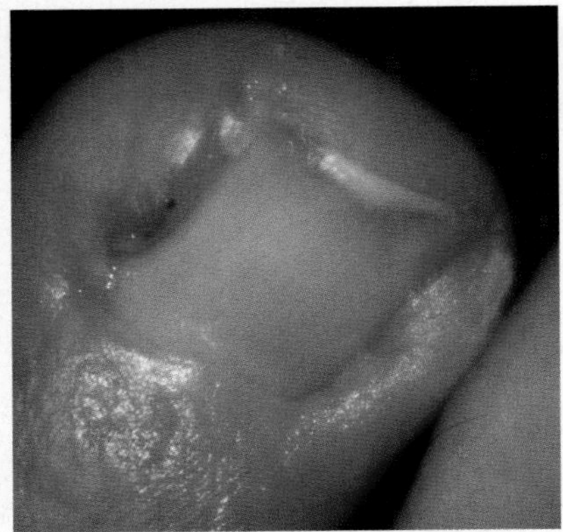

Figure 24-18 Chronic paronychia.

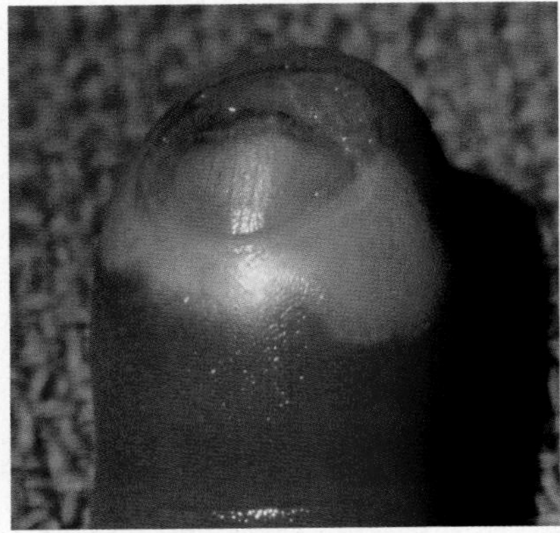

Figure 24-19 Paronychia.

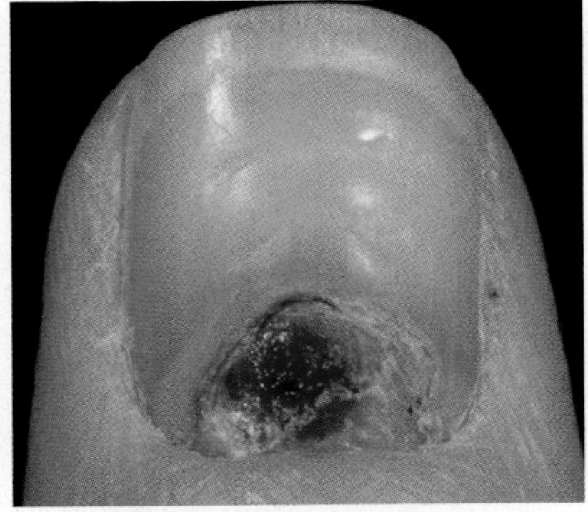

Figure 24-20 Pyogenic granuloma.

skin psoriasis will often experience these nail disorders. Nail psoriasis can also affect the nail bed, causing it to develop yellowish to reddish spots underneath the nail plate, which are called salmon patches. Onycholysis is also much more prevalent in people with nail psoriasis. When all of these symptoms are present on the nail unit at the same time, nail psoriasis becomes a likely cause of the client's problem nails and the client should be referred to a physician for diagnoses.

Paronychia (payr-uh-NIK-ee-uh) is a bacterial inflammation of the tissues surrounding the nail (Figure 24-18). Pus and swelling are usually seen in the skin fold adjacent to the nail plate.

Individuals who work with their hands in water, such as dishwashers and bartenders, or who must wash their hands continually, such as health care workers and food processors, are more susceptible, since their hands are often very dry or chapped from excessive exposure to water, detergents, and so on. This makes them much more likely to develop infections.

Toenails, because they spend a lot of time in a warm, moist environment, are often more susceptible to paronychia infections as well (Figure 24-19). Use moisturizing hand lotions to keep skin healthy and keep feet clean and dry.

Pyogenic granuloma (py-oh-JEN-ik gran-yoo-LOH-muh) is a severe inflammation of the nail in which a lump of red tissue grows up from the nail bed to the nail plate (Figure 24-20).

Tinea pedis is the medical term for fungal infections of the feet. These infections can occur on the bottoms of the feet and often appear as a red itchy rash in the spaces between the toes, most often between the fourth and fifth toe. Sometimes there is a small degree of scaling of the skin. Clients should be advised to wash their feet every day and dry them completely. This will make it difficult for the infection to live or grow. Advise clients to wear cotton socks and change them at least twice per day. They should also avoid wearing the same pair of shoes each day, since it can take up to 24 hours for a pair of shoes to completely dry. Over-the-counter antifungal powders can help keep feet dry and may help speed healing (Figure 24-21).

Onychomycosis (ahn-ihkoh-my-KOH-sis) is a fungal infection of the nail plate (Figure 24-22). A common form is whitish patches that can be

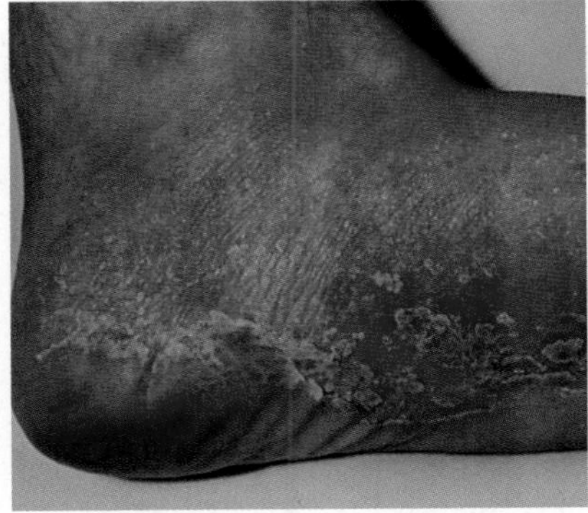

Figure 24-21 Tinea pedis.

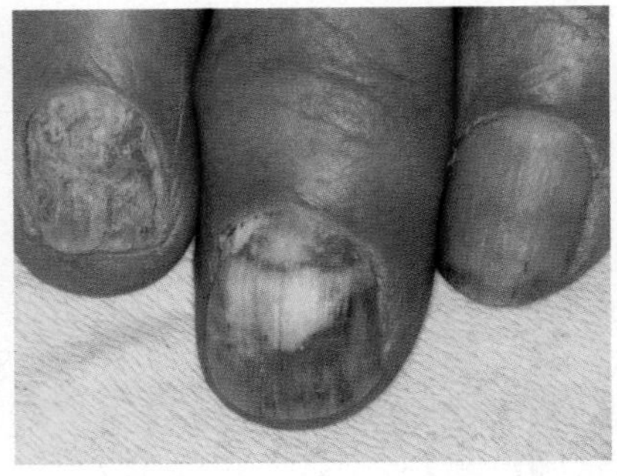

Figure 24-22 Onychomycosis.

scraped off the surface of the nail. Another common type of infection shows long whitish or pale yellowish streaks within the nail plate. A third common form causes the free edge of the nail to crumble and may even affect the entire plate. These types of infection often invade the free edge and spread toward the matrix.

Did You Know

To learn more about the natural nail and understand more about infections and disorders, be sure to read *Nail Structure and Product Chemistry,* second edition, by Douglas Schoon (Delmar/Thomson Learning, 2005).

REVIEW QUESTIONS

1. What conditions do fungal organisms favor for growth?
2. Name two common causes of onycholysis.
3. In what situation should a nail service not be performed?
4. What is *Pseudomonas aeruginosa*? Why is it important to learn about it?
5. Name at least eight nail disorders and describe their appearance.
6. What is the most effective way to avoid transferring infections among your clients?

CHAPTER GLOSSARY

Beau's lines	Visible depressions running across the width of the natural nail plate.
bruised nails	Condition in which a blood clot forms under the nail plate, forming a dark purplish spot, usually due to injury.
corrugations	Wavy ridges caused by uneven nail growth; usually result of illness or injury.
eggshell nails	Noticeably thin, white nail plate that is more flexible than normal.
furrows	Depressions in the nail that run either lengthwise or across the nail; result from illness, injury, stress or pregnancy.
hangnail or agnail	Condition in which the eponychium or other living tissue surrounding the nail plate becomes split or torn.
infected finger	Redness, pain, swelling, or pus; refer to physician.
leukonychia spots	Whitish discoloration of the nails, usually caused by injury to the matrix area; white spots.
melanonychia	Darkening of the fingernails or toenails; may be seen as a black band under or within the nail plate, extending from the base to the free edge.
nail disorder	Condition caused by an injury or disease of the nail unit.
nail psoriasis	Condition that affects the surface of the natural nail plate, causing it to appear rough and pitted, as well as causing reddish spots on the nail bed and onycholysis.

CHAPTER GLOSSARY

nail pterygium	Abnormal conditions that occurs when the skin is stretched by the nail plate; usually caused by serious injury or allergic reaction.
onychatrophia	Atrophy or wasting away of the nail; caused by injury or disease.
onychauxis (hypertrophy)	Overgrowth in thickness of the nail; caused by local infection, internal imbalance, or may be hereditary.
onychia	Inflammation of the nail matrix with shedding of the nail.
onychocryptosis	Ingrown nails.
onychogryposis	Thickening and increased curvature of the nail.
onycholysis	Loosening of the nail without shedding.
onychomadesis	The separation and falling off of a nail from the nail bed; can occur on fingernails and toenails.
onychomycosis	Fungal infection of the natural nail plate.
onychophagy	Bitten nails.
onychophosis	Growth of horny epithelium in the nail bed.
onychoptosis	Periodic shedding of one or more nail.
onychorrhexis	Split or brittle nails that also have a series of lengthwise ridges giving a rough appearance to the surface of the nail plate.
onychosis	Any deformity disease of the natural nails.
paronychia	Bacterial inflammation of the tissues around the nail; pus, thickening, and brownish discoloration of the nail plate.
plicatured nail	A type of highly curved nail plate often caused by injury to the matrix, but may be inherited; also called "folded nail".
Pseudomonas aeruginosa	One of several common bacteria that can cause nail infection.
pterygium	Forward growth of the cuticle.
pyogenic granuloma	Severe inflammation of the nail in which a lump of red tissue grows up from the nail bed to the nail plate.
ridges	Vertical lines running the length of the natural nail plate, usually related to normal aging.
tile-shaped nails	Increased crosswise curvature throughout the nail plate.
tinea pedis	Medical term for fungal infections of the feet.
tinea (ringworm)	Reddened patches of small blisters; slight or severe itching.
tinea unguium	Whitish patches on the nail that can be scraped off or long yellowish streaks within the nail substance.
trumpet nails (pincer nails)	Edges of the nail plate curl around to form the shape of a trumpet or cone around the free edge.

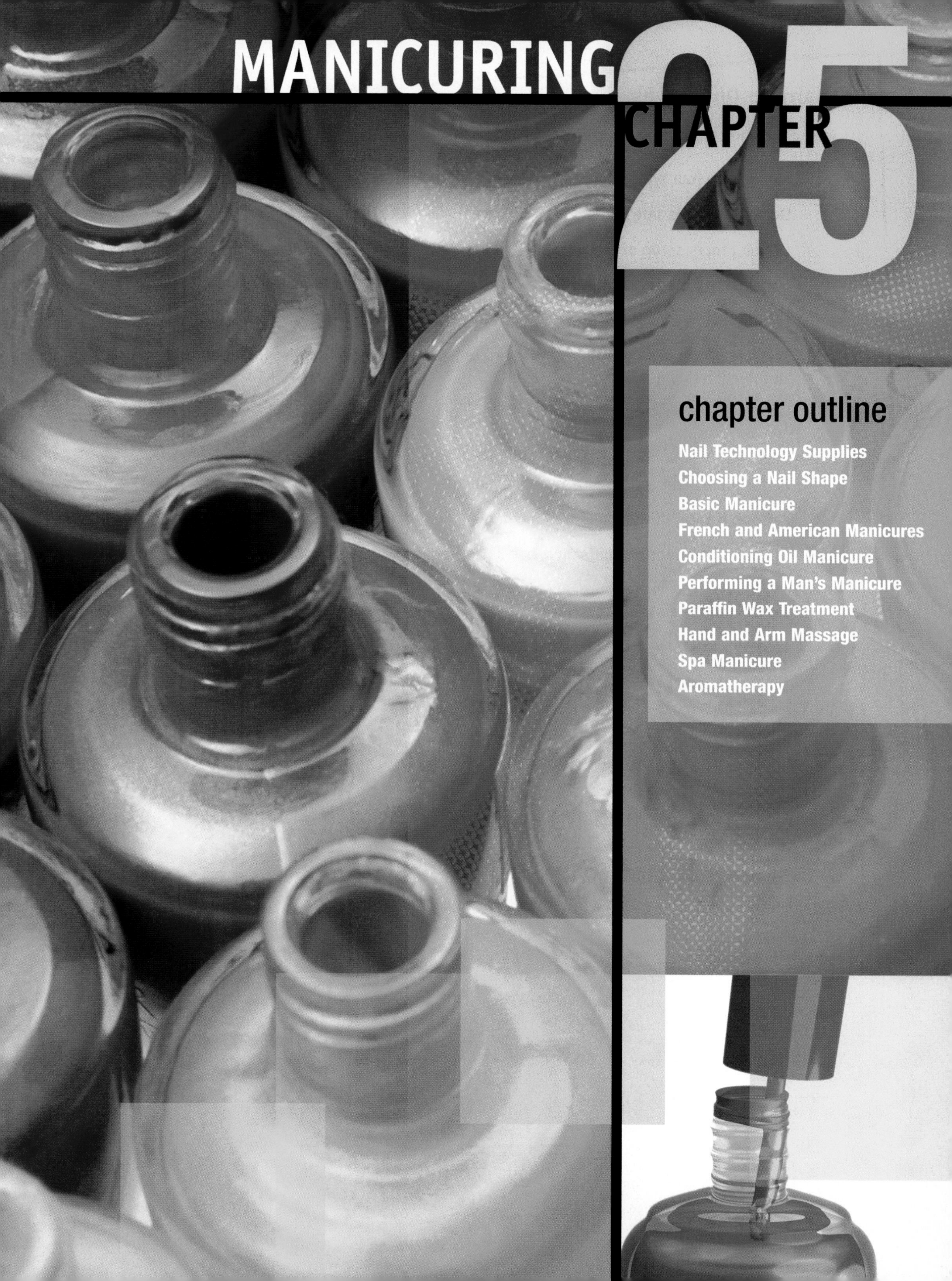

MANICURING

CHAPTER 25

chapter outline

Learning Objectives

After completing this chapter, you will be able to:

- Identify the four types of nail implements and/or tools required to perform a manicure.
- Demonstrate the safe and correct handling of nail implements and tools.
- Exhibit proper setup of a manicuring table.
- Demonstrate the necessary three-part procedure requirements for nail services.
- Identify the five basic nail shapes.
- Perform a basic and conditioning oil manicure incorporating all safety, sanitation, and disinfection requirements.
- Demonstrate the correct technique for the application of nail polish.
- Perform the five basic nail polish applications.
- Perform the hand and arm massage movements associated with manicuring.
- Perform a paraffin-wax hand treatment.
- Display all sanitation, disinfection, and safety requirements essential to nail and hand care services.
- Define and understand aromatherapy.
- Identify carrier oils and understand their use.
- Understand how aromatherapy can be incorporated into a service.

Key Terms

Page number indicates where in the chapter the term is used.

aromatherapy pg. 692

bevel pg. 659

chamois buffer pg. 661

dimethyl urea hardeners pg. 666

effleurage pg. 690

essential oils pg. 692

formaldehyde hardeners pg. 665

mild abrasive pg. 664

oval nail pg. 668

petrissage kneading movement pg. 691

pledgets pg. 663

pointed nail pg. 668

protein hardener pg. 665

pumice powder pg. 664

reinforcing-fiber hardeners pg. 665

round nail pg. 668

square nail pg. 668

squoval nail pg. 668

The importance of having well-manicured nails and hands has become a significant part of our culture for both men and women. It is one of the fastest-growing services requested in a salon. Once you have learned the basic knowledge and mastered the fundamental techniques in this chapter, you will be on your way to becoming a professional and providing these much-requested services.

NAIL TECHNOLOGY SUPPLIES

As a professional, it is imperative that you learn to work with the tools required for this service, and incorporate all safety, sanitation, and disinfection specifications during any procedure. The four types of nail technology tools that you will incorporate into your services include the following:

- Equipment
- Implements
- Materials
- Professional nail cosmetic products

EQUIPMENT

Equipment includes all permanent tools used to perform nail services that are not implements.

MANICURE TABLE WITH ADJUSTABLE LAMP

Most standard manicuring tables include a drawer (for storing properly sanitized and disinfected implements and professional products), and an attached adjustable lamp. The lamp should have a 40- to 60-watt incandescent bulb or a true-color fluorescent bulb. The heat from a higher-wattage incandescent or halogen bulb can interfere with the proper curing of artificial nail enhancement products. Do not rely on your light source to warm your client's hands. Warm client's hands by placing them on a warming pad or adjusting the temperature of the salon.

PROFESSIONAL'S CHAIR AND CLIENT'S CHAIR

The professional's chair should be selected for ergonomics, comfort, durability, and easy cleaning (sanitizing). The client's chair must be durable, comfortable, and easy to clean. For the comfort of all clients, select a client chair that can be raised and lowered, does not have arms on the sides, and supports the back so that the client's arms can rest on the nail table without stretching.

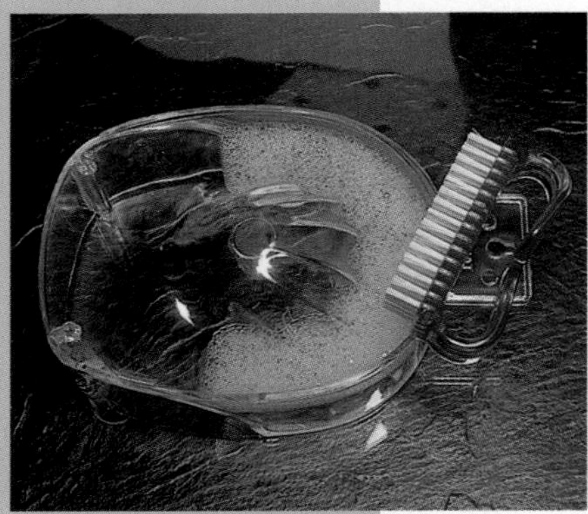

Figure 25-1 Fingerbowl filled with warm water and liquid soap, with nail brush.

FINGERBOWL

A fingerbowl is specifically designed for soaking the client's fingers in warm water with liquid soap or moisturizing soak product added. A fingerbowl can be made from materials such as plastic, metal, or glass, and should be durable and easy to sanitize after use on each client (Figure 25-1).

DISINFECTION CONTAINER

A disinfection container is a receptacle with a cover that is large enough to hold a liquid disinfectant solution in which the implements requiring disinfection can be completely immersed. Complete immersion is an important requirement. Even the handles of all the implements must be completely submerged. Containers that do not allow the entire implement, including handles, to be submerged are not adequate or acceptable for professional salons. Total immersion of the implements during disinfection is a requirement of the federal Environmental Protection Agency (EPA). Disinfectant containers come in a number of shapes, sizes, and materials. They must have a lid, which is used to keep the disinfectant solution from becoming contaminated when not in use. Some containers are equipped with a tray—lifting the tray by a handle removes implements from the solution, without contamination of the solution or implements. After removing the implements from the disinfectant container, they should be rinsed and/or air dried in accordance with the manufacturer's instructions. It is important to remember that disinfectants must never be allowed to come in contact with the skin. If your disinfectant container does not have a lift tray, always remove the implements using tongs or tweezers. Never allow your fingers to come in contact with disinfectant solution, as this contaminates the solution and damages the skin. Never place any used implements into the disinfectant container until they have been properly cleaned. Implements cannot be disinfected unless they are first properly sanitized. Remember, cleaning is the most important step, and it must occur before disinfection begins (Figure 25-2).

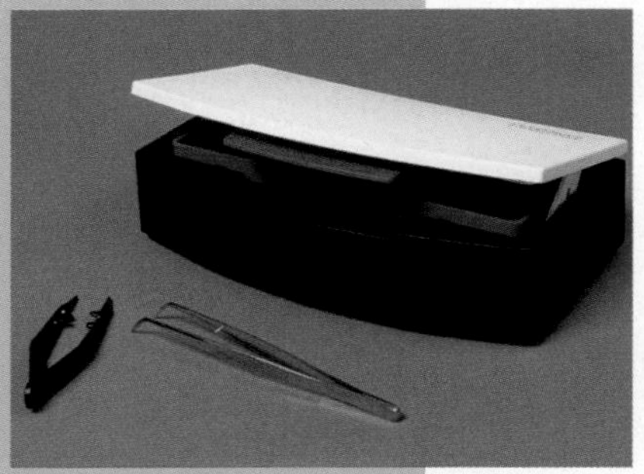

Figure 25-2 Disinfection container.

CLIENT'S ARM CUSHION

An 8-inch by 12-inch cushion for this purpose, specially made for manicuring, can be used. A towel that is folded to cushion size may also be used. Of course, a fresh clean towel must be used for each appointment.

WIPE CONTAINER

This container holds clean absorbent cotton or lint-free wipes.

SUPPLY TRAY

The tray holds cosmetics such as polishes, polish removers, and creams. It should be durable, balanced, and easy to clean.

ULTRAVIOLET OR ELECTRIC NAIL POLISH DRYER

A nail polish dryer is an optional item designed to shorten the time necessary for the client's nail polish to dry. Electric dryers have heaters that blow warm air onto the nail plates to speed evaporation of solvents from nail polishes, causing them to harden more quickly. Ultraviolet or other light bulb type nail polish dryers also create warm air to speed drying and work in the same fashion as electric dryers.

IMPLEMENTS

Implements are tools used to perform your services. In general, all implements must be properly cleaned and disinfected prior to use on another client. Some are considered disposable, and therefore must be thrown away after a single use.

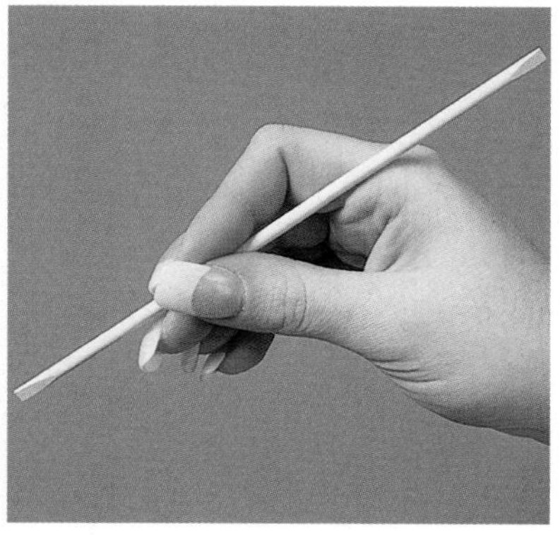

Figure 25-3 Wooden pusher.

WOODEN PUSHER

Use the wooden pusher to remove cuticle tissue from the nail plate or to clean under the free edge. Hold the stick as you would a pencil. *If you drop a wooden pusher on the floor, it must be discarded.* It is a disposable implement, and not intended for reuse. You may also use a wooden pusher to apply cosmetics by wrapping a small piece of cotton around the end (Figure 25-3). *The cotton on your wooden pusher must be changed after each use.*

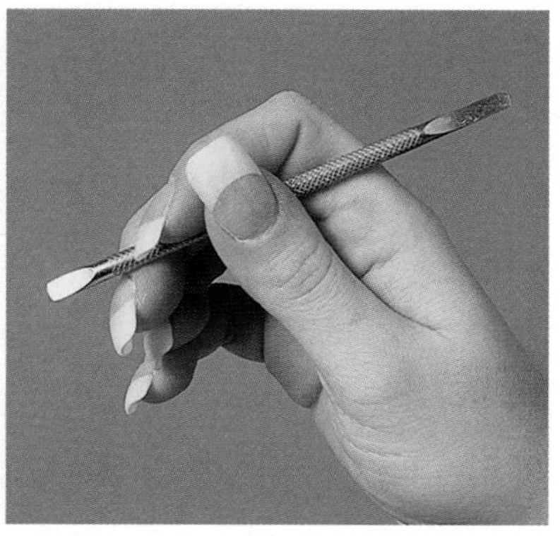

Figure 25-4 Metal pusher.

METAL PUSHER

The metal pusher, incorrectly called a cuticle pusher, is actually used to push back the eponychium, but can also be used to gently scrape cuticle tissue from the natural nail plate. Hold the metal pusher the way you hold a pencil. The spoon end is used to loosen and push back the eponychium. If you have rough or sharp edges on your pusher, use an abrasive file to dull them. This prevents digging into the nail plate or damaging the protective barrier created by the eponychium and cuticle. These devices must be properly sanitized and disinfected before use on a client. Also, use them with great care. If used improperly, they can damage the nail unit and lead to infections of the matrix or tissue surrounding the nail plate (Figure 25-4).

ABRASIVE NAIL FILES AND BUFFERS

Abrasive nail files and buffers are available in many different types and grits, such as firm, rigid, supporting cores to padded and very flexible cores, and grits ranging from less than 180 to over 240 per centimeter. A rule of thumb is the lower the grit, the larger the abrasive particles on the board and the more aggressive its action. Therefore, lower-grit boards (less than 180 grit) are relatively aggressive and will quickly reduce the thickness of any surface. Lower-grit boards also produce deeper and more visible scratches on the surface than do higher-grit boards. Therefore, lower-grit boards must be used with greater care, since they can cause more damage. Medium-grit abrasives (180 to 240 grit or higher) are used to smooth and refine surfaces. Fine-grit abrasives are in the category of 240 and higher grits. They are designed for buffing, polishing, and removing very fine scratches. Abrasive boards and buffers typically have one, two, or three different grit surfaces, depending on type and style. Coarse grit should not be used directly on the surface of the natural nail since it can create excessive thinning and damage. Coarse-grit abrasives must be used with great care, since they may create serious damage to the nail unit, if not used correctly. It is best to stick with medium- or fine-grit abrasives while performing a manicure.

To **bevel** the nail, hold the board at a 45-degree angle and file, using gentle pressure, on the top or underside of the nail.

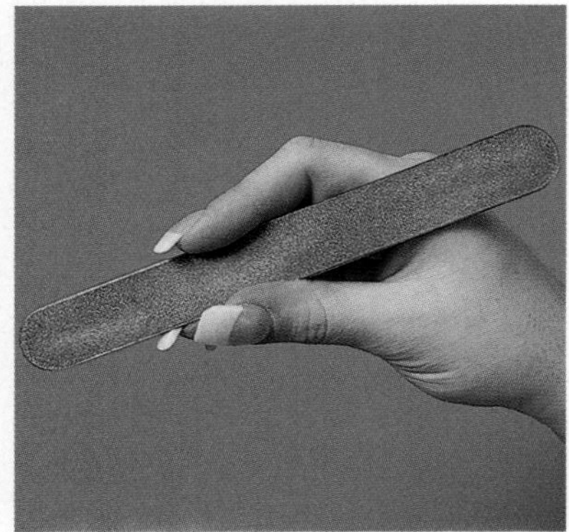

Figure 25-5 Abrasive nail file.

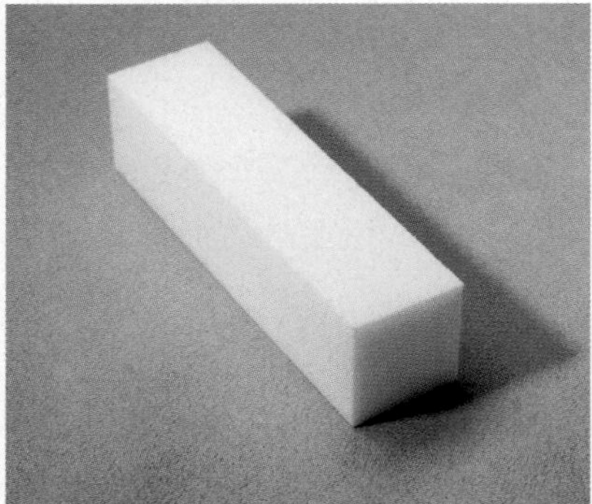

Figure 25-6 Four-way abrasive block.

Many abrasive boards and buffers can be sanitized and disinfected. Check with the manufacturer to see if the abrasive of your choice can be disinfected. All abrasives must be cleaned and disinfected before reuse on another client. Abrasives that cannot survive the sanitizing and disinfection process without being damaged or rendered ineffective are considered disposable and must be discarded after use on a single client.

It is never a good idea to store abrasives or other implements in a plastic bag or other sealed container. Airtight storage containers can promote bacterial growth. These containers create the perfect environment for pathogens to grow and multiply before your client's next appointment. Always store your clean and disinfected abrasives in a clean, unsealed container that will protect them from contamination by dust and other debris, while still allowing air to circulate freely (Figures 25-5 and 25-6).

NIPPER

A nipper is used to carefully trim away tags of dead skin. Never use the nipper to cut, rip, or tear any living tissue. Never use the nipper to trim or cut away the proximal nail fold (eponychium). To use the nippers, hold them in the palm of your hand with the blades facing the eponychium. Place your thumb on one handle and three fingers on the other handle, with your index finger on the screw to help guide the blade. They are multi-use tools that must be properly cleaned and disinfected before use on every client. It is wise to have several sets available so that you have a clean and disinfected pair ready for clients while the others are being processed (Figure 25-7).

TWEEZERS

Tweezers can be used for a wide range of uses, including lifting small bits of debris from the nail plate or removing implements from disinfectant solutions. Tweezers are multi-use tools that must be properly cleaned and disinfected since they may come in contact with a client's skin or nails.

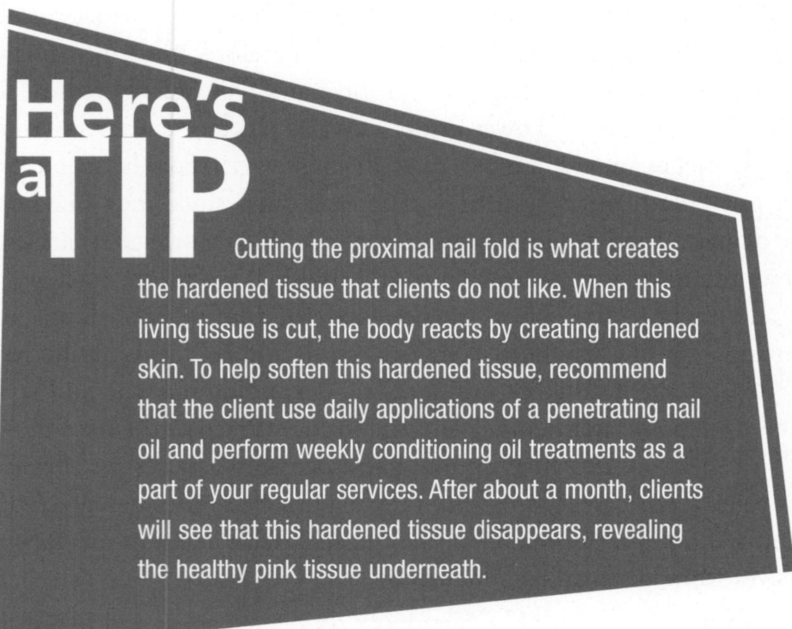

Here's a TIP

Cutting the proximal nail fold is what creates the hardened tissue that clients do not like. When this living tissue is cut, the body reacts by creating hardened skin. To help soften this hardened tissue, recommend that the client use daily applications of a penetrating nail oil and perform weekly conditioning oil treatments as a part of your regular services. After about a month, clients will see that this hardened tissue disappears, revealing the healthy pink tissue underneath.

NAIL BRUSH

A nail brush is used to clean fingernails and to remove dust and debris with warm soapy water. Hold the nail brush with the bristles turned down and away from you. Place your thumb on the handle side of the brush that is facing you, and place your fingers on the other side. These brushes must be properly sanitized and disinfected before use on a client. The safest way to do this is to have a basket or container of nail brushes that are clean and disinfected near the sink. After each client uses a clean nail brush to scrub their nails, it must be placed in a separate storage container. Used nail brushes can be kept in a disinfectant container in the bathroom after clients scrub their nails. At the end of the day, remove all of the brushes and clean and disinfect them correctly. Allow the nail brushes to air dry on a clean towel.

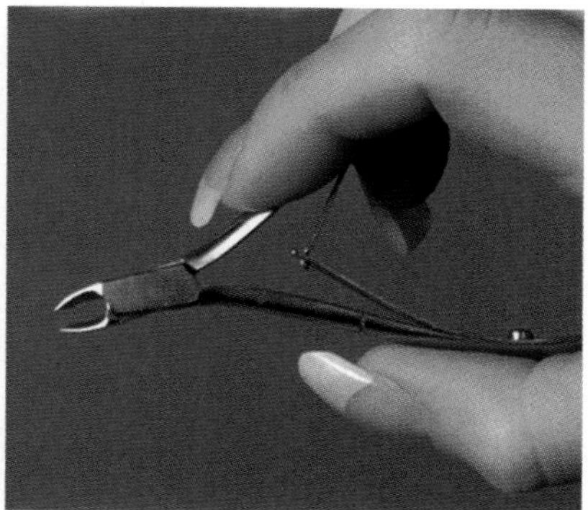

Figure 25-7 Nippers.

CHAMOIS BUFFER

The **chamois** (SHAM-ee) **buffer** is used to add shine to the nail and to smooth out wavy ridges on nails. Be guided by your instructor on how to hold the chamois buffer. Check with your instructor to determine whether chamois buffers are allowed by your state regulations (Figures 25-8 and 25-9).

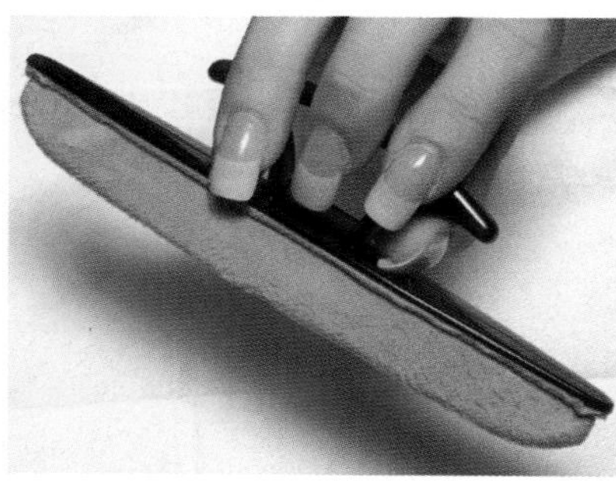

Figure 25-8 Holding a nail buffer.

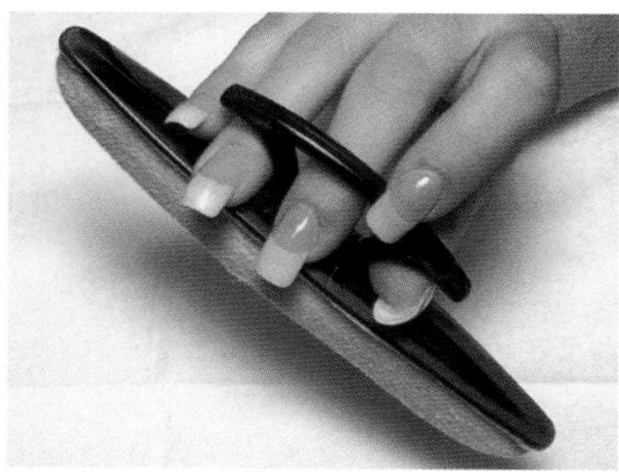

Figure 25-9 Alternative way to hold a nail buffer.

THREE-WAY BUFFER

A new abrasive technology is a buffer that replaces the chamois and creates a beautiful shine on actual nail plates or artificial nails. These buffers do not require the use of dry buffing powders and produce an equally high shine with much less effort and mess.

NAIL CLIPPERS

Nail clippers are used to shorten the nail plate. If your client's nail plates extend very far past the free edge, clipping them short will save filing time. They are multi-use, so they must be properly sanitized and disinfected before use on every client.

SANITATION AND DISINFECTION FOR IMPLEMENTS AND TOOLS

It is a good idea to have at least two complete sets of implements and abrasives ready and waiting, so that you will always have a completely clean and disinfected set for each client, with no waiting between appointments. If you have only one set of implements, remember that it takes approximately 20 minutes to properly clean and disinfect implements after each use. An overview of sanitation and disinfection of implements and tools follows. (For a more complete discussion, see Chapter 5.)

1. **Wash with warm water.** Thoroughly wash all implements/tools by scrubbing with liquid soap and warm water, and then rinse away all traces of soap with warm running water. All visible debris must be removed before proceeding to the next step.
2. **Fully immerse.** All non-disposable multi-use tools or implements must be completely and fully immersed in a disinfection container that is filled with an appropriate disinfectant solution which is approved by your state board regulations and properly prepared

according to the manufacturer's instructions. Follow the disinfectant manufacturer's instructions for the required disinfection time.

3. **Rinse and dry.** Rinse the implements (if required), and then air dry or dry with a clean towel when you remove them from the disinfection container.
4. **Store properly.** Store clean and disinfected tools or implements in a clean container and sanitary manner. Never store them in sealed containers or plastic bags. One appropriate method is to wrap them in a clean dry towel that has been taped or tied closed to prevent re-contamination of the implements via dust or other debris. Your instructor may be able to provide you with other valuable ideas and suggestions for storing implements that meet these guidelines. Remember, never allow your fingers to come into contact with a disinfectant solution.

MATERIALS

Some materials and supplies that are used during a manicure are designed to be disposable and must be replaced for each client. These items are considered to be "non-disinfectable."

DISPOSABLE TOWELS OR TERRY CLOTH TOWELS

A fresh, clean terry cloth towel or a disposable towel is used to cover the client's armrest cushion before each manicure. Another fresh towel must be used to dry the client's hands after soaking in the fingerbowl. Other terry cloth or lint-free disposable towels are used to wipe spills that may occur around the fingerbowl. Fresh towels are an example of materials that can be properly cleaned, but do not require the disinfection procedures necessary to ensure the safety of implements or abrasives.

BRUSHES AND APPLICATORS

Any brush or applicator that comes into contact with client's nails or skin, must be properly sanitized and disinfected before use on another client. If they cannot be properly cleaned and disinfected, they must be disposed of after a single use. Check with the manufacturer if you are unsure whether a brush or applicator can be properly sanitized and disinfected. One exception to this rule would be brushes used in products that are not capable of becoming contaminated with bacteria, such as alcohol, nail polish, artificial nail monomers or ultraviolet gels, nail primers, dehydrators, and bleaches, among others. Since these products cannot harbor pathogen growth, and are therefore considered to be "self-disinfecting," these brushes do not need to be sanitized and disinfected between each use. However, a brush used to apply penetrating nail oil to the nail plate would be considered unsanitary, since these products can become contaminated with bacteria if the brush is placed back into the product.

COTTON BALLS, PADS, OR PLEDGETS

Lint-free, plastic-back fiber or cotton pads are often used to remove nail polish. These are preferred over cotton balls since the plastic backing protects nail professionals' fingertips from overexposure to drying solvents and other chemicals.

Cotton can be wrapped around the end of a wooden pusher to remove nail polish from areas that are hard to reach. It can also be used for applying other nail cosmetics, such as cuticle removers. Small fiber-free squares known as **pledgets** can also be used.

PLASTIC OR METAL SPATULAS

A plastic or metal spatula must be used for removing nail cosmetics from their respective containers. If a spatula comes into contact with your skin or the client's skin, it must be properly cleaned and disinfected before being used again. This will prevent contamination of your products. Never use the same spatula to remove unlike products from different containers. Never use your fingers to remove cosmetics from a container, as they can contaminate cosmetics and may help to spread infections. A closed contaminated container of nail cosmetics is a perfect place for bacteria from fingers to grow. Cosmetic products that contain water can provide perfect growth opportunities for pathogens. All containers should be closed when not in use to avoid contamination.

TRASH CONTAINERS

A metal trash container with a self-closing lid that is operated by a foot pedal should be located next to your workstation. This type of container is one of the best ways to prevent excessive odors and vapors in the salon. The trash container should be lined, and should be closed when not in use. It must be emptied at the end of each workday before you leave or when necessary.

PROFESSIONAL NAIL COSMETIC PRODUCTS

As a professional, you need to know how to properly use each nail cosmetic and what ingredients it contains. You must know how to properly apply each cosmetic and how to avoid causing or aggravating a client's skin allergies or sensitivities. This section provides a basic understanding of several professional tools. For more detailed information on products and ingredients, see *Nail Structure and Product Chemistry,* second edition, by Douglas Schoon (Thomson Delmar Learning, 2005).

SOAP

Soap is used to clean the professional's and client's hands before a service begins. It is also mixed with warm water and used in the finger bowl as a manicure soak. Liquid soaps are recommended and preferred because bar soap harbors bacteria and can become a breeding place for pathogens.

POLISH REMOVER

Removers are used to dissolve and remove nail polish. These products contain solvents such as acetone or ethyl acetate. Oil is sometimes added to offset the drying effect of these products. Products claiming to be "non-acetone" generally contain either ethyl acetate or methyl ethyl ketone. Like acetone, both are safe for this application. Acetone works more quickly and is a better solvent than the other types of removers. Non-acetone removers will not dissolve wrap resins as quickly as acetone, so they are preferred when removing nail polish from wrap types of nail enhancements. Both acetone and non-acetone polish removers can be used safely. As with all products, be sure to read and follow the manufacturer's instructions for use.

NAIL CREAMS AND PENETRATING NAIL OILS

These products are designed to soften dry skin around the nail plate and to increase the flexibility of natural nails. They are especially effective on nails that appear to be brittle or dry. Nail creams contain ingredients designed to seal the surface and hold in the moisture found in the skin. Penetrating nail oils are designed to absorb into the nail plate (or surrounding skin) and increase flexibility. These oils will also help seal in valuable moisture. Typically, oils that can penetrate the nail plate or skin will have longer-lasting effects than creams, but both can be highly effective and useful for clients, especially as daily-use home care products.

CUTICLE REMOVERS

Cuticle removers are designed to loosen and dissolve dead tissue from the nail plate so that it can be more easily and thoroughly removed from the nail plate. These products typically contain 2- to 5-percent sodium or potassium hydroxide plus glycerin or other moisturizing ingredients to counteract the skin-drying effects of the remover. Since these products typically contain a significant amount of alkaline ingredients, they can be very drying/damaging to living tissue in the absence of proper care. Thus, removers must be used in strict accordance with the manufacturer's directions, and skin contact must be avoided where possible. Excessive exposure of the eponychium can cause skin dryness, splitting, and hangnails.

NAIL BLEACH

Apply nail bleach to the nail plate and under the free edge to remove yellow surface discoloration or stains (e.g., tobacco stains). Usually these products contain hydrogen peroxide or some other keratin-bleaching agent. Always use these products exactly as directed by the manufacturer to avoid damaging the natural nail plate or surrounding skin. Since these products can be corrosive to soft tissue, take care to limit skin contact.

PUMICE POWDER

Pumice powder (PUM-iss) is used with the chamois buffer to create additional shine on the surface of the nail plate. Pumice powder is a **mild abrasive** (ah-BRAY-sihv), which polishes fine scratches from the surface of the plate.

COLORED POLISH, ENAMEL, LACQUER, OR VARNISH

Colored coatings applied to the natural nail plate are variously known as polish, enamel, lacquer, or varnish. These are different marketing terms used to describe the same types of products containing similar ingredients. "Polish" is a generic term describing any type of solvent-based colored film applied to the nail plate for the purpose of adding color or special visual effects (e.g., sparkles). It is usually applied in two coats, but sheer colors may require only one coat. Colored polish contains a solution of nitrocellulose in a mixture of volatile solvents, such as toluene or ethyl acetate. Once the solvents evaporate, a solid film is left behind to secure the color to the nail plate. The "drying time" is largely determined by the amount and type of solvents used, as well as the temperature of the salon and the client's hands. In general, products with a thicker viscosity will contain fewer solvents and appear to dry more quickly. Thinner viscosity products contain more solvents and are slower drying. However, products that dry more quickly will often harden in the container more quickly as well. To avoid wasting products and prevent this from occurring, always keep the caps of nail polish bottles tightly sealed. This is your best defense against preventing premature evaporation of solvents. *Care must be taken not to get nail bleach on skin because it can cause skin dryness and irritation.*

CAUTION

All base coats and top coats, as well as nail polishes, are highly flammable.

BASE COAT

The base coat creates a colorless layer on the natural nail that improves adhesion of polish. Base coats also prevent polish from imparting a yellowish staining or other discoloration to the natural nail plate. These products usually rely on resins which act as an anchor for polish. Like nail polishes, base coats contain solvents designed to evaporate. After evaporation a sticky, adhesion promoting film is left behind on the surface of the nail plate. Base coats are also important to use on artificial nails, since they will help prevent surface staining from polishes.

NAIL HARDENER

Nail hardeners are used to either improve the surface hardness or durability of weak or thin nail plates. They can also prevent splitting or peeling of the nail plate. Several basic types of nail hardener are described below.

Protein hardener is a combination of clear polish and protein, such as collagen. These provide a clear, hard coating on the surface of the nail, but do not change or affect the natural nail plate itself. Collagen and protein are very large molecules and cannot absorb into the nail plate.

Reinforcing-fiber hardeners contain fibers such as nylon, but also cannot absorb into the nail plate. Therefore, the protection they provide comes from the coating itself. These products can be used on any type of natural nail.

Formaldehyde hardeners contain up to 5 percent formaldehyde, but typically they are between ¾ and 1% formaldehyde. Formaldehyde creates bridges or cross-links between the keratin strands that make up the natural nail, thereby making the plate much stiffer and more resistant to bending. These products are useful for thin and weak nail plates, but should never be applied to plates that are already very hard, rigid, and/or brittle. Formaldehyde hardeners can make brittle nails become so rigid that they may split and shatter. Also, formaldehyde hardeners must be kept off the skin because they can cause adverse skin reactions. If signs of excessive brittleness or splitting, discoloration of the nail bed, development of pterygium, or other adverse skin reactions occur, discontinue use. Once clients have achieved the desired effects with this type of hardener, they should discontinue use until the nails begin to grow out again. In other words, use as needed until clients reach the desired goal and then discontinue use until the product is needed again.

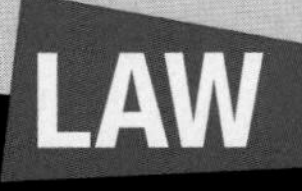

Material safety data sheets, commonly referred to as MSDS, provide valuable safe-handling information about the products, as well as first aid and proper storage information. Salons must carry an MSDS for every professional product in use. They must be kept on file or in a notebook with easy access for staff to use as a reference. The company or distributor from which you order professional products is required by law to provide you with appropriate MSDS. Your instructor can explain the importance of MSDS and how to read them.

Dimethyl urea hardeners use dimethyl urea (DMU) and also add cross-links to the natural nail plate, but unlike hardeners containing formaldehyde, they do not cause adverse skin reactions. These hardeners do not work as quickly as formaldehyde-containing hardeners, but they will not over-harden the nails and are much less likely to cause skin sensitivity.

TOP COAT

Top coats are applied over colored polish to prevent chipping and to add a shine to the finished nail. These contain ingredients that create hard shiny films after the solvent has evaporated. Typically the main ingredients are acrylic or cellulose-type film formers.

NAIL POLISH DRYERS

These products designed to hasten the drying of nail polishes are typically either applied with a dropper, a brush or sprayed on to the surface of the polish. These promote rapid drying by pulling solvents from the nail polish, causing the colored film to form more quickly. These products can dramatically shorten the dry time and will reduce the risk of smudging.

HAND CREAM AND LOTION

Hand lotion or cream adds a finishing touch to a manicure. Since they soften and smooth the hands, they make the skin and finished manicure look as beautiful as possible. Hand cream helps the skin retain moisture, so hands are less prone to becoming dry or cracked. Hand creams or lotions can be used in conjunction with warming mitts or paraffin dips to speed penetration into the skin.

NAIL CONDITIONERS

Nail conditioners contain ingredients to reduce brittleness of the nail plate and moisturize the surrounding skin. They should be applied as directed by the manufacturer, but they are especially useful when applied at night before bedtime.

BASIC TABLE SETUP

It is important that your manicure table is sanitary and properly equipped with implements, materials, and the cosmetic products needed to perform the service. Everything you need during a service should be at your fingertips. Having an orderly table will save you time and give your client more confidence in your abilities. Suggested placement of supplies on the manicuring table appears below. Since regulations regarding table setup vary from state to state, be guided by your instructor. To set up your table, use Procedure 25-1.

PROCEDURE 25-1

BASIC TABLE SETUP

1. **Clean table.** Clean manicure table and drawer with an appropriate or approved disinfectant cleaner.
2. **Prepare arm cushion.** Wrap your client's arm cushion with a clean terry cloth or disposable towel. Place the cushion in the middle of the table so that it extends toward the client and the end of the towel extends in your direction.
3. **Fill disinfectant container.** Ensure that your disinfection container is filled with clean disinfectant solution at least 20 minutes before your first manicure of the day. Use any disinfectant solution approved by your state board regulations, but make sure that you use it *exactly* as directed by the manufacturer. Also make sure that you change the disinfectant every day or whenever it becomes cloudy or visibly contaminated with debris. Nothing bothers a client or inspector more than seeing implements taken from a disinfectant jar filled with a cloudy, "dirty-looking" liquid. Put yourself in your client's shoes and put your best foot forward. If you are going to practice sanitation and disinfection, do it right. Do not just go through the motions!

   Put all disinfectable implements into the disinfection container, but only after they have been thoroughly washed and all visible debris has been removed. Place the disinfection container to your right if you are right-handed, or to your left if you are left-handed.
4. **Place products.** Place the professional products that you will use during the service (except polish) on the right side of the table behind your disinfection container (if left-handed, place on left).
5. **Place abrasives.** Place the abrasives and buffers of your choice on the table to your right (if left-handed, to your left).
6. **Place fingerbowl.** Place the fingerbowl and brush in the middle or to the left of the table, toward the client. The fingerbowl should not be moved from side to side of the manicure table. It should stay where you place it for the duration of your manicure.
7. **Prepare for waste disposal.** Tape or clip a plastic bag to the right side of table (if left-handed, tape to left side), if a metal trash receptacle with a self-closing lid is not available. This is used for depositing used materials during your manicure. These bags *must* be emptied after each client departs to prevent product vapors from escaping into the salon air.
8. **Place polishes.** Place polishes to the left (if left-handed, place on right).
9. **Prepare drawer.** The drawer can be used to store the following items for immediate use: extra cotton or cotton balls in their original container or in a fresh plastic bag, abrasives, buffers, nail polish dryer, and other supplies. Never place used materials in your drawer. Only completely sanitized and disinfected implements stored in an unsealed container (to protect them from dust and re-contamination) and extra materials or professional product should be placed in the drawer. Your drawer should always be organized and clean (Figure 25-10).

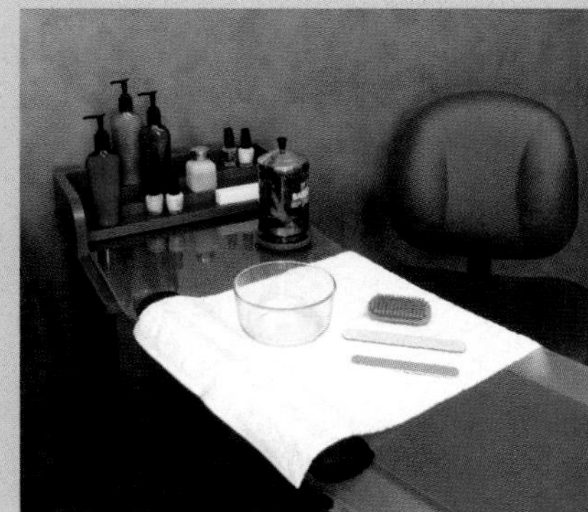

Figure 25–10 Basic table setup. Your instructor's table setup may vary from this one, and is equally correct.

CHOOSING A NAIL SHAPE

After the client consultation, you will discuss the shape and color of nails that your client prefers. Keep the following considerations in mind: shape of the hands, length of fingers, shape of the cuticle area, hobbies, recreational activities, and type of work. The length and shape of the nail plate should reflect all of these considerations. Generally it is recommended that the shape of the nail plate enhance the overall shape of the fingertip (Figure 25-11). The five basic shapes that customers prefer are discussed below.

The **square nail** is completely straight across with no rounding at the edges. You should recommend a length for nails based on your consultation.

The **squoval nail** has a square free edge that is rounded off and should extend only slightly past the fingertip. This shape is sturdy because the width of the nail is not altered and there is no square edge to break off. Clients who work with their hands—on a typewriter, computer, or assembly line—may need shorter, squoval nails.

The **round nail** should be slightly tapered and extend just a bit past the tip of the finger. Round nails are the most common choice for male clients because of their natural shape.

The **oval nail** is an attractive and more conservative nail shape that fits most women's hands. The oval shape is similar to a squoval nail with even more rounded corners. Professional clients who have their hands on display (e.g., business people, teachers, or sales people) may want longer oval nails.

The **pointed nail** is suited to thin hands with narrow nail beds. The nail is tapered somewhat longer than usual to emphasize and enhance the slender appearance of the hand; however, these nails are weaker, break more easily, and are more difficult to maintain. They should be recommended to fashion-conscious people who do not need the strongest, most durable shape of nail enhancements.

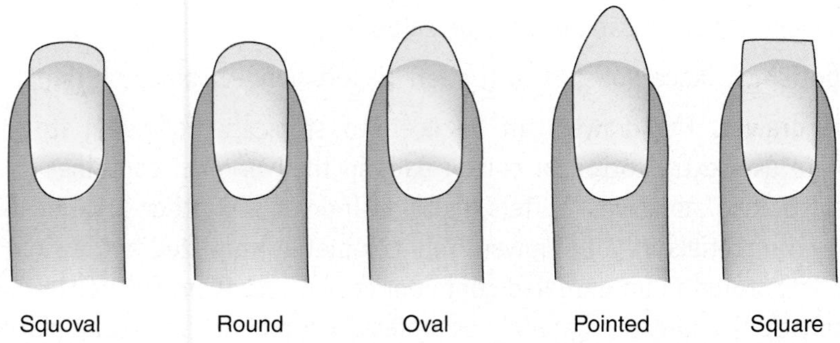

Figure 25-11 The five basic nail shapes: squoval, round, oval, pointed, and square.

BASIC MANICURE

THREE-PART PROCEDURE

It is easy to keep track of what you are doing if you break your procedures down into three individual parts. These three parts are pre-service, actual service performed, and post-service/recommendations.

1. Pre-service
    - Complete pre-service sanitation according to Procedure 25-3.
    - Greet your client with a smile (Figure 25-12).
    - Have client remove jewelry and place it in a safe, secure place.
    - Have your client wash and dry her or his hands using a liquid soap and clean terry cloth or disposable towel.
    - The client should already have filled out the information on the consultation form. At this stage, you can use this information to perform a client consultation and fill out the client service form. These forms are used to record responses from clients and record your observations before and after the service. Before beginning, always check the nails and skin area to make sure that they are healthy and that the service you are providing is appropriate. If there is a reason that the service cannot be performed, explain the reason to the client, and when appropriate suggest that he or she seek medical attention. All of this information should then be recorded on the client service form. If there are no potential issues observed, continue with the service.
2. Actual service performed
    - *During* the actual manicure, talk with your clients about the products that you are using, and suggest the products available for purchase to maintain their nails and skin care between appointments.
    - *Before* the polish application, ask your client to replace jewelry, locate necessary keys, pay for the service and retail products, and put on any outer clothing such as a sweater or jacket. By suggesting that your client complete these steps ahead of the polish application, chances of smudging the polish once the application is completed decreases.
3. Post-service
    - Complete post-service procedure according to Procedure 25-4.

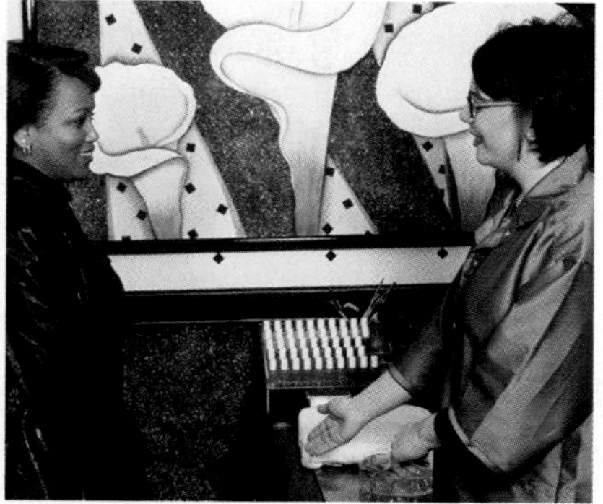

Figure 25-12 Greet your client with a smile.

HANDLING BLOOD DURING A MANICURE

On occasion, a client can be cut and blood is drawn. It could happen from careless use of a nipper or abrasive file. When this occurs, the first thing you must consider is your own safety and that of your client. Using proper sanitation and disinfection techniques is a sure way to guarantee safety. Should you accidentally cut a client, do not panic. Instead, follow the steps in Procedure 25-2.

PROCEDURE 25-2

HANDLING BLOOD DURING A MANICURE

1. **Put on gloves.** Immediately put on gloves and inform your client of what has occurred. Apologize and proceed.
2. **Apply pressure.** Apply slight pressure to the area with cotton and then clean with an antiseptic.
3. **Stanch bleeding.** If the bleeding does not stop, have the client hold the cotton to the wound or use a bandage to secure it in place for a few more minutes until the bleeding stops.
4. **Complete service.** If appropriate, continue and complete the service, avoiding the area where the injury occurred.
5. **Discard used materials.** Properly dispose of any blood-contaminated absorbent materials and abrasive files used during the service by sealing them inside a plastic bag and place this bag in the trash can. Blood-contaminated materials must be "double-bagged." Your instructor will inform you of proper disposal methods or techniques required by your state regulations.
6. **Clean table and disinfect implements.** Properly clean and disinfect all implements in accordance with your regulatory oversight agency.
7. **Remove gloves and wash hands.** Once you have removed your gloves, wash your hands for at least 30 seconds using a liquid soap and warm running water.

Always remember to use the Universal Precautions established by the Occupational Safety and Health Administration when handling items exposed to blood or other body fluids (see Chapter 5). Be guided by your instructor for your state's mandatory requirements and procedures for disinfecting any implements that have come into contact with blood or other body fluids.

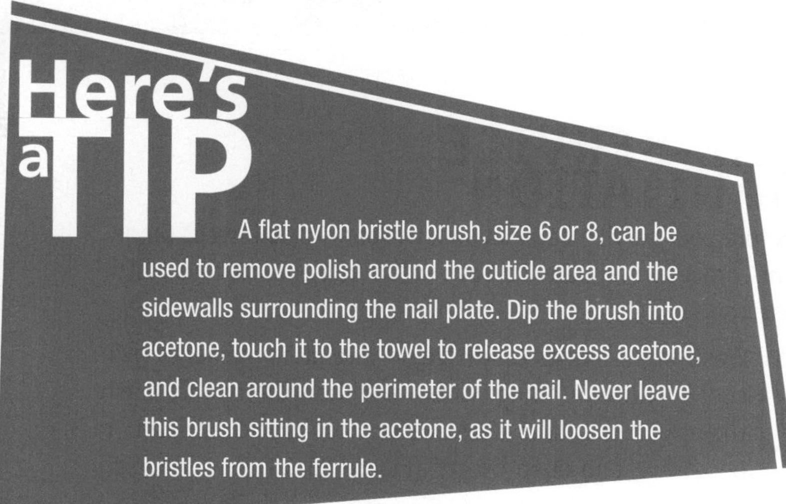

FINISHING THE NAILS

The following points provide guidelines for the proper application of nail finishes.

Nail strengthener/hardener (optional). Apply this before the base coat if the client requests this service, and if her nail plates are thin and weak.

Base coat. Always apply a base coat to keep polish from staining the artificial or natural nails, and to help colored polish adhere to the nail plate.

Colored polish. Apply two coats of colored polish. Complete your first color coat on both hands before starting the second coat. If you get polish on the skin surrounding the nail plate, use a cotton-tipped wooden pusher saturated with polish remover to clean it off. Never use a polish corrector pen because they are unsanitary.

Top coat. Apply one coat of top coat to prevent chipping and to give nails a glossy, finished appearance.

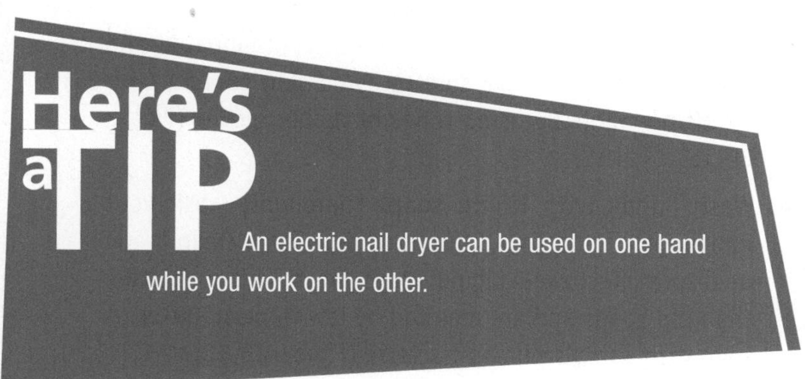
Here's a TIP
A flat nylon bristle brush, size 6 or 8, can be used to remove polish around the cuticle area and the sidewalls surrounding the nail plate. Dip the brush into acetone, touch it to the towel to release excess acetone, and clean around the perimeter of the nail. Never leave this brush sitting in the acetone, as it will loosen the bristles from the ferrule.
An electric nail dryer can be used on one hand while you work on the other.

PROCEDURE 25-3

PRE-SERVICE SANITATION

Before your service begins you must perform the steps below. This procedure applies to both salon implements and multi-use tools.

1. **Wash implements (sanitize).** Rinse all implements with cool or warm running water, and then thoroughly wash them with soap and warm water. Brush grooved items if necessary, and open hinges (Figure 25-13).
2. **Rinse implements in water.** Rinse away all traces of soap with cool or warm running water. The presence of soap in most disinfectants can cause them to become inactive. Soap is most easily rinsed off in warm, but not hot water. Hotter water will not work any better and can be damaging to hands. Dry thoroughly with a clean or disposable towel. Your implements are now properly sanitized and ready for disinfection (Figure 25-14).
3. **Immerse implements.** It is extremely important that your implements be completely clean before placing them into the disinfectant solution. If you do not, your disinfectant may become contaminated and rendered ineffective. Immerse implements in an appropriate disinfection container holding an EPA-registered disinfectant for the required time (usually 10 minutes). If it is cloudy, the solution has been contaminated and must be replaced. Make sure to avoid skin contact with all disinfectants by using tongs or rubber gloves (Figure 25-15).
4. **Wash hands with liquid soap.** Thoroughly wash your hands with liquid soap, rinse, and dry with a clean fabric or disposable towel. Liquid soaps are far more sanitary than bar soaps and are required by law in most states. A soap dish can also breed bacteria (Figure 25-16).
5. **Rinse and dry implements.** Remove implements from disinfectant solution with tongs or while wearing rubber gloves, rinse well in water, and wipe dry with a clean fabric or disposable towel to prevent rust (Figure 25-17).

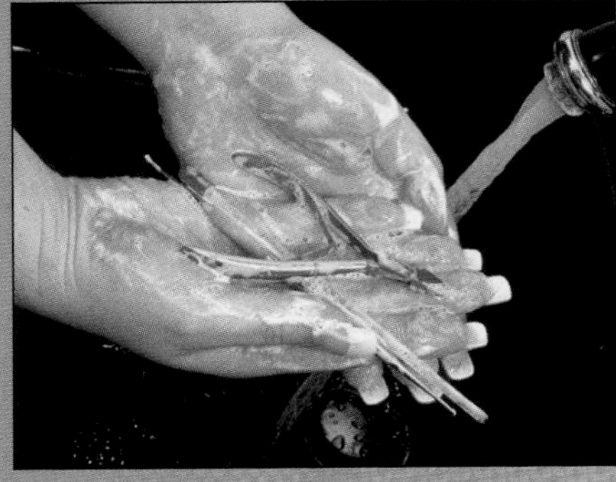

Figure 25-13 Wash implements.

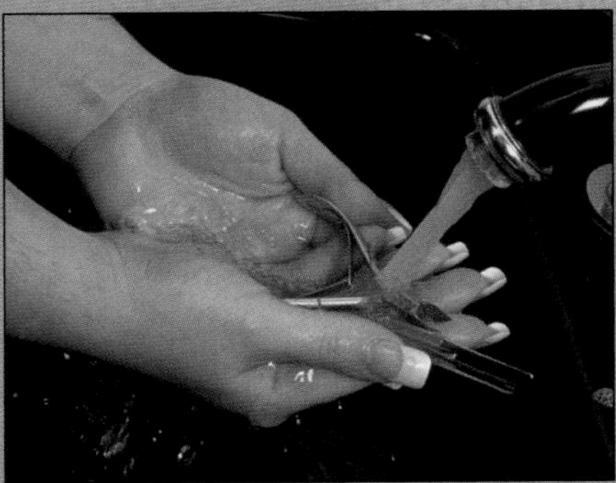

Figure 25-14 Rinse implements in clear water.

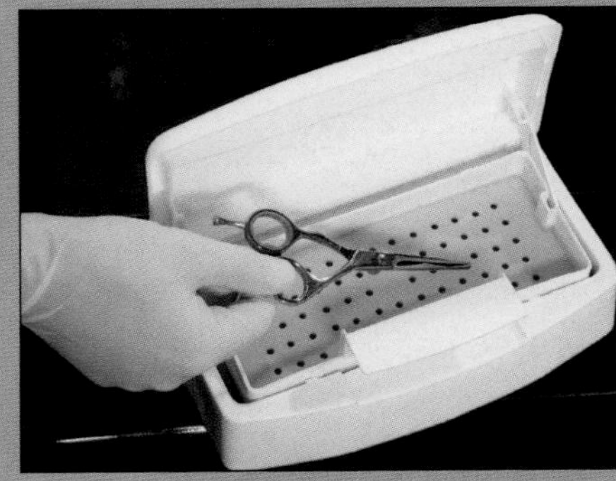

Figure 25-15 Immerse implements in disinfectant.

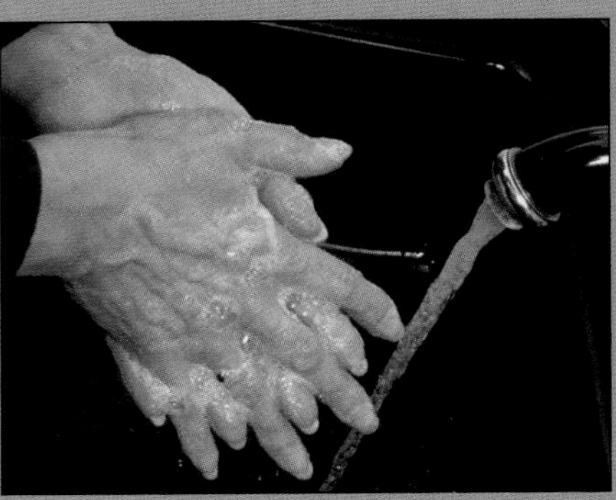

Figure 25-16 Wash hands with a liquid soap.

6. **Follow approved storage procedure.** Follow your regulatory oversight agency's requirements for storage of properly sanitized and disinfected manicuring implements. The regulations will tell you to store sanitized and disinfected implements in unsealed containers, or to keep them in a cabinet sanitizer until ready for use (Figure 25-18). Never store your implements in airtight containers. This will prevent them from properly drying and can create an environment that will foster bacterial growth.
7. **Sanitize table.** To sanitize, wipe manicuring table with cleaning solution (Figure 25-19).
8. **Disinfect surface.** To disinfect a surface that comes in contact with the client's skin, spray surface with any EPA-registered disinfectant or equivalent that is allowed by your state regulations for use in disinfecting large surfaces. Allow the surface to remain wet for 10 minutes and wipe dry, and then spray again and let air dry (Figure 25-20).
9. **Prepare the client's cushion.** Put a clean towel over your manicuring cushion. Be sure to use a clean towel for each client (Figure 25-21).
10. **Refill disposable materials.** Put a new wooden pusher stick, cotton balls, and other disposable materials on your manicuring table. These materials are discarded after use on *one* client (Figure 25-22).
11. **Use hand sanitizers.** Clients like to see that you practice sanitation. Make a ceremony of this and they will trust you. After your clients have thoroughly washed their hands, you can offer them a waterless hand sanitizer gel or wipe for their hands. You can do so as well. Be sure to make an effort to regularly rehydrate your hands, as repeated use of hand sanitizers can cause skin dryness (Figure 25-23). It is very important to remember that these products cannot and do not replace proper hand washing. Proper hand washing is a vital part of the service and it cannot be skipped or ignored. Clients must properly wash their hands before and after the service, and you must properly wash your hands between each customer. *Now you are ready to begin your service.*

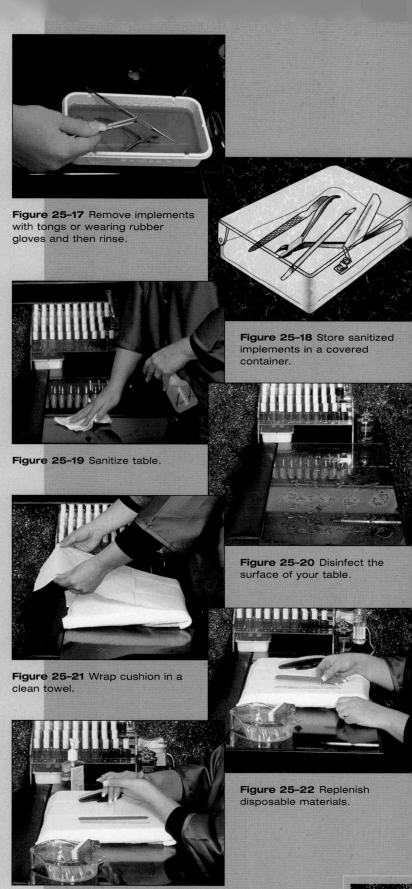

Figure 25-17 Remove implements with tongs or wearing rubber gloves and then rinse.

Figure 25-18 Store sanitized implements in a covered container.

Figure 25-19 Sanitize table.

Figure 25-20 Disinfect the surface of your table.

Figure 25-21 Wrap cushion in a clean towel.

Figure 25-22 Replenish disposable materials.

Figure 25-23 Use sanitizing hand wash.

PROCEDURE 25-4

PERFORMING A BASIC MANICURE

Begin working with the hand that is *not* the client's favored hand. The favored hand will need to soak longer, because it is used more often. In brief, if the client is left-handed, begin with the right hand; if the client is right-handed, begin with the left hand.

During the manicure, talk with your client about the products and procedures you are using. Suggest additional products that the client will need to maintain the manicure between salon visits. These products might include nail or skin treatments, polish, lotion, top coats, and so on. **Note:** This procedure is written for a right-handed client.

1. **Remove polish.** Begin with your client's left hand, little finger. Saturate cotton ball or plastic-backed cotton pad with polish remover. Hold saturated cotton on nail while you silently count to 10. The old polish will now remove easily from the nail plate with a stroking motion toward the free edge. If all polish is not removed, repeat this step until all traces of polish are gone. It may be necessary to put cotton around the tip of a wooden pusher and use it to clean polish away from the nail fold area. Repeat this procedure on each finger (Figure 25-24).

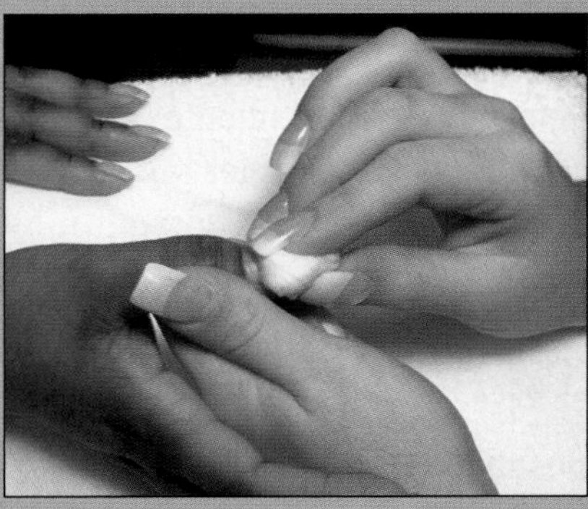

Figure 25-24 Remove polish.

Here's a TIP

Roll a piece of cotton between your hands before you use it. This keeps loose cotton fibers from sticking to the nail or finger. An alternative way to remove nail polish is to moisten small pieces of cotton, called *pledgets* (PLEJ-ets), with nail polish remover and put them on all the nails at the same time.

2. **Shape the nails.** Using your abrasive board, shape the nails as you and the client have agreed. Start with the left hand, little finger, holding it between your thumb and index finger. Do not use less than a medium-grit (180) abrasive file to shape the natural nail. File from the right side to the center of the free edge and from the left side to the center of the free edge (Figure 25-25). To lessen the chance of developing ingrown nails, do not file into the corners of the nails (Figure 25-26). File each hand from the little finger to the thumb. Never use a sawing back and forth motion when filing the natural nail, as this can disrupt the nail plate layers and cause splitting and peeling.

   Never file nails that have been soaking in water. Water will absorb into the nail plate and make it softer and more easily broken or split during filing. If the nails need to be shortened, they can be cut with nail clippers. This will save time during the filing process.

3. **Soften the eponychium and cuticles.** After filing the nails on the left hand, place the fingertips in the fingerbowl to soak and soften the eponychium (living skin) and cuticle (dead tissue on the nail plate) while you file the nails on the right hand.

4. **Clean nails.** Brushing the nails and hands with a nail brush cleans fingers and helps remove pieces of debris from the nails. Remove the left hand from the fingerbowl and brush the fingers with your nail brush. Use downward strokes, starting at the first knuckle and brushing toward the free edge (Figure 25-27).

5. **Dry hand.** Dry the hand with the end of a fresh towel. Make sure you dry between the fingers. As you dry, gently push back the eponychium (Figure 25-28).

6. **Apply cuticle remover.** Use a cotton-tipped wooden or metal pusher or cotton swab to apply cuticle remover to the cuticle on each nail plate of the left hand (Figure 25-29). Take care to avoid getting this type of product on living skin, since it can cause dryness or irritation. Spread evenly, and avoid using so much that it runs into the soft tissue. Cuticle removers soften skin by dissolving it, so that they are inappropriate for regular skin contact, especially with your own skin. Typically, these products have

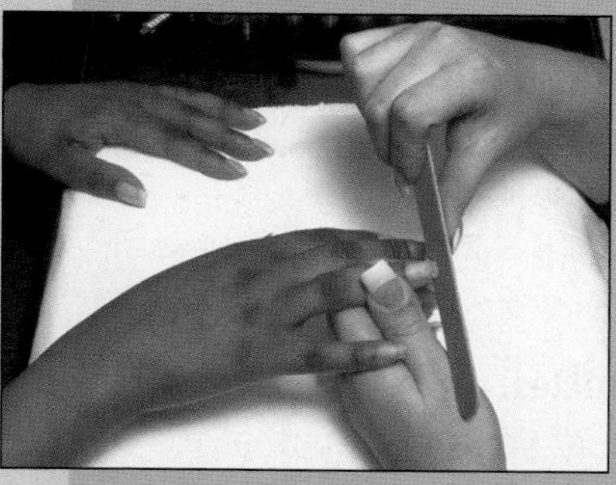

Figure 25-25 Shape nails.

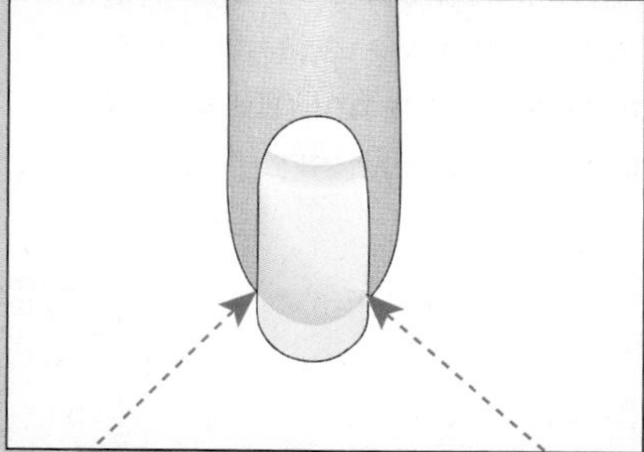

Figure 25-26 Do not file into the corners of the nail.

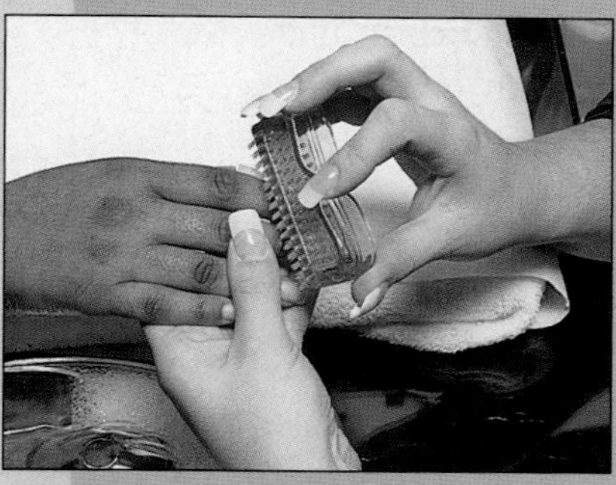

Figure 25-27 Clean nails.

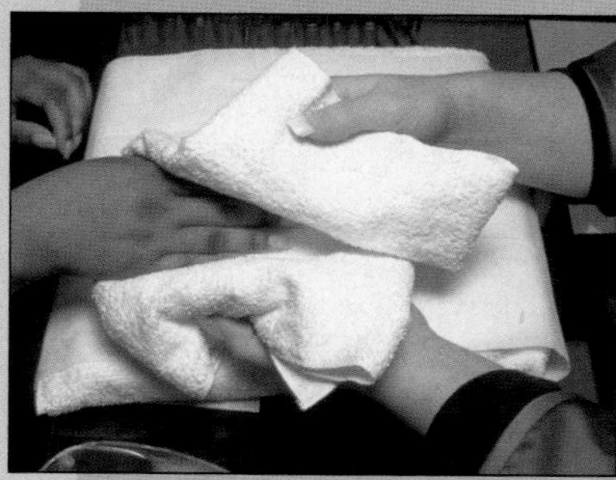

Figure 25-28 Dry hand.

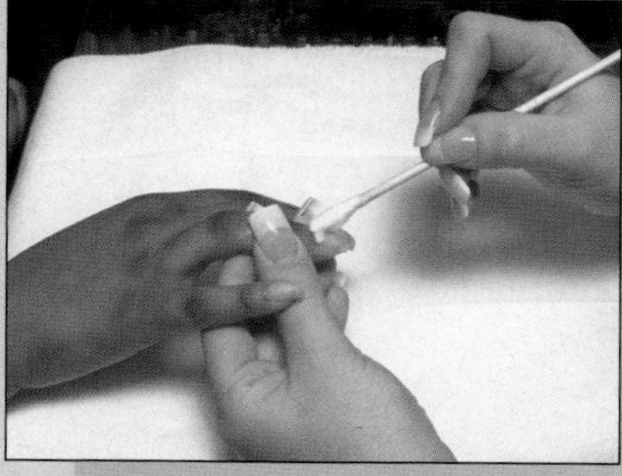

Figure 25-29 Apply cuticle remover.

a pH of 12 or higher and are corrosive. After leaving the product on for the manufacturer's recommended length of time, the cuticle will be easily removed from the nail plate with a wooden pusher or other implement designed for such purposes.

7. **Loosen and remove cuticles.** Use your wooden pusher or the spoon end of your metal pusher to gently push and lift cuticle tissue off each nail plate of the left hand (Figure 25-30). Use a circular movement to help lift dead, tightly adhering tissue. Now place the right hand into the fingerbowl to soak while you continue to work on your client's left hand (Figure 25-31).
8. **Clip away dead tags of skin.** Use nippers to remove any loosely hanging tags of skin (hangnails). Never rip or tear the living skin, since this can damage skin and may lead to infection (Figure 25-32).
9. **Clean under free edge.** Carefully clean under the free edge using a cotton swab or cotton-tipped wooden pusher. Cleaning too aggressively in this area can break the hyponychium seal under the free edge and cause onycholysis. Remove right hand from the fingerbowl. Hold the left hand over the fingerbowl and brush one last time to remove bits of debris and traces of cuticle remover. It is important to make sure that all traces of cuticle remover are washed from the skin, as remnants can lead to dryness and/or irritation. Then, let the client rest the left hand on the towel (Figure 25-33).
10. **Repeat Steps 5 to 9 on the right hand.**
11. **Bleach nails (optional).** If the client's nails are yellow, you can bleach them with a nail bleach designed specifically for this purpose. Apply the bleaching agent to the yellowed nail with a cotton-tipped orangewood stick. Be careful not to brush bleach on your client's skin, because it may cause irritation.

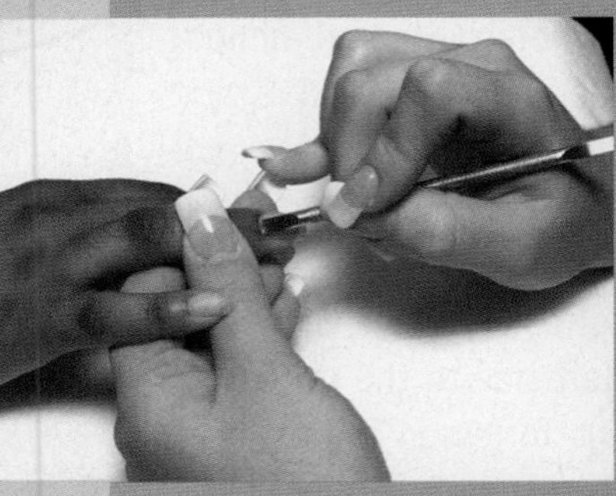

Figure 25-30 Loosen and remove the cuticle from the nail plate.

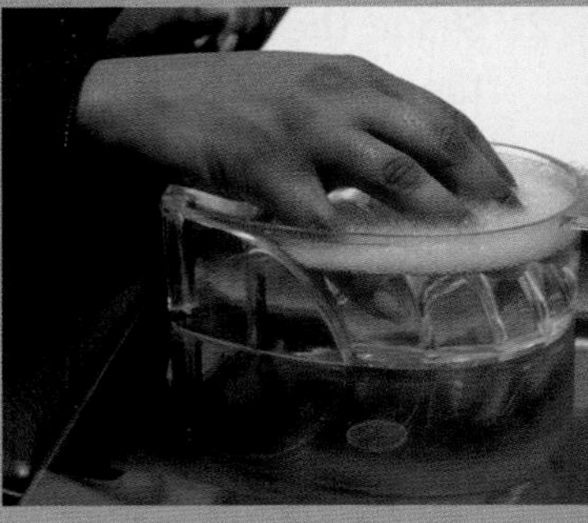

Figure 25-31 Soak hand.

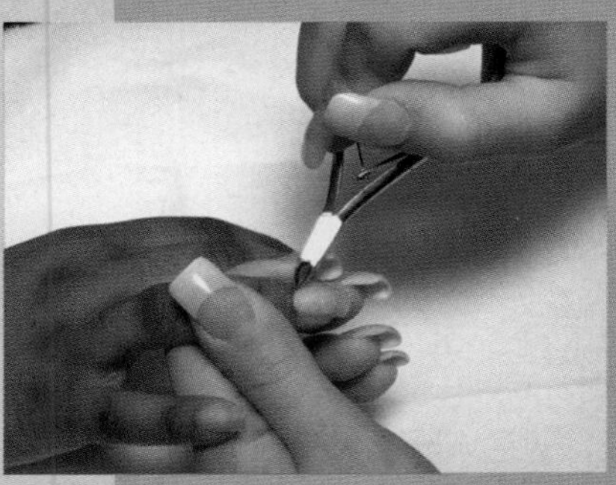

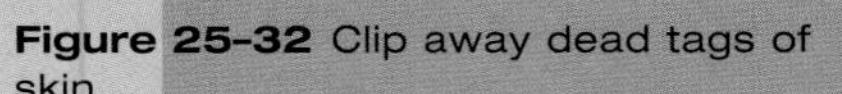

Figure 25-32 Clip away dead tags of skin.

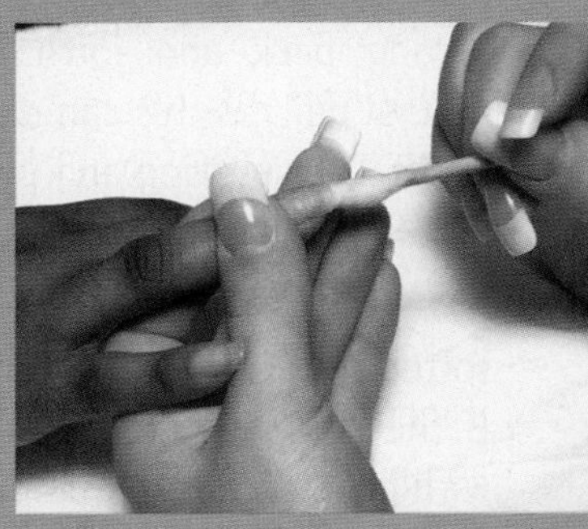

Figure 25-33 Clean under free ed

CAUTION

When pushing back the eponychium, take care not to use too much force or pressure since damage to this area could harm the nail matrix.

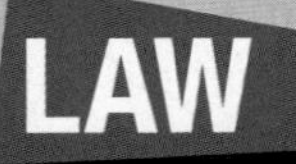

LAW

State or province regulations do not permit nail professionals to cut or ni living skin. This practice can lead to serious skin infections and injury.

Repeat application if nails are extremely yellow. You may need to bleach certain clients' nails several times, as all of the yellow stain or discoloration may not fade after a single service. You should plan to repeat the procedure when the client receives the next manicure. Surface stains are removed more easily than those that travel deep into the nail plate. Yellow discoloration that goes deep into the nail plate will never be completely removed by nail bleaches. These products work best for surface stains (e.g., tobacco).

12. **Buff with a high-shine buffer.** Use a high-shine buffer to smooth out surface scratches and give the natural nail a brilliant shine (Figures 25-34 and 25-35).
13. **Apply nail oil.** Use a cotton-tipped wooden pusher, cotton swab, or an eyedropper to apply nail oil to each nail plate. Start with the little finger, left hand, and massage oil into the nail plate and surrounding skin using a circular motion (Figure 25-36).
14. **Bevel nails.** To bevel (BEH-vel) the underside of the free edge, hold a medium-grit abrasive board at a 45-degree angle, and file with an upward stroke. This removes any rough edges or cuticle particles. A fine-grit abrasive board or buffer may also be used (Figure 25-37).
15. **Apply lotion and massage.** Applying hand lotion is the finishing touch for any manicure, but should be done before you apply the polish, since it may interfere with proper adhesion. You can use the lotion to massage your client's hands and arms. (Follow the steps for hand and arm massage in Procedures 25-10 and 25-11.)
16. **Remove traces of oil.** You must remove all traces of lotion or oil from the nail plate before proceeding, or the polish will not adhere as well. Use a small piece of cotton saturated with alcohol or polish remover, and scrub the nail plate clean as if you were removing a stubborn red nail polish. Do not forget to clean under the free edge of the nail plate to remove any remaining massage lotion. The cleaner you get the nail plate, the better the polish will adhere to the nail plate.
17. **Choose a color.** If your client is undecided about the color of the nail polish, help the client to choose one. Suggest a shade that complements the skin tone. If the manicure and polish are for a special occasion, pick a color that matches the client's clothing or the holiday season. Generally, darker shades are appropriate for fall and winter, and lighter shades are better for spring and summer.

    Always have a wide variety of nail polish colors available. Before applying polish, you may ask your client to pay for the service, put on any jewelry, sweater, or jacket, and get out car keys. This will avoid smudges to the freshly applied polish.

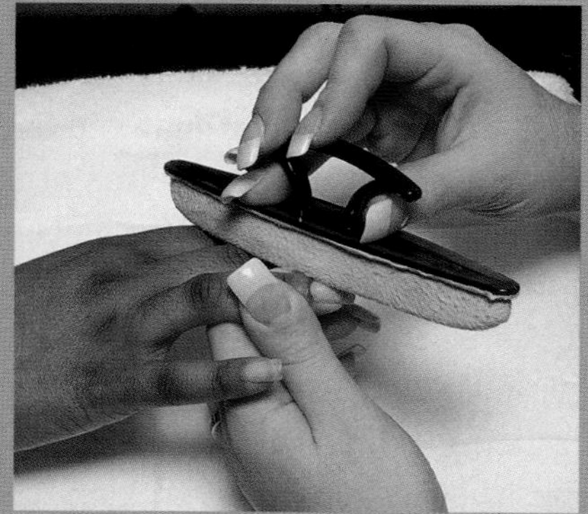

Figure 25-34 Buff nails.

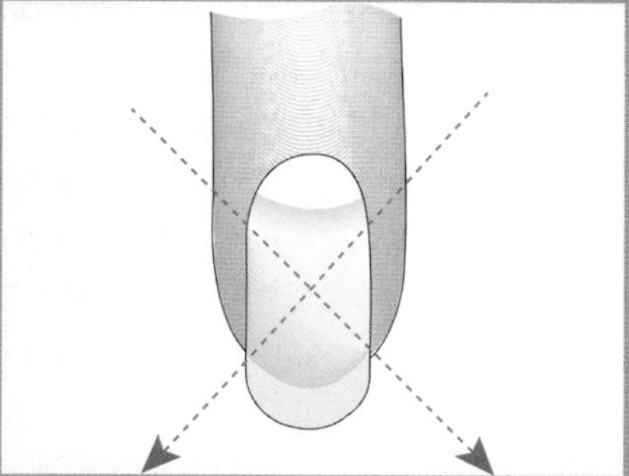

Figure 25-35 Buff nail in an "X" pattern with downward strokes.

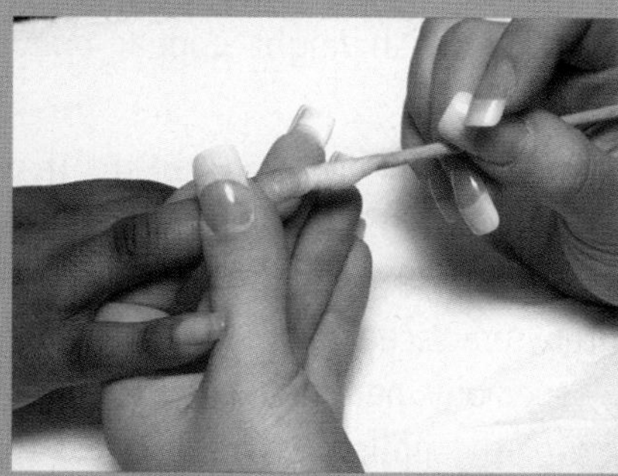

Figure 25-36 Apply cuticle oil.

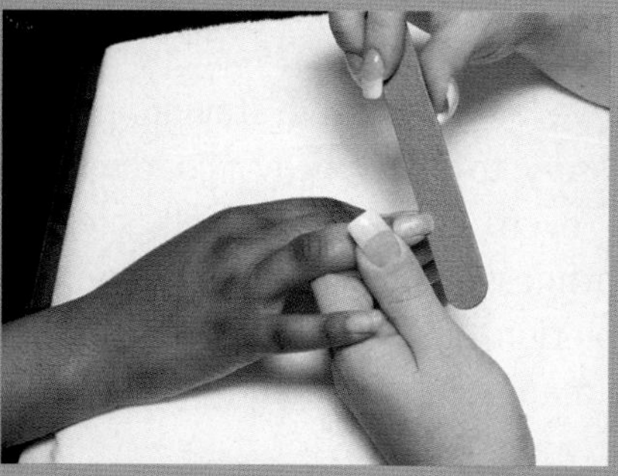

Figure 25-37 Bevel nail.

18. **Apply polish.** The greatest success in applying nail polish is best achieved by using four coats. The first, the base coat, is followed by two coats of polish color and one application of top coat to give a protective seal. The techniques are the same for applying all polishes, base coats, or top coats. Never shake your polish bottles. Shaking will cause air bubbles to form and make the polish application rough and appear irregular. Gently roll the polish bottles between your palms to thoroughly mix.

    When applying, remove the brush from the bottle and wipe it on the inside of the neck of the bottle to remove excess polish. You should have a bead of polish on the end of the brush. There should be enough polish on the brush to add one layer of polish to the nail plate without having to dip the brush back into the polish bottle, unless the nail plate is unusually long. Hold the brush at approximately a 30- to 35-degree angle. Place it 1/16 inch away from the cuticle area, starting in the center of the nail. Brush toward the free edge of the nail. Use the same technique for the entire nail. If you go back and dab at any spots that you missed, the polish might appear uneven on the nail.

    When applying the colored polish, if you miss a small area on your client's nail you can cover this area before you apply the second coat, but definitely practice covering the entire nail each time, especially near the cuticle area to avoid a shadow of the polish. In addition to the finished nail appearance, the purpose of using multiple layers of product when applying polish is to provide the best longevity and durability of the service. By building layer upon layer, you will improve adhesion and staying power. It is not necessary to apply heavy coatings. Instead, use thin even coats. This will create maximum smoothness and minimum drying time. On completion of the polish application, the polish should appear smooth and even on the nails.

Here's a TIP

Excessive downward pressure or low-grit abrasives can generate excessive heat on the nail bed. This can lead to a friction burn that could result in onycholysis and possible infection. If your client is feeling heat or a sharp burning sensation as you file, you should lighten the downward pressure and/or use a less aggressive (higher-grit) abrasive. The client should not feel burning sensations on their nail beds as you file.

Here's a TIP

When applying an iridescent or frosted polish, it is imperative to make sure that the strokes are parallel to the sidewalls of the nail.

PROCEDURE 25-5

POST-SERVICE PROCEDURES

The steps below should be followed after any nail service.

1. **Schedule next appointment.** Set up date, time, and services for your client's next appointment. Write the information on your business card and give it to the client.
2. **Advise client.** Advise client about proper home maintenance for their service. For example, if they have long nails or nail extensions, advise them to take care when opening doors or file cabinet drawers. If the service was a pedicure, advise them of the importance of wearing properly fitted and comfortable shoes.
3. **Promote product sales.** Depending on the service provided, there may be a number of retail products that you should recommend for the client to take home. This is the time to do so.
4. **Clean work area.** Clean your work area and properly dispose of all used materials.
5. **Disinfect implements.**
6. **Record service information.** Record service information, observations, and product recommendations on the client service form.

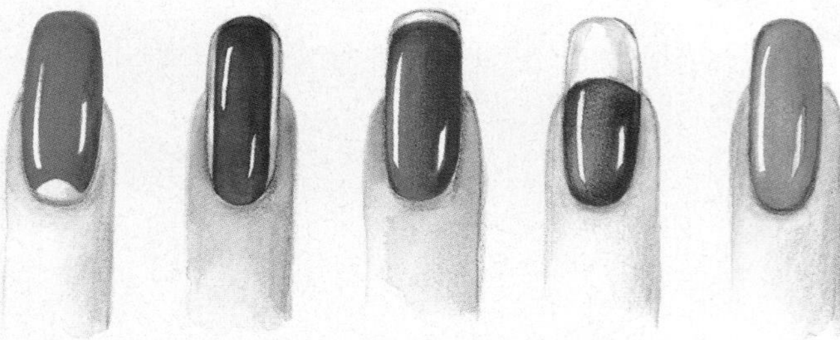

Figure 25-38 Five polish options: half moon or lunula, slimline or free walls, hairline tip, free edge, or full coverage.

FIVE TYPES OF POLISH APPLICATION

Once you have mastered the techniques necessary to apply polish correctly and expertly, you can focus on creating the following five types of polish applications (Figure 25-38).

Full coverage. Entire nail plate is polished.

Free edge. The free edge of the nail is unpolished. This helps to prevent polish from chipping.

Hairline tip. The nail plate is polished and 1⁄16-inch is removed from the free edge. This prevents polish from chipping.

Slim-line or free walls. Leave 1⁄16-inch margin on each side of nail plate. This makes a wide nail appear narrow.

Half-moon or lunula. A half-moon shape, the lunula, at the base of the nail is unpolished.

Polishing is very important. It is the last step in a perfect manicure and the last thing your client sees between visits. When your client looks at his or her nails polished perfectly, they will admire them, and you for doing a great job (Figure 25-39).

FRENCH AND AMERICAN MANICURES

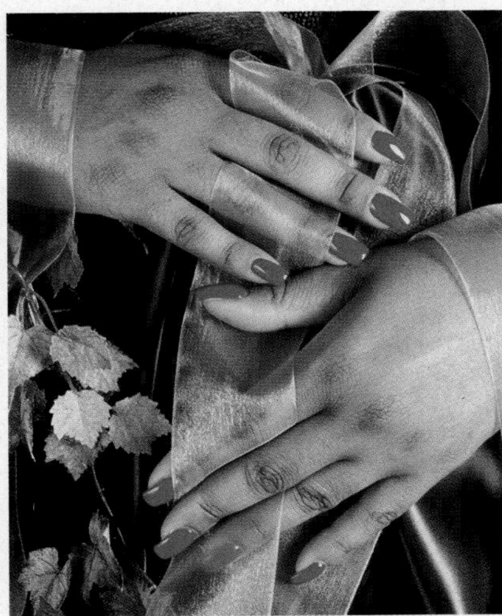

Figure 25-39 Finished manicure.

French polish applications, as well as American polish applications, are very popular and often requested in the salon. These polish techniques create nails that appear clean and can have a natural appearance. They provide a good base for endless service designs that can be enhanced with the use of hand-painted art, air-brushing, rhinestones, pearls, or stripping tape. The French manicure usually has a dramatic white on the free edge of the nail, where the American manicure calls for a more subtle white. Perform the basic manicuring procedures up to the polish application then begin Procedure 25-6.

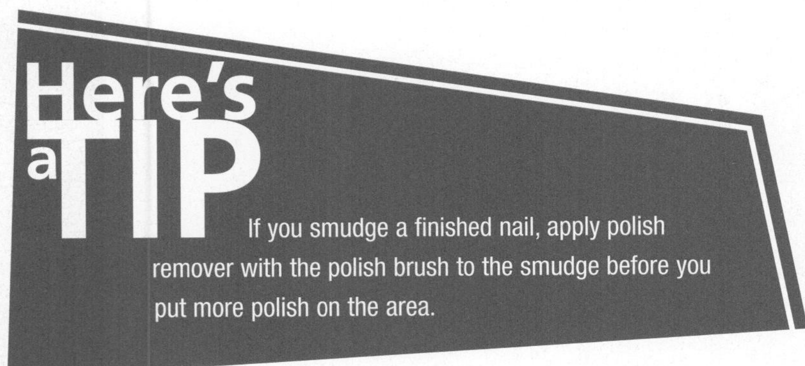

Here's a TIP

If you smudge a finished nail, apply polish remover with the polish brush to the smudge before you put more polish on the area.

PROCEDURE 25-6

PERFORMING FRENCH AND AMERICAN MANICURES

1. **Apply base coat.** Apply a base coat to the nail. The base coat can be applied under the free edge as well. If the nail has pitting, striations, or ridges, use a ridge-filling base coat to mask these imperfections and provide a smooth surface for the polish. Ridge-filling base coats contain an opaque colorant that fills in and hides these minor surface defects.
2. **Apply white polish.** Apply white polish to the free edge by starting at one side (usually left side of nail) and sweeping across toward the center of the free edge on a diagonal line. Repeat this on the right side of the nail. This will form a "V" shape. Some clients like this look. If not, fill the open top of the "V," so that you have an even line across the free edge. White may be applied under the free edge. Allow the white polish to dry (Figures 25-40 to 25-42).
3. **Apply translucent polish.** Apply a sheer white, pink, natural, or peach color polish from the base to the free edge. Be careful not to get any on the eponychium. Most clients will prefer a pink shade, but choose the color according to skin tone and client preference. This is an important and valuable service that you can provide to your clients and they will love you for it.
4. **Apply top coat.** Apply a top coat over the entire nail plate and under the free edge (if applicable to situation) (Figure 25-43).

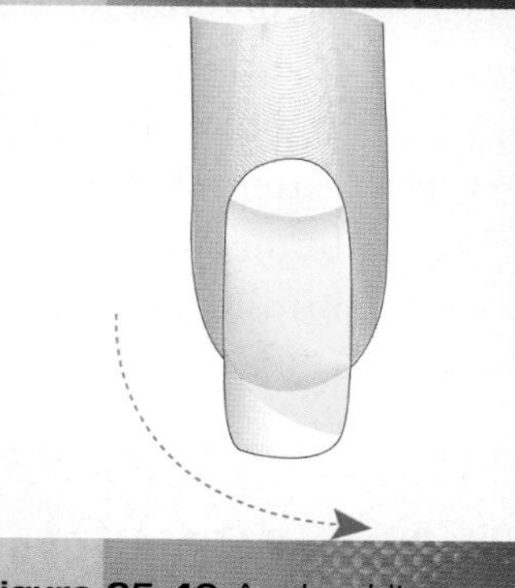

Figure 25-40 Apply white polish on free edge from the left side of the nail to the center.

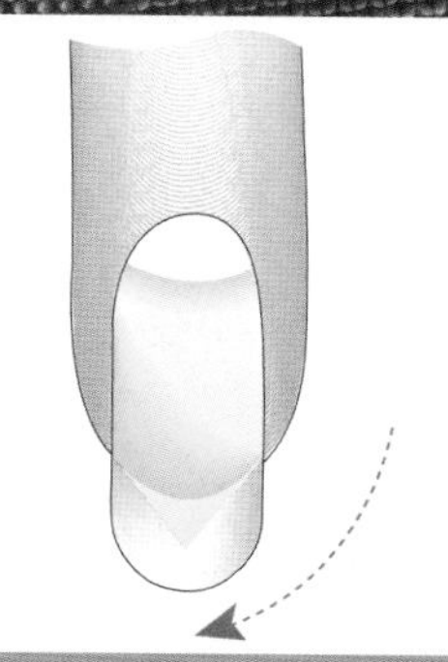

Figure 25-41 Apply white polish on free edge from the right side of the nail to the center.

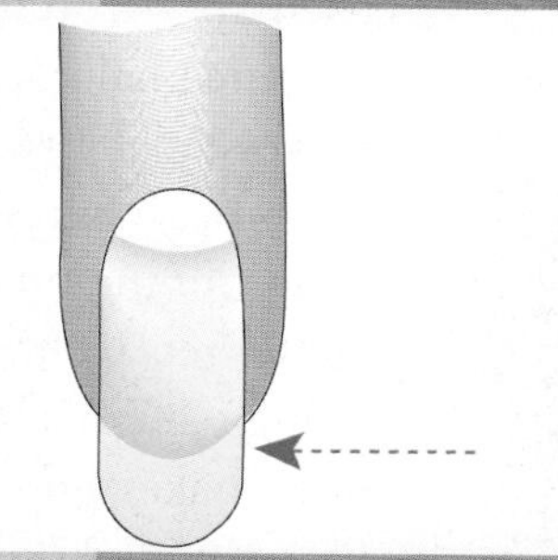

Figure 25-42 Fill in "V" with white polish.

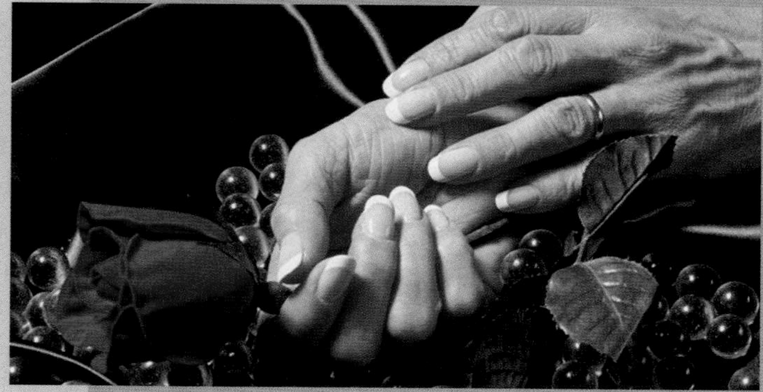

Figure 25-43 Finished French manicure

Here's a TIP

Buy an artist color wheel and learn about the theory of color. You can use what you learn to help clients select complementary colors that match their skin tone. Color theory is fun and easy to learn, and this knowledge will benefit you in many ways, including with cosmetics and fashions.

CONDITIONING OIL MANICURE

A conditioning oil manicure is recommended for clients who have ridged and brittle nails or dry skin around the nail plate. It improves the hand and nail plate condition and leaves the skin soft. Warm oil treatments are extremely beneficial to clients who are hard on their nails, such as nail biting and or activities resulting in plates that split, shatter, or become brittle or overly rigid (See Procedure 25-7).

PERFORMING A MAN'S MANICURE

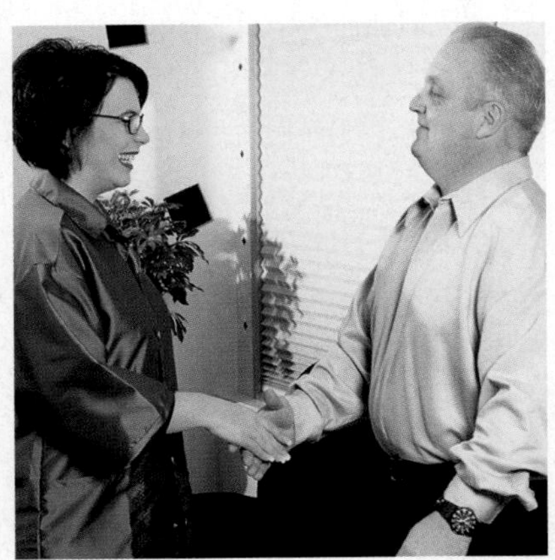

Figure 25-46 Greet client with a handshake.

Men are becoming increasingly aware of the importance of having well-groomed nails and hands. Consequently, many seek services offered by a professional nail professional. A man's manicure is executed using the same procedures as described previously for the basic manicure or the conditioning oil treatment. Follow each of the steps but *omit the colored polish;* replace this step with either clear polish or buffing the nails with a high-shine abrasive buffer. Upon arrival, greet the client with a handshake and escort him to your station (Figure 25-46). Next, consult with the client to determine the type of service that he is requesting, and then complete the client information form. Evaluate the client's current nail condition to determine what products are needed (Figure 25-47).

Begin the service by removing old polish if present from a previous manicure, and shaping the nails. The most common and requested shape for men's nails is round, but always ask whether he has a preference. Next, wash and dry the nails and hands, and carefully apply cuticle remover, following standard procedure. Most men will need a little more work done on their cuticle areas and eponychium than women. If the client prefers, the manicure procedure can be shortened at this point by buffing the nails with an abrasive buffer to add shine (Figure 25-48).

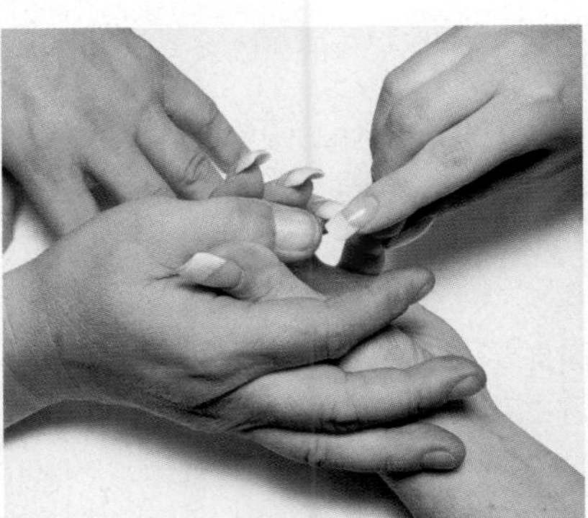

Figure 25-47 Evaluate client's nails.

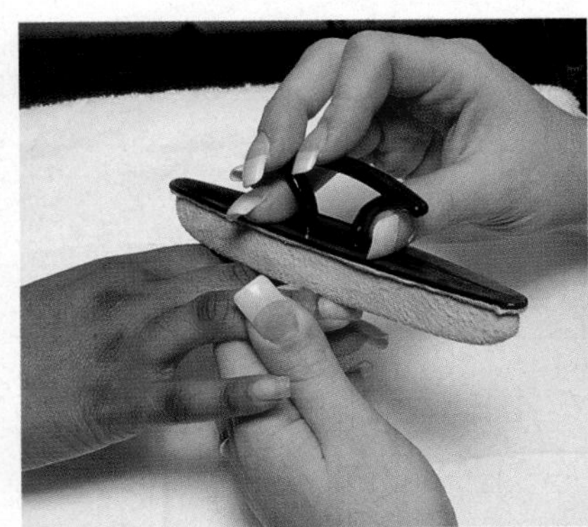

Figure 25-48 Buff nails with an abrasive buffer.

PROCEDURE 25-7

PERFORMING A CONDITIONING OIL MANICURE

1. **Perform pre-service sanitation and table setup.**
2. **Begin manicure.** Begin working with the hand that is not the client's favored hand. It is important to remember that during the procedure you should talk with your client about the professional products you recommend for them to use between salon visits.
3. **Remove old polish.**
4. **Shape nails.** Shape the nails on the hand that is not the client's favored hand.
5. **Apply oil.** Apply a penetrating, conditioning nail oil with a cotton swab or eye dropper, and massage it into nail plate and surrounding skin. Explain the benefits of this step to your clients and tell them that daily use of the professional product that you recommend will be greatly beneficial and will preserve the manicure until the next salon visit.
6. **Apply lotion.** Apply hand lotion to your hand and spread it over the client's hand, arm, and elbow. This will give you enough lotion for the massage.
7. **Proceed with hand and arm massage.** Follow the steps for hand and arm massage described in Procedures 25-10 and 25-11.
8. **Remove cuticle tissue from nail plate.** Use a wooden pusher covered with cotton or a metal pusher to gently push back the eponychium.
9. **Remove tags of dead skin.** Use nippers to trim away any tags and dead skin. Take great care not to rip or tear living tissue as this could increase the risk of infection. Let the client rest the hand on a clean terry cloth or disposable towel.
10. **Repeat on other hand.** Proceed with Steps 7 through 9, and distribute lotion on each hand after these steps.
11. **Remove excess lotion.** If necessary, take a warm terry cloth towel and wipe off excess lotion, or have client wash hands.
12. **Remove oil.** Remove all traces of oil and lotion from the surface of the nail plate. Saturate cotton in alcohol or polish remover and vigorously wipe off oil and lotion from nail plates. This is an important step, so perform it well. This step removes only oils remaining on the surface; beneficial oils that absorbed into the nail plate during your treatment are not removed.

13. Apply polish.

14. Complete manicure post-service. Make recommendations to client for take-home products.

ADD-ON SERVICE

If the client needs a deep nail conditioning treatment, the following add-on service may be performed. First, saturate a cotton ball with a penetrating and conditioning nail oil and press it against the nail plate. Second, wrap the entire finger and cotton ball with a piece of tinfoil large enough to seal the bottom just below the first finger joint. The foil will secure the oil-saturated cotton against the nail plate. This technique utilizes the body's own heat to warm the oil to a toasty 98°F. Oil this warm will penetrate more quickly than oil at room temperature and will condition the nail plate more deeply (Figures 25-44 and 25-45).

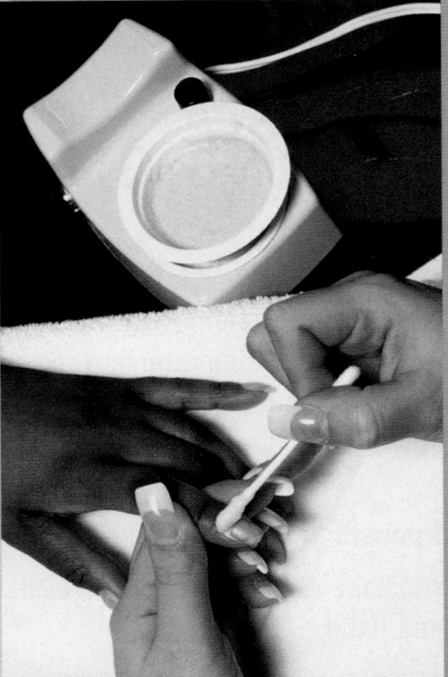

Figure 25-44 Apply nail oil with cotton swab or eye dropper, and then massage into skin.

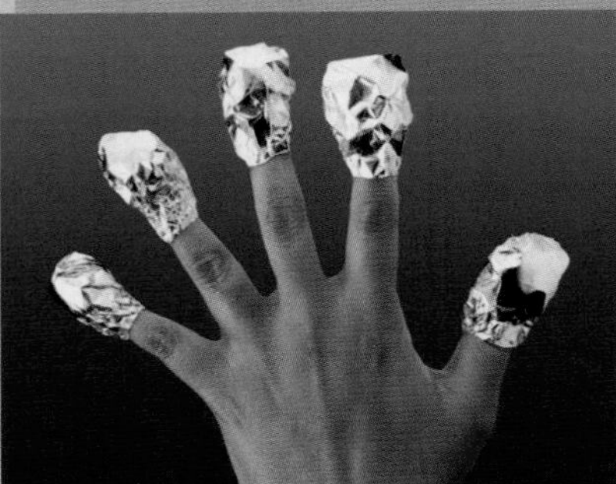

Figure 25-45 Deep nail conditioning treatment.

After cleansing and shaping nails, apply hand lotion and massage the hands and lower arms (Figure 25-49). A citrus- or spice-scented hand cream is recommended over a flowery scent for the male client. If a polish application is requested, apply a base coat and a clear satin top coat, followed with nail polish dryer (Figure 25-50).

The man's manicure is complete (Figure 25-51).

With today's emphasis on good grooming, more and more men are interested in taking care of their nails. Even so, they are not aware of their options. Alert the male public to your nail services by advertising in the business and sports pages of local publications. Since most men are new to nail care, do not forget to include a brief written description of what the services entail and a summary of benefits. You may also want to distribute flyers at local gyms, athletic stores, and other places where men gather. Probably your best option is to sell gift certificates to your female clients for their boyfriends and husbands, especially around the holidays. The men may not come in until after the holidays when you are not as busy and could use the new clientele. To make men feel more at home in your chair, have men's magazines on hand and be careful that your decor is unisex. Staying open later or opening earlier makes it easier for both working men and women to schedule appointments.

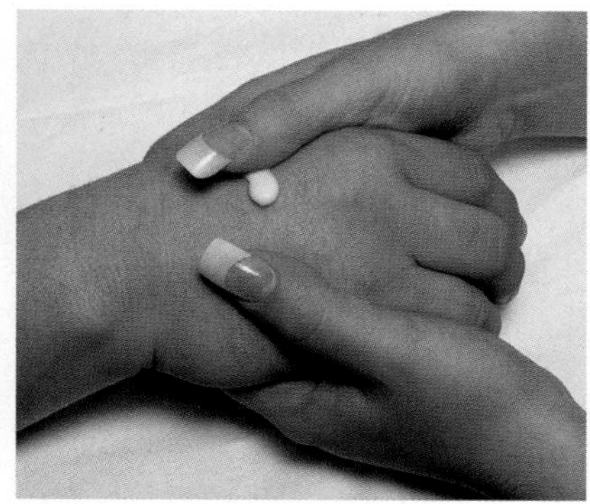

Figure 25-49 Apply hand lotion.

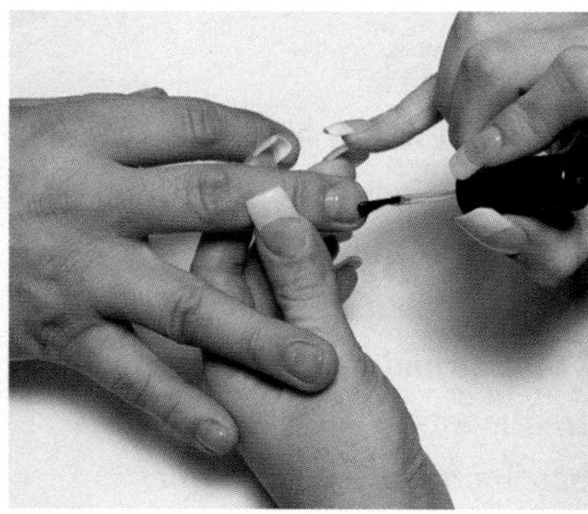

Figure 25-50 Polish with a matte or satin polish, if preferred.

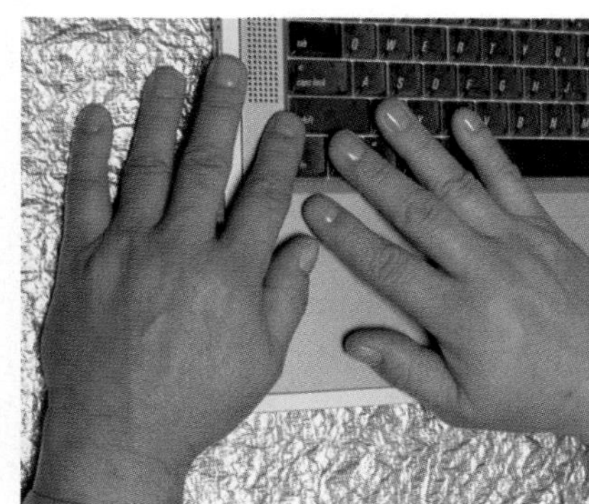

Figure 25-51 Finished man's manicure.

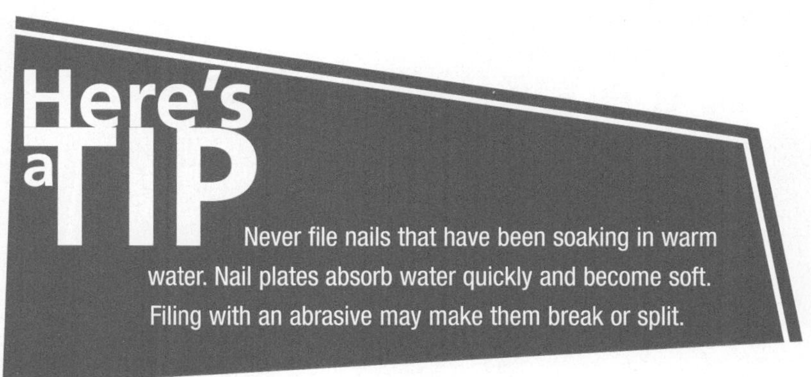

Never file nails that have been soaking in warm water. Nail plates absorb water quickly and become soft. Filing with an abrasive may make them break or split.

PARAFFIN WAX TREATMENT

Paraffin wax treatments work by trapping moisture in the skin while the heat causes skin pores to open. Besides opening the pores, heat from the warm paraffin increases blood circulation. This is considered a luxurious add-on service and can be safely performed on most clients.

Paraffin is a petroleum by-product that has excellent sealing properties to hold in moisture. Special units are utilized to melt solid wax into a liquid and then maintained at a temperature generally between 125° and 130°F. When using this treatment only use the equipment that is designed specifically for this use. Never try to heat the wax in anything other than the proper equipment. This can be very dangerous and may result in painful skin burns or a fire.

If proper procedures are followed, paraffin will not adversely affect artificial nail enhancements or natural nails. Be guided by your instructor and your state regulations because some states require the service to be performed before the manicure.

CAUTION

Read and follow all operating instructions that come with your paraffin heating unit. Generally, you should avoid giving paraffin treatments to anyone who has impaired circulation or skin irritations such as cuts, burns, rashes, warts, or eczema. Senior citizen clients may be more sensitive to heat, because of medications or age-related thinning of the skin. Place a small patch of wax on the client's skin to see if the temperatures can be tolerated by these individuals.

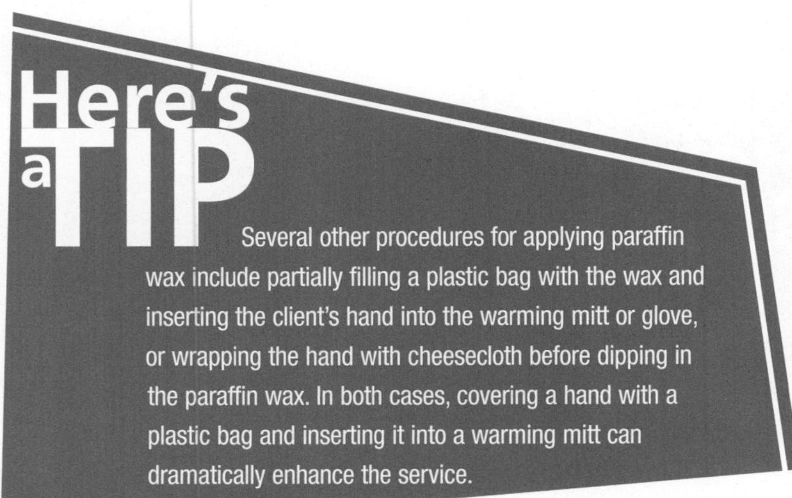

Here's a TIP

Several other procedures for applying paraffin wax include partially filling a plastic bag with the wax and inserting the client's hand into the warming mitt or glove, or wrapping the hand with cheesecloth before dipping in the paraffin wax. In both cases, covering a hand with a plastic bag and inserting it into a warming mitt can dramatically enhance the service.

PROCEDURE 25-8

PARAFFIN WAX TREATMENT BEFORE MANICURE

The paraffin wax treatment presented in Procedure 25-8 is performed before a basic manicure (Figure 25-52).

1. Perform pre-service sanitation and table setup.
2. Check to ensure that client's hands are free from open wounds, diseases, or disorders. If it is safe to perform the procedures, continue with the service. Assure clients that they are receiving a sanitary service. Never use this option as a way of avoiding hand washing (Figure 25-53).
3. Apply moisturizing lotion or penetrating oil to client's hands and gently massage into the skin.
4. Test the temperature of the wax.
5. Position the hand for the dipping procedure (Figure 25-54). The palm should be flat with the wrist slightly bent and the fingers slightly apart.
6. Aid the client in dipping one hand into the wax up to the wrist for about 3 seconds. Remove. Allow the wax to solidify before dipping again (Figure 25-55).
7. Repeat this process three to five times.
8. Wrap the hands in plastic wrap or insert them into plastic gloves before inserting them into a warming mitt (Figure 25-56).
9. Repeat this procedure on the other hand.
10. Allow the paraffin to remain on the hands for approximately 5 to 10 minutes.
11. To remove the paraffin, with plastic gloves still on the client's hand, start at the wrist, massage the client's hands gently to loosen the wax, and peel the paraffin from the hands (Figure 25-57).
12. Properly dispose of the used paraffin. It is unsanitary to reuse paraffin.
13. Begin the manicuring procedure.

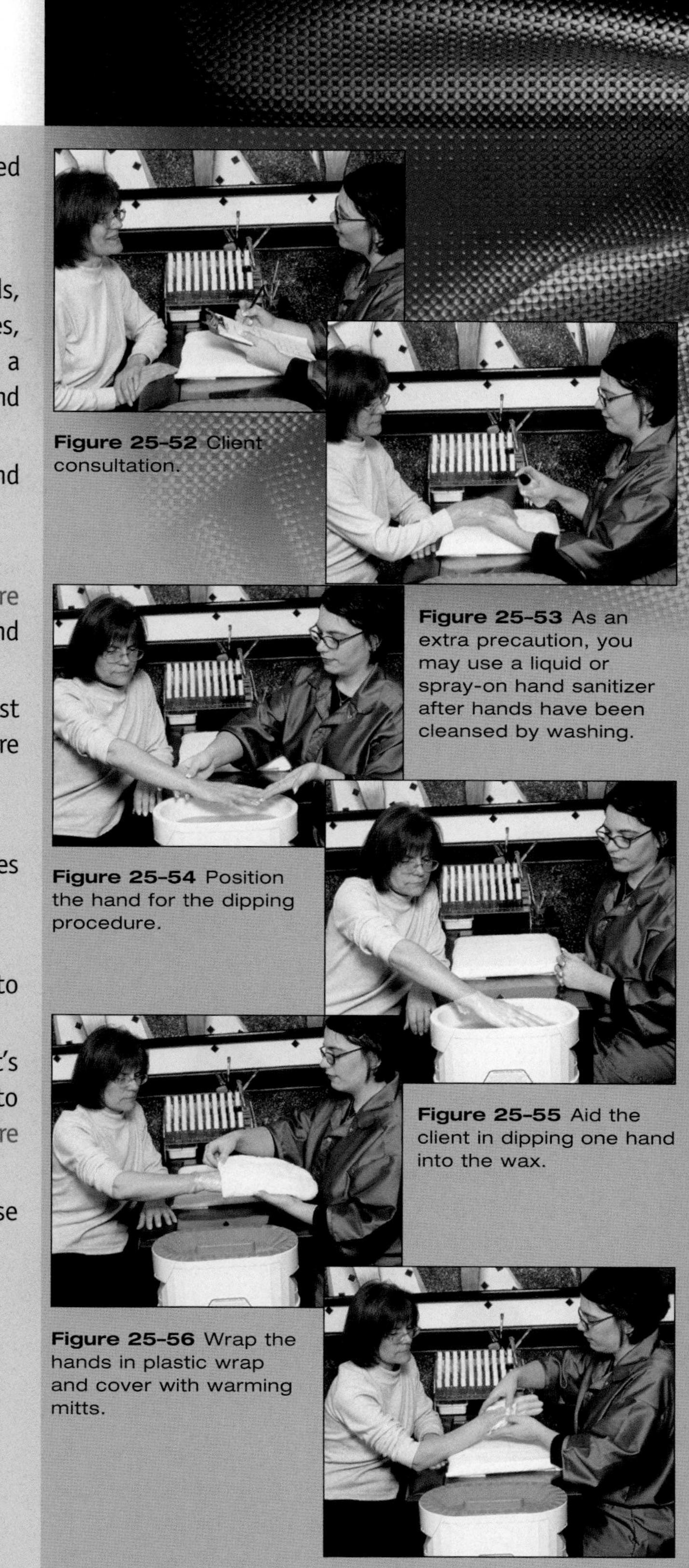

Figure 25-52 Client consultation.

Figure 25-53 As an extra precaution, you may use a liquid or spray-on hand sanitizer after hands have been cleansed by washing.

Figure 25-54 Position the hand for the dipping procedure.

Figure 25-55 Aid the client in dipping one hand into the wax.

Figure 25-56 Wrap the hands in plastic wrap and cover with warming mitts.

Figure 25-57 To remove the paraffin, start at the wrist, massage lightly to loosen wax, and peel paraffin or unwrap plastic wrap from hand.

PROCEDURE 25-9

PARAFFIN WAX TREATMENT DURING MANICURE

The process presented in Procedure 25-9 occurs during a manicure.

Be guided by your instructor for the amount of time the hands should be left in the paraffin wax.

1. Perform pre-service sanitation and table setup.
2. Remove old polish and shape the nails to the desired shape. If any repairs are needed, complete the procedures for necessary repairs before proceeding with the manicure.
3. Apply moisturizer to client's hands and gently massage into skin.
4. Complete Steps 4 to 12 in Procedure 25-8.
5. Proceed with the manicuring procedure.

HAND AND ARM MASSAGE

A hand and arm massage is a service that can be offered with all types of manicures. This service is included in all spa manicures, and can be performed on most clients.

A massage is one of the client's high priorities during the manicure, as most clients look forward to the soothing and relaxing effects. The massage manipulations should be executed with rhythmic and smooth movements, never leaving the client's arm or hand untouched during the procedure.

During the manicure it is suggested that the massage be performed after the basic manicure procedure, just before the polish application. After performing a massage, it is essential that the nail plate be thoroughly cleansed to ensure that it is free from any residue such as oil, cream, wax, or lotion. You can use alcohol or nail polish remover to cleanse the nail plate.

Hand and arm massage is optional during a basic manicure, but incorporating this special, relaxing service to the client will be advantageous to the professional. This will show the client that you are giving them 100 percent of your time, knowledge, and service.

CAUTION

Do not **provide a massage service if the client has high blood pressure or a heart condition, or has had a stroke. Massage increases circulation and may be harmful to such a client. Have client consult a physician first. Be very careful to avoid vigorous massage of joints if your client has arthritis or joint injury. Talk with your client throughout the massage, and adjust your touch to the client's needs.**

Here's a TIP

Before performing hand and arm massage, make sure that you are sitting in a comfortable position and not stretching or leaning forward toward your customer. While giving the customer a massage, you must take care to ensure that your posture is correct and relaxed. Sitting or working in an uncomfortable or strained position can cause back, neck, and shoulder injuries. If this is done repeatedly, it could lead to cumulative trauma disorders (CTDs) and possibly permanent injury.

PROCEDURE 25-10

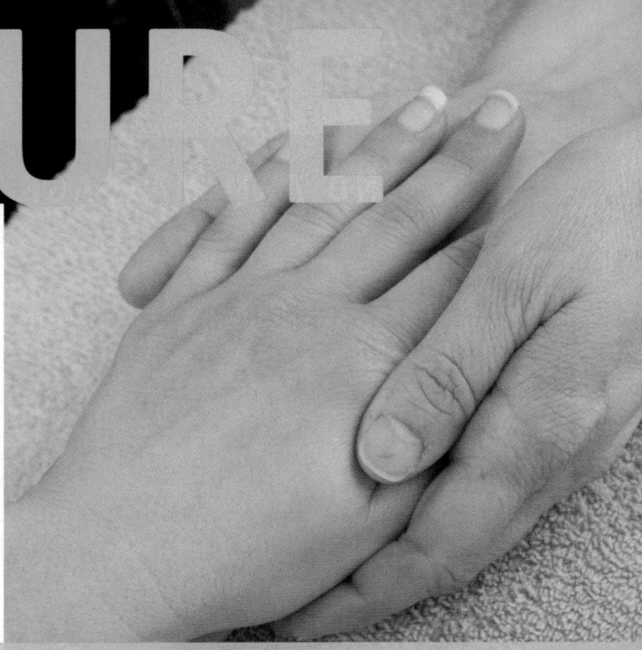

HAND MASSAGE

1. **Relaxer movement.** This is a form of massage known as "joint movement." At the beginning of the hand massage, the client has already received hand lotion or cream. Place the client's elbow on a cushion covered with a clean towel. With one hand, brace the client's arm.

   With your other hand, hold the client's wrist and bend it back and forth slowly, 5 to 10 times, until you feel that the client has relaxed (Figure 25-58).
2. **Joint movement on fingers.** Bring the client's arm down, brace the arm with the left hand, and with your right hand start with the little finger, holding it at the base of the nail. Gently rotate fingers to form circles. Work toward the thumb, about three to five times on each finger (Figure 25-59).
3. **Circular movement in palm.** This is **effleurage** (EF-loo-rahzh)—light stroking that relaxes and soothes. Place the client's elbow on the cushion and, with your thumbs in the client's palm, rotate in a circular movement in opposite directions (Figure 25-60).
4. **Circular movement on wrist.** Hold the client's hand with both of your hands, placing your thumbs on top of client's hand, and your fingers below the hand. Move your thumbs in a circular movement in opposite directions from the client's wrist to the knuckle on back of the client's hand. Move up and down, three to five times. The last time that you rotate up, wring the client's wrist by bracing your hands around the wrist and gently twisting in opposite directions. This is a form of friction massage movement that is a deep rubbing action and very stimulating (Figure 25-61).
5. **Circular movement on back of hand and fingers.** Now rotate down the back of the client's hand using your thumbs. Rotate down the little finger and the client's thumb, and gently squeeze off at the tips of client's fingers. Go back and rotate down the ring finger and index finger, gently squeezing off. Now do the middle finger and squeeze off at the tip.

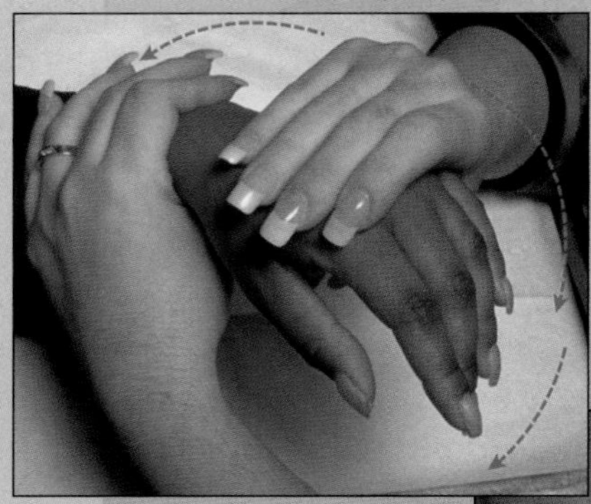

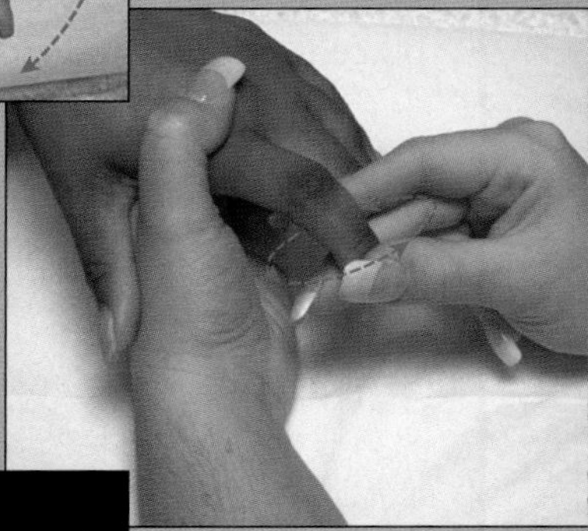

Figure 25-58 Relaxer movement.

Figure 25-59 Joint movement on fingers.

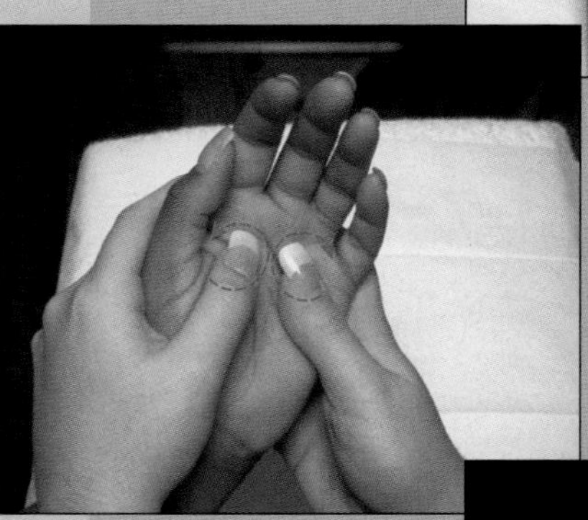

Figure 25-60 Circular movement or effleurage.

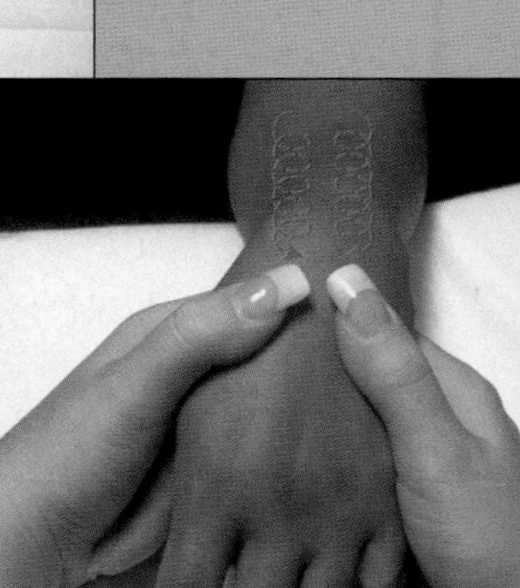

Figure 25-61 Circular movement on wrist.

PROCEDURE 25-11

ARM MASSAGE

1. **Distribute lotion or cream.** Apply a small amount of lotion or cream to the client's arm and work it in. Work from the client's wrist toward the elbow, except on the last movement; work from the elbow to wrist, and then squeeze off at fingertips as you did at the end of the hand massage. Apply more lotion if necessary (Figure 25-62).
2. **Effleurage on arms.** Put the client's arm on the table, bracing the arm with your hands. Hold your client's hand palm up in your hand. Your fingers should be under the client's hand, and your thumbs side by side in your client's palm. Rotate your thumbs in opposite directions, starting at the client's wrist and working toward the elbow. When you reach the elbow, slide your hand down the client's arm to the wrist and rotate back up to the elbow three to five times. Turn the client's arm over and repeat three to five times on the top side of arm (Figure 25-63).
3. **Wringing/friction movement.** A friction massage involves deep rubbing to the muscles. Bend the client's elbow so the arm is horizontal in front of you, with the back of the hand facing up. Place your hands around the arm with your fingers facing the same direction as the arm, and gently twist in opposite directions as you would wring out a washcloth from wrist to elbow. Do this up and down the forearm three to five times (Figure 25-64).
4. **Kneading movement.** This technique is called the **petrissage** (PE-tre-sahza) **kneading movement.** It is very stimulating and increases blood flow. Place your thumb on the top side of the client's arm so that they are horizontal. Move them in opposite directions, from wrist to elbow and back down to the wrist. This squeezing motion moves flesh over bone and stimulates the arm tissue. Do this three to five times (Figure 25-65).
5. **Rotation of elbow—friction massage movement.** Brace the client's arm with your left hand and, apply lotion to the elbow. Cup elbow with your right hand and rotate your hand over the client's elbow. Do this three to five times. To finish the elbow massage, move your left arm to the top of the client's forearm. Gently slide both hands down the forearm from the elbow to the fingertips as if climbing down a rope. Repeat this three to five times (Figure 25-66).

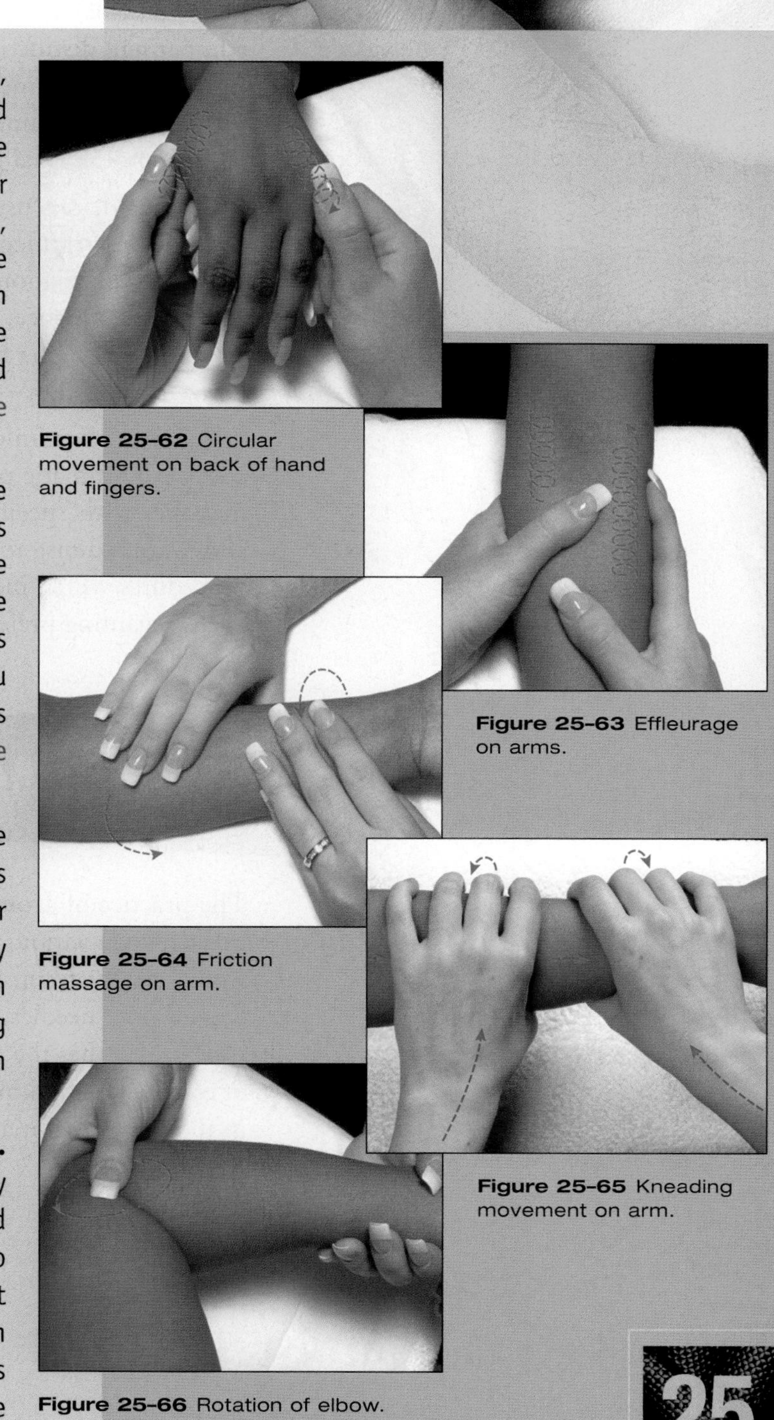

Figure 25-62 Circular movement on back of hand and fingers.

Figure 25-63 Effleurage on arms.

Figure 25-64 Friction massage on arm.

Figure 25-65 Kneading movement on arm.

Figure 25-66 Rotation of elbow.

SPA MANICURE

Spa manicures are fast becoming a much-requested and desired salon service, but they are more advanced than basic manicures. Professionals who advance their education and knowledge necessary for implementing this service may find this area to be very lucrative, as well as more beneficial to your clients. Spa manicures encompass not only extensive knowledge of nail care but skin care as well. They are known for their pampering, distinctive results, and skin-care-based methods. All spa manicures should include a relaxing massage and some form of exfoliation for not only polishing and smoothing, but also for enhancing penetration of your professional products.

Spa manicures usually come with unique and distinctive names that describe the treatment with imagination and flair. For example, "The Rose Garden Rejuvenation Manicure" incorporates the use of rose oils and rose petals for ambience. The "Alpha Hydroxy Acid Manicure" incorporates the use of an alpha hydroxy acid-based product for exfoliation and skin rejuvenation.

Additional techniques that may be incorporated into a spa manicure consist of aromatic paraffin dips; aromatherapy; aromatic hand and arm massages with specifically recommended oils and lotions; hand masks; and warm, moist towel applications. When performing any advanced procedures which include any oils or cosmetics, always check with your client regarding preferences and allergies.

AROMATHERAPY

The practice of **aromatherapy** involves the use of **essential oils** that are extracted via various forms of distillation from seeds, bark, roots, leaves, wood, and/or resin. Each part produces a different aroma. For instance, Scotch pine needles, resin, and wood each yield a different aroma. The time of day that the plant was harvested also changes the aroma. The use of essential oils is limitless. Tables 25-1 to 25-4 are provided to assist you in the use of essential oils as a cosmetology practitioner.

ESSENTIAL OILS	DESCRIPTION
Lavender	Herbaceous (having the characteristics of an herb), overall first-aid oil, antiviral and antibacterial, boosts immunity, antidepressant, anti-inflammatory, relaxant, balance, and antispasmodic
Chamomile	Fruity, anti-inflammatory, digestive, relaxant, PMS, soothes frayed nerves, migraine, stamina, and antidepressant
Marjoram	Herbaceous, antispasmodic, anti-inflammatory, headaches, comfort, menstrual cramps, and antiseptic
Rosemary	Camphoraceous (from the wood or bark of the camphor tree), stimulating to circulation, relieves pain, and decongestant
Tea tree	Camphoraceous, antifungal, and antibacterial
Cypress	Coniferous (mostly from evergreen trees with cones, such as pine) astringent, stimulating to circulation, and antiseptic
Peppermint	Minty, digestive, clears sinuses, antiseptic, energy, decongestant, and stimulant
Eucalyptus	Camphoraceous, decongestant, antiviral, antibacterial, and stimulant
Bergamot	Citrus aroma, antidepressant, antiviral, antibacterial, water retention, and anti-inflammatory
Geranium	Floral, balancing to mind and body, tranquility, antifungal, and anti-inflammatory

Table 25-1 Ten Basic Essential Oils

CARRIER OILS	DESCRIPTION
Sweet almond oil	An excellent lubricant that is softening to the skin; a medium- to light-weight multipurpose massage or skin oil
Sunflower seed oil	Highly lubricating and softening, medium- to light-weight oil, and highly resistant to degradation from oxygen and light
Apricot oil	Especially for prematurely aged, dry skin; a light-weight massage oil
Avocado oil	Recommended for dull and dehydrated skin, a medium- to heavy-weight oil
Grapeseed oil	A very popular, light-weight massage oil with a fine texture and little odor
Jojoba oil	A natural oil that resembles the structure of skin's sebum, giving it excellent penetration and moisturizing properties; also an excellent carrier oil
Olive oil	An excellent natural oil that contains squalene, a component of skin sebum

Table 25-2 Carrier Oils

DESIRED RESULT	CHOOSING AN AROMA Useful Oils
Calming	Lavender, rosemary, sandalwood, ylang ylang, vetiver
Ambience	Vanilla, cinnamon, orange, pine, jasmine, lavender, bayberry, rose, cherry, lemon
Energy	Eucalyptus, orange, peppermint, geranium, spearmint, jasmine, lemon, fennel
Invigorating	Spearmint, peppermint, lemon, rosemary
Stress relief	Lavender, chamomile, vetivert
Clear minds	Rosemary, cypress
Romance	Ylang ylang, sandalwood, jasmine
Foot odor	Sage, baking powder
Bactericide	Cinnamon, clove, lemon, eucalyptus, lavender, pine, grapefruit, lime
Cuts and scrapes	Tea tree, lavender, eucalyptus
Barber's rash	Lemongrass, peppermint, geranium
Nail infection	Tea tree
Oily skin	Bergamot, geranium, clary sage, petigrain, cedarwood

Table 25-3 Choosing an Aroma

DESIRED RESULT	RECIPES FOR MANICURES AND PEDICURES
Nail strengthening	20 drops lemon, 15 drops carrot oil, 13 drops grapeseed oil, 13 drops rosemary, 13 drops avocado oil. Blend together and keep in light-sensitive bottle. Use on client after nails have been polished by adding one drop around cuticle and allowing it to absorb into the matrix.
Cuticle softener	15 drops carrot oil, 12 drops peppermint, 12 drops eucalyptus, 2 oz jojoba oil. Blend together and keep in light-sensitive bottle. Use one drop on each nail and massage well into the cuticle.
Age deterrent (spot reduction)	15 drops lemon, 10 drops lime, 5 drops rosemary, 5 drops lavender, 1 drop spearmint, 1 oz grape-seed oil. Blend together and keep in light-sensitive bottle. Use 2 to 3 drops on back of hands, not on nails. Gently massage back of hand for 3 to 4 minutes to see fading of discoloration within 4 to 5 treatments.
Decadent manicure	¼ cup heavy cream, 10 drops of pure or blended essential oil of your choice, 1 bowl of fragrant salts for aroma only, a few candles, spa music in background. Light candles and prepare aromatics. Place hands in heavy cream and essential oils and let soak for 5 to 10 minutes. Proceed with normal manicure. Wipe off nails before applying polish.
Dry and cracked heels on feet	10 drops rose, 5 drops chamomile, 5 drops geranium, 5 drops pettigraine oil. Blend ingredients and keep in light-sensitive bottle. Add 8 to 10 drops to the pedicure water before adding anything else. Soak feet for 10 minutes. Proceed with pedicure. Before massage, add 3 to 4 drops on each heel and massage until completely penetrated.
Swollen feet	15 drops lavendar, 15 drops chamomile, 15 drops rosemary, 15 drops fennel, 4 oz jojoba oil. Blend ingredients and keep in light-sensitive bottle. Use about 25 to 30 drops as a massage oil for a thorough massage. Have client elevate feet for 10 to 15 minutes above the heart.
Decadent pedicure	1 to 2 cups heavy cream, 25 drops of pure or blended essential oil of your choice or 3 fragrant salt crystals in the pedicure bath, 1 bowl of fragrant salts for aroma only (or candle if permitted), spa background music. Light candles and/or prepare aromatics. Place feet in heavy cream mixture and let soak for 5 to 50 minutes. Proceed with normal pedicure. Wipe off toes before applying polish.

Table 25-4 Recipes for Manicures and Pedicures

REVIEW QUESTIONS

1. List the four types of nail implements or tools used in manicuring.
2. Describe the procedures for sanitizing and disinfecting implements.
3. Briefly describe the procedures for handling blood in a salon.
4. Describe the procedure for a basic manicure table setup.
5. List two types of polish remover.
6. Why is having a material safety data sheet for all the products used in a salon important?
7. List the five basic nail shapes.
8. What special factors should be considered when selecting the nail shape?
9. List and discuss the three-part procedure sequence required in manicuring.
10. Describe the correct procedures for polish application.
11. What is the purpose of a conditioning oil treatment?
12. Discuss the basic differences between a female manicure and a male manicure.
13. What are the benefits of a paraffin wax treatment?
14. List the suggested procedures for performing a paraffin wax treatment.
15. Name five hand and arm massage techniques.
16. What is aromatherapy?
17. How are essential oils used?
18. List five basic essential oils and their uses.

CHAPTER GLOSSARY

aromatherapy	Use of aromatic fragrances to induce relaxation; therapy through aroma.
bevel	To slope the free edge of the nail surface to smooth any rough edges.
chamois buffer	Implement that holds a disposable chamois cloth that is used to add shine to the nail and to smooth out wavy ridges on nails.
dimethyl urea hardeners	Hardeners that use dimethyl urea (DMU) and add crosslinks to the natural nail plate but do not cause adverse skin reactions.
effleurage	Light, continuous-stroking massage movement applied with fingers and palms in a slow and rhythmic manner.
essential oils	Oils used in aromatherapy that are extracted via diverse forms of distillation from seeds, bark, roots, leaves, woods, and resin.
formaldehyde hardeners	Contain up to 5 percent formaldehyde and create bridges or cross-links between the keratin strands that make up the natural nail, making the plate much stiffer and more resistant to bending.
mild abrasive	Substances used for smoothing nails and skin (e.g., pumice).
oval nail	Nail shape that is similar to squoval with even more rounded corners. This shape is attractive for most women's hands.
petrissage kneading movement	Kneading movement in massage performed by lifting, squeezing, and pressing the tissue.
pledgets	Small, fiber-free cotton squares often used by nail professionals to remove polish.
pointed nail	Nail shape suited to thin hands with narrow nail beds. The shape is tapered and somewhat longer than usual.
protein hardener	A combination of clear polish and protein, such as collagen, that provide a clear hard coating on the surface of the nail.
pumice powder	White or grayish powdered abrasive derived from volcanic rock, used for smoothing and polishing.
reinforcing-fiber hardeners	Contain fibers such as nylon, and protect the nail by coating the natural nail.
round nail	Nail shape that is slightly tapered and extends just a bit past the tip of the finger. This natural looking shape is common for male clients.
square nail	Nail shape that is completely straight across with no rounding at the edges. The length of the nail can vary.
squoval nail	Nail shape with a square free edge that is rounded off and extends just slightly past the tip of the finger.

PEDICURING

CHAPTER 26

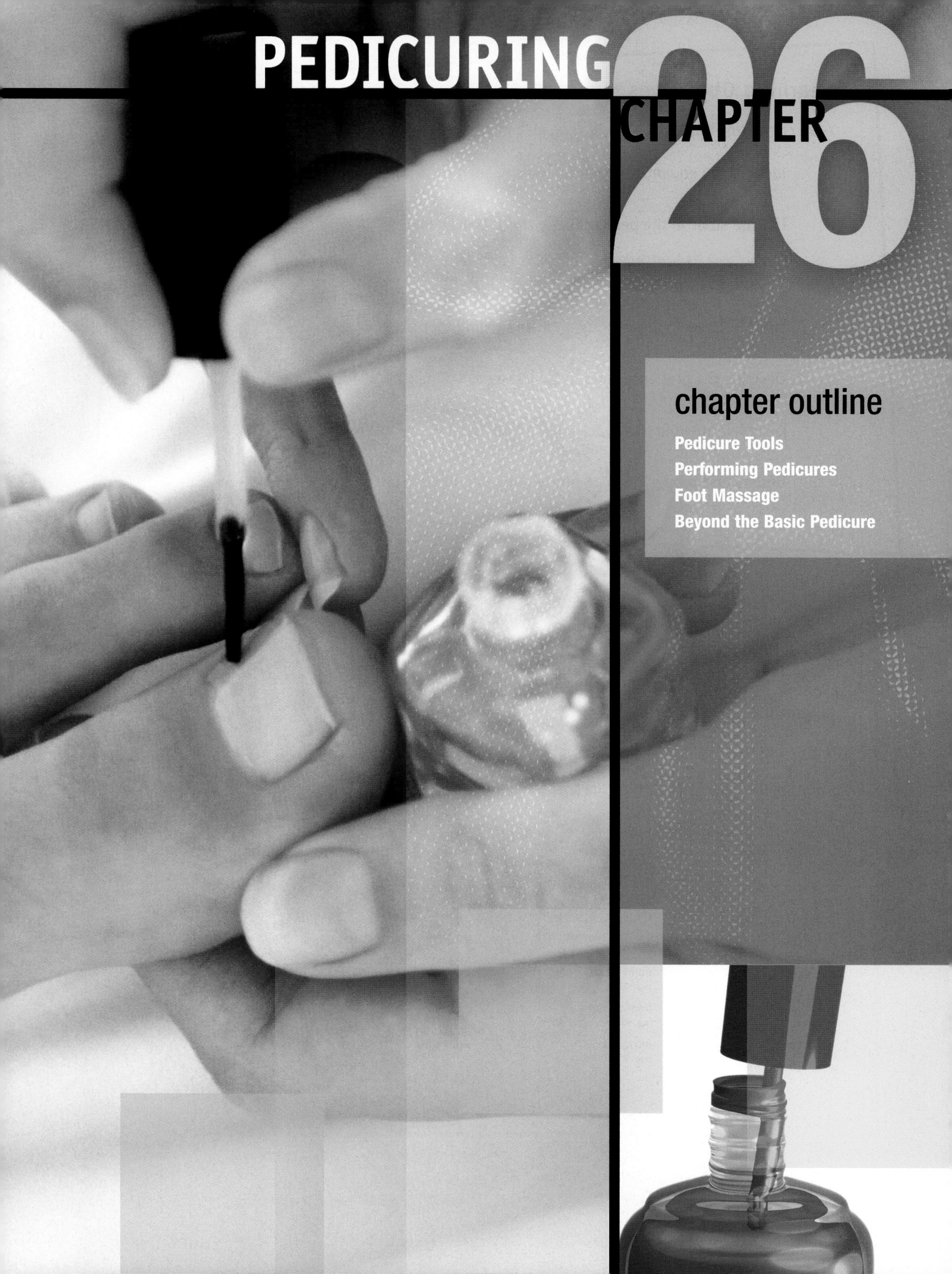

chapter outline

Learning Objectives

After completing this chapter, you will be able to:

- Identify the equipment and materials needed for a pedicure and explain.
- List the steps in the pedicure pre-service procedure.
- Demonstrate the proper procedures and precautions for a pedicure.
- Describe the proper technique to use in filing toenails.
- Describe the proper technique for trimming the nails.
- Demonstrate your ability to perform foot massage properly.
- Understand proper cleaning and disinfecting of pedicure equipment.

Key Terms

Page number indicates where in the chapter the term is used.

abrasive nail file pg. 701

abrasive scrubs pg. 714

callus softeners pg. 715

curette pg. 700

cuticle removers pg. 714

exfoliating scrubs pg. 719

foot files or *paddles* pg. 701

foot lotion, oil, or cream pg. 699

foot soaks pg. 713

friction movement pg. 712

hand movements pg. 705

liquid soap pg. 699

masques pg. 715

massage oils pg. 714

massage preparations pg. 714

nail rasp pg. 700

nippers pg. 701

paraffin baths pg. 715

pedicure pg. 699

pedicure slippers pg. 700

tapotement pg. 705

toe separators pg. 699

toenail clippers pg. 700

The information in this chapter will show you the pedicuring skills you need to care for clients' feet, toes, and toenails. A **pedicure** includes trimming, shaping, exfoliating skin and polishing toenails as well as foot massage. Pedicures are a standard service performed by cosmetologists. They are a basic part of good foot care and hygiene. They are particularly important for clients who are joggers, dancers, cosmetologists, or anyone who spends a lot of time standing on their feet. Once the client experiences the comfort, relaxation, and value of a good pedicure they will return for more. In short, pedicure services are for just about everyone, but different clients will have different needs. For example, not all clients will want or need a full pedicure service.

Some clients only need a professional nail trimming. Do not limit yourself. Tailor your pedicure service to meet the needs of your entire clientele. Talk to your clients about getting monthly pedicures to ensure healthy happy feet, as they are in constant use and need routine maintenance. Proper foot care through pedicuring improves both personal appearance and basic foot comfort.

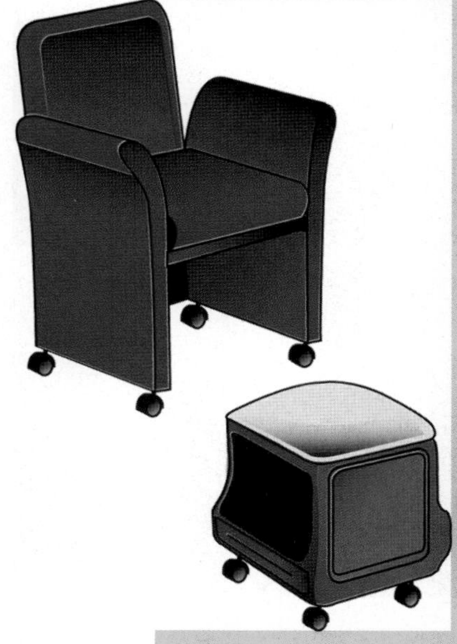

Figure 26-1 Pedicure station including client's chair, footrest, and pedicuring stool.

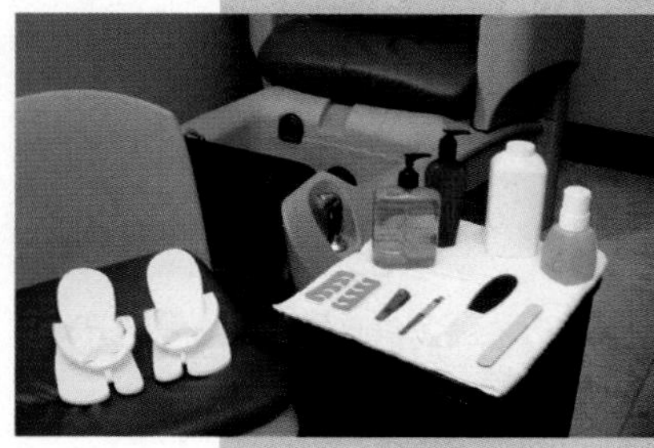

Figure 26-2 Supplies needed for pedicure.

PEDICURE TOOLS

PEDICURE SUPPLIES

You will need the following supplies in addition to your standard manicure setup to perform pedicures (Figures 26-1 and 26-2).

- **Toe separators.** Foam rubber toe separators or cotton are used to keep toes apart while polishing the nails.
- **Liquid soap.** Liquid soap for pedicuring contains a mild detergent for cleansing the feet.
- **Foot lotion, oil, or cream.** Lotions, oils, and creams are an important part of the service and are used to condition and moisturize feet. They are also used for performing a foot massage.

Here's a TIP

When making an appointment for a pedicure, suggest that your client wear open-toed shoes or sandals so that polish will not smear, and caution clients not to shave their legs within 24 hours before the pedicure. In the pedicure area, post a sign cautioning clients about shaving their legs. Tiny microscopic abrasions from shaving increase the risk of stinging, irritation, or infection.

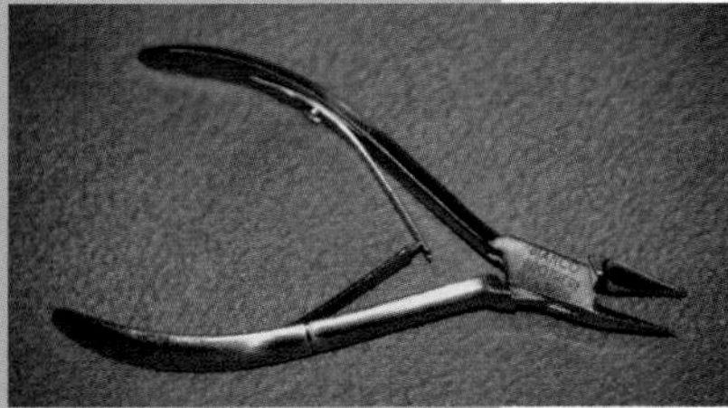

Figure 26-3 5-½ inch nail nippers with straight jaws.

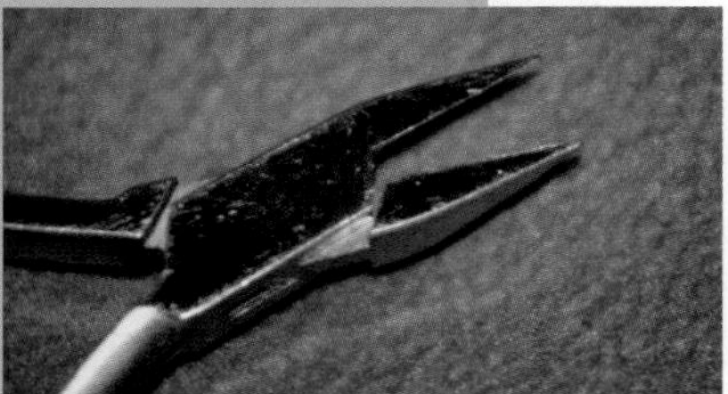

Figure 26-4 Close-up of jaws of nail nipper.

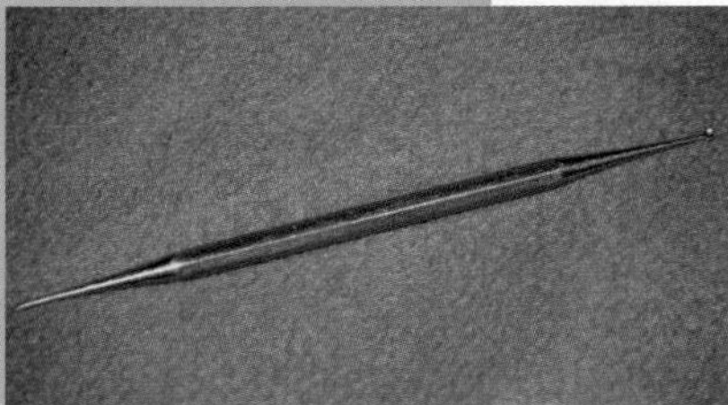

Figure 26-5 Double-ended curette.

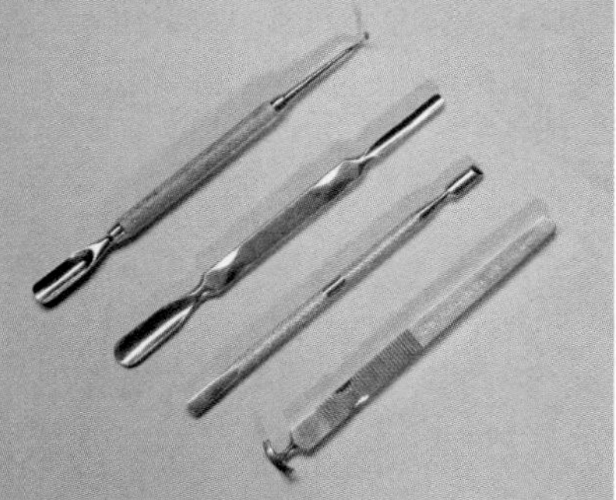

Figure 26-6 Close-up of curette.

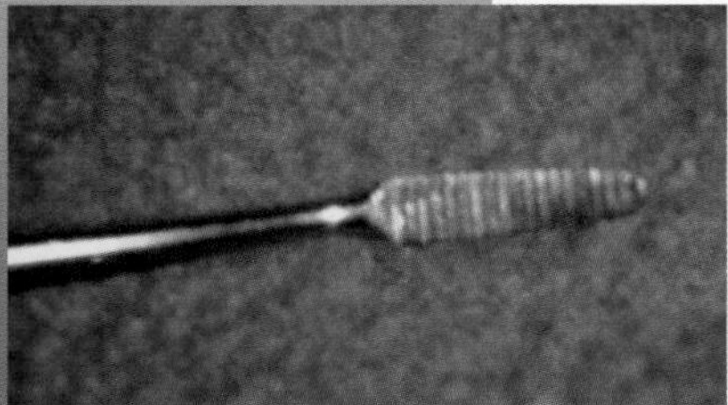

Figure 26-7 Close-up of nail rasp.

- **Pedicure slippers.** Disposable paper or foam slippers are needed for clients who have not worn open-toed shoes and want to avoid smudging toenail polish.

PEDICURE IMPLEMENTS

The use of high-quality, professional implements by the cosmetologist is very important. High-quality instruments will last many years and make the job easy. This is particularly true when it comes to working on the foot. Improper implements can easily cause injury to toenails and the soft tissues of the foot. For your client's safety, only use implements and equipment made specifically for performing professional pedicures. Described below are some basic implements that you will need.

TOENAIL CLIPPERS

Use only professional implements made for cutting toenails. **Toenail clippers** are not just larger than fingernail clippers; they are specifically designed for toenails.

These clippers come with either curved or straight jaws (Figures 26-3 and 26-4). The best clippers have jaws that come to a fairly fine point. Clippers with blunt points are difficult to use in the small corners of highly curved nail plates.

CURETTES

A **curette** is a small instrument shaped like an ice cream scooper that, if carefully used, allows for more efficient removal of debris from the nail folds and cuticle area (Figures 26-5 and 26-6). Properly used, the curette is the ideal instrument for pedicures, especially around the edges of the great toenail plate. A double-ended curette, which has a 0.06-inch (1.5-millimeter) diameter on one end and a 0.1-inch (2.5-millimeter) diameter on the other, is recommended. Some are made with a small hole, which makes the curette easier to clean after use. The curette must never be used to "cut out" tissue or debris that is strongly adhering to living tissues. The cosmetologist must never use curettes with sharp edges, as these can seriously injure clients. Only curettes with dull edges are safe and appropriate.

NAIL RASP

This **nail rasp** is a metal file designed to be used in a specific fashion. Rasps are designed to file in one direction. The filing surface of the instrument is about ⅛ inch wide and about ¾ inch long (Figure 26-7). It is attached to a straight or angled metal handle. The angled file is recommended because it is easier to use along the nail groove, where the nail plate meets the living side-wall tissue. This instrument smoothes the edges of the nail plate along the nail groove. It should be placed in the nail groove against the free edge of the nail plate.

The file is then gently pulled along the edge of the nail toward the end of the toe. This will smooth any rough edges of the nail plate that may have been produced during the trimming or curetting procedures. This process may be repeated a number of times to ensure that no rough edges remain along the nail margin.

The nail rasp, like the curette, is mainly used along the side wall of the nail plate on the great toenail. The lesser toenails do not usually require filing along their sidewalls. Removing sharp edges along the nail plate edge reduces the possibility of the nail plate digging into the soft tissues and creating an ingrown nail. As you become proficient in the use of this file you will find it to be an invaluable and time-saving instrument. Properly used, it will add the professional finishing touch required in the care of toenails.

ABRASIVE NAIL FILES

To file the free edge of the toenails and, in some cases, to thin them, an **abrasive nail file** is an excellent instrument (Figure 26-8). For some toenails, coarse-grit abrasives are needed, but for most, a medium grit will work best. Abrasive files are made of many types of abrasive materials, including aluminum oxide, diamond chips, and nickel. Nickel and diamond abrasive files do not fill up with nail debris as quickly as other types during use.

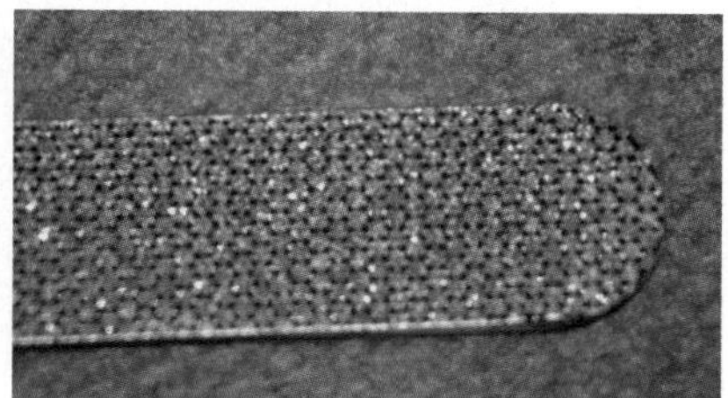

Figure 26-8 Close-up of an abrasive nail file.

FOOT FILES (PADDLES)

Foot files or **paddles** are larger than those designed for fingernails and toenails. These large sanding files are designed to reduce dry, flaky skin and smooth foot calluses. They come in many different grits and shapes (Figure 26-9). Foot files must be properly cleaned and disinfected between each use or disposed of after a single use, if the manufacturer has not designed them to be disinfectable. In general, if an abrasive file cannot survive proper cleaning and disinfection procedures without being rendered unusable, it must be considered disposable. Foot paddles with disposable and replaceable abrasive surfaces are also available.

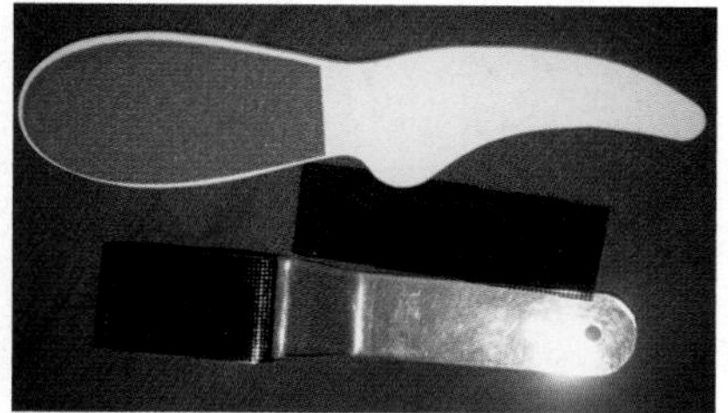

Figure 26-9 Abrasive foot paddle.

NIPPERS

Nippers can be used to remove dead tags of skin, but take great care to avoid cutting, tearing, or ripping living tissue. Avoid using nippers on clients who are diabetic since the risk of infection from accidental injury is great. Also, avoid using nippers on clients with psoriasis since injury to the toenail unit can create new psoriasis lesions where the damage occurs.

PEDICURE EQUIPMENT

This section is focused on equipment necessary to provide pedicure services. As with implements, high-quality, comfortable, and easy-to-use equipment will be cost effective, and also will help to promote your services. If you are uncomfortable and awkward while performing your services, you may end up injuring your back, neck, arms, wrists, or shoulders. In addition, if you are relaxed, then your client will relax and enjoy the pedicure.

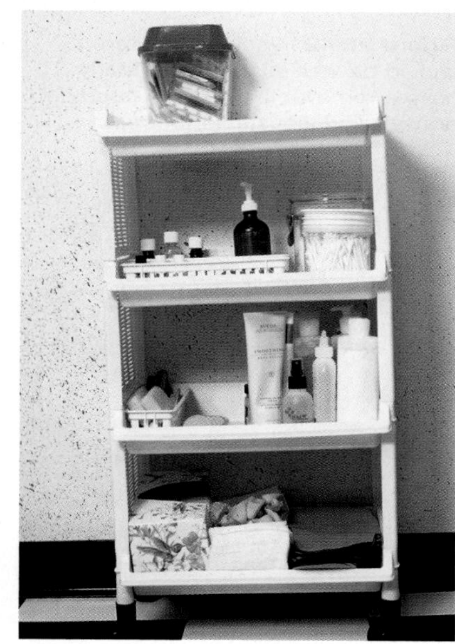

Figure 26-10 A portable pedicure cart has a place for the foot bath, storage area for supplies, and an adjustable footrest.

PEDICURE CARTS

These carts are a useful way to keep your supplies organized (Figure 26-10). Pedicure carts are available in many different designs and from many manufacturers. The carts have drawers and shelves for organized storage of implements and pedicure products. Some of these units even

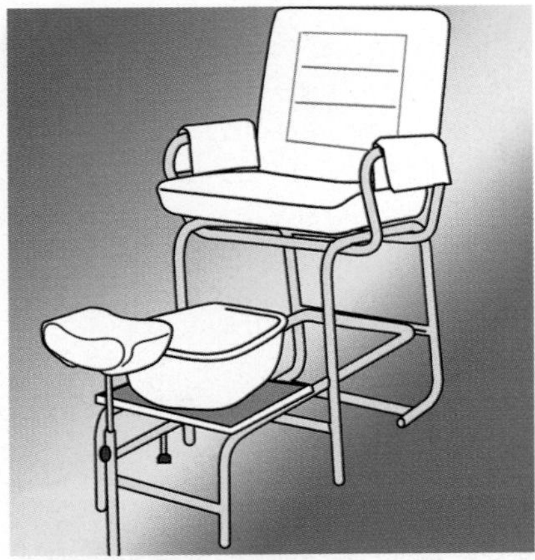

Figure 26-11 A customized type of pedicure station, well-built and affordable. It has an adjustable footrest and a place for the water bath.

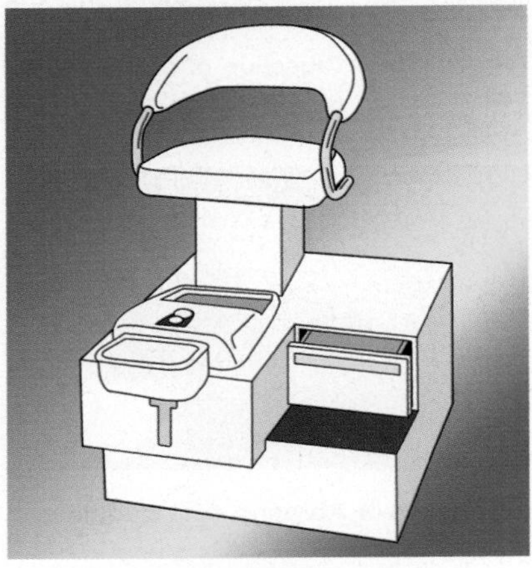

Figure 26-12 Pedicure centers should be well constructed. Many have a removable foot bath, storage drawer, and adjustable footrest.

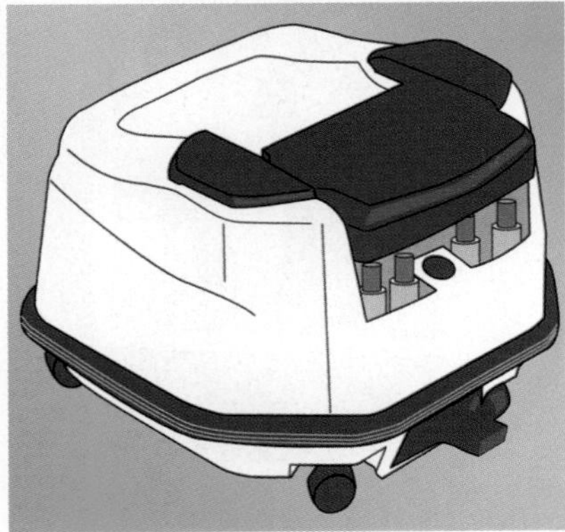

Figure 26-13 A fully self-contained portable foot basin.

include a space for the footbath. Most units are designed to be compact so that they take up very little space.

WATER BATHS

These useful and transportable devices can be purchased in a wide variety of sizes, shapes, and prices. Water baths must be manually filled and emptied after each client service.

If you use the portable type, be sure to have a comfortable chair or lounge in a private or semi-private area for the client to sit in while receiving the pedicure. In addition, your chair should be adjustable, so that you can work at a comfortable height and reduce the risk of back strain.

More customized pedicure units with a built-in removable foot bath are available (Figures 26-11 and 26-12). They are constructed with both the client and the cosmetologist in mind, as they add to the service and are more ergonomically designed, making it much easier for the cosmetologist to perform the pedicure. A portable pedicure cart has a place for the foot bath and storage area for supplies.

Portable foot basins with built-in, motorized whirlpool action that can be filled from the sink are also available (Figure 26-13). After the service, they are drained by pumping the water back into the sink drain. These units have built-in footrests and areas for storing pedicure materials. The gentle massaging action of the whirlpool adds an extra touch to the service.

The ultimate pedicure foot bath is the fully plumbed pedicure basin chair or "throne" (Figure 26-14). These units are not portable; they are attached to both hot and cold water as well as to a drain. If a floor drain is not available, a pump option can be purchased to pump the water to an available sink.

Also available are units with a built-in massage feature as well as a warmer in the client chair, which adds to the client's relaxation.

No matter which water bath unit you use, be sure that your seat fits both you and the unit. Look for a stool or chair that is adjustable for height and provides good lower back support. Such seats are more ergonomic, and will help prevent back pain or injury.

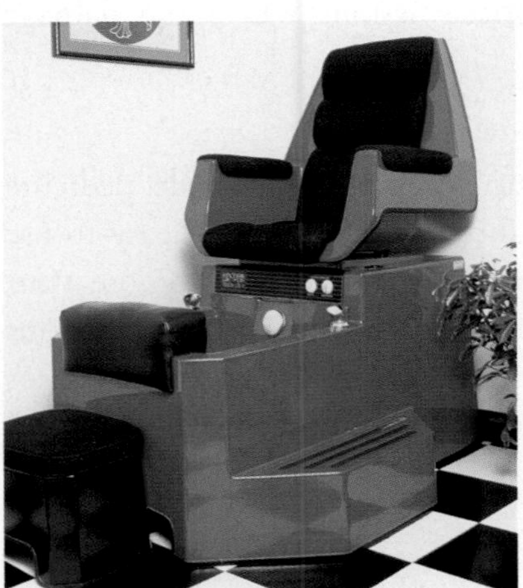

Figure 26-14 A fully-plumbed throne-type pedicure unit comes with many options including a massage unit built into the client chair.

PERFORMING PEDICURES

As with other procedures, a pedicure involves three parts: the pre-service, the pedicure procedure, and the post-service. In the pre-service you will clean and disinfect your implements, greet your client, and do a client consultation. Next you will perform the steps involved in the actual procedure. Then, in the post-service, you will schedule another appointment for your client, make recommendations and sell the beneficial retail products you discussed during the service, clean your area, and sanitize and disinfect all disinfectable implements and abrasives.

PEDICURE PRE-SERVICE

Your pedicure area should be close to a sink so that it is convenient for filling the pedicure baths with water. Follow the steps in Procedure 26-1.

BASIC PEDICURE SERVICE

When using a manufacturer's product line, you should follow all recommendations and suggested procedures, because they have been tested and found to enhance the effectiveness of the product line. You should time the individual steps of the pedicure based on the time suggested by the manufacturer to complete the entire service economically and efficiently. Do not give the client the feeling of being rushed, but develop your procedures so that there are no wasted motions. Have your implements and products within easy reach (Figure 26-15). There should be no distractions for you or the client during the pedicure. You should always understand and keep in mind your client's goals and expectations for the service. Make clients feel that you have nothing more to do than to take care of their needs. Talk to them if they wish to talk, but if they want to drift off, allow them the peace and tranquility they are seeking.

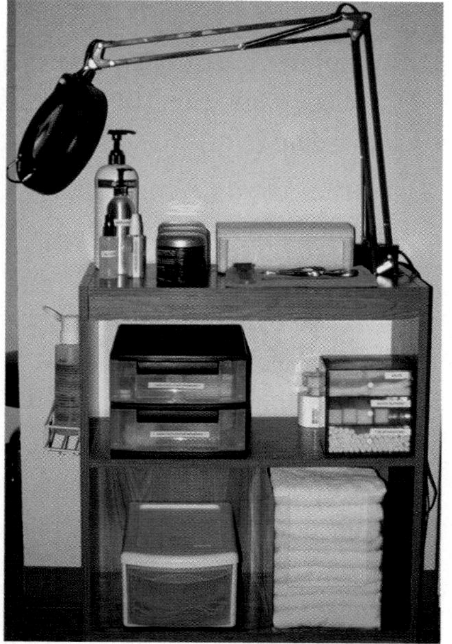

Figure 26-15 A portable pedicure supply cart containing all the instruments and supplies for a pedicure.

Be gentle, but firm, when handling the foot. A gentle, light touch can produce a tickling sensation, which is not at all relaxing. In fact, this may cause the client to become tense and pull away from the cosmetologist during the service. Many people normally cannot stand having their feet touched, but will accept and tolerate a firm, comfortable grip on the foot (Figure 26-16).

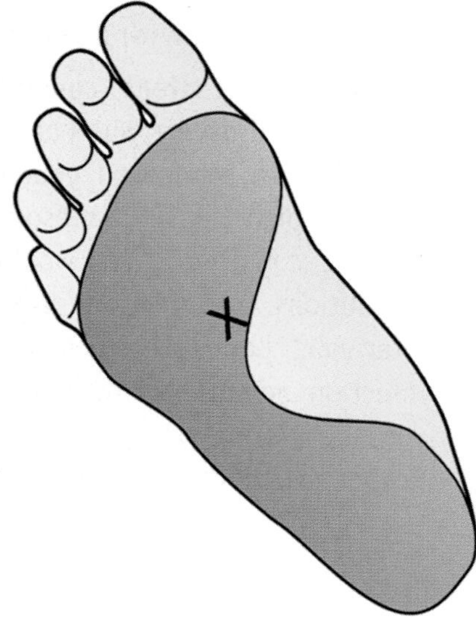

Figure 26-16 "X" marks the spot—Applying pressure to this area will often have a calming effect on ticklish or apprehensive clients.

In most instances, when working on the foot, it should be grasped between the thumb and fingers at the mid-tarsal area. This accomplishes two things:

- It "locks" the foot, making it rigid. When the foot is not locked, it is flexible and loose. Locking also allows the practitioner to place the thumb or index finger at the point on the bottom of the foot where the two skin creases meet on the ball. This spot is usually located at the beginning of the longitudinal arch.
- Applying a firm grip at this point has a calming effect on clients and overcomes any apprehension about someone touching their feet.

PROCEDURE 26-1

PRE-SERVICE FOR PEDICURE

1. **Complete pre-service sanitation.** Complete your pre-service sanitation and disinfection procedure (this procedure is described in Procedure 25-3).
2. **Station set up.** Your station should be set up to include a comfortable and ergonomically correct pedicuring stool/chair, client's chair, and a footrest for your client.
3. **Arrange towels.** Spread one terrycloth towel on the floor in front of client's chair to place feet during the pedicure. Put another towel over the footrest. This will be used to dry the feet.
4. **Set up standard manicure table.** Set up your standard manicuring table for use while doing pedicures. You will also need to add toe separators, an abrasive foot file or paddle, toenail clippers, liquid soap, foot lotion, oil, or cream, a rapid nail dryer, and pedicure slippers.
5. **Fill basin with warm water.** Add a measured amount of liquid soap to the bath (follow manufacturer's directions).
6. **Greet your client with a smile.**
7. **Complete the client consultation.** Check for nail disorders and decide whether it is safe and appropriate to perform a service on your client. Determine if the client is diabetic, or has psoriasis or other signs of a medical condition that would warrant taking extra precautions. If infection or inflammation is present, refer your client to her or his physician. If any signs of infection are present, you must not perform a pedicure—you are risking your professional license if you do! Record the client's responses and your observations.

The actual pedicure procedure can be divided into five basic steps: the soak, nail care, skin care, massage, and nail polishing. Each of these steps is distinct from the other. Depending on client needs, some steps may not be necessary. For example, some clients may only need nail care. This will take less time than a more complete treatment. If you have a great massage technique, clients may want only the soak and a massage to relieve tension and stress after a day's work. Others may want the full treatment, since they are there to be pampered. Remember to be innovative and creative when it comes to your pedicure services.

During the pedicure procedure, talk with your client about the products that are needed to maintain the service between salon visits. You might recommend polish, top coat, and foot lotion or cream.

PEDICURE POST-SERVICE

The steps in Procedure 26-3 should be followed after every pedicure service.

DISINFECTING FOOT SPAS

Foot spas should be cleaned and disinfected after every service and at the end of the working day. In addition, extra cleaning and disinfecting are recommended on a biweekly schedule. Post-client, daily, and biweekly steps are presented in Procedure 26-4.

CAUTION

Be sure the floor around the pedicure area is dry because wet floors are slippery. You or your clients can fall. When water is spilled, wipe it up immediately. The same holds true for slippery oils, lotions, or creams. You must always be on guard to ensure your client's safety. That's your job as a salon professional!

FOOT MASSAGE

Massage is defined in medical dictionaries as "a method of manipulation of the body by rubbing, pinching, kneading, tapping, etc." The art of massage has probably been around since the beginning of time. Most of us enjoy being touched, and the art of massage takes touching to a higher, even therapeutic level. Foot massage during a pedicure stimulates blood flow and is relaxing to the client.

The following basic forms of **hand movements** are utilized in therapeutic massage:

- Light or hard stroking movements called **effleurage**
- Compression movements called **petrissage,** which include kneading, squeezing, and friction
- In percussion or **tapotement** (tah-POT-mynt), sides of hands strike skin in rapid succession

Effleurage relaxes muscles, and improves circulation to the small, surface blood vessels. Petrissage helps to increase movement by stretching muscles and tendons. Tapotement is also a technique for improving circulation.

There are a number of massage styles and techniques. No matter what technique you use, perfect it so that it becomes second nature to you.

PROCEDURE 26-2

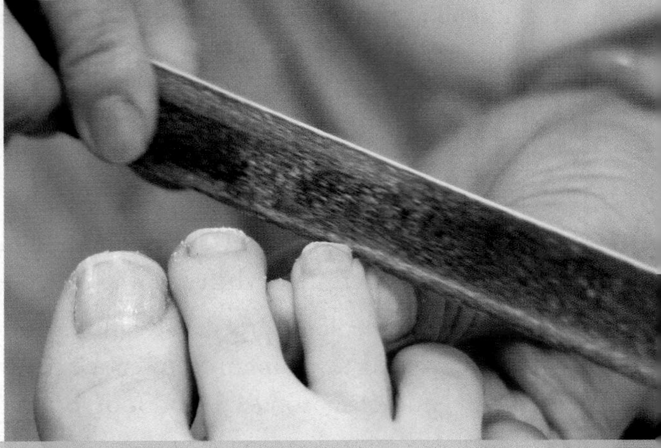

PERFORMING A BASIC PEDICURE

1. **Remove shoes and socks.** Ask your client to remove shoes, socks, and hose, and roll pant legs to the knees.
2. **Soak feet.** Put client's feet in soap bath for 5 minutes to soften and clean the feet before you begin the pedicure (Figure 26-17).
3. **Dry feet thoroughly.** Make sure you dry between the toes. Ask client to place both feet on the towel you have placed on the floor (Figure 26-18).
4. **Remove existing polish.** Remove polish from the little toe on left foot working towards the big toe. Repeat with the right foot (Figure 26-19).
5. **Clip nails.** Carefully clip the toenails of the left foot so that they are even with the end of the toe (Figure 26-20). Do not clip nails too short. Take care not to break the hyponychium, an important part of the seal that protects the toenail unit from infection.

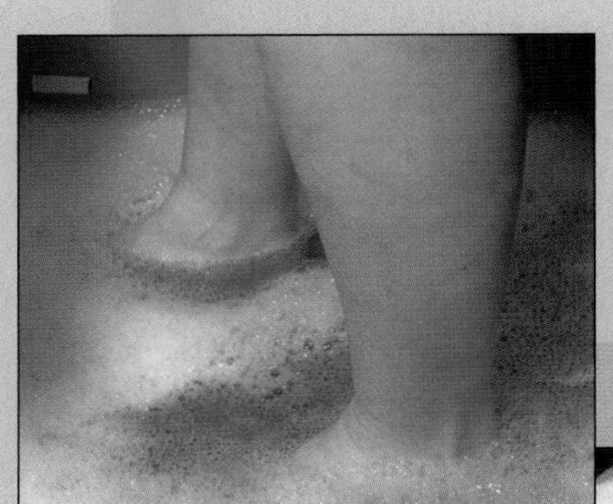

Figure 26-17 Soak feet for 5 minutes to soften and cleanse skin.

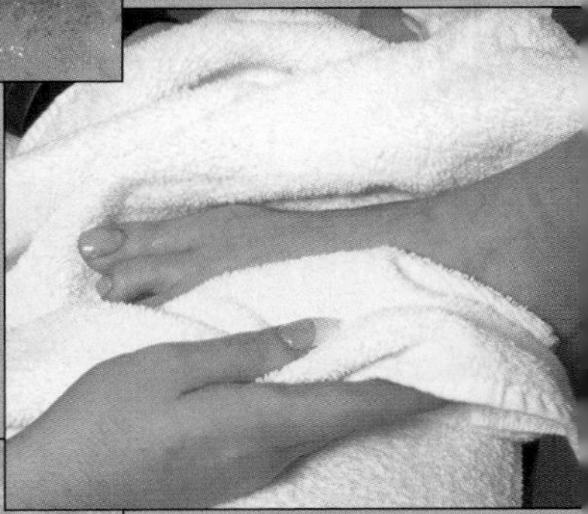

Figure 26-18 Dry feet thoroughly.

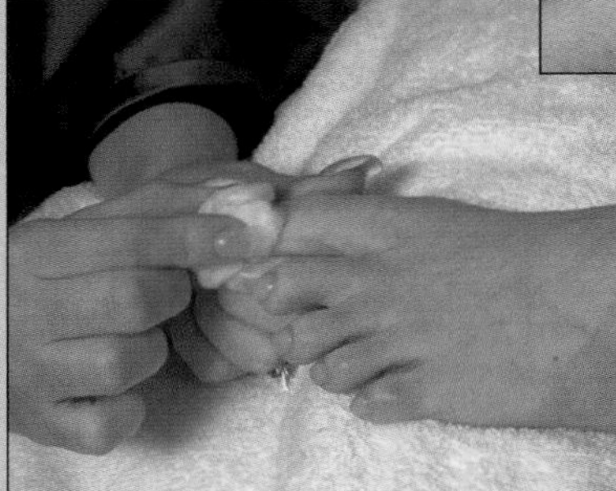

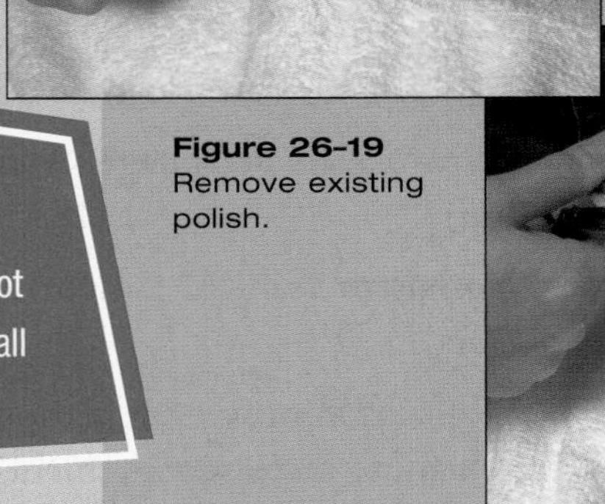

Figure 26-19 Remove existing polish.

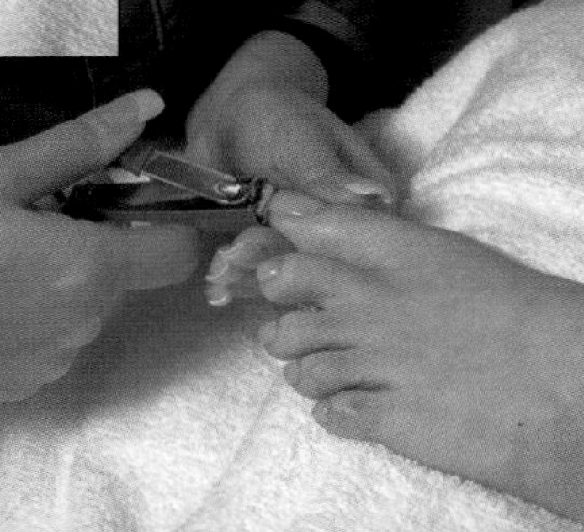

Figure 26-20 Carefully clip toenails.

Here's a TIP

Add a few drops of aromatherapy oil to the foot bath to excite the client's senses and enhance the overall experience.

6. **File nails.** Carefully file the nails of the left foot with an appropriate abrasive file. File them straight across, rounding them slightly at the corners to conform to the shape of the toes. Smooth rough edges with the fine side of an abrasive file (Figure 26-21). Repeat this step on the other foot.
7. **Use foot file.** Use foot file on the ball and heel of foot to smooth dry skin and calluses. Do not try to completely remove a client's calluses. Removing this protective layer and can lead to blisters, irritation, or infections (Figure 26-22).
8. **Rinse foot.** Place the left foot in foot bath.
9. **Repeat Steps 7 and 8 on the right foot.**
10. **Brush nails.** While the left foot is in the foot bath, brush nails with nail brush. Remove the foot and dry thoroughly (Figure 26-23).
11. **Apply cuticle remover.** Use a new cotton-tipped wooden pusher or eye dropper to apply cuticle remover to the left foot. Begin with the little toe and work toward the big toe (Figure 26-24).
12. **Removing cuticle tissue.** When performing a pedicure, do not push back the eponychium. Feet are more susceptible to infections and pushing back the eponychium (or cutting) can increase the risk of serious infections on feet. This is especially important for clients with diabetes or psoriasis. Carefully remove the cuticle tissue using a wooden or metal pusher taking care not to break the important seal it creates between the nail plate and eponychium. Use a nipper to carefully remove any loose tags of dead skin, but do not cut, rip, or tear the living skin, since this too could lead to serious infections (Figure 26-25).

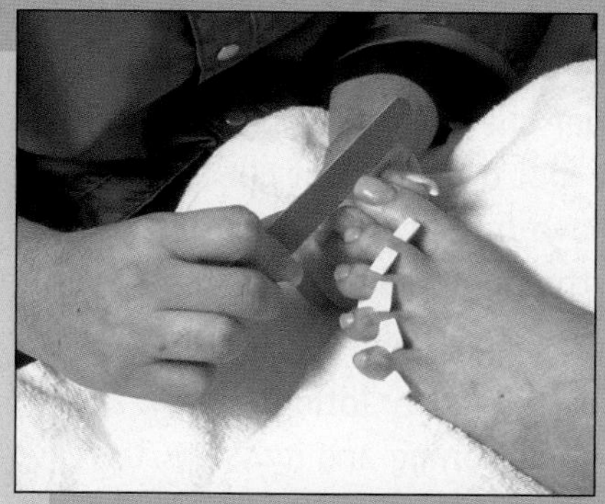

Figure 26-21 File nails.

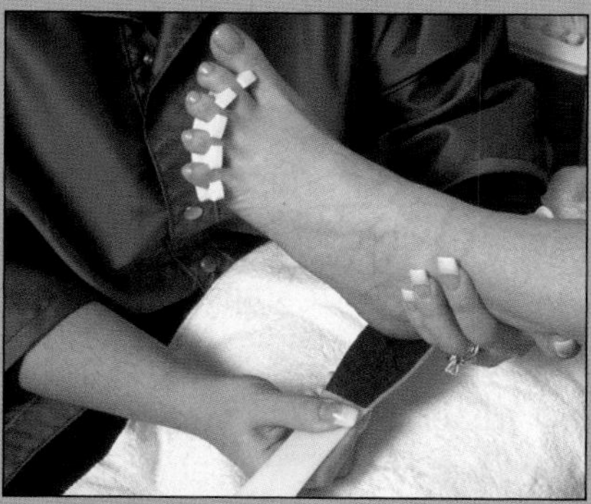

Figure 26-22 Use foot file.

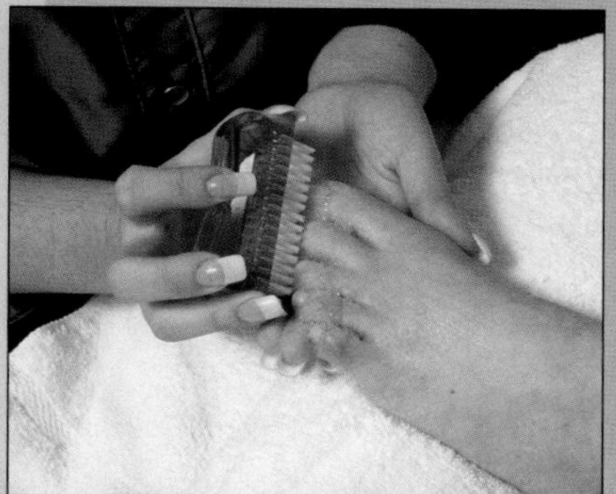

Figure 26-23 Brush nails.

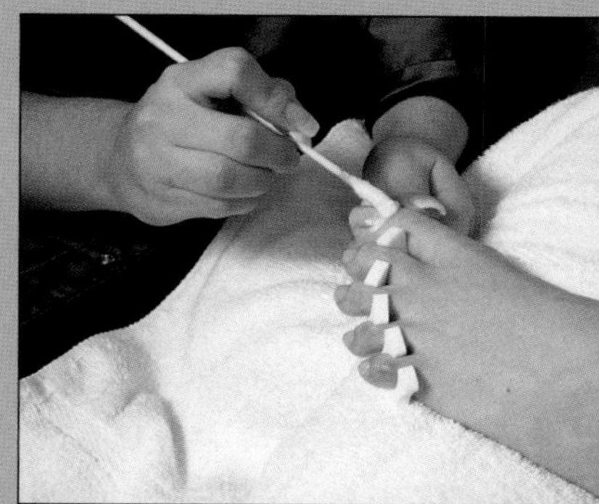

Figure 26-24 Apply cuticle remover.

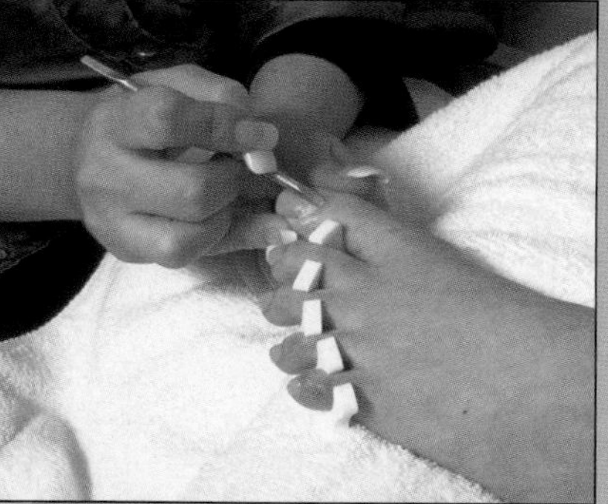

Figure 26-25 Carefully remove dead cuticle tissue from the nail plate.

13. **Brush toenails.** Ask your client to dip left foot into foot bath. With the left foot over the foot bath, brush with nail brush to remove bits of debris and cuticle remover. Dry the foot thoroughly and place foot on towel.
14. **Apply lotion, cream, or oil.** Apply lotion, cream, or oil to the foot for skin conditioning and massage. Use a firm touch to avoid tickling your client's feet (Figure 26-26).
15. **Massage foot.** Perform foot massage on the left foot. Then place foot on a clean towel on the floor. (See "Foot Massage" section in this chapter.)
16. Proceed with Steps 10 to 15 on the right foot.
17. **Remove traces of lotion.** Remove traces of lotion, cream, or oil from toenails of both feet with a small piece of cotton or plastic-backed cotton pad that has been saturated with polish remover.
18. **Apply polish.** Insert the toe separators. Apply base coat, two coats of color, and top coat to toenails. Spray with rapid polish dryer to prevent smudging of the polish. Place feet on a towel to dry (Figure 26-27).

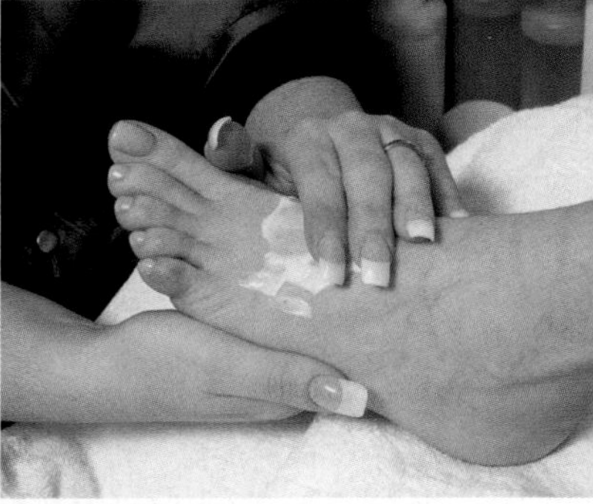

Figure 26-26 Apply lotion.

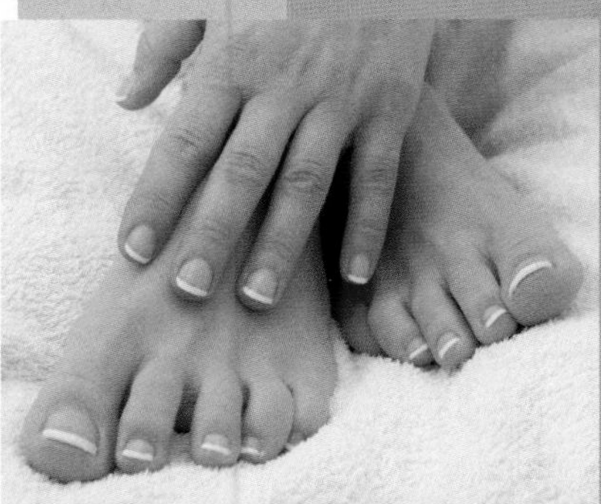

Figure 26-27 Finished pedicure.

LAW

Never use a razor or other sharp device to cut calluses from the feet. These are potentially dangerous devices that must never be used by cosmetologists, especially on diabetic clients. It is not legal in any state for a cosmetologist to perform medical procedures. Using a razor is prohibited and can cause you to lose your license.

Here's a TIP

Toe separators can be used to hold the toes apart while filing or applying cuticle remover, if preferred.

PROCEDURE 26-3

POST-SERVICE PROCEDURES

1. **Make another appointment.** Schedule another pedicure appointment for your client.
2. **Advise client.** Advise client about proper foot care. For example, remind the client that wearing tight shoes and very high heels can cause problems with the feet.
3. **Recommend take home products.** Suggest that your client purchase and use the professional products that you have discussed during the pedicure or recommend at the end of the service. Products such as polish, foot lotions or creams, skin moisturizers, softeners, cooling gels, powders, and top coats help to maintain the pedicure until the next service.
4. **Clean and disinfect pedicure basin.** After every pedicure, disinfect the pedicure basin as instructed in Procedure 26-4.
5. **Clean your table.** Clean and disinfect implements and multi-use tools (e.g., abrasives). Typically this step requires 20 minutes of proper cleaning and disinfection before implements or the pedicure basin can be used on the next client. Return your table to its basic setup.

Here's a TIP

Think that you don't have 10 minutes between pedicures to disinfect? Before reaching for the massage lotion, clean the basin and fill with water and disinfectant solution. The disinfectant can remain in the basin while you complete the pedicure. This keeps you on schedule and shows the client that you are providing safe services.

26-4 DISINFECTING FOOT SPAS

AFTER EVERY CLIENT

1. **Drain and remove.** Drain all water and remove all foreign matter (contaminants) from the foot spa.
2. **Clean surfaces.** Clean the surfaces and walls of the foot spa with soap or detergent and rinse with clean, clear water.
3. **Disinfect.** Disinfect with a regulatory oversight agency-approved disinfectant and according to the manufacturer's instructions.
4. **Rinse and dry.** Rinse and wipe dry with a clean towel.

PROCEDURE AT THE END OF WORKING DAY

1. **Remove and clean screen.** Remove the screen and clean all debris trapped behind the screen of the foot spa.
2. **Wash screen.** Wash the screen and inlet with soap or detergent and clean, clear water. Then totally immerse in regulatory oversight agency approved-disinfectant, according to the manufacturer's instructions.
3. **Flush system.** Flush the system with low-sudsing soap and warm water for 10 minutes. Then rinse, drain, and let air-dry.

BIWEEKLY PROCEDURE

1. **Follow the daily procedure, and fill the spa with bleach solution.** After following the recommended daily cleaning procedure described above, fill the foot spa tub (5 gallons) with water and 4 teaspoons of 5% bleach solution.
2. **Circulate solution.** Circulate the solution through the foot spa system for 10 minutes.
3. **Soak in solution.** Let the solution sit overnight (at least 6 to 10 hours).
4. **Drain and flush.** The following morning, in advance of the first customer, drain and flush the system.

CAUTION

Never place client's feet water that contains a disinfectant. This can cau injury to client's skin!

Study and practice various methods to individualize the massage for clients. During this part of the pedicure, be keenly aware of your client's needs and meet those requirements by giving a massage that fulfills them. They will likely be back for more!

The amount of pressure applied during the massage should be only as deep as is comfortable for you and your client. Ask the client whether she or he would like more or less pressure. Be aware of the parts of the massage that the client needs or enjoys most and put greater emphasis in these areas. Sit in a comfortable and unstrained position and keep your wrists straight in order to reduce the risk of injury to your back, shoulders, arms, wrists, and hands. Do not favor your dominant or strongest hand; always remembering to use both hands equally. Pay attention to your own body's positioning and make sure you are working ergonomically. For example, avoid leaning toward or stretching to reach your client's feet. Sit in a comfortable and relaxed position.

Although it important to give your client the best possible service, it's more important to keep yourself healthy during the process and avoid injuries caused by strain or repetitive motion. Take a minute to stretch before and after a pedicure to keep your body limber and more resistant to injury. Stretching is not just for athletes; it can help everyone if done regularly.

Attention to these finer details will always make your massage stand out from others and will keep your body healthy at the same time.

FOOT MASSAGE TECHNIQUES

The following techniques and illustrations provide directions for massage of the left foot.

- **Relaxer movement to the joints of the foot.** Rest client's foot on footrest or stool. Grasp the leg just above the ankle with your left hand. This will brace the client's leg and foot. Use your right hand to hold left foot just beneath the toes and rotate foot in a circular motion (Figure 26-28).
- **Effleurage on top of foot.** Place both thumbs on top of foot at the instep. Move your thumbs in circular movements in opposite directions down the center of the top of the foot. Continue this movement to the toes. Keep one hand in contact with foot or leg, firmly slide one hand at a time back to the instep and rotate back down to the toes. This is a relaxing movement. Repeat three to five times (Figure 26-29).
- **Effleurage on heel (bottom of foot).** Use the same thumb movement that you did in the

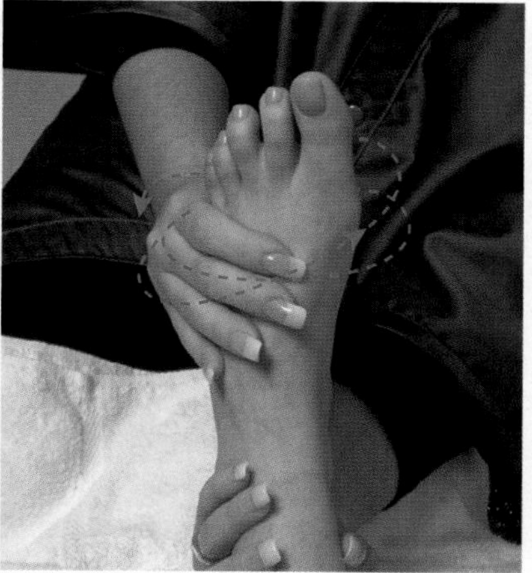

Figure 26-28 Relaxer movement to joints of the foot.

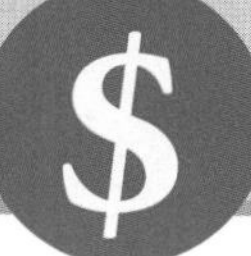

BUSINESS TIP: PUSHING PEDICURES DURING COLD WEATHER

It's relatively easy to sell pedicures during the summer—the weather is warm and clients want their bare or sandal-clad feet in tip-top shape. But in the winter, feet are bundled up in layers of socks and shoes or boots. Many clients forget about foot care, because they do not see their feet as much. Pedicures should be promoted as therapy for the feet, because they are an important part of good grooming and a preventive health aid. Like other parts of the body, feet can suffer from extreme dryness and cracking. Remind clients that feet are in daily use and they need routine maintenance for both men and women, especially during the winter months. Monthly pedicures during the winter keep feet healthy and happy.

CAUTION

For clients who have high blood pressure or a heart condition, or who have had a stroke, massage may be harmful because it increases circulation. Have the client consult a physician before you perform this service.

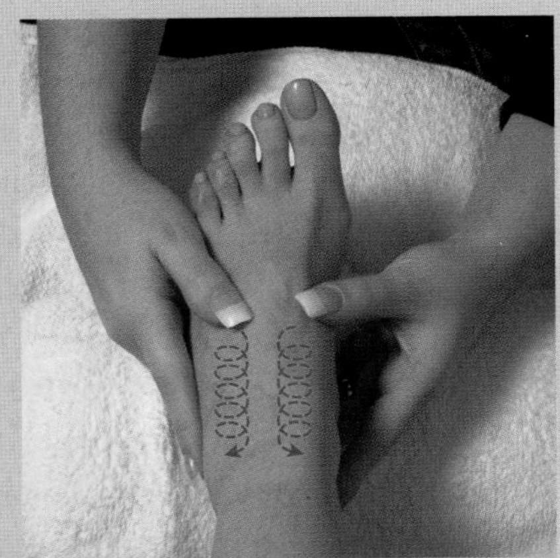

Figure 26-29 Effleurage on top of foot.

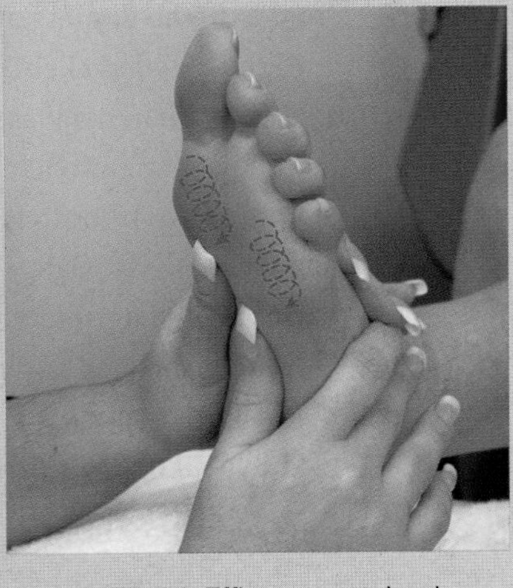

Figure 26-30 Effleurage on heel.

previous massage technique. Start at the base of the toes and move from the ball of the foot to the heel, rotating your thumbs in opposite directions. Slide hands back to the top of the foot. This is a relaxing movement. Repeat three to five times (Figure 26-30).

- **Effleurage movement on toes.** Start with the little toe, using the thumb on top and the index finger on the bottom of foot. Hold each toe and rotate with your thumb. Start at the base of the toe and work toward the end of the toes. This is relaxing and soothing. Repeat three to five times (Figure 26-31).
- **Joint movement for toes.** Start with the little toe and make a figure eight with each toe. Repeat three to five times (Figure 26-32).
- **Thumb compression** or **friction movement.** Make a fist with your fingers, keeping your thumb out. Apply firm pressure with your thumb and move your fist up the heel toward the ball of the foot. Work from the left side of foot and back down the right side toward the heel. As you massage over the bottom of the foot, check for any nodules or bumps. If you find one, be very gentle because the area may be tender. This movement stimulates the blood flow and increases circulation (Figure 26-33).
- **Metatarsal scissors (a petrissage massage movement, or kneading).** Place your fingers on top of the foot along the metatarsal bones with your thumb underneath the foot. Knead up and down along each bone by raising your thumb and lower fingers to apply pressure. This promotes flexibility and stimulates circulation. Repeat three to five times (Figure 26-34).
- **Fist twist compression (friction movement, deep rubbing).** Place your left hand on top of the foot and make a fist with your right hand. Your left hand will apply pressure while your right hand twists around the bottom of the foot. This helps stimulate circulation. Repeat three to five times up and around foot (Figure 26-35).

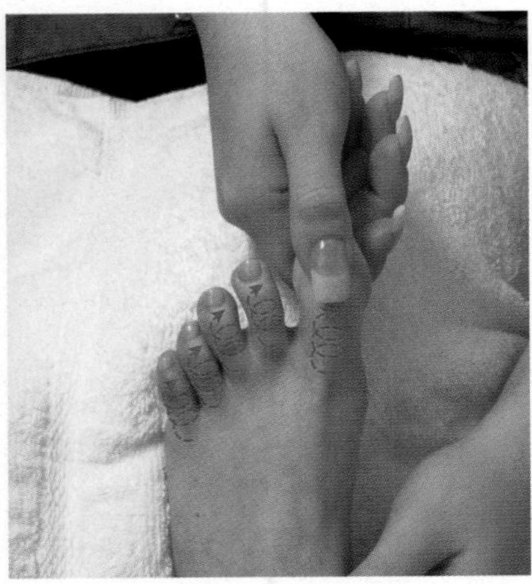

Figure 26-31 Effleurage on toe.

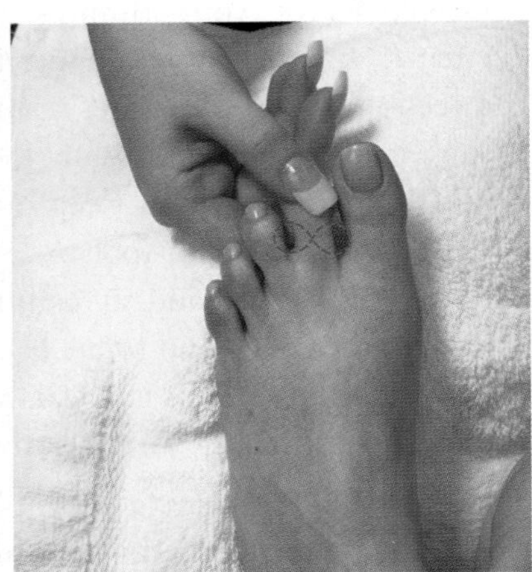

Figure 26-32 Joint movement for toes.

- **Effleurage on instep.** Place your fingers at the ball of the foot. Move your fingers in circular movements in opposite directions. Massage to the end of each toe, gently squeezing the tip of each toe (Figure 26-36).
- **Percussion or tapotement movement.** Use fingertips to perform percussion or tapotement movements to lightly tap over the entire foot to complete a massage.

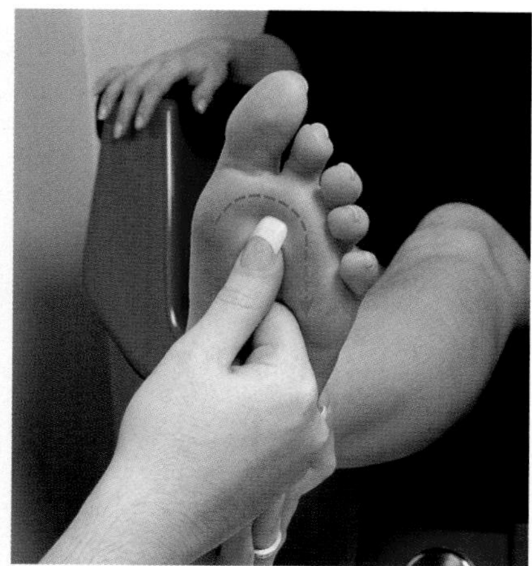
Figure 26-33 Thumb compression—"friction movement."

BEYOND THE BASIC PEDICURE

The basic step-by-step pedicure procedure is a necessary learning tool to help you master a valuable service. There is, however, much more information to come to enable you to go beyond the basics. The products, implements, and equipment you will need to perform a pedicure are an important part of the service. When you become more proficient and begin to customize a pedicure, the following information will be indispensable in helping you accomplish customization.

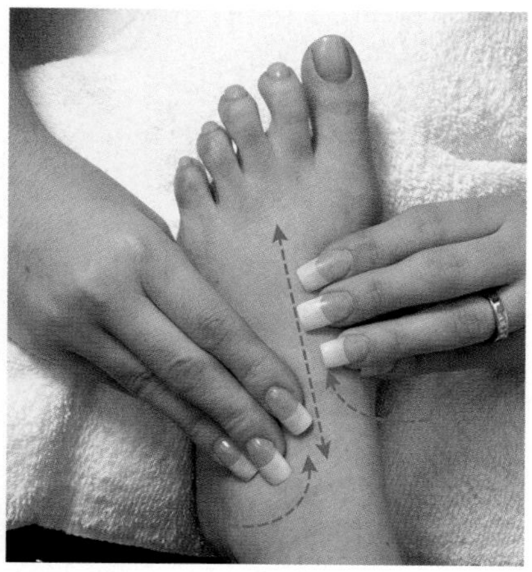
Figure 26-34 Metatarsal scissors.

Just as there are "systems" for nail enhancement products, so are there pedicure systems or lines available from many manufacturers of professional nail products. These manufacturers produce a complete line of products for the professional pedicure. It is recommended that you check out all of these lines. Compare them with each other and decide for yourself which is best for your clients. The educational support and commitment of the company are important in making this decision.

The basic types of products necessary for the pedicure service are abrasive scrubs, soaks, massage preparations, and cuticle removers. Each of the types is discussed below.

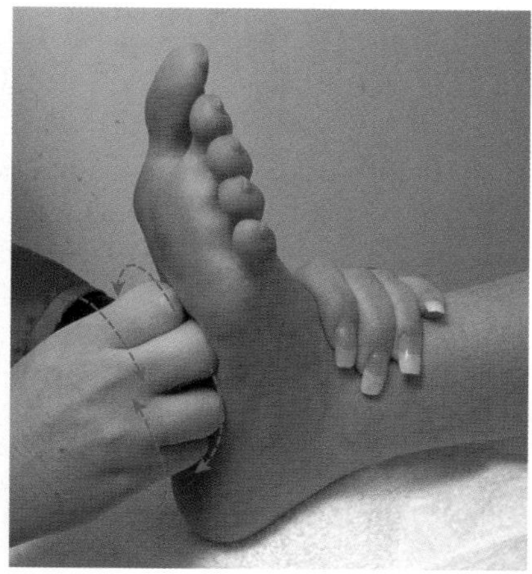
Figure 26-35 Fist twist compression.

Foot soaks are products used in the pedicure bath to soften the skin. A good soak must contain a gentle but effective soap to thoroughly clean and deodorize the feet. Antibacterial soaps are no more effective than soaps whose labels do not make antibacterial claims. Therefore, do not choose a product simply because it is "antibacterial." Like all soaps, the main function of so-called antibacterial soaps is to make bacteria so slippery that they slide off the skin. All soaps then are antibacterial, whether or not their manufacturers make this claim.

Dead Sea salts, which are often found in foot-soak products, contain many types of salt including sodium, calcium, and magnesium salts. All are thought to be highly beneficial to the skin. Professionally formulated products are recommended because they are designed to properly cleanse the foot without being overly harsh to the skin. Other ingredients may include natural oils used for their moisturizing and/or aromatherapy qualities. The soak sets the stage for the rest of the pedicure, so be sure to

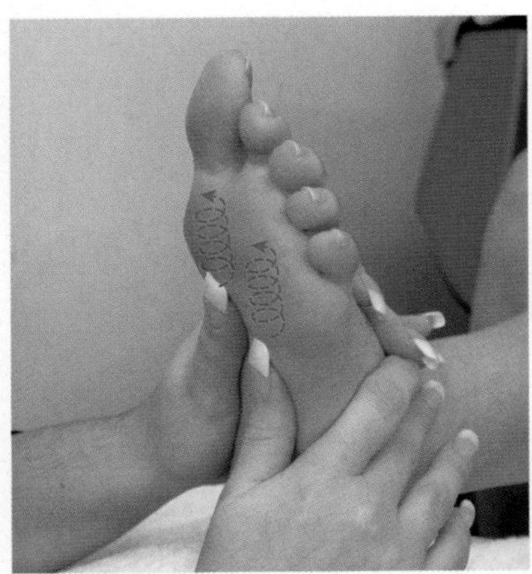

Figure 26-36 Effleurage on instep.

use a high-quality product and start your pedicure service on a positive note.

Beware of misleading product claims. There is no additive or soak that is added to the water during a pedicure that kills pathogens and replaces your obligation to clean and disinfect the foot spa after the pedicure. Any chemical that is strong enough to kill pathogens is not safe for contact with skin. Disinfectants must **never** be placed in the foot bath with the client's feet.

Abrasive scrubs are used to help remove and smooth dry flaky skin and calluses. They are usually creams or lotions that contain an abrasive powder as the exfoliating agent. These are used to remove dry, flaky skin and leave it feeling smoother and more moisturized. Avoid excessive use of abrasive scrubs since they can damage the client's skin. Abrasive scrubs can also remove the living skin from the hands of the cosmetologist, if the product is used many times during a short period of time. If hands become sore from repeated services, consider finding a gentler product or wearing gloves while using the abrasive scrub.

Sea sand, ground apricot kernels, pumice, quartz crystals, and plastic beads are all exfoliating agents found in pedicure scrubs. Essential aroma oils, beneficial extracts, and moisturizers that help to condition the skin, may also be found in scrub preparations.

Massage preparations consist of oils, creams, and lotions used to lubricate, moisturize, and invigorate the skin. They allow the hands of the cosmetologist to glide soothingly over the skin during the massage part of the pedicure. They also help to promote a general feeling of relaxation and well-being in the client. Most quality **massage oils** are a blend of therapeutic oils, which help promote skin health.

Aromatherapy oils may also be incorporated for their relaxing and calming effects. Tea tree oil is often included for its antiseptic properties, as well as its medicinal fragrance. Cosmetologists, like some massage therapists, may wish to formulate their own massage oil. Some massage therapy supply stores have base massage oils to which different essential oils can be added. A number of massage oils can be formulated in this manner to match individual client needs, and thus give a customized quality to the pedicure. Preparing only small quantities of these blends (i.e., the amount required for the service) is recommended because formulating larger amounts of these oils must be done under very clean (hygienic) conditions or the blends could become contaminated with bacteria and rapidly spoil.

Cuticle removers are designed to soften cuticles for removal from the nail plate. These products are highly alkaline and corrosive substances that are capable of dissolving cuticles or other tissues within a very short period of time. Since these products are so fast acting, they must not be left on the nail plate for any longer than recommended by the product manufacturer, usually 1 to 2 minutes. If left on longer than recommended, serious damage can occur to the nail plate and/or surrounding skin. Improper use can also result in dryness and splits in the eponychium and side walls.

Cuticle removers must only be applied to the nail plate, and contact with living skin must be avoided. These products must be completely rinsed off after use to avoid skin irritation. If not thoroughly removed, residues on the nail plate can also cause lifting. Cosmetologists should avoid prolonged or repeated skin contact with these products, and safety eyewear should be worn to prevent accidental eye exposure. Any highly alkaline substances can be potentially dangerous if accidentally splashed in the eye or used incorrectly, so read the directions and follow them exactly.

ADD-ON PRODUCTS

Add-ons are used to enhance and expedite the pedicure experience. Professional-strength **callus softeners** are offered to help soften and smooth calluses, especially on heels and over pressure points. These products are applied directly to the callus and allowed to soak in for a short period of time to soften the hard tissue, making them easier to remove with abrasive boards, blocks, or paddles.

These products usually contain either sodium hydroxide or lactic acid, both powerful callus-softening agents. Sodium hydroxide is highly alkaline (usually pH 12 or higher). Lactic acid is an alpha hydroxy acid; products formulated with lactic acid are acidic (usually pH 4 or less). In both cases, it is very important to read and understand the manufacturer's instructions and use the product exactly as directed.

Products containing either sodium hydroxide or lactic acid should be considered potentially hazardous to eyes, and safety glasses should be worn whenever using or pouring them. Be sure to wash your hands before touching your face or eye area. Used improperly, these types of products can cause severe burns to the client's skin and may cause irritation to the cosmetologist's hands with repeated exposure. Used correctly, they can be very safe and effective.

Masques are usually composed of mineral clays, moisturizing agents, skin softeners, aromatherapy oils, and beneficial extracts. They are applied to the skin and left in place for 5 minutes. These skin treatments are typically highly valued by clients.

Hot **paraffin baths** for the feet are an excellent addition to the pedicure. The paraffin bath stimulates circulation, and the deep heat helps to reduce inflammation and promote circulation to the affected joints. Apply moisturizing lotions, creams, or oils to the skin, and use the paraffin to seal them in, allowing the heat to speed penetration of beneficial ingredients.

Aromatherapy oils can also be incorporated into the paraffin bath. Clients feel pampered and the hot paraffin wax service adds to the relaxation of the pedicure experience.

Do *not* provide this service to clients with impaired foot circulation, loss of feeling, or other diabetic-related problems. The hot wax may cause burns or skin breakdown in these situations.

CAUTION

Hot wax services should not be provided to clients with poor circulation or to diabetic clients without a doctor's release.

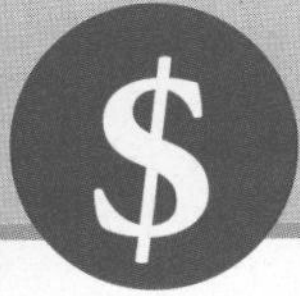

BUSINESS TIP: SERVICE FOR THE ELDERLY

The elderly also need care and maintenance for their feet on a year-round basis. A substantial proportion of the elderly population cannot reach their feet and need help in their foot care maintenance. It is estimated that 40 million Americans suffer from some form of arthritis. Many of them cannot reach their feet or cannot squeeze the nail nippers. They need proper foot care that a good cosmetologist can provide. Cosmetologists who offer pedicure services for this segment of the population will be doing these individuals a great favor, and will find plenty of willing clients in need of their services.

Other items necessary for the best-ever pedicure could include the following:

- Pedicure slippers—Disposable paper or foam slippers are needed for those clients who have not worn open-toed shoes.
- Pedicure sandals—Sandals with toe separators incorporated in their design can be purchased by clients and brought in every time they have a pedicure.

FULL-SERVICE PEDICURE

The full-service pedicure presented in Procedure 26-5 includes a variety of "extras" and add-ins that were not part of the basic pedicure described previously.

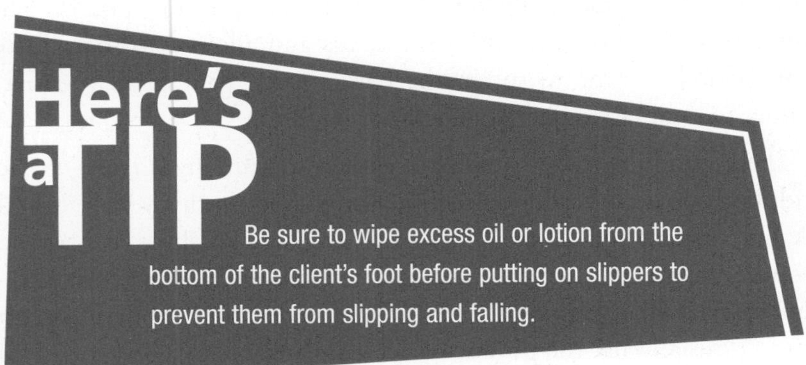

Here's a TIP
Be sure to wipe excess oil or lotion from the bottom of the client's foot before putting on slippers to prevent them from slipping and falling.

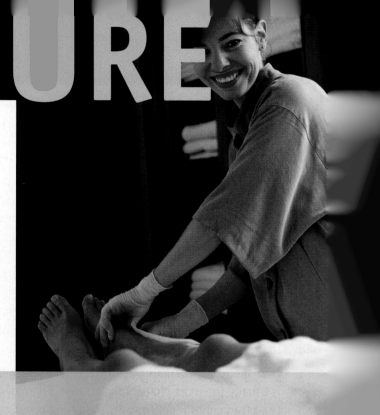

THE FULL-SERVICE PEDICURE

1. **The soak.** This service starts the procedure. It is important to soften and prepare the skin for what is to follow. The water must not exceed 104°F; use a thermometer to ensure that it is the proper temperature. Place the soaking product into the water according to the manufacturer's recommendation. Allow the client to soak for approximately 5 minutes to clean the foot and soften the skin. You have time during this part of the service to make sure everything you will need for the rest of the pedicure is in its proper place. Then you will not have to search for a needed item in the middle of the pedicure process, which looks very unprofessional to your clients.
2. **Nail care.** Remove one foot from the bath and dry it with a towel.
   (a) Remove polish. Remove any existing nail polish from the toenails.
   (b) Apply cuticle remover. At this point apply cuticle remover and/or callus softeners where needed. Applying the remover at this point will give the product time to work while you care for the nails.
   (c) Use curette. Next, the curette is used to gently push the soft tissue folds away from the walls of the lateral nail plate (Figure 26-37). This allows you to visually inspect the nail plate so that it can be trimmed without injuring the client. If there is extra buildup of debris between the nail plate and surrounding tissue, gently remove it with the curette. To use this instrument, place the rounded side of the spoon toward the wall of living skin. A gentle scooping motion is then used along the nail plate to remove any loose debris. A gentle pressure is all that is necessary to accomplish the removal of the built-up debris. The pressure of this debris is quite uncomfortable if left in place. You may need to repeat this scooping motion several times to adequately remove enough of the loose debris. Take care not to overdo it. *Do not* use this instrument to dig into the soft tissues along the nail fold. These living tissues are delicate and are easily injured. Any debris attached to the soft tissue that is not easily removed in the manner described must be removed by a medical doctor or podiatrist. If the tissue is inflamed, such as an ingrown toenail, refer the client to a qualified medical doctor or podiatrist.

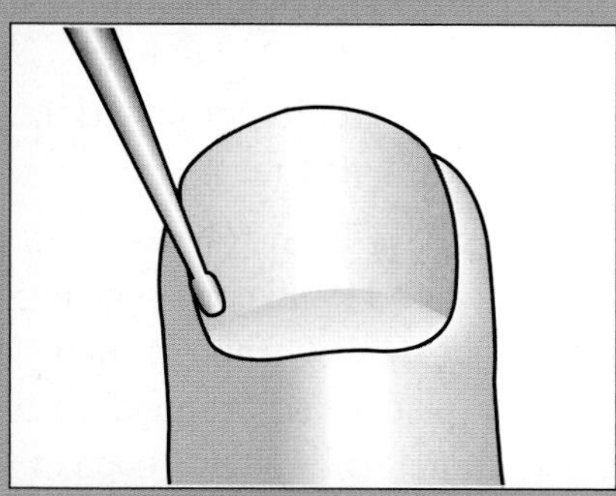

Figure 26-37 The curette is used to gently push the soft tissue away from the nail plate.

(d) Trim toenails. The nails should now be carefully trimmed using the toenail clippers. The clippers are used like a pair of scissors (Figure 26-38). The nail is trimmed in a number of small cuts to avoid flattening it out and injuring the hyponychium during the process. Place the clipper over the free nail edge and slightly tilt the top of the clipper back toward the nail plate. This reduces the possibility of cutting the soft tissues of the hyponychium under the free edge (Figure 26-39). Give the clipper a slight squeeze before actually cutting the nail. The reaction of the client to this squeeze will tell you if you are cutting too deep and are against living tissue. If you get a reaction, reposition the clipper on the nail and start the process over.

Trim the lesser toenails straight across. The big toenail is usually the most challenging to trim. The nail groove can often contain debris, lint, soap, and other material that has built up over time. Trim the great toenail just as described for the lesser toes, but pay particular attention to the side-wall area. Do not leave any rough edges or "hooks" that can catch on soft tissue. These can create an opportunity for infections. Remove these rough edges with a nail rasp.

After the nails have been trimmed with the clipper, go back with the curette and gently remove any debris left along the side walls. This is done, as previously described, by placing the cupped part of the curette against the lateral nail wall and edge of the nail. Gently draw the curette along the nail plate. This process may have to be repeated several times. In most instances, an adequate amount of the debris will be removed, thereby relieving the pressure and making the client comfortable. During this process, also recheck the nail plate along the side-wall areas for rough edges or "hooks" left behind after trimming.

(e) Remove cuticle tissue. The curette is also used to remove cuticle tissue from the top of the nail plate (Figure 26-40). The eponychium should not be pushed back on the toenails. Any small break in the seal created by the cuticle and eponychium may increase the risk of infection. To remove the cuticle tissue very carefully, draw the curette over the plate away from the eponychium in a sweeping "C" type motion from the nail fold toward the center of the nail plate.

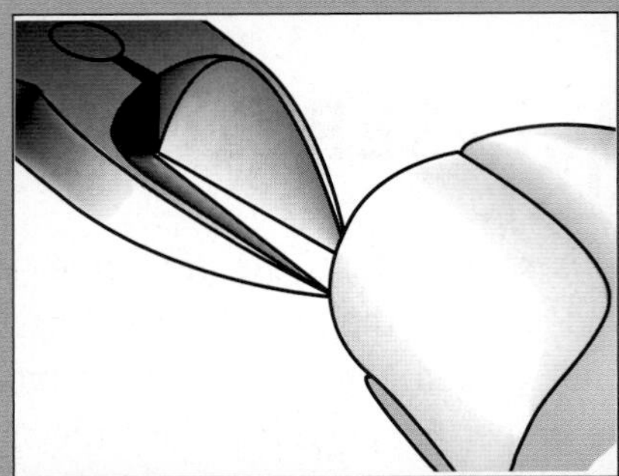

Figure 26-38 The nail nippers are used like a pair of scissors.

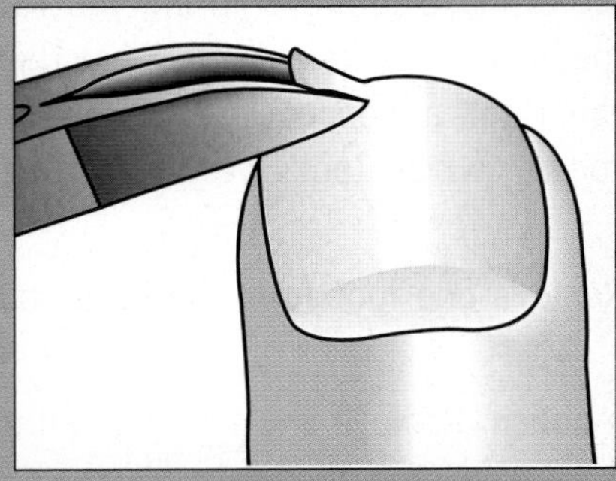

Figure 26-39 Trim the nail at a 45-degree angle. Note the tilt of the nipper, which reduces the possibility of injury to underlying soft tissue.

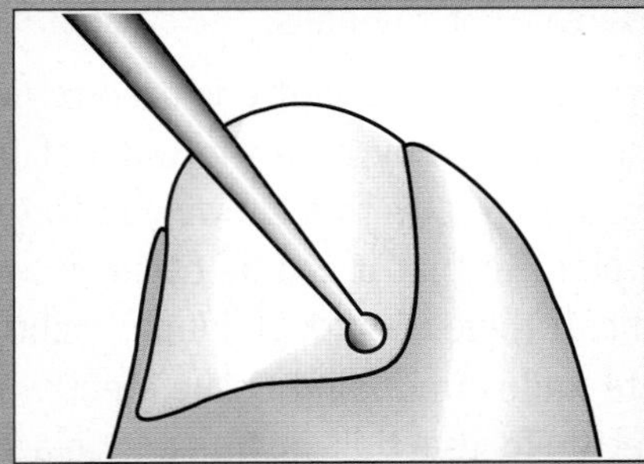

Figure 26-40 The curette is also used to remove the cuticle tissue from the surface of the nail plate.

This motion is then repeated from the opposite side of the nail plate. You may need to repeat these motions a number of times to remove all of the cuticle tissue from the top of the nail plate. Be careful not to cut or injure the eponychium during this process.

(f) Smooth edges of nail plate. The small nail rasp is then used to smooth the edges of the nail plate along the nail grooves (Figure 26-41). The rasp is made for this purpose. It is narrow and will only file the nail in one direction. It can be used to remove, smooth, and round off any sharp points or edges. Do not probe with the rasp, but instead gently draw it along the edge of that portion of the nail plate that you have just trimmed. Small, short strokes with the file from back to front will accomplish the task.

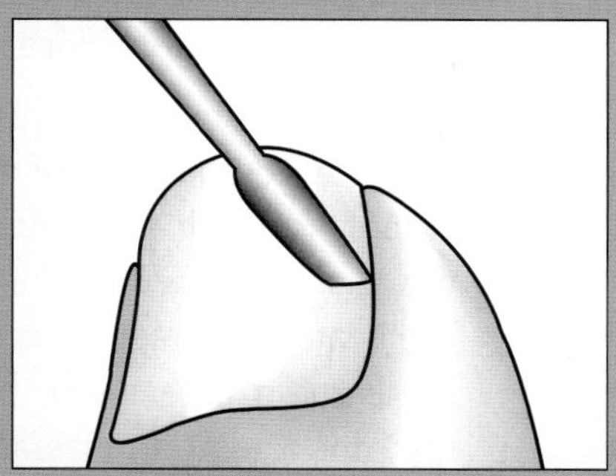

Figure 26-41 The small nail file or rasp is used to gently smooth and remove any rough edges or hooks left behind after the trimming process.

(g) Smooth remainder of nail. The abrasive file should then be used to finally shape and smooth the rest of the nail. If the nail is very thick, a file can be used to slightly thin the nail plate.

(h) Repeat process on other foot. After completing the nail service on one foot, place it back in the foot bath and repeat the process described above on the other foot. The entire nail-trimming process should take approximately 15 minutes.

3. **Skin care.** At this point, the skin has been softened by the solution in which it is soaking. The thicker areas of callus have been softened with the professional-strength callus softeners during the nail-trimming procedure.

   (a) Exfoliate. **Exfoliating scrubs** can now be used to remove dry or scaly skin. One foot is again removed from the bath and the scrub is liberally applied. Using a massaging motion, scrub the dry skin off the foot. Use extra pressure (which creates more friction) on the heels and other areas where more callus and dry skin build up.

   (b) Smooth calluses. During this process, the abrasive foot paddle is used to smooth and reduce the thicker areas of callus. Remember that callus protects the underlying skin from irritation and is there for a purpose. Remove only enough to make the client comfortable. Calluses should be softened and smoothed—not excessively thinned or removed. You may need to educate your client about callus formation and the protective function it provides. Also discuss products for home use to help soften and condition calluses between salon appointments.

   (c) Rinse. The foot is then rinsed in the bath. Do not forget to clean between the toes. These areas are often missed.

   (d) Apply masque. If a skin masque product is to be used, this is a good time to apply it. After rinsing and cleaning the foot, apply the masque according to the manufacturer's recommendations. Afterwards, wrap the foot in a clean towel and place it on the footrest.

   (e) Scrub and treat calluses on other foot. The abrasive scrubbing and callus smoothing process is then completed on the other foot. The entire process should take approximately 10 minutes. At this point, approximately 35 minutes have been used for the pedicure. You may wish to allow the client to relax with the mask product (if used) for another 5 minutes. This will leave 20 minutes for the massage and polish.

A hot wax service may also be added instead of a skin masque as a separate add-on part of the pedicure. The wax must be applied in accordance with the manufacturer's instructions. Lotions, creams, or oils can be applied to the foot before application of the paraffin wax. The heat will increase penetration of the ingredients into the skin. After the paraffin is removed, the residual product left on the skin can be used for a relaxing massage. After applying the wax, a plastic bag is placed over the foot and the foot is placed into a terrycloth boot or wrapped in a towel. The process is repeated on the other foot, and then the client should be allowed to relax for 5 minutes. Like all add-on services, hot wax and masque application take more time, require special equipment, and provide more benefit to the client. Therefore, you should charge extra for these services. Your time and services are very valuable, so do not be afraid or hesitant to charge for them.

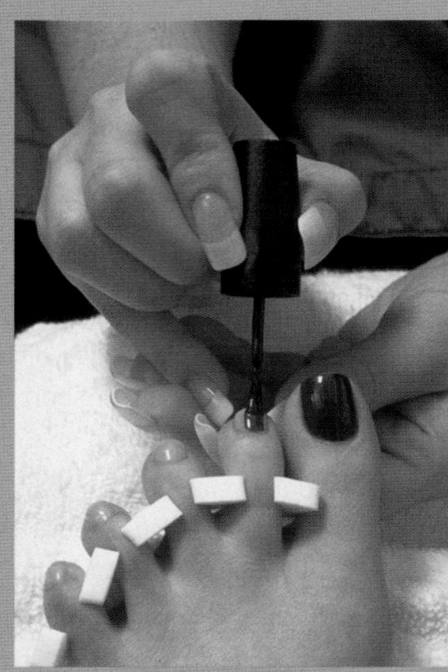

Figure 26-42 Apply nail polish after thoroughly cleaning the nail plate.

4. **Massage.** Massage is a part of the professional pedicure where the cosmetologist can excel. This is what the client has been looking forward to and often enjoys the most. A good massage will make the client come back again for another pedicure. The cosmetologist who perfects a good massage technique will build a good reputation. Massage aids relaxation, which is one of the most important reasons for giving a massage. Massage will give the client a sense of well-being and has a tremendous calming effect that reduces stress. The massage also promotes increased circulation and muscle relaxation in the lower extremities (see the "Foot Massage" section of this chapter).
5. **Apply nail polish (optional).** After the massage, if the client desires, nail polish should be applied according to manufacturer's recommendations. Insert toe separators during this procedure. Removing all traces of massage products from the toenails with polish remover is necessary to ensure that the polish adheres. Apply base coat, two coats of polish, and a topcoat (Figure 26-42). Place feet on a towel and allow the polish to dry. A rapid nail polish dryer can speed up this process.
6. **Post-pedicure procedures.** Follow Procedure 26-3. Once the client has left, sanitize (wash with soap and water) the equipment and implements used for the pedicure and then completely immerse the clean instruments and abrasives into the disinfectant solution. If you are performing many pedicures, you may need two sets of implements. One set can be disinfecting while you use the other set on your client. Properly clean and disinfect your pedicure tub as directed by your state regulations. Your instructor will provide you with specific details on these requirements. This is an extremely important step that must not be forgotten; otherwise, clients are exposed to risk of infection. Take this responsibility seriously, and be sure to properly clean and disinfect all pedicure equipment, implements, and so on.

REVIEW QUESTIONS

1. Name five pedicure supplies.
2. List the steps in the pedicure pre-service.
3. Describe the proper technique to use when filing toenails.
4. Describe the proper technique for trimming toenails.
5. List the steps in the pedicure post-service.
6. Name and describe six foot massage techniques.
7. Explain why calluses should never be removed.
8. Why must you be especially careful when giving a pedicure to a diabetic client?

CHAPTER GLOSSARY

abrasive nail file	A thin elongated board with a rough surface, used to file the free edge of the nails.
abrasive scrubs	Slightly abrasive products containing softening agents or oils to penetrate dry, flaky skin and calluses that need to be smoothed during a pedicure.
callus softeners	Helps soften and smooth calluses, especially on heels and over pressure points.
curette	Small, spoon-shaped instrument used for cleaning debris from the edges of nail plate.
cuticle removers	Products designed to soften cuticles for removal from the nail plate.
exfoliating scrubs	Preparations used to remove dry or scaly skin on the feet and legs.
foot files* or *paddles	Large abrasive files used to smooth and reduce thicker areas of calluses.
foot lotion, oil, or cream	Products used to condition and moisturize the feet; also used for performing a foot massage.
foot soaks	Products containing gentle soaps, moisturizers, and so on, that are used in a pedicure bath to cleanse and soften the skin.
friction movement	Firm pressure applied to the bottom of the foot using thumb compression to work from side to side and toward the heel.
hand movements	Movements used in therapeutic massage.

CHAPTER GLOSSARY

liquid soap	Used in pedicuring, contains a mild detergent for cleansing the feet.
masques	Usually composed of mineral clays, moisturizing agents, skin softeners, aromatherapy oils, and beneficial extracts.
massage oils	Blend of oils used to lubricate, moisturize, and invigorate the skin during a massage.
massage preparations	Oils, creams, and lotions used to lubricate, moisturize, and invigorate the skin.
nail rasp	Metal file with an edge that can file the nail plate in only one direction.
nippers	Instrument used for manicures and pedicures to trim tags of dead skin.
paraffin baths	Used to stimulate circulation and to reduce inflammation and promote circulation to the affected joints.
pedicure	Standard service performed by cosmetologists that includes care and massage of feet and trimming, shaping, and polishing toenails.
pedicure slippers	Disposable paper or foam slippers are needed for those clients who have not worn open-toed shoes.
tapotement	Massage movement using a short, quick hacking, slapping, or tapping technique.
toe separators	Foam rubber toe separators or cotton are used to keep toes apart while polishing the nails.
toenail clippers	Professional instruments with curved or straight jaws used for cutting toenails.

NAIL TIPS, WRAPS, & NO-LIGHT GELS

CHAPTER 27

chapter outline

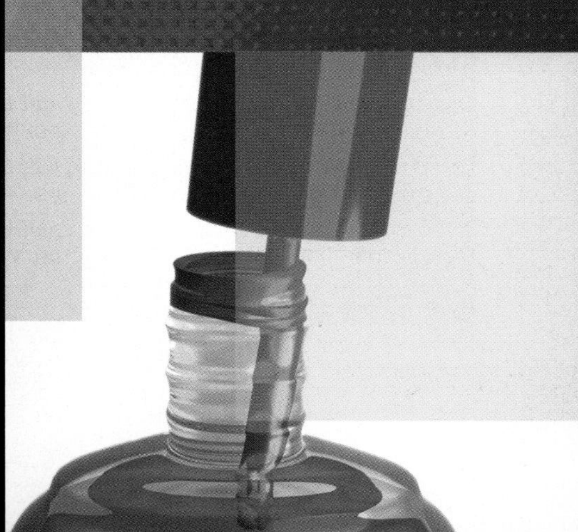

Learning Objectives

After completing this chapter, you will be able to:

- Identify the supplies needed for nail tips and explain why they are needed.
- Identify the three types of nail tips.
- Demonstrate the proper procedure and precautions to use in applying nail tips.
- Demonstrate the proper removal of tips.
- List four kinds of nail wraps and what they are used for.
- Explain benefits of using silk, linen, fiberglass, and paper wraps.
- Demonstrate the proper procedures and precautions used in fabric wrap application.
- Describe the maintenance of fabric wrap. Include a description of the 2-week and 4-week rebalance.
- Explain how to use fabric wrap for crack repairs.
- Demonstrate the proper procedure and precautions for fabric wrap removal.
- Define no-light gels.
- Demonstrate the proper procedures for applying no-light gels.

Key Terms

Page number indicates where in the chapter the term is used.

abrasive board **pg. 725**
ABS **pg. 725**
activator **pg. 733**
buffer block **pg. 725**
fabric wraps **pg. 733**
fiberglass **pg. 733**
linen **pg. 733**
nail tip **pg. 725**
nail tip adhesive **pg. 725**
nail wraps **pg. 726**
no-light gel **pg. 744**
overlay **pg. 725**
paper wraps **pg. 733**
repair patch **pg. 735**
silk **pg. 733**
stress strip **pg. 735**
tip cutter **pg. 729**
wrap resin **pg. 726**

One of the most popular services that a cosmetologist can offer clients is the opportunity to wear beautifully cared for nails in almost an endless variety of length and strength. In many cases, this is accomplished by the use of a **nail tip,** a plastic, premolded nail shaped from a tough polymer made from acrylonitrile butadiene styrene **(ABS)** or tenite acetate. Nail tips are adhered to the natural nail to add extra length and to serve as support for a nail enhancement product. Tips are combined with another service, such as a fabric wrap, overlay, or sculptured nail extensions. Nail tips are not long-wearing and can break easily without reinforcement, which is called an **overlay.** Overlays are acrylic (methacrylate) liquid and powder, wraps, or UV gels applied over a tip for added strength. These tips serve as a support for nail enhancement products. Sculpting a nail requires more technical skill, so nail tips were created to serve as a "canvas" to create beautiful nails. In this chapter, you will learn the correct way to apply nail tips.

NAIL TIPS

This section begins with a list of supplies required for nail tip application. Procedures for nail tip application pre-service, nail tip application, post-service nail tip application, and removing nail tips follow.

SUPPLIES FOR NAIL TIPS

In addition to the materials on your basic manicuring table, you will need the supplies listed below for nail tip application (Figure 27-1).

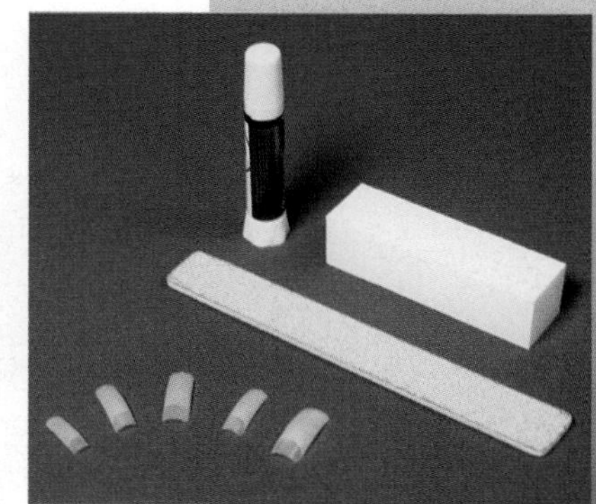

Figure 27-1 Supplies needed for tip application.

Abrasive board. Rough surface that is used to shape or smooth the nail and remove surface shine. They come in many shapes, sizes, and colors.

Buffer block. Lightweight rectangular block that is abrasive and used to buff nails.

Nail tip adhesive. The bonding agent used to secure the nail tip to the natural nail. These adhesives are made from cyanoacrylate monomer. Adhesives can be purchased in either tubes or brush-on containers and are available in several viscosities. Viscosity refers to the thickness of the adhesive. For instance, "gelled" adhesives are the thickest, and require more time to dry than fast-setting adhesives that set up in about 5 seconds. These adhesives usually come in a tube with a pointed applicator tip, a one-drop applicator, or as a brush-on. Use care when opening adhesive containers—always point the opening away from your face and not in the direction of your client. Cosmetologists should always protect their eyes when using and handling nail tip adhesives. Even the smallest amount of glue in the eyes may cause serious injury. Cosmetologists should always wear safety eyewear when using and handling nail tip adhesives.

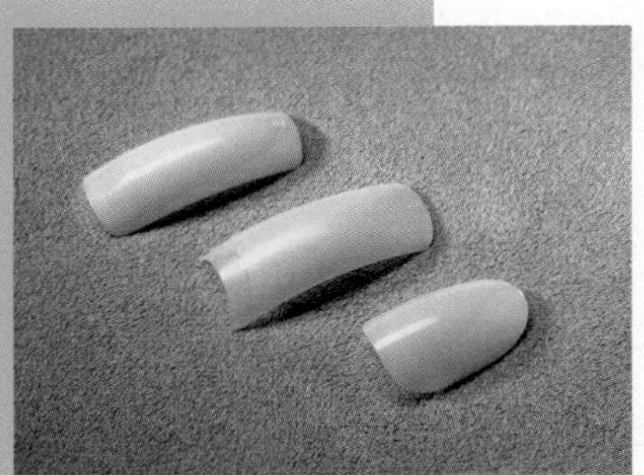

Figure 27-2 Tip with full well, tip with half well, and well-less tip.

Nail tips. Many tips have a shallow depression called a "well" that serves as the point of contact with the nail plate. The position stop is the point where the free edge of the nail meets the tip where it is adhered to the nail. Nail tip types include partial well, full well, and well-less (no well at all) (Figure 27-2). The nail tip should never cover more than one-third of the natural nail plate. Nail tips are available in many sizes, colors, and shapes so that it is easier to fit each client with precisely the right size and shape tip. Tips can be purchased in containers of 100 to 500, as well as in various individual refill sizes. With a wide assortment, it is easier to fit each client with precisely the right size and shape of tip.

NAIL TIP APPLICATION PRE-SERVICE

Before application of any type of nail tip, prepare yourself and your client with the steps in Procedure 27-1.

NAIL TIP APPLICATION

During the application, Procedure 27-2, discuss products such as polish, top coat, and hand lotion or cream that will help your client maintain the service between salon visits.

NAIL TIP APPLICATION POST-SERVICE

See Procedure 27-3.

NAIL TIP REMOVAL

Sometimes one or more tips have to be removed due to improper application. Tips that have adhered to the nail plate can cause damage if removed improperly, so be careful. Use a tip remover or acetone when performing Procedure 27-4.

NAIL WRAPS

Nail wraps are types of nail enhancements made by using a nail-size piece of cloth or paper bonded to the top of the nail plate with **wrap resin.** The heart of a nail wrap system, the wrap resin is what gives these systems their unique properties. Nail wrap systems can be used to lengthen the natural nail, but are most often used as coatings or "overlays" on the natural nail plate and on nail tips. Wrap resins are made from cyanoacrylate monomers, and are closely related to chemicals used to create other types of artificial nail enhancements. Nail wraps are used to

PROCEDURE 27-1

NAIL TIP APPLICATION PRE-SERVICE

1. **Complete pre-service sanitation and disinfection procedure** (this procedure is described in Procedure 25-3).
2. **Set up your standard manicuring table.** Add abrasive boards, buffer blocks, nail adhesive, nail dehydrator, and nail tips to your table.
3. **Greet your client and ask that she wash her hands with soap and warm running water.** Thoroughly dry the client's hands with a clean fabric or disposable towel.
4. **Perform client consultation, using a client consultation form to record responses and observations.** Check for nail disorders or unhealthy conditions, and decide whether it is safe and appropriate to perform a service on this client. If the client should not receive service, explain your reasons and refer the client to a doctor, if appropriate.

PROCEDURE 27-2

NAIL TIP APPLICATION

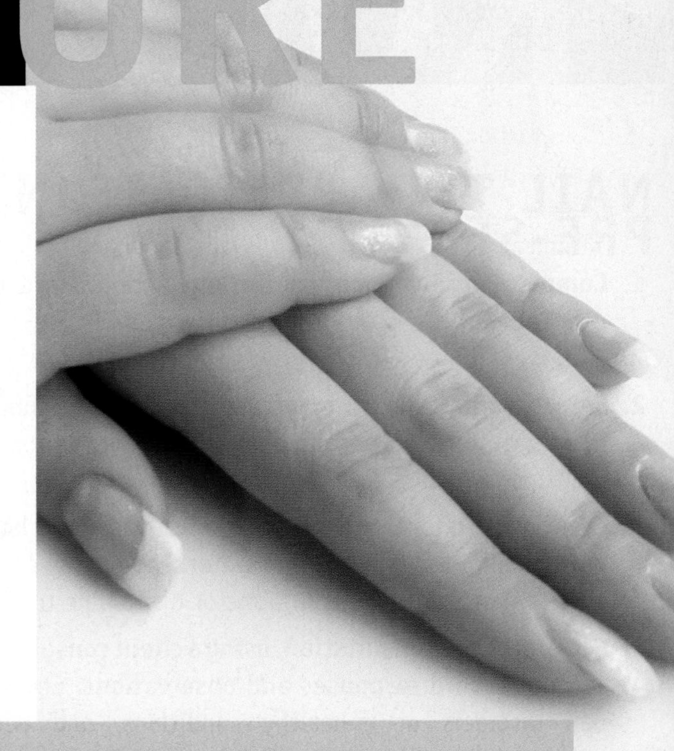

1. **Remove existing polish.** Begin with your client's little finger on the left hand, and work toward the thumb. Then repeat on the right hand.
2. **Push back eponychium.** Gently push back the eponychium. Use a new cotton-tipped wooden or metal pusher to gently push back the eponychium.
3. **Remove cuticle tissue.** Carefully remove the cuticle tissue from the nail plate using a cuticle remover and a wooden or metal pusher/curette. Do not remove cuticle beyond the line of skin created by the eponychium.
4. **Buff nail to remove shine.** Buff very lightly over the nail plate with a medium-fine abrasive (180 grit or higher) to remove the shine caused by natural oil and contaminants on the surface of the nail plate (Figure 27-3). Do not use a coarse abrasive, and be careful to avoid applying excessive pressure. The goal is to remove only the shine and as little nail plate thickness as possible. Remove the dust with a nailbrush by stroking from the cuticle area toward the free edge.
5. **Size tips.** Take time to ensure that you are choosing properly sized tips for your client's nail plate. Make sure that the tips you choose exactly cover the nail plate from side wall to side wall. Do not make the mistake of using a tip that is narrower than the nail plate. This can cause the tip to crack at the sides or split down the middle. Rather than attempting to force a too-small tip to the nail, it is better to use a slightly larger tip, and then apply an abrasive board to tailor the fit. If the tip does not fit exactly from side to side, oversize the tip (choose the next size larger—the smaller the number, the larger the tip), and use your abrasive board to customize the fit. The tip must never cover more than one-third the length of the nail plate (Figure 27-4). You should also trim and bevel the well area, which can save you blending time after you apply the tip. Nail tips that are pre-beveled require much less filing on the natural nail after application. This also cuts down the potential for damage to the natural nail. Put all of the pre-tailored and -sized tips on a towel, in the order of finger position.

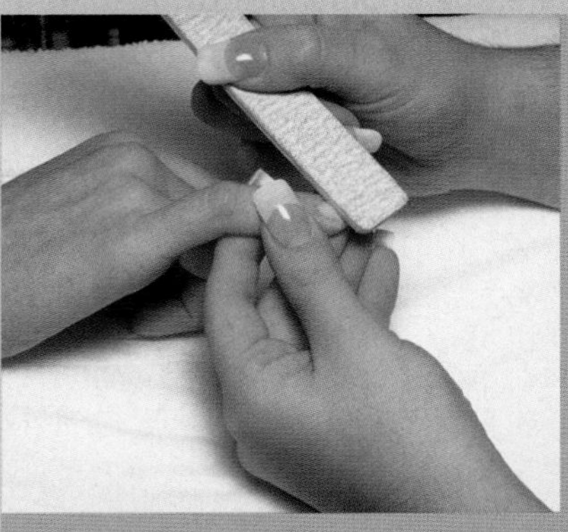

Figure 27-3 Carefully remove the oily shine from nails.

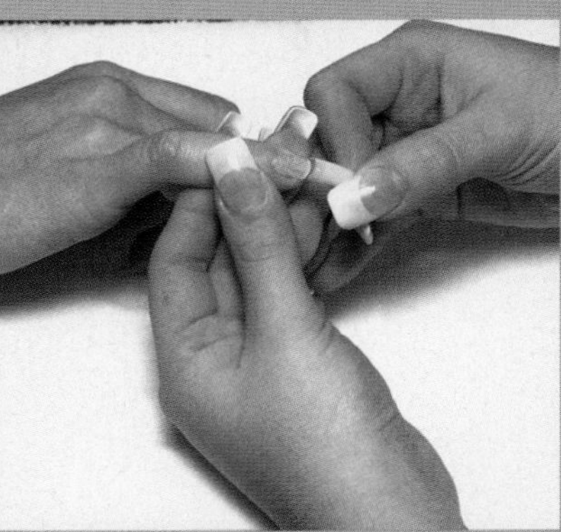

Figure 27-4 Size tips.

6. **Apply nail dehydrator/cleanser.** Use a cotton-tipped wooden pusher or spray to apply nail dehydrator/cleanser to nails. This step can help improve adhesion, especially on clients with naturally oily skin. Begin with the little finger on the left hand (Figure 27-5).
7. **Apply adhesive.** Place enough adhesive on the nail plate to cover the area where the tip will be placed, or apply the adhesive to well of tip. Do not apply too much—less is more when it comes to nail tip adhesives! Do not let adhesive run onto the skin. Apply adhesive from the middle of the nail plate to free edge (Figure 27-6).
8. **Slide on tips.** Remember the *stop, rock, and hold procedure.* Find the stop against the free edge at a 45-degree angle. Rock the tip on slowly. Hold the tip in place for 5 to 10 seconds until the adhesive has hardened (Figure 27-7). You may also apply the adhesive to the well area of the tip. This may ensure that there are fewer air bubbles trapped in the adhesive. This technique also works on well-less tips, followed by positioning on the nail plate and holding it in place for 5 to 10 seconds until the adhesive hardens.
9. **Trim nail tip.** Trim the nail tip to desired length using a **tip cutter** or large nail clippers. Cut from one side to the other. Do not use fingernail or toenail clippers. Cutting the tip with these types of clippers will weaken the tip and cause it to crack (Figure 27-8).
10. **Finish blending tip.** Your pre-blended tips will still need additional blending to make them match with the surface of the natural nail plate. Take great care because this step can cause damage to the natural nail plate, if done improperly. Use a medium- to fine-grit block buffer file (180 grit or higher) to

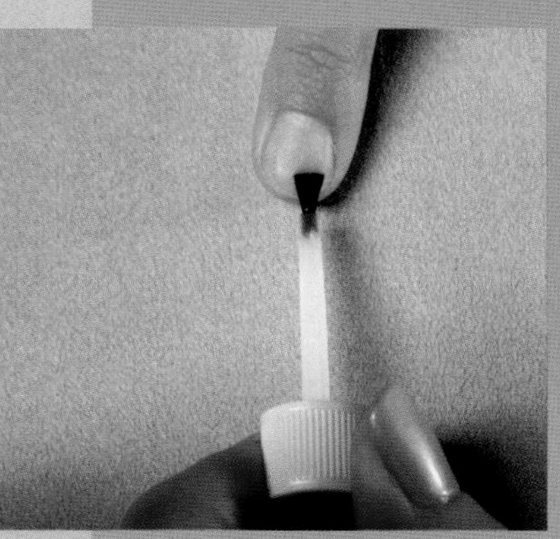

Figure 27-5 Apply nail dehydrator.

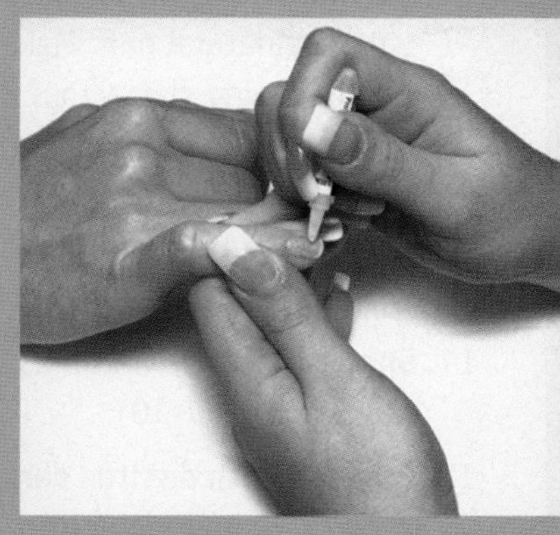

Figure 27-6 Apply adhesive.

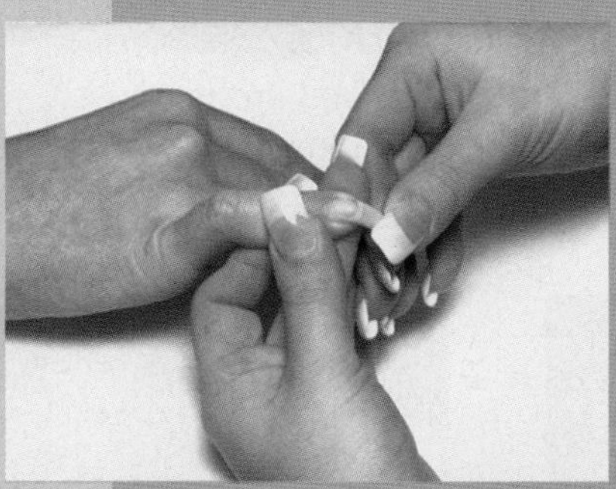

Figure 27-7 Slide on tips.

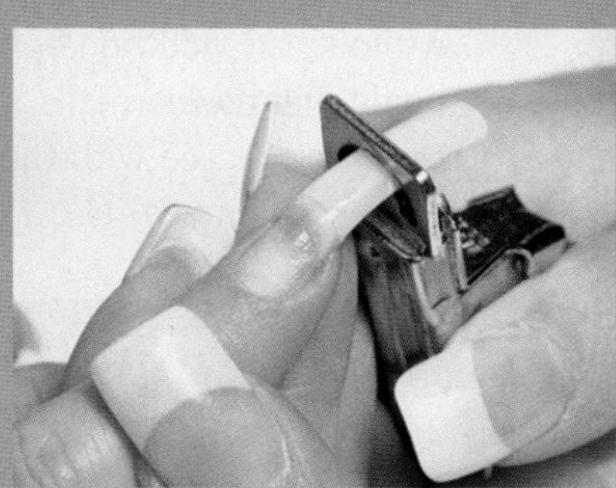

Figure 27-8 Trim nail tip.

CAUTION

If you accidentally touch or contaminate the freshly prepped natural nail, you must clean it again and reapply nail dehydrator.

carefully smooth the contact area down until it is flush with the natural nail. Make sure to keep your buffer (or board) laying flat across the surface of the nail plate at all times. Never hold the file at an angle because the edge of the abrasive may gouge the nail plate and damage it. After you finish, use the abrasive to remove the shine from the rest of the tip (Figure 27-9).

11. **Shape nail.** Use an abrasive to shape the new, longer nail (Figure 27-10).
12. **Proceed with desired service.** Your nail tip application process is now complete. Although your client's tips blend with the natural nails, tips should not be worn without an additional nail service such as wraps, liquid and powder nails, or UV gel nails. You are now ready to proceed with the service that your client has chosen (Figure 27-11).

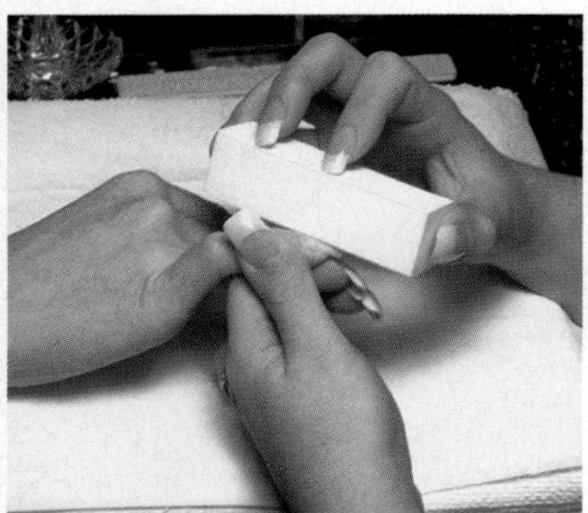

Figure 27-9 Buff tip and blend.

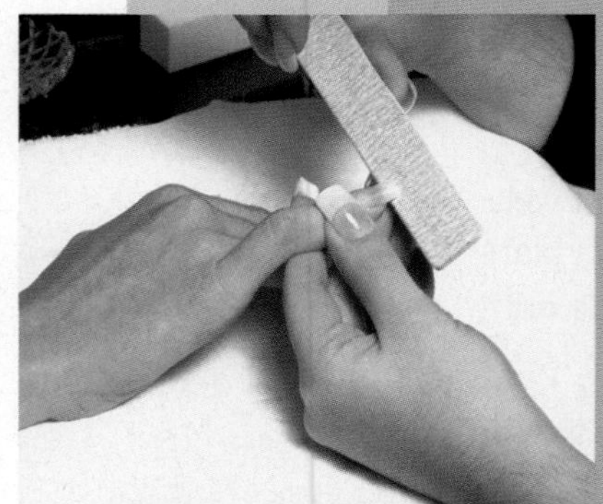

Figure 27-10 Shape tip.

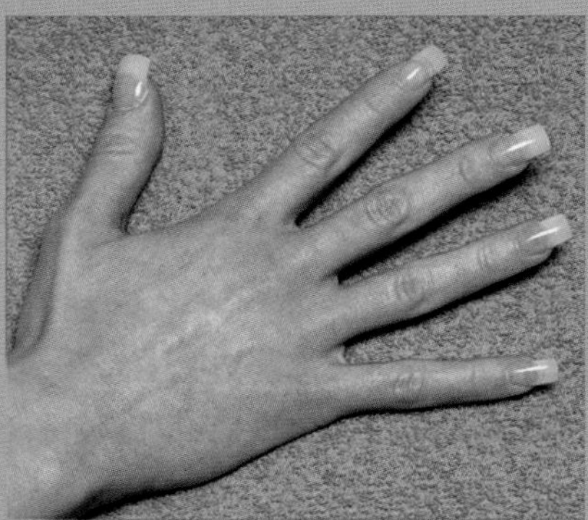

Figure 27-11 Finished tip application.

PROCEDURE 27-3

NAIL TIP APPLICATION POST-SERVICE

1. **Make another appointment.** Schedule another appointment with your client to return in 2 or 3 weeks to have the nails manicured and rebalanced, and possibly for a pedicure as well.
2. **Recommend take-home products.** Suggest professional products that you believe your client would benefit from, such as polish, top coat, and hand lotions, among others. These are valuable maintenance tools for clients to have at home and they will appreciate your professional recommendation.
3. **Clean up around your table.** Take the time to restore the basic setup of your table, re-stock supplies, and make sure that all caps are tight.
4. **Discard used materials.** Place all used materials in the trash receptacle.
5. **Clean your table, and then sanitize and disinfect implements and multiuse tools, such as abrasive implements.** Perform complete pre-service sanitation and disinfection procedures. Implements need to be cleaned and disinfected before they can be used on the next client, and this procedure will take about 20 minutes.

PROCEDURE 27-4

NAIL TIP REMOVAL

1. **Soak tips and nails.** Place enough remover in a small glass bowl to cover nails. Soak for a few minutes.
2. **Slide off the nail tip.** Use a new wooden pusher to slide off the softened nail tip. Be careful not to pry the nail tip off because you can cause damage to the nail unit.
3. **Buff nail.** Gently buff the natural nail with a fine buffer to remove any adhesive residue.
4. **Reapply nail tip as directed.**
5. **Proceed to desired service.**

CAUTION

Never nip off the nail tip! This may lead to damage of the nail unit and/or the important seals that guard and protect against infection.

repair or strengthen natural nails or to create nail extensions. Wraps can be cut from a swatch of cloth, rolls of fabric, or a piece of paper to fit a client's nail size and shape, or they can be purchased pre-cut. Pre-cut overlays have an adhesive backing.

Fabric wraps are made from silk, linen, or fiberglass. **Silk** is a thin natural material with a tight weave that becomes transparent when wrap resin is applied. A silk wrap is lightweight and has a smooth appearance when applied to the nail. **Linen** is a closely woven, heavy material. It is much thicker and bulkier than other types of wrap fabrics. Wrap resins do not penetrate linen as easily as silk or fiberglass. Because it is opaque, even after adhesive is applied, a colored polish must be used to cover it completely. Linen is used because it is considered the strongest wrap fabric. A **fiberglass** wrap is a very thin synthetic mesh with a loose weave. The loose weave makes it easy to use and for adhesive to penetrate, which improves adhesion. Even though fiberglass is not as strong as linen or silk, it can create a durable nail enhancement. **Paper wraps** are made of very thin paper. Paper was one of the very first materials used to create wraps. They are quite simple to use, but do not have the strength and durability of fabric wraps. For this reason, paper wraps are considered a temporary service.

FABRIC WRAPS

SUPPLIES

In addition to the materials on your basic manicuring table, you will need the items listed below (Figure 27-12).

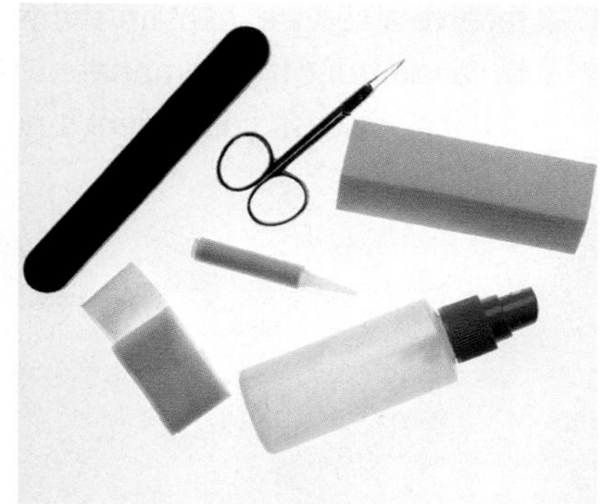

Figure 27-12 Materials necessary for fabric wrap application.

- **Fabric.** Small swatches of linen, silk, or fiberglass material can be cut to fit a client's nail size and shape. You may also find pre-cut wrap material with adhesive backing.
- **Nail tip adhesive.** Adhesives are used to secure the nail tip or fabric to the natural nail. The adhesive usually comes in a tube with a pointed applicator tip called an *extender tip* or in brush-on form. When working with wrap resins, be sure to protect your eyes with protective eyewear and offer them to your client as well.
- **Wrap resin** and **activator.** Resin and its hardening activator are used for application to the fabric. The manufacturer's instructions for using these products may differ slightly from the general guidelines presented below. **Activators** speed up the curing process of resins and adhesives. When used incorrectly, they may cause a heat spike that can be uncomfortable to the client and could even cause nail bed damage. You must always use products in accordance with the manufacturer's instructions. Also, your instructor may present slightly different techniques that are equally correct.
- **Small scissors.** Use small and sharp scissors for cutting fabric.
- **Nail buffer or adhesive.**
- **Small piece of plastic or tweezers.**

NAIL WRAP PRE-SERVICE

Use the preparation steps in Procedure 27-5 for all nail wrap procedures.

PROCEDURE 27-5

NAIL WRAP PRE-SERVICE

1. Perform the pre-service sanitation and disinfection procedure for nail wraps (this procedure is described in Procedure 25-3).
2. Set up a standard manicuring table. Add fabric, wrap resin and activator, small scissors, nail buffer, and a small square of thin plastic sheeting to your table.
3. Greet your client and ask her to wash her hands with liquid soap and to rinse thoroughly with warm running water. Dry hands and nails thoroughly with a clean fabric or disposable towel.
4. Perform a client consultation, using a client consultation form to record the responses and your observations. Check for nail disorders. Decide if the client's nails and hands are healthy enough for you to perform a service. If the client has a nail or skin disorder and must not receive a service, explain the reasons and refer the client to a doctor, if appropriate. If you proceed with the service, discuss your client's needs and expectations.

NAIL WRAP APPLICATION

During the application procedure, discuss with your client the professional products that will be useful or beneficial for the client to help maintain the service between salon visits. See Procedure 27-6.

NAIL WRAP POST-SERVICE

Follow this post-service for all nail wrap services. See Procedure 27-7.

NAIL WRAP MAINTENANCE, REMOVAL, AND REPAIR

Nail wraps need regular maintenance to keep them looking fresh. In this section, you will learn how to rebalance fabric wraps after 2 weeks and after 4 weeks. You will also learn how to remove nail wraps and how to perform crack repairs.

NAIL WRAP REBALANCE

Nail wraps are rebalanced with additional resin after 2 weeks, and with resin and new fabric rebalances after 4 weeks.

TWO-WEEK FABRIC WRAP MAINTENANCE

After 2 weeks use the following procedure to maintain nail wraps. You will need to add wrap resin, accelerator, and an abrasive buffer or board to your standard table setup. See Procedure 27-8.

FOUR-WEEK FABRIC WRAP MAINTENANCE

After 4 weeks, use the following maintenance procedure to apply fabric and wrap resin to new growth. You will need wrap resin, abrasive buffer or board, fabric, small scissors, and wrap resin accelerator, in addition to your standard table setup. See Procedure 27-9.

FABRIC WRAP REPAIRS

Small pieces of fabric can be used to strengthen a weak point in the nail or repair a break in the nail. A **stress strip** is a strip of fabric cut to ⅛ inch.

The strip is applied to the weak point of the nail, using the 4-week maintenance procedure. A **repair patch** is a piece of fabric that is cut so that it completely covers the crack or break in the nail. Use the 4-week fabric wrap maintenance procedure to apply your repair patch.

FABRIC WRAP REMOVAL

Be careful not to damage the nail plate when removing fabric wraps. See Procedure 27-10.

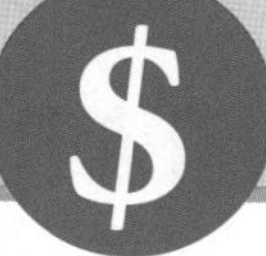

BUSINESS TIP: HOST NAIL FASHION NIGHTS

The person who coined the phrase "seeing is believing" must have known that people are more likely to purchase something familiar. To acquaint customers firsthand with the latest manicure looks, try hosting a nail fashion night. For an admission fee of $10.00 to $16.00, you showcase the latest nail looks by giving each attendee a manicure—using the season's most popular fashion colors and hottest new products, of course. To top off the evening, offer each client a nail care fashion kit comprised of trial-sized products and a gift certificate for 16 percent off the next nail care purchase or service. Spending an entire night focused on the products creates a buzz about them and shows clients how to use them. The sample size gets them hooked and the gift certificate gives them an incentive to return to you.

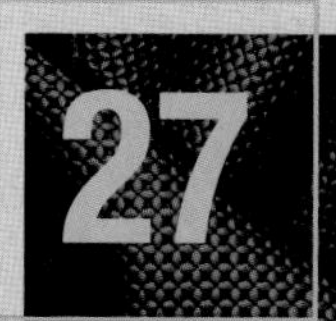

PROCEDURE 27-6

NAIL WRAP APPLICATION

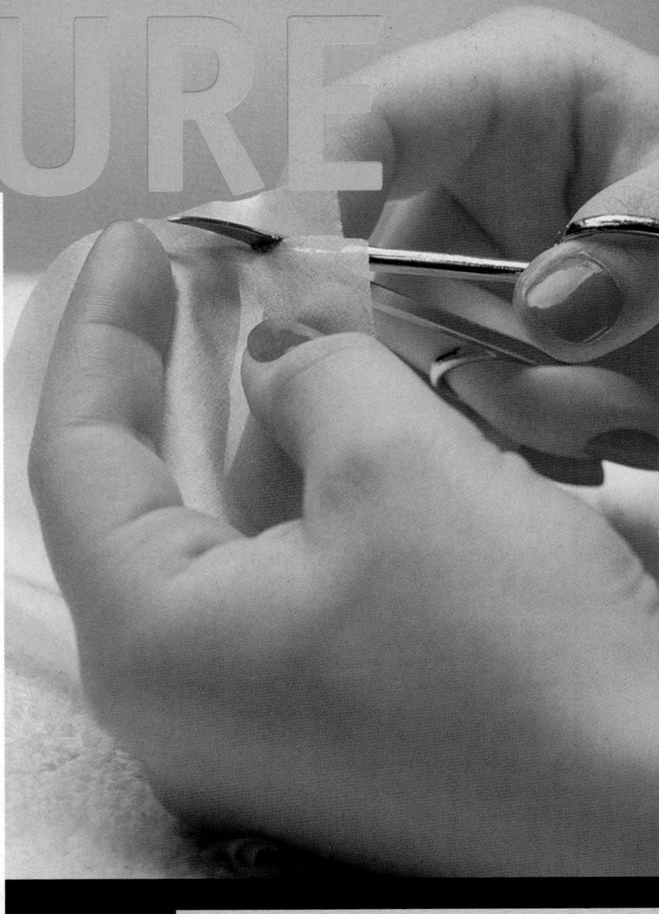

1. **Remove existing polish.** Begin with the client's little finger on the left hand. Saturate a cotton ball or plastic-backed pad with polish remover. If client is already wearing fabric wrap nails, use nonacetone remover to avoid damaging them. Hold saturated cotton on the nail while you silently count to 10. Wipe away the existing polish from the nail plate with a stroking motion towards the free edge. If all polish is not removed, repeat this step until traces of polish are gone. It may be necessary to put cotton around the tip of a new wooden pusher and use it to clean polish away from the sidewall and cuticle areas. Repeat this procedure on each finger of both hands.
2. **Clean nails.** Dip nails in a fingerbowl filled with warm water and liquid soap. Then use a nail brush to clean nails over the fingerbowl. Rinse nails briefly in clear water or have the client wash at the sink. If the client's natural nails are thin or weak, it is recommended that you do not soak the nails in water before you apply a nail wrap. Natural nails are porous and absorb water, which can reduce the longevity of a fabric wrap service.
3. **Push back the eponychium and remove cuticle tissue from plate.** Use the same cotton-tipped wooden pusher, with new cotton applied to the tip, to gently push back eponychium. Use a light touch because the eponychium has not been soaked in water and will be less flexible. Use a wooden pusher stick or a curette to gently remove the cuticle tissue from the nail plate.
4. **Remove the oily shine.** Lightly buff the nail plate with a medium-fine abrasive (240 grit) to remove shine caused by the oil found on the natural nail plate. Do not use a coarse file, and be careful not to apply very much pressure. Remove only the oily shine and avoid removing layers from the natural nail plate. Nail wraps can be performed over natural nails or over a set of nail tips. If you are using nail tips, you should use your abrasive to shape the free edges of the natural nails to match the shape of the nail tip to the stop point.
5. **Apply nail dehydrator.** Spray or wipe a nail dehydrator onto the nail plate. The dehydrator will remove moisture from the surface, and thus will help improve adhesion. Wiping the dehydrator with a plastic-backed cotton pad on the nail plate has the added benefit of removing any remaining natural oil, even on clients with oily skin.

CAUTION

Do not use the same wooden pusher stick on more than one client. They are not disinfectable and are considered single-use items.

6. **Apply nail tips if desired.**
7. **Cut fabric.** Cut fabric to the approximate width and shape of the nail plate or nail tip. Be careful to keep the dust and oils from your fingers from contaminating the adhesive-backed fabric. This could prevent the fabric from adhering to the nail (Figure 27-13).
8. **Apply fabric adhesive.** If you are using a non-adhesive-backed fabric, you will need to apply a drop of adhesive to the center of the nail. Remember to keep adhesive off the skin. Besides potentially damaging your client's skin, this could cause the wrap to lift or separate from the nail plate (Figure 27-14).
9. **Apply fabric.** Gently fit fabric over the nail plate, 1⁄16 inch away from the side wall or eponychium. Press to smooth it onto the nail plate, using a small piece of thick plastic (Figure 27-15).
10. **Trim fabric.** Use small scissors to trim fabric 1⁄16 inch away from side walls and free edge. Trimming fabric slightly smaller than the nail plate prevents fabric from lifting and separating from the nail plate (Figure 27-16).

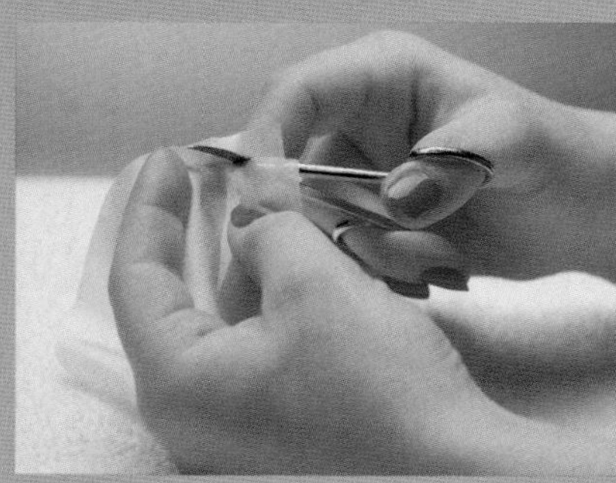

Figure 27-13 Cut fabric.

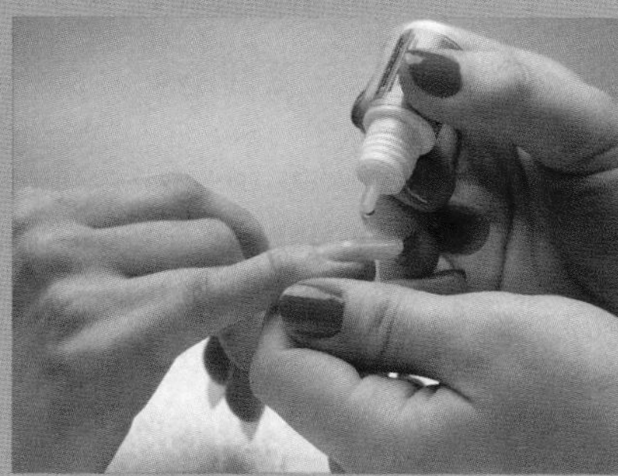

Figure 27-14 Apply fabric adhesive if using non-adhesive-backed fabric.

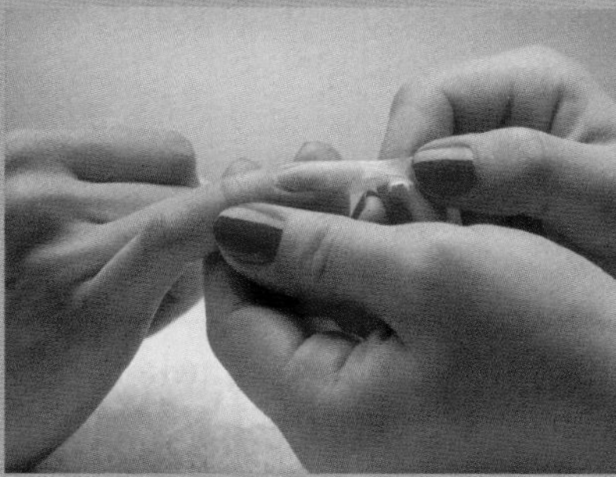

Figure 27-15 Apply fabric.

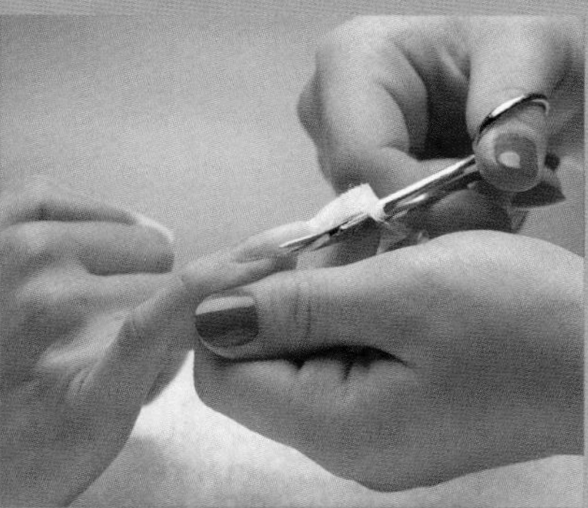

Figure 27-16 Trim fabric.

Here's a TIP

Using a 6-inch × 4-inch piece of flexible plastic sheet to press fabric onto the nail plate will prevent the transfer of oil and debris from your fingers. Wrap resin will not easily penetrate fibers that are contaminated with oil, and those strands become visible in the clear coating. Thus, it is best not to touch them more than you must. Changing to an unused portion of the plastic for each finger is necessary.

11. **Apply wrap resin.** Draw a thin-coat of wrap resin down the center of the nail using the extender tip to apply. Do not touch the skin. The adhesive will penetrate the fabric and adhere to the nail surface (Figure 27-17). Use the plastic again to make sure that the resin is evenly distributed and there are no bubbles or areas of bare fabric.
12. **Apply wrap resin accelerator.** Spray, brush, or drop on wrap resin accelerator designed for the wrap resin of your choice. Use according to wrap resin manufacturer's instructions. Keep wrap resin accelerator off the skin to prevent overexposure to the product (Figure 27-18).
13. **Apply second coat of wrap resin.** Apply and spread wrap resin with extender tip. Seal free edge with wrap resin by running the extender tip on the edge of the nail tip to prevent lifting.
14. **Apply second coat of wrap resin accelerator.**
15. **Shape and refine nails.** Use medium-fine abrasive (240 grit) to shape and refine the wrap nail.
16. **Buff wrap nail.** Apply nail oil and buff to a high shine with fine (350 grit or higher) buffer. Use the buffer to smooth out rough areas in the fabric. Do not buff excessively or for too long. Overbuffing can wear through the wrap and weaken it (Figure 27-19).
17. **Remove traces of oil.** Send your client to thoroughly wash at the sink with a nail brush, liquid soap, and warm running water, to remove not only oils, but any dust or other contaminants.
18. **Apply polish** (Figure 27-20).

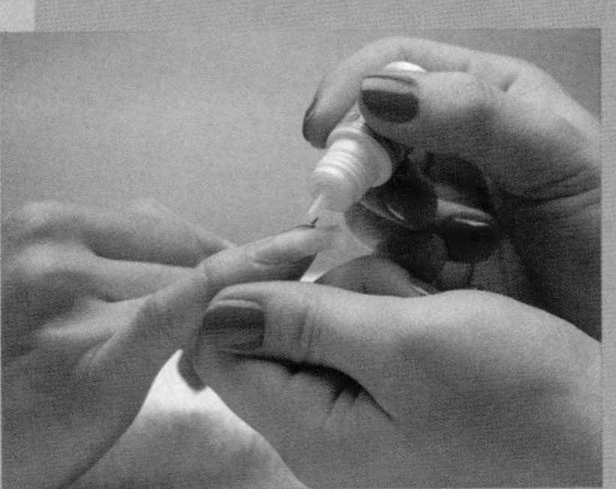

Figure 27-17 Apply adhesive.

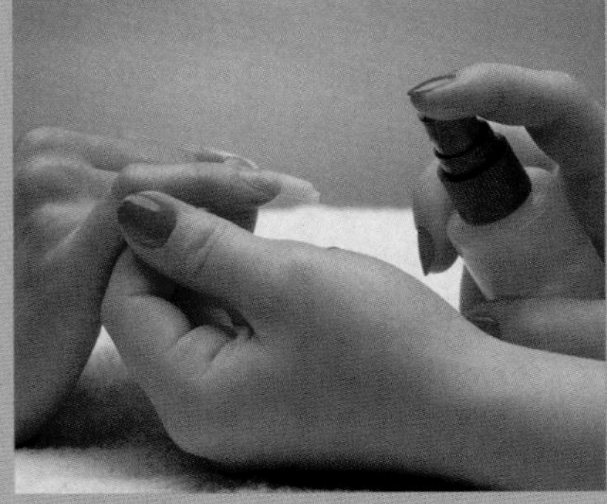

Figure 27-18 Apply wrap resin accelerator.

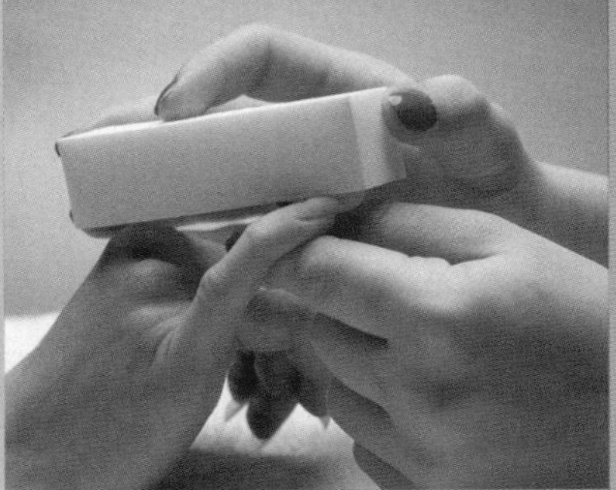

Figure 27-19 Buff tip.

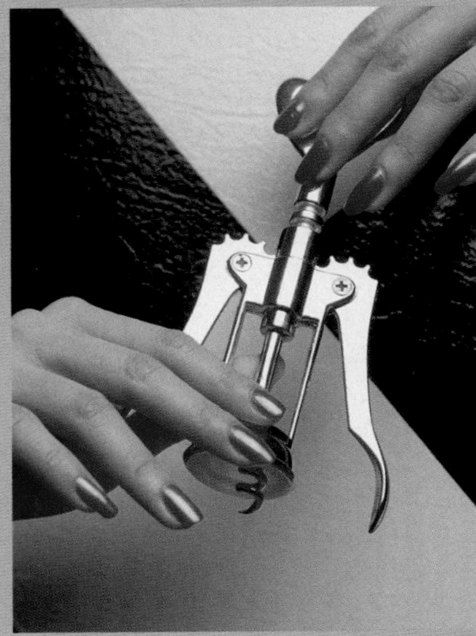

Figure 27-20 Finished fabric wraps.

PROCEDURE 27-7

NAIL WRAP POST-SERVICE

1. **Make another appointment.** Schedule another appointment with your client to maintain the nail wrap that she has just received or for another service.
2. **Recommend take-home products.** Suggest professional products that you believe your client would benefit from. Polish, top coat, and hand lotions, among others, are valuable maintenance tools for them to have and they will appreciate your professional recommendation.
3. **Clean up around your table.** Take the time to restore the basic setup of your table, re-stock on supplies, and make sure that all products are tightly capped.
4. **Clean extender tips.** To clean clogged extender tips, place them in a covered glass jar with acetone. Poke a clean toothpick through the hole.
5. **Store fabric.** Store fabric in a resealable plastic bag to protect it from dust and other debris.
6. **Discard used materials.** Place all used and disposable materials in a covered waste receptacle.
7. **Clean your table, and then sanitize and disinfect implements and/or multi-use tools, such as abrasive implements.** Perform complete pre-service sanitation and disinfection procedures. Implements need to be cleaned and disinfected before they can be used on the next client, and this procedure will take about 20 minutes.

PROCEDURE 27-8

TWO-WEEK FABRIC WRAP MAINTENANCE

1. **Complete nail wrap pre-service.**
2. **Remove existing polish.** Use a nonacetone polish remover to avoid damaging nail wraps.
3. **Clean natural nails.**
4. **Push back eponychium and carefully remove cuticle tissue from the nail plate.**
5. **Lightly file the nail plate to remove oily shine.**
6. **Apply nail dehydrator.**
7. **Apply wrap resin to new nail growth area.** Brush on or apply a small amount of wrap resin to the area of new nail growth. Spread the resin with the extender tip, taking care to avoid touching the skin.
8. **Apply wrap resin accelerator.** Follow the manufacturer's instructions.
9. **Apply wrap resin to entire nail plate.** Apply a second coat of wrap resin to the entire nail plate to strengthen and reseal the nail wrap.
10. **Apply wrap resin accelerator.**
11. **Shape and refine nail wrap.** Use medium-fine abrasive over the surface of the nail wrap to remove any high spots and/or other imperfections.
12. **Buff nail wraps.** Apply nail oil and buff to a high shine with a fine buffer (350 grit or higher).
13. **Apply hand lotion and massage hand and arm.**
14. **Remove traces of oil.** Use a small piece of cotton or plastic-backed cotton pad to remove all traces of oil from the nail so that polish will adhere.
15. **Apply polish.**
16. **Complete nail wrap post-service.**

PROCEDURE 27-9

FOUR-WEEK FABRIC WRAP MAINTENANCE

1. **Complete nail wrap pre-service.**
2. **Remove existing polish.** Use a nonacetone polish remover to avoid damaging wraps.
3. **Clean nails.** Use a nail brush, liquid soap, and warm running water.
4. **Push back the eponychium and gently remove the cuticle.**
5. **Buff nail to remove shine.** Lightly buff the nail plates with a medium-fine (240-grit) abrasive to remove the shine created by natural oil, and to remove any small pieces of fabric that may have lifted since the last service. Buff the end of the wrap until smooth, without scratching or damaging the natural nail plate. Carefully refine the nail until there is no obvious line of demarcation between new growth and fabric wrap. Avoid damaging the natural nail with the abrasive. Do not file into the natural nail surface.
6. **Apply nail dehydrator.** Apply nail dehydrator to nails with a cotton-tipped wooden pusher, cotton pad with a plastic backing, brush, or spray. Begin with the little finger on the left hand and work toward the thumb. Repeat on the right hand.
7. **Cut fabric.** Cut a piece of fabric large enough to cover the new growth area and slightly overlap the old wrap fabric.
8. **Apply wrap resin to regrowth area.** Apply a small amount of wrap resin to the fill area. Spread throughout the new growth area with the extender tip or fill in the area with brush-on adhesive. Avoid touching the skin (Figure 27-21).
9. **Apply fabric.** Gently fit fabric over new growth area and smooth (Figure 27-22).

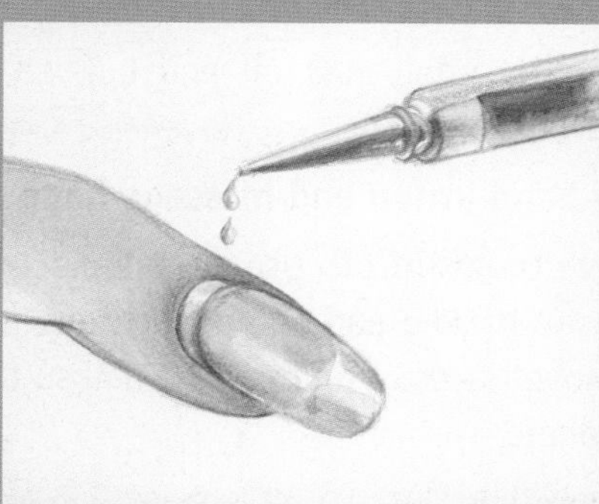

Figure 27-21 Apply wrap resin to regrowth area.

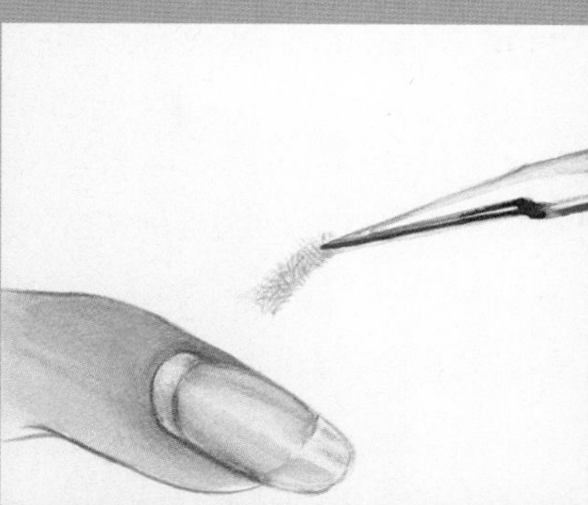

Figure 27-22 Apply fabric.

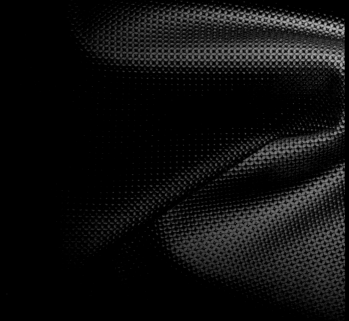

10. **Apply wrap resin.** Apply another small amount of wrap resin, again avoiding the skin.
11. **Apply wrap resin accelerator.** Spray, brush, or drop on the wrap resin accelerator to dry the wrap resin more quickly. Use as instructed by the manufacturer of the wrap resin.
12. **Apply wrap resin.** Apply a second coat of wrap resin to regrowth area.
13. **Apply second coat of wrap resin accelerator.**
14. **Apply wrap resin to entire nail.** Apply a thin coat of wrap resin to entire nail to strengthen and seal wrap.
15. **Apply wrap resin accelerator.**
16. **Shape and refine nail.** Use medium-fine abrasive (240 grit) over surface of nail to remove any high spots or other imperfections. Carefully avoid the skin around the eponychium and side walls so that you do not cause cuts or damage.
17. **Buff nails.** Apply nail oil and buff to a high shine with a buffer.
18. **Apply hand lotion and massage hand and arm.**
19. **Remove traces of oil.** Use a small piece of cotton ball or plastic-backed pad and nonacetone polish remover to remove traces of oil from the nail so that the polish will adhere.
20. **Apply polish.**
21. **Complete nail wrap post-service.**

PROCEDURE 27-10

FABRIC WRAP REMOVAL

1. **Complete nail wrap pre-service.**
2. **Soak nails.** Put enough acetone in a small glass bowl to cover the nail wrap. Immerse client's wraps in the bowl and soak for a few minutes. The acetone should be approximately $^{1}/_{2}$ inch above the nail wraps.
3. **Slide off softened nail wraps.** Use a wood or metal pusher to slide softened wraps away from nail plate.
4. **Buff natural nail.** Gently buff natural nails with a fine buffer (240 grit) to remove the wrap resin.
5. **Condition skin.** Condition the skin surrounding the nail plate with nail oils or lotions designed for this purpose.

NO-LIGHT GELS

A **no-light gel** is a thicker-viscosity cyanoacrylate monomer. This gel-like material can be applied with a brush like nail polish, or with the bottle itself to spread a thin coat of product onto the entire nail plate. The gels are called "no-light" because they do not require a UV light to harden them as do UV-gel products. To harden no-light gels, a small amount of activator is dispensed atop the enhancement. The activator can be brushed or sprayed on the surface to cause the product to cure. The following procedure is designed to show how no-light gels are applied. For actual application, you will need to follow the manufacturer's instructions.

SUPPLIES

In addition to the materials in your basic manicuring setup, you will need the following items: no-light gel and manufacturer-recommended activator, buffer block, nail tips, and adhesive.

NO-LIGHT GEL APPLICATION

Procedure 27-11 is designed to show how no-light gels are applied. For actual application, you will need to follow the manufacturer's instructions.

NO-LIGHT GELS AND FIBERGLASS/SILK FABRIC

No-light gels can also be used with fiberglass or silk fabrics. Layering no-light gel and fiberglass or silk in a sandwich effect can create a durable nail enhancement. The fabric is used between the first and second coat of no-light gel.

1. **Pre-cut fiberglass or silk sections in no greater than ¼-inch wide and ½-inch long strips.** Adjust and trim length of strips accordingly to size of the client's nail plates. Avoid excess overhanging material.
2. **Place a section of fiberglass or silk material diagonally across wet no-light gel.** Use a wooden pusher to carefully position it in place. Place the first strip from the upper left corner to lower right corner of the nail, slightly above the stress area. Position the second strip from the upper right corner to the lower left corner of the nail, forming an "X."
3. **Activate and follow with the second coat of gel.** Activate and finish as you would according to the no-light gel application procedure.

PROCEDURE 27-11

NO-LIGHT GEL APPLICATION

1. **Complete no-light gel application pre-service.**
2. **Remove existing polish.** Begin with your client's left hand, little finger, and work toward the thumb. Then repeat on the right hand.
3. **Clean finger nails.** Ask the client to dip nails in a fingerbowl filled with liquid soap. Then use a nail brush to clean nails over fingerbowl. Rinse thoroughly in clean water to remove soapy residues that can lead to lifting.
4. **Push back eponychium and carefully remove cuticle from the nail plate.** Use a cotton-tipped wooden or metal pusher to gently push back the eponychium, and then apply cuticle remover. Use as directed by the manufacturer, and carefully remove cuticle tissue from the nail plate.
5. **Remove oily shine from natural nail surface.** Lightly buff nail plate with medium-fine (240-grit) abrasive to remove the natural oil that causes the shine on the surface of the nail plate.
6. **Apply nail tips if desired.** If your client requires nail tips, apply them according to the procedure described earlier in this chapter.
7. **Apply nail dehydrator.** Apply nail dehydrator to nails with cotton-tipped wooden pusher, cotton pad with plastic backing, brush, or spray. Begin with the little finger on the left hand and work toward the thumb.
8. **Apply no-light gel.** Following the manufacturer's instructions, use brush to paint on gel or use the bottle to spread a thin coat of gel onto the entire nail. Apply gel to the five nails of one hand, leaving a tiny free margin between the product and skin to avoid lifting.
9. **Cure no-light gel with activator.** Following the instructions of the no-light gel product manufacturer, spray or brush no-light gel activator onto the enhancement.
10. **Repeat Steps 7, 8, and 9 on the right hand.**
11. **Apply second coat of no-light gel, if required.** With no-light gels, a second application of gel may not be necessary. Follow your manufacturer's directions for correct application.
12. **Shape and refine nails.** Shape and refine the entire surface of the nail with a medium-fine abrasive (240 grit). Use a light touch to remove any imperfections.
13. **Buff nail.** Buff nail with a fine buffer (350 grit or higher) to shine. If polish is not to be worn, a high shine buffer can be used.
14. **Apply nail oil.** Rub nail oil into surrounding skin and nail surface.
15. **Apply hand cream and massage hand and arm.**
16. **Clean nail enhancements.** Ask client to dip nails in a fingerbowl filled with liquid soap. Then use a nail brush to clean nails over fingerbowl. Rinse with water and dry thoroughly with a clean disposable towel.
17. **Apply nail polish.**
18. **Complete post-service.**

REVIEW QUESTIONS

1. List the four supplies, in addition to your basic manicuring table, that you need for nail tip application.
2. Name the three types of nail tips.
3. What is the maximum amount or portion of natural nail plate that should be covered by a nail tip?
4. Briefly describe the procedure for a nail tip application.
5. Describe how to pre-blend the nail tip.
6. Describe how to avoid damaging the natural nail during the tip-blending process.
7. Describe the procedure for the removal of nail tips.
8. Describe the stop, rock, and hold procedure.
9. Explain why it is important to ensure that tips fit the client properly.
10. Why should nippers not be used for removing tips?
11. List five types of nail wraps.
12. Explain the benefits of using each of the three types of fabric used to create nail wraps.
13. Describe the procedure for fabric wrap application.
14. Explain how a fabric wrap is used as a crack repair.
15. Describe how to remove fabric wraps and what to avoid.
16. Why are paper wraps not as durable as fabric wraps?
17. What is the purpose of a nail dehydrator?
18. What is the purpose of a wrap resin accelerator?
19. What type of monomer is used to make wrap resins?
20. What is the main difference between performing a wrap resin 2-week rebalance and a 4-week rebalance?

CHAPTER GLOSSARY

abrasive board	Thin, elongated board with a rough surface.
ABS	Acrylonitrile butadiene styrene.
activator	A product used to speed up the curing process of resins and adhesives.
buffer block	Lightweight, rectangular abrasive block.
fabric wraps	Nail wraps made of silk, linen, or fiberglass.
fiberglass	Very thin synthetic mesh with a loose weave.

CHAPTER GLOSSARY

linen	Closely woven, heavy material used for nail wraps.
nail tip	Artificial nail made of ABS or tenite acetate polymer that is adhered to the natural nail to add length.
nail tip adhesive	Liquid or gel-like product made from cyanoacrylate monomer, and used to secure a nail tip to the natural nail.
nail wraps	Nail-size pieces of cloth or paper that are bonded to the top of the nail plate with nail adhesive; often used to repair or strengthen natural nails or nail tips.
no-light gel	Thickened cyanoacrylate monomers.
overlay	Acrylic (methacrylate) liquid and powder, wraps, or UV gels applied over a tip for added strength.
paper wraps	Temporary nail wraps made of very thin paper. Not nearly as strong as fabric wraps.
repair patch	Piece of fabric cut to completely cover a crack or break in the nail during a 4-week fabric wrap maintenance procedure.
silk	Thin, natural material with a tight weave that becomes transparent when adhesive is applied.
stress strip	Strip of fabric, ⅛ inch long, applied during a 4-week fabric wrap rebalance to repair or strengthen a weak point in a nail enhancement.
tip cutter	Implement similar to a nail clipper, designed especially for use on nail tips.
wrap resin	An adhesive used over the fabric wrap, to adhere it to the nail extension or nail plate.

28 CHAPTER ACRYLIC (METHACRYLATE) NAILS

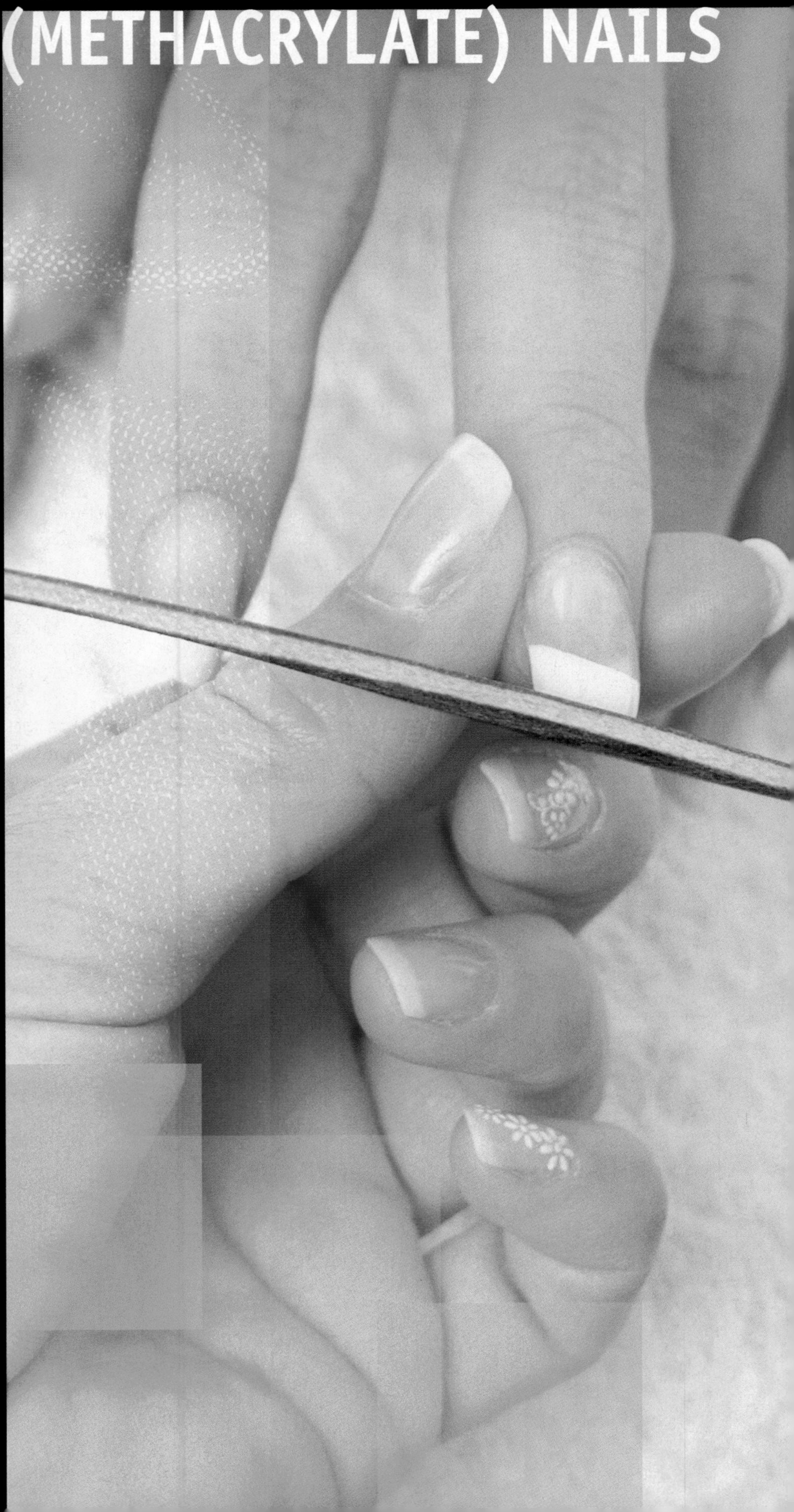

chapter outline

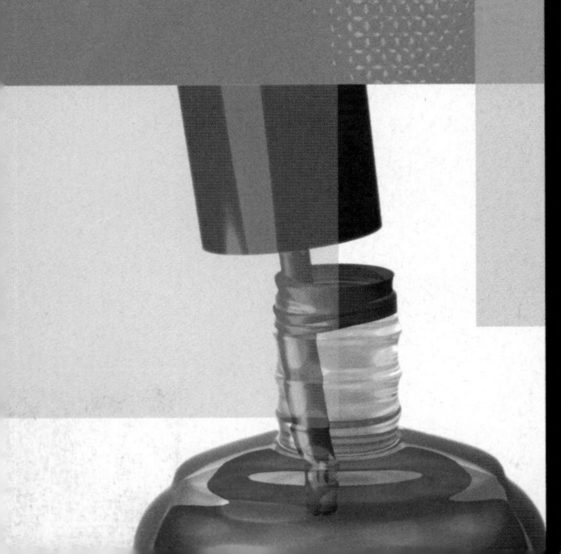

Learning Objectives

After completing this chapter, you will be able to:

- **Explain acrylic (methacrylate) nail enhancement chemistry and how it works.**
- **List the supplies needed for acrylic (methacrylate) nail enhancements application.**
- **Demonstrate the proper procedures for applying acrylic (methacrylate) nail enhancements using forms over tips, and on natural nails.**
- **Practice safety precautions involving the application of nail primers.**
- **Describe the proper procedure for maintaining healthy acrylic (methacrylate) nail enhancements.**
- **Perform regular rebalance procedures and repairs.**
- **Implement the proper procedure for removing acrylic (methacrylate) nail enhancements.**
- **Explain how the application of odorless acrylic (methacrylate) products differs from the application of traditional acrylic (methacrylate) products.**

Key Terms

Page number indicates where in the chapter the term is used.

acrylic (methacrylate) monomer liquid **pg. 753**

acrylic (methacrylate) nail enhancements **pg. 752**

acrylic (methacrylate) polymer powder **pg. 753**

catalyst **pg. 751**

chain reaction **pg. 751**

dappen dish **pg. 755**

dust masks & protective gloves **pg. 755**

initiators **pg. 751**

mix ratio **pg. 753**

nail dehydrator **pg. 753**

nail forms **pg. 754**

nail primer **pg. 753**

odorless acrylic (methacrylate) products **pg. 767**

polymer **pg. 750**

polymerization **pg. 751**

rebalancing **pg. 767**

safety eyewear **pg. 755**

***Editor's Note:** Nail enhancements based on mixing liquids and powders together are commonly referred to as "acrylic" (a-KRYL-yk) nails. It might surprise you to discover the real definition of "acrylic," since for many years this word has actually been used incorrectly by the nail enhancement industry. The term "acrylic" actually refers to an entire family of thousands of different substances, but all share important, closely related features. Acrylics are used to make a wide range of things including contact lenses, cements for mending broken bones, Plexiglas windows, and even makeup and other cosmetics. Surprisingly, all artificial nail enhancement products are based almost entirely on ingredients that come from the acrylic family. For example, the ingredients in two-part liquid and powder enhancement systems belong to a sub-branch of the acrylic family called "methacrylates." In other words, "acrylic" is a very general term for a large group of ingredients. Liquid and powder artificial nail enhancement products are based on the methacrylates (METH-ah-cry-latz) subcategory. You can see some similarity in the spelling of the terms, which indicates that they are from the same chemical family or group. To avoid further confusion, you will find that the two-part liquid and powder enhancement system in this book will be referred to as acrylic (methacrylate) nails.*

Acrylic (methacrylate) nail enhancements are created by combining monomer (MON-oh-mehr) liquid and **polymer** (POL-i-mehr) powder; thus the common name "liquid and powder"system. "Mono" means "one" and "mer" stands for "units," so a monomer is one unit called a "molecule." "Poly" means "many," so polymer means "many units" or many molecules. This is important to remember, since you will hear these terms many times throughout your career.

"LIQUID AND POWDER" NAIL ENHANCEMENTS

Liquid and powder products can be applied in three basic ways:

1. Applied to the natural nail as a protective overlay
2. Over a nail tip
3. Sculpted to extend the natural nail using a flexible form

A natural hair brush is the best device to use in applying these products. The brush is immersed in the monomer liquid. The natural hair bristles absorb and hold the monomer like a reservoir. The tip of the brush is then touched to the surface of the dry polymer powder, and as the monomer liquid absorbs the polymer powder, a small bead of product forms. This small bead is then carefully placed on the nail surface and molded into shape with the brush. The liquid portion is usually based on ethyl methacrylate monomer, but often contains other monomers used as customizing additives. It may seem strange to learn that polymer powder is also made mostly from ethyl methacrylate monomer. The polymer powder is made using a special chemical reaction called **polymerization** (POL-i-mehr-eh-za-shun). In this process, trillions of monomers are linked together to create long chains. These long chains create the tiny beads of polymer powder used to create certain types of artificial nails.

During the production of the polymer, the powder forms into tiny beads of slightly varying sizes. These are poured through a series of special screens that sort the beads by size. The ones that are the right size are separated and then mixed with other special additives and colorants. The final mixture is packaged and sold as acrylic (methacrylate) polymer powder. It is a surprisingly high-tech process that requires very special manufacturing equipment, lots of quality control, and scientific know-how to do it right.

Special additives are blended into both the liquid and powder. These additives ensure complete set or cure, maximum durability, color stability, and shelf life, among other attributes. It is these special "custom" additives that make different products work and behave differently. The polymer powders are usually blended with pigments and colorants to create a wide range of shades, including pinks, whites, and milky translucents, as well as reds, blues, greens, purples, yellows, oranges, browns, and even jet black.

When liquid is picked up by a brush and mixed with the powder, the bead that forms on the end of the brush quickly begins to harden. It is then put into place with other beads and shaped into place as they harden. In order for this process to begin, the monomers and polymers require special additives called catalysts (KAT-a-list) and initiators. A **catalyst** is an additive designed to speed up chemical reactions. Catalysts are added to the monomer liquid and used to control the set or curing time. In other words, when the monomer liquid and polymer powder are combined, the catalyst (in the liquid) helps control the set-up or hardening time. How? The catalyst energizes and activates the initiators. The **initiators** start a **chain reaction** that leads to the creation of fantastically long polymer chains. It is actually the initiators found in the powder that (once activated) will spring into action and start causing monomer molecules to permanently link together into these long polymer chains. This is another example of the polymerization process discussed above, except this time, its actually occurring on the fingernail. The polymerization process begins the second the liquid in the brush picks up powder from the container and forms a bead. Creating polymers can be thought of as a chain reaction, much like many dominos lined up and set on their edges—tap the first domino, it hits the next, and so on. This is how polymers form. Once the monomers join together to create a polymer, they do not detach from each other easily.

The initiator that is added to the polymer powder is called benzoyl peroxide (BPO). It is the same ingredient used in over-the-counter acne medicine, except that it has a different purpose in nail enhancement products. BPO is used to start the chain reaction that leads to curing (hardening) of the nail enhancement. There is much less BPO in nail powders than in acne treatments. Diverse nail enhancement products often use different amounts of BPO, since the polymer powders are designed to work specifically with a certain monomer liquid. Some monomer liquids require more BPO to properly cure than others. This is why it is very important to use the polymer powder that was designed for use with the monomer liquid that you are using. Using the wrong powder can create nail enhancements that are not properly cured and may lead to service breakdown or could increase the risk of your clients developing a skin irritation or sensitivity. To learn more about how these products work and how to troubleshoot problems, see *Nail Structure and Product Chemistry,* second edition, by Douglas Schoon (Thomson Delmar Learning, 2005).

ACRYLIC (METHACRYLATE) NAIL ENHANCEMENTS USING FORMS

Today's acrylic (methacrylate) polymer powders come in many colors, including variations of basic pink, white, clear, and natural. These colors can be used alone or blended to create everything from customized shades of pink to match or enhance the color of your client's nail beds to bold primaries or pastels that can be used to create a wide range of designs and patterns. With these powders you can create unique colors or designs that can be locked permanently in the artificial nail. They offer a wonderful way to customize your services or to express your artistry and creativity.

Acrylic (methacrylate) overlays and nail enhancements can be created with a single color powder, if the client wears nail polish all the time. Or they can be created by using a pink or natural colored powder over the nail bed or a natural or soft white powder to replicate a natural-nail free edge. A stark white powder can be use to create the French manicure look. The finished nail enhancement can be polished with nail polish or buffed to a high-gloss shine for a more natural look. These types of services are extremely versatile and highly durable, which partially explains their great popularity.

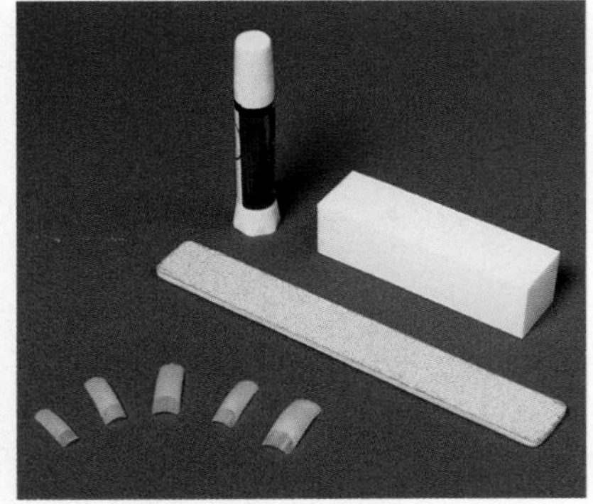

Figure 28–1 Materials needed for application of acrylic (methacrylate) nail enhancements.

SUPPLIES FOR ACRYLIC (METHACRYLATE) NAIL ENHANCEMENTS

Acrylic (methacrylate) nail enhancements are created by combining acrylic (methacrylate) monomer liquid with polymer powder. In addition to the supplies in your basic manicuring setup, you will need the items listed below (Figure 28-1).

- **Acrylic (methacrylate) monomer liquid.** The monomer liquid will be combined with acrylic (methacrylate) polymer powder to form the sculptured nail. The amount of monomer liquid and polymer powder used to create a bead is called the **mix ratio.** A bead mix ratio can be best described as "dry," "medium," or "wet." If equal amounts of liquid and powder are used to create the bead, it is called a "dry bead." If twice as much liquid as powder is found in the bead, it is called a "wet bead." Halfway between these two is a "medium" bead, which consists of 50 percent more liquid than powder. In general, medium beads are the ideal mix ratio for working with monomer liquids and polymer powders. Mix ratio typically ensures proper set and maximum durability of the nail enhancement. For instance, if too much or too little flour is added when making cookies, the cookies will be dry and crumbly (too much) or too soft and gooey (too little). The same holds true for monomer liquids and polymer powders. If too much powder is picked up in the bead, the enhancement will cure incorrectly and may lead to brittleness and/or discoloration. If too little powder is used, the nail enhancement can become weak, and the risk of clients developing skin irritation and sensitivity may increase.

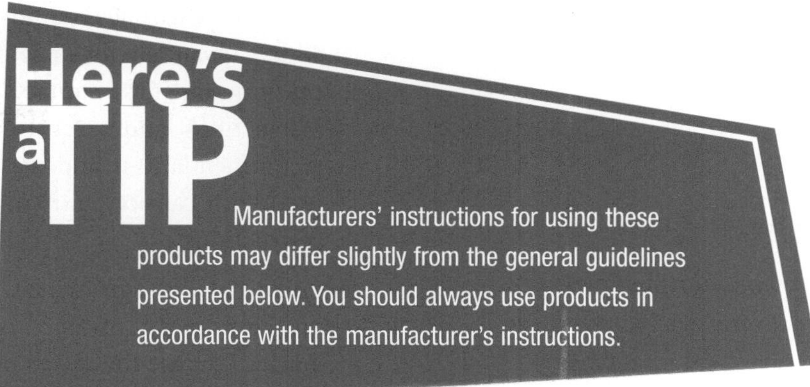

Here's a TIP
Manufacturers' instructions for using these products may differ slightly from the general guidelines presented below. You should always use products in accordance with the manufacturer's instructions.

- **Acrylic (methacrylate) polymer powder.** Polymer powder in white, clear, natural, pink, and many other colors is available. The color(s) you choose will depend on the nail enhancement method you are using.
- **Nail dehydrator.** Apply liberally to natural nail plate only and avoid skin contact. Nail dehydrators remove surface moisture and tiny amounts of oil left on the natural nail plate, both of which can block adhesion. This step is a great way to help prevent lifting of the artificial nail enhancements.
- **Nail primer.** Many kinds of nail primers are available today. Acid-based primer (methacrylic acid) was once widely used to enhance the adhesion of enhancements to the natural nail. Since this type of nail primer is corrosive to the skin and potentially dangerous to eyes, "acid free" and "nonacid" primers were developed and are in wide use today. These alternatives work as well as or better than acid-based nail

Here's a TIP

Hand sanitizers do not clean the hands. They cannot remove dirt or debris from hands. They only kill some of the bacteria on skin, not all of it. But, they do give clients peace of mind. Clients like to see cosmetologists using hand sanitizers and many clients prefer to use them as well. Keep a high-quality, professional hand sanitizer at your station and offer some to your clients. Let them see you using it, and they will have a greater degree of confidence in the cleanliness of your services. But do not let them replace hand washing—there is no replacement for that.

CAUTION

Acid-based nail primers are very effective but can cause serious, and sometimes irreversible, damage to the skin and eyes. Never use acid-based nail primer or any other on corrosive material without protective gloves and safety eyewear.

primers. Since they are not corrosive to the skin or eyes, they have an added advantage. Even so, all nail primer products must be used with caution, and skin contact must be avoided. Read the manufacturer's instructions and refer to the respective MSDS for safe handling recommendations and instructions. Acid-based nail primers must be used with caution and strictly in accordance with the manufacturer's instructions.

For acid-based nail primers: Using a tiny applicator brush, insert the brush tip into the nail primer. Touch the brush tip to the edge of the bottle's neck to release the excess primer back into the bottle. With a relatively dry brush, using a light dotting action, carefully dab the brush tip to the center of the properly prepared natural nail. The acid-based primer will spread out and cover the nail plate. Do not use too much product to avoid running into the skin and causing burns or injury. *Be sure to read the label for the manufacturer's suggested use and precautions.*

For nonacid and acid-free nail primers: Using the applicator brush, insert brush into the nail primer. Wipe off excess from the brush, and using a slightly damp brush, ensure that the nail plate is completely covered. Avoid using too much product to avoid running into the skin and causing skin irritation or sensitivity. The brush should hold enough product to treat two or three nails before dipping back into the container. Be sure the entire nail plate is covered. Also, read the label for the manufacturer's suggested application procedures and precautions.

- **Abrasives.** Select a medium grit (180 to 240) for natural nail preparation and initial shaping. Choose a medium grit for smoothing, and a fine buffer (350 grit or higher) for final buffing. A three-way buffer is used to create a high shine on the enhancement when no polish is worn. If you avoid putting the product on too thickly, a 180 grit is usually enough to shape the nail enhancement. Avoid using coarser (lower-grit) abrasives on freshly applied enhancement product, since they can damage the freshly created nail enhancement. Acrylic (methacrylate) nail enhancements take 24 to 48 hours to reach peak strength. Using overly coarse abrasives or aggressive techniques on freshly applied enhancement products of any type must be avoided.

Here's a TIP

The best way to dispose of small amounts of liquid monomer is to mix them with small amounts of the corresponding powder designed to cure them. (This is safe for volumes less than a half-ounce of monomer liquid, as well as ounces, quarts, or gallons.) They should never be disposed of in the trash or down the drain. Tiny amounts left in a dappen dish can be wiped out with a paper towel and disposed of in a metal trash can with a self-closing lid, as long as skin contact is avoided during the process and the trash is disposed of several times during the day so that vapors do not escape into the salon air.

- **Nail forms.** These are placed under the free edge and used to extend the nail enhancements beyond the fingertip for additional length. These nail forms are often made of paper/mylar coated with adhesive backs, or pre-shaped plastic or aluminum. Each of these forms is disposable, excepting aluminum forms, which can be properly cleaned and disinfected.

- **Nail tips.** These are pre-formed nail extensions made from ABS or tenite acetate plastic, and are available in a wide variety of shapes, styles, and colors, such as natural, white, and clear (see Chapter 27 for more information and instructions).
- **Nail adhesive.** There are many types of nail adhesives used for securing nail tips to the natural nails, but they are all based on cyanoacrylate monomers. Each type uses different, customized additives to enhance set times, strength, and other properties. It is chiefly the special additives that a manufacturer chooses that make these adhesives different from each other.

  Choose a small size (4 to 6 grams maximum) because these adhesives have a short shelf life and can expire within 6 months after the date of purchase, depending on usage and storage conditions. To obtain the maximum shelf life, be sure to close the cap securely, set upright, and store out of direct sunlight and at room temperature between 60° to 85°F. If you do not, the nail adhesive may harden in the tube and will have to be discarded.
- **Dappen dish.** The monomer liquid and polymer powder are each poured into a special holder called a dappen dish. These dishes must have narrow openings to minimize evaporation of the monomer into the air. Do not use open-mouth jars or other containers with large openings. These will dramatically increase evaporation of your liquid and can allow the product to be contaminated with dust and other debris. Your dappen dish must be covered with a tightly fitting lid when not in use. Each time the brush is dipped into the dappen dish, the remaining monomer is contaminated with small amounts of polymer powder. So *never* pour the unused portion of monomer back into the original container. Empty the monomer from your dappen dish after the service and wipe it clean with a disposable towel. Avoid skin contact with monomer during this process to avoid skin irritation or sensitivity. Wipe clean with acetone, if necessary, before storing in a dust-free location.
- **Nail brush.** The best brush for use with these types of procedures is composed of sable hair. Synthetic and less expensive brushes do not pick up enough monomer liquid or do not release the liquid properly. Choose the brush shape and size with which you feel the most comfortable. Avoid overly large brushes, since they can hold excessive amounts of liquid that may dilute the enhancement product and lead to service breakdown. They also increase the risk of accidentally touching the client's skin with liquid monomer and may increase the risk of developing skin irritation or sensitivities.
- **Safety eyewear.** Safety eyewear should be used to protect eyes from flying objects or accidental splashes. There are many types and styles to choose from. You can get more information by searching the Internet, or contacting a local optometrist, who can also help you with both nonprescription and prescription safety eyewear.
- **Dust masks and protective gloves.** Dust masks are designed to be worn over the nose and mouth to prevent inhalation of excessive

amounts of dusts. They provide no protection from vapors. Both disposable and multiuse varieties of protective gloves can be purchased. Many types of materials are used to make these gloves. For many nail salon-related applications, gloves made of "nitrile" polymer work best.

ACRYLIC (METHACRYLATE) NAIL ENHANCEMENTS PRE-SERVICE

Before application of any type of acrylic (methacrylate) nail enhancement, prepare yourself and your client with the steps below.

1. **Complete the pre-service sanitation and disinfection procedure, described in Chapter 25.**
2. **Set up your standard manicuring table.** Add the additional supplies needed to perform this service to your table. Always have enough supplies to prevent running out while performing the service.
3. **Greet the client and direct her to wash her hands with liquid soap and warm running water.** Be sure to dry hands thoroughly with a clean disposable towel.
4. **Perform a client consultation, using a client consultation form to record responses and observations.** Check for nail disorders to determine if it is safe and appropriate to perform a service on this client. If the client must not receive a service, explain your reasons and refer her to a doctor, if necessary. Record any skin or nail disorders, allergies, and so on. Make notes concerning the client's nail habits—for instance, is the client a nail biter, does the client pick at her own nails, or does she do heavy lifting in her daily routine? Also make brief notations about the performance of the client's enhancements, if she is wearing them. Record specific information about the service, such as acrylic (methacrylate) overlay with polish or pink and white acrylic (methacrylate) nail with glossy top coat, and make a note of the client's choice in polish color.

You are now ready to begin Procedure 28-1.

PROCEDURE 28-1

APPLICATION OF ACRYLIC (METHACRYLATE) NAIL ENHANCEMENTS USING FORMS

1. **Clean nails and remove existing polish.** Begin with your client's little finger on the left hand, and work toward the thumb. Then repeat on the right hand (Figure 28-2). Ask the client to put her nails in a fingerbowl with liquid soap. Then use a nail brush to clean nails over the fingerbowl. Thoroughly rinse with clean water to remove soap residues, which can cause lifting.
2. **Push back eponychium and carefully remove cuticle from the nail plate.** Use a cotton-tipped wooden or metal pusher to gently push back the eponychium, and then apply the cuticle remover. Use as directed by the manufacturer, and carefully remove cuticle tissue from the nail plate.
3. **Remove oily shine from natural nail surface.** Lightly buff the nail plate with medium-fine (240 grit) abrasive to remove the natural oil that causes the shine on the surface of the nail plate (Figure 28-3).
4. **Apply nail dehydrator.** Apply nail dehydrator to nails with cotton-tipped wooden pusher, cotton pad with a plastic backing, brush, or spray. Begin with the little finger on the left hand and work toward the thumb (Figure 28-4).
5. **Position nail form.** Position nail form on nail plate. If you are using disposable forms, peel a nail form from its paper backing and, using the thumb and index finger of each of your hands, bend the form into an arch to fit the client's natural nail shape. Slide the form into place and press adhesive backing to the sides of the finger. Check to see that the form is snug under the free edge and level with the natural nail.

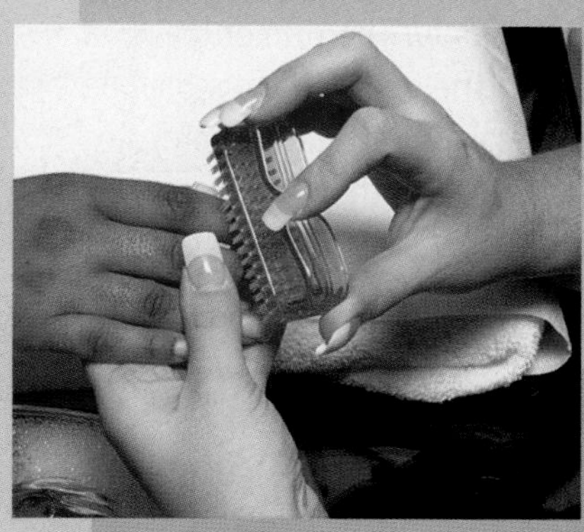

Figure 28-2 Clean nails.

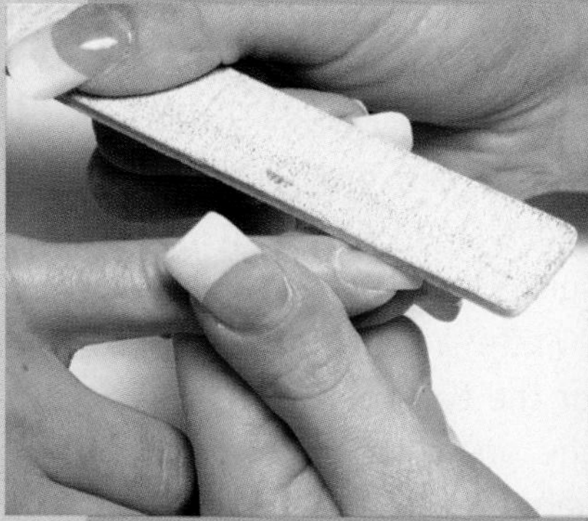

Figure 28-3 Buff natural nails to remove shine.

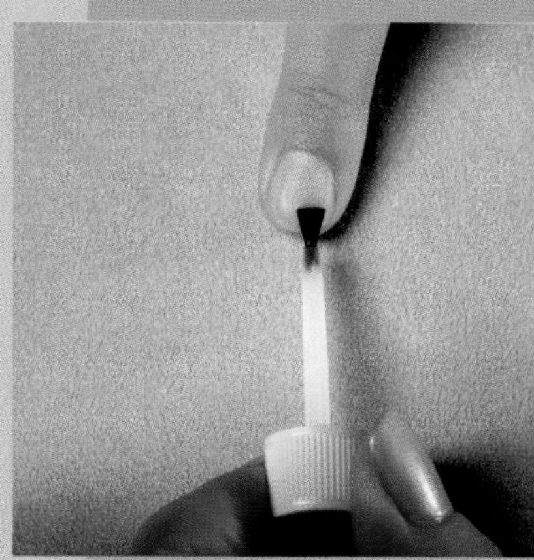

Figure 28-4 Apply nail dehydrator.

If you are using multiuse forms, slide the form into place making sure the free edge is over the form and that it fits snugly. Be careful not to cut into the hyponychium under the free edge. Tighten the form around the finger by squeezing lightly (Figure 28-5).

6. **Apply nail primer.** Apply nail primer by touching the brush tip to the edge of the bottle's neck to release the excess primer back into the bottle. Using a light dotting action, dab the brush tip to the prepared natural nail only. The primer leaves a residue molecule behind. The open-ended molecule connects with the acrylic (methacrylate) molecules to form a better bond to each other. Always follow the manufacturer's directions.

   Allow nail primer to dry thoroughly. Never apply nail enhancement product over wet nail primer, since this can cause product discoloration and service breakdown. Avoid overuse of nail primers (Figures 28-6 and 28-7).

7. **Prepare monomer liquid and polymer powder.** Pour acrylic (methacrylate) liquid and powder into separate dappen dishes. If you are using the two-color method, you will need three dappen dishes—one for the white tip powder; one for the clear, natural, or pink powder; and one for the acrylic (methacrylate) monomer liquid. (Throughout this chapter, pink and white acrylic [methacrylate] powders are used for the two-color method. Your client may select the one-color method or may pick a clear or natural powder, or when you are in the salon you can offer a custom-blended pink shade to match the client's skin tones.)

8. **Dip brush in monomer liquid.** Dip brush fully in the monomer liquid and wipe on the edge of the container to remove the excess (Figure 28-8).

9. **Form product bead.** Dip the tip of the same brush into the acrylic (methacrylate) polymer powder and rotate slightly. You will pick up a bead of product—and it should have a medium consistency, not runny or wet—that is large enough for shaping

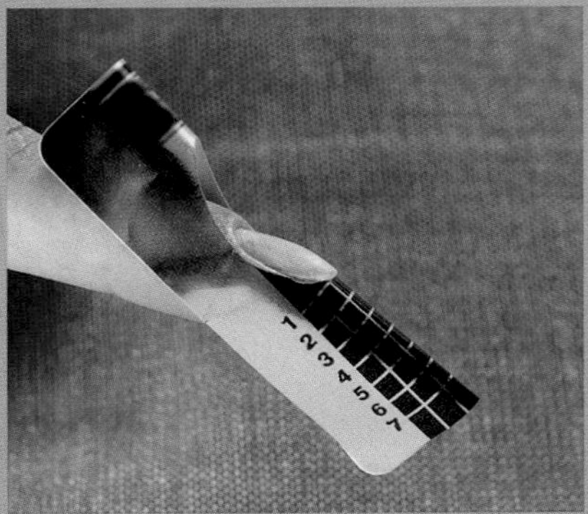

Figure 28-5 Position nail form.

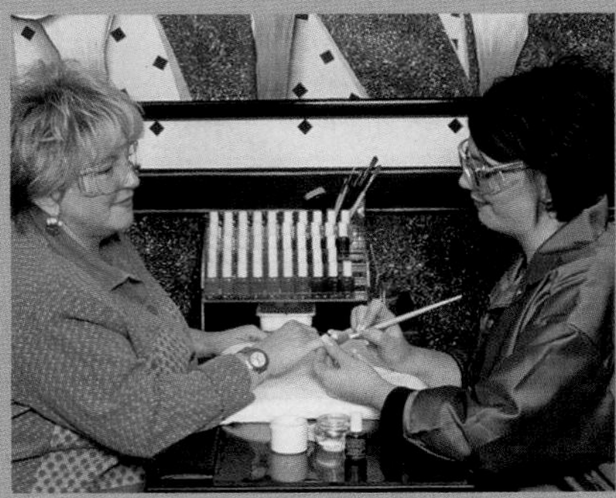

Figure 28-6 Always wear safety glasses when applying acid-based nail primer.

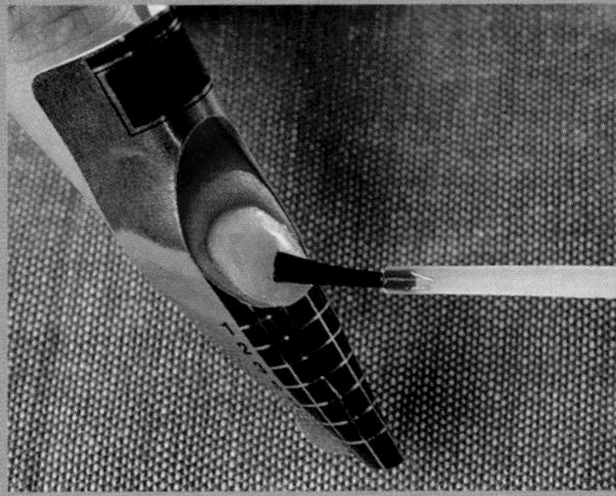

Figure 28-7 Carefully dot on acid-based primer. Allow to spread. Avoid overuse.

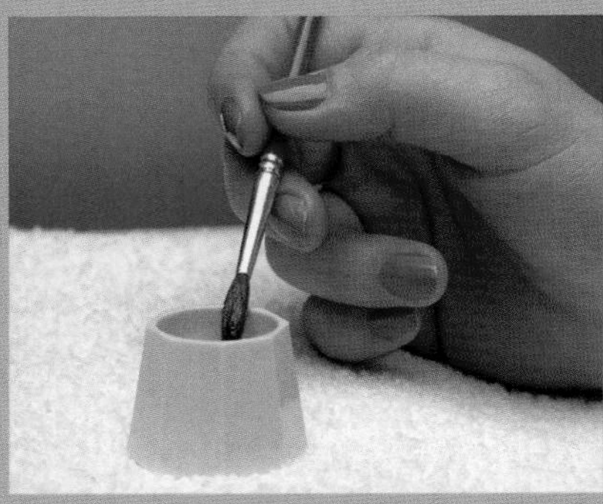

Figure 28-8 Dip brush into monomer liquid.

the entire free-edge extension. If this is too large a bead to properly shape, using two smaller beads may be easier. If you are using the two-color acrylic (methacrylate) method, use the white powder at this point (Figure 28-9).

10. **Place bead of product.** Place the bead on the nail form at the point where the free edge joins the nail form (Figures 28-10 and 28-11).
11. **Shape free edge.** Use the middle portion of your sable brush to press and smooth the product to shape the enhancement in the free edge area. Do not "paint" the enhancement product onto the nail. Pressing and smoothing produces a more natural-looking nail. Keep side wall lines parallel, and avoid widening the tip beyond the natural width of the nail plate. If you are using the two-color nail enhancement method, create a natural-looking shape with the white powder to produce the French manicure look (Figures 28-12 and 28-13).
12. **Place second bead of product.** Pick up a second bead of product of medium consistency and place it on the natural nail below the last bead and next to the free edge line in the center of nail.
13. **Shape second bead of product.** Press and smooth product toward the side walls, making sure that the product is very thin around all the edges

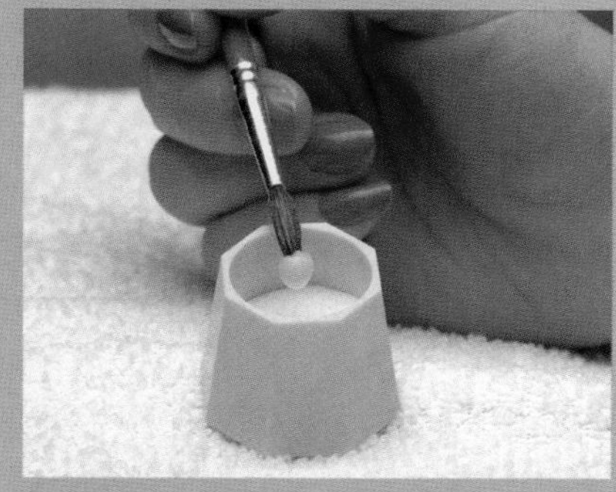

Figure 28-9 Form a bead of product.

Here's a TIP

Do not touch primed area of the nail with your brush until you apply enhancement product on the area. The enhancement may become discolored where wet nail primer touches the product, and this can also lead to lifting.

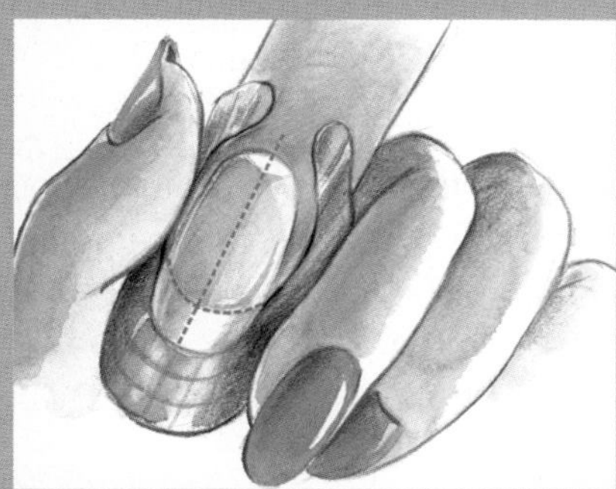

Figure 28-10 The center line and free edge of the nail.

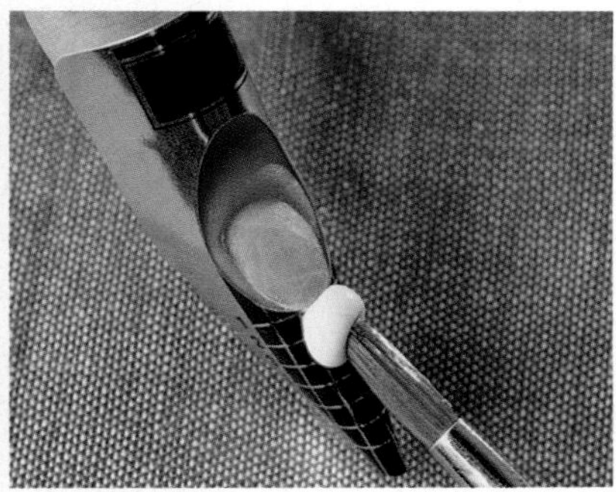

Figure 28-11 Place bead of product on nail form.

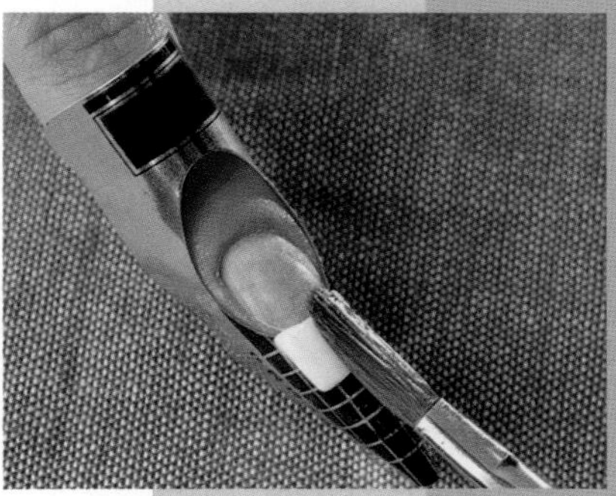

Figure 28-12 Shape white bead(s) into a natural looking "smile line."

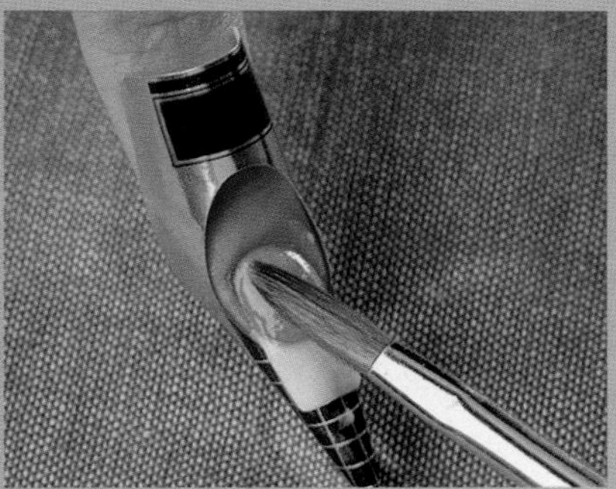

Figure 28-13 Press product bead flat, keeping brush flat to nail, and then smooth it into shape.

(Figure 28-14). Leave a tiny free margin between the product placement and skin. Avoid placing the product too close to the skin, or it may cause it to lift away from the nail plate and may increase the chance of causing skin irritation or sensitivity. If you are using a two-color acrylic (methacrylate) product, use the pink powder in this step (Figure 28-15). Make sure to use a medium consistency. Avoid working too wet.

14. **Apply product bead.** Pick up smaller bead of pink polymer powder with your brush and place at base of the nail plate, leaving a tiny free margin between it and the skin. Use the brush to press and smooth these beads over entire nail plate. Glide brush over nail to smooth out imperfections. Enhancement product application near eponychium, side wall, and free edge must be thin for a natural-looking nail (Figure 28-16).
15. **Apply product to remaining nails.** Repeat steps 5 through 14 on remaining nails.
16. **Remove nail forms.** When nail enhancements are thoroughly hardened, loosen forms and slide them off. Nail enhancements are hard enough to file and shape if they make a clicking sound when lightly tapped with a brush handle.
17. **Shape nail enhancements.** Use medium abrasive (180 to 240 grit) to shape the free edge and to remove imperfections. Glide abrasive over each

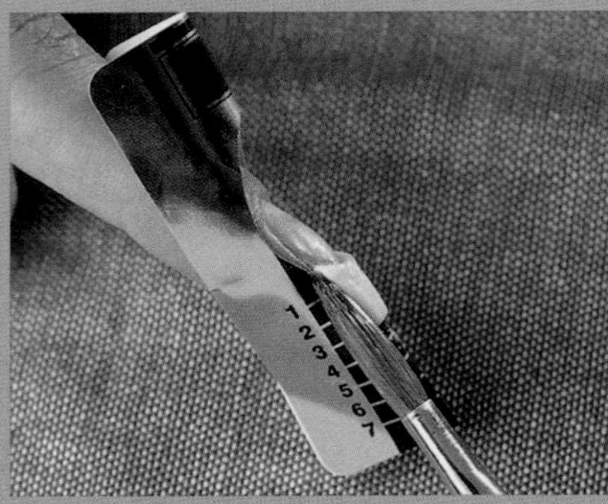

Figure 28-14 Check side walls to be sure that they are even and parallel.

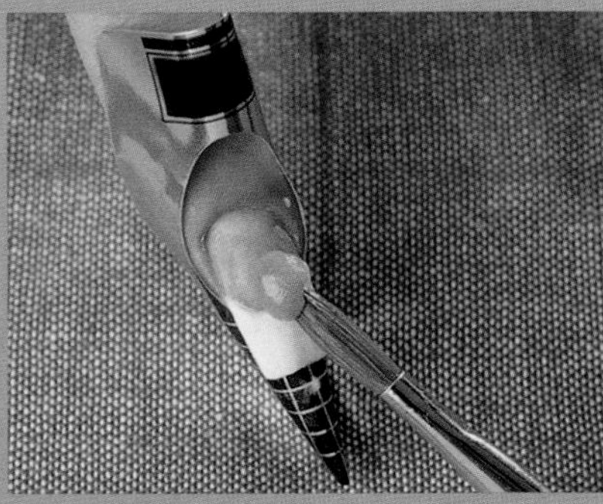

Figure 28-15 Place bead above smile line onto natural nail.

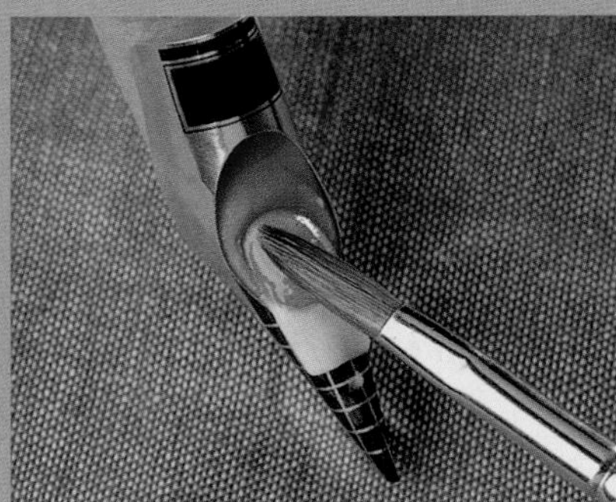

Figure 28-16 Shape second bead of product, and then press and smooth into place.

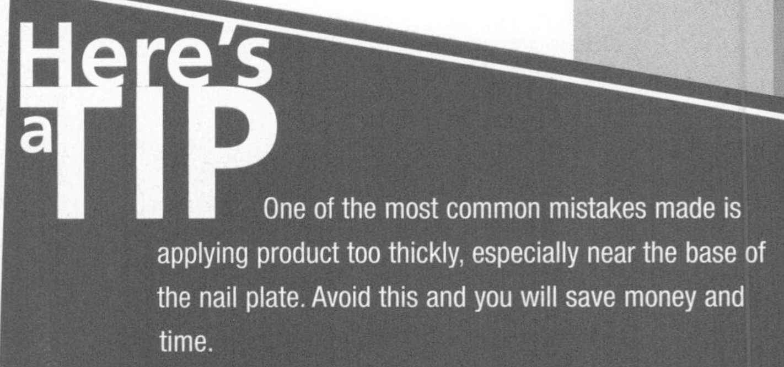

Here's a TIP

One of the most common mistakes made is applying product too thickly, especially near the base of the nail plate. Avoid this and you will save money and time.

nail with long sweeping strokes to further shape and perfect the enhancement surface. Thin the product near the base of all nail plates, free edges, and side walls (Figure 28-17).

18. **Buff nail enhancements.** Buff the enhancement with a fine-grit buffer (350 grit or higher) until entire surface is smooth (Figures 28-18 to 28-21); use a high-shine buffer if polish is not to be worn.

19. **Apply nail oil.** Use a cotton-tipped wooden pusher or an eyedropper to apply nail oil to the skin surrounding the nail plate, and massage briefly to speed penetration (Figure 28-22).

20. **Apply hand cream and massage hand and arm.**

21. **Clean nail enhancements.** Ask client to wash with soap and use a nail brush to clean her nail enhancements. Thoroughly rinse with water to remove all soap residues that may cause lifting. Dry thoroughly with a clean disposable towel. If your client selected the two-color method, her acrylic (methacrylate) nail enhancements are finished.

22. **Apply nail polish.** If your client selected one-color acrylic (methacrylate) nail enhancements, apply the selected nail polish (Figure 28-23).

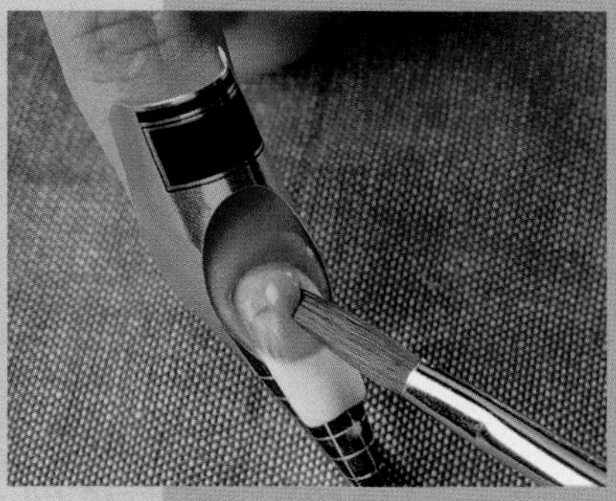

Figure 28-17 Apply smaller beads of product near the base of the nail plate and leave a tiny free margin between the product and the skin.

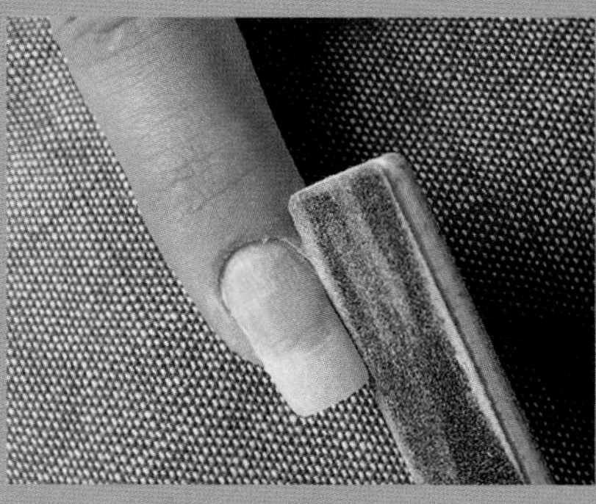

Figure 28-18 File the two side walls evenly and parallel with each other.

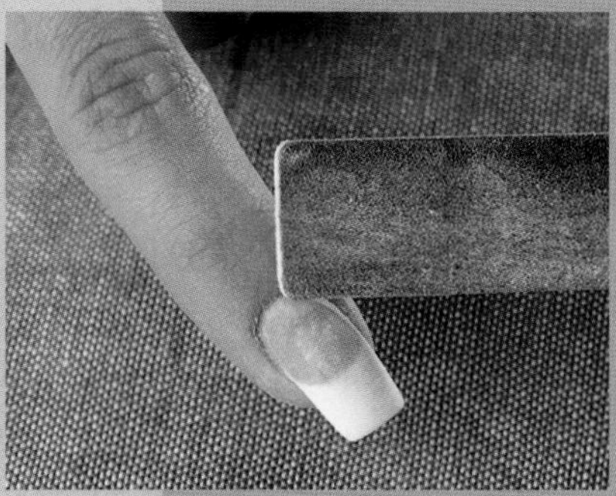

Figure 28-19 Smooth and thin.

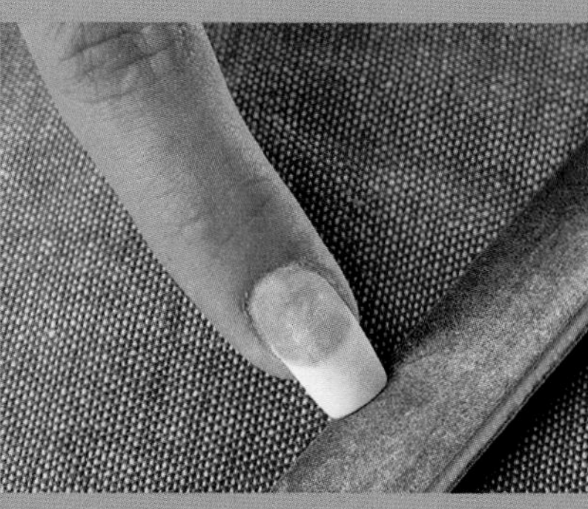

Figure 28-20 Shape and contour.

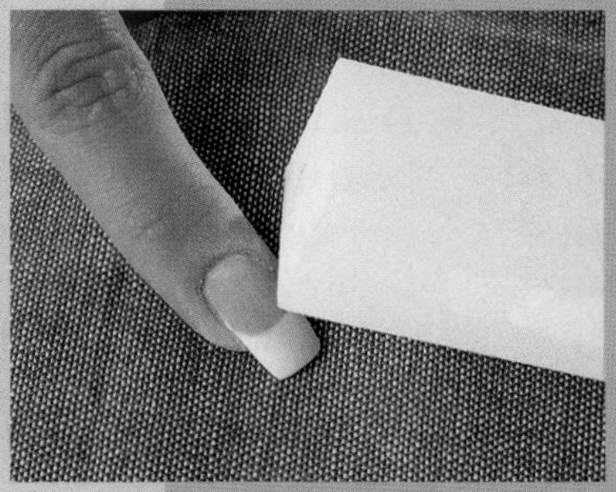

Figure 28-21 Buff entire surface with a fine-grit buffer (350 grit or higher), and then a high-shine buffer if desired.

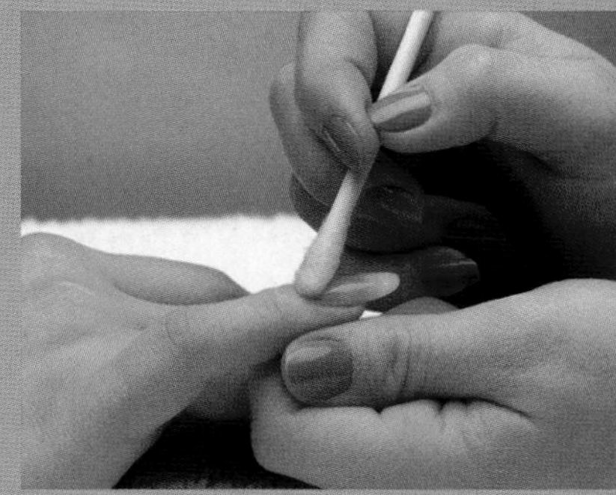

Figure 28-22 Apply nail oil.

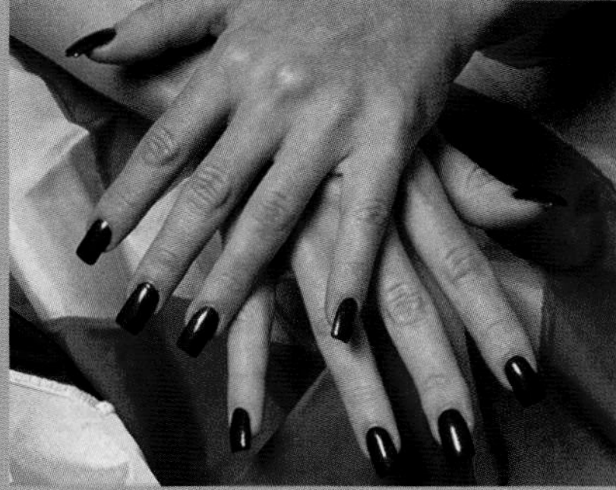

Figure 28-23 Finished nail enhancements.

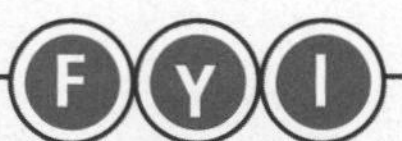

Avoid wiping your brush too rapidly or hard against a table towel. This can press hairs against the sharp edge of the metal ferrule that holds the hairs in place and cut them off.

ACRYLIC (METHACRYLATE) NAIL POST-SERVICE

1. **Make another appointment.** Schedule another appointment with your client for maintaining her nail enhancements. A rebalance will be necessary in 2 or 3 weeks, depending on how quickly the nails grow. Encourage your client to return for a basic manicure between rebalance appointments if the acrylic (methacrylate) nail enhancements are polished.
2. **Take-home product recommendations.** Suggest professional products that you believe your client would benefit from, such as polish, top coat, and hand lotions. These are valuable maintenance tools for clients, and they will appreciate your professional recommendation.
3. **Clean up around your table.** Take the time to restore the basic setup of your table, restock supplies, and make sure all caps are tight.
4. **Clean brush.** Clean brush according to the manufacturer's instructions. Never pull out bristles of the brush because you may loosen the remaining bristles. Clip one stray hair if necessary, but never trim bristles because you may ruin the accuracy of the brush. Do not allow the brush to sit in acetone or brush cleaner. Generally, it is better to clean the brush in monomer liquid. Brush cleaners and acetone can dry out the hairs and make them brittle. Never immerse any application brush into any liquid disinfecting solution—this can cause product contamination and lead to service breakdown.
5. **Store acrylic products.** Store acrylic powders in covered containers. Store all primers and acrylic liquids in a cool, dark area. Do not store products near heat.
6. **Discard used materials.** Never save used monomer liquid that has been removed from the original container. Use on one client only. To dispose of small amounts of leftover monomer, carefully pour it into a highly absorbent paper towel and then place it in a plastic bag. Avoid skin contact with the liquid monomer and never pour the monomer directly into the plastic bag! Should skin contact occur, wash hands with liquid soap and water. After all used materials have been collected, seal them in a plastic bag and discard it in a closed waste receptacle. It is important to remove items soiled with enhancement product from your manicuring station after each client. This will help maintain the quality of your salon's air. Dispose of these items according to local rules and regulations.
7. **Clean your table, and then clean and disinfect implements and multiuse tools, such as abrasives and implements**. Perform complete pre-service sanitation and disinfection procedures. Implements need to be cleaned and disinfected before they can be used on the next client, and this procedure will take about 20 minutes. See Procedure 28-2.

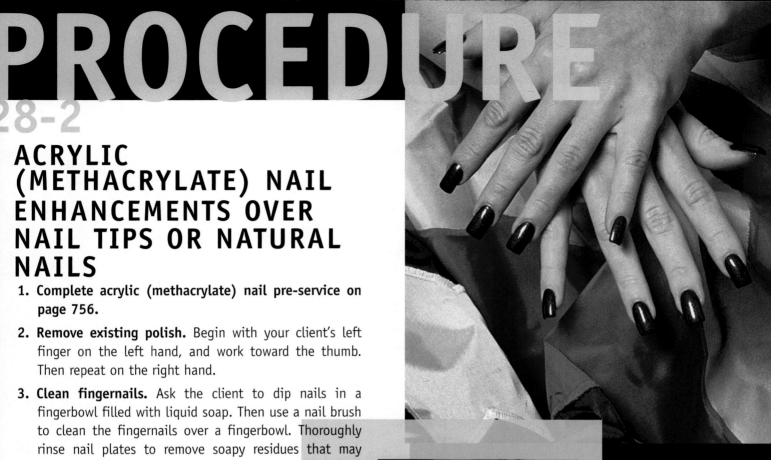

PROCEDURE 28-2

ACRYLIC (METHACRYLATE) NAIL ENHANCEMENTS OVER NAIL TIPS OR NATURAL NAILS

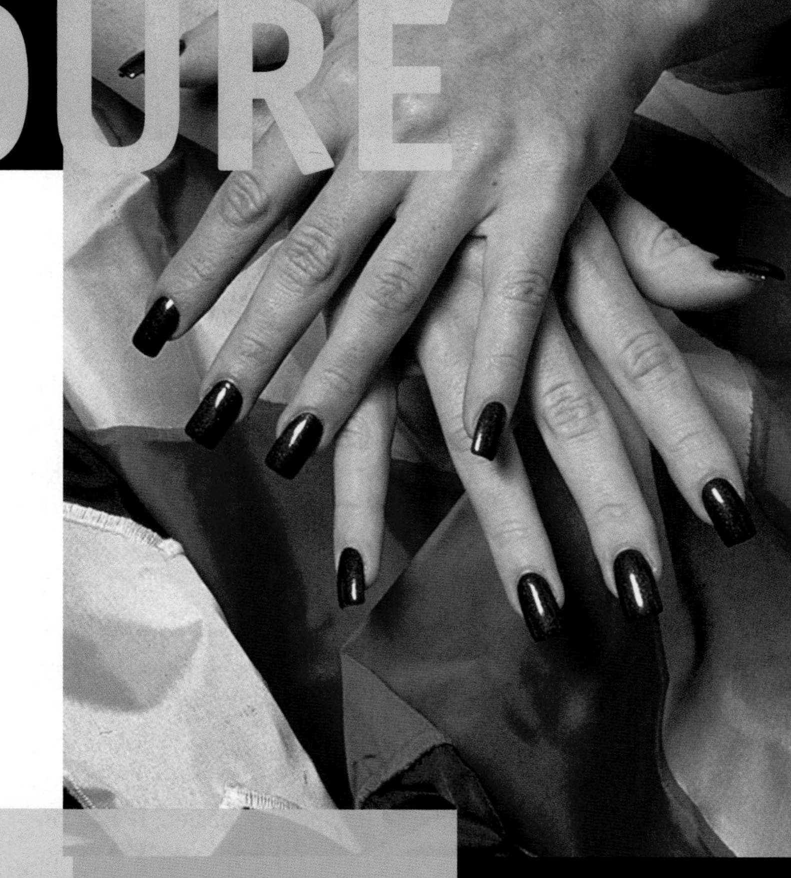

1. **Complete acrylic (methacrylate) nail pre-service on page 756.**
2. **Remove existing polish.** Begin with your client's left finger on the left hand, and work toward the thumb. Then repeat on the right hand.
3. **Clean fingernails.** Ask the client to dip nails in a fingerbowl filled with liquid soap. Then use a nail brush to clean the fingernails over a fingerbowl. Thoroughly rinse nail plates to remove soapy residues that may cause lifting. Dry thoroughly with a clean disposable towel.
4. **Push back eponychium and carefully remove cuticle from the nail plate.** Use a cotton-tipped wooden or metal pusher to gently push back the eponychium, and then apply cuticle remover. Use as directed by the manufacturer, and carefully remove cuticle tissue from the nail plate.
5. **Buff nail plate to remove oily shine.** Buff the nail plate with medium-fine abrasive (240 grit) to remove the shine caused by natural oil on the surface of the nail plate. Avoid over-filing of the nail plate.
6. **Apply nail dehydrator.** Apply nail dehydrator to nails with cotton-tipped wooden or metal pusher, plastic-backed cotton pad, brush, or spray. Begin with the little finger on the left hand and work toward the thumb.
7. **Apply tips.** Apply tips if your client desires them and cut to the appropriate length, using the technique described in Chapter 27. Cut tip to desired length (Figure 28-24).
8. **Apply nail primer.** Apply nail primer as previously described, and follow the manufacturer's directions. Allow nail primer to dry thoroughly. Never apply nail enhancement product over wet nail primer, since this can cause product discoloration and service breakdown. Avoid overuse of nail primers. Apply primer to the natural nail, and avoid putting it on the nail tips unless instructed by the manufacturer of the nail primer.

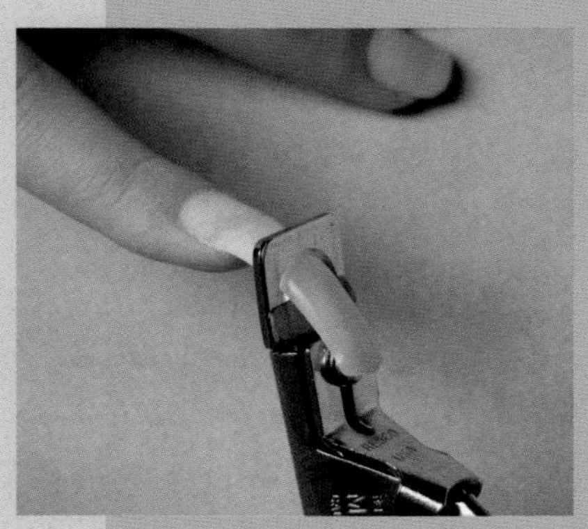

Figure 28-24 Cut tip to desired length.

9. **Prepare acrylic (methacrylate) liquid and powder.** Pour monomer liquid and polymer powder into separate small dappen dishes. If you are using the two-color system, you will need three dappen dishes—one for the white tip powder, one for the pink powder, and one for the monomer liquid.
10. **Dip brush into monomer liquid.** Dip brush fully into the monomer liquid and wipe on the edge of the container to remove the excess.
11. **Form product bead.** Dip the tip of the same brush into the acrylic (methacrylate) polymer powder and rotate slightly. You will pick up a bead of product, and it should have a medium consistency, not runny or wet, that is large enough for shaping the entire free-edge extension. If it is too large to properly shape, two smaller beads may be easier. If you are using the two-color acrylic method, use the white powder at this point.
12. **Place bead of product on free edge.** Place product bead on the free edge of the tip or natural nail (Figure 28-25).
13. **Shape free edge.** Use the middle portion of your sable brush to press and smooth the product to shape the enhancement's free edge. Do not "paint" the product onto the nail. Pressing and smoothing produce a more natural-looking nail. Keep side wall lines parallel, and avoid widening the tip beyond the natural width of the nail plate. If you are using the two-color method, create a natural-looking shape with the white powder to produce the French manicure look (Figure 28-26).
14. **Place second bead of acrylic on free edge.** Use medium consistency and place it on the nail plate below the first bead and next to the free edge line in the center of the nail (Figure 28-27).
15. **Shape second bead of product.** Press and smooth product to side walls, making sure that the product is very thin around all edges. Leave a tiny free margin between the product placement and skin. Avoid placing the product too close to the skin, or the product may lift away from the nail plate, and may

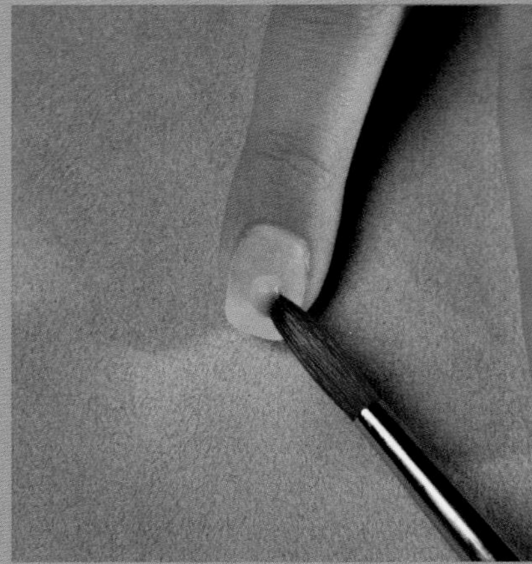

Figure 28-25 Place bead of product on free edge.

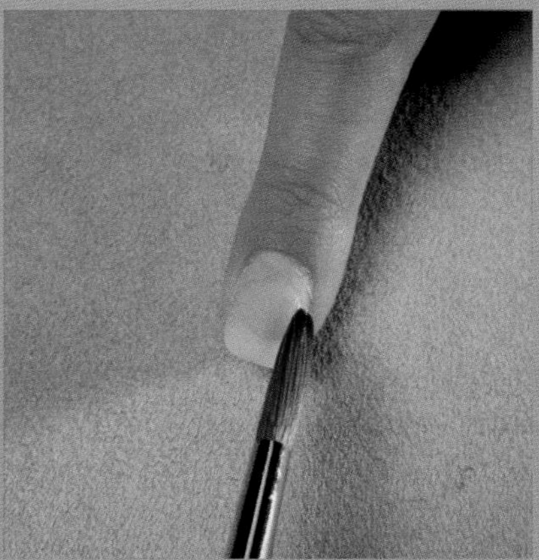

Figure 28-26 Press and smooth the bead over stress zone.

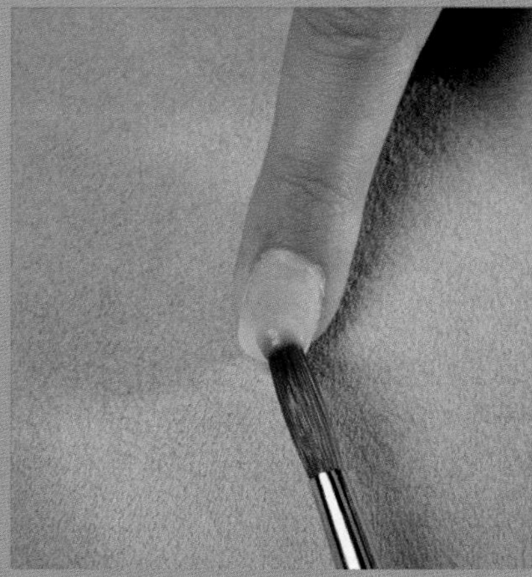

Figure 28-27 Place second bead of product on nail plate.

also increase the chance of the client developing a skin irritation or sensitivity. If you are using a two-color product, use the pink powder in this step (Figure 28-28). Make sure to use a medium consistency that is not too wet.

16. **Apply product beads.** Pick up smaller beads of pink polymer powder with your brush and place them at the base of the nail plate, leaving a tiny free margin between the product and the skin. Use the brush to press and smooth these beads over the entire nail plate. Glide the brush over the nail to smooth out imperfections. Product application near the eponychium, side wall, and free edge must be thin for a natural-looking nail. For the two-color method, use pink powder to create the beads (Figures 28-29 to 28-31).

17. **Shape and refine nail enhancement.** Use medium abrasive (180 to 240 grit) to shape the free edge and to remove imperfections. Then refine with medium-fine abrasive (240 grit) (Figure 28-32).

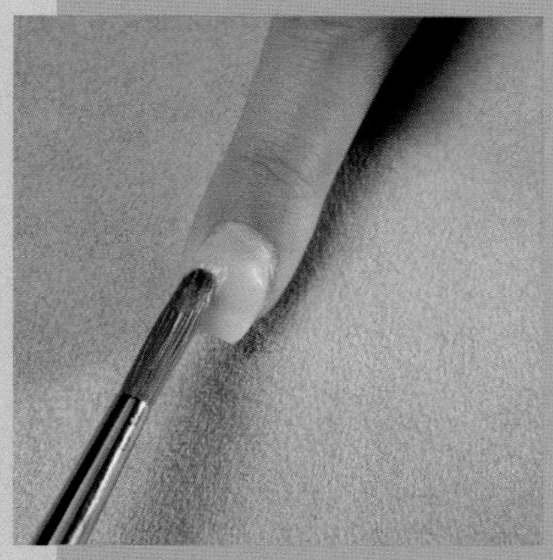

Figure 28-28 Press and smooth second bead.

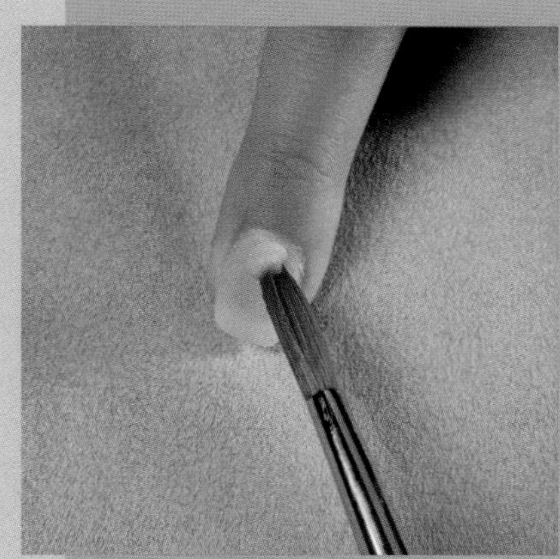

Figure 28-29 Apply smaller beads near the base of the nail plate.

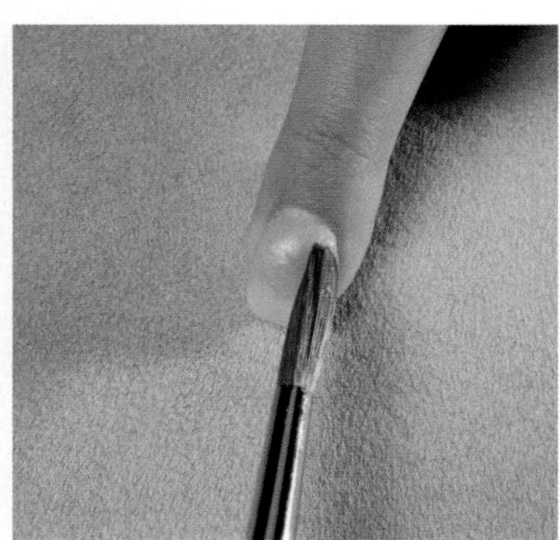

Figure 28-30 Press and smooth smaller beads at base of nail plate. Leave a tiny free margin and avoid skin contact with product.

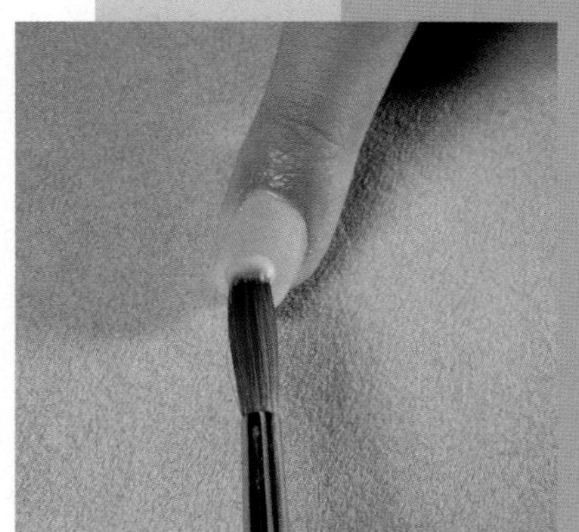

Figure 28-31 Press and smooth the bead over stress zone.

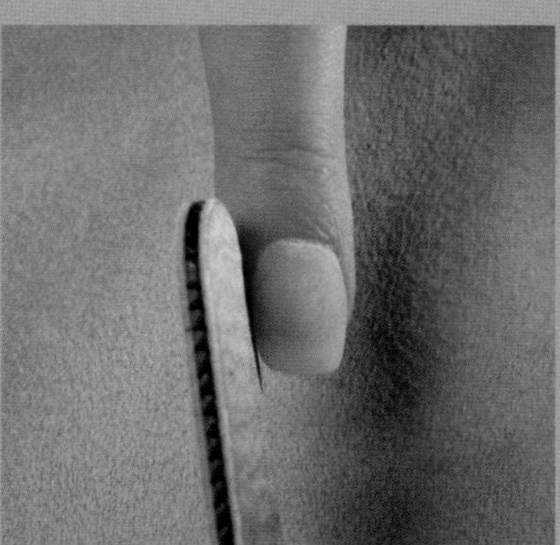

Figure 28-32 Shape and contour free edge.

18. **Buff nail enhancement.** Buff the nail enhancement with fine-grit buffer (350 grit or higher) until the entire surface is smooth (Figure 28-33), or use a high-shine buffer if nail with polish is to be worn.
19. **Apply nail oil.** Rub nail oil into the surrounding skin and nail enhancement, and massage briefly to speed penetration.
20. **Apply hand cream and massage hand and arm.**
21. **Clean nail enhancements.** Ask client to dip nail enhancements in a fingerbowl filled with liquid soap and water. Then use nail brush to clean nails over fingerbowl. Thoroughly rinse with clean water to remove soap residues that may cause lifting. Dry thoroughly with a clean disposable towel. If your client selected the two-color method, the nail enhancements are finished.
22. **Apply nail polish.** Polish one-color nail enhancements (Figure 28-34).
23. **Complete acrylic (methacrylate) enhancement post-service procedure described on page 762.**

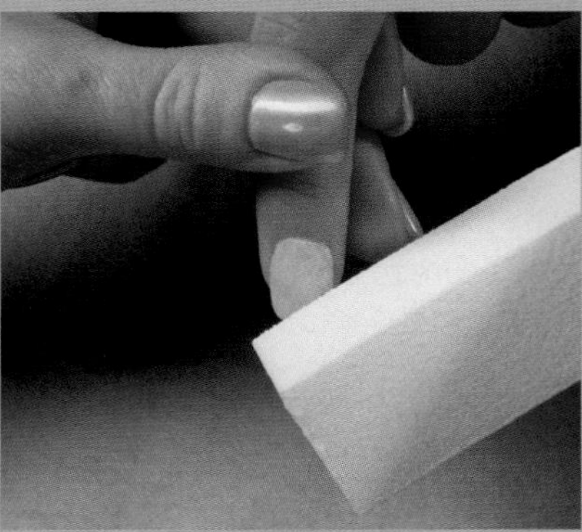

Figure 28-33 Buff nail enhancement.

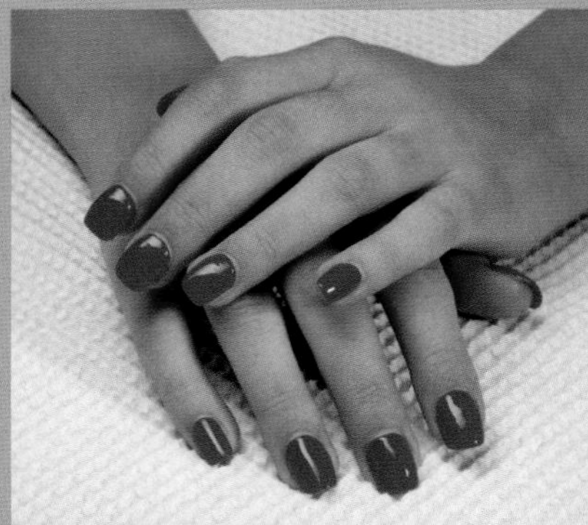

Figure 28-34 Finished artificial nail enhancements.

CAUTION

Check your nail primer daily for clarity to ensure that it does not become contaminated with nail dusts and other floating debris, which can dramatically reduce primer effectiveness. Avoid using nail primers that are visibly contaminated with floating debris.

MAINTENANCE AND REMOVAL OF ACRYLIC (METHACRYLATE) NAIL ENHANCEMENTS

Regular maintenance helps prevent nail enhancements from lifting or cracking. If the nail enhancements are not properly maintained, they have a greater tendency to lift and break, which increases the risk of the client developing an infection and other problems. For this reason, a full and proper rebalance must be performed every 2 to 3 weeks, depending on how fast the client's nails grow. If cracks occur, they should be repaired as soon as possible for the same reason. When the client no longer wishes to wear nail enhancements (for whatever reason), they should be removed as soon as possible as well. Steps for rebalancing, crack repair, and removal are found in Procedures 28-3 through 28-5.

REBALANCING

Rebalancing is a method for maintaining the beauty, durability, and longevity of artificial nail enhancements. Learning how to properly rebalance is a critical skill for you to learn, if you wish to be a successful cosmetologist. Do not let clients go too long without having a proper rebalance, or you will have many more repairs to perform when they return. Proper rebalancing is both safe and gentle to the nail unit, and will not result in injury or damage. In rebalancing, the nail is thinned down, the apex of the nail will be removed, and the entire nail enhancement is reduced in thickness. Use Procedure 28-3 for performing a rebalance.

CRACK REPAIR

Crack repair is the addition of enhancement product to repair cracks. Advantages to performing repairs as soon as possible after cracks occur are similar to those for rebalancing. Follow Procedure 28-4 for this maintenance technique.

REMOVAL

When the client requests nail enhancement removal this should be performed as soon as possible. Among other things, professional removal prevents natural nail bed damage. For this technique, see Procedure 28-5 on page 771.

ODORLESS ACRYLIC (METHACRYLATE) PRODUCTS

Odorless acrylic (methacrylate) products have the same chemistry as all other monomer liquid and polymer powder products. But rather than use ethyl acrylic (methacrylate), these products rely on monomers that have little odor.

PROCEDURE 28-3

ACRYLIC (METHACRYLATE) NAIL ENHANCEMENT REBALANCE

1. **Complete acrylic (methacrylate) nail enhancement application pre-service on page 756.**
2. **Remove existing polish.**
3. **Smooth ledge between new growth and acrylic nail.** Using a medium-coarse abrasive (120 to 180 grit), carefully smooth down the ledge of the existing product until it is flush with the new growth of nail plate. Do not dig into or damage the natural nail plate with your abrasive.
4. **Refine entire nail enhancement.** Hold the medium abrasive (180 to 240 grit) flat and glide it over entire nail enhancement to reshape, refine, and thin out the free edge until the white tip appears translucent. Take care not to damage the client's skin with the abrasive.
5. **Buff nail enhancement.** Use a fine-grit buffer (350 grit or higher) to buff the product, and smoothly blend it into new growth area without damaging the natural nail plate.
6. **Blend areas of lifting.** Use a medium-abrasive (180 to 240 grit) file to smooth out any areas of product that may be lifting or forming pockets. Do not file into the natural nail plate.
7. **Clean nail enhancements.** Use a fingerbowl filled with warm water and liquid soap and a nail brush to gently wash nails. Do not soak nails. Rinse well with clean water to remove soap residues that may cause lifting.
8. **Push back eponychium and carefully remove cuticle from the nail plate.** Use a cotton-tipped wooden or metal pusher to gently push back the eponychium, and then apply cuticle remover. Use as directed by the manufacturer, and carefully remove cuticle tissue from the nail plate.
9. **Remove oily shine from natural nail surface.** Lightly buff the nail plate with medium-fine abrasive (240 grit) to remove the natural oil.
10. **Apply nail dehydrator.** Apply nail dehydrator to nails with cotton-tipped wooden or metal pusher, plastic-backed cotton pad, brush, or spray.

11. **Apply nail primer.** Apply nail primer as previously described, and follow manufacturer's directions. Allow primer to dry thoroughly. Avoid applying nail enhancement product over wet primer, since this can cause product discoloration and service breakdown. Avoid overusing nail primer.
12. **Prepare acrylic (methacrylate) liquid and powder.** Pour acrylic (methacrylate) liquid and powder into separate dappen dishes.
13. **Place beads of enhancement product.** Pick up one or more small pink powder beads of enhancement product and place them on the new growth area. Only pink or natural powder is required if nail polish is to be worn.
14. **Shape beads of enhancement product.** Use the middle of the brush to press and smooth the product into place.
15. **Place beads of enhancement product.** Pick up one or more small beads of pink powder and place them at the center of the nail plate.
16. **Shape beads of enhancement product.** Use the brush to smooth these beads over the entire nail enhancement. Glide the brush over the nail to smooth out imperfections. Enhancement product application near the eponychium, side wall areas, and free edge must be extremely thin for a natural-looking nail. If you are using a two-color product, use the pink powder in this step. Carefully push a product up against the edge of the newly re-created white smile line. Be sure to leave a tiny free margin between the nail enhancement product and skin.
17. **Shape nail enhancements.** Allow the nails to harden. Nails are hard when they make a clicking sound when lightly tapped with a brush handle. Use a coarse-medium grit abrasive (120 to 180 grit) to shape the free edge and apex, and remove any imperfections. Use medium-fine abrasive to glide over the nail enhancement with long sweeping strokes to further shape and perfect the nail surface. Taper the nail shape toward the eponychium, free edge, and side walls, making it thin at all edges.
18. **Buff nail enhancement.** Smooth the entire surface of the nail using a fine buffer (350 grit or higher) until it is smooth. Use a high-shine buffer, if desired, and nail polish will not be worn.
19. **Apply nail oil.** Apply nail oil into surrounding skin and nail enhancement surface using a cotton-tipped wooden pusher or eyedropper, and massage briefly to speed penetration.
20. **Apply hand cream and massage hand and arm.**
21. **Thoroughly clean nail enhancements.**
22. **Apply nail polish.**
23. **Complete acrylic (methacrylate) nail enhancement application post-service as seen on page 762.**

CAUTION

Do not use a nipper to clip away loose nail enhancement product. Nipping may perpetuate the lifting problem and can damage the nail plate. If lifting is excessive, soak off the enhancement and start fresh with a new nail application.

ACRYLIC (METHACRYLATE) NAIL ENHANCEMENT CRACK REPAIR

1. **Complete acrylic (methacrylate) nail application pre-service on page 756.**
2. **Remove existing polish.**
3. **File crack in nail enhancement.** File a "V" shape into the crack or file flush to remove crack.
4. **Clean nail enhancements.** Ask client to wash hands with liquid soap. Thoroughly rinse nails in clean water to remove soap residues that may cause lifting. Dry thoroughly with a clean disposable towel.
5. **Apply nail dehydrator.** Apply nail dehydrator to nails using a cotton-tipped wooden pusher, plastic-backed cotton pad, brush, or spray.
6. **Apply nail primer.** Apply nail primer as previously instructed, following all the manufacturer's instructions and precautions.
7. **Apply nail form.** If the crack is large, apply a nail form for added support.
8. **Prepare monomer liquid and polymer powder.** Pour liquid and powder into separate dappen dishes.
9. **Place beads of enhancement product.** Pick up one or more small beads of product, and apply them to the cracked area. If you are using the two-color system, be sure to use the correct color of polymer powder.
10. **Shape beads of enhancement product.** Press and smooth the enhancement product to fill the crack. Be careful not to let the product seep under form.
11. **Place additional beads of enhancement product.** Apply additional beads, if needed, to fill in the crack or reinforce the rest of the nail. Shape the enhancement and allow it to harden.
12. **Remove the form (if used).**
13. **Reshape nail enhancement using a medium abrasive (180 to 240 grit).**
14. **Buff until smooth.** Use a fine abrasive (350 grit or higher). Use a high-shine buffer, if desired.
15. **Clean nail enhancements.**
16. **Apply nail oil to skin and enhancement, and massage in for more rapid penetration.**
17. **Apply hand cream and massage hand and arm.**
18. **Clean nail enhancements thoroughly.**
19. **Apply nail polish.**
20. **Complete acrylic (methacrylate) enhancement application post-service on page 762.**

PROCEDURE 28-5

ACRYLIC (METHACRYLATE) NAIL ENHANCEMENT REMOVAL

1. **Fill bowl with acetone or manufacturer-recommended product remover.** Fill glass bowl with enough acetone or product remover to cover higher than client's enhancements.
2. **Soak nail enhancements.** Soak client's nail enhancements for 20 to 30 minutes, or as long as needed to remove the enhancement product. Refer to the manufacturer's directions and precautions for nail enhancement product removal.
3. **Remove nail enhancement.** Use a wooden or metal pusher to gently push off the softened nail. Repeat until all have been removed. Do not pry off with nippers, as this will damage the natural nail plate. Avoid removing enhancements from the acetone or product remover, or they will quickly re-harden, making them more difficult to remove.
4. **Buff natural nails.** Gently buff natural nail with a fine buffer (350 grit or higher) to remove product residue. Do not thin or damage the natural nail by over-buffing.
5. **Condition skin.** Condition surrounding skin with hand lotion.

Here's a TIP

Nail plates may appear to be thinner after enhancements have been removed. This is generally because there is more moisture in the natural nail plate, which makes them more flexible. It is not an indication that the nail plates have been weakened by the nail enhancement. This excess flexibility will be lost as the natural nails lose moisture over the next 24 hours, and the nail plates will seem to be more rigid and thick.

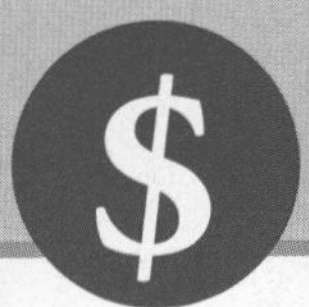

BUSINESS TIP: CELEBRATE THE HOLIDAYS

Take advantage of gift-giving holidays such as Christmas, Chanukah, St. Valentine's Day, Secretary's Day, and Mother's Day to provide your customers with professional products that were designed for you to retail. It's easy to make lots of extra money during the holidays. Decorate festively to encourage clients to consider shopping for presents, and offer a wide range of gifts that customers can conveniently buy while they are in the salon for appointments. Try creating two or three festive packages with different product combinations and sizes, priced from $5.00 to $15.00. People buy these for stocking stuffers or to give them as office or church/synagogue gifts. They will thank you for making their shopping easier and for your professional product recommendations. Also, don't forget to offer gift certificates in all denominations.

Although these products are called "odorless," they do have a slight odor. Generally, if a monomer liquid does not produce a strong enough odor that others in the salon can detect its presence, it is considered to be an "odorless product." Those that create a slight odor in the salon are called "low odor."

In general, odorless products must be used with a dry mix ratio (equal parts liquid and powder in bead). If used too wet, the risk of the client developing skin irritation or sensitivity will increase. This mix ratio creates a "snowy-appearing" bead on your brush. Multiple circular motions in the powder with a brush may be needed to create a bead with the proper mix ratio. Lift your brush and tap gently to remove excess powder from the product bead. Once the product bead is placed on the nail, it will slowly form into a firm glossy bead that will hold its shape until pressed and smoothed with the nail brush. Wipe your brush frequently to avoid the product sticking to the hairs. Never re-wet the brush with monomer. This will dilute the enhancement product already placed on the nail and will create the wrong mix ratio, which can lead to product discoloration, service breakdown, and increased risk of skin irritation and sensitivity. Without re-wetting your brush, use it to shape and smooth the surface to perfection.

Odorless products harden more slowly, which creates the tacky layer called the "inhibition layer." Once the enhancement has hardened, this layer can be removed using alcohol, acetone, or a manufacturer-recommended product. It is always best to use a plastic-backed cotton pad to avoid skin contact with the inhibition layer, since repeated contact with this layer can lead to skin irritation and sensitivity. This layer can also be filed away, but avoid skin contact with these freshly filed particles.

COLORED ACRYLIC (METHACRYLATE) POWDERS

Polymer powders are now available in a wide range of colors that mimic almost every shade available in nail polish. Nail artistry with acrylic (methacrylate) nails is limited only by your imagination. Some cosmetologists use colors to go beyond the traditional pink and white French manicure combinations and offer custom blended colors to their clients. They maintain recipe cards so that they can reproduce these custom blends on demand. This new technique allows cosmetologists to create customized nail enhancements that your clients cannot get from anyone else. As with all customized techniques, clients are willing to pay a few dollars more for the special service.

REVIEW QUESTIONS

1. Describe the origin of acrylic nail chemistry and what makes it work.
2. List the supplies needed for nail enhancement application.
3. Describe the procedures for application of nail enhancements using forms and using tips, and as an overlay on natural nails.
4. Describe precautions that must be taken to safely apply acid-based nail primers. What must be avoided?
5. Describe how catalysts work and explain where they are found in acrylic (methacrylate) nail enhancement systems.
6. Describe how accelerators work and explain where they are found in acrylic (methacrylate) nail enhancement systems.
7. Describe how to perform a rebalance on nail enhancements using monomer liquid and polymer powder.
8. Describe the proper procedure for removing nail enhancements.
9. Explain how the application of odorless enhancement products differs from the application of traditional acrylic (methacrylate) nail products based on ethyl acrylic (methacrylate).
10. Explain why it is important to use the powder that was designed for the liquid monomer that you are using.

CHAPTER GLOSSARY

acrylic (methacrylate) monomer liquid	The liquid that will be combined with acrylic (methacrylate) polymer powder to form the sculptured nail.
acrylic (methacrylate) nail enhancements	Created by combining acrylic (methacrylate) monomer liquid with polymer powder.
acrylic (methacrylate) polymer powder	Powder in white, clear, pink, and many other colors that will be combined with acrylic (methacrylate) monomer liquid to form the sculptured nail.
catalyst	Substance that speeds up chemical reactions between monomer liquid and polymer powder.
chain reaction	Process that joins monomers to create very long polymer chains; also called "polymerization reaction."
dappen dish	A special container used to hold the monomer liquid and polymer powder.
dust masks and protective gloves	Designed to be worn over the nose and mouth to prevent inhalation of excessive amounts of dusts.
initiators	Energized and activated by catalyst; initiators start the chain reaction.
mix ratio	The amount of monomer liquid and polymer powder used to create a bead.
nail dehydrator	Substance used to remove surface moisture and tiny amounts of oil left on the natural nail plate, both of which can block adhesion.
nail forms	Often made of paper/mylar coated with adhesive backs, or pre-shaped plastic or aluminum; placed under the free edge and used to extend the nail enhancements beyond the fingertip for additional length.
nail primer	Used to enhance the adhesion of enhancements to the natural nail.
odorless acrylic (methacrylate) products	Nail enhancement products that are slightly different from acrylic (methacrylate) products, and are considered "no odor" or "low odor."
polymer	Substance formed by combining many small molecules (monomers) into very long chain-like structures.
polymerization	Chemical reaction that creates polymers; also called curing or hardening.
rebalancing	Method for maintaining the beauty, durability, and longevity of the nail enhancement.
safety eyewear	Used to protect eyes from flying objects or accidental splashes.

CHAPTER 29 UV GELS

chapter outline

Learning Objectives

After completing this chapter, you will be able to:

- **Describe the chemistry and main ingredients of UV gels.**
- **Identify the supplies needed for UV gel application.**
- **Demonstrate the proper procedures for maintaining UV gel services using forms over tips and on natural nails.**
- **Describe the one-color and two-color methods for applying UV gels.**
- **Explain how to safely and correctly remove UV gels.**

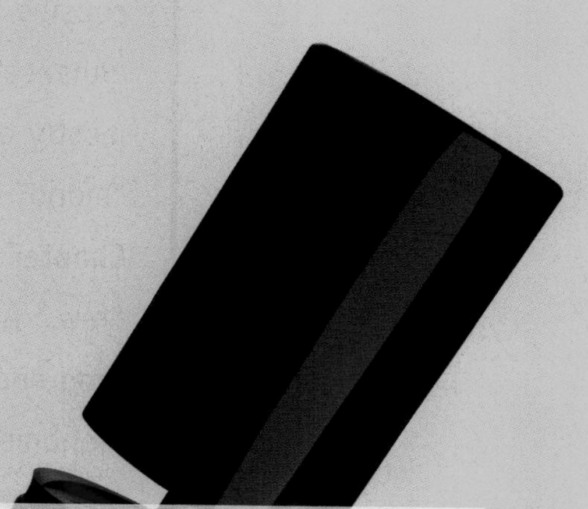

Key Terms

Page number indicates where in the chapter the term is used.

inhibition layer
pg. 781

oligomer
pg. 776

one-color method
pg. 780

two-color method
pg. 780

urethane acrylate or *urethane methacrylate*
pg. 776

UV gels
pg. 776

UV gel primer
pg. 777

UV gel lamps
pg. 777

UV lightbulbs
pg. 777

wattage
pg. 777

This chapter introduces **UV gels** as an alternative method for an artificial nail enhancement service. Nail enhancements based on UV curing chemistry are not traditionally thought of as being "acrylics," but they are. Like wrap resins, adhesives, and methacrylate nail enhancements, UV gel enhancements rely on ingredients from the acrylic family. Their ingredients are part of a subcategory of this family and are called "acrylates," whereas wrap resins are from the subcategory called "cyanoacrylates," and monomer liquid/polymer powder nail enhancements are from the same category called "methacrylates."

Although most UV gels are made from "acrylates," new UV gel technologies have been recently developed that use their cousins, the "methacrylates." Like wraps and methacrylate nail enhancements, UV gels can also contain monomers, but they rely mostly on a related form called an oligomer. Remember the terms "mono" meaning "one" and "poly" meaning "many" described in Chapter 28. Now we will add a new term, "oligo," which means "few." An **oligomer** is a short chain of monomers that is not long enough to be considered a polymer. Since nail enhancement monomers are liquids and polymers are solids, it is not surprising that oligomers are in between. Oligomers are often thick, gel-like, and sticky. Traditionally, UV gels rely on a special type of acrylate called a **urethane acrylate,** while newer UV gel systems use **urethane methacrylates.**

UV gels can be easy to apply, file, and maintain. They also have the advantage of having very little odor. Although they are not as durable as methacrylate nail enhancements, UV gels can create beautiful, long-lasting nail enhancements. The application process differs from other types of nail enhancements. After the nail plate is properly prepared, each layer of product applied to the natural nail, nail tip, or form requires exposure to UV light to cure or harden. The UV light required for curing comes from a special lamp designed to emit the proper type of UV light.

APPLICATION OF UV GEL NAIL ENHANCEMENTS

In addition to the materials in your basic manicuring setup, you will need the following items:

- **UV gel lamps.** UV gel lamps are designed to produce the correct amount of UV light needed to properly cure UV gel nail enhancement products. UV gels are usually packaged in small opaque pots or squeeze tubes to protect them from UV light. Even though UV light is invisible to the eye, it is found in sunlight and tanning lamps. Also, both "true-color" and "full-spectrum" bulbs emit a significant amount of UV light. If the UV gel product is exposed to these types of ceiling or table lamps, its shelf life may be shortened, causing the product to harden in its container.

It is important to know that wattage does not indicate how much UV light a UV lamp will emit. **Wattage** is a measure of how much electricity the bulb consumes, much like miles per gallon tell you how much gasoline it will take to drive your car a certain distance. Miles per gallon will not tell you how fast the car can go, just like wattage does not indicate how much UV light a lamp will produce. Depending on their circuitry, different lamps and bulbs produce greatly differing amounts of UV light. For these reasons, it is important to use the UV lamp that was designed for the selected UV gel product. Use the lamp that was specifically designed for that UV gel product and you will have a much greater chance of success and fewer problems.

- **UV lightbulbs.** UV lightbulbs will stay blue for years, but after a few months of use they may produce too little UV light to properly cure the enhancement. Typically, UV bulbs must be changed two or three times per year, depending on use of the UV lamp. If bulbs are not changed regularly, service breakdown, skin irritation, and sensitivity become more likely to occur.

For more interesting and useful information about UV gel enhancement products, see *Nail Structure and Product Chemistry,* second edition, by Douglas Schoon (Thomson Delmar Learning, 2005).

- **Brush.** Synthetic brushes with small, flat, square bristles to hold and spread the UV gel.
- **UV gel primer.** Primers are designed specifically to improve adhesion of UV gels to the natural nail plate. Use UV gel primers as instructed by the manufacturer of the UV gel product that you are using and heed all recommendations and precautions.
- **Nail tips.** Use nail tips recommended for use with UV gel nail enhancement systems.
- **Nail dehydrator.** Removes surface moisture and tiny amounts of oil left on the natural nail plate, both of which can block adhesion. This step is a great way to help prevent lifting of nail enhancements.

- **Nail adhesive.** There are many types of nail adhesives for securing preformed nail tips to natural nails. Select a type best suited for the work that you are doing. For example, do not purchase large-size containers, unless you can use them up fairly quickly. Even though you can usually save money by purchasing professional products in bulk amounts, nail adhesives only have a shelf life of 6 months or less, depending on your usage. One way to improve shelf life is to close the cap securely, and store at 60° to 85° Fahrenheit.
- **Abrasive files and buffers.** Select a medium abrasive (180 to 240 grit) for natural nail preparation. Choose a medium-fine abrasive (240 grit) for smoothing, and a fine buffer (350 grit or higher) for finishing. A high-shine buffer can also be used if desired, and nail polish is not to be worn.

UV GEL APPLICATION PRE-SERVICE

1. **Complete the pre-service sanitation and disinfection procedure in Chapter 25.**
2. **Prepare your workstation with everything you need at your fingertips.** Set up your standard manicuring table. Add the additional supplies needed to perform the services to your table. Always have enough supplies to prevent running out while performing the service.
3. **Greet your client with a smile.** Then ask the client to wash hands with liquid soap and rinse with warm running water. You must also wash your hands. Both you and the client must dry hands thoroughly with a clean disposable towel.
4. **If this is your client's first appointment, a client consultation form should be prepared.** Mark the date of the service. This is important in the scheduling of future appointments. Record any skin or nail disorders and allergies, and determine if it is safe and appropriate to perform this service on the client. If the client is a nail biter or does heavy work as a daily routine, write a brief notation. Record any specific information about the service you will perform, such as UV gel overlay without polish, and if polish is preferred, record the client's color preference. This will help keep you in touch with your client's needs.
5. **If this is a return visit, perform client consultation, using the consultation form to record responses and observations.** Check for nail disorders and decide whether it is safe and appropriate to perform a service on this client. If the client cannot receive a service, explain your reasons and refer the client to a doctor, if appropriate.

LIGHT-CURED GEL APPLICATION

After completing the pre-service steps, use Procedure 29-1 to apply light-cured gel enhancements.

PROCEDURE 29-1

LIGHT-CURED GEL APPLICATION

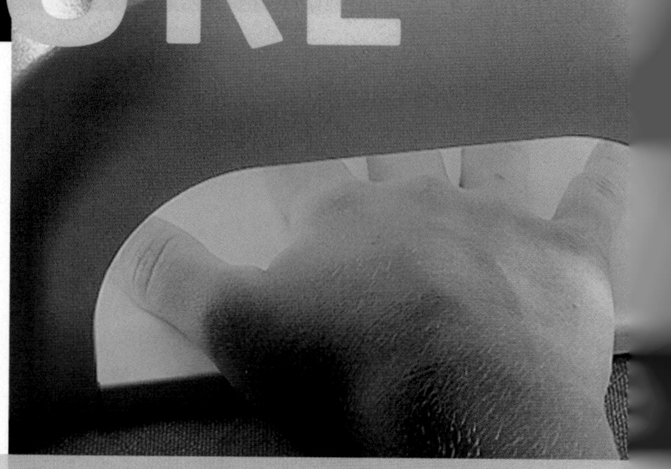

1. **Clean nails and remove existing polish.** Begin with your client's little finger on the left hand, and work toward the thumb. Then repeat on the right hand. Ask the client to place nails into a finger bowl with liquid soap. Then use a nail brush to clean nails over the fingerbowl. Thoroughly rinse with clean water to remove soap residues that can cause lifting.
2. **Push back eponychium and carefully remove cuticle from the nail plate.** Use a cotton-tipped wooden or metal pusher to gently push back eponychium, and then apply cuticle remover to the nail plate. Use as directed by the manufacturer, and carefully remove cuticle tissue from the nail plate.
3. **Remove oily shine from natural nail surface.** Lightly buff nail plate with medium-fine (240-grit) abrasive to remove the natural oils that cause the shine on the surface of the nail plate.
4. **Apply nail dehydrator.** Apply nail dehydrator to nails with cotton-tipped wooden pusher, plastic-backed cotton pad, brush, or spray. Begin with the little finger on the left hand and work toward the thumb (Figures 29-1 and 29-2).
5. **Apply nail tips if desired.** If your client requires nail tips, apply them according to the procedure described in Chapter 27. Be sure to shorten and shape tip prior to application of the UV gel. During the procedure, the UV gel overlaps the tip's edge to prevent lifting. During the filing process, the seal can be broken, allowing the UV gel to peel or lift. Be careful not to break this seal (Figure 29-3).

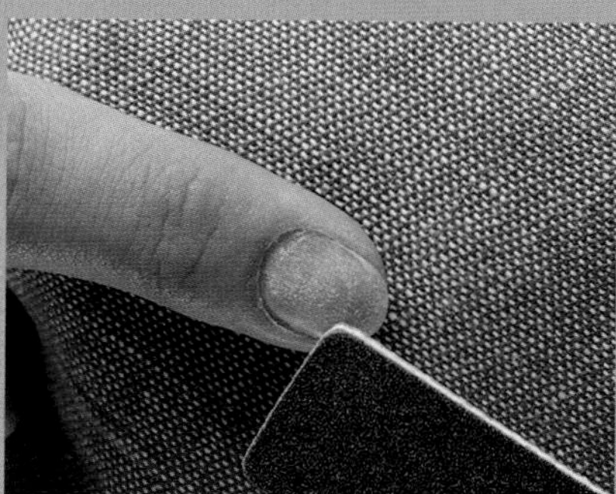

Figure 29-1 Remove oily shine from natural nail using vertical strokes.

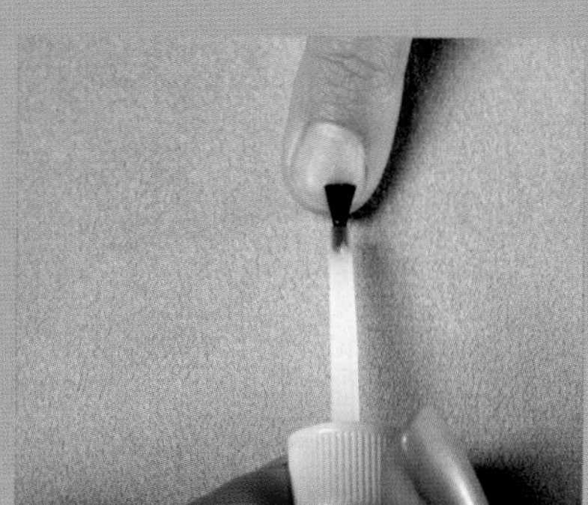

Figure 29-2 Apply nail plate dehydrator.

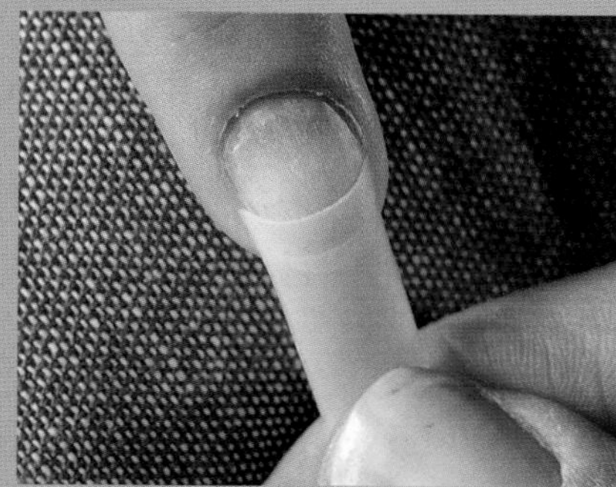

Figure 29-3 Select nail tip for proper fit, and then trim and shape prior to UV gel application.

6. **Natural nail preparation.** Follow the manufacturer's instructions for natural nail preparation. Your success as a professional depends on your ability to properly prepare the nail plate for services. This is a very important step, so do it well. Insert the applicator brush into the nail primer. Wipe off excess from brush, and using a slightly damp brush, ensure that the nail plate is completely covered. Avoid using too much product to prevent running into the skin, which can increase the risks of developing skin irritation or sensitivity (Figure 29-4).
7. **Apply first UV gel (base coat gel).** Firmly brush UV gel onto entire nail surface including free edge. Keep UV gel from touching the eponychium or side walls. Leave a tiny free margin between the UV gel enhancement product and the skin to reduce the risk of the client developing skin irritation or sensitivity. Apply to client's left hand from pinky to pointer (Figure 29-5). If performing a **one-color method—**that is, nail polish will be worn—you may use a clear, or natural color UV gel. If performing a **two-color method,** you should use a pink or natural color UV gel at this stage.
8. **Cure first UV gel (base coat gel).** Properly position the hand in the UV lamp for the required cure time as defined by the manufacturer (Figure 29-6). Always cure each layer of the UV gel for the time required by the manufacturer's instructions. Curing for too little time can result in service breakdown, skin irritation, and/or sensitivity. Improper positioning of the hands inside the lamp can also cause improper curing.
9. **Repeat steps 7 and 8 on the right hand.** Then repeat the same steps for both thumbs.
10. **Apply second UV gel (building UV gel).** Apply a small amount of UV gel over the properly cured first layer. Carefully pull the UV gel across the first layer, and smooth it into place. Avoid patting the brush or pressing too hard. Brush the UV gel over and around the free edge to create a seal. Avoid touching the skin under the free edge to prevent

a TIP

The procedure recommended for applying curing UV gel varies from one manufacturer to anot Some systems recommend applying UV gel to four one hand and curing, and then repeating this proce the other hand before applying and curing UV gel o thumbnails. Be sure to follow the instructions recon by the manufacturer of the system that you are usi

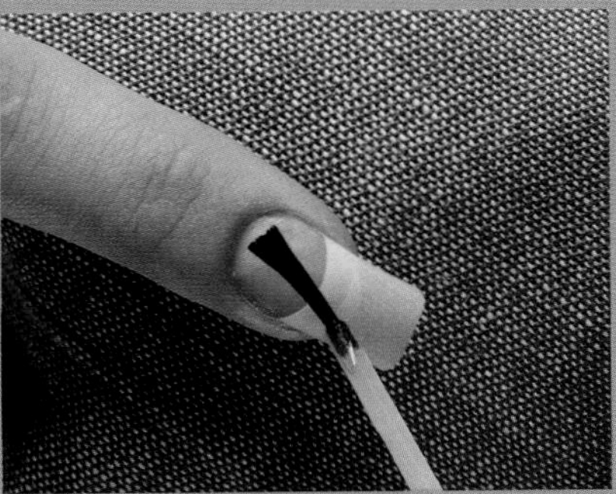

Figure 29-4 Carefully apply nail primer to the natural nail and avoid skin contact.

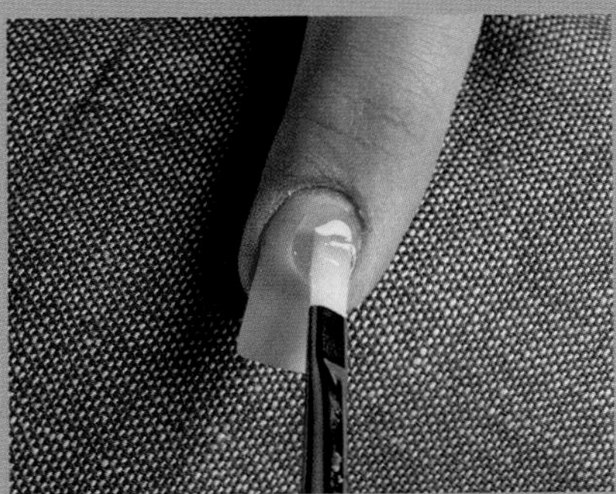

Figure 29-5 Apply first UV gel (base coat UV gel).

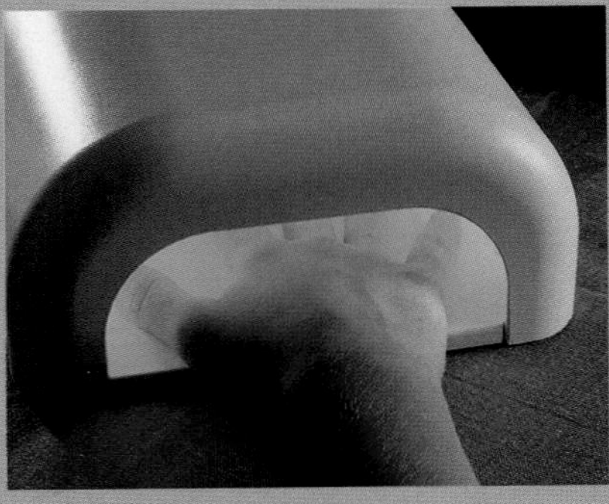

Figure 29-6 Cure in UV lamp for the required time.

skin irritation and sensitivity. Repeat this application process for the other four nails on the client's left hand from pinky to pointer. If performing a one-color method, you will use the same colored UV gel as before. If performing a two-color method, use white gels to create a smile line at the free edge. Then apply pink UV gel over remainder of the nail plate, leaving a tiny free margin between the UV gel and skin.

11. **Cure second UV gel (builder UV gel).** Properly position the hand in the UV lamp for the manufacturer's required cure time.
12. **Repeat steps 10 and 11 on the right hand, and then repeat the same steps for both thumbs.**
13. If required, another layer of the second UV gel (builder UV gel) may be applied. Repeat steps 11 and 12 for both hands (Figures 29-7 and 29-8).
14. **Remove inhibition layer.** UV gels cure with a tacky surface called an **inhibition layer.** This layer can be removed by filing with a medium abrasive (180 to 240 grit) or with alcohol, acetone, or other suitable remover on a plastic-backed cotton pad to avoid skin contact. Prolonged or repeated skin contact with the inhibition layer may cause skin irritation or sensitivity. Avoid placing your arm in fresh filings from UV gel enhancements (Figure 29-9).
15. **Check nail contours.** UV gel nails are softer, so they file very easily. Using a medium abrasive (180 to 240 grit), refine the surface contour. File carefully near the side walls and eponychium to avoid injuring the client's skin (Figure 29-10).

Here's a TIP

During the procedure, keep the brush and UV gel away from sunlight, UV gel lamps, and full-spectrum table lamps to prevent them from hardening.

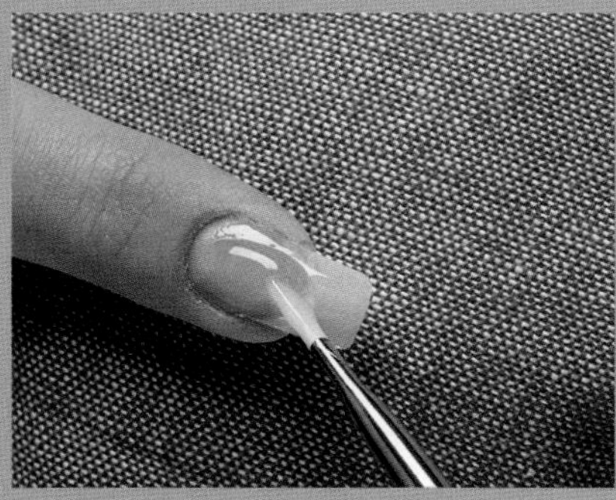

Figure 29-7 Apply second UV gel (building UV gel).

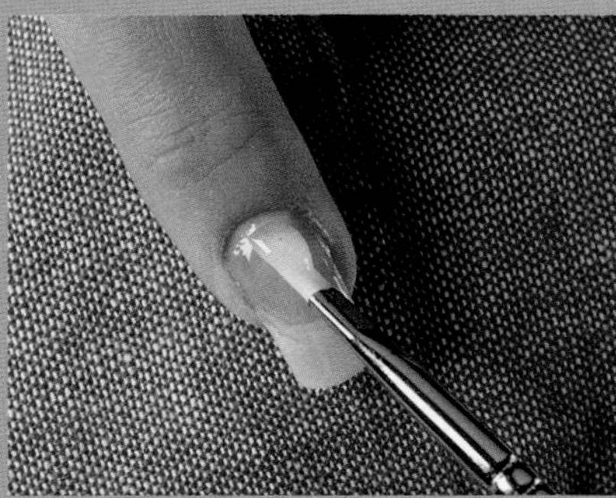

Figure 29-8 Dispense a smaller amount of UV gel.

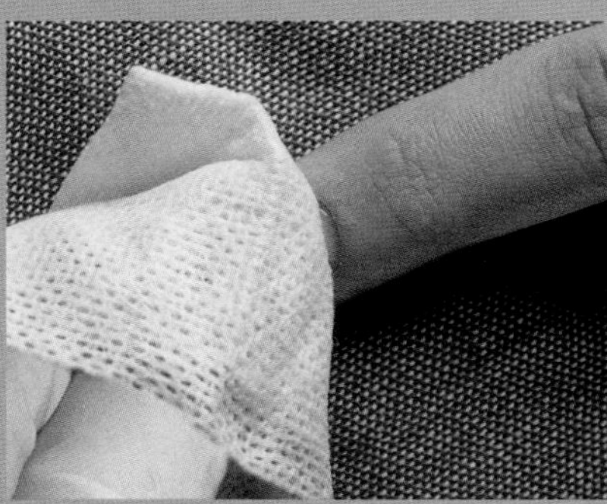

Figure 29-9 Remove inhibition layer with plastic-backed cotton pad.

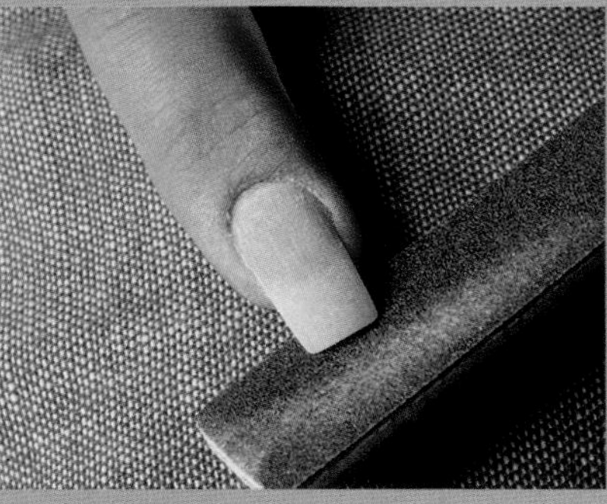

Figure 29-10 File, shape, and contour entire surface.

Bevel down, stroking the file at a 45-degree angle from the top center dome to free edge. Check the free edge thickness and even out imperfections with gentle strokes with the abrasive.

16. **Remove dust.** Remove dust and filings with a disinfectable nylon brush. Be sure to properly clean and disinfect these brushes between each client, as required by your state regulations. Your instructor will advise you about these requirements (Figure 29-11).

17. **Apply third UV gel (sealer or finisher UV gel).** Apply a small amount of the third UV gel (sealer or finisher UV gel). Starting from base of the nail plate, stroke toward the free edge, using polish-style strokes and covering the entire nail surface. Be sure to wrap this final layer under the natural nail's free edge to seal the coating and provide additional protection. Avoid touching the client's skin.

18. **Repeat step 11, then continue on right hand and both thumbs.**

19. **Remove the inhibition layer.** Remove this layer if required. Avoid skin contact.

20. **Apply nail oil.** Rub nail oil into surrounding skin and nail surface (Figure 29-12).

21. **Apply hand lotion and massage hand and arm.**

22. **Clean nail enhancements.** Ask the client to dip nail enhancements into a fingerbowl filled with liquid soap. Then use nail brush to clean enhancements over fingerbowl. Thoroughly rinse with water to remove soap residues that can cause polish to lift. Dry thoroughly with a clean disposable towel.

23. **Apply nail polish** (Figure 29-13).

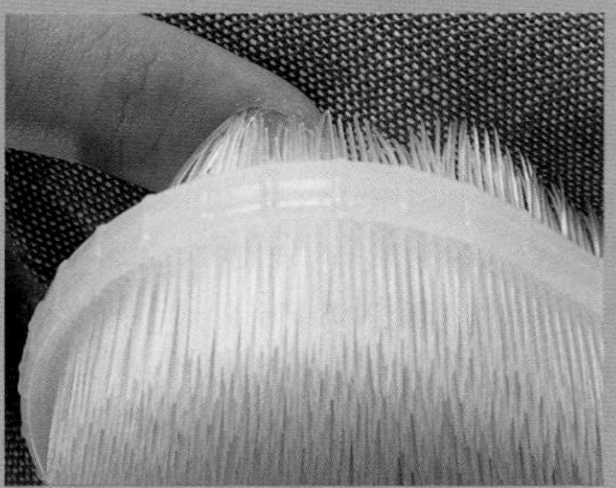

Figure 29-11 Remove dust and filings with a disinfectable nylon brush.

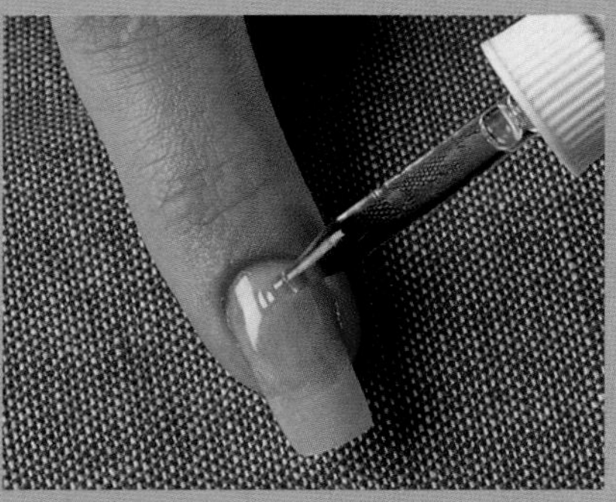

Figure 29-12 Apply nail oil and massage into nail to speed penetration.

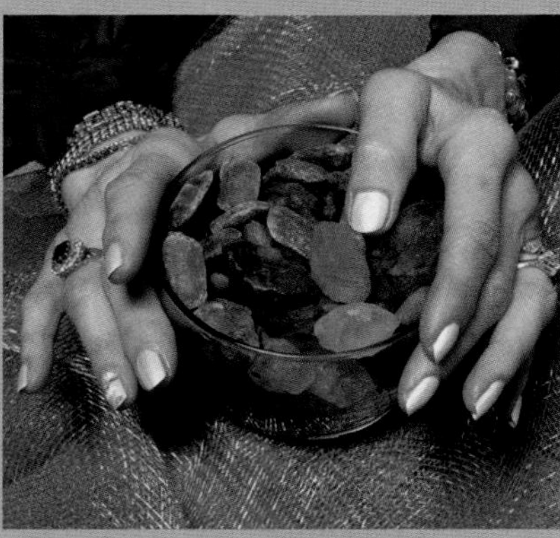

Figure 29-13 Apply polish for finished look.

UV GEL APPLICATION POST-SERVICE

Your UV gel service is complete. Follow the post-service procedure described below.

1. **Make another appointment.** Schedule another appointment with the client to maintain nail enhancements. A rebalance will be necessary in 2 or 3 weeks, depending on how quickly the nails grow. Encourage your client to return for a basic manicure between rebalance appointments if the UV gel enhancements are polished.
2. **Recommend take-home products.** Suggest professional products that you believe your client would benefit from, such as polish, nail oil, top coat, and hand lotion, among others. These are valuable maintenance tools and they will appreciate your professional recommendation.
3. **Clean up around your table.** Take the time to restore the basic setup of your table, restock supplies, and make sure that all caps are tight.
4. **Clean brush.** Clean brush according to manufacturer's instructions. Keeping it away from UV light sources will make cleaning much easier and will prevent you from ruining your brush.
5. **Discard used materials.** Dispose of waste materials. After all used materials have been collected, seal them in a plastic bag and discard it in a self-closing waste receptacle. It is important to remove items soiled with enhancement product from your manicuring station after each client. This will help maintain the quality of your salon's air. Dispose of these items according to your local rules and regulations.
6. **Clean your table, and then clean and disinfect implements and multiuse tools, such as abrasives.** Perform complete pre-service sanitation and disinfection procedures. Implements need to be cleaned and disinfected before they can be used on the next client, and this procedure will take about 20 minutes.

UV GEL APPLICATION OVER FORMS

Some clients wish to lengthen nail enhancements beyond the free edge. Procedure 29-2 demonstrates the technique for achieving longer nail enhancements with UV gels.

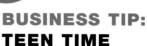

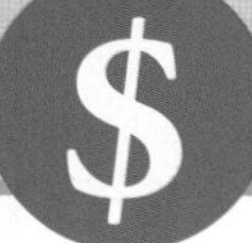

BUSINESS TIP: TEEN TIME

Take advantage of teenagers' interests in good grooming by introducing them to professional nail care. Some great promotion suggestions include a 20-percent discount on all prom and graduation nail services. Contact local schools to see when these events take place, and then spread the word by advertising the promotion in high school newspapers 6 to 8 weeks ahead of time.

Another option is to hold a "back-to-school night." Decorate the salon in fun colors, provide refreshments, and invite teens to pay a $10.00 registration fee for a night of nail education and fashion manicures, plus a take-home bag of trial-sized products. Many professionals report success with discounted nail extensions offered to the cheerleading squad, sports manicures to the volleyball team, or even a "good-grade discount" for any teen earning a 3.0 or higher grade point average.

MAINTENANCE AND REMOVAL OF UV GEL NAIL ENHANCEMENTS

UV gel enhancements must be rebalanced every 2 to 3 weeks as described previously in Chapter 28, depending on how fast the client's nails grow. Use a medium abrasive file (180 to 240 grit) to thin and shape the enhancement. Be careful not to damage the natural nail plate with the abrasive.

REMOVING UV GEL NAIL ENHANCEMENTS

Read and follow the manufacturer's recommended procedure to remove UV gel nails. UV gel enhancements can be more quickly removed by carefully reducing the thickness with a medium-coarse abrasive (120 to

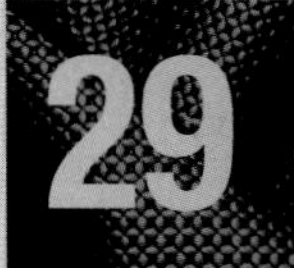

PROCEDURE 29-2

APPLICATION OF UV GEL OVER FORMS

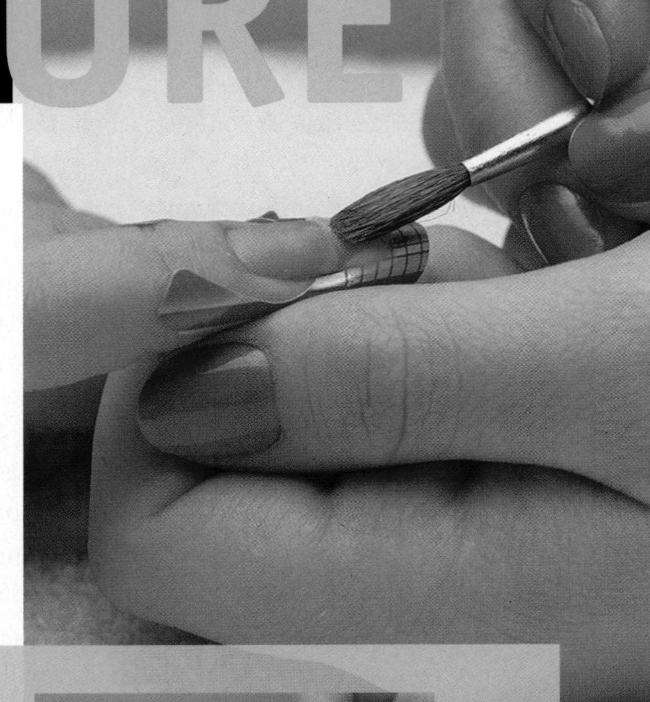

1. **Complete UV gel application pre-service.** Place UV gel supplies, including nail forms, on your manicuring table.
2. **Apply nail forms.** Fit forms onto all ten fingers just as described in Chapter 28. Remember to clean and disinfect multi-use forms, if disposable forms are not used. Clear plastic forms are sometimes used to allow UV light to penetrate from the underside for more complete curing of the free edge (Figure 29-14).
3. **Apply first UV gel (base coat UV gel).** Brush UV gel onto free edge of the form and create a free edge. Add more UV gel to cover the remainder of the natural nail. Keep UV gel from touching eponychium or side walls. Use the same color of gel that was previously used in this step.
4. **Cure first UV gel (base coat gel).** Properly position the hand in the UV lamp for the cure time required by the manufacturer (Figure 29-15). Always cure each layer of the UV gel for the time required by the manufacturer's instructions.
5. **Repeat steps 3 and 4 on the right hand.** Then repeat the same steps for both thumbs.
6. **Apply second UV gel (building UV gel).** Apply a small amount of UV gel over the properly cured first layer. Pull it across the first layer and smooth. Avoid touching the skin. Repeat this application process for the other four nails on the client's left hand from pinky to pointer. If performing a one-color method, you may use a clear, pink, or natural-color UV gel. If performing a two-color method, you should use a pink or natural-color UV gel over the nail bed area and a white UV gel to create a smile line.
7. **Properly position hand and cure UV gel for the required time.**
8. **Carefully remove nail forms.**
9. **Shape free edge.** Use a medium abrasive (180 to 240 grit) to shape the free edge of the enhancement.

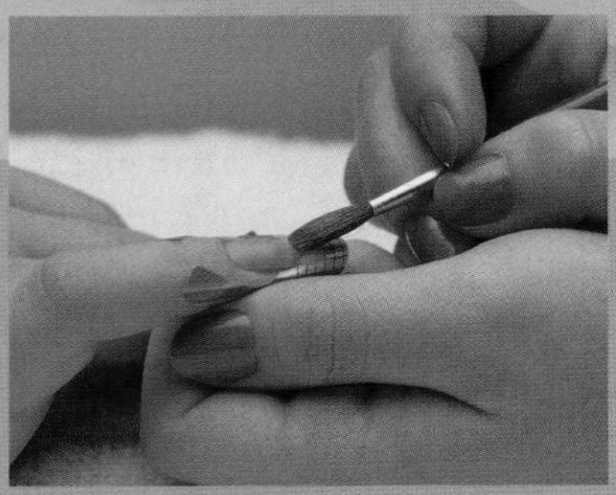

Figure 29-14 Apply UV gel to natural nail and form.

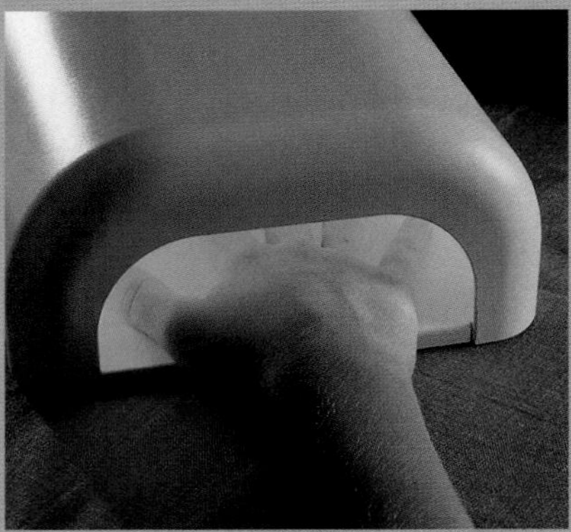

Figure 29-15 Cure UV gel as specified.

10. **Apply second UV gel (building UV gel).** If required, apply second UV gel over the entire nail enhancement and cure properly (Figure 29-16).
11. **Remove inhibition layer.** This layer can be removed by filing with a medium abrasive (180 and 240 grit) or with alcohol, acetone, or other suitable remover on a plastic-backed cotton pad to avoid skin contact. Avoid skin contact with the inhibition layer.
12. **Check nail contours.** Using a medium abrasive (180 to 240 grit), refine the surface contour.
13. **Remove dust.** Remove dust and filings with a disinfectable nylon brush.
14. **Apply third UV gel (sealer or finisher).** Apply a small amount of the third UV gel (sealer or finisher UV gel). Starting from the base of the nail plate, stroke toward the free edge using polish-style strokes, covering the entire nail surface. Be sure to wrap this final layer under the natural nail's free edge to seal the coating and provide additional protection. Avoid touching the client's skin underneath the free edge with UV gel.
15. **Cure UV nail.** Properly cure UV nail enhancement as recommended.
16. **Remove inhibition layer.** Remove this layer if required. Avoid skin contact.
17. **Repeat step 12.**
18. **Apply nail oil.** Rub nail oil into surrounding skin and nail surface.
19. **Apply hand lotion and massage hand and arm.**
20. **Clean nail enhancements.** Ask client to dip nails into a fingerbowl filled with liquid soap. Then use a nail brush to clean nails over the fingerbowl. Thoroughly rinse with water and dry thoroughly with a clean disposable towel.
21. **Apply nail polish if desired.**
22. **Complete UV gel application post-service.**

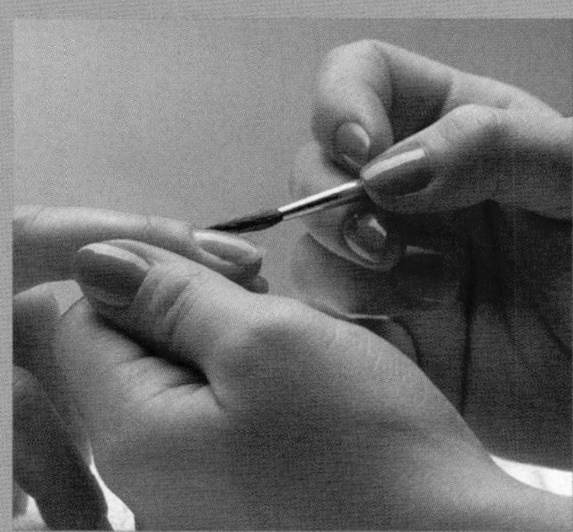

Figure 29-16 Apply UV gel to entire nail without nail form.

180 grit) before soaking in acetone or product remover. Once the enhancement begins to soften, gently scrape it from the nail plate with a wooden pusher.

Follow up with a gentle buffing of the natural nail using a fine buffer (350 grit or higher). This will remove product residue and smooth the nail plate. Condition surrounding skin with nail oil and lotion or follow with a manicure.

REVIEW QUESTIONS

1. Describe the chemistry of UV gel nail enhancements, and how they differ from other types of enhancements. How are their major ingredients different and how are they the same?
2. Identify the supplies needed for UV gel nail enhancement application.
3. Demonstrate the proper procedures for applying UV gel nail enhancements using forms.
4. Why is it important to use the proper UV lamp with the UV gel of your choice?
5. Explain how UV gels are safely and correctly removed.
6. What does wattage mean in terms of UV gel lights?
7. What is the tacky layer called on the surface of UV gel nails?
8. What precaution must be taken when removing a tacky layer from a UV gel nail?
9. What are oligomers and why are they important to UV gel nail enhancements?
10. What types of oligomers are used in UV gels?

CHAPTER GLOSSARY

inhibition layer	Tacky surface left on the nail once a UV gel has cured.
oligomer	Short chain of monomers that is not long enough to be considered a polymer.
one-color method	Gel is applied over the entire surface of the nail.
two-color method	Two different colors of gel are applied to the surface of the nail, in different places, as in a French manicure.
urethane acrylate **or** ***urethane methacrylate***	Main ingredient used to create UV gel nail enhancements.
UV lightbulbs	Special bulbs that emit UV light to cure UV gel nail enhancements.
UV gels	Types of nail enhancement products that harden when exposed to a UV light.
UV gel primer	Product designed specifically to improve adhesion of UV gels to the natural nail plate.
UV gel lamps	Specialized electronic devices that power and control UV lights to cure UV gel nail enhancements.
wattage	Measure of how much electricity a light bulb consumes.

BUSINESS SKILLS

PART 6

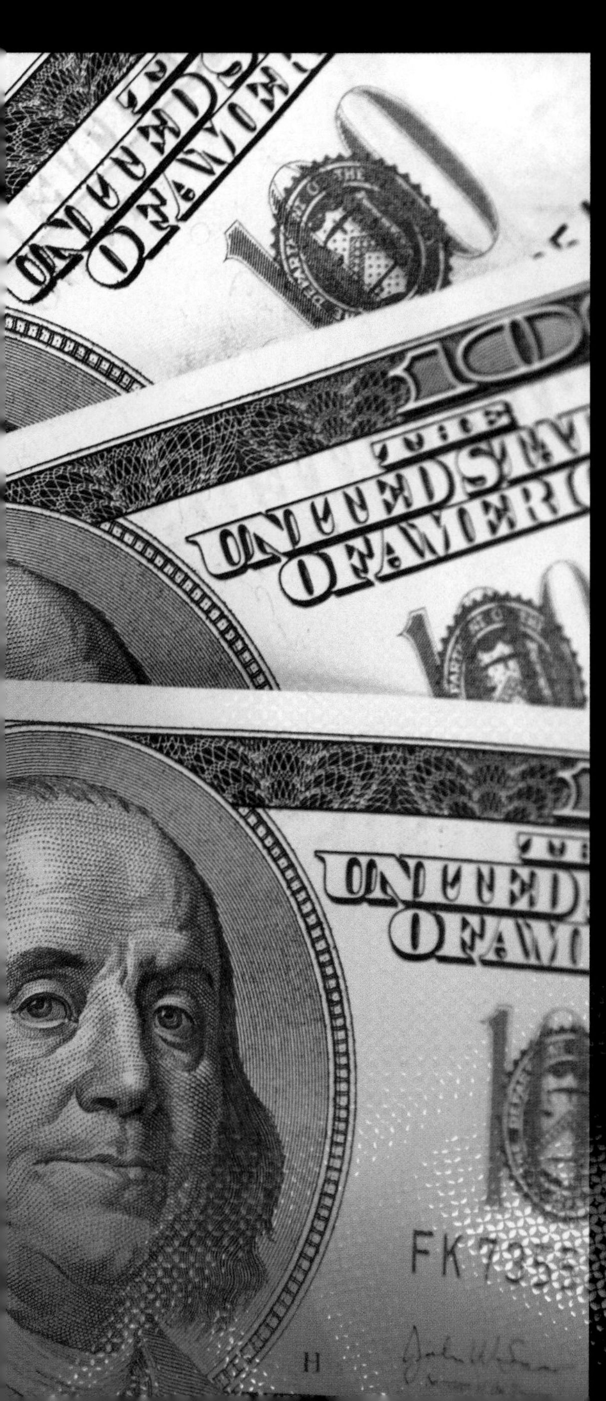

30

CHAPTER SEEKING EMPLOYMENT

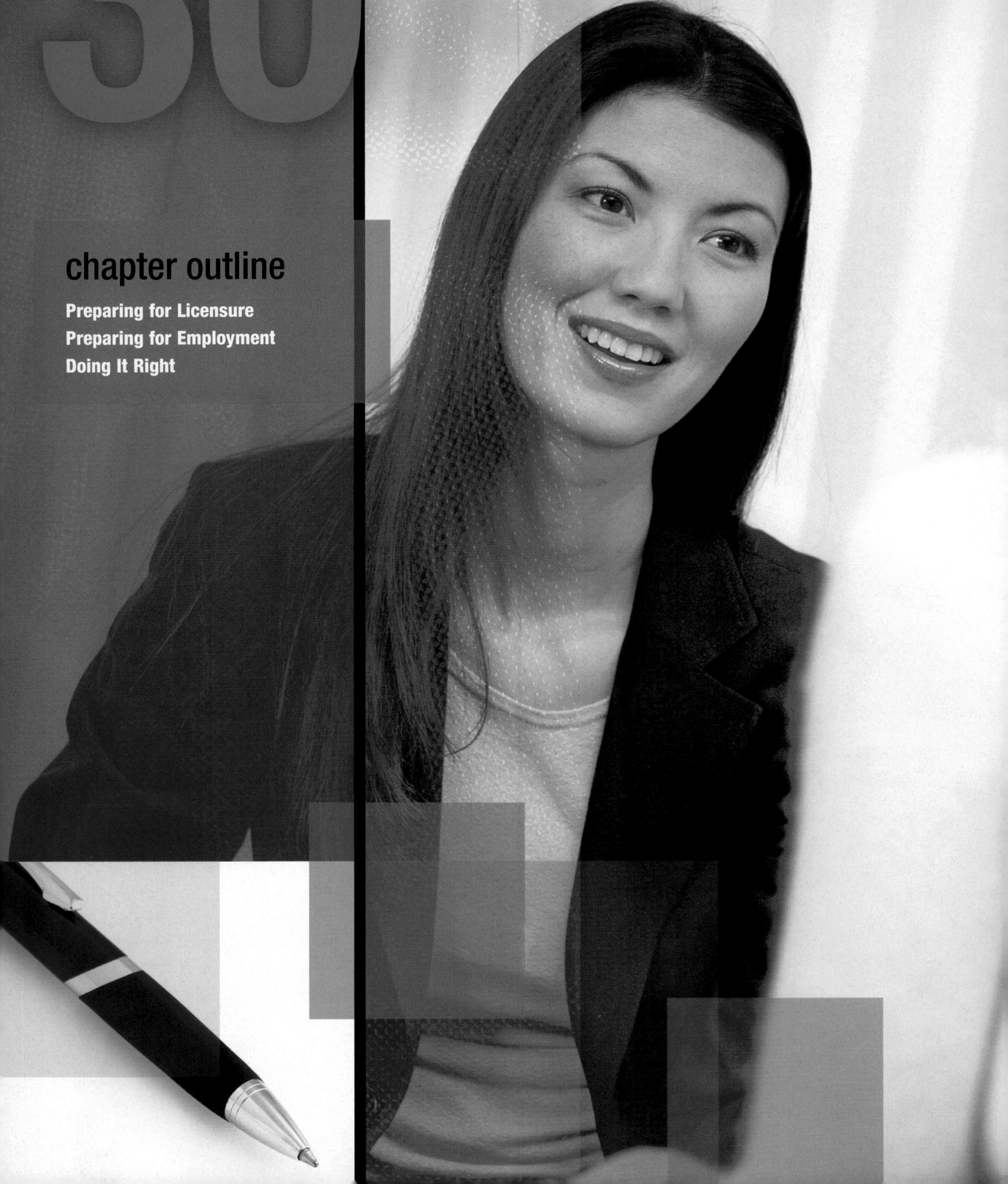

chapter outline

Preparing for Licensure
Preparing for Employment
Doing It Right

Learning Objectives

After completing this chapter, you will be able to:

- **Discuss the essentials of becoming test-wise.**
- **Explain the steps involved in preparing for employment.**
- **List and describe the various types of salon businesses.**
- **Write an achievement-oriented resume and prepare an employment portfolio.**
- **Explain how to explore the job market and research potential employers.**
- **Be prepared to complete an effective employment interview.**

Key Terms

Page number indicates where in the chapter the term is used.

deductive reasoning
pg. 794

employment portfolio
pg. 805

resume
pg. 801

test-wise
pg. 792

transferable skills
pg. 803

work ethic
pg. 799

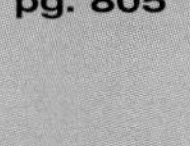

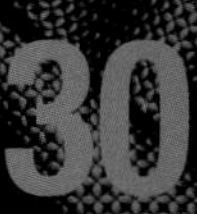

There are plenty of great jobs out there for energetic, hardworking, talented people. If you look at the top professionals in the field, you will find they were not born successful; they achieved success through self-motivation, energy, and persistence. Like you, these practitioners began their careers by enrolling in cosmetology school. They were the ones who used their time wisely, planned for the future, went the extra mile, and drew on a reservoir of self-confidence to meet any challenge. They owe their success to no one but themselves, because they created it. If you want to enjoy this same success, you must prepare for the opportunities that await you.

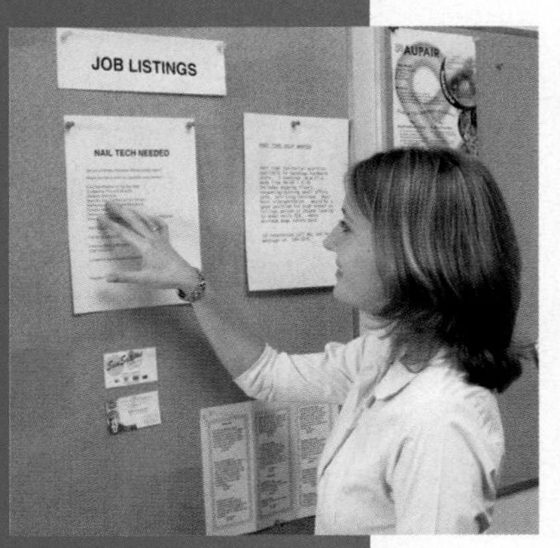

Figure 30-1 Job listings are often posted on the school bulletin board.

No matter what changes occur in the economy, there are often more jobs available for entry-level cosmetology professionals than there are people to fill them. This is a tremendous advantage for you. It does not mean, however, that you do not have to thoroughly research the job market in your chosen area before committing to your first job (Figure 30-1). If you make the right choice, your career will be on the road to success. If you make the wrong choice, it will not be a tragedy, but it may cause unnecessary delay.

PREPARING FOR LICENSURE

Before you can obtain the career position you are hoping for, you must first pass your state licensing examination and secure the required credentials. Many factors will affect how well you perform during that licensing examination and on tests in general. They include your physical and psychological state; your memory; time management; and the skills you have developed in reading, writing, note taking, test taking, and general learning.

Of all the factors that will affect your test performance, the most important is your mastery of course content. Even if you feel that you have truly learned the material, though, it is still very beneficial to have strong test-taking skills. Being **test-wise** means understanding the strategies for successfully taking tests.

PREPARING FOR THE TEST

A test-wise student begins to prepare for taking a test by practicing good study habits and time management that are such an important part of effective studying. These habits include the following:

- Having a planned, realistic study schedule
- Reading content carefully and becoming an active studier
- Keeping a well-organized notebook
- Developing a detailed vocabulary list
- Taking effective notes during class
- Organizing and reviewing handouts
- Reviewing past quizzes and tests
- Listening carefully in class for cues and clues about what could be expected on the test

In addition, there are other, more holistic (having to do with the "whole you") hints to keep in mind.

- Make yourself mentally ready and develop a positive attitude toward taking the test.
- Get plenty of rest the night before the test.
- Dress comfortably.
- Anticipate some anxiety (feeling concerned about the test results may actually help you do better).
- Avoid cramming the night before an examination.

ON TEST DAY

After you have taken all the necessary steps to prepare for your test, there are a number of strategies you can adopt on the day of the exam that may be helpful (Figure 30-2).

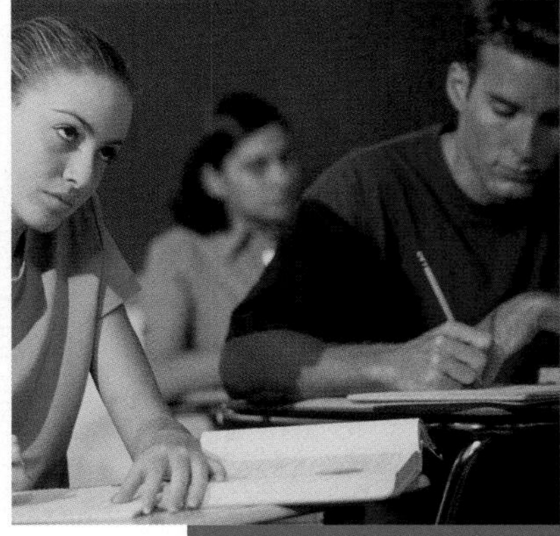

Figure 30-2 Candidates taking an in-house school exam.

1. Relax and try to slow down physically.
2. If possible, review the material lightly the day of the exam.
3. Arrive early with a self-confident attitude; be alert, calm, and ready for the challenge.
4. Read all written directions, and listen carefully to all verbal directions before beginning.
5. If there are things you do not understand, do not hesitate to ask the examiner questions.
6. Skim the entire test before beginning.
7. Budget your time to ensure that you have plenty of opportunity to complete the test; do not spend too much time on any one question.
8. Wear a watch so that you can monitor the time.
9. Begin work as soon as possible, and mark the answers in the test booklet carefully, but quickly.
10. Answer the easiest questions first in order to save time for the more difficult ones. Quickly scanning all the questions first may clue you in to the more difficult questions.
11. Mark the questions you skip so that you can find them again later.
12. Read each question carefully to make sure that you know exactly what the question is asking, and that you understand all parts of the question.

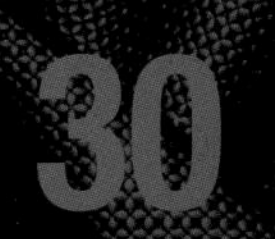

13. Answer as many questions as possible. For questions that you are unsure of, guess or estimate.
14. Look over the test when you are done to ensure that you have read all questions correctly, and have answered as many as possible.
15. Make changes to answers only if there is a good reason to do so.
16. Check the test booklet carefully before turning it in (for instance, you might have forgotten to put your name on it!).

DEDUCTIVE REASONING

Another technique that students should learn to use for better test results is called **deductive reasoning.** Deductive reasoning is the process of reaching logical conclusions by employing logical reasoning.

Some strategies associated with deductive reasoning follow.

Eliminate options known to be incorrect. The more answers you can eliminate as incorrect, the better your chances of identifying the correct one.

Watch for key words or terms. Look for any qualifying conditions or statements. Keep an eye out for such words and phrases as: **usually, commonly, in most instances, never, always**, and the like.

Study the stem (the basic question or problem). It will often provide a clue to the correct answer. Look for a match between the stem and one of the choices.

Watch for grammatical clues. For instance, if the last word in a stem is "an," the answer must begin with a vowel rather than a consonant.

Looking at similar or related questions. They may provide clues.

In answering essay questions, watch for words such as **compare, contrast, discuss, evaluate, analyze, define,** or **describe** and develop your answer accordingly.

In reading-type tests that contain long paragraphs followed by several questions, read the questions first. This will help identify the important elements in the paragraph.

UNDERSTANDING TEST FORMATS

There are a few additional tips that all test-wise learners should know, especially with respect to the state licensing examination. Keep in mind, of course, that the most important strategy of test taking is to **know your material.** With that said, however, consider the following tips on the various types of question formats.

TRUE/FALSE

- Watch for qualifying words **(all, most, some, none, always, usually, sometimes, never, little, no, equal, less, good, bad).** Absolutes **(all, none, always, never)** are generally *not* true.
- For a statement to be true, the *entire* statement must be true.
- Long statements are more likely to be true than short statements. It takes more detail to provide truthful, factual information.

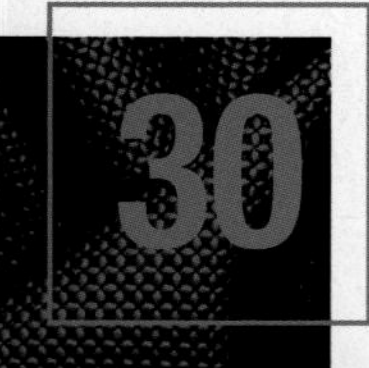

MULTIPLE CHOICE

- Read the entire question carefully, including all the choices.
- Look for the best answer; more than one choice may be true.
- Eliminate incorrect answers by crossing them out (if taking the test on the test form).
- When two choices are close or similar, one of them is probably right.
- When two choices are identical, both must be wrong.
- When two choices are opposites, one is probably wrong, and one is probably correct, depending on the number of other choices.
- "All of the above" types of responses are often the correct response.
- Pay special attention to words such as **not, except,** and **but**.
- Guess if you do not know the answer (provided that there is no penalty).
- The answer to one question may be in the stem of another (Figure 30-3).

MATCHING

- Read all items in each list before beginning.
- Check off items from the brief response list to eliminate choices.

FINAL EXAM

1. The study of the hair is called:
   a. hairology
   b. dermatology
   c. trichology
   d. biology

2. Hair is not found on the palms of the hands, soles of the feet, lips, and:
   a. neck
   b. eyelids
   c. ankles
   d. wrists

3. The technical term for eyelash hair is:
   a. cilia
   b. barba
   c. capilli
   d. supercilia

4. Hair is composed chiefly of:
   a. oxygen
   b. keratin
   c. melanin
   d. sulfur

5. The two main divisions of the hair are the hair root and:
   a. hair shaft
   b. follicle
   c. papilla
   d. bulb

6. The hair root is located:
   a. above the skin surface
   b. below the skin surface
   c. under the cuticle
   d. within the cortex

7. The hair root is encased by a tubelike depression in the skin known as the:
   a. bulb
   b. arrector pili
   c. papilla
   d. follicle

8. The club-shaped structure that forms the lower part of the hair root is the:
   a. arrector pili
   b. bulb
   c. papilla
   d. hair shaft

Figure 30-3 Sample of a multiple-choice test.

ESSAYS

- Organize your answer according to the cue words in the question.
- Think carefully and outline your answer before you begin writing.
- Make sure that what you write is complete, accurate, relevant to the question, well organized, and clear.

Remember that even though you may understand test formats and effective test-taking strategies, this does not take the place of having a complete understanding of the material on which you are being tested. In order to be successful at taking tests, you must follow the rules of effective studying and be thoroughly knowledgeable of the exam content for both the written and the practical examination.

In order to be better prepared for the practical portion of the examination, the new graduate should follow these tips:

- Practice the correct skills required in the test as often as you can.
- Participate in "mock" licensing examinations, including the timing of applicable examination criteria.
- Familiarize yourself with the content contained in the examination bulletins sent by the licensing agency.
- Make certain that all equipment and implements are clean, sanitary, and in good working order prior to the exam.
- If allowed by the regulatory or licensing agency, observe other practical examinations prior to taking yours.
- If possible, locate the examination site the day before the exam to ensure that you are on time for the actual exam.
- As with any exam, listen carefully to the examiner's instructions and follow them explicitly.
- Focus on your own knowledge, and do not allow yourself to be concerned with what other test candidates are doing.
- Follow all sanitation and safety procedures throughout the entire examination.

PREPARING FOR EMPLOYMENT

When you chose to enter the field of cosmetology, your primary goal was to find a good job after being licensed. Now you need to reaffirm that goal by reviewing a number of important questions.

- What do you really want out of a career in cosmetology?
- What particular areas within the beauty industry are the most interesting to you?
- What are your strongest practical skills, and in what ways do you wish to use them?
- What personal qualities will help you have a successful career?

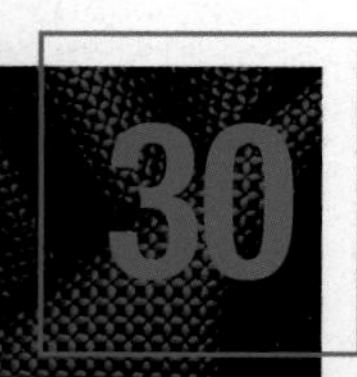

One way that you can answer these questions is to make a copy of, and then complete the Personal Inventory of Characteristics and Skills (Figure 30-4). After you have completed this inventory and identified the areas that need further attention, you can then determine where to focus the remainder of your training. In addition, you should have a better idea of what type of establishment would best suit you for your eventual employment.

During your training, you may have the opportunity to network with various industry professionals who are invited to be guest speakers. Be prepared to ask them questions about what they like least and most in their current positions. Ask them for any tips they might have that will assist you in your search for the right establishment. In addition, be sure to take advantage of your institution's in-house placement assistance program when you begin your employment search (Figure 30-5).

Your willingness to work hard is a key ingredient to your success. The commitment you make now in terms of time and effort will pay off later in the workplace, where your energy will be appreciated and rewarded. Having enthusiasm for getting the job done can be contagious, and when everyone works hard, everyone benefits. You can begin to develop this enthusiasm by establishing good work habits as a student.

ACTIVITY

For 1 week, keep a daily record of your performance in the following areas, and ask a few of your fellow students to provide feedback as well.

- Positive attitude
- Professional appearance
- Punctuality
- Regular class and clinic attendance
- Diligent practice of newly learned techniques
- Interpersonal skills
- Teamwork
- Helping others

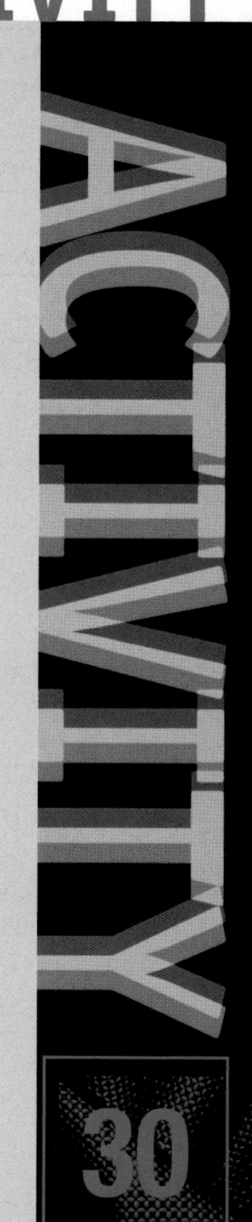

INVENTORY OF PERSONAL CHARACTERISTICS

PERSONAL CHARACTERISTIC	Exc.	Good	Avg.	Poor	Plan for Improvement
Posture, Deportment, Poise					
Grooming, Personal Hygiene					
Manners, Courtesy					
Communications Skills					
Attitude					
Self-Motivation					
Personal Habits					
Responsibility					
Self-esteem, Self Confidence					
Honesty, Integrity					
Dependability					

INVENTORY OF TECHNICAL SKILLS

TECHNICAL SKILLS	Exc.	Good	Avg.	Poor	Plan for Improvement
Hair shaping/cutting					
Hairstyling					
Haircoloring					
Texture Services, Perming					
Texture Services, Relaxing					
Manicuring, Pedicuring					
Artificial Nail Extensions					
Skin Care, Facials					
Facial Makeup					
Other					

After analyzing the above responses, would you hire yourself as an employee in your firm? Why or why not?
State your short-term goals that you hope to accomplish in 6 to 12 months:
State your long-term goals that you hope to accomplish in 1 to 5 years:

Ask yourself: Do you want to work in a big city or small town? Are you compatible with a sophisticated, exclusive salon or a trendy salon? Which clientele are you able to communicate with more effectively? Do you want to start out slowly and carefully or do you want to jump in and throw everything into your career from the starting gate? Will you be in this industry throughout your working career or is this just a stopover? Will you only work a 30 or 40 hour week or will you go the extra mile when opportunities are available? How ambitious are you and how many risks are you willing to take?

Figure 30-4 Inventory of personal characteristics and technical skills.

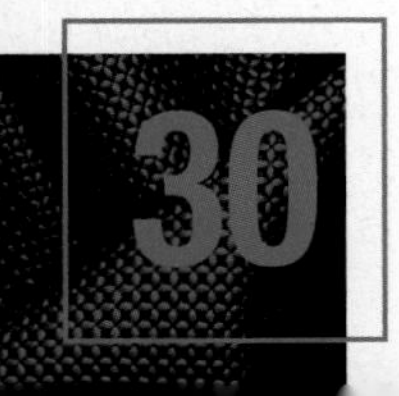

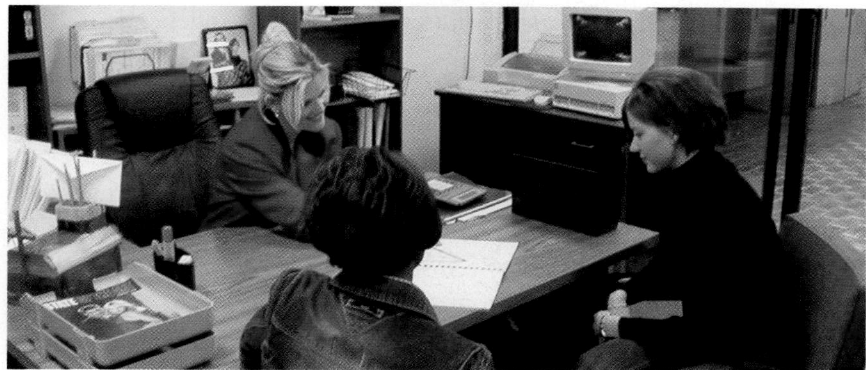

Figure 30-5 Your school advisor can help you find employment.

HOW TO GET THE JOB YOU WANT

There are several key personal characteristics that will not only help you get the position you want, but will help you keep it. These characteristics include the points listed below.

Motivation. This means having the drive to take the necessary action to achieve a goal. Although motivation can come from external sources—parental or peer pressure, for instance—the best kind of motivation is internal.

Integrity. When you have integrity, you are committed to a strong code of moral and artistic values. Integrity is the compass that keeps you on course over the long haul of your career.

Good technical and communication skills. While you may be better in either technical or communication skills, you must develop both to reach the level of success you desire.

Strong work ethic. In the beauty business, having a strong **work ethic** means taking pride in your work, and committing yourself to consistently doing a good job for your clients, employer, and salon team.

Enthusiasm. Try never to lose your eagerness to learn, grow, and expand your skills and knowledge.

A SALON SURVEY

In the United States alone, the professional salon business numbers nearly 313,000 establishments. These salons employ more than 1,604,000 active cosmetology professionals. This year, like every year, thousands of cosmetology school graduates will find their first position in one of the types of salons described below.

SMALL INDEPENDENT SALONS

Owned by an individual or two or more partners, this kind of operation makes up the majority of professional salons. The average independent salon has three styling chairs, but many have as many as 40 styling stations. Usually, the owners are hair practitioners who maintain their own clientele while managing the business. There are nearly as many types of independent salons as there are owners. Their image, decor, services, prices, and clientele all reflect the owner's experience and taste. Depending on the owner's willingness to help a newcomer learn and

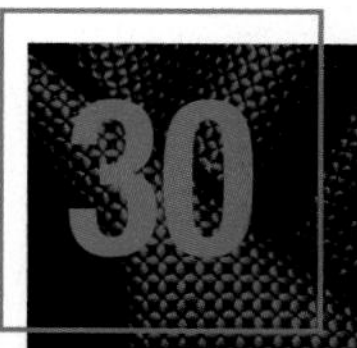

grow, a beginning stylist can learn a great deal in an independent salon while also earning a good living.

INDEPENDENT SALON CHAINS

These are usually chains of five or more salons that are owned by one individual or two or more partners. Independent salon chains range from basic hair salons to full-service salons and day spas, and offer everything from low-priced to very high-priced services.

In large, high-end salons, practitioners can advance to specialized positions in color, nail care, skin care, or other chemical services. Some larger salons also employ education directors and style directors, and practitioners are often hired to manage particular locations.

LARGE NATIONAL SALON CHAINS

These companies operate salons throughout the country, and even internationally. They can be budget or value priced, haircut only or full service, mid-price or high end. Some salon chains operate within department store chains. Management and marketing professionals at the corporate headquarters make all the decisions for each salon, such as size, decor, hours, services, prices, advertising, and profit targets. Many newly licensed cosmetology professionals seek their first jobs in national chain salons because of the secure pay and benefits, additional paid training, management opportunities, and corporate advertising. Because the chains are large and widespread, employees have the added advantage of being able to transfer from one location to another.

FRANCHISE SALONS

Another form of chain salon organization, this one has a national name and consistent image and business formula throughout the chain. Franchises are owned by individuals who pay a fee to use the name; these individuals then receive a business plan and can take advantage of national marketing campaigns. Such decisions as size, location, decor, and prices are determined in advance by the parent company. Franchises are generally not owned by practitioners, but by investors who seek a return on their investment.

Franchise salons commonly offer employees the same benefits as corporate-owned chain salons.

BASIC VALUE-PRICED OPERATIONS

Often located in busy, low-rent shopping center strips that are anchored by a nearby supermarket or other large business, these outlets depend on a high volume of walk-in traffic. They hire recent cosmetology graduates and generally pay them by the hour, sometimes adding commission-style bonuses if individual sales pass a certain level. Haircuts are usually reasonably priced and practitioners are trained to work fast with no frills.

MID-PRICED FULL-SERVICE SALONS

These salons offer a complete menu of hair, nail, and skin services and retail products. Successful mid-priced salons promote their most profitable

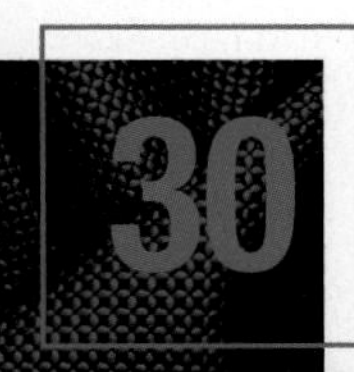

services and typically offer "service and retail packages" to entice haircut-only clients. They also run strong marketing programs to encourage client returns and referrals. These salons train their professional styling team to be as productive and profitable as possible. If you are inclined to give more time to each client during the consultation, you may like working in a full-service salon. Here you will have the opportunity to build a relationship with clients that may extend over time.

HIGH-END "IMAGE" SALONS OR DAY SPAS

This type of business employs well-trained practitioners and salon assistants who offer higher-priced services to clients that are filled with luxurious extras such as a 5-minute head, neck, and shoulder massage as part of the shampoo and luxurious spa manicures and pedicures. Most high-end salons are located in trendy, upscale sections of large cities; others may be located in elegant mansions, high-rent office and retail towers, or luxury hotels and resorts. Clients expect a high level of personal service, and such salons hire practitioners whose technical expertise, personal appearance, and communication skills meet their high standards (Figure 30-6).

BOOTH RENTAL ESTABLISHMENTS

Booth renting (also called chair rental) is possibly the least expensive way of owning one's own business. For a detailed discussion of booth rental, see Chapter 32.

RESUME DEVELOPMENT

A **resume** is a written summary of your education and work experience. It tells potential employers at a glance what your achievements and accomplishments are. Here are some basic guidelines to follow when preparing your professional resume.

- Keep it simple. Limit it to one page if possible.
- Print it on good-quality white, buff, or gray bond paper.
- Include your name, address, phone number, and e-mail address on both the resume and your cover letter.
- List recent, relevant work experience.
- List relevant education and the name of the institution from which you graduated, as well as relevant courses attended.

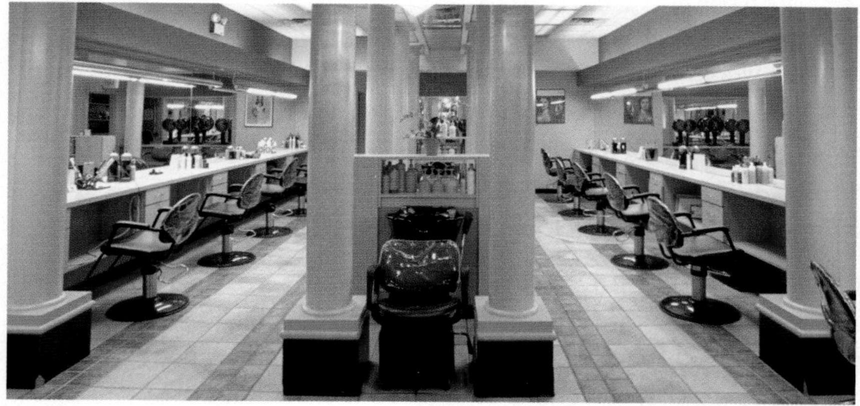

Figure 30-6 A high-end salon.

- List your abilities and accomplishments.
- Focus on information that is relevant to the position you are seeking.

The average time that a potential employer will spend scanning your resume before deciding whether to grant you an interview is about 20 seconds. That means you must market yourself in such a manner that the reader will want to meet you. Never make the mistake of detailing your previous duties and responsibilities. Rather, focus your achievements. Accomplishment statements should always enlarge your basic duties and responsibilities. The best way to do this is to add numbers or percentages whenever possible. You might ask yourself the following questions:

- How many regular clients do I serve?
- How many clients do I serve weekly?
- What was my service ticket average?
- What was my client retention rate?
- What percentage of my client revenue came from retailing?
- What percentage of my client revenue came from color or texture services?

This type of questioning can help you develop accomplishment statements that will interest a potential employer. There is no better time for you to achieve significant accomplishments than while you are in school. Even though your experience may be minimal, you must still present evidence of your skills and accomplishments. This may seem a difficult task at this early stage in your working career, but by closely examining your training performance, extracurricular activities, and the full- or part-time jobs you have held, you should be able to create a good, attention-getting resume. For example, consider the following questions:

- Did you receive any honors during your course of training?
- Were you ever selected "student of the month"?
- Did you receive special recognition for your attendance or academic progress?
- Did you win any cosmetology-related competitions while in school?
- What was your attendance average while in school?
- Did you work with the student body to organize any fundraisers? What were the results?

Answers to these types of questions may indicate your people skills, personal work habits, and personal commitment to success (Figure 30-7).

Since you have not yet completed your training, you still have the opportunity to make some of the examples listed above become a reality before you graduate. Positive developments of this nature while you are still in school can do much to improve your resume.

THE DO'S AND DON'TS OF RESUMES

You will save yourself from many problems and a lot of disappointment right from the beginning of your job search, if you keep a clear idea in your mind of what to do and what not to do when it comes to creating a resume. Here are some of the do's:

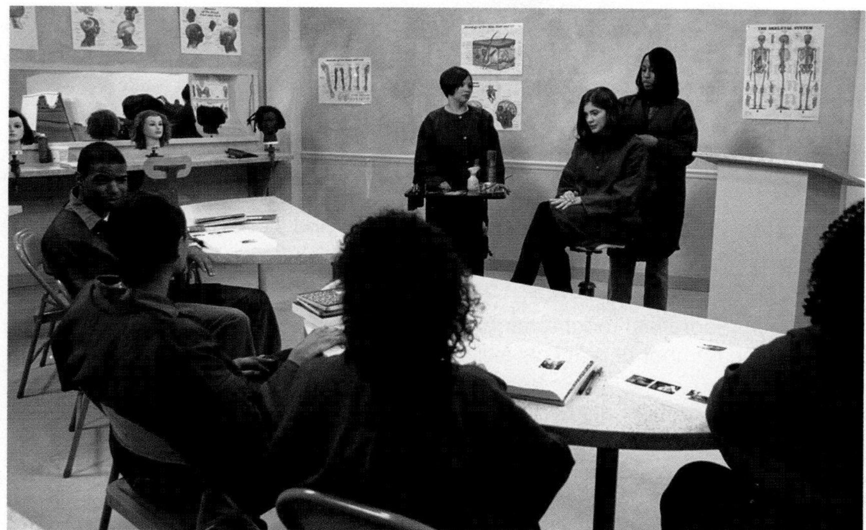

Figure 30-7 Excelling in school can help you build a good resume.

Make it easy to read. Use concise, clear sentences and avoid "overwriting" or flowery language.

Know your audience. Use vocabulary and language that will be understood by your potential employer.

Keep it short. Make sure the overall length does not exceed two pages. One page is preferable.

Stress accomplishments. Emphasize past accomplishments and the skills you used to achieve them.

Focus on career goals. Highlight information that is relevant to your career goals and the position you are seeking.

Emphasize transferable skills. Transferable skills are the skills you have already mastered at other jobs that can be put to use in a new position.

Use action verbs. Begin accomplishment statements with action verbs such as **achieved, coordinated, developed, increased, maintained,** and **strengthened**.

Make it neat. A poorly structured, badly typed resume does not reflect well on you.

And now for the don'ts to watch out for:

Avoid salary references. Don't state your salary history or reason for leaving your former employment.

Don't stretch the truth. Misinformation or untruthful statements usually catch up with you.

Don't include personal references. Potential employers are really only interested in references that can speak about your professional ability.

Don't expect too much. Don't have unrealistic expectations of what your resume can accomplish.

Review Figure 30-8, which represents an achievement-oriented resume for a recent graduate of a cosmetology course. But keep in mind that you

MARY CURL
143 Fern Circle
Anytown, USA 12345
(123) 555-1234

A cosmetologist with honors in attendance and practical skills who is creative, artistic, and works well with people of all ages.

ACCOMPLISHMENTS/ABILITIES

Academics — Achieved an "A" average in theoretical requirements and excellent ratings in practical requirements; Exceeded the number of practical skills required for graduation.

Sales — Named "Student of the Month" for best attendance, best attitude, highest retail sales, and most clients served; Increased chemical services to 30 percent of my clinic volume by graduation. Achieved a client ticket average comparable to $33.00 in the area salon market.

Increased retail sales of cosmetics by over 18 percent during part-time employment at local department store.

Client Retention — Developed and retained a personal client base of over 75 individuals of all ages, both male and female.

Image Consulting — Certified as an Image Consultant who aids in providing full salon services to all clientele.

Administration — Supervised a student "salon team" that developed a business plan for opening a twelve chair, full service salon; project earned an "A" and was recognized for thoroughness, accuracy, and creativity.

As President of the student council, organized fund raising activities including car washes, bake sales, and yard sales which generated enough funds to send 19 students to a regional hair show.

Externship — Trained one day weekly at the salon for ten weeks under the state approved student externship program.

Special Projects — Reorganized school facial room for more efficiency and client comfort.

Organized the school dispensary which increased inventory control and streamlined operations within the clinic.

Catalogued the school's library of texts, books, videos and other periodicals by category and updated the library inventory list.

EXPERIENCE

Salon Etc. — Spring 2006
Student Extern in all Phases of Cosmetology

Macy's — Summer 2006
Retail Sales, Cosmetics

Food Emporium — 2004-2005
Cashier

EDUCATION

Graduate, New Alamo High School, 2004
Graduate, Milady Career Institute of Cosmetology, August 2006
Licensed as Cosmetologist, September 2006

Figure 30–8 An achievement-oriented resume.

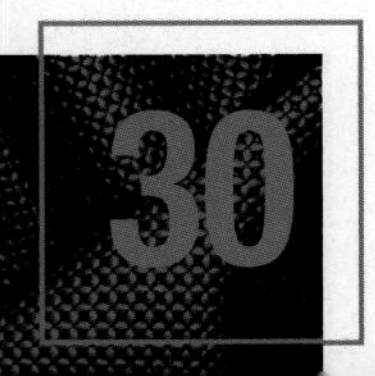

are much more than the sum of your parts. It just may take a while before someone recognizes that.

EMPLOYMENT PORTFOLIO

As you prepare to work in the field of cosmetology, an **employment portfolio** can be extremely useful. An employment portfolio is a collection, usually bound, of photos and documents that reflect your skills, accomplishments, and abilities in your chosen career field (Figure 30-9).

While the actual contents of the portfolio will vary from graduate to graduate, there are certain items that have a place in any portfolio.

A powerful portfolio includes:

- Diplomas, including high school and cosmetology school
- Awards and achievements received while a cosmetology student
- Current resume, focusing on accomplishments
- Letters of reference from former employers
- Summary of continuing education and/or copies of training certificates
- Statement of membership in industry and other professional organizations
- Statement of relevant civic affiliations and/or community activities
- Before-and-after photographs of services that you have performed on clients or models
- Brief statement about why you have chosen a career in cosmetology
- Any other information that you regard as relevant

Once you have assembled your portfolio, ask yourself whether it accurately portrays you and your career skills. If it does not, identify what needs to be changed. If you are not sure, run it by a neutral party for feedback about how to make it more interesting and accurate. This kind of feedback is also useful when creating a resume. The portfolio, like the resume, should be prepared in a way that projects professionalism.

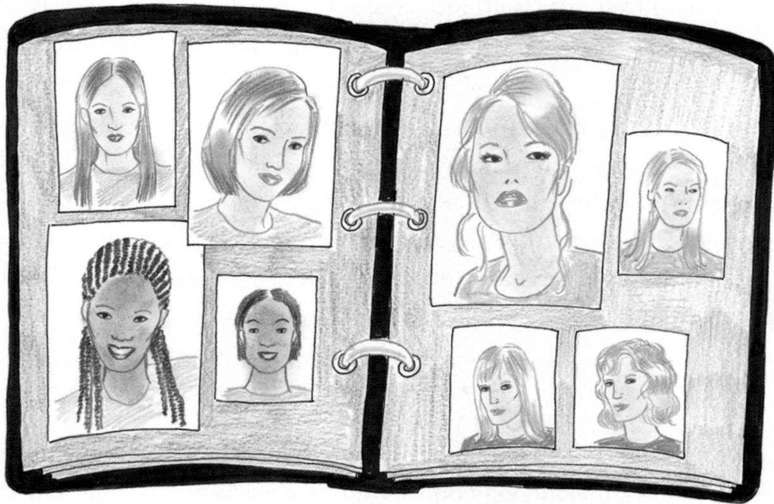

Figure 30-9 Before-and-after photos in an employment portfolio.

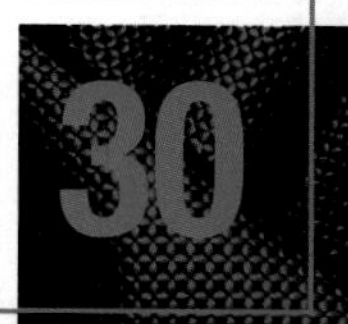

- Nothing should be handwritten. All summaries and letters should be typed.
- For ease of use, you may want to separate sections with tabs.
- When writing about why you chose a career in cosmetology, you might include a statement that explains what you love about your new career, a description of your philosophy about the importance of teamwork and how you see yourself as a contributing team member, and a description of methods you would try in an effort to increase service and retail revenue.

TARGETING THE ESTABLISHMENT

One of the most important steps in the process of job hunting is narrowing your search. Listed below are some points to keep in mind about targeting potential employers.

- **Accept that you probably will not begin in your dream job.** Few people are so lucky.
- **Do not wait until graduation to begin your search.** If you do, you may be tempted to take the first offer you receive, instead of carefully investigating all possibilities before making a decision.
- **Locate a salon that serves the type of clients you wish to serve.** Finding a good fit with the clients and staff is critical from the outset of your career.
- **Make a list of area salons or establishments.** The Yellow Pages will be your best source for this. If you are considering relocating to another area, your local library will probably have out-of-state phone directories to help you compile your list. You may also access *www.anywho.com* on the Internet for a complete listing of businesses throughout the United States.
- **Follow newspapers, television, and radio for salon advertising.** Get a feel for what market each salon is targeting.

FIELD RESEARCH

A great way to find out about jobs is to actually get out there and use your eyes, ears, and any other sense that can help you gather information. A highly effective technique that you should learn is called "networking."

Networking allows you to establish contacts that may eventually lead to a job, and helps you gain valuable information about the workings of various establishments. If possible, make contact with salons while you are still a student. You might even make contact as a salon customer yourself. When you are ready to network, your first contact should be by telephone, and you should follow these guidelines:

1. Use your best telephone manner. Speak with confidence and self-assurance.
2. Ask to speak to the owner, manager, or personnel director.
3. State your name and explain that you are preparing to graduate from school in your chosen field.

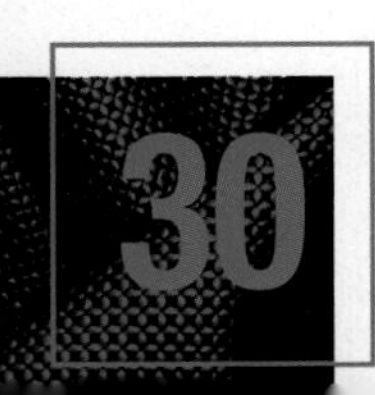

4. Explain that you are researching the local salon market for potential positions, and that you need just a few minutes to ask a few questions.
5. If the person is receptive to your phone call, ask whether the salon is in need of any new practitioners, and how many the salon currently employs.
6. Ask if you can make an appointment to visit the salon to observe sometime during the next few weeks. If the salon representative is agreeable, make an appointment and confirm it with a typewritten or handwritten note on good-quality paper (Figure 30-10).

Remember that a rejection is not a negative reflection on you. Many professionals are too busy to make time for this kind of networking. The good news is that you are bound to discover many genuinely kind people who remember what it was like when they started out, and are willing to devote a bit of their time to help others who are beginning their careers.

THE SALON VISIT

When you visit the salon, take along a checklist to ensure that you observe all the key areas that might ultimately affect your decision making. The checklist will be similar to the one used for field trips that you probably have taken to area salons while in school. Keep the checklist on file for future reference so that you can make informed comparisons among establishments (Figure 30-11).

After your visit, always remember to write a brief note thanking the salon representative for his or her time (Figure 30-12). Even if you did not like the salon, or would never consider working there, it is important to send a thank-you note (Figure 30-13).

Never burn your bridges. Instead, build a network of contacts who have a favorable opinion of you.

ARRANGING THE EMPLOYMENT INTERVIEW

After you have graduated and completed the first two steps in the process of securing employment—targeting and observing salons—you are ready to pursue employment in earnest. The next step is to contact the

Dear Ms. (or Mr.) ______________________,

I appreciate the time you spent with me on the phone earlier today. I am looking forward to meeting with you and visiting your salon next Friday at 2:00 p.m. I am eager to observe your salon and staff at work. If you should need to reach me before that time for any reason, my home phone number is _______________, and my email address is _______________. See you on Friday.

Sincerely,
(your name)

Figure 30-10 Sample appointment confirmation note.

SALON VISIT CHECKLIST

When you visit a salon, observe the following areas and rate them from 1 to 5, with 5 considered being the best.

_____ **SALON IMAGE:** Is the salon's image consistent and appropriate for your interests? Is the image pleasing and inviting? What is the decor and arrangement? If you are not comfortable or if you find it unattractiive, mark the salon off your list of employment possibilities.

_____ **PROFESSIONALISM:** Do the employees present the appropriate professional appearance and behavior? Do they give their clients the appropriate levels of attention and personal service or do they act as if work is their time to socialize?

_____ **MANAGEMENT:** Does the salon show signs of being well managed? Is the phone answered promptly with professional telephone skills? Is the mood of the salon positive? Does everyone appear to work as a team?

_____ **CLIENT SERVICE:** Are clients greeted promptly and warmly when they enter the salon? Are they kept informed of the status of their appointment? Are they offered a magazine or beverage while they wait? Is there a comfortable reception area? Are there changing rooms, attractive smocks?

_____ **PRICES:** Compare price for value. Are clients getting their money's worth? Do they pay the same price in one salon but get better service and attention in another? If possible, take home salon brochures and price lists.

_____ **RETAIL:** Is there a well-stocked retail display offering clients a variety of product lines and a range of prices? Do the stylists and receptionist (if applicable) promote retail sales?

_____ **IN-SALON MARKETING:** Are there posters or promotions throughout the salon? If so, are they professionally made and do they reflect contemporary styles?

_____ **SERVICES:** Make a list of all services offered by each salon and the product lines they carry. This will help you decide what earning potential stylists have in each salon.

SALON NAME: ______________________________

SALON MANAGER: ______________________________

Figure 30–11 Salon visit checklist.

Dear Ms. (or Mr.) ____________________,

I appreciate having had the opportunity to observe your salon/spa in operation last Friday. Thank you for the time you and your staff gave me. I was impressed by the efficient and courteous manner in which your stylists served their clients. The atmosphere was pleasant and the mood was positive. Should you ever have an opening for a professional with my skills and training, I would welcome the opportunity to apply. You can contact me at the address and phone number listed below. I hope we will meet again soon.

Sincerely,

(your name, address, telephone)

Figure 30–12 Sample thank-you note.

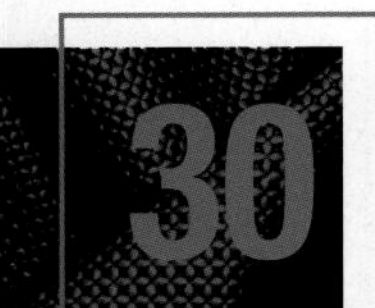

Dear Ms. (or Mr.) ______________________,

I appreciate having had the opportunity to observe your salon in operation last Friday. I know how busy you and all your staff are, and want to thank you for the time that you gave me. I hope my presence didn't interfere with the flow of your operations too much. I certainly appreciate the courtesies that were extended to me by you and your staff. I wish you and your salon continued success.

Sincerely,
(your name)

Figure 30–13 Thank-you note to a salon at which you do not expect to seek employment.

Your Name
Your Address
Your Phone Number

Ms. (or Mr.) ______________________,
Salon Name
Salon Address

Dear Ms. (or Mr.) ______________________,

We met in August when you allowed me to observe your salon and staff while I was still in cosmetology training. Since that time, I have graduated and have received my license. I have enclosed my resume for your review and consideration.
I would very much appreciate the opportunity to meet with you and discuss either current or future career opportunities at your salon.
I was extremely impressed with your staff and business, and I would like to share with you how my skills and training might add to your salon's success.
I will call you next week to discuss a time that is convenient for us to meet. I look forward to meeting with you again soon.

Sincerely,
(your name)

Figure 30–14 Sample resume cover letter.

establishments that you are most interested in by sending them a resume with a cover letter requesting an interview.

Mark your calendar for a time when it would be suitable to make a follow-up call to this letter. A week is generally sufficient. When you call, try to schedule an interview appointment. Keep in mind that some salons may not have openings, and may not be granting interviews at this time. When this is the case, be polite and ask them to keep your resume on file

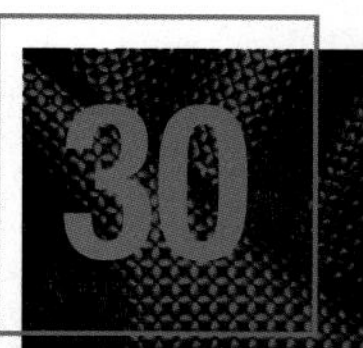

should an opening arise in the future. Be sure to thank them for their time and consideration.

INTERVIEW PREPARATION

When preparing for an interview, make sure that you have all the necessary information and materials in place (Figure 30-15), including the following items:

1. **Identification.**
    - Social Security number
    - Driver's license number
    - Names, addresses, and phone numbers of former employers
    - Name and phone number of the nearest relative not living with you

Here's a TIP

When you call a salon to make an appointment for an interview, you may be told that they are not hiring at the time, but would be happy to conduct an interview for future reference. Never think that this would be a waste of time.

Take advantage of the opportunity. Not only will it give you valuable interview experience, but may provide opportunities that otherwise you would miss. There is such a thing as love at first sight!

PREPARING FOR THE INTERVIEW CHECKLIST

RESUME COMPOSITION

1. Does it present your abilities and what you have accomplished in your jobs and training?
2. Does it make the reader want to ask, "How did you accomplish that?"
3. Does it highlight accomplishments rather than detailing duties and responsibilities?
4. Is it easy to read? Is it short? Does it stress past accomplishments and skills?
5. Does it focus on information that is relevant to your own career goals?
6. Is it complete and professionally prepared?

PORTFOLIO CHECKLIST

_____ Diploma, secondary, and post-secondary
_____ Awards and achievements while in school
_____ Current resume focusing on accomplishments
_____ Letters of reference from former employers
_____ List of, or certificates from, trade shows attended while in training
_____ Statement of professional affiliations (memberships in cosmetology organizations, etc.)
_____ Statement of civic affiliations and/or activities
_____ Before and after photographs of technical skills services you have performed
_____ Any other relevant information

Ask: Does my portfolio portray me and my career skills in the manner that I wish to be perceived? If not, what needs to be changed?

Figure 30-15 Preparing for the interview checklist.

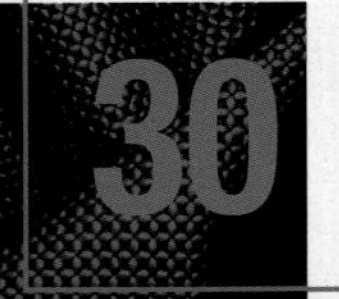

2. **Interview wardrobe.** Your appearance is crucial, especially since you are applying for a position in the image and beauty industry (Figure 30-16). It is recommended that you obtain one or two "interview outfits." You may be requested to return for a second interview; hence the need for the second outfit. Consider the following points:
   - Is the outfit appropriate for the position?
   - Is it both fashionable and flattering to your shape and personality?
   - Are your accessories both fashionable and functional (e.g., not noisy or so large that they interfere with performing services)?
   - Are your nails meticulously groomed and do they say something about your abilities as a cosmetologist?
   - Is your hairstyle current? Does it flatter your face and your overall style?
   - Is your makeup current? Does it flatter your face and your overall style?
   - (For men:) Are you clean shaven, or is your beard properly trimmed?
   - Is your perfume or cologne subtle?
   - Are you carrying either a handbag or briefcase, but not both?
3. **Supporting materials.**
   - **Resume.** Even if you have already sent one, take another copy with you.
   - **Facts and figures.** Have ready a list of names and dates of former employment, education, and references.
   - **Employment portfolio.**
4. **Answers to anticipated questions.** Certain questions are typically asked during an interview. It would be a good idea to reflect on your answers ahead of time. You might even consider role-playing an interview situation with friends, family, or fellow students. Typical questions include the following:
   - What did you like best about your training?
   - Are you punctual and regular in attendance?
   - Will your school director or instructor confirm this?
   - What skills do you feel are your strongest?
   - What areas do you consider to be less strong?
   - Are you a team player? Please explain.
   - Do you consider yourself flexible? Please explain.
   - What are your career goals?
   - What days and hours are you available for work?
   - Do you have your own transportation?
   - Are there any obstacles that would prevent you from keeping your commitment to full-time employment?
   - What assets do you believe that you would bring to this salon and this position?

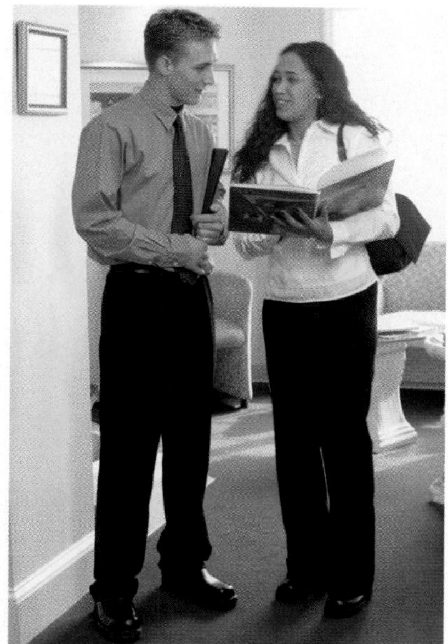

Figure 30-16 Dressed for an interview.

- Who is the most interesting person you have met in your work and/or education experience? Why?
- How would you handle a problem client?
- How do you feel about retailing?
- Would you be willing to attend our company training program?
- Describe ways that you provide excellent customer service.
- Please share an example of consultation questions that you might ask a client.
- What steps do you take to build your business and ensure that clients return to see you?

5. **Be prepared to perform a service.** Some salons require applicants to perform a service in their chosen discipline as part of the interview. Be sure to confirm whether this is a requirement. If it is, make sure that your model is appropriately dressed and properly prepared for the experience, and that you take the requisite supplies.

THE INTERVIEW

On the day of the interview, try to make sure that nothing occurs that will keep you from completing the interview successfully. There are certain behaviors you should practice in connection with the interview itself.

- Always be on time or, better yet, early. If you are unsure of the location, find it the day before so there will be no reason for delays.
- Project a warm, friendly smile. Smiling is the universal language.
- Walk, sit, and stand with good posture.
- Be polite and courteous.
- Do not sit until asked to do so, or until it is obvious that you are expected to do so.
- Never smoke or chew gum, even if one or the other is offered to you.
- Do not come to an interview with a cup of coffee, a soft drink, snacks, or anything else to eat or drink.
- Never lean on or touch the interviewer's desk. Some people do not like their personal space invaded without an invitation.
- Try to project a positive first impression by appearing as confident and relaxed as you can (Figure 30-17).
- Speak clearly. The interviewer must be able to hear and understand you.
- Answer questions honestly. Think about the question and answer carefully. Do not speak before you are ready, and not for more than 2 minutes at a time.
- Never criticize former employers.
- Always remember to thank the interviewer at the end of the interview.

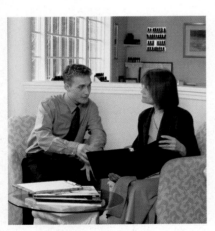

Figure 30-17 Interview in progress.

Another critical part of the interview comes when you are invited to ask the interviewer questions of your own. You should think about those questions ahead of time and bring a list if necessary. Doing so will show that you are organized and prepared. Some questions that you might consider include the following:

- Is there a job description? May I review it?
- Is there a salon manual?
- How frequently does the salon advertise?
- How long do practitioners typically work here?
- Are employees encouraged to grow in skills and responsibility? How so?
- Does the salon offer continuing education opportunities?
- Is there room for advancement? If so, what are the requirements for promotion?
- What benefits does the salon offer, such as paid vacations, personal days, and medical insurance?
- What is the form of compensation?
- When will the position be filled?
- Should I follow up on your decision, or will you contact me?

Do not feel that you have to ask all of your questions. The point is to create as much of a dialogue as possible. Be aware of the interviewer's reactions and make note of when you have asked enough questions. By obtaining the answers to at least some of your questions, you can compare the information you have gathered about other salons, and then choose the one that offers the best package of income and career development.

Remember to write a thank-you note. It should simply thank the interviewer for the time he or she spent with you. Close with a positive statement that you want the job (if you do). If the interviewer's decision comes down to two or three possibilities, the one expressing the most desire may be offered the position. Also, if the interviewer suggests that you call to learn about the employment decision, then by all means do so.

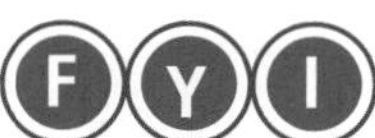

Many women find it difficult to afford the two or three outfits necessary to project a confident and professional image when going out into the workplace. Fortunately, several nonprofit organizations have been formed to address this need. These organizations receive donations of clean, beautiful clothes in good repair from individuals and manufacturers. These are then passed along to women who need them. For more information, visit Wardrobe for Opportunity at *http://www.wardrobe.org,* and Dress for Success at *http://www.dressforsuccess.org.*

LEGAL ASPECTS OF THE EMPLOYMENT INTERVIEW

Over the years, a number of issues have arisen about questions that may or may not be included in an employment application or interview, including **race/ethnicity, religion,** and **national origin.** Generally, there should be no questions in any of these categories. Additional categories are listed below.

Age or date of birth. It is permissible to ask the age if the applicant is younger than 18. Age should not be relevant in most hiring decisions, so date-of-birth questions prior to employment are improper.

Disabilities or physical traits. The Americans with Disabilities Act prohibits general inquiries about health problems, disabilities, and medical conditions.

Drug use or smoking. Questions regarding drug or tobacco use are permitted. In fact, the employer may obtain the applicant's agreement to be bound by the employer's drug and smoking policies and to submit to drug testing.

ACTIVITY

Find a partner among your fellow students and role-play the employment interview. Each of you can take turns as the applicant and the employer. After each session, conduct a brief discussion regarding how it went, that is, what worked and what didn't work. Discuss how the process could be further improved. Bear in mind that a role-play activity will never predict exactly what will occur in a real interview. However, the process will assist you in being better prepared for that important event in your employment search.

Citizenship. Employers are not allowed to discriminate because an applicant is not a U.S. citizen.

It is important to recognize that not all potential employers will understand that they may be asking improper or illegal questions. If you are asked any of these questions, you may choose to answer them or not. You might simply respond that you believe the question is irrelevant to the position you are seeking, and that you would like to focus on your qualities and skills that are suited to the job and the mission of the establishment.

THE EMPLOYMENT APPLICATION

Any time that you are applying for any position, you will be required to complete an application, even if your resume already contains much of the requested information. Your resume and the list you have prepared prior to the interview will assist you in completing the application quickly and accurately.

You may want to fill out the sample form in Figure 30-18 in preparation for your employment interviews (Figure 30-18). The form each salon uses may be different, but it will probably request similar information.

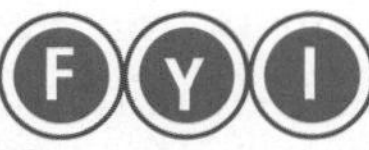

These are examples of illegal questions as compared to legal questions:

Illegal Questions	**Legal Questions**
How old are you?	**Are you over the age of 18?**
Please describe your medical history.	**Are you able to perform this job?**
Are you a U.S. citizen?	**Are you authorized to work in the United States?**
What is your native tongue?	**In which languages are you fluent?**

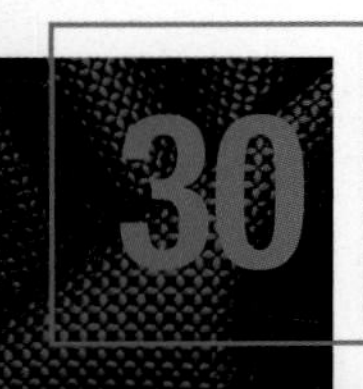

EMPLOYMENT APPLICATION

Applicants are considered for all positions, and employees are treated during employment without regard to race, color, religion, sex, national origin, age, marital or veteran status, medical condition or handicap.

PERSONAL INFORMATION

SS#__________ Phone__________ Date__________

Last name__________ First__________ Middle__________

Present street address City State Zip

Permanent street address City State Zip

If related to anyone employed here, state name:__________

Referred to salon by:__________

EMPLOYMENT DESIRED

Position__________

Date you can start__________ Salary Desired__________

Current Employer__________

May we contact?__________

Ever applied with this company before?__________ Where?__________ When?__________

EDUCATION

Name/location of School	Years Completed	Subjects Studied

Subject of special study or research work:

What foreign languages do you speak fluently?

Read fluently:__________

Write fluently:__________

US Military Service Rank Present Membership

In Nat'l Guard/Reserve

Figure 30-18 Typical job application form.

Activities (other than religious) Civic, Athletic, Fraternal, etc. (Exclude organizations for which the name or character might indicate race, creed, color or national origin of its members).

FORMER EMPLOYMENT

List below last four employers, beginning with the most recent one first.

DATE: Month/Year	Name, Address of Employer	Salary	Position	Reason For Leaving
From:				
To:				
From:				
To:				
From:				
To:				
From:				
To:				

REFERENCES

Give below the names of three persons not related to you whom you have known at least one year.

Name	Address	Business	Years Known

PHYSICAL RECORD

Please list any defects in hearing, vision, or speech that might affect your job performance.

In case of emergency, please notify:

Name Address Telephone

I authorize investigation of all statements contained in this application. I understand that misrepresentation or omission of facts called for is cause for dismissal if hired.

Signature______________________ Date______________

Figure 30-18, cont'd

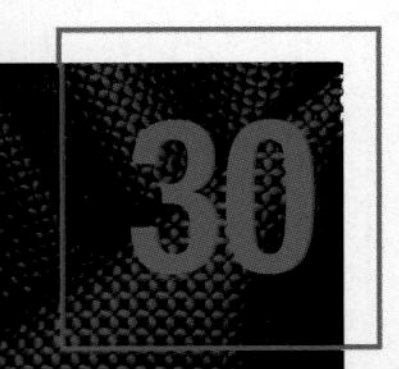

DOING IT RIGHT

You are ready to set out on your exciting new career as a professional cosmetologist. The right way to proceed is by learning important study and test-taking skills early and applying them throughout your program.

Think ahead to your employment opportunities and use your time in school to develop a record of interesting, noteworthy activities that will make your resume exciting. When you compile a history that shows how you have achieved your goals, your confidence will build and your ambitions will grow.

Always take one step at a time. Be sure to take the helpful preliminary steps that we have discussed when preparing for employment.

Develop a dynamic portfolio. Keep your materials, information, and questions organized in order to ensure a high-impact interview.

Once employed, take the necessary steps to learn all that you can about your new position and the establishment you will be serving. Read all you can about the industry. Attend trade shows and take advantage of as much continuing education as you can manage. Become an active participant in making this great industry even better. See Chapter 31 to learn some great strategies for ensuring your career success.

REVIEW QUESTIONS

1. What is the most important way that a learner can do well on any test?
2. Explain deductive reasoning.
3. List eight steps that learners should take prior to the examination to improve results.
4. List at least 12 strategies that learners can use on the day of the examination for improved results.
5. When considering a statement on a true/false test, why are long statements more likely to be true than shorter statements?
6. Name and describe at least five types of salon businesses.
7. List up to eight strategies that you will find helpful when writing your resume.
8. List at least six things that you should avoid when developing your resume.
9. List several items that should be included in your professional portfolio.
10. Briefly summarize the preliminary things that you should consider before beginning your salon search.
11. In your own words, explain what can be accomplished by visiting a salon prior to an employment interview.
12. Why are thank-you notes important even if you visit a salon where you do not wish to become employed?
13. List 12 important interview behaviors that you should practice.

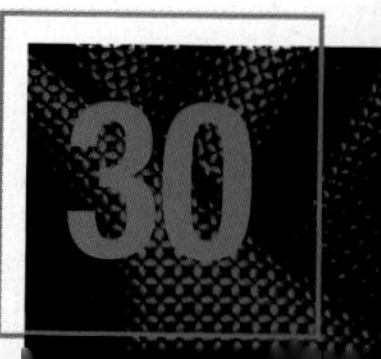

CHAPTER GLOSSARY

deductive reasoning	Process of reaching logical conclusions by employing logical reasoning.
employment portfolio	Collection, usually bound, of photos and documents that reflect your skills, accomplishments, and abilities in your chosen career field.
resume	Written summary of a person's education and work experience.
test-wise	Having a complete and thorough knowledge of the subject matter, and understanding the strategies for taking tests successfully.
transferable skills	Skills mastered at other jobs that can be put to use in a new position.
work ethic	Taking pride in your work, and committing yourself to consistently doing a good job for your clients, employer and salon team.

ON THE JOB

CHAPTER 31

chapter outline

Moving from School to Work
Out in the Real World
Managing Your Money
Discover the Selling You
On Your Way

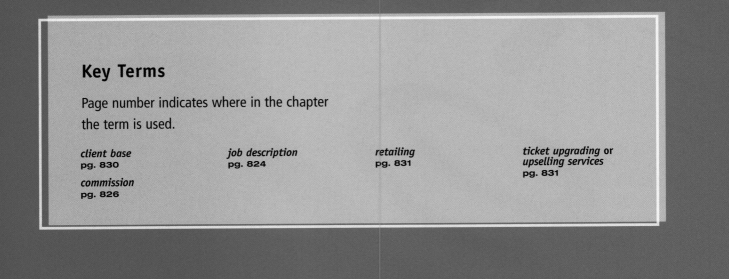

Learning Objectives

After completing this chapter, you will be able to:

- Describe the qualities that help a new employee succeed in a service profession.
- List the habits of a good salon team player.
- Explain the function of a job description.
- Describe three different ways in which salon professionals are compensated.
- Create a personal budget.
- List the principles of selling products and services in the salon.
- List the most effective ways to build a client base.

Key Terms

Page number indicates where in the chapter the term is used.

client base
pg. 830

commission
pg. 826

job description
pg. 824

retailing
pg. 831

ticket upgrading or *upselling services*
pg. 831

Congratulations! You have worked hard in cosmetology school, passed your state's licensing exam, and have been offered your first job in the field. Now, more than ever, you need to prioritize your goals, and commit to personal rules of conduct and behavior. These goals and rules should guide you throughout your career. If you let them do so, you can always expect to have work, and enjoy all the freedom that your chosen profession can offer (Figure 31-1).

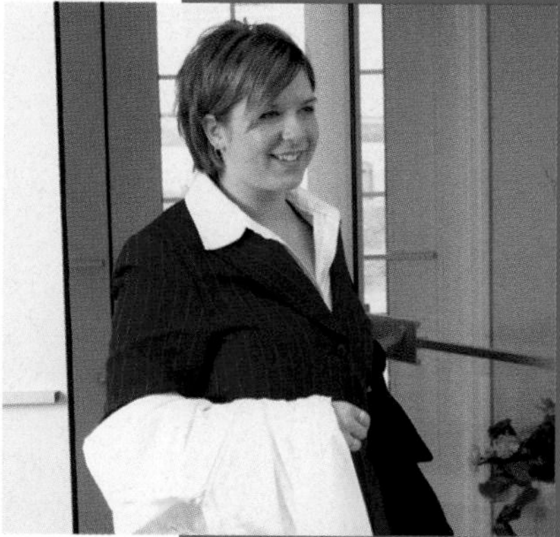

Figure 31-1 Getting off to a good start.

MOVING FROM SCHOOL TO WORK

Making the transition from school to work can be difficult. While you may be thrilled to have a job, working for a paycheck brings with it a number of duties and responsibilities that you may not have thought about.

Cosmetology school is a forgiving environment. You are given the chance to do a certain procedure over and over again until you get it right. Making and fixing mistakes is an accepted part of the process, and your instructors and mentors are there to help you. Schedules can be adjusted if necessary, and you are given some leeway in the matter of juggling your personal life with the demands of your schooling.

When you become the employee of a salon, however, you will be expected to put the needs of the salon and its clients ahead of your own. This means that you must always be on time for your scheduled shifts, and be prepared to perform whatever services or functions are required of you, regardless of what is happening in your personal life. If someone comes to you with tickets for a concert on Saturday, for instance, you cannot just take the day off. To do so would definitely inconvenience your clients, who might even decide not to return to the salon. It could also burden your coworkers, who, if asked to take on your appointments, might feel resentful. In short, one practitioner's selfish and immature decision can create problems for the entire salon.

OUT IN THE REAL WORLD

Many students believe they should be rewarded with a high-paying job, and doing only the kinds of services they wish to do, as soon as they graduate from cosmetology school. Well, welcome to the world. It does not work out that way, at least not for most people. In a job, you may be asked to do work or perform services that are not your first choice. The good news, however, is when you are really working "in the trenches," you are learning every moment, and there is no substitute for that kind of experience.

The important thing is to be honest with yourself as you evaluate your skills, in order to best determine which type of position is right for you. If you need help and direction in sorting out the issues around the various workplaces you are considering, ask your instructor for advice.

THRIVING IN A SERVICE PROFESSION

The first thing to remember when you are in a service business is that your work revolves around serving your clients. Some people have a hard time with the idea of customer service, because they feel that it is demeaning in some way. While it is true that there will always be some clients who do not treat people with respect, the majority of people you will encounter will truly appreciate the work you do for them. They will look forward to seeing you, and will show their appreciation for your hard work with their loyalty. Never let the negativity of a few affect your overall outlook.

Here are some points that will help guide you as you serve your clients.

Put others first. You will have to quickly get used to putting your own feelings or desires aside, and putting the needs of the salon and the client first. This means doing what is expected of you, unless you are physically unable to do so.

Be true to your word. Choose your words carefully and honestly. Be someone who can be counted on to tell the truth, and to do what you say you will do.

Be punctual. Scheduling is central to the salon business. Getting to work on time is not only respectful of your clients, but also your coworkers who will have to handle your clients if you are late.

Be grateful. Remember that it is an honor to have a job that will provide you and your family with financial stability. If you become unhappy with your salon, look for another job and move on before you start acting out in an ungrateful, disrespectful manner.

Be a problem solver. No job or situation comes without its share of problems. Be someone who recognizes problems promptly, and finds ways to resolve them constructively.

Be respectful. Although you may not like or agree with the salon manager or her rules, you must give her the benefit of the doubt. If you find that you really cannot come to terms with the salon's rules, then it is time for you to find a new job before your anger takes over.

Be a lifelong learner. A valued employee is one who intends to keep on learning. Thinking that you will never need to learn anything more once you are out of school is immature and limiting. Your career might go in all kinds of interesting directions, depending on what new things you learn. This applies to everything in your life. Besides learning new technical skills, you should continue gaining more insight into your own behavior, and how to better deal with people, problems, and issues.

SALON TEAMWORK

Working in a salon requires that you practice and perfect your people skills. A salon is very much a team environment. To become a good team player, you should do the following things:

Strive to help. Be concerned not only with your own success, but also with the success of others. Stay a little later, or come in a little earlier, to help out a teammate.

Pitch in. Be willing to help with whatever needs to be done in the salon—from folding towels to making appointments—when you are not busy servicing clients (Figure 31-2).

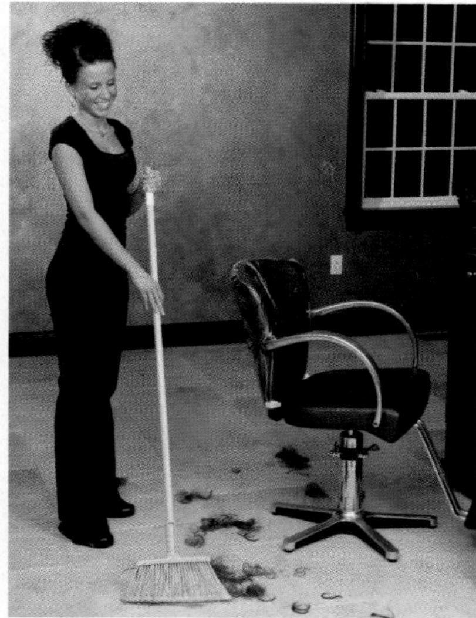

Figure 31-2 Pitch in wherever you're needed.

Share your knowledge. Be willing to share what you know. This will make you a respected member of any team.

Remain positive. Given the stress of a typical salon, there will be lots of opportunities for you to become negative, or to have conflicts with your teammates. Resist all temptations to give in to maliciousness and gossip.

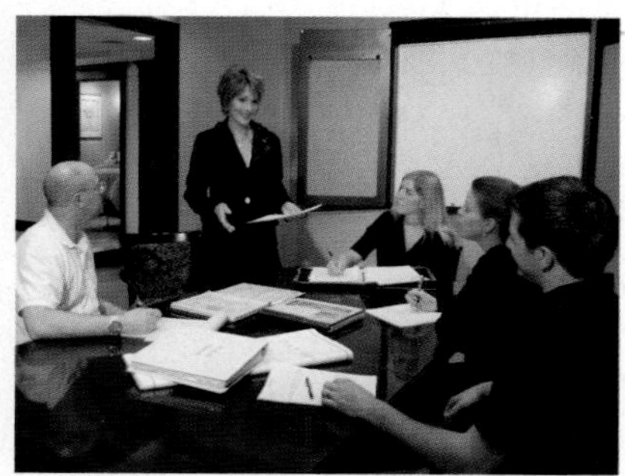

Figure 31-3 Staff meetings are essential for building a loyal team.

Become a relationship builder. Just as there are different kinds of people in the world, there are different types of relationships within the world of the salon. You do not have to be someone's best friend in order to build a good working relationship with that person.

Be willing to resolve conflicts. The most difficult part of being in a relationship is when conflict arises. A real teammate is someone who knows that conflict and tension are bad for the people who are in it, those who are around it, and the salon as a whole. Conflict is also a natural part of life. If you can work constructively toward resolving conflict, you will always be a valued member of the team.

Be willing to be subordinate. No one starts at the top. Keep in mind that beginners almost always start out lower down in the pecking order.

Be sincerely loyal. Loyalty is vital to the workings of a salon. Practitioners need to be loyal to the salon and its management. Management needs to be loyal to the staff and clients. Ideally, clients will be loyal to the practitioner and the salon. As you work on all the team-building characteristics, you will start to feel a strong sense of loyalty building up within you (Figure 31-3).

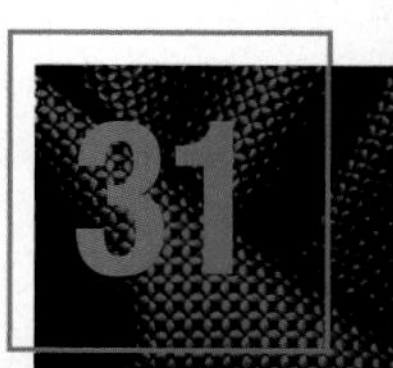

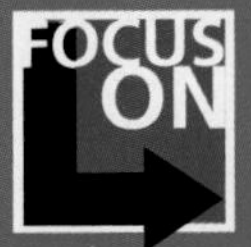

Focus on . . . The Team

Always put the team first. While each individual may be concerned with getting ahead and being successful, a good teammate knows that no one can be successful alone. The only way you can truly be successful is for the entire salon to be successful!

THE JOB DESCRIPTION

When you take a job, you will be expected to behave appropriately, perform services asked of you, and conduct your business professionally. In order to do this to the best of your abilities, you should be given a **job description**, a document that outlines all the duties and responsibilities of a particular position in a salon or spa. Many salons have a pre-printed job description that they can give you. If you find yourself at a salon that does not use job descriptions, you may want to write one for yourself. You can then present this to your salon manager for review, to ensure that both of you have a good understanding of what is expected of you.

Once you have your job description, be sure you understand it. While reading it over, make notes and jot down any questions you may want to ask your manager. When you assume your new position, you are agreeing to do everything as it is written down in the job description. If you are unclear about something, or need more information, it is your responsibility to ask.

Remember, you will be expected to fulfill all of the functions listed in the job description. How well you do this will influence your future at the salon, as well as your financial rewards in the years to come.

In crafting a job description, the best salons cover their bases. They make sure to outline not only the duties and responsibilities of the job, but also the attitudes that they expect their employees to have, and the opportunities that are available to them. Figure 31-4 shows some highlights from a well-written job description. This is just one example. Like the salons that generate them, job descriptions come in all sizes and shapes, and feature a variety of requirements, benefits, and incentives.

COMPENSATION PLANS

When you assess a job offer, your first concern will probably be around the issue of compensation, or what you will actually get paid for your work. Compensation varies from one salon to another. There are, however, three standard methods of compensation that you are likely to encounter: salary, commission, and salary plus commission.

SALARY

Being paid an hourly rate is usually the best way for a new salon professional to start out, since that person will most likely not have an established clientele for a while. An hourly rate is generally offered to a new practitioner, and is usually based on the minimum wage. Some salons offer an hourly wage that is slightly higher than the minimum wage to encourage new practitioners to take the job and stick with it. In this situation, if you earn $10 per hour and you work 40 hours, you will be paid $400 that week. If you work more hours, you will get more pay. If you work less hours, you will get less pay. Regular taxes will be taken out of your earnings.

Remember: If you are offered a set salary each week, in lieu of an hourly rate, it must be equal to at least minimum wage, and you are entitled to overtime pay if you work more than 40 hours per week. The only exception would be if you were in an official salon management position.

Job Description: Assistant

Every assistant must have a cosmetology license as well as the determination to learn and grow on the job. As an assistant you must be willing to cooperate with coworkers in a team environment, which is most conducive to learning and having a good morale among all employees. You must display a friendly yet professional attitude toward coworkers and clients alike.

Excellent time management is essential to the operation of a successful salon. An assistant should be aware of clients who are early and late or stylists who are running ahead or behind in their schedule. You should be prepared to assist in these situations, and to change your routine if necessary. Keep the receptionist and stylists informed about clients who have entered the salon. Be prepared to stay up to an hour late when necessary. Always keep in mind that everyone needs to work together to get the job done.

The responsibilities of an assistant include:

1. Greeting clients by offering them a beverage, hanging up coats, and informing the receptionist and stylist that they have arrived.
2. Shampooing and conditioning clients.
3. Assisting stylists on the styling floor.
4. Assisting stylists in services that require extra help, such as dimensional coloring.
5. Cleaning stations and mirrors, including hand-held mirrors.
6. Keeping the styling stations and back bars well stocked with appropriate products.
7. Notifying the salon manager about items and supplies that need to be reordered.
8. Making sure the shampoo sink and drain are always clean and free of hair.
9. Keeping the makeup display neat and clean.
10. Keeping the retail area neat and well stocked.
11. Keeping the bathroom and dressing room neat, clean, and stocked.
12. Performing housekeeping duties such as: emptying trash receptacles, cleaning haircolor from the floor, keeping the lunch room and dispensary neat and clean, helping with laundry, dusting shelves, and maintaining sanitary bathrooms.
13. Making fresh coffee when necessary.
14. Training new assistants.

Continuing Education

Your position as assistant is the first step toward becoming a successful stylist. In the beginning, your training will focus on the duties of an assistant. Once you have mastered those, your training will focus on the skills you will need as a stylist. As part of your continuing education in the salon you will be required to:

- attend all salon classes
- attend our special Sunday Seminars
- acquire all professional tools necessary for training at six weeks (shears, brushes, combs, clips, etc.)

Advancement

Upon successful completion of all required classes and seminars, and your demonstration of the necessary skills and attitudes, you will have the opportunity to advance to the position of Junior Stylist. This advancement will always depend upon your perfomance as an assistant, as well as the approval of management. Remember: how quickly you achieve your goals in this salon is up to you!

Figure 31-4 An example of a job description.

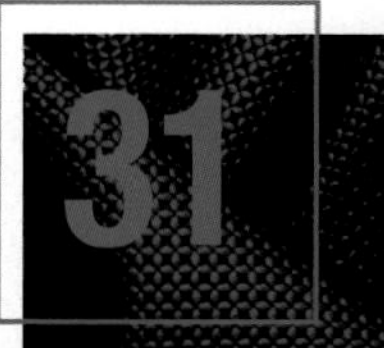

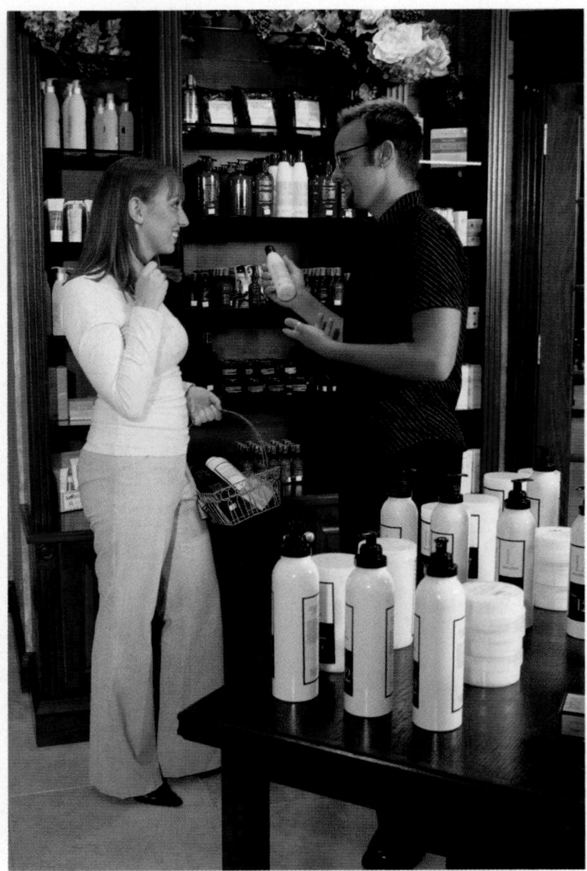

Figure 31-5 Commissions on retail sales boost income.

COMMISSION

A **commission,** a percentage of the revenue that the salon takes in, is usually offered to practitioners once they have built up a loyal clientele. A commission payment structure is very different from an hourly wage in that any money you are paid is a direct result of the total amount of service dollars you generate for the salon. Commissions are paid based on percentages of your total service dollars, and can range anywhere from 25 to 60 percent, depending on your length of time at the salon, your performance level, and the benefits that are part of your employment package. For example, at the end of the week, when you add up all the services that you have performed, your total is $1,000. If you are at the 50-percent commission level, then you would be paid $500 (before taxes). Keep in mind that until you have at least 2 years of servicing clients under your belt, you may not be able to make a living on straight commission compensation.

SALARY PLUS COMMISSIONS

A salary-plus-commission structure is another common way to be compensated in the salon business. It basically means that you receive both a salary and a commission. This kind of structure is often used to motivate practitioners to perform more services, thereby increasing their productivity. For example, imagine that you earn an hourly wage that is equal to $300 per week, and you perform about $600 worth of services every week. Your salon manager may offer you an additional 25% commission on any services you perform over your usual $600 per week. Or perhaps you receive a straight hourly wage, but you can receive as much as a 15% commission on all the retail products you sell. You can see how this kind of structure quickly leads to significantly increased compensation (Figure 31-5).

TIPS

When you receive satisfactory service at a hotel or restaurant, you are likely to leave your server a tip. It has become customary for salon clients to acknowledge beauty professionals in this way, too. Some salons have a tipping policy; others have a no-tipping policy. This is determined by what the salon feels is appropriate for its clientele.

The usual amount to tip is 15% of the total service ticket. For example, if a customer spends $50, then the tip might be 15% of that, or $7.50. Tips are income in addition to your regular compensation, and must be tracked and reported on your income tax return. Reporting tips will be beneficial to you if you wish to take out a mortgage or another type of loan and want your income to appear as strong as it really is.

As you can see, there are a number of ways to structure compensation for a salon professional. You will probably have the opportunity to try each of these methods at different points in your career. When deciding whether a certain compensation method is right for you, it is important to be aware of what your monthly expenses are, and to have a personal financial budget in place. Budget issues are addressed later in this chapter.

EMPLOYEE EVALUATION

The best way to keep tabs on your progress is to ask for feedback from your salon manager and key coworkers. Most likely, your salon will have a structure in place for evaluation purposes. Commonly, evaluations are scheduled 90 days after hiring, and then once a year after that. But you should feel free to ask for help and feedback any time you need it. This feedback can help you improve your technical abilities, as well as your customer service skills.

Ask a senior practitioner to sit in on one of your client consultations, and to make note of areas where you can improve. Ask your manager to observe your technical skills, and to point out ways you can perform your work more quickly and more efficiently. Have a trusted coworker watch and evaluate your skills when it comes to selling retail products. All of these kinds of evaluations will benefit your learning process enormously.

FIND A ROLE MODEL

One of the best ways to improve your performance is to model your behavior after someone who is having the kind of success that you wish to have. Watch other practitioners in your salon. You will easily be able to identify who is really good, and who is just coasting along. Focus on the skills of the ones who are really good. What do they do? How do they treat their clients? How do they treat the salon staff and manager? How do they book their appointments? How do they handle their continuing education? What process do they use when formulating color, or deciding on product? What is their attitude toward their work? How do they handle a crisis? Conflicts?

Go to these professionals for advice. Ask for a few minutes of their time, but be willing to wait for it because in a busy salon, it may not be easy to find time to talk during the day. If you are having a problem, explain your situation, and ask if they can help you see things differently. Be prepared to listen and not argue your points. Remember that you asked for help, even when what they are saying is not what you want to hear. Thank them for their help, and reflect on the advice you have been given.

A little help and direction from skilled, experienced coworkers will go a long way toward helping you achieve your goals.

MANAGING YOUR MONEY

Although a career in the beauty industry is very artistic and creative, it is also a career that requires financial understanding and planning. Too many cosmetology professionals live for the moment, and do not plan for their futures. They may end up feeling cheated out of the benefits that their friends and family in other careers are enjoying.

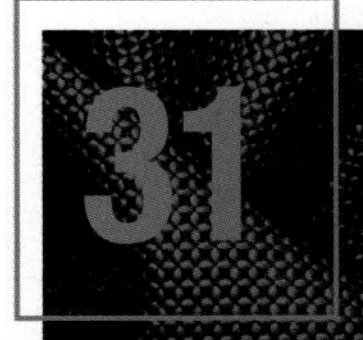

In a corporate structure, the human resources department of the corporation handles a great deal of the employee's financial planning for them. For example, health and dental insurance, retirement accounts, savings accounts, and many other items may be automatically deducted and paid out of the employee's salary. Most beauty professionals, however, must research and plan for all of those things on their own. This may seem difficult, but in fact it is a small price to pay for the kind of freedom, financial reward, and job satisfaction that a career in cosmetology can offer. And the good news is that managing money is something everyone can learn to do.

MEETING FINANCIAL RESPONSIBILITIES

In addition to making money, responsible adults are also concerned with paying back their debts. Throughout your life and your career, you will undoubtedly incur debt in the form of car loans, home mortgages, or student loans. While it is easy for some people to merely ignore their responsibility in repaying these loans, it is extremely irresponsible and immature to accept a loan and then shrug off the debt. Not paying back your loans is called "defaulting," and it can have serious consequences regarding your personal and professional credit. The best way to meet all of your financial responsibilities is to know precisely what you owe, and what you earn, so that you can make informed decisions about where your money goes.

PERSONAL BUDGET

It is amazing how many people work hard and earn very good salaries, but never take the time to create a personal budget. Many people are afraid of the word "budget" because they think that it will be too restrictive on their spending, or they have to be mathematical geniuses in order to work with a budget. Thankfully, neither of these fears is rooted in reality.

You can create a personal budget that ranges from being extremely simple to extremely complex. It all depends on what your needs are. At the beginning of your career, a simple budget should be sufficient. To get started, take a look at the worksheet in Figure 31-6. It lists the standard monthly expenses that most people have to budget. It also includes school loan repayment, savings, and payments into an individual retirement account (IRA).

Keeping track of where your money goes is one step toward making sure that you always have enough. It also helps you to plan ahead and save for bigger expenses such as a vacation, your own home, or even your own business. All in all, sticking to a budget is a good practice to follow faithfully for the rest of your life.

GIVING YOURSELF A RAISE

Once you have taken some time to create, use, and work with your personal budget, you may want to look at ways in which you can generate greater income for yourself. You might automatically jump to the most obvious sources, such as asking your employer for a raise, or asking for a

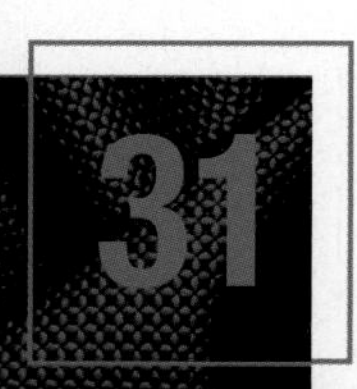

Personal Budget Worksheet

A. Expenses

1.	My monthly rent (or share of the rent) is	$__________
2.	My monthly car payment is	__________
3.	My monthly car insurance payment is	__________
4.	My monthly auto fuel/upkeep expenses are	__________
5.	My monthly electric bill is	__________
6.	My monthly gas bill is	__________
7.	My monthly health insurance payment is	__________
8.	My monthly entertainment expense is	__________
9.	My monthly bank fees are	__________
10.	My monthly grocery expense is	__________
11.	My monthly dry cleaning expense is	__________
12.	My monthly personal grooming expense is	__________
13.	My monthly prescription/medical expense is	__________
14.	My monthly telephone is	__________
15.	My monthly student loan payment is	__________
16.	My IRA payment is	__________
17.	My savings account deposit is	__________
18.	Other expenses:	__________
	TOTAL EXPENSES	$__________

B. Income

1.	My monthly take-home pay is	__________
2.	My monthly income from tips is	__________
3.	Other income:	__________
	TOTAL INCOME	$__________

C. Balance

Total Income (B)	__________
Minus Total Expenses (A)	__________
BALANCE	$__________

Figure 31-6 A budget worksheet.

higher percentage of commission. While these tactics are certainly valid, you will also want to think about other ways to increase your income, such as the following:

Spending less money. Although it may be difficult to reduce your spending, it is certainly one way to increase the amount of money that is left over at the end of the month. These dollars can be used to invest or save.

Increasing service prices. Although it will probably take some time before you are in a position to increase your service prices, once you have fully mastered all the services that you are performing, and you have a loyal **client base,** there is nothing wrong with increasing your prices every year or two, as long as you do so by a reasonable amount. Do a little research to determine what your competitors are charging for similar services, and increase your fees accordingly.

ACTIVITY

Go through the budget worksheet and fill in the amounts that apply to your current living and financial situation. If you are unsure of the amount of an expense, put in the amount you have averaged over the past 3 months, or give it your best guess. For your income, you may need to have 3 or 4 months of employment history in order to answer, but fill in what you can.

SEEK PROFESSIONAL ADVICE

Just as you will want your clients to seek out your advice and services for their hair care needs, sometimes it is important for you to seek out the advice of experts, especially when it comes to your finances. You can research and interview financial planners who will be able to give you advice on reducing your credit card debt, on how to invest your money, and on retirement options. You can speak to the officers at your local bank who may be able to suggest bank accounts that offer you greater returns or flexibility with your money, depending on what you need.

When seeking out advice from other professionals, be sure not to take anyone's advice without carefully considering whether the advice makes sense for your particular situation and needs. Before you buy into anything, be an informed consumer about other people's goods and services.

- How do your expenses compare to your income?
- What is your balance after all your expenses are paid?
- Were there any surprises for you in this exercise?
- Do you think that keeping a budget is a good way to manage money?
- Do you know of any other methods people use to manage money?

DISCOVER THE SELLING YOU

Another area that touches on the issue of you and money is selling. As a salon professional, you will have enormous opportunities to sell retail products and upgrade service tickets. **Ticket upgrading,** or **upselling services,** is the practice of recommending and selling additional services to your clients that may be performed by you or other practitioners licensed in a different field (Figure 31-7). **Retailing** is the act of recommending and selling products to your clients for at-home haircare. These two activities can make all the difference in your economic picture. The following dialogue is an example of ticket upgrading. In this scene, Judy, the practitioner, suggests an additional service to Ms. King, her client, who has just had her hair styled for a wedding she will be attending that evening.

Read the script yourself and change the words to make them fit your personality. Then try it the next time you feel that an additional service could help one of your clients.

Judy: I'm really glad you like your new hairstyle. It will be perfect with the dress you described. Don't you just love formal weddings?

Ms. King: I don't know. To tell you the truth, I don't get dressed up all that often, and putting the look together was harder than I thought it would be.

Judy: Yes, I know what you mean. Are you all set with your makeup for tonight, Ms. King? It would be a shame to have a beautiful new dress and gorgeous hair, and then have to worry about your makeup.

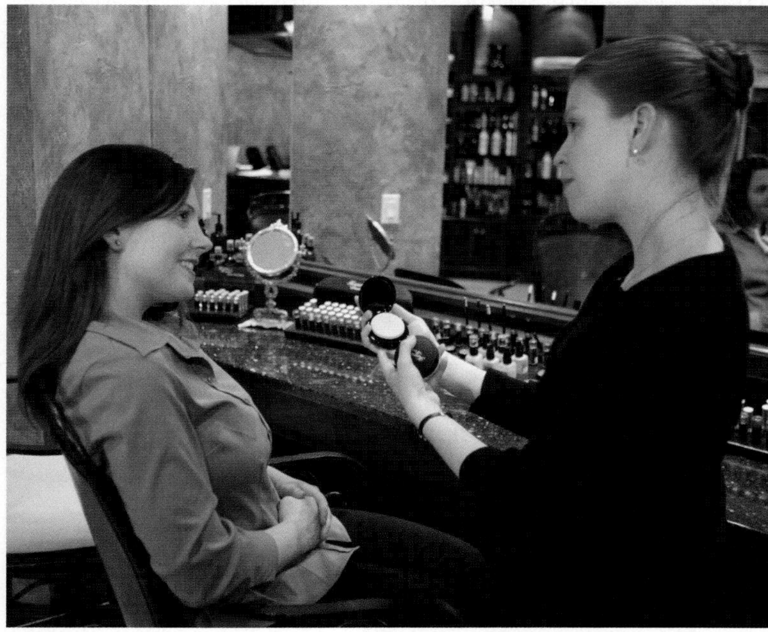

Figure 31-7 This client may wish for a makeup service as well as hairstyling.

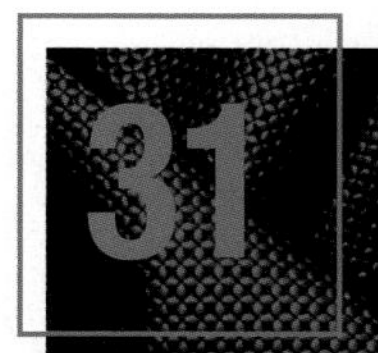

Ms. King: Well, actually, I was sort of wondering about that. I'm wearing this long black dress and I'm not really sure what the best look is for the occasion. Got any ideas?

Judy: Well, as you know, my specialty is hair care, but we have an excellent makeup artist right here on staff who's available for a consultation. You might want to make an appointment with her and she can do your makeup for you. I don't know if you've ever had a professional do it before, but it's a real treat, and it only costs $25. Plus they throw in a small lipstick to take with you. Shall I get her for you?

Ms. King: Definitely. That sounds terrific!

Judy: You know, since this is such an important occasion, you may want to consider having Marie, one of our nail techs, manicure your nails as well. That will ensure that your total look is the best it can be.

Ms. King: I think that's a great idea. Thanks for the suggestion!

PRINCIPLES OF SELLING

Some salon professionals shy away from sales. They think that it is scary, being pushy, or beneath them. A close look at how selling works can set your mind at ease. Not only can you become very good at selling once you understand the principles behind it, but also feel good about providing your clients with a valuable service.

To be successful in sales, you need ambition, determination, and a good personality. The first step in selling is to sell yourself. Clients must like and trust you before they will purchase beauty services, cosmetics, skin or nail care items, shampoos and conditioners, or other merchandise.

Remember, every client who enters the salon is a potential purchaser of additional services or merchandise. Recognizing the client's needs and preferences lays the foundation for successful selling.

To become a proficient salesperson, you must be able to apply the following principles of selling:

- Be familiar with the merits and benefits of the various services and products that you are trying to sell, and recommend only those that the client really needs.
- Adapt your approach and technique to meet the needs and personality of each client. Some clients may prefer a "soft sell" that involves informing them about the product, without stressing that they purchase it. Others are comfortable with a "hard-sell" approach that focuses emphatically on why a client should buy the product.
- Be self-confident when recommending products for sale. You become confident by knowing about the products you are selling, and by believing that they are as good as you say they are.
- Generate interest and desire in the customer by asking questions that determine a need.
- Never misrepresent your services or products. Making unrealistic claims will only lead to your client's disappointment, and will make it unlikely that you will ever be able to sell to that client again.

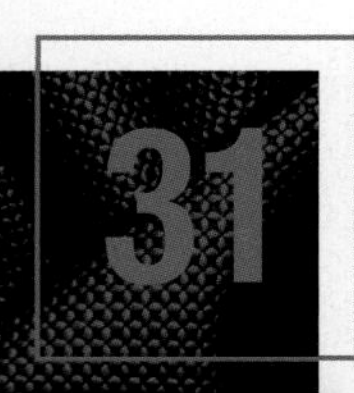

- Do not underestimate the client's intelligence, or her knowledge of her own beauty regimen or particular needs.
- To sell a product or service, deliver your sales talk in a relaxed, friendly manner and, if possible, demonstrate use (Figure 31-8).
- Recognize the right psychological moment to close any sale. Once the client has offered to buy, quit selling. Do not oversell, except to praise the client for the purchase and to assure her that she will be happy with it.

THE PSYCHOLOGY OF SELLING

Most people have reasons for doing what they do, and when you are selling something, it is your job to figure out the reasons that might motivate a person to buy. When dealing with salon clients, you will find that their motives for buying salon products vary widely. Some may be concerned with issues of vanity (they want to look better). Some are seeking personal satisfaction (they want to feel better about themselves). Others need to solve a problem that is bothersome (they want to spend less time maintaining their nails).

Sometimes, a client may inquire about a product or service, but may still be undecided or doubtful. In this type of situation, you can help the decision along by offering honest and sincere advice. When you explain a beauty service to a client, address the results and benefits of that service. Always keep in mind that the best interests of the client should be your first consideration. You will need to know exactly what your client's needs are, and you need to have a clear idea as to how those needs can be fulfilled. Refer to the sample dialogues in this section—one involves ticket upgrading, and the other involves retailing, both of which demonstrate effective selling techniques.

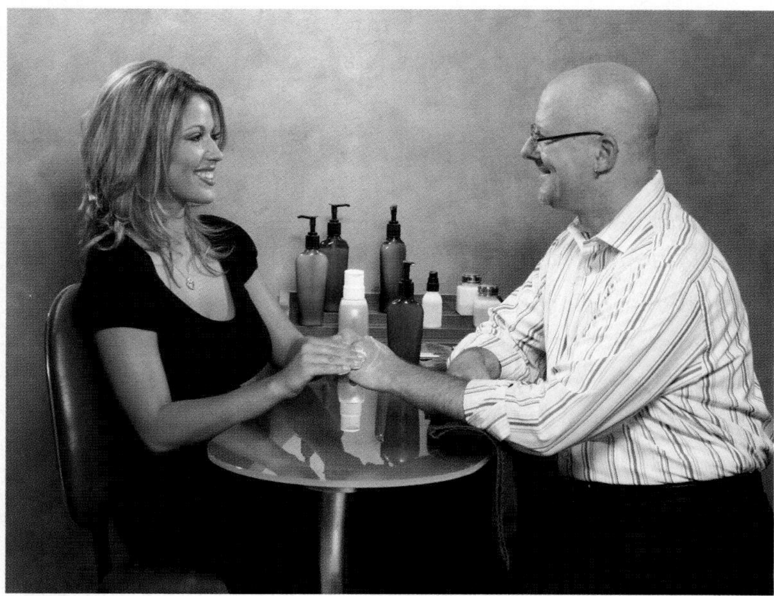

Figure 31-8 Demonstrate a product's benefits.

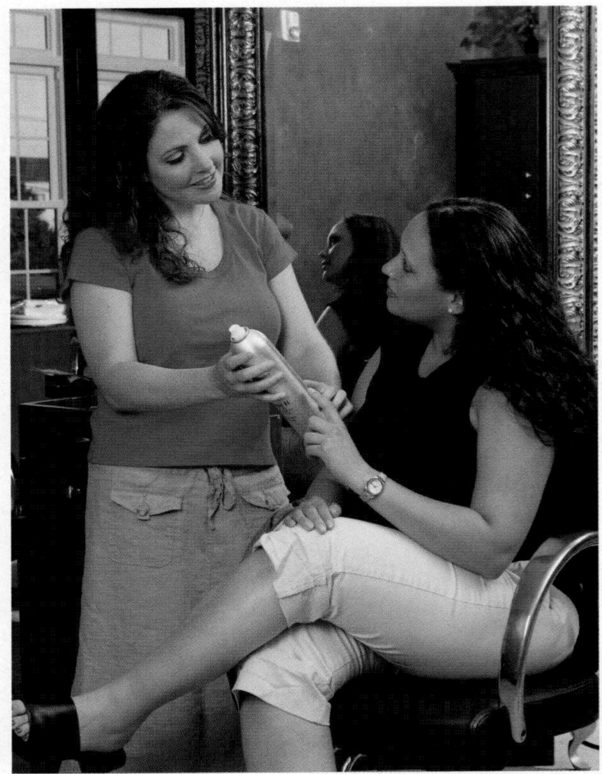
Figure 31-9 Place the product in the client's hands.

Here are a few tips on how to get the conversation started on retailing products:

- Ask every client what products they are using for home maintenance of their nails, hands, and feet.
- Place products in the client's hands whenever possible, or have them in view (Figure 31-9).
- Advise the client about how the recommended service will provide personal benefit (more manageable hairstyling or longer-lasting nail polish, for instance).
- Keep retail areas clean, well lit, and appealing.
- Inform clients of any promotions and sales that are going on in the salon.
- Be informed about the merits of using a professional product as opposed to generic store brands.

While you realize that retailing products is a service to your clients, you may not be sure how to go about it. Imagine the following scenes and see how Lisa, the practitioner, highlights the benefits and features of a product to her client, Ms. Steiner. Note that price is not necessarily the "bottom line."

SCENARIO 1: NAIL CLIENT

Ms. Steiner: I just love the way you do my nails. How do you always make my cuticles and hands look like they're in such good shape?

Lisa: I always use a penetrating cuticle oil on your cuticles, Ms. Steiner. It's a wonderful product and one you should be using on your cuticles every day. I also use the lotion made by the same company.

Ms. Steiner: Is that the lotion you use with the great lavender scent?

Lisa: I love that light lavender scent too. It's a really great moisturizing lotion that we swear by—it's fabulous for treating dry and even chapped skin. I use it on my pedicure clients too, and it soothes that dry, rough skin that can accumulate on feet, especially in dry winter weather. Do you use any lotion at home after your shower or after having your hands in water?

Ms. Steiner: Yeah, I do, something I picked up in the grocery store one day. But it's very runny, not thick like your lotion.

Lisa: Oh, well our lotion is very rich and emollient because it has been especially formulated to stay on your hands and feet and moisturize them throughout the day.

Ms. Steiner: Yeah, well, nothing really makes much of a difference in this weather.

Lisa: Well, I can tell you that I have several clients who are using this lotion at home, and every one of them comes back in and raves about how much better their skin feels and how their dry flaky skin has gone away!

ACTIVITY

Pick a partner from class and role-play the dynamics of a sales situation. Take turns being the customer and the practitioner. Evaluate each other on how you did, with suggestions about where you can improve. Then try this exercise with someone else, as no two customers are the same.

Ms. Steiner: Really?

Lisa: Yes. You may want to give it a try yourself and see how it works for you. It's available at the front when you check out. I'll grab you a bottle of lotion and the cuticle oil product, so you can look at them while I finish up your service.

Ms. Steiner: Great!

HOW TO EXPAND YOUR CLIENT BASE

Once you have mastered the basics of good service, take a look at some marketing techniques that will expand your client base, or those customers that keep coming back to you for services. These are only a few suggestions; there are many others that may work for you. The best way to decide which techniques are most effective is to try several.

Birthday cards. Ask clients for their birthday information (just the month and day, not the year) on the client consultation card, and then use it as a tool to get them into the salon again. About 1 month prior to the client's birthday, send a card with a special offer. Make it valid only for the month of their birthday.

Provide consistently good service. It seems basic enough, but it is amazing how many professionals work hard to get clients, and lose them because they rush through a service and leave them feeling dissatisfied. Providing good-quality service must always be your first concern.

Be reliable. Always be courteous, thoughtful, and professional. Be at the salon when you say you will be there, and do not keep clients waiting (Refer to Chapter 4 for tips on how to handle the unavoidable times when you are running late). Give your clients the hair length and style they ask for, not something else. Recommend a retail product only when you have tried it yourself, and you know what it can and cannot do.

Be respectful. When you treat others with respect, you become worthy of respect yourself. Being respectful means that you do not gossip or make fun of anyone or anything related to the salon. Negative energy brings everyone down, especially you.

Be positive. Become one of those people who always sees the glass as half full. Look for the positive in every situation. No one enjoys being around a person who is always unhappy.

Be professional. Sometimes, a client may try to make your relationship more personal than it ought to be. It is in your best interest, and your client's best interest, not to cross that line. Remember that your job is

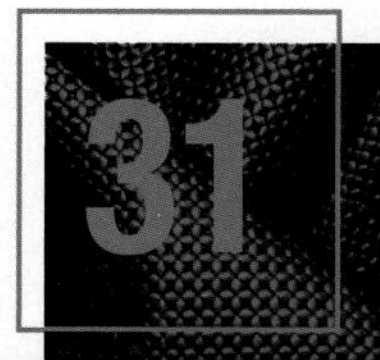

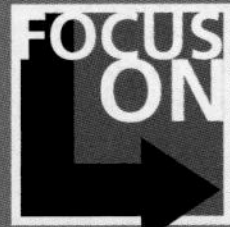

Focus on . . . Retailing

For quick reference, keep these five points in mind when selling:

1. Establish rapport with the client.
2. Determine the client's needs.
3. Recommend products/services based on these needs.
4. Emphasize benefits.
5. Close the sale.

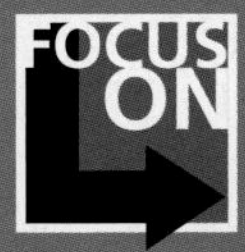

Focus on . . . The Goal

Always remember that success does not just come to you; you make it happen. How? By being a team player, having a positive attitude, and keeping a real sense of commitment to your work foremost in your mind.

to be the client's beauty advisor, not a psychiatrist, a marriage counselor, or a buddy.

Business card referrals. Make up a special business card with your information on it, but leave room for a client to put her name on it as well. If your client is clearly pleased with your work, give her several cards. Ask her to put her name on them, and to refer her friends and associates to you. For every card you receive from a new customer with her name on it, give her 10% off her next salon service, or a complementary added service to her next appointment. This gives the client lots of motivation to recommend you to others, which in turn, helps build up your clientele (Figure 31-10).

Local business referrals. Another terrific way to build business is to work with other businesses in your area. Look for clothing stores, florists, gift shops, and other small businesses near your salon. Offer to have a card swap and commit to referring your clients to them when they are in the market for goods or services that your neighbors can provide, if they will do the same for you. This is a great way to build a feeling of community among local vendors, and to reach new clients you may not be able to otherwise.

Public speaking. Make yourself available to speak to local women's groups, the PTA, organizations for young men and women, and anywhere else that will put you in front of people in your community who are all potential clients. Put together a short program (20 to 30 minutes) in which, for example, you might discuss professional appearance with emphasis in your chosen field and other grooming tips for people looking for jobs or who are already employed.

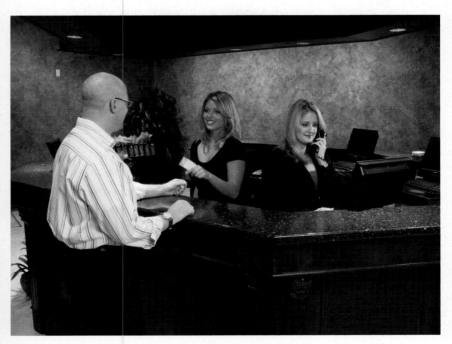

Figure 31-10 Referral cards help build your client base.

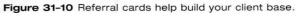

REBOOKING CLIENTS

The best time to think about getting your client back into the salon is while she is still in your salon. It may seem a little difficult to assure your client that you are concerned with her satisfaction on this visit while you are talking about her next visit, but, in fact, the two go together. The best way to encourage your client to book another appointment before she leaves is to simply talk with her, ask questions, and listen carefully to her answers.

During the time that you are working on a client's hair, for instance, talk about the condition of her hair, her hairstyling habits at home, and the benefits of regular or special salon maintenance. You might raise these issues in a number of ways.

SCENARIO 2: COLOR CLIENT

"Mrs. Rivera, When I cut your hair today I noticed that you need a color retouch. Shall I book a retouch for your next visit?"

SCENARIO 3: HAIRCUTTING CLIENT

"Your son is getting married next month? How wonderful. Have you thought about having a clear glazing so your hair will be bright and shiny and will look as beautiful as the rest of you in that new dress you told me about? I can set up an appointment for the day before the wedding."

Again, you will want to listen carefully to what your clients are telling you during their visit, because they will often give the careful listener many good clues as to what is happening in their lives. That will open the door to discussing their next appointment.

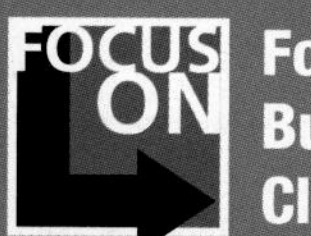

Focus on . . . Building Your Client Base

Some professionals believe that the more time they spend with their clients performing services, the better the service will be. Not so! Your client should be in the salon only as long as is necessary for you to adequately complete a service.

Be aware of how much time it takes you to perform various services and then schedule accordingly. As you become more and more experienced, you should see a reduction in the amount of time it takes you to perform these services. That means clients wait less, you can increase the number of services you can provide in a day, and the increase in services naturally increases your income.

ON YOUR WAY

Your first job in the beauty industry will most likely be the most difficult. Getting started in this business means being on a big learning curve for a while. Be patient with yourself as you transition from the "school you" to the "professional you." Always remember that in your work life, as in everything else you do, practice makes perfect. You will not know everything you need to know right at the start, but be confident in the fact that you are graduating from cosmetology school with a solid knowledge base. Make use of the many generous and experienced professionals you will encounter, and let them teach you the tricks of the trade. Make the commitment to perfecting your technical and customer service skills.

Above all, always be willing to learn. If you let the concepts that you have learned in this book be your guide, you will enjoy your life and reap the amazing benefits of a career in cosmetology (Figure 31-11).

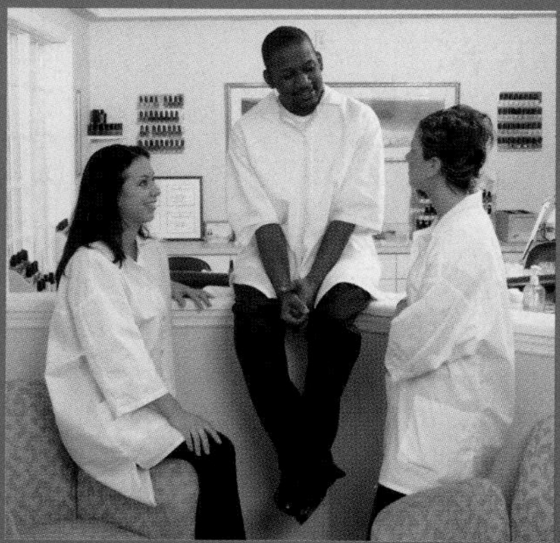

Figure 31-1 1 Make career satisfaction your goal.

REVIEW QUESTIONS

1. What should you look for in a salon to determine whether it is right for you?
2. List seven rules of conduct that help a new employee succeed in a service profession like cosmetology.
3. List six habits of a good team player.
4. Explain how a job description is used by the salon and by the employee.
5. What are the three most common methods of salon compensation?
6. Complete a personal budget and explain why managing your personal finances is important to your success.
7. Name at least six principles of selling retail products in the salon.
8. List the important personal characteristics that help you build a client base.
9. Explain at least three different activities that you can undertake to expand your client base.

CHAPTER GLOSSARY

client base	Customers who are loyal to a particular cosmetologist.
commission	Percentage of revenue that a salon takes in from sales earmarked for practitioner.
job description	Document that outlines all duties and responsibilities of a particular position in a salon or spa.
retailing	Act of recommending and selling products to your clients for at-home hair care.
ticket upgrading* or *upselling services	Practice of recommending and selling additional services to clients.

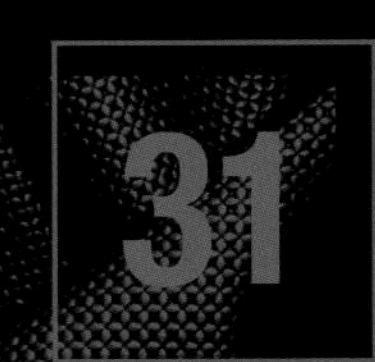

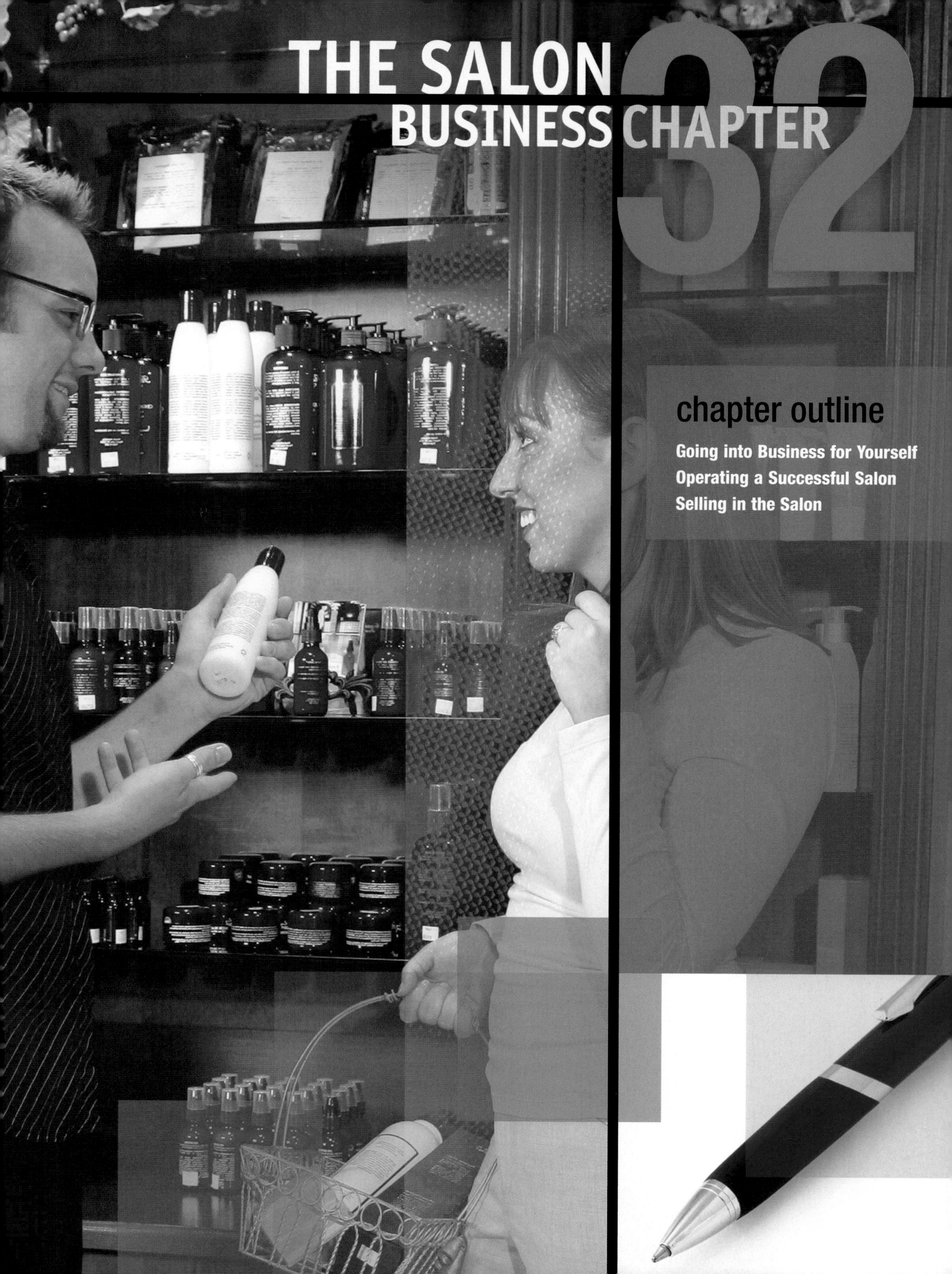

THE SALON BUSINESS CHAPTER 32

chapter outline

Learning Objectives

After completing this chapter, you will be able to:

- List the two ways in which you may go into business for yourself.
- List the factors to consider when opening a salon.
- Name and describe the types of ownership under which a salon may operate.
- Explain the importance of keeping accurate business records.
- Discuss the importance of the reception area to a salon's success.
- Demonstrate good salon telephone techniques.
- List the most effective forms of salon advertising.

Key Terms

Page number indicates where in the chapter the term is used.

booth rental
pg. 842

business plan
pg. 843

business regulations and laws
pg. 843

capital
pg. 844

consumption supplies
pg. 848

corporations
pg. 844

demographics
pg. 843

insurance
pg. 843

partnership
pg. 844

personnel
pg. 849

record-keeping
pg. 843

retail supplies
pg. 848

salon operation
pg. 843

salon policies
pg. 843

sole proprietor
pg. 844

written agreements
pg. 843

As you become more proficient in your craft and your ability to manage yourself and others, you may decide to become an independent booth renter, or even a salon owner. While this may seem like an easy thing to do, being a successful business person requires experience, a genuine love of people, and solid business management skills. To become a successful entrepreneur, you will need to commit to always being a student of business. You will also have to learn how to attract practitioners and clients to your business, and maintain their loyalty over long periods of time. Remember: The better prepared you are, the greater your chances of success (Figure 32-1).

Many books have been written on each of the topics touched on in this chapter, so be prepared to read and research your business idea extensively before making any final decisions. The following information is only meant to be a general overview of the salon business.

GOING INTO BUSINESS FOR YOURSELF

If you reach a point in your life when you feel that you are ready to become your own boss, you will have two main options to consider: (1) owning your own salon, or (2) renting a booth in an existing salon. Both options have their pros and cons.

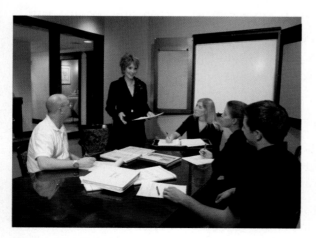

Figure 32-1 Opening your own salon or spa is a big step.

32

BOOTH RENTAL

Booth rental has become so popular that it is now practiced in over 50% of all salons in the United States. Currently, it is legal in every state except Pennsylvania, where there is a law prohibiting booth rental, and New Jersey where the state board does not recognize booth rental as an acceptable method of doing business. Many people see booth rental, or renting a station in a salon (also known as chair rental), as a more desirable alternative to owning a salon. In a booth rental arrangement, a practitioner generally:

- Rents a station or workspace in a salon from the salon owner
- Is solely responsible for his or her own clientele, supplies, record-keeping, and accounting
- Pays the salon owner a weekly fee for use of the booth
- Becomes his/her own boss for a very small amount of money
- Maintains expenses that are fairly low

Booth rental is a desirable situation for many practitioners who have large, steady clienteles, and do not have to rely on the salon to keep busy. Unless you are at least 70% booked all the time, however, it may not be advantageous to rent a booth.

Although it may sound like a good option, booth renting has its share of obligations, such as:

- Keeping records for income tax purposes and other legal reasons
- Paying all taxes, including higher Social Security (double that of an employee)
- Carrying adequate malpractice insurance and health insurance
- Maintaining inventory
- Managing the purchase of products and supplies
- Budgeting for advertising, or offering incentives to ensure a steady influx of new clients
- Paying for all education
- Working in an independent atmosphere where teamwork usually does not exist, and salon standards are interpreted on an individual basis

As a booth renter, you will not enjoy the same benefits as an employee of a salon would, such as paid days off or vacation time. Remember, when you are not working, you do not get paid.

OPENING YOUR OWN SALON

Like climbing Mount Everest, and all the physical and mental challenges that it entails, opening your own salon is a huge undertaking. Regardless of the type of salon you hope to open, there are some basic factors that you should consider carefully, such as the following:

1. **Location.** Having good visibility and accessibility are two of the most important factors in predicting the success of a business. The location that you select should reflect your target market, have access to plenty

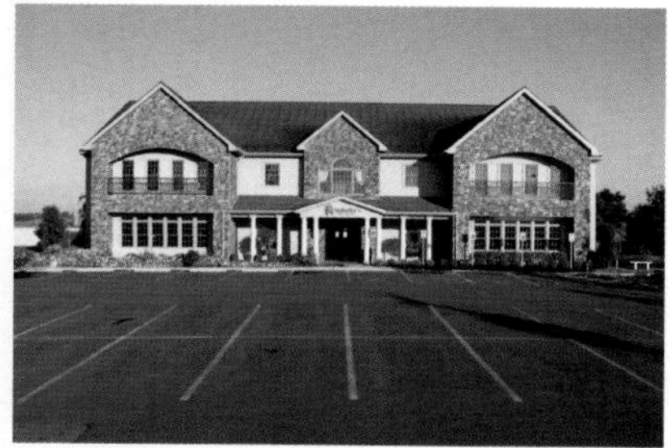

Figure 32-2 Location. Location. Location. Your salon should have good visibility, plenty of parking, and high pedestrian traffic.

of parking, and should be far enough away from competing salons to avoid too much competition (Figure 32-2).

2. **Written agreements.** Before you open a salon, you must develop a **business plan,** a written description of your business as you see it today, and as you foresee it in the next 5 years (detailed by year). If you wish to obtain financing, it is essential that you have a business plan in place first. The plan should include a general description of the business and the services that it will provide; area **demographics** (e.g., average income in your proposed area, average cost of services, number of salons within a 5-mile radius); expected salaries and cost of related benefits; an operations plan that includes pricing structure and expenses such as equipment, supplies, repairs, advertising, taxes, and insurance; and projected income and overhead expenses for up to 5 years. A certified public accountant (CPA) can be invaluable in helping you gather accurate financial information. The Chamber of Commerce in your proposed area typically has information on area demographics.

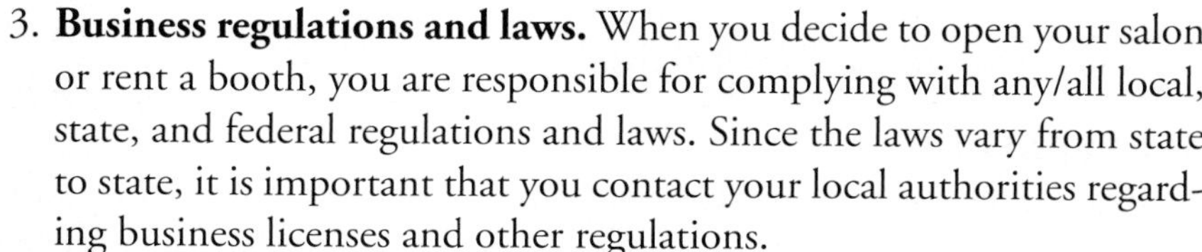

3. **Business regulations and laws.** When you decide to open your salon or rent a booth, you are responsible for complying with any/all local, state, and federal regulations and laws. Since the laws vary from state to state, it is important that you contact your local authorities regarding business licenses and other regulations.
4. **Insurance.** When you open your business, you will need to purchase insurance that covers malpractice, property liability, fire, burglary and theft, and business interruption. You will need to have disability policies as well. Make sure that your policies cover you for all the monetary demands you will have to meet on your lease.
5. **Salon operation.** You must know and comply with all federal Occupational Safety and Health Administration (OSHA) guidelines, including those that require the ingredients of cosmetic preparations be available for employees. OSHA requires Material Safety Data Sheets (MSDS) for this purpose.
6. **Record-keeping.** You will need to keep accurate and complete records of all financial activities in your business.
7. **Salon policies.** Even small salons and booth renters should have policies that they adhere to. These ensure that all clients and associates are being treated fairly and consistently.

TYPES OF SALON OWNERSHIP

A salon can be owned and operated by an individual, partnership, or corporation. Before deciding which type of ownership is most desirable for your situation, research each thoroughly. There are excellent reference tools available, and you can also consult a small business attorney for advice.

INDIVIDUAL OWNERSHIP

If you like to make your own rules, and are responsible enough to meet all the duties and obligations of running a business, individual ownership may be the best arrangement for you.

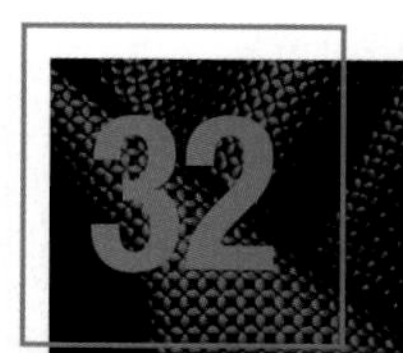

The **sole proprietor:**

- Is the owner and, most often, the manager of the business
- Determines policies, and has the last say in decision making
- Assumes expenses, receives profits, and bears all losses

PARTNERSHIP

Partnerships may mean more opportunity for increased investment and growth. They can be magical if the right chemistry is struck, or they can be disastrous if you find yourself linked with someone you wish you had known better in the first place.

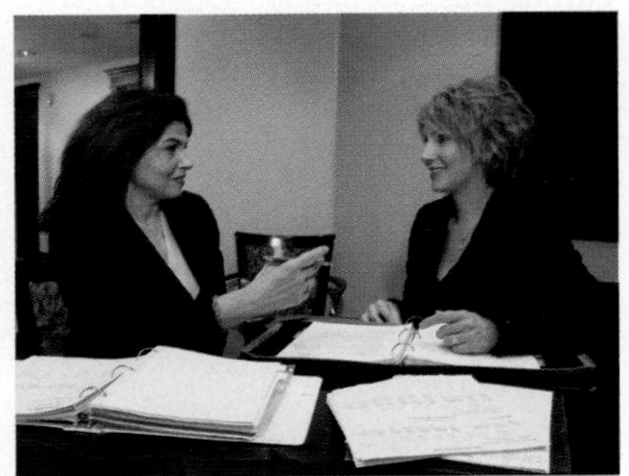

Figure 32-3 Partners share the work and the responsibilities.

In a **partnership** two or more people:

- Share ownership, although not necessarily equally. One reason for going into a partnership arrangement is to have more **capital** for investment; another is to have help running your operation.
- Pool their skills and talents, making it easier to share work, responsibilities, and decision making (Figure 32-3).
- Assume the other's unlimited liability for debts.

CORPORATION

Incorporating is one of the best ways that a business owner can protect her or his personal assets. Most people choose to incorporate solely for this reason, but there are other advantages as well. For example, the corporate business structure saves you money in taxes, provides greater business flexibility, and makes raising capital easier. It also limits your personal financial liability if your business accrues unmanageable debts or otherwise runs into financial trouble.

Characteristics of corporations follow:

- **Corporations** raise capital by issuing stock certificates or shares.
- Stockholders (people or companies that purchase shares) have an ownership interest in the company. The more stock they own, the bigger that interest becomes.
- You can be the sole stockholder (or shareholder), or have many stockholders.
- Corporate formalities, such as director and stockholder meetings, are required to maintain a corporate status.
- Income tax is limited to the salary that you draw, and not the total profits of the business.
- Corporations cost more to set up and run than a sole proprietorship or partnership. For example, there are the initial formation fees, filing fees, and annual state fees.
- A stockholder of a corporation is required to pay unemployment insurance taxes on his or her salary, whereas a sole proprietor or partner is not.

PURCHASING AN ESTABLISHED SALON

Purchasing an existing salon could be an excellent opportunity, but, as with anything else, you have to look at all sides of the picture. If you choose to buy an established salon, seek professional assistance from an accountant and a business lawyer (Figure 32-4). In general, any agreement to buy an established salon should include the following:

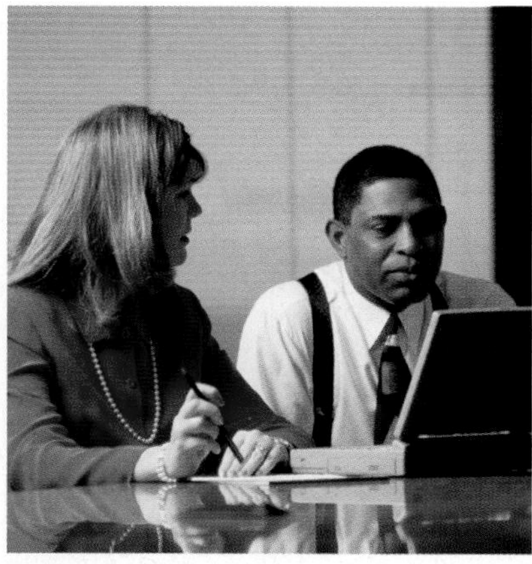

Figure 32-4 A lawyer specializing in leases and business sales is a good source of professional advice.

- Written purchase and sale agreement to avoid any misunderstandings between the contracting parties.
- Complete and signed statement of inventory (goods, fixtures, and the like) indicating the value of each article.
- If there is a transfer of a note, mortgage, lease, and bill of sale, the buyer should initiate an investigation to determine whether there are defaults in the payment of debts.
- Identity of owner.
- Use of the salon's name and reputation for a definite period of time.
- Disclosure of any and all information regarding the salon's clientele, and its purchasing and service habits.
- Noncompete agreement stating that the seller will not work in, or establish a new salon, within a specified distance from the present location.

DRAWING UP A LEASE

In most cases, owning your own business does not mean that you own the building that houses your business. When renting or leasing space, you must have an agreement between yourself and the building's owner that has been well thought out and well written. The lease should specify clearly who owns what, and who is responsible for which repairs and expenses. You should also secure the following:

- Exemption of fixtures or appliances that might be attached to the salon so that they can be removed without violating the lease.
- Agreement about necessary renovations and repairs, such as painting, plumbing, fixtures, and electrical installation.
- Option from the landlord that allows you to assign the lease to another person. In this way, obligations for the payment of rent are kept separate from the responsibilities of operating the business, should you decide to bring in another person or owner.

PROTECTION AGAINST FIRE, THEFT, AND LAWSUITS

- Ensure that your business has adequate locks, fire alarm system, and burglar alarm system.
- Purchase liability, fire, malpractice, and burglary insurance, and do not allow these policies to lapse while you intend to remain in business.
- Become thoroughly familiar with all laws governing cosmetology, and with the sanitary codes of your city and state.
- Keep accurate records of the number of employees, their salaries, lengths of employment, and Social Security numbers as required by

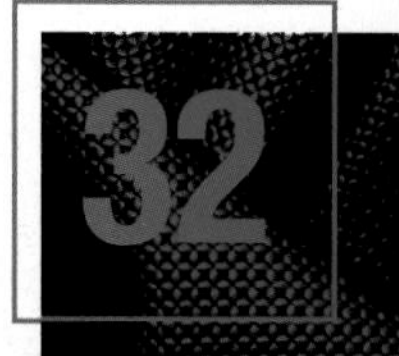

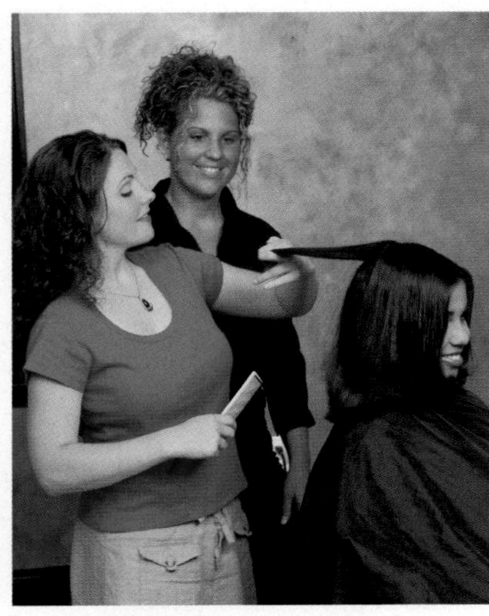

Figure 32-5 Coaching a new practitioner.

various state and federal laws that monitor the social welfare of workers.

- Ignorance of the law is no excuse for violating it. Always check with your regulatory agency if you have any questions about a law or regulation.

BUSINESS OPERATIONS

Whether you are an owner or a manager, there are certain skills that you must develop in order to successfully run a salon. To run a people-oriented business, you need the following:

- An excellent business sense, aptitude, good judgment, and diplomacy
- Knowledge of sound business principles

Because it takes time to develop these skills, you would be wise to establish a circle of contacts—business owners, including some salon owners—that can give you advice along the way. Consider joining a local entrepreneurs group, or your city's Chamber of Commerce, to extend the reach of your networking.

Smooth business management depends on the following factors:

- Sufficient investment capital
- Efficiency of management

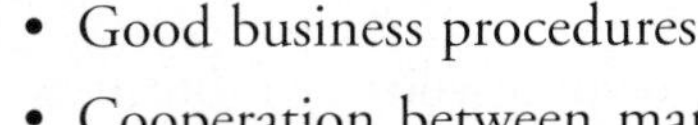

- Good business procedures
- Cooperation between management and employees
- Trained and experienced salon personnel (Figure 32-5)
- Excellent customer service delivery
- Proper pricing of services (Figure 32-6)

STYLES BY DOTTI

Haircuts	
Designer cuts for women	$40
Men's cut	$25
Children's cut	starting at $15
Formal updos	starting at $45
Haircolor Services	
Virgin application, single-process	starting at $40
Color retouch	starting at $35
Double-process	starting at $55
Dimensional highlighting (full head)	$75
Dimensional highlighting (partial head)	$60
Texture Services	
Customized perming	starting at $80
Spiral perm	starting at $100
Includes complimentary home maintenance product.	

Figure 32-6 Typical salon price list.

ALLOCATION OF MONEY

As a business operator, you must always know where your money is being spent. A good accountant and an accounting system are indispensable. The figures in Table 32-1 serve as a guideline, but may vary depending on locality.

THE IMPORTANCE OF RECORD-KEEPING

Good business operations require a simple and efficient record system. Proper business records are necessary to meet the requirements of local, state, and federal laws regarding taxes and employees. Records are of value only if they are correct, concise, and complete. Proper bookkeeping methods include keeping an accurate record of all income and expenses. Income is usually classified as receipts from services and retail sales.

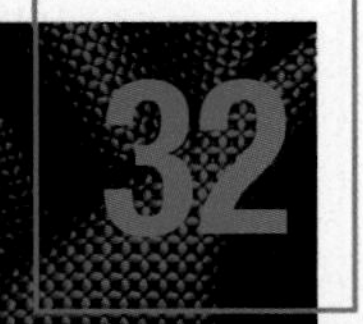

EXPENSES	Percent of Total Gross Income
Salaries and commissions (including payroll taxes)	53.5
Rent	13.0
Supplies	5.0
Advertising	3.0
Depreciation	3.0
Laundry	1.0
Cleaning	1.0
Light and power	1.0
Repairs	1.5
Insurance	.75
Telephone	.75
Miscellaneous	1.5
Total expenses	85.0
Net profit	15.0
Total	100.0

Table 32-1 Average Expenses for Salons in the United States

Expenses include rent, utilities, insurance, salaries, advertising, equipment, and repairs. Retain check stubs, canceled checks, receipts, and invoices. A professional accountant or a full-charge bookkeeper is recommended to help keep records accurate. (A "full-charge bookkeeper" means someone who is trained to do everything from record sales and payroll, to generating a profit-and-loss statement.)

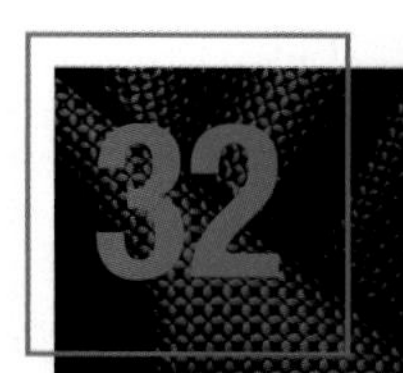

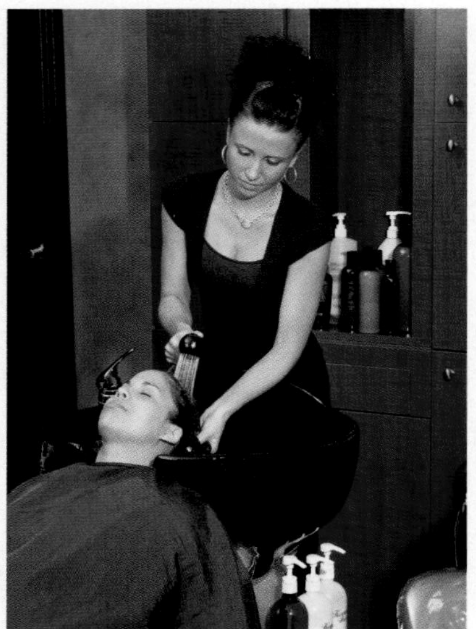
Figure 32-7 Consumption supplies for each shampoo station.

PURCHASE AND INVENTORY RECORDS

The purchase of inventory and supplies should be closely monitored. Purchase records help maintain a perpetual inventory, which prevents overstocking or shortage of needed supplies, and also alerts you to any incidents of pilfering (petty theft by employees). These records also help establish the net worth of the business at the end of the year.

Keep a running inventory of all supplies, and classify them according to their use and retail value. Those to be used in the daily business operation are **consumption supplies** (Figure 32-7). Those to be sold to clients are **retail supplies.**

SERVICE RECORDS

Always keep service records or client cards that describe treatments given, and merchandise sold to each client. Either a card file system or software program will serve this purpose. All service records should include the name and address of the client, the date of each purchase or service, the amount charged, products used, and results obtained. Clients' preferences and tastes should also be noted. For more information on filling out these cards, and for examples of a client record card, see Chapter 4.

OPERATING A SUCCESSFUL SALON

The only way to guarantee that you will stay in business and have a prosperous salon is to take excellent care of your clients. Clients visiting your salon should feel that they are being well taken care of, and that they always look forward to their next visit. To accomplish this, your salon must be physically attractive, well organized, smoothly run, and, above all, sparkling clean.

PLANNING THE SALON'S LAYOUT

One of the most exciting opportunities ahead of you is planning and constructing the best physical layout for the type of salon you envision. Maximum efficiency should be the primary concern. For example, if you are opening a low-budget salon offering quick service, you will need several stations, and a small- to medium-sized reception area since clients will be moving in and out of the salon fairly quickly. Your retail area may also be on the small side, since your clients may not have a lot of disposable income to spend on retail products (Figure 32-8).

However, if you are opening a high-end salon or luxurious day spa where clients expect the quality of the service to be matched by the environment, you will want to plan for more room in the waiting area. You may, in fact, choose to have several areas in which clients can lounge between services and enjoy beverages or light snacks. Some upscale salons feature small coffee bars that lend an air of sophistication to the environment. Others offer quiet, private areas where clients can pursue business activities such

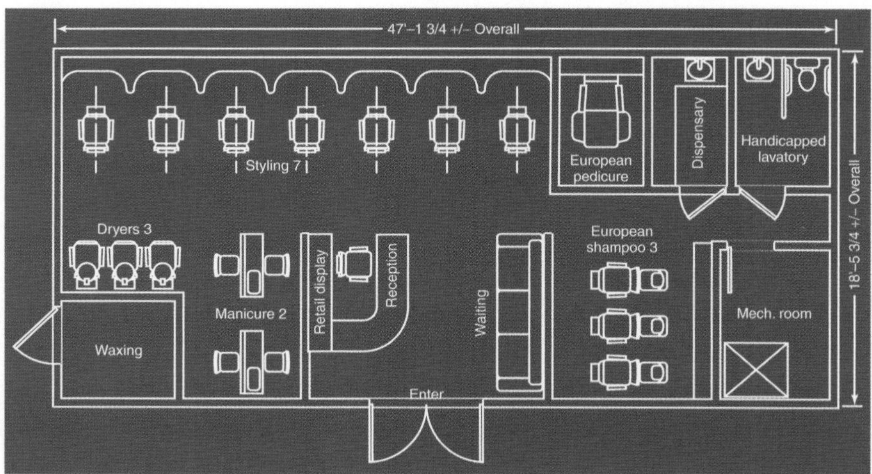

Figure 32-8 Layout for a typical salon.

as phone work or laptop activities between services. The retail area should be spacious, inviting, and well lit.

Layout is crucial to the smooth operation of a salon. Once you have decided the type of salon that you wish to run, seek the advice of an architect with plenty of experience in designing salons. For renovations, a professional equipment and furniture supplier will be able to help you (Figure 32-9).

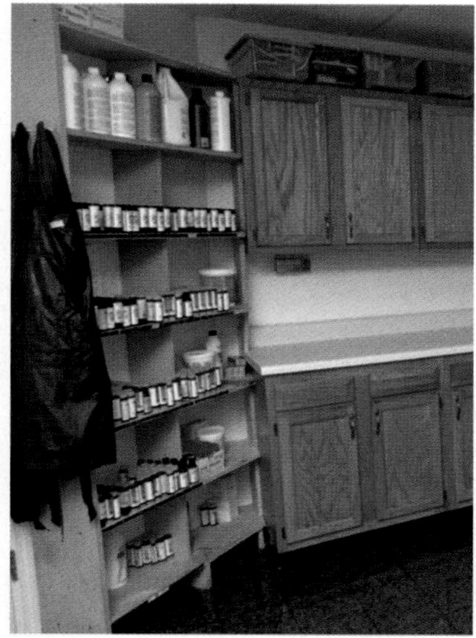

Figure 32-9 Salon dispensary.

PERSONNEL

The size of your salon will determine the size of your staff. Large salons and day spas require receptionists, hair practitioners, nail technicians, shampoo persons, colorists, massage therapists, estheticians, and hair removal specialists.

Smaller salons have some combination of these **personnel** who perform more than one type of service. For example, the practitioner might also be the colorist and texture specialist. The success of a salon depends on the quality of the work done by the staff.

When interviewing potential employees, consider the following:

- Level of skill (What is their educational background? When was the last time they attended an educational event?)
- Personal grooming (Do they look like you would want their advice on your personal grooming?)
- Image as it relates to the salon (Are they too progressive, or too conservative for your environment?)
- Overall attitude (Do they seem more negative than positive in their responses to your questions?)
- Communication skills (Are they able to understand your questions? Can you understand their responses?)

Making good hiring decisions is crucial. Undoing bad hiring decisions is painful for all involved, and can be more complicated than you might expect.

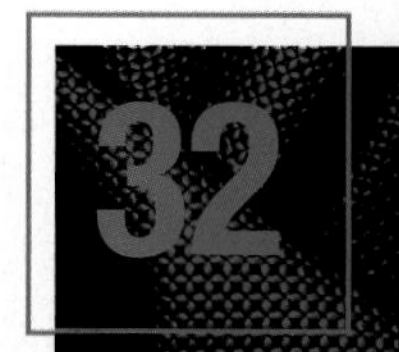

PAYROLL AND EMPLOYEE BENEFITS

In order to have a successful business, one in which everyone feels appreciated and is happy to work hard and service clients, you must be willing to share your success with your staff whenever it is financially feasible to do so. You can do this in a number of ways.

- Make it your top priority to meet your payroll obligations. In the allotment of funds, this comes first.
- Whenever possible, offer hardworking and loyal employees as many benefits as possible. Either cover the cost of these benefits, or at least make them available to employees and allow them to decide if they can cover the cost themselves.
- Provide staff members with a schedule of employee evaluations. Make it clear what is expected of them if they are to receive pay increases.
- Create and stay with a tipping policy. It is a good idea both for your employees and your clients to know exactly what is expected.
- Put your entire pay plan in writing.
- Create incentives by giving your staff opportunities to earn more money, prizes, or tickets to educational events and trade shows.

Create salon policies and stick to them. Everyone in the salon should be governed by the same rules, including you!

ACTIVITY

What would your "dream salon" look like? Try your hand at designing a salon that would attract the kinds of clients you want, offer the services you would like to specialize in, and provide an efficient, comfortable working environment for cosmetology professionals.

Draw pictures, use word pictures, or try a combination of both. Pay attention to practical requirements, but feel free to dream a little, too. Skylights? Fountains? An employee exercise room? You name it. It's your dream (Figure 32-10)!

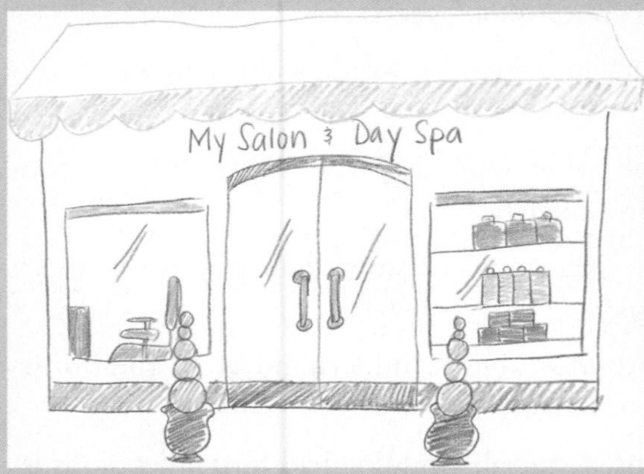

Figure 32-10 What does your dream salon look like?

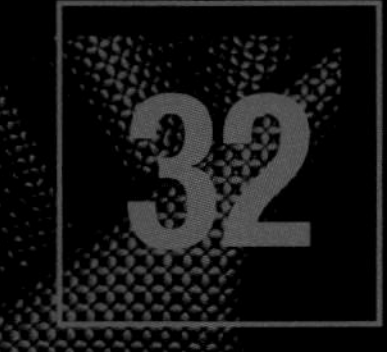

MANAGING PERSONNEL

As a new salon owner, one of your most difficult tasks will be managing your staff. But this can also be very rewarding. If you are good at managing others, you can make a positive impact on their lives, and their ability to earn a living. If managing people does not come naturally, do not despair. People can learn how to manage other people, just as they learn how to drive a car or perform hair services. Keep in mind that managing others is a serious job. Whether it comes naturally to you or not, it takes time to become comfortable with the role.

There are many excellent books, both in and out of the professional salon industry, that you can use as resources for managing employees and staff. Spend an afternoon online or at your local bookstore researching the topic and purchasing materials that will educate and inform you. Once you have a broad base of information, you will be able to select a technique or style that best suits your personality and that of your salon.

THE FRONT DESK

Most salon owners believe that the quality and pricing of services are the most important elements of running a successful salon. Certainly these are crucial, but too often the front desk—the "operations center"—is overlooked. The best salons employ professional receptionists to handle the job of scheduling appointments and greeting clients.

THE RECEPTION AREA

First impressions count, and since the reception area is the first thing clients see, it needs to be attractive, appealing, and comfortable. This is your salon's "nerve center," where your receptionist will sit, retail merchandise will be on display, and the phone system is centered.

Make sure that the reception area is stocked with business cards, and a prominently displayed price list that shows at a glance what your clients should expect to pay for various services.

THE RECEPTIONIST

Second only in importance to your practitioners is your receptionist. A well-trained receptionist is the "quarterback" of the salon, and will be the first person the client sees on arrival. The receptionist should be pleasant, greet each client with a smile, and address her or him by name. Efficient, friendly service fosters goodwill, confidence, and satisfaction.

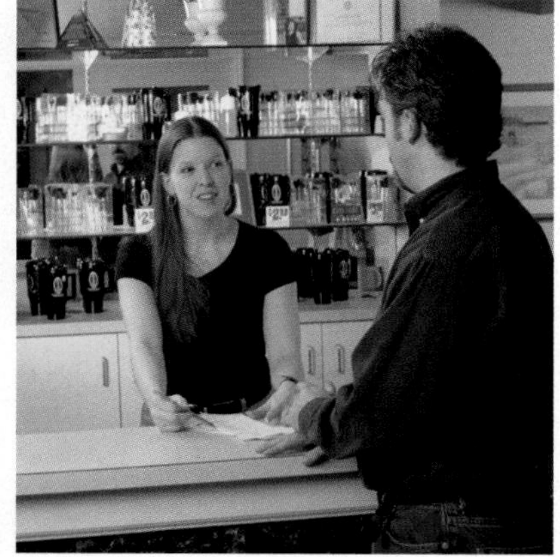

Figure 32–11 A good receptionist is key to a salon's success.

In addition to filling the crucial role of greeter, the receptionist handles other important functions, including answering the phone, booking appointments, informing the practitioner that a client has arrived, preparing the daily appointment information for the staff, and recommending other services to the client. The receptionist should have a thorough knowledge of all retail products carried by the salon so that she or he can also serve as a salesperson and information source for clients (Figure 32-11).

During slow periods, it is customary for the receptionist to perform certain other duties and activities, such as straightening up the reception area and maintaining inventory and daily reports. The receptionist should

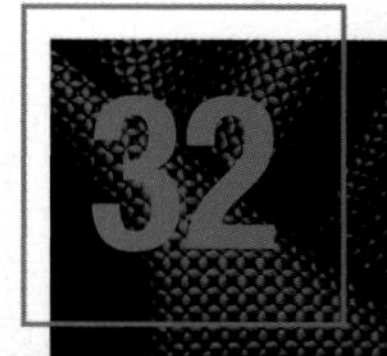

also reserve these slow times for making any necessary personal calls, or otherwise being away from the front desk.

BOOKING APPOINTMENTS

One of the most important duties the receptionist has is booking appointments. This must be done with care, as services are sold in terms of time on the appointment page. Appointments must be scheduled to make the most efficient use of everyone's time. Under ideal circumstances, a client should not have to wait for a service, and a practitioner should not have to wait for the next client.

Booking appointments may be the main job of the receptionist, but when she is not available, the salon owner or manager, or any of the practitioners, can help with scheduling. Therefore, it is important for each person in the salon to understand how to book an appointment and how much time is needed for each service. Regardless of who actually makes the appointment, anyone who answers the phone or deals with clients must have a pleasing voice and personality.

In addition, the receptionist must have the following qualities:

- Attractive appearance
- Knowledge of the various services offered
- Unlimited patience with both clients and salon personnel

APPOINTMENT BOOK

The appointment book helps practitioners arrange time to suit their clients' needs. It should accurately reflect what is taking place in the salon at any given time. In most salons, the receptionist prepares the appointment schedule for staff members; in smaller salons, each person may prepare his own schedule (Figure 32-12).

The appointment book may be an actual hardcopy book that is located on the reception desk, or it may be a computerized appointment book that is easily accessed through the salon's computer system.

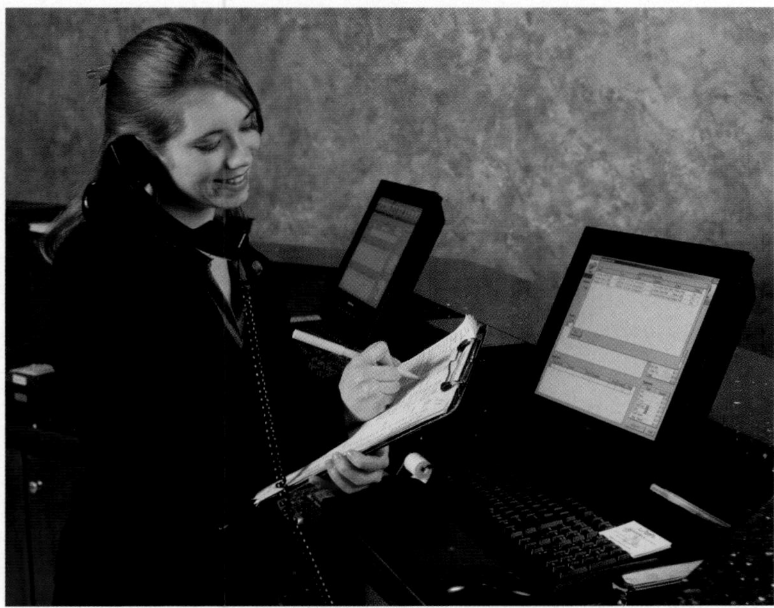

Figure 32-12 Computerized appointment book.

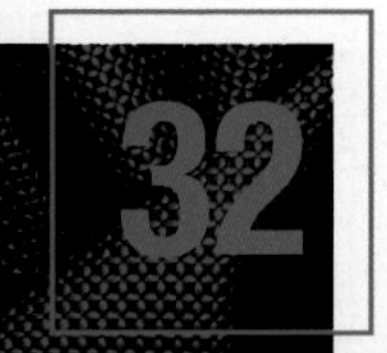

USE OF THE TELEPHONE IN THE SALON

An important part of the business is handled over the telephone. Good telephone habits and techniques make it possible for the salon owner and practitioners to increase business and improve relationships with clients and suppliers. With each call, a gracious, appropriate response will help build the salon's reputation.

GOOD PLANNING

Because it can be noisy, business calls to clients and suppliers should be made at a quiet time of the day, or from a telephone placed in a quieter area of the salon.

When using the telephone, you should:

- Have a pleasant telephone voice, speak clearly, and use correct grammar. A "smile" in your voice counts for a lot.
- Show interest and concern when talking with a client or a supplier.
- Be polite, respectful, and courteous to all, even though some people may test the limits of your patience.
- Be tactful. Do not say anything to irritate the person on the other end of the line.

INCOMING TELEPHONE CALLS

Incoming phone calls are the lifeline of a salon. Clients usually call ahead for appointments with a preferred practitioner, or they might call to cancel or reschedule an appointment. The person answering the phone should develop the necessary telephone skills to handle these calls. In addition, some guidelines for answering the telephone are discussed below.

When you answer the phone, say, "Good morning [afternoon or evening], Milady Salon. May I help you?" or "Thank you for calling Milady Salon. This is Jane speaking. How may I help you?" Some salons require that you give your name to the caller. The first words you say tell the caller something about your personality. Let callers know that you are glad to hear from them.

Answer the phone promptly. On a system with more than one line, if a call comes in while you are talking on another line, ask to put the person on hold, answer the second call, and ask that person to hold while you complete the first call. Take calls in the order in which they are received.

If you do not have the information requested by a caller, either put the caller on hold and get the information, or offer to call the person back with the information as soon as you have it.

Do not talk with a client standing nearby while you are speaking with someone on the phone. You are doing a disservice to both clients.

BOOKING APPOINTMENTS BY PHONE

When booking appointments, take down the client's first and last name, phone number, and service booked. Many salons call the client to confirm the appointment 1 or 2 days before it is scheduled.

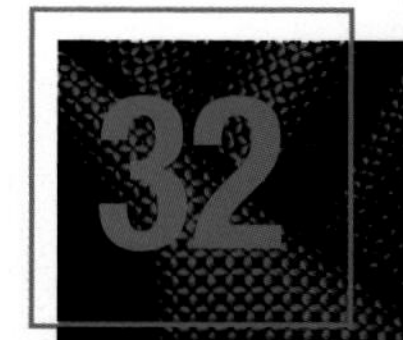

You should be familiar with all the services and products available in the salon and their costs, as well as which cosmetology professionals perform specific services such as color correction. Be fair when making assignments. Try not to schedule six appointments for one practitioner and only two for another.

However, if someone calls to ask for an appointment with a particular cosmetology professional on a particular day and time, every effort should be made to accommodate the client's request. If the practitioner is not available when the client requests, there are several ways to handle the situation:

- Suggest other times that the practitioner is available.
- If the client cannot come in at any of those times, suggest another practitioner.
- If the client is unwilling to try another practitioner, offer to call the client if there is a cancellation at the desired time.

HANDLING COMPLAINTS BY TELEPHONE

Handling complaints, particularly over the phone, is a difficult task. The caller is probably upset and short-tempered. Respond with self-control, tact, and courtesy, no matter how trying the circumstances. Only then will the caller be made to feel that she has been treated fairly.

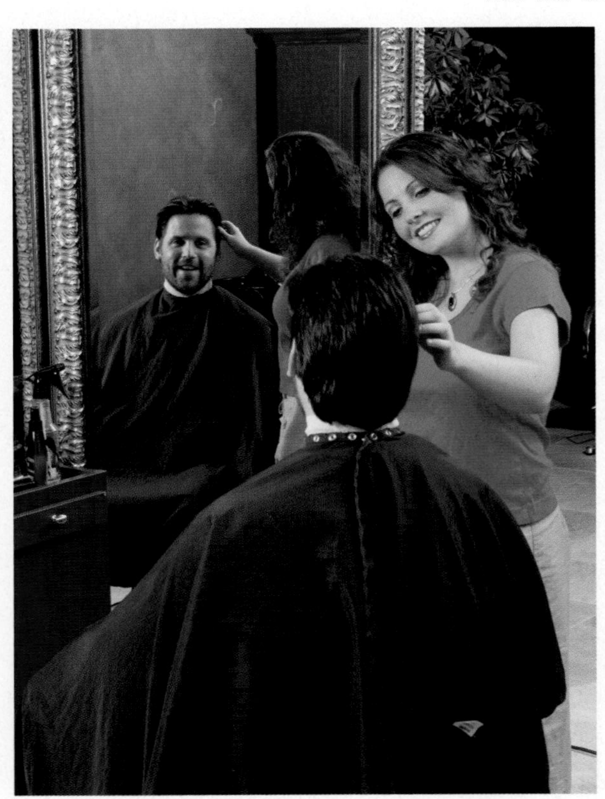

Figure 32-13 Customer satisfaction is your best advertising.

The tone of your voice must be sympathetic and reassuring. Your manner of speaking should convince the caller that you are really concerned about the complaint. Do not interrupt the caller. After hearing the complaint in full, try to resolve the situation quickly and effectively.

ADVERTISING

A new salon owner will want to get the business up and running as soon as possible to start earning some revenue, and begin to pay off debts. One of the first things the new salon owner should consider is how to advertise the salon. It is important to understand the many aspects of advertising.

Advertising includes all activities that promote the salon favorably, from a newspaper ad to radio spots, to a charity event such as a fashion show that the salon participates in. Advertising must attract and hold the attention of readers, listeners, or viewers to create a desire for a service or product.

A satisfied client is the very best form of advertising, because she will refer your salon to friends and family. So make your clients happy (Figure 32-13)!

If you have some experience developing ads, you may decide to do your own advertising. If, however, you need help, you can hire a small local agency or ask a local newspaper or radio station to help you produce the ad. As a general rule, an advertising budget should not exceed 3 percent of your gross income. Plan well in advance

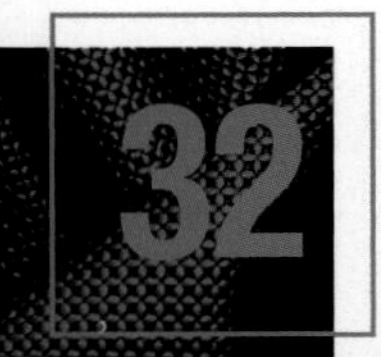

for holidays and special yearly events such as proms, New Year's Eve, or the wedding season.

Here are some advertising venues that may prove fruitful for you.

- Newspaper ads and coupons, or coupon books (Figure 32-14).
- Direct mail to mailing lists and your current salon client list.
- Classified advertising in the local phone book or Yellow Pages directory.
- Email newsletters and discount offers to all clients who have agreed to receive such mailings. Always include an "unsubscribe" link.
- Website offerings.
- Giveaway promotional items such as combs, emery boards, key chains, refrigerator magnets, or calendars.
- Window displays that feature and attract attention to the salon and your retail products.
- Radio advertising.
- Television advertising.

Spring Specials
at
The Manor Day Spa

Celebrate the coming of spring!
Let us pamper you with one of our new deluxe packages

The Getaway:	Swedish massage, facial, manicure, pedicure, makeup, haircut and styling (includes complimentary lunch)	$200
The Refresher:	deep cleansing facial, makeup, haircut and styling	$100
Body Sensations:	aromatherapy massage, facial, makeup	$75
Tips and Toes:	spa manicure, hot stones pedicure	$55

Feb. 15 through May 15 only

Deep conditioning treatment with every haircolor service!
Call now to reserve an hour, two hours, or a whole day
of relaxation and pampering at the Manor.

Bring in this ad to receive a 5% discount on any service.

The Manor Day Spa, 123 Main Street, Hometown, USA 12345
(300-555-1111)

Open Tuesday - Friday 10-6,
Saturday 10-4

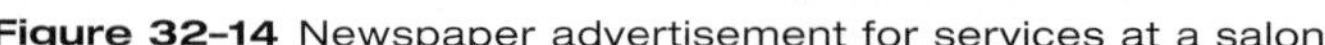

Figure 32-14 Newspaper advertisement for services at a salon.

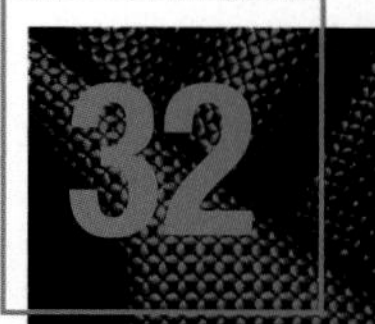

- Community outreach by volunteering at women's and men's clubs, church functions, political gatherings, charitable affairs, and on TV and radio talk shows.
- Client referrals.
- Contacting clients who have not been in the salon for a while.
- Telemarketing to tell your customers about products and services. (You need permission in advance to do this.)
- Videos may be used in the salon to promote your salon and its goods.

SELLING IN THE SALON

An important aspect of the salon's financial success revolves around the sale of additional salon services and take-home or maintenance products. Whether you own or manage a large salon with several employees, or you are a booth renter with only yourself to worry about, adding services or retail sales to your service ticket means additional revenue. Beauty professionals, in general, seem to feel uncomfortable about having to make sales of products or additional services. It is important to work at overcoming this feeling. When practitioners are reluctant to sell, it is often because they carry a negative stereotype of salespeople—pushy or aggressive—and they do not want to be seen this way themselves. While there are salespeople like that, remember that there are also very helpful and knowledgeable sales professionals who make customer care their top priority. These people play a major role in the lives of their customers, and are very valuable to them because they offer good advice (Figure 32-15).

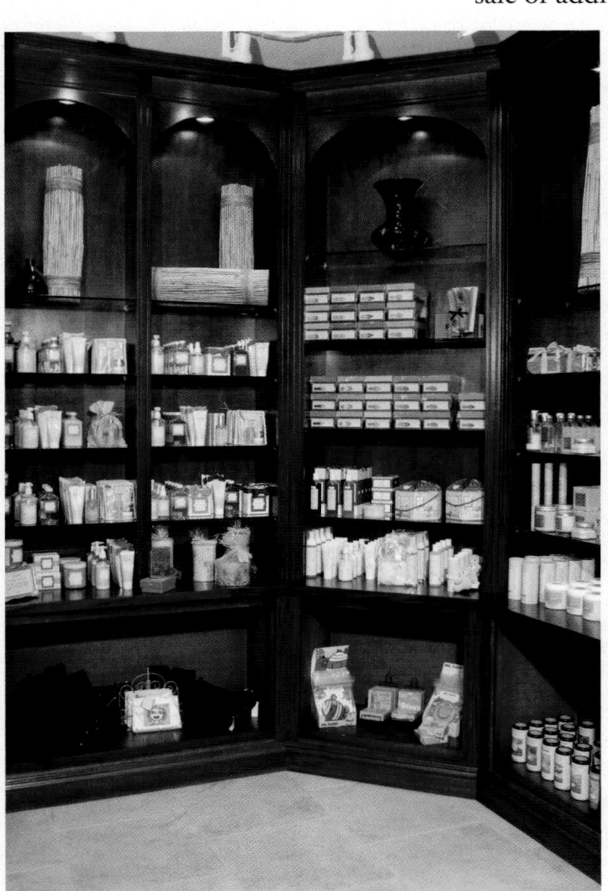

Figure 32-15 Selling retail products benefits everyone.

REVIEW QUESTIONS

1. What are the two ways in which you may go into business for yourself?
2. List five factors to consider when opening a beauty salon.
3. Name three types of ownership under which a business may operate.
4. What purpose do accurate records serve?
5. What two types of supplies make up a beauty salon's inventory?
6. Why is the reception area of a salon important?
7. Why is the receptionist called the "quarterback" of the salon?
8. Explain the elements of good telephone technique.
9. List six different kinds of advertising.
10. What is the best form of advertising? Why?

CHAPTER GLOSSARY

booth rental	Renting a booth or station in a salon (also known as chair rental).
business plan	Written plan of a business, as it is seen in the present and envisioned in the future.
business regulations and laws	The rules of any/all local, state, and federal agencies you must comply with when you decide to open your salon or rent a booth.
capital	Money needed to start a business.
consumption supplies	Supplies used in daily business operation structure controlled by one.
corporation	Ownership structure controlled by one or more stockholders.
demographics	Information about the size, average income, and buying habits of the population.
insurance	A means of guaranteeing protection or safety for malpractice, property liability, fire, burglary and theft, and business interruption.
partnership	Business structure in which two or more people share ownership, although not necessarily equally.
personnel	Employees; staff.
record-keeping	The maintaining of accurate and complete records of all financial activities in your business.
retail supplies	Supplies sold to clients.
salon operation	Knowing and complying with all Federal Occupational Safety and Health Administration (OSHA) guidelines, including those that require the ingredients of cosmetic preparations be available for employees.
salon policies	The rules or regulations adopted by a salon to ensure that all clients and associates are being treated fairly and consistently.
sole proprietor	Individual owner and manager of a business.
written agreements	Documents such as a business plan, which is a written description of your business as you see it today, and as you foresee it in the next 5 years.

A SPECIAL MESSAGE FROM ROBERT CROMEANS
INTERNATIONAL ARTISTIC DIRECTOR OF PAUL MITCHELL SYSTEMS

USE YOUR TIME WISELY

Many times in school, all we're focused on is getting out. The reality is that we need to focus every single day on making the right choices so that we can be the best beauty professional possible.

One thing that I remember from being a student is the idle time, the down time, and if there's anything I wish I had done differently, it's this: I wish I had done more techniques and services while still in school.

So instead of taking off till three o'clock, or hanging out and waiting for somebody to come in to teach you something, you should be focusing on creating more opportunities to practice every type of hair, skin, and nail service.

FORM GOOD HABITS

Many times we think that when we're in school, we can dress or act a certain way. But these are the first habits that you're going to form in your new profession. So why not start forming habits now that will change your whole attitude when you get into the industry? Your professional life starts when you walk into school. From day one, you are a cosmetologist. Think forward to the end result—you want to be a good cosmetologist. You don't want to be mediocre. That means that you dress up, you apply makeup, and if you don't like makeup, be a nurse. You're in the beauty business. Do not treat school like a backstage rehearsal. Treat school like you're on stage. Start being the person you want to be while you're in cosmetology school.

SEEK MENTORS

While I was in cosmetology school, I picked a few mentors who helped me. The first was a company, Paul Mitchell, which may not sound like it's a mentorship, but the reality is, companies can give common knowledge to an industry. I think it's very important to use a company as a mentor for information and ideas.

Being connected into something bigger is just smart business. The business values are the enterprise it operates on. So find a company to believe in by looking out in the industry to see what inspires you, what seems to make the most connection to you.

EXPLORE THE POSSIBILITIES

I think the most important thing for new cosmetologists is to find the right salon environment to work in. Start today on your homework—targeting salons you want to work for. We want you to stay in the business. There are far too few cosmetologists, and we want to keep each and every one of you and show you how to make it.

Look around and pick one or two salons you'd like to work in—not when you think you're going to take your licensing exam, not when you plan to graduate, but many months before. Many of these salons would like to meet you in advance.

You could already be working in there after hours, not doing hair but just serving coffee and water. That way you can start to feel the vibe, start to see what professional haircare is truly about.

Communication, connecting with people, is the key. Start while you're in school.

Young kids sometimes say to me, "I'm working through school. What do I do?" I tell them the best thing to do is wait tables, because by waiting tables you get to blend with lots of different types of people, and you're there to serve them. It's very similar to cosmetology—not that we're waiters or waitresses, we're professionals, but with a human attitude. We're not working on mannequins. We're working on human beings, and our job is to make them feel beautiful inside and out.

LEARN THE BUSINESS

Business may seem like the farthest thing from your mind while you're in school. I'm not talking about balancing your checkbook; I'm talking about starting to understand business as it applies to professional beauty.

Business skills can be learned, and the information is out there. It's on websites, in industry journals and in Milady business books; even the large companies are a source. Remember, the point here is that you have to accelerate your education, and the way you accelerate is not by studying harder, but by doing more. That will make a tremendous difference.

CONTINUE TO LEARN

Advanced education is one of the most important things you can do, while in school and definitely when you're first beginning. DVDs are a good way to learn because you can fast forward, stop and go back, or watch it again a day later and find those missing clues that didn't make sense the first time. Websites like *www.behindthechair.com* are an incredible way to get information and ideas. A friend of mine, Winn Claybaugh, tapes interviews with successful beauty professionals and markets them as the Master Series. You want to sign up for those because the people he interviews will give you tons of working tools.

Distributors do some of the most important education for our industry. They're at the local level, so you don't have to be tied into a national program. Distributors are looking for people like you. My first connection with Paul Mitchell was via one of my distributors in Memphis, who started utilizing me for local classes while I was in beauty school. Make a point of getting to as many of their local events as you can. It's not a case of which company you love; anybody who is teaching at the level you're at right now will help you, either by showing you what to do or, in some cases, what not to do. Either way it's learning, and the quicker you can eliminate mistakes based on watching other people, the better.

There is so much going on, so get out and look around. Don't just look at the education you want; look at where in the world you haven't been yet. Find the education and make that your point of reference. You'll get to see other places, like the Italian streets, and it will make you think differently about style in America. Everybody in America has a certain way of thinking about Europe, and in Europe everybody wants everything American. Even in Japan they want a piece of America. You've taken on a license that gives you the language we all speak, the language of professional beauty. So get a passport and get ready. It's all about education, travel, having fun, and making money.

I want to be the first to congratulate you and welcome you into our incredible industry. You know the things we must do together to make things happen. Zig Zeigler, one of my favorite motivational speakers, said it the best: "If you do the things you ought to do when you ought to do them, the day comes when you get to do what you want to do when you want to do it." So pick your mentors, pick a target, and start thinking of school as a place where you learn your skills and develop a good work ethic.

Develop the habit of working hard in school; that will make things so easy when you become an employee of a salon because you'll fit right in. You'll already be up to speed. The thing about this industry that will blow your mind is how quickly you get to move closer to your goal. If you focus every day on taking a step in that direction, in no time at all you will realize your first goal—and then, my friends, you get to move on to the second one.

See you at a trade show soon!

APPENDIX A

BARBER STYLING

Scali-Sheahan, Maura T. *Milady's Standard Professional Barbering, 4E.* 1-4018-7395-2.

*Milady's Standard Professional Barbering: Student Exam Review, 4E.*1-4018-7396-0.

Milady's Standard Professional Barbering: Student Workbook, 4E. 1-4018-7399-5.

BASIC COSMETOLOGY

Milady's Standard Cosmetologia. 1-4180-4960-3.

Hayden, Thomas, and James Williams. Milady's Black Cosmetology. 0-87350-3775.

BASIC COSMETOLOGY SUPPLEMENTS

Milady's Standard Cosmetology Exam Review. 1-4180-4943-3.

Milady's Standard Cosmetology Study Guide: The Essential Companion. 1-4180-4940-9.

Milady's Standard Cosmetology Student CD-ROM. 1-4180-4945-X

Milady's Standard Cosmetology Study Summary for Chinese. 1-4018-1085-3.

Milady's Standard Cosmetology Study Summary for Korean. 1-4018-1084-5.

Milady's Standard Cosmetology Study Summary for Vietnamese. 1-4018-1083-7.

Milady's Standard Cosmetology Theory Workbook. 1-4180-4941-7.

Milady's Standard Cosmetology Practical Workbook.

1-4180-4942-5.

Milady's Situational Problems for Cosmetology Students. 1-4180-4944-1.

Beatty, Deborah. *Preparing for the Practical Exam: Cosmetology.* 1-4018-1532-4.

Milady's Situational Problems for the Cosmetology Student (Spanish edition). 1-4180-4954-6.

Guia de Estudios de Cosmetologia: La Acompanante Esencial. 1-4180-4951-4.

Libro de Ejercicios de Cosmetologia Teorico Revisado. 1-4180-4953-0

Libro de Ejericios de Cosmetologia Practico Revisado. 1-4180-4952-2.

Repaso del Examen de Cosmetologia. 1-4180-4955-7.

BUSINESS/CAREER

Capellini, Steve. *Massage Therapy Career Guide for Hands-on Success, 2E.* 1-4180-1051-0.

Cotter, Louise and Francis London DuBose. *The Transition: How to Become a Salon Professional.* 1-56253-263-4.

D'Angelo, Janet. *Spa Business Strategies: A Plan for Success.* 1-4018-8164-5

Edgerton, Leslie. *Managing Your Business: Milady's Guide to the Salon.* 1-56253-084-4.

Gambino, Henry J. *SalonOvations' Marketing and Advertising for the Salon.* 1-56253-262-6.

Hoffman, Lee. *Salon Dialogue for Successful Results.* 1-56253-3223.

Kilmer, Beverly. *Staffing Policies and Procedures.* 1-56253-314-2.

Maurer, Gretchen. *The Business of Bridal Beauty.* 1-56253-338-X.

Oppenheim, Robert. *101 Salon Promotions.* 1-56253-358-4.

Phillips, Carol. *In the Bag: Selling in the Salon.* 1-56253-236-7.

Salon Training International. *Assistant Training Tools (Manual & CD's).* ISBN: 1-4180-7331-8.

Booth Renters: Management System (Manual). ISBN: 1-4180-7333-4.

Bottom Line Results. ISBN: 0-9650-7770-5.

Front Desk Management System (Manual). ISBN: 1-4180-7330-X.

Passion: A Salon Professionals Handbook for Building a Successful Business. ISBN: 0-9650-7778-0.

Payday (3 CD's). ISBN: 0-9650-7779-9.

Recruiting for Excellence (CD/Handbook). ISBN: 0-9650-7773-X.

Salon Management Tools (Manual). ISBN: 1-4180-7329-6.

The Coaching Solution 2.0 (CD). ISBN: 1-4180-7335-0.

The Profit Factor (CD/Handbook). ISBN: 0-9650-7775-6.

Tezak, Edward. *Successful Salon Management for Cosmetology Students, 5E.* 1-56253-679-6.

Ventura, Judy. *Salon Promotions: Creative Blueprints for Success.* 1-56253-350-9.

Wiggins, Joanne L. *Milady's Guide to Owning and Operating a Nail Salon.* 1-56253-201-4.

ESTHETICS

Milady's Standard Fundamentals for Estheticians, 9E. 9E. 1-56253-836-5.

Milady's Standard Comprehensive Training for Estheticians. 1-56253-805-5.

Lees, Mark. *Skin Care: Beyond the Basics, 3E.* 1-4180-1234-3.

Skin Care: Beyond the Basics Workbook, 3E. 1-4180-1950-X.

Hill, Pamela. *Advanced Face and Body Treatments for the Spa.* 1-4018-8172-6.

Advanced Hair Removal. 1-4018-8174-2.

Botox, Dermal Fillers, and Sclerotherapy. 1-4018-8169-6.

Common Drugs and Side Effects: A Handbook for the Aesthetician. 1-4018-8172-6.

Common Skin Diseases: A Handbook for the Aesthetician. 1-4018-8170-2.

Creating Profitability in the Medical Spa. 1-4018-8167-X.

Ensuring an Optimal Outcome in Skin Care. 1-4018-8178-8.

Medical Terminology: A Handbook for the Skin Care Specialist. 1-4018-8171-8.

Microdermabrasion. 1-4018-8176-9.

Peels and Peeling Agents. 1-4018-8177-7.

Permanent Makeup: Tips and Techniques. 1-4018-8173-4.

The Cosmetic Surgery Patient: The Aesthetician's Role. 1-4018-8168-8.

Arroyave, Efrain. *Understanding Cosmetic Procedures: Surgical and Non-Surgical.* 1-4018-9745-2.

Bickmore, *Helen. Milady's Hair Removal Techniques: A Comprehensive Manual.* 1-4018-1555-3.

Deitz, Sallie. *The Clinical Esthetician: An Insider's Guide to Succeeding in a Medical Office.*1-4018-1788-2.

Gambino, Henry J. *Modern Esthetics: A Scientific Source for Estheticians.* 1-56253-043-7.

Place, Stan Campbell. *The Art and Science of Professional Makeup.* 0-87350-361-9.

Poignard, Renee. *Milady's Waxing Made Easy: A Step-by-Step Guide.* 1-56253-171-9.

Rayner, Victoria. *Clinical Cosmetology: A Medical Approach to Esthetics Procedures.* 1-56253-056-9.

Thrower, Angelo P. *Black Skin Care for the Practicing Professional.* 1-56253-352-5.

HAIRCOLORING

Foley, Mark. *Double Your Haircolor Income in 20 Days.* ISBN: 1-4018-4461-8.

Rangl, Deborah. *Milady's Standard Hair Coloring Manual and Activities Book.* 1-56253-356-8.

Warren, Roxy. *Haircoloring in Plain English: A Practical Guide for Professionals.* 1-56253-357-6.

HAIRCUTTING/HAIRSTYLING

Bailey, Diane Carol. *Natural Hair Care and Braiding.* 1-56253-316-9.

Cotter, Louise. *Mature Elegance: Styles and Techniques for Mature Clients.* 1-56253-339-8.

Jones, Jamie Rines. *SalonOvations' Braids and Updos Made Easy.* 1-56253-318-5.

Milady's Standard System of Salon Skills: Hairdressing Student Course Book. 1-56253-398-3.

SalonOvations' The Multicultural Client: Cuts, Styles, and Chemical Services. 1-56253-178-6.

Scali-Sheahan, Maura. *Milady's 18 Men's Styles.* 1-56253-177-8.

Young, Kenneth. *Milady's 28 Black Styles.* 1-56253-042-9.

Milady's 28 Styles. 1-56253-070-4.

Milady's Razor Cutting. 1-56253-180-8.

MASSAGE

Beck, Mark. *Theory and Practice of Therapeutic Massage, 4E.* 1-4018-8029-0 (HC), 1-4018-8030-4 (SC), 1-4018-8031-2 (Workbook).

NAILS

Milady's Standard Nail Technology, 5E. 1-4180-1615-2.

Milady's Standard Nail Technology Exam Review. 1-4180-1624-1.

Milady's Standard Nail Technology Student Workbook. 1-4180-1622-5.

Milady's Standard Nail Technology Study Summary for Chinese. 1-4018-1187-6.

Milady's Standard Nail Technology Study Summary for Korean. 1-4018-1186-8.

Milady's Standard Nail Technology Study Summary for Vietnamese. 1-4180-1626-8.

Preparing for the Practical Exam: Nail Technology. 1-4018-1757-2.

Milady's Standard Tecnologia de Unas. 1-4180-1644-6.

Milady's Standard Nail Technology Spanish Study Resource. 1-4180-1629-2.

Anthony, Elizabeth. *SalonOvations' Airbrushing for Nails.* 1-56253-270-7.

Bigan, Tammy. *Nail Art and Design.* 1-56253-118-2.

McCormick, Janet. *Spa Manicuring.* 1-56253-460-2.

Mix, Godfrey. *The Salon Professional's Guide to Foot Care.* 1-56253-332-0.

Peters, Vicki. *SalonOvations' Nail Q and A Book.* 1-56253-266-9.

Schoon, Douglas D. *Milady's Nail Structure and Product Chemistry, 2E.* 1-4018-6709-X.

VIDEOS

Beck, Mark F. *Milady's Massage Fundamentals Video Series.* 1-56253-750-4.

Hair Structure and Chemistry Simplified Video. 1-4018-0868-9.

Jones, Jamie Rines. *Braids and Updos Video Series:*

Advanced Braiding Made Easy. 0-87350-241-8.

Braiding Made Easy. 0-87350-650-2.

French Braiding Made Easy. 0-87350-459-3.

More Updos Made Easy. 1-56253-379-7.

Ribbon Braiding Made Easy. 1-56253-377-0.

Updos Made Easy. 1-56253-378-9.

Nelson, Dennis G. *Safety and Health in the Salon Training System.* 1-56253-709-1.

FOR THE INSTRUCTOR

Beatty, Deborah. *Preparing for the Practical Exam: Instructor's Manual.* 1-4018-1756-4.

Lees, Mark. *Skin Care Beyond the Basics 3E: Workbook Answer Key* 1-4180-1951-8.

Halal, John. *Hair Structure and Chemistry Simplified Course Management Guide.* 1-56253-632-X.

Milady's Hair Removal Techniques Course Management Guide 1-4018-4524-X.

Milady's Master Educator Program Leaders Manual 1-56253-583-8.

Milady's Master Educator Program Videos on DVD 1-4180-2926-2.

Milady's Standard Comprehensive Training for Estheticians Leaders Manual 1-56253-808-X.

Milady's Standard Comprehensive Training for Estheticians Workbook Answer Key 1-4018-3659-3.

Milady's Standard Comprehensive Training for Estheticians Video Library 1-56253-809-8.

Milady's Standard Comprehensive Training for Estheticians Video Library on DVD 1-4180-2928-9.

Milady's Standard: Comprehensive Training for Estheticians Leader's Manual with CTB. 1-56253-808-X.

Milady's Standard Cosmetology Course Management Guide. 1-4180-4937-9.

Milady's Standard Cosmetology Course Management Guide CD-ROM 1-4180-4938-7.

Milady's Standard Cosmetology Instructor Support Slides 1-4180-4939-5.

Milady's Standard Cosmetology DVD Series 1-56253-905-1.

Milady's Standard Cosmetology Procedure Posters 1-4018-3743-3.

Milady's Standard Cosmetology Admissions Video 1-56253-906-X.

Milady's Standard Cosmetology Student CD-ROM NETWORK Version 1-4180-4946-8.

Milady's Standard Cosmetology Supplement Sampler Demo 1-4180-6137-9.

Milady's Standard Fundamentals for Estheticians Course Management Guide 1-56253-838-1.

Milady's Standard Fundamentals for Estheticians Course Management Guide CDROM 1-4018-4882-6.

Milady's Standard Fundamentals for Estheticians Instructor Support Slides 1-4018-4082-5.

Milady's Standard Fundamentals for Estheticians Procedure Posters 1-4018-3899-5.

Milady's Standard Nail Technology Course Management Guide, 5E. 1-4180-1618-7.

Milady's Standard Nail Technology Course Management Guide CD-ROM 1-4180-1619-5.

Milady's Standard Nail Technology DVD Series 1-4180-5460-7.

Milady's Standard Nail Technology Instructor Support Slides 1-4180-1621-7.

Milady's Standard Nail Technology Procedure Posters 1-4018-3900-2.

Milady's Standard Nail Technology Student CD-ROM NETWORK Version 1-4180-1628-4.

Milady's Standard Professional Barbering Course Management Guide, 4E. 1-4018-7398-7.

Milady's Standard Professional Barbering Course Management Guide CD-ROM 1-4018-7400-2.

Milady's Standard Professional Barbering Instructor Support Slides. 1-4018-7403-7.

Milady's Standard System of Salon Skills: Hairdressing Image Library, CD-ROM. 1-56253-559-5.

Milady's Standard System of Salon Skills: Hairdressing Leader's Manual. 1-56253-399-1.

Milady's Standard System of Salon Skills Support Tools, CD-ROM. 1-56253-665-6.

Milady's Standard System of Salon Skills Video Library 1-56253-400-9.

Milady's Theory and Practice of Therapeutic Massage IML, 4E. 1-4018-8032-0.

Successful Salon Management for Cosmetology Students, 5E Answer Key. 1-56253-681-8.

VIDEOS/DVDS

Barnes, Letha. *Milady's Master Educator Program, 2002. (Instructor's package)* 1-56253-735-0.

Jones, Jamie Rines. *Braids & Updos Made Easy: The Long Hair System.* 0-82738-730-X.

_____. *Braids & Updos Made Easy: The Training Package.* 0-82738-729-6.

Milady's Soft Skills: Interpersonal Skills for the Beauty Industry. 1-4018-9940-4.

Milady's Standard: Comprehensive Training for Estheticians System DVDs. 1-4180-2928-9.

Milady's Standard: Cosmetology DVD Series. 1-56253-905-1.

Milady's Standard Professional Barbering DVD Series. 1-4018-8015-0.

Milady's Standard System of Salon Skills: Hairdressing. (Instructor's package) 1-56253-401-7.

Milady's Standard Nail Technology DVD's. 1-4180-5460-7.

Whitten, Cheryl. *Step-by-Step Makeup Videos on DVD.* 1-4180-2927-0.

FOR REFERENCE

Balhorn, Linda A. *The Professional Model's Handbook.* 0-87350-376-7.

Chesky, Sheldon R., Isabel Christina, and Richard B. Rosenberg. *Playing It Safe: Milady's Guide to Decontamination, Sterilization, and Personal Protection.* 1-56253-179-4.

Halal, John. Milady's *Hair Care Products Ingredients Dictionary.* 1-56253-919-1.

Hess, Shelley. *SalonOvations' Guide to Aromatherapy.* 1-56253-313-4.

SalonOvations' Professional's Reflexology Handbook. 1-56253-334-7.

Levine, Karen. *A Survival Guide for Cosmetologists: Tips from the Trenches.* 1-4018-1545-6.

Michalun, Natalia. *Milady's Skin Care and Cosmetic Ingredients Dictionary, 2E.* 1-56253-660-5.

Milady's Illustrated Cosmetology Dictionary, 2E. 1-56253-667-2.

Miller, Erica. *SalonOvations' Day Spa Operations.* 1-56253-255-3.

_____. *SalonOvations' Day Spa Techniques.* 1-56253-261-8.

_____. *SalonOvations' Shiatsu Massage.* 1-56253-264-2.

Nelson, Dennis. *Safety and Health in the Salon Training System.* 1-56253-709-1.

Schoon, Douglas. *HIV/AIDS and Hepatitis: Everything You Need to Know to Protect Yourself and Others.* 1-56253-175-1.

MAGAZINES

American Salon
Official publication of the National Cosmetology Association (NCA)
Subscriptions: (218) 723-9477

Beauty Store Business
Subscriptions: (800) 624-4196
PO Box 16087 North Hollywood, CA 91615
www.beautystorebusiness.com

Canadian Hairdresser
Subscriptions: (416) 923-1111
11 Spadina Road Toronto, Ont.
Canada M5R 2S9
www.canhair.com

Day Spa
Subscriptions: (800) 624-4196
PO Box 15757 North Hollywood, CA 01615
www.dayspamag.com

Dermascope
Subscriptions: (972) 226-2309
2611 N. Beltline Rd., Suite 101 Sunnyvale, TX 75182
www.dermascope.com

Les Nouvelles Esthetiques
Subscriptions: (800) 471-0229
306 Alcazar Ave.
Coral Gables, FL 33134
www.lneonline.com

Modern Salon
Subscriptions: www.modernsalon.com
PO Box 1414 Lincolnshire, IL 60069

NailPro
Subscriptions: (800) 624-4196
PO Box 17017 North Hollywood CA 91615
www.nailpro.com

Nails
Subscriptions: (888) NAILS-44
PO Box 1067 Skokie, IL 60076

Salon News
Subscriptions: (800) 477-6411
PO Box 5035 Brentwood, TN 37024-5035

Salon Today
Subscriptions: (800) 808-2623 ext. 305 400
Knightsbridge Parkway Palatine, IL 60069
www.modernsalon.com

Skin, Inc.
Subscriptions: (800) 469-7445
3625 S. Schmale Road Carol Stream, IL 60188-2787

WEB SITES

www.beautynet.com
Virtual salon for hair, skin, and nail care.

www.beautytech.com
Trade show schedule, continuing education calendar, message center (to trade information), information specifically for nail technicians, cosmetologists, and salon owners.

www.behindthechair.com
BTC Bookstore, up-to-date products and trends, find a job, post a job.

www.careersinbeauty.com
Resource for students: news, events, scholarships, and more.

www.cosmeticworld.com
Daily supplement to the leading weekly newsletter for cosmetics and fragrance industry.
Beauty On-line, an online magazine; *American Salon,* inside look at the beauty business; list of salons in the U.S.; window shopping; more.

www.milady.com
Milady's Web site: information on books, audio, and video tapes, computer software programs, The Career Institute.

www.ybn.com
Resource for students to prepare for business success in the beauty industry.

APPENDIX B: ASSOCIATIONS

Accrediting Commission of Career Schools and Colleges of Technology (ACCSCT)
2101 Wilson Blvd., Suite 302
Arlington, VA 22201 (703) 247-4212
www.accsct.org

Allied Beauty Association (ABA)
450 Matheson Blvd. East, Units 46 & 47
Mississauga, Ont.
Canada L4Z 1R5 (905) 568-0158
www.abacanada.com

American Association of Cosmetology Schools (AACS)
15825 N. 71st St., Suite 100
Scottsdale, AZ 85254-1521 (800) 831-1086
www.beautyschools.org

American Association for Esthetics Education (AAEE)
401 N. Michigan Ave.
Chicago, IL 60611-4267 (312) 245-1570 www.chicagomidwestbeautyshow.com/MEMBERSHIP/AmericanAssociationforEstheticsEducation

American Health & Beauty Aids Institute (AHBAI)
401 N. Michigan Ave., #2200
Chicago, IL 60611-4267 (312) 644-6610
www.ahbai.org

Barbers International (BI)
2708 Pine Street
Arkadelphia, AR 71923 (866) 698-6463
www.barbersinternational.com

The Cosmetic, Toiletry, and Fragrance Association
1101 17th St. NW, Suite 300
Washington, DC 20036 (202) 331-1770
www.ctfa.org

Cosmetology Advancement Foundation (CAF)
PO Box 811 FDR Station
New York, NY 10150-0811 (212) 750-2412
www.cosmetology.org

Cosmetology Educators Association (CEA)
11811 N. Tatum Blvd., Suite 1085
Phoenix, AZ 85028-1625 (800) 831-1086
www.oneroof.org

Cosmetology Industry Association of British Columbia (CIABC)
899 West 8th Avenue
Vancouver, British Columbia Canada V5Z 1E3 (604) 871-0222
www.cabccanada.com

The Day Spa Association
310 17th Street
Union City, NJ 07087 (201) 865-2065
www.dayspaassociation.com

Independent Cosmetic Manufacturers and Distributors (ICMAD)
1220 W. Northwest Highway
Palatine, IL 60067 (800) 334-2623
www.icmad.org

Intercoiffure
11 bis, rue Jean Goujon 75008 Paris, France
www.intercoiffure.net

International Guild of Hair Removal Specialists (IGHRS)
1918 Bethel Road
Columbus, Ohio 43220 (800) 830-3247
www.ighrs.org

International Nail Technicians Association (INTA)
2035 Paysphere Circle
Chicago, IL 60674 (312) 321-5161 www.chicago-midwestbeautyshow.com/MEMBERSHIP/InternationalNailTechniciansAssociation

National Association of Barber Boards of America (NABBA)
2703 Pine Street
Arkadelphia, AR 71923 (501) 682-2806
www.nationalbarberboards.com

National Accrediting Commission of Cosmetology Arts & Sciences (NACCAS)
4401 Ford Ave., Suite 1300
Alexandria, VA 22302 (703) 527-7600
www.naccas.org

National Beauty Culturists League
25 Logan Circle NW
Washington, D.C. 20005-3725 (202) 332-2695
www.nbcl.org

National Coalition of Estheticians, Manufacturers/Distributors and Associations (NCEA)
484 Spring Avenue
Ridgewood, NJ 07450-4624 (201) 670-4100
www.ncea.tv

National Cosmetology Association (NCA)
401 N. Michigan Ave.
Chicago, IL 60611-4267 (312) 245-1595
www.ncacares.org

National-Interstate Council of State Boards of Cosmetology (NIC)
7622 Briarwood Circle
Little Rock, AR 72205 (501) 227-8262
www.nictesting.org

Professional Beauty Association
15825 N. 71st Street, Suite 100
Scottsdale, AZ 85254 (800) 468-2274
www.probeauty.org

Society of Permanent Cosmetic Professionals
69 North Broadway
Des Plaines, IL 60016 (847) 635-1330
www.spcp.org

SkillsUSA (Vocational Industrial Clubs of America, Inc.)
PO Box 3000
Leesburg, VA 20177-0300 (703) 777-8810
www.skillsusa.org

GLOSSARY/INDEX

A

B

C

21st century, 8
1901-1910, 6–7
1920's, 7
1930's, 7
1940's, 7–8
1951-2000, 7–8
Chinese, 4
Egyptians, 4
the Greeks, 5
Middle Ages, 5
Renaissance, 5–6
the Romans, 5
Victorian Age, 6

Couperose (coo-per-ros), European term describing areas of diffuse redness and dilated red capillaries, 569

Cowlick, tuft of hair that stands straight up, 150

Cranium (KRAY-nee-um), an oval, bony case that protects the brain, 91

Cream masks, mask treatments for dry skin that do not harden or dry on the face, 573

Creative capability, 17

Creative Nail Design, 8

Croquignole (KROH-ken-ohl) perms, perms in which the hair strands are wrapped at an angle perpendicular to the perm rod, in overlapping concentric layers, 7, 434

Cross-checking, parting the haircut in the opposite way from which you cut it, to check for precision of line and shape, 259

Crown, area of the head between the apex and back of the parietal ridge, 245

Crust, dead cells that form over a wound or blemish while it is healing; an accumulation of sebum and pus, sometimes mixed with epidermal material, 537

CTFA. *See* Cosmetic, Toiletry, and Fragrance Association

Curette, small, spoon-shaped instrument used for cleaning debris from the edges of nail plate, 700

Curl, hair that is wrapped around the roller; also called circle, 317

Curl re-forming, 470–473
procedure, 471–473
safety precautions, 470

Curvature perm, 450–451

Curvature perm wrap, perm wrap in which partings and bases radiate throughout the panels to follow the curvature of the head, 443

Curved lines, lines on an angle, used to soften a design, 198

Cuticle (KYOO-ti-kul) (nail), dead tissue that adheres to the nail plate, 135
removal, 714–715

Cuticle (KYOO-ti-kul) (hair), outermost layer of hair, consisting of a single, overlapping layer of transparent, scale-like cells, 143
hair, 143

Cuticle removers, products designed to soften cuticles for removal from the nail plate, 714

Cutting line, angle at which the fingers are held when cutting, and ultimately the line that is cut; also known as finger angle, finger position, cutting position, cutting angle, 246

Cutting specialist, 9

Cyst (SIST), closed, abnormally developed sac containing fluid, semifluid, or morbid matter, above or below the skin, 536

Cytoplasm (sy-toh-PLAZ-um), all the protoplasm of a cell except that which is in the nucleus; the watery fluid that contains food material necessary for growth, reproduction, and self-repair of the cell, 88

D

Dandruff, 158–159, 224

Dappen dish, a special container used to hold the monomer liquid and polymer powder, 755

DC. *See* Direct current

DeCaprio, Noel, 8

Deductive reasoning, process of reaching logical conclusions by employing logical reasoning, 794

Deep peroneal nerve, a nerve that extends down the front of the leg, behind the muscles. It supplies impulses to these muscles and also to the muscles and skin on the top of the foot and adjacent sides of the first and second toes, 103

Deep-conditioning treatments, chemical mixtures of concentrated protein and the heavy cream base of a moisturizer; used to provide treatments when an equal degree of moisturizing and protein treatment is required, 226

Deltoid (DEL-toyd), large triangular muscle covering the shoulder joint that allows the arm to extend outward and to the side of the body, 98

Demipermanent haircolor, also called no-lift, deposit-only color. Formulated to deposit, but not lift (lighten) natural hair color. Demipermanent colors are able to deposit without lifting because they are less alkaline than permanent colors and are mixed with a low-volume developer, 486

Demographics, information about the size, average income, and buying habits of the population, 840

Dendrites (DEN-dryts), tree-like branching of nerve fibers extending from a nerve cell; short nerve fibers that carry impulses toward the cell, 100

Depilatory, substance, usually a caustic alkali preparation, used for the temporary removal of superfluous hair by dissolving it at the skin surface level, 552

Depressor labii inferioris muscle (dee-PRES-ur LAY-bee-eye in-FEER-ee-orus), muscle surrounding the lower lip; depresses the lower lip and draws it to one side, 97

Dermal papilla (puh-PIL-uh), small, cone-shaped elevation located at the base of the hair follicle that fits into the hair bulb, 143

Dermatitis, 537–538, 541–542

Dermatitis, inflammatory condition of the skin, 538

Dermatitis (dur-muh-TY-tis) venenata, also known as contact dermatitis. An eruptive skin infection caused by contact with irritating substances such as chemicals or tints, 541–542

Dermatologist, physician engaged in the science of treating the skin, including its structures, functions, and diseases, 121

Dermatology, medical branch of science that deals with the study of skin and its nature, structure, functions, diseases, and treatment, 125

Dermis (DUR-mis), underlying or inner layer of the skin; also called the derma, corium, cutis, or true skin, 122

Design texture, wave pattern, 199

Desincrustation (des-inkrus-TAY-shun), process used to soften and emulsify grease deposits (oil) and blackheads in the hair follicles, 186

Detergents, 77

Developer, oxidizing agent that, when mixed with an oxidation haircolor, supplies the necessary oxygen gas to develop color molecules and create a change in hair color, 488

Diagnosis, determining the nature of a disease or infection, 63

Diagonal lines, lines positioned between horizontal and vertical lines, 197, 245

Diamond face, 208

E

F

G

H

Holidays, 772
Honesty, 49
Horizontal lines, lines parallel to the floor or horizon; creates width in hair design, 197, 245
Hormones, secretions produced by one of the endocrine glands and carried by the bloodstream or body fluid to another part of the body to stimulate a specific activity, 108
Hubbard, Elizabeth, 6
Human immunodeficiency virus (HIV), 64
Human relations, 35–37
golden rules, 37
Humectants (hew-MECK-tents), substances that absorb moisture or promote the retention of moisture, 225, 572
Humerus (HYOO-muh-rus), uppermost and largest bone in the arm, extending from the elbow to the shoulder, 93
Hydrogen bonds, weak physical side bonds that are the result of an attraction between opposite electrical charges; easily broken by water, as in wet setting, or heat, as in thermal styling, and re-form as the hair dries or cools, 145, 427
Hydrogen peroxide developers, 488
Hydrophilic (hy-drah-FIL-ik), capable of combining with or attracting water, 171, 222
Hydroxide neutralization, does not involve oxidation or rebuilding disulfide bonds. The neutralization of hydroxide relaxers neutralizes (deactivates) the alkaline residues left in the hair by the relaxer. The pH of hydroxide relaxers is so high that the hair remains at an extremely high pH, even after thorough rinsing, 460
Hydroxide relaxers, very strong alkalis with a pH over 13. The hydroxide ion is the active ingredient in all hydroxide relaxers, 459–460
types, 460–461
Hyoid (HY-oyd) bone, u-shaped bone at the base of the tongue that supports the tongue and its muscles; also called "adam's apple," 92
Hyperhidrosis (hy-per-hy-DROH-sis), excessive sweating, caused by heat or general body weakness, 538
Hypertrichosis (hi-pur-trih-KOH-sis) (hirsuties) (hur-SOO-shee-eez), condition of abnormal growth of hair, characterized by the growth of terminal hair in areas of the body that normally grow only vellus hair, 156
Hypertrophy (hy-PUR-truh-fee), abnormal growth of the skin, 540
Hyponychium (hy-poh-NIK-eeum), the slightly thickened layer of skin that lies beneath the free edge of the nail plate, 135

I

Immiscible, not capable of being mixed, 170
Immunity, ability of the body to destroy and resist infection, 66
Implements
for makeup, 612–613
for pedicures, 700
Inactive electrode, opposite pole from the active electrode, 185
Indentation, the point where curls of opposite directions meet, forming a recessed area, 318
Individual retirement account (IRA), 828
Infected finger, redness, pain, swelling, or pus; refer to physician, 648
Infection, 56–83. *See also* Hair; Nails; Scalp
contagious, 64
control, 60
decontamination, 66–79
local, 64
principles of prevention, 60–66
professional salon image, 80–81
regulation, 56–59
Infection, invasion of body tissue by pathogenic bacteria, 63
Infectious, infection that can be spread from one person to another person or from one infected body part to another, 64
Inferior labial (LAY-bee-ul) artery, supplies blood to the lower lip, 106
Inflammation, body's response to injury or infection with redness, heat, pain, and swelling, 63
Infraorbital (in-frah-OR-bih-tul) artery, supplies blood to the muscles of the eye, 107
Infraorbital (in-frah-OR-bih-tul) nerve, affects the skin of the lower eyelid, side of the nose, upper lip, and mouth, 101
Infrared rays, invisible rays that have longer wavelengths, penetrate deeper, and produce more heat than visible light, 188
Infratrochlear (in-frah-TRAHK-lee-ur) nerve, nerve that affects the membrane and skin of the nose, 100
Inhalation (in-huh-LAY-shun), the breathing in of air, 109
Inhibition layer, tacky surface left on the nail once a UV gel has cured, 781
Initiators, energized and activated by catalyst; initiators start the chain reaction, 751
Inorganic chemistry, study of substances that do not contain carbon, 166
Insertion, part of the muscle at the more movable attachment to the skeleton, 95
Instant conditioners, conditioners that either remain on the hair for a very short period (1 to 5 minutes) or are left in the hair during styling ("leave-in" conditioners), 226
Insulator (IN-suh-layt-ur) or nonconductor, substance that does not easily transmit electricity, 181
Insurance, a means of guaranteeing protection or safety for malpractice, property liability, fire, burglary and theft, and business interruption, 840
Integration hairpiece, hairpiece with an opening in the base through which the client's own hair is pulled to blend with the hair (natural or synthetic) of the hairpiece, 413
Integrity, 21
Integument (in-TEG-yuh-ment), largest and fastest growing organ of the body; composed of the hair, skin, and nails, 142
Integumentary system, the skin and its accessory organs, such as the oil and sweat glands, sensory receptors, hair, and nails, 109
Interior guideline, guideline that is inside the haircut rather than on the perimeter, 273
Interior, inner or internal part, 247
Internal carotid artery, supplies blood to the brain, eyes, eyelids, forehead, nose, and internal ear, 106
Internal jugular (JUG-yuh-lur) vein, vein located at the side of the neck to collect blood from the brain and parts of the face and neck, 107
Interview, 807–814
checklist, 810
conducting, 812–813
legal aspects, 813–814
preparation, 810–812
Intestines, 89
Inverted triangle face, 208
Invisible or inverted braid, three-strand braid produced by overlapping the strands of hair on top of each other, 374

J

K

L

M

N

O

P

Q

R

S

T

U

V

W

Willatt, Arnold F., 7
Work ethic, taking pride in your work and committing yourself to consistently doing a good job for your clients, employer; and salon team, 799
Work surfaces, disinfection procedure, 73
Wrap resin, an adhesive used over the fabric wrap to adhere it to the nail extension or nail plate, 726
Wringing, vigorous movement in which the hands, placed a little distance apart on both sides of the client's arm or leg and working downward, apply a twisting motion against the bones in the opposite direction, 578
Wrinkles, 633
Written agreements, documents such as a business plan, which is a written description of your business as you *see* it today, and as you foresee it in the next 5 years, 843

Y

Yellowed hair, 518

Z

Zygomatic (zy-goh-MAT-ik) nerve, affects the muscles of the upper part of the cheek, 101
Zygomatic/malar (zy-goh-MAT-ik) bones, form the prominence of the cheeks; cheekbones, 92
Zygomaticus (zy-goh-MAT-ih-kus), muscles extending from the zygomatic bone to the angle of the mouth; elevate the lip, as in laughing, 97

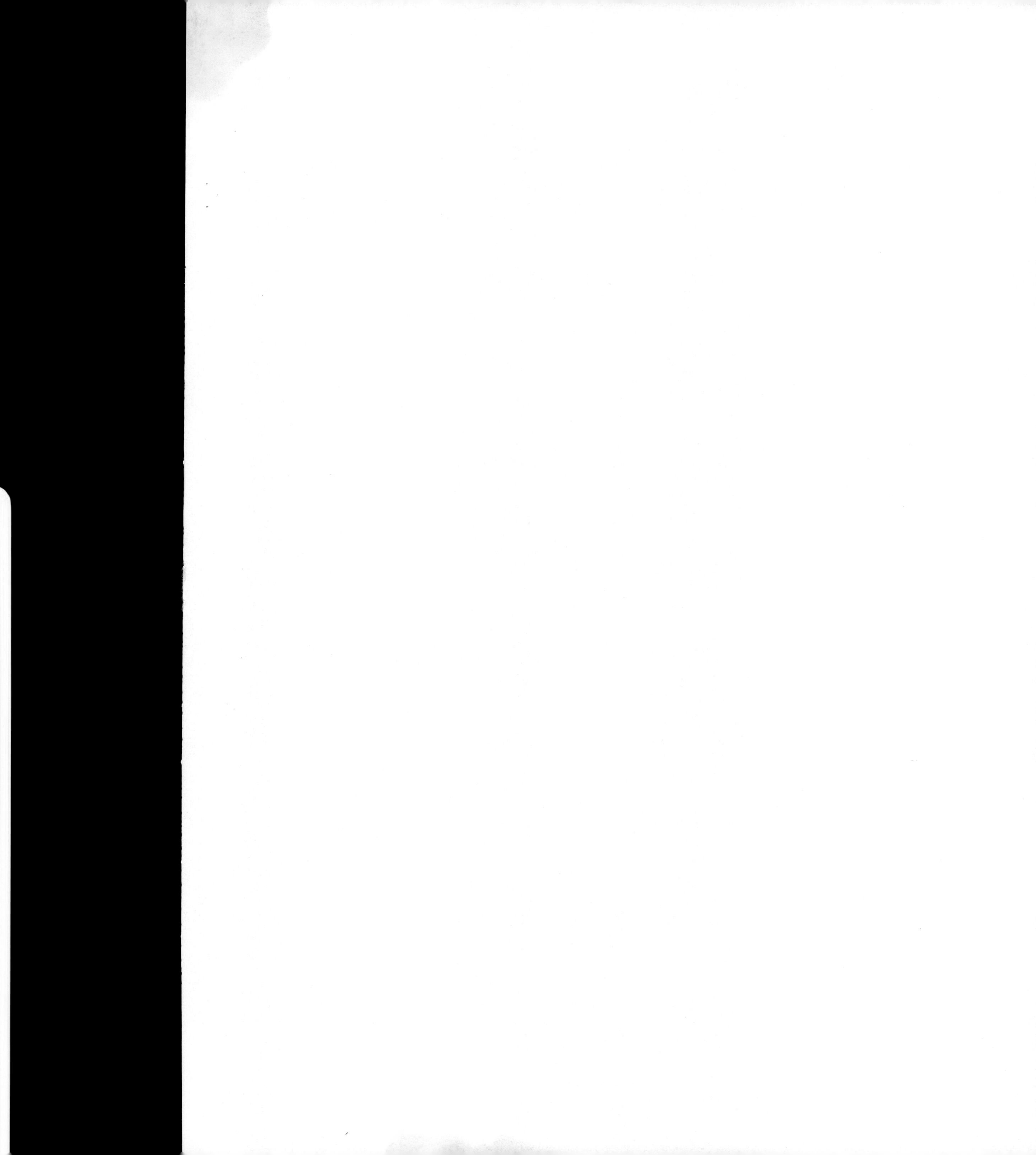

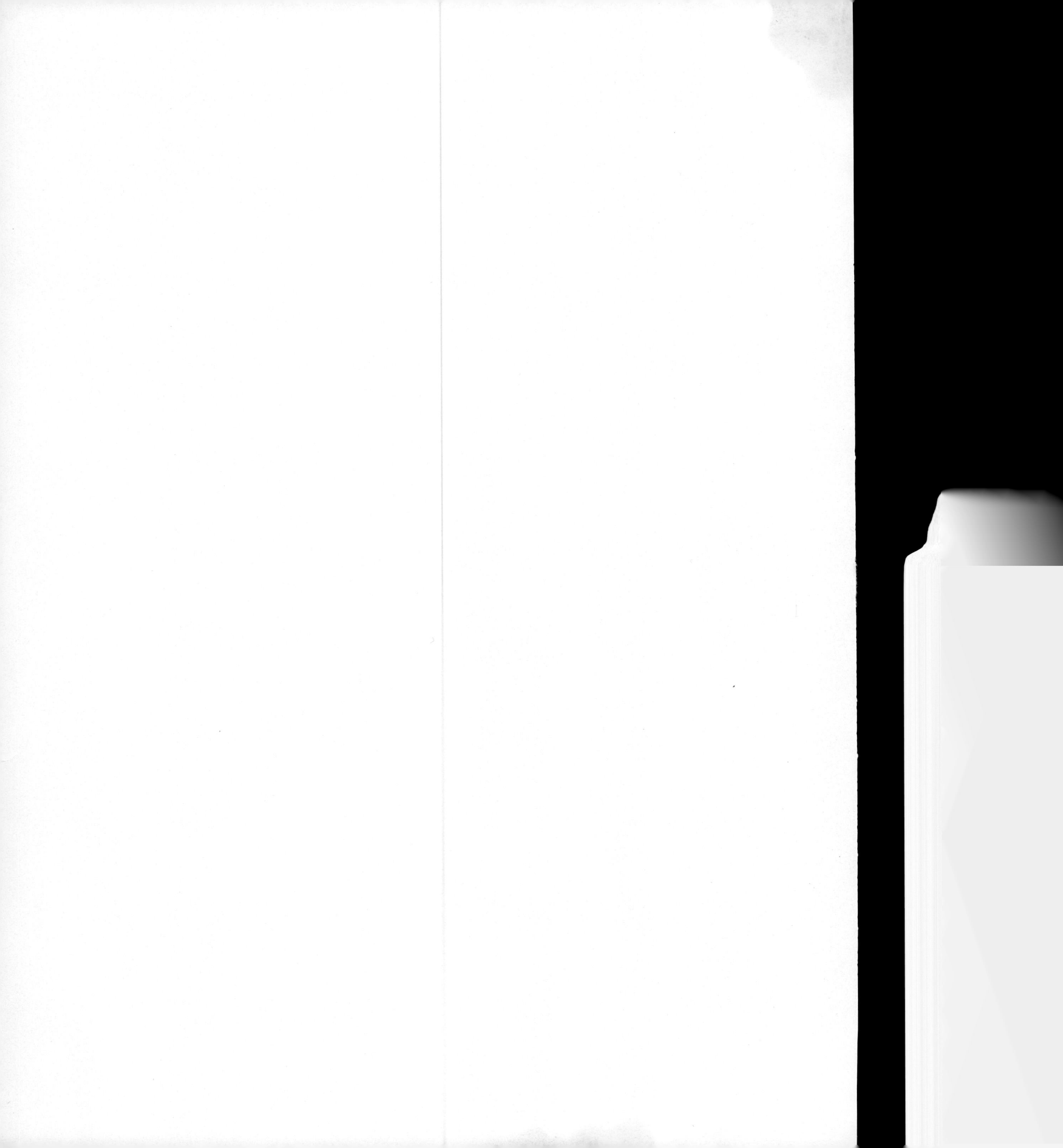